Basic Skills in Interpreting Laboratory Data

Fifth Edition

Mary Lee, PharmD, BCPS, FCCP

Vice President

Chief Academic Officer

Pharmacy, Optometry, and Health Science Education

Midwestern University

Professor, Pharmacy Practice

Midwestern University Chicago College of Pharmacy

Downers Grove, Illinois

American Society of Health-System Pharmacists®

Any correspondence regarding this publication should be sent to the publisher, American Society of Health-System Pharmacists, 7272 Wisconsin Avenue, Bethesda, MD 20814, attention: Special Publishing.

The information presented herein reflects the opinions of the contributors and advisors. It should not be interpreted as an official policy of ASHP or as an endorsement of any product.

Because of ongoing research and improvements in technology, the information and its applications contained in this text are constantly evolving and are subject to the professional judgment and interpretation of the practitioner due to the uniqueness of a clinical situation. The editors, contributors, and ASHP have made reasonable efforts to ensure the accuracy and appropriateness of the information presented in this document. However, any user of this information is advised that the editors, contributors, advisors, and ASHP are not responsible for the continued currency of the information, for any errors or omissions, and/or for any consequences arising from the use of the information in the document in any and all practice settings. Any reader of this document is cautioned that ASHP makes no representation, guarantee, or warranty, express or implied, as to the accuracy and appropriateness of the information contained in this document and specifically disclaims any liability to any party for the accuracy and/or completeness of the material or for any damages arising out of the use or non-use of any of the information contained in this document.

Director, Special Publishing: Jack Bruggeman
Acquisitions Editor: Robin Coleman
Editorial Project Manager: Ruth Bloom
Production Editor: Kristin Eckles
Cover and Page Design: Carol Barrer

Library of Congress Cataloging-in-Publication Data

Basic skills in interpreting laboratory data / [edited by] Mary Lee. -- 5th ed.
    p. ; cm.
Includes bibliographical references and index.
ISBN 978-1-58528-343-9
I. Lee, Mary (Mary Wu-Len) II. American Society of Health-System Pharmacists.
[DNLM: 1. Clinical Laboratory Techniques. 2. Reference Values. QY 25]
616.07'5--dc23

2012040827

ISBN 978-1-58528-343-9

DEDICATION

This book is dedicated to Scott Traub, the originator of *Basic Skills in Interpreting Laboratory Data*. He saw the need for this textbook, had the vision to create the first edition, and edited the second edition.

Mary Lee

CONTENTS

ACKNOWLEDGMENTS

The authors and I would like to acknowledge all of the careful and selfless work of the many chapter reviewers; Dr. John Kennedy, our clinical laboratory/pathologist expert reviewer of the entire book; and the Special Publishing staff at ASHP, including Jack Bruggeman, Robin Coleman, Ruth Bloom, and Kristin Eckles, for their technical assistance. We also express our gratitude to our families who supported us through this project.

Mary Lee

PREFACE

In January 2011, the American Society of Health-System Pharmacists (ASHP) invited me to serve as editor for the third time for *Basic Skills in Interpreting Laboratory Data*. Based on the revisions to the fourth edition, the book was well received and was becoming a popular educational tool among colleges of pharmacy in the United States and at international programs. What an honor for me to work on this project again!

The authors, many of whom have traveled along with me on my professional path, are experienced pharmacists and/or faculty at prestigious colleges of pharmacy and medicine. They participate in medication therapy management in their practices, supervise residents and other postdoctoral students in training, and publish widely. They know how to teach, and how to teach well. As you use this book, their depth of experience shows in the clarity of the content and the practical examples in the cases that demonstrate how to apply a laboratory test result to a particular patient's diagnosis, treatment, or drug therapy monitoring plan. A few new authors have joined the team, and we are grateful for their fresh approach, insights, and expertise.

The fifth edition includes several enhancements over previous editions. We have revised the template for the Quickview tables at the end of each chapter to make the content easier to understand. This table format is the same as that used in ASHP's *Interpreting Laboratory Data: A Point-of-Care Guide*. In addition, all of the abbreviations used throughout the book have been consolidated into one master list in the front; this should increase the convenience of finding the explanation of each abbreviation. Our eagle-eye pathologist consultant, Dr. John Kennedy, has standardized all the normal value ranges for the laboratory test results to mirror those used in *Harrison's Principles of Internal Medicine*, which reduces some of the variation in normal lab value ranges between this book and other textbooks. Finally, in many of the chapters the cases have been updated or changed.

What has been preserved in the fifth edition are the same chapter topics; discussion of commonly used laboratory tests for each major organ system and how they are used for screening, diagnosis, treatment, or monitoring response to treat; patient cases that highlight application of test results; and learning points that summarize important concepts at the end of each chapter. This book is designed to be a companion to commonly used pharmacotherapeutic textbooks; therefore, the emphasis is on covering laboratory tests that are used for management of diseases discussed in those textbooks.

When using this book, readers should be aware of the following guidelines:

- All laboratory tests are organized into one of three sections: Concepts (chapters 1–6), Body Systems (chapters 7–18), and Special Populations (chapters 19–21).
- Readers can find the most appropriate chapter by checking the Table of Contents or the Index.
- To look up a specific laboratory test, it is most efficient to check the Index.
- For each laboratory test, we have included a short description of how measurement of this laboratory test is related to normal physiologic processes or the pathophysiology of the disease, common diseases or medications that might increase or decrease laboratory test results, and how to interpret an abnormal laboratory result.
- We have minimized redundancy in the descriptions of laboratory tests where appropriate. For example, prostate specific antigen is covered in Chapter 22: Common Medical Disorders of Aging Males—Clinical and Laboratory Test Monitoring, but it is not covered in Chapter 19: Cancers and Tumor Markers.

- For certain diseases, other types of tests—including **radiographs, scans**, and **electrocar-diograms**—are used. We have described **how these other tests are used for diagnosis,** management, and monitoring of selected diseases as **appropriate.**

This book differs from many classic textbooks on **clinical laboratory tests** in that the focus is on clinical interpretation of laboratory test results as they apply to individual patients. If the reader is seeking an in-depth description of the assay **methodology of a particular laboratory** test, rare disease or medication-related causes of abnormal laboratory test results, or causes of in vitro interferences with a particular laboratory test, **then this is not the** appropriate resource to use. Chapter 3: Primer on Drug Interferences **with Test Results** includes a listing of alternative reference resources that would be **best for those purposes.**

As you use this book, the authors' and reviewers' **commitment to ensure that this book** provides accurate, clinically pertinent, and up-to-date information will be clearly evident.

Mary Lee
May 2013

CONTRIBUTORS

Editor

Mary Lee, PharmD, BCPS, FCCP
Vice President, Chief Academic Officer
Pharmacy, Optometry, and Health Science
    Education
Midwestern University
Professor, Pharmacy Practice
Midwestern University Chicago College of
    Pharmacy
Downers Grove, Illinois

Contributors

Val Adams, PharmD, FCCP, BCOP
Associate Professor of Pharmacy
College of Pharmacy
University of Kentucky
Lexington, Kentucky

Brian Altman, PharmD
Albany College of Pharmacy and Health
    Sciences, 2012
Longmeadow, Massachusetts

Amber L. Beitelshees, PharmD, MPH, FAHA
Assistant Professor
Department of Medicine
University of Maryland, Baltimore
Baltimore, Maryland

Brady Blackorbay
Doctor of Pharmacy Candidate
School of Pharmacy
University of Wisconsin-Madison
Madison, Wisconsin

Jill S. Borchert, PharmD, BCPS, FCCP
Professor and Vice-Chair, Pharmacy Practice
Midwestern University Chicago College of
    Pharmacy
Downers Grove, Illinois

Candace S. Brown, MSN, PharmD
Professor of Clinical Pharmacy, Obstetrics &
    Gynecology, and Psychiatry
University of Tennessee Health Science Center
Memphis, Tennessee

Rodrigo M. Burgos, PharmD
Clinical Assistant Professor
College of Pharmacy
University of Illinois at Chicago
Chicago, Illinois

Lingtak-Neander Chan, PharmD, BCNSP
Associate Professor
School of Pharmacy
University of Washington
Seattle, Washington

Rosane Charlab, PhD
Genomics Group, Office of Clinical
    Pharmacology
Office of Translational Sciences
Center for Drug Evaluation and Research
U.S. Food and Drug Administration
Silver Spring, Maryland

Peter A. Chyka, PharmD
Professor and Executive Associate Dean
College of Pharmacy, Knoxville Campus
The University of Tennessee Health Science
    Center
Knoxville, Tennessee

Samir Y. Dahdal, MD, FACC
Clinical Assistant Professor of Medicine
Medical Director, General Cardiology Practice
The University of Arizona Medical Center
Tucson, Arizona

**Wafa Y. Dahdal, PharmD, BCPS
    (AQ Cardiology)**
Director of International Programs
Associate Director of Professional Development
American College of Clinical Pharmacy
Lenexa, Kansas
Adjunct Clinical Professor
Department of Pharmacy Practice
College of Pharmacy
University of Illinois at Chicago
Chicago, Illinois

Lea E. Dela Peña, PharmD, BCPS
Associate Professor, Pharmacy Practice
Midwestern University Chicago College of
    Pharmacy
Downers Grove, Illinois

Philip F. DuPont, MD, PhD
Adjunct Professor
Department of Pathology
Chicago College of Osteopathic Medicine
Midwestern University
Downers Grove, Illinois
Department of Biology
Benedictine University
Lisle, Illinois

Sharon M. Erdman, PharmD
Clinical Professor of Pharmacy Practice
Purdue University School of Pharmacy
Wishard Health Services
Indianapolis, Indiana

Paul Farkas, MD, FACP, AGAF
Chief of Gastroenterology
Mercy Hospital
Assistant Clinical Professor of Medicine
Tufts University School of Medicine
Springfield, Massachusetts

Paul R. Hutson, PharmD, BCOP
Associate Professor, Pharmacy Practice
School of Pharmacy
University of Wisconsin
Madison, Wisconsin

Ashley M. Johnson, PharmD
Clinical Pharmacist
St. Mary's Hospital
Madison, Wisconsin

Min J. Joo, MD, MPH, FCCP
Assistant Professor of Medicine
Department of Medicine
University of Illinois at Chicago
Chicago, Illinois

Kathy E. Komperda, PharmD, BCPS
Associate Professor, Pharmacy Practice
Midwestern University Chicago College of
   Pharmacy
Downers Grove, Illinois

**Donna M. Kraus, PharmD, FAPhA,
FPPAG, FCCP**
Associate Professor of Pharmacy Practice
Departments of Pharmacy Practice and
   Pediatrics
Colleges of Pharmacy and Medicine
University of Illinois at Chicago
Chicago, Illinois

Alan Lau, PharmD, FCCP
Professor and Director, International Clinical
   Pharmacy Education
College of Pharmacy
University of Illinois at Chicago
Chicago, Illinois

Mary Lee, PharmD, BCPS, FCCP
Vice President, Chief Academic Officer
Pharmacy, Optometry, and Health Science
   Education
Midwestern University
Professor, Pharmacy Practice
Midwestern University Chicago College of
   Pharmacy
Downers Grove, Illinois

Janis J. MacKichan, PharmD, FAPhA
Professor and Vice Chair
Department of Pharmacy Practice
Northeast Ohio Medical University
Rootstown, Ohio

Patrick J. Medina, PharmD, BCOP
Associate Professor of Pharmacy
University of Oklahoma College of Pharmacy
Oklahoma City, Oklahoma

Anastasia L. Roberts, PharmD, BCPS
Assistant Professor of Pharmacy Practice
St. Louis College of Pharmacy
St. Louis, Missouri

Keith A. Rodvold, PharmD, FCCP, FIDSA
Professor of Pharmacy Practice and Medicine
College of Pharmacy
University of Illinois at Chicago
Chicago, Illinois

Joanna Sampson, MD
Baystate Medical Center
Springfield, Massachusetts

**Terry L. Schwinghammer, PharmD, FCCP,
FASHP, FAPhA, BCPS**
Professor and Chair
Department of Clinical Pharmacy
School of Pharmacy
West Virginia University
Morgantown, West Virginia

Roohollah Sharifi, MD, FACS
Section Chief of Urology
University of Illinois College of Medicine
Chicago, Illinois

Barry Slitzky, MD
Senior Clinical Instructor
Tufts University School of Medicine
Springfield, Massachusetts

Karen J. Tietze, PharmD
Professor of Clinical Pharmacy
Department of Pharmacy Practice and
    Pharmacy Administration
Philadelphia College of Pharmacy
Philadelphia, Pennsylvania

**Dominick P. Trombetta, PharmD, BCPS,
    CGP, FASCP**
Associate Professor, Pharmacy Practice
Wilkes University
Wilkes-Barre, Pennsylvania

**Eva M. Vivian, PharmD, MS, CDE,
    BC-ADM, FAADE**
Clinical Associate Professor
School of Pharmacy
University of Wisconsin-Madison
Madison, Wisconsin

Michelle J. Washington, BS, PharmD
Clinical Pharmacist
ExcelleRx, Inc.
Memphis, Tennessee

**Lori A. Wilken, PharmD, BCACP, TT-S,
    AE-C**
Clinical Assistant Professor, Ambulatory Care
Department of Pharmacy Practice
University of Illinois at Chicago
Chicago, Illinois

REVIEWERS

Eric G. Boyce, PharmD
Associate Dean for Academic Affairs & Professor
    of Pharmacy Practice
Thomas J. Long School of Pharmacy & Health
    Sciences
University of the Pacific
Stockton, California

Joseph Bubalo, PharmD, BCPS, BCOP
Oncology Clinical Pharmacy Specialist
Assistant Professor of Medicine
Oregon Health & Science Hospital & Clinics
Portland, Oregon

Katie S. Buehler, PharmD, BCPS
Assistant Professor of Pharmacy Practice
St. Louis College of Pharmacy
St. Louis, Missouri

**Vince Colucci, PharmD, BCPS(AQ-Card),
    CPP**
Professor, Department of Pharmacy Practice
The University of Montana, CHPBS
Missoula, Montana

**Susan Cornell, BS, PharmD, CDE, FAPhA,
    FAADE**
Assistant Director of Experiential Education
Associate Professor of Pharmacy Practice
Midwestern University Chicago College of
    Pharmacy
Downers Grove, Illinois

**Emily R. Hajjar, PharmD, BCPS,
    BCACP, CGP**
Associate Professor
Jefferson School of Pharmacy
Thomas Jefferson University
Philadelphia, Pennsylvania

**Evelyn R. Hermes-DeSantis, PharmD,
    BCPS**
Clinical Professor
Pharmacy Practice & Administration
Rutgers, The State University of New Jersey
Director Drug Information Service
Robert Wood Johnson University Hospital
New Brunswick, New Jersey

Tudy Hodgman, PharmD, FCCM, BCPS
Clinical Coordinator/Critical Care Specialist
Northwest Community Hospital
Associate Professor, Pharmacy Practice
Critical Care Residency Director
Midwestern University Chicago College of
    Pharmacy
Downers Grove, Illinois

Arthur I. Jacknowitz, MSc, PharmD
Professor and Distinguished Chair Emeritus
School of Pharmacy
Robert C. Byrd Health Sciences Center
West Virginia University
Morgantown, West Virginia

Samantha Karr, PharmD, BCPS, BCACP
Assistant Professor of Pharmacy Practice
College of Pharmacy–Glendale
Midwestern University
Glendale, Arizona

John L. Kennedy, MD
Lead Pathologist
Pathology and Laboratory Medicine Service
Jesse Brown VA Medical Center
Clinical Associate Professor
Department of Pathology
University of Illinois at Chicago
Chicago, Illinois

Lisa J. Killam-Worrall, PharmD, BCPS
Director of Experiential Education
Associate Professor of Pharmacotherapy
University of North Texas System College of
    Pharmacy
University of North Texas Health Science Center
Fort Worth, Texas

Julie M. Koehler, PharmD, FCCP
Associate Dean for Clinical Education &
    External Affiliations
Professor of Pharmacy Practice
College of Pharmacy & Health Sciences
Butler University
Ambulatory Care Clinical Pharmacist
Methodist Hospital of Indiana University Health
Indianapolis, Indiana

Taimour Langaee, MSPH, PhD
Research Associate Professor
Graduate Coordinator
Director, Center for Pharmacogenomics
    Genotyping Core Lab
College of Pharmacy
University of Florida
Gainesville, Florida

Catherine M. Oliphant, PharmD
Associate Professor of Pharmacy Practice
College of Pharmacy
Idaho State University
Meridian, Idaho

Nancy D. Ordonez, PharmD, BCPS
Assistant Dean for Experiential Programs
College of Pharmacy
University of Houston
Houston, Texas

Frank P. Paloucek, BS, PharmD, DABAT, FASHP
Director, Residency Programs
Clinical Associate Professor in Pharmacy
    Practice
Department of Pharmacy Practice
College of Pharmacy
University of Illinois at Chicago
Chicago, Illinois

Tracy Pettinger, PharmD, BCPS
Clinical Assistant Professor
College of Pharmacy
Idaho State University
Pocatello, Idaho

Theresa Prosser, PharmD, BCPS, AE-C, FCCP
Professor of Pharmacy Practice
St. Louis College of Pharmacy
St. Louis, Missouri

William Spruill, PharmD, FASHP, FCCP
Professor
Clinical and Administrative Pharmacy
College of Pharmacy
University of Georgia
Athens, Georgia

Holli Temple, PharmD, BCPS, CGP
Clinical Assistant Professor
College of Pharmacy
University of Texas at Austin
Austin, Texas

Timothy J. Todd, PharmD
Associate Professor of Pharmacy Practice
Midwestern University Chicago College of
    Pharmacy
Downers Grove, Illinois

ABBREVIATIONS

1,25-DHCC	1,25-dihydroxycholecalciferol
17-OHP	17 alpha-hydroxyprogesterone
2,3 DPG	2,3-diphosphoglycerate
25-HCC	25-hydroxycholecalciferol
3SR	self-sustained sequence replication
5-HT	serotonin
6-AM	6-acetylmorphine
6MWT	6-minute walk test
A-G6PD	glucose-6 phosphate dehydrogenase variant
A1c	glycosylated hemoglobin
A2M	alpha 2-macroglobulin
ABG	arterial blood gas
ACA	anticentromere antibody
ACC	American College of Cardiology
ACCF	American College of Cardiology Foundation
ACCP	American College of Clinical Pharmacy
ACCP	anticyclic citrullinated peptide
ACE	angiotensin-converting enzyme
ACE-I	angiotensin-converting enzyme inhibitor
ACPA	anticitrullinated protein antibody
ACR	American College of Rheumatology
ACS	acute coronary syndrome
ACT	activated clotting time
ACT	alpha 1-antichymotrypsin
ACTH	adrenocorticotropic hormone (corticotropin)
ADA	American Diabetes Association
ADAM	androgen deficiency in aging males
ADCC	antibody-dependent cellular cytotoxicity
ADH	antidiuretic hormone
ADME	**a**bsorption, **d**istribution, **m**etabolism, **e**xcretion
ADP	adenosine diphosphate
AFB	acid-fast bacilli
AFP	alpha fetoprotein
AHA	American Heart Association
AIDS	acquired immunodeficiency syndrome
ALK	anaplastic lymphoma kinase
ALL	acute lymphoblastic leukemia
ALP	alkaline phosphatase
ALT	alanine aminotransferase
AMA	antimitochondrial antibody
AMI	acute myocardial infarction
AML	acute myelogenous leukemia
ANA	antinuclear antibody
ANCA	antineutrophil cytoplasmic antibody
ANF	atrial natriuretic factor
ANP	atrial natriuretic peptide
anti-CCP	anti-cyclic citrullinated peptide
anti-HAV IgG	IgG antibody against hepatitis A virus
anti-HAV IgM	IgM antibody against hepatitis A virus
anti-HBc	antibody to hepatitis B core antigen
anti-HbeAg	antibody to hepatitis B extracellular antigen
anti-HBs	antibody to hepatitis B surface antigen

anti-HCV	antibody against HCV antigen
anti-HD	antibody against hepatitis D
APC	activated protein C
APC	antigen-presenting cell
ApoB	apolipoprotein B
APS	antiphospholipid antibody syndrome
aPTT	activated partial thromboplastin time
ARB	angiotensin receptor blocker
ASA	aspirin
ASCO	American Society of Clinical Oncology
AST	aspartate aminotransferase
AT	antithrombin
ATP	adenosine triphosphate
ATP-K	adenosine triphosphate potassium
ATP	Adult Treatment Panel
ATP III	Adult Treatment Panel III
ATS	American Thoracic Society
AUA	American Urological Association
AUC	area under the (serum concentration time) curve
AV	atrioventricular
AVP	arginine vasopressin
B&B	Brown and Brenn
B_2M	beta-2-microglobulin
BAL	bronchial alveolar lavage; bronchoalveolar lavage
BAMT	blood assay for *Mycobacterium tuberculosis*
BBT	basal body temperature
BCG	Bacille Calmette-Guérin
bDNA	branched-chain DNA
BGMK-hDAF	buffalo green monkey kidney cell line
BHI	brain heart infusion
BHR	bronchial hyper-responsiveness
BID	twice daily
BMI	body mass index
BMP	basic metabolic panel
BNP	brain natriuretic peptide
BP	blood pressure
BPH	benign prostatic hyperplasia
BPSA	benign prostate-specific antigen
BPT	bronchial provocation testing
BRAF	v-Raf murine sarcoma viral oncogene homolog B1
BSA	body surface area
BSL	biosafety level
BT	bleeding time
BUN	blood urea nitrogen
C. difficile	*Clostridium difficile*
C3	complement protein 3
C4	complement protein 4
CA	cancer antigen
CA	carbonic anhydrase
CABG	coronary artery bypass graft
CA_{corr}	corrected serum calcium level
CAD	coronary artery disease

CAH	congenital adrenal hyperplasia
CAN2	ChromID Candida agar
cANCA	cytoplasmic antineutrophil cytoplasmic antibody
CAP	College of Pathologists
CAP	community-acquired pneumonia
CAT	computerized axial tomography
CA_{uncorr}	uncorrected serum calcium level (or actual measured total serum calcium)
CBC	complete blood count
CCFA	cycloserine cefoxitin fructose agar
CCNA	cell cytotoxicity neutralization assay
CCP	cyclic citrullinated peptide
CCR5	chemokine coreceptor 5
cCRP	cardiac C-reactive protein
CCT	cardiac computed tomography
cd	candela
CD	clusters of differentiation
CDC	Centers for Disease Control and Prevention
CDR	complementarity-determining regions
CE	capillary electrophoresis
CEA	carcinoembryonic antigen
CEDIA	cloned enzyme donor immunoassay
CF	complement fixation
CFTR	cystic fibrosis transmembrane conductance regulator
CFU, cfu	colony-forming units
CFW	calcofluor white
CH_{50}	complement hemolytic 50%
CHD	coronary heart disease
CHF	congestive heart failure
CI	chemical ionization
CIS	combined intracavernous injection and stimulation
CK	creatine kinase
CK-MB	creatine kinase isoenzyme MB
CK1	creatine kinase isoenzyme 1
CK2	creatine kinase isoenzyme 2
CK3	creatine kinase isoenzyme 3
CKD	chronic kidney disease
CLIA-88	Clinical Laboratory Improvement Amendments of 1988
CLIA	Clinical Laboratory Improvement Amendments
CLL	chronic lymphocytic leukemia
CLSI	Clinical and Laboratory Standards Institute
cm	centimeter
CMA	cornmeal agar
CML	chronic myelogenous leukemia
CMP	comprehensive metabolic panel
CMR	cardiac magnetic resonance
CMV	cytomegalovirus
CNA	colistin-nalidixic acid
$C_{normalized}$	normalized total concentration
CNP	c-type natriuretic peptide
CNS	central nervous system
CO	carbon monoxide
CO	cardiac output

CO_2	carbon dioxide
CO-Hgb	carboxyhemoglobin
COP	colloid osmotic pressure
COPD	chronic obstructive pulmonary disease
CPE	cytopathic effect
CPK	creatine phosphokinase
CPPD	calcium pyrophosphate dihydrate
cPSA	complexed PSA
CrCl	creatinine clearance
CREST	syndrome characterized by <u>c</u>alcinosis, <u>R</u>aynaud disease, <u>e</u>sophageal motility disorder, <u>s</u>clerodactyly, and <u>t</u>elangiectasias
CRH	corticotrophin-releasing hormone
CRP	C-reactive protein
CSF	cerebrospinal fluid
$C_{ss, avg}$	average steady-state concentration
CT	computed tomography
cTnC	cardiac-specific troponin C
cTnI	cardiac-specific troponin I
CX	circumflex
CXCR4	CXC chemokine coreceptor
CYP	cytochrome P450 drug metabolizing enzymes
CYP2C19	cytochrome P450 2C19 enzyme
CYP2D6	cytochrome P450 2D6 enzyme
CYP3A4	cytochrome P450 3A4 enzyme
CYP450	cytochrome P450 enzyme
CZE	capillary zone electrophoresis
D5W	5% dextrose in water
DAT	direct agglutination test
DAT	direct antibody test
DCCT	Diabetes Control and Complications Trial
DCP	des-gamma-carboxyprothrombin
DDAVP	desmopressin
DDT	dichlorodiphenyltrichloroethane
DFA	direct fluorescent antibody
DHA	docosahexaenoic acid
DHEA	dehydroepiandrostenedione
DHEAS	dehydroepiandrosterone sulfate
DI	diabetes insipidus
DIC	disseminated intravascular coagulation
DIM	dermatophyte identification medium
DKA	diabetic ketoacidosis
dL	deciliter
DLCO	diffusing capacity of the lung for carbon monoxide
DM	diabetes mellitus
DNA	deoxyribonucleic acid
DNP	dendroaspis natriuretic peptide
DO_2	oxygen delivery
DPD	dihydropyrimidine dehydrogenase
DPP-4	dipeptidyl peptidase-4
dsDNA	double-stranded DNA
DST	dexamethasone suppression test
DTI	direct thrombin inhibitor

DTM	dermatophyte test medium
EBM	esculin base medium
EBV	Epstein-Barr virus
ECD	energy coupled dye
ECG	electrocardiogram
ECMO	extracorporeal membrane oxygenation
ECT	ecarin clotting time
ECW	extracellular water
ED	emergency department
EDTA	ethylenediaminetetraacetic acid
EGFR	epidermal growth factor receptor
eGFR	estimated glomerular filtration rate
EI	electron ionization
EIA	enzyme immunoassay
EIB	exercise- or exertion-induced bronchospasm
EKG	electrocardiogram
ELISA	enzyme-linked immunosorbent assay
ELVIS	enzyme-linked virus-inducible system
EM	electron microscopy
EMB	eosin methylene blue
EMIT	enzyme-multiplied immunoassay technique
EOF	electroosmotic force
EPA	eicosapentaenoic acid
EPS	expressed prostatic secretions
ER	estrogen receptor
ERS	European Respiratory Society
ERV	expiratory reserve volume
ESA	erythrocyte-stimulating agent
ESBL	extended-spectrum beta-lactamase
ESC	European Society of Cardiology
ESI	electrospray ionization
ESR	erythrocyte sedimentation rate
Etest®	epsilometer test
ETIB	enzyme-linked immunoelectrotransfer blot
EU	ELISA units
EUCAST	European Committee on Antimicrobial Susceptibility Testing
EULAR	European League Against Rheumatism
FA	fluorescent antibody
Fab	fraction antigen-binding
FAB	fast atom bombardment
FAB	French-American-British
FACS	fluorescence-activated cell sorting
FALS	forward-angle light scattering
FANA	fluorescent antinuclear antibody
FDA	Food and Drug Administration
FDP	fibrin degradation product
FEF_{25-75}	forced expiratory flow at 25% to 75% of vital capacity
FEF	forced expiratory flow
FE_{Na}	fractional excretion of sodium
FENO	fractional exhaled nitric oxide
$FEV_{0.5}$	forced expiratory volume in 0.5 second
FEV_1	forced expiratory volume in 1 second

FISH	fluorescence in situ hybridization
FITC	fluorescein isothiocyanate
fL	femtoliter
FM	Fontana-Masson
FN	false negative
FP	false positive
FPG	fasting plasma glucose
FPIA	fluorescence polarization immunoassay
fPSA	free prostate specific antigen
FRC	functional residual capacity
FSH	follicle-stimulating hormone
FTA-ABS	fluorescent treponemal antibody absorption
FVC	forced vital capacity
FWR	framework regions
g	gram
G-CSF	granulocyte colony–stimulating factor
G6PD	glucose-6 phosphate dehydrogenase
GA	gestational age
GADA	glutamic acid decarboxylase autoantibodies
GC	gas chromatography
GC-MS	gas chromatography and mass spectrometry
GERD	gastroesophageal reflux disease
GF	Gridley fungus
GFR	glomerular filtration rate
GGT, GGTP	gamma-glutamyl transferase; gamma-glutamyl transpeptidase
GHB	gamma-hydroxybutyrate
GI	gastrointestinal
GIP	glucose-dependent insulinotropic peptide
GLC	gas liquid chromatography
GLP-1	incretin hormones glucagon-like peptide-1
GLUT	glucose transporter
GM-CSF	granulocyte/macrophage colony-stimulating factor
GMS	Gomori methenamine silver
GnRH	gonadotropin-releasing hormone
GOLD	Global Initiative for Chronic Obstructive Lung Disease
gp	glycoprotein
GTF	glucose tolerance factor
H&E	hematoxylin and eosin
H. Pylori	Helicobacter pylori
HAAg	hepatitis A antigen
HAP	hospital-acquired pneumonia
HAV	hepatitis A virus
Hb	hemoglobin
HbA1c	glycosylated hemoglobin
HBcAg	hepatitis B core antigen
HBeAg	hepatitis B extracellular antigen
HBsAg	hepatitis B surface antigen
HBV	hepatitis B virus
HCG, hCG	human chorionic gonadotropin
HCO_3^-	bicarbonate
HCT, Hct	hematocrit
HCV	hepatitis C virus

HDAg	hepatitis D antigen
HDL	high-density lipoprotein
HDL-C	high-density lipoprotein cholesterol
HDV	hepatitis D virus
HER-1	human epidermal growth factor receptor 1
HER-2	human epidermal growth factor receptor 2
HEV	hepatitis E virus
HGA	human granulocytic anaplasmosis
Hg, Hgb	hemoglobin
HHS	hyperosmolar hyperglycemia state
HIPA	heparin-induced platelet activation
HIT	heparin-induced thrombocytopenia
HIV	human immunodeficiency virus
HIV-1	human immunodeficiency virus type 1
HLA	human leukocyte antigen
HLAR	high-level aminoglycoside resistance
HME	human monocytic ehrlichiosis
HMG-CoA	hydroxymethylglutaryl-coenzyme A
HMWK	high-molecular weight kininogen
HPA	hypothalamic pituitary axis
HPF	high-power field
HPLC	high-performance (or pressure) liquid chromatography
HPV	human papillomavirus
HR	heart rate
hr	hour
hs-CRP	high-sensitivity C-reactive protein
HSG	hysterosalpingogram, hysterosalpingography
hsTnI	high-sensitivity troponin I
hsTnT	high-sensitivity troponin T
HSV	herpes simplex virus
Ht	height
I	intermediate
IA	immunoassay
IA-2A	insulinoma-associated-2 autoantibodies
IAA	insulin autoantibodies
IAT	indirect antibody test
IBW	ideal body weight
IC	inspiratory capacity
IC_{50}	inhibitory concentration 50%
ICA	immunochromatographic assay
ICA	islet cell cytoplasmic autoantibodies
ICTV	International Committee on Taxonomy of Viruses
ICU	intensive care unit
ICW	intracellular water
ID	immunodiffusion
IDC	International Diabetes Center
IDL	intermediate-density lipoproteins
IDMS	isotope dilution mass spectrometry
IFA	immunofluorescence assay; indirect fluorescent antibody
IFN-γ	interferon gamma
IgA	immunoglobulin A
IgD	immunoglobulin D

IgE	immunoglobulin E
IgG	immunoglobulin G
IgM	immunoglobulin M
IHC	immunohistochemistry
IHD	ischemic heart disease
IIEF	International Index of Erectile Function
IIM	idiopathic inflammatory myopathy
IMA	inhibitory mold agar
INR	international normalized ratio
IP	interphalangeal
iPSA	inactive PSA
IPSS	International Prostate Symptom Score
IRMA	immunoradiometric assay
IRV	inspiratory reserve volume
ISE	ion-selective electrode
ISI	International Sensitivity Index
ITP	idiopathic thrombocytopenic purpura
IV	intravenous
JIA	juvenile idiopathic arthritis
JRA	juvenile rheumatoid arthritis
k	constant of proportionality
K	kelvin
K_{corr}	corrected serum potassium level
KDOQI	Kidney Disease Outcome Quality Initiative
kg	kilogram
KIMS	kinetic interaction of microparticles in solution
Km	Michaelis constant
KOH	potassium hydroxide
KRas	V-Ki-ras2 Kirsten rat sarcoma viral oncogene homolog
K_{uncorr}	uncorrected serum potassium level (or actual measured serum potassium)
L	liter
LA	latex agglutination
La/SSB	La/Sjögren syndrome B
LAD	left anterior descending
LBBB	left bundle branch block
LC	liquid chromatography
LCR	ligase chain reaction
LDH	lactate dehydrogenase
LDH1	lactate dehydrogenase isoenzyme 1
LDH2	lactate dehydrogenase isoenzyme 2
LDH3	lactate dehydrogenase isoenzyme 3
LDH4	lactate dehydrogenase isoenzyme 4
LDH5	lactate dehydrogenase isoenzyme 5
LDL	low-density lipoprotein
LDL-C	low-density lipoprotein cholesterol
LE	lupus erythematosus
LFT	liver function test
LH	luteinizing hormone
LHRH	luteinizing hormone–releasing hormone
LMP	last menstrual period
LMWH	low molecular weight heparin
$Lp\text{-}PLA_2$	lipoprotein-associated phospholipase A_2

LSD	lysergic acid diethylamide
LTA	light transmittance aggregometry
LUTS	lower urinary tract symptoms
LVEF	left ventricular ejection fraction
m	meter
m^2	meters squared
MAbs	monoclonal antibodies
Mac	MacConkey
MAC	membrane attack complex
MAC	*Mycobacterium avium* complex
MALDI	matrix-assisted laser desorption/ionization
MALDI-TOF	matrix-assisted laser desorption ionization time-of-flight
MAP	mitogen-activated protein
MAT	microscopic agglutination
MBC	minimum bactericidal concentration
MBP	mannose-binding protein
mcg	microgram
MCH	mean corpuscular hemoglobin
MCHC	mean corpuscular hemoglobin concentration
MCP	metacarpophalangeal
MCT	medium chain triglycerides
MCTD	mixed connective tissue disease
MCV	mean corpuscular volume
MDMA	3,4-methylenedioxy-N-methamphetamine (Ecstasy)
MDR	multidrug resistant
MDRD	Modification of Diet in Renal Disease
MDx	molecular diagnostics
mEq	milliequivalent
mg	milligram
MHA	Mueller-Hinton agar
MHA-TP	microhemagglutination *Treponema pallidum*
MHC	major histocompatibility complex
MI	myocardial infarction
MIC	minimum inhibitory concentration
MIC_{50}	MIC value representing 50% of a bacterial population
MIC_{90}	MIC value representing 90% of a bacterial population
MIF	microimmunofluorescence
min	minute
mL	milliliter
mm	millimeter
mm^3	cubic millimeter
mmol	millimole
MoAB	monoclonal antibody
mol	mole
MOTT	mycobacteria other than tuberculosis
MPO	myeloperoxidase
MPV	mean platelet volume
MRI	magnetic resonance imaging
mRNA	messenger ribonucleic acid
MRO	medical review officer
MRSA	methicillin-resistant *Staphylococcus aureus*
MS	mass spectrometry

MSSA	methicillin-susceptible *Staphylococcus aureus*
MTP	metatarsophalangeal
NA	nucleic acid
NAAT	nucleic acid amplification test
NACB	National Academy of Clinical Biochemistry
NAEPP	National Asthma Education Prevention Program
NASBA	nucleic acid sequence-based amplification
NASH	nonalcoholic steatohepatitis
NCCB	nondihydropyridine calcium channel blocker
NCEP	National Cholesterol Education Program
ng	nanogram
NHL	Non-Hodgkin lymphoma
NK cells	natural killer (T) lymphocytes
NNRTI	non-nucleoside reverse transcriptase inhibitor
NNS	number needed to screen
NQMI	non Q-wave myocardial infarction
NRTI	nucleoside reverse transcriptase inhibitor
NSAID	nonsteroidal anti-inflammatory drug
NSCLC	non-small-cell lung cancer
NSTEMI	non-ST-segment elevation myocardial infarction
NT-proBNP	N-terminal-proBNP
NTM	nontuberculous mycobacteria
NYHA	New York Heart Association
OA	osteoarthritis
OAT	organic anion transport
OCT	organic cation transport
OGTT	oral glucose tolerance test
OSHA	Occupational Safety and Health Administration
P	serum creatinine concentration
$P_1G_1O_1$	one live birth, one pregnancy, no spontaneous or elective abortions
P-gp	P-glycoprotein
$PaCO_2$	arterial partial pressure of carbon dioxide
PAI1	plasminogen activator inhibitor 1
pANCA	perinuclear antineutrophil cytoplasmic antibody
PaO_2	arterial partial pressure of oxygen
PAS	periodic acid-Schiff
PBC	primary biliary cirrhosis
PBMC	peripheral blood mononuclear cell
PBP	penicillin-binding protein
$PC_{20}FEV_1$	provocation concentration of the bronchoconstrictor agent that produces a 20% reduction in FEV_1
PCA	postconceptional age
PCI	percutaneous coronary intervention
pCO_2	partial pressure of carbon dioxide (in an arterial blood gas)
PCOS	polycystic ovary syndrome
PCP	phencyclidine
PCR	polymerase chain reaction
PDA	potato dextrose agar
PE	phycoerythrin
PEA	phenylethyl alcohol
PEFR	peak expiratory flow rate
PET	positron emission tomography

PF3	platelet factor 3
PF4	platelet factor 4
PFA	potato flake agar
PFT	pulmonary function test
pg	picogram
PG	prostaglandin
PG_2	prostacyclin
pH	power of hydrogen or hydrogen ion concentration
Ph	Philadelphia
PICU	pediatric intensive care unit
PID	pelvic inflammatory disease
PIP	proximal interphalangeal
PKU	phenylketonuria
PMA	postmenstrual age
PMN	polymorphonuclear leukocyte
PNA	postnatal age
PO	per os (by mouth)
pO_2	partial pressure of oxygen
POC	point-of-care
POCT	point-of-care testing
PPAR	peroxisome proliferator-activated receptor
PPD	purified protein derivative
PPG	postprandial glucose
PPI	proton pump inhibitor
PR	progesterone receptor
PR3	proteinase 3
PRN	as needed
PSA	prostate specific antigen
PSAD	prostate specific antigen density
PSB	protected specimen brush
PSM	patient self-management
PST	patient self-testing
PT	prothrombin time
PTCA	percutaneous transluminal coronary angioplasty
PTH	parathyroid hormone
q	every
Q	perfusion
QC	quality control
QID	four times daily
qPCR	real-time polymerase chain reaction
QRS	electrocardiograph wave; represents ventricular depolarization
QwMI	Q-wave myocardial infarction
R	resistant
R-CVA	right cerebral vascular accident
RA	rheumatoid arthritis
RAAS	renin-angiotensin-aldosterone system
RADT	rapid antigen detection test
RAEB	refractory anemia with excess blasts
RAIU	radioactive iodine uptake test
RALS	right-angle light scattering
RBC	red blood cell
RBF	renal blood flow

RCA	right coronary artery
RDW	red cell distribution width
RF	rheumatoid factor
RhMK	rhesus monkey kidney
RI	reticulocyte index
RIA	radioimmunoassay
RIBA	recombinant immunoblot assay
RIDTs	rapid influenza diagnostic tests
RNA	ribonucleic acid
RNP	ribonucleoprotein
Ro/SSA	Ro/Sjögren syndrome A antibody
RPF	renal plasma flow
RPR	rapid plasma reagin
RR	respiratory rate
RSA	rapid sporulation agar
RSV	respiratory syncytial virus
RT	reverse transcriptase; reverse transcription
RT-PCR	reverse-transcriptase polymerase chain reaction
RV	residual volume
S	susceptible
S:P ratio	saliva:plasma concentration ratio
SA	sinoatrial
SAMHSA	Substance Abuse and Mental Health Services Administration
SAT	serum agglutination test
SBA	sheep blood agar
SBT	serum bactericidal test
Scl_{70}	scleroderma-70 or DNA topoisomerase I antibody
SCr	serum creatinine
SD	standard deviation
SDA	Sabouraud dextrose agar
SDA	strand displacement amplification
sec	second
SGE	spiral gradient endpoint
SGLT	sodium glucose cotransporters
SHBG	sex hormone-binding globulin
SI	International System of Units
SIADH	syndrome of inappropriate antidiuretic hormone
SLE	systemic lupus erythematosus
Sm	Smith antibody
SMBG	self-monitoring blood glucose
SNP	single nucleotide polymorphism
SnRNP	small nuclear ribonucleoprotein particle
SPECT	single-photon emission computed tomography
SPEP	serum protein electrophoresis
SRA	C-serotonin release assay
ssDNA	single-stranded DNA
SSRI	selective serotonin reuptake inhibitor
STD	sexually transmitted disease
STEMI	ST segment elevation myocardial infarction
SV	stroke volume
SVC	slow vital capacity
SvO_2	mixed venous partial pressure of oxygen

T_3	triiodothyronine
T_4	thyroxine
TAT	turnaround time
TB	tuberculosis
TBG	thyroxine-binding globulin
TBI	total body irradiation
TBPA	thyroid-binding prealbumin
TBW	total body water
TBW	total body weight
TC	total cholesterol
TCA	tricyclic antidepressant
TDM	therapeutic drug monitoring
TEE	transesophageal echocardiography
TF	tissue factor
TFPI	tissue factor pathway inhibitor
TG	triglyceride
TIBC	total iron-binding capacity
TID	three times daily
TJC	The Joint Commission
TK	tyrosine kinase
TKI	tyrosine kinase inhibitor
TLA	total laboratory automation
TLC	therapeutic lifestyle changes
TLC	thin layer chromatography
TLC	total lung capacity
TMA	transcription mediated amplification
TN	true negative
TnC	troponin C
TNF	tumor necrosis factor
TnI	troponin I
TnT	troponin T
TP	true positive
TP	tube precipitin
tPA	tissue plasminogen activator
TPMT	thiopurine methyltransferase
TR	therapeutic range
TRH	thyrotropin-releasing hormone
TRUS	transrectal ultrasound of the prostate
TSB	trypticase soy broth
TSH	thyroid-stimulating hormone
TST	tuberculin skin test
TT	thrombin time
TTE	transthoracic echocardiography
TTP	thrombotic thrombocytopenic purpura
TTP	total testing process
TV	tidal volume
TXA_2	thromboxane A_2
type 1 DM	type 1 diabetes mellitus
type 2 DM	type 2 diabetes mellitus
U	urinary creatinine concentration
U_1RNP	uridine-rich ribonuclear protein
UA	unstable angina

UCr	urine creatinine
UFC	urine-free cortisol
UFH	unfractionated heparin
UGT1A1	uridine diphosphate glucuronyl transferase
UKPDS	United Kingdom Prospective Diabetes Study
ULN	upper limit of normal
uNGAL	urine neutrophil gelatinase associated lipocalcin
uPA	urokinase plasminogen activator
UTI	urinary tract infection
V	total urine volume collected
V	ventilation
V	volt
VAP	ventilator-associated pneumonia
VC	vital capacity
Vd	volume of distribution
VDRL	Venereal Disease Research Laboratory
VKORC1	vitamin K epoxide reductase complex subunit 1
VLDL	very low-density lipoprotein
V_{max}	maximum rate of metabolism
VO_2	oxygen consumption
VRE	vancomycin-resistant enterococci
VTE	venous thromboembolism
vWF	von Willebrand factor
VZV	varicella zoster virus
WB	western blot
WBC	white blood cell
WHO	World Health Organization
WNL	within normal limits
Wt	weight
WT	wild type
yr	year

CHAPTER 1

DEFINITIONS AND CONCEPTS

KAREN J. TIETZE

This chapter is based, in part, on the second edition chapter titled "Definitions and Concepts," which was written by Scott L. Traub.

Objectives

After completing this chapter, the reader should be able to

- Differentiate between accuracy and precision

- Distinguish between quantitative, qualitative, and semiqualitative laboratory tests

- Define reference range and identify factors that affect a reference range

- Differentiate between sensitivity and specificity, and calculate and assess these parameters

- Identify potential sources of laboratory errors and state the impact of these errors in the interpretation of laboratory tests

- Identify patient-specific factors that must be considered when assessing laboratory data

- Discuss the pros and cons of point-of-care and at-home laboratory testing

- Describe a rational approach to interpreting laboratory results

Laboratory testing is used to detect disease, guide treatment, monitor response to treatment, and monitor disease progression. However, it is an imperfect science. Laboratory testing may fail to identify abnormalities that are present (false negatives [FNs]) or identify abnormalities that are not present (false positives, [FPs]). This chapter defines terms used to describe and differentiate laboratory tests and describes factors that must be considered when assessing and applying laboratory test results.

DEFINITIONS

Many terms are used to describe and differentiate laboratory test characteristics and results. The clinician should recognize and understand these terms before assessing and applying test results to individual patients.

Accuracy and Precision

Accuracy and *precision* are important laboratory quality control measures. Laboratories are expected to test analytes with accuracy and precision and to document the quality control procedures. Accuracy of a quantitative assay is usually measured in terms of an analytical performance, which includes accuracy and precision. *Accuracy* is defined as the extent to which the mean measurement is close to the true value. A sample spiked with a known quantity of an analyte is measured repeatedly; the mean measurement is calculated. A highly accurate assay means that the repeated analyses produce a mean value that is the same as or very close to the known spiked quantity. Accuracy of a qualitative assay is calculated as the sum of the true positives (TPs) and true negatives (TNs) divided by the number of samples tested (accuracy = [(TP + TN) ÷ number of samples tested] × 100%). *Precision* refers to assay reproducibility (i.e., the agreement of results when the specimen is assayed many times). An assay with high precision means that the methodology is consistently able to produce results in close agreement. The accuracy of those results is another question.

Analyte

The *analyte* is the substance measured by the assay. Some substances, such as phenytoin and calcium, are bound extensively to proteins such as albumin. Although the unbound fraction elicits the physiological or pharmacological effect (bound substances are inactive), most routine assays measure the total substance (bound plus unbound). The free fraction may be assayable, but the assays are not routine. Therefore, the reference range for total and free substances may be quite different. For example, the reference range is 10–20 mcg/mL for total phenytoin, 1–2 mcg/mL for free phenytoin, 9.2–11.0 mg/dL for total serum calcium, and 4.0–4.8 mg/dL for free (also called ionized) calcium.

Some analytes exist in several forms and each has a different reference range. These forms are referred to as fractions, subtypes, subforms, isoenzymes, or isoforms. Results for the total and each form are reported. For example, bilirubin circulates in conjugated and unconjugated subforms as well as bound irreversibly to albumin (delta bilirubin). *Direct bilirubin* refers to the sum of the conjugated plus the delta forms; *indirect bilirubin* refers to the unconjugated form. Lactate dehydrogenase (LDH) is separated electrophoretically into five different isoenzymes: LDH1, LDH2,

MINICASE 1

Assays for Detecting Noroviruses

IN 411 PATIENTS WITH ACUTE GASTROENTERITIS SYMPTOMS, fecal specimens were tested for norovirus with a standard real-time reverse transcription-polymerase chain reaction (RT-PCR) molecular assay and a new immunochromatographic assay.[2] The new immunochromatographic assay provides very rapid results but may not be as sensitive as standard molecular assays.

Question: After reviewing the following results, what conclusions can be made about the clinical performance of the new immunochromatographic assay?

Immunochromatographic Assay Results (n=411):

True Positives	52	**True Negatives**	342
False Positives	1	**False Negatives**	16

Discussion: Calculate sensitivity, specificity, predictive value of a positive test, and the predictive value of a positive and negative test.

Sensitivity = (TP ÷ [TP + FN]) × 100% = (52 ÷ [52 + 16]) × 100% = 76.5%

Specificity = (TN ÷ [FP +TN]) × 100% = (342 ÷ [342 + 1]) × 100% = 99.7%

Predictive value of positive test = (TP ÷ [TP + FP]) × 100% = (52 ÷ [52 + 1]) × 100% = 98.1%

Predictive value of negative test = (TN ÷ [TN + FN]) × 100% = (342 ÷ [342 + 16]) × 100% = 95.5%

In this study, the new immunochromatographic assay had high specificity but low sensitivity as compared to a standard real-time RT-PCR assay. The new immunochromatographic assay may be useful for the rapid detection of norovirus infections, but it is not sensitive enough to rule out norovirus infection in those with negative test results.

LDH3, LDH4, and LDH5. Creatine kinase (CK) exists in three isoforms: CK1, CK2, and CK3.

Biomarker

A *biomarker* (biological marker) is a marker (not necessarily a quantifiable laboratory parameter) defined by the National Institutes of Health as "A characteristic that is objectively measured and evaluated as an indicator of normal biological processes, pathogenic processes, or pharmacologic responses to a therapeutic intervention.[1] Biomarkers are used to diagnose and stage disease (i.e., determine the extent of disease), assess disease progression, or assess response to therapeutic interventions. Tumor markers are biomarkers used to identify the presence of some cancers, to stage disease, or to assess patient response to drug and nondrug cancer treatments. Many biomarkers are common laboratory parameters. For example, glycosylated hemoglobin A1c (HbA1c) is used to assess long-term glucose control in people with diabetes.

Noninvasive Versus Invasive Tests

A *noninvasive test* is a procedure that examines fluids or other substances (e.g., urine and exhaled air) obtained without using a needle, tube, device, or scope to penetrate the skin or enter the body. An invasive test is a procedure that examines fluids or tissues (e.g., venous blood and skin biopsy) obtained by using a needle, tube, device, or scope to penetrate the skin or enter the body. *Invasive tests* pose variable risk depending on the method of specimen collection (e.g., pain and bruising associated with venipuncture) and are less convenient than noninvasive tests.

Predictive Value

The *predictive value*, derived from a test's sensitivity, specificity, and prevalence (incidence) of the disease in the population being tested, is used to assess a test's reliability (Table 1-1). As applied to a positive test result, the predictive value indicates the percent of positives that are TPs. For a test with equal sensitivity and specificity, the predictive value of a positive result increases as the incidence of the disease in the population increases. For example, the glucose tolerance test has a higher predictive value for diabetes in women who are pregnant than in the general population. A borderline abnormal serum creatinine concentration has a higher predictive value for kidney disease in patients in a nephrology unit than in patients in a general medical unit. The lower the prevalence of disease in the population tested, the greater the chance that a positive test result is in error. The predictive value may also be applied to negative results. As applied to a negative test result, the predictive value indicates the percent of negatives that are TNs (refer to Minicase 1).

Qualitative Tests

A *qualitative test* is a test whose results are reported as either positive or negative without further characterization of the degree of positivity or negativity. Exact quantities may be measured in the lab but are still reported qualitatively using predetermined ranges. For example, a serum or urine pregnancy test is reported as either positive or negative; a bacterial wound culture is reported as either positive for one or more specific microorganisms or reported as no growth; a urine toxicology drug screen is reported as either positive or negative for specific drugs; and an acid-fast stain for *Mycobacterium* is reported as either positive or negative.

Quantitative Tests

A *quantitative test* is a test whose results are reported as an exact numeric measurement (usually a specific mass per unit measurement) and assessed in the context of a reference range of values. For example, serum potassium is reported in milliequivalents per liter, creatinine clearance is reported in milliliters per minute, and LDH is reported in units per liter. Some test results are reported as titers (dilutions). For example, a serum antinuclear antibody titer of 1:160 is usually associated

TABLE 1-1. Relationship of Sensitivity, Specificity, Disease Prevalence, and Predictive Value of Positive Test (the predictive value of a positive test increases as the disease prevalence and sensitivity and specificity of the test increase)

SENSITIVITY AND SPECIFICITY (%)	PREVALENCE (%)	PREDICTIVE VALUE OF POSITIVE TEST (%)
95	0.1	1.9
	1	16.1
	2	27.9
	5	50
	50	95
99	0.1	9
	1	50
	2	66.9
	5	83.9
	50	99

Predictive value of positive test = [TP ÷ (TP + FP)] × 100%.
Predictive value of negative test = [TN ÷ (TN + FN)] × 100%.
Disease prevalence = (TP + FN) ÷ number of patients tested.
TP = diseased persons detected by test (true positives).
FP = nondiseased persons positive to test (false positives).
FN = diseased persons not detected by test (false negatives).
TN = nondiseased persons negative to test (true negatives).

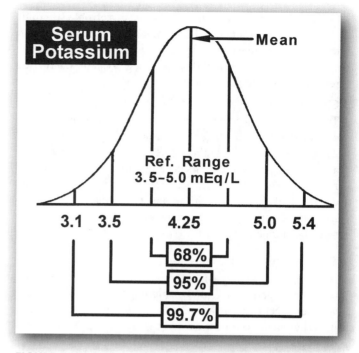

FIGURE 1-1. Gaussian (random) value distribution with a visual display of the area included within increments of standard deviation (SD) above and below the mean: ±1 SD = 68% of total values; ±2 SD = 95% of total values; and ±3 SD = 99.7% of total values.

with active systemic lupus erythematosus (LE) or other autoimmune diseases, though some patients may have "low titer" disease with titers of 1:40 or 1:80.

Reference Range

The *reference range* is a statistically-derived numerical range obtained by testing a sample of individuals assumed to be healthy. The upper and lower limits of the range are not absolute (i.e., normal versus abnormal), but rather points beyond which the probability of clinical significance begins to increase. The term *reference range* is preferred over the term *normal range*.[3] The reference population is assumed to have a Gaussian distribution with 68% of the values within one standard deviation (SD) above and below the mean, 95% within ±2 SD, and 99.7% within ±3 SD (Figure 1-1).

The reference range for a given analyte is usually established in the clinical laboratory as the mean or average value plus or minus two SDs. Acceptance of the mean ±2 SD indicates that one in 20 normal individuals will have test results outside the reference range (2.5% have values below the lower limit of the reference range and 2.5% have values above the upper limit of the reference range). Accepting a wider range (e.g., ±3 SD) includes a larger percentage (97.5%) of normal individuals but increases the chance of including individuals with values only slightly outside of a more narrow range, thus decreasing the sensitivity of the test.

Qualitative laboratory tests are either negative or positive and without a reference range; any positivity is considered abnormal. For example, any amount of serum acetone,

porphobilinogen, or alcohol is considered abnormal. The presence of glucose, ketones, blood, bile, or nitrate in urine is abnormal. The results of the Venereal Disease Research Laboratory (VDRL) test, the LE prep test, tests for red blood cell (RBC) sickling, and the malaria smear are either positive or negative.

Factors That Influence the Reference Range

Many factors influence the reference range. Reference ranges may differ between labs depending on analytical technique, reagent, and equipment. The initial assumption that the sample population is normal may be false. For example, the reference range is inaccurate if too many individuals with covert disease (i.e., no signs or symptoms of disease) are included in the sample population. Failure to control for physiologic variables (e.g., age, gender, ethnicity, body mass, diet, posture, and time of day) introduces many unrelated factors and may result in an inaccurate reference range. Reference ranges calculated from nonrandomly distributed (non-Gaussian) test results or from a small number of samples may not be accurate.

Reference ranges may change as new information relating to disease and treatments becomes available. For example, the National Cholesterol Education Program's (NCEP) Third Report of the Expert Panel on Detection, Evaluation, and Treatment of High Blood Cholesterol in Adults (Adult Treatment Panel III or ATP III), released in 2001, includes recommendations to lower and more closely space reference range cutoff points for low-density lipoprotein cholesterol (LDL-C), high-density lipoprotein cholesterol (HDL-C), and triglycerides

(TGs).[4] The availability of more sensitive thyrotropin (thyroid-stimulating hormone [TSH]) assays and the recognition that the original reference population data was skewed has led some clinicians to conclude that there is a need to establish a revised reference range for this analyte.[5]

Critical Value

The term *critical value* refers to a result that is far enough outside the reference range that it indicates impending morbidity (e.g., potassium <2.8 mEq/L). Because laboratory personnel are not in a position to consider mitigating circumstances, a responsible member of the healthcare team is notified immediately on discovery of a critical value test result. Critical values may not always be clinically relevant, however, because the reference range varies for the reasons discussed above.

Semiquantitative Tests

A *semiquantitative test* is a test whose results are reported as either negative or with varying degrees of positivity but without exact quantification. For example, urine glucose and urine ketones are reported as negative or 1+, 2+, 3+; the higher numbers represent a greater amount of the measured substance in the urine, but not a specific concentration.

Sensitivity

The *sensitivity* of a test refers to the ability of the test to identify positive results in patients who actually have the disease (TP rate).[6,7] Sensitivity assesses the proportion of TPs disclosed by the test (Table 1-2). A test is completely sensitive (100% sensitivity) if it is positive in every patient who actually has the disease. The higher the test sensitivity, the lower the chance of a false-negative result; the lower the test sensitivity, the higher the chance of a false-negative result. However, a highly sensitive test is not necessarily a highly specific test (see below).

Highly sensitive tests are preferred when the consequences of not identifying the disease are serious; less sensitive tests may be acceptable if the consequence of a false negative is less significant or if low sensitivity tests are combined with other tests. For example, inherited phenylalanine hydroxylase deficiency (phenylketonuria or PKU) results in increased phenylalanine concentrations. High phenylalanine concentrations damage the central nervous system and are associated with mental retardation. Mental retardation is preventable if PKU is diagnosed

and dietary interventions initiated before 30 days of age. The phenylalanine blood screening test, used to screen newborns for PKU, is a highly sensitive test when testing infants at least 24 hours of age.[8] In contrast, the prostate specific antigen (PSA) test, a test commonly used to screen men for prostate cancer, is highly sensitive at a low PSA cutoff value but highly specific only at a high PSA cutoff value.[9] Thus, PSA cannot be relied on as the sole prostate cancer screening method.

Sensitivity also refers to the range over which a quantitative assay can accurately measure the analyte. In this context, a sensitive test is one that can measure low levels of the substance; an insensitive test cannot measure low levels of the substance accurately. For example, a digoxin assay with low sensitivity might measure digoxin concentrations as low as 0.7 ng/mL. Concentrations below 0.7 ng/mL would not be measurable and would be reported as "less than 0.7 ng/mL" whether the digoxin concentration was 0.69 ng/mL or 0.1 ng/mL. Thus this relatively insensitive digoxin assay would not differentiate between medication nonadherence with an expected digoxin concentration of 0 ng/mL and low concentrations associated with inadequate dosage regimens.

Specificity

Specificity refers to the percent of negative results in people without the disease (TN rate).[6,7] Specificity assesses the proportion of TNs disclosed by the test (Table 1-2); the lower the specificity, the higher the chance of a false-positive result. A test with a specificity of 95% for the disease in question indicates that the disease will be detected in 5% of people without the disease. Tests with high specificity are best for confirming a diagnosis because the tests are rarely positive in the absence of the disease. Several newborn screening tests (e.g., PKU, galactosemia, biotinidase deficiency, congenital hypothyroidism, and congenital adrenal hyperplasia) have specificity levels above 99%.[10] In contrast, the PSA test is an example of a test with low specificity. The PSA is specific for the prostate but not specific for prostate carcinoma. Urethral instrumentation, prostatitis, urinary retention, prostatic needle biopsy, and benign prostatic hyperplasia elevate the PSA. The erythrocyte sedimentation rate (ESR) is another nonspecific test; infection, inflammation, and plasma cell dyscrasias increase the ESR.

Specificity as applied to quantitative laboratory tests refers to the degree of cross-reactivity of the analyte with other substances in the sample. For example, vitamin C cross-reacts with glucose in some urine tests (e.g., Clinitest®), falsely elevating the urine glucose test results. Quinine may cross-react with or be measured as quinidine in some assays, falsely elevating reported quinidine concentrations.

Specimen

A *specimen* is a sample (e.g., whole blood, venous blood, arterial blood, urine, stool, sputum, sweat, gastric secretions, exhaled air, cerebrospinal fluid, or tissues) that is used for laboratory analysis. Plasma is the watery acellular portion of blood. Serum is the liquid that remains after the fibrin clot is removed from plasma. While some laboratory tests are performed only on plasma (e.g., renin activity and adrenocorticotropic hormone

TABLE 1-2. Calculation of Sensitivity and Specificity

Screening Test Result	Diseased	Not Diseased	Total
Positive	TP	FP	TP + FP
Negative	FN	TN	FN + TN
Total	TP + FN	FP + TN	TP + FP + FN + TN

Sensitivity = [TP ÷ (TP + FN)] × 100%.

Specificity = [TN ÷ (FP + TN)] × 100%.

TP = diseased persons detected by test (true positives).

FP = nondiseased persons positive to test (false positives).

FN = diseased persons not detected by test (false negatives).

TN = nondiseased persons negative to test (true negatives).

[ACTH] concentration) or serum (e.g., serum electrophoresis and acetaminophen concentration), other laboratory tests can be performed on either plasma or serum (e.g., aldosterone, potassium, and sodium concentrations).

LABORATORY TEST RESULTS

Units Used in Reporting Laboratory Results

Laboratory test results are reported with a variety of units. For example, four different units are used to report serum magnesium concentration (1.0 mEq/L = 1.22 mg/dL = 0.5 mmol/L = 12.2 mg/L). Additionally, the same units may be reported in different ways. For example, mg/dL, mg/100 mL, and mg% are equivalent units. Enzyme activity is usually reported in terms of units, but the magnitude varies widely and depends on the methodology. Rates are usually reported in volume per unit of time (e.g., creatinine clearance is measured in mL/min or L/hr), but the ESR is reported in mm/hr and coagulation test results are reported in seconds or minutes. This lack of standardization is confusing and may lead to misinterpretation of the test results.

The International System of Units (Système Internationale d'Unités, or SI) was created about 40 years ago to standardize quantitative units worldwide.[11] Four base units and symbols are designated: length (meter, m), mass (kilogram, kg), time (second, s), and substance (mole, mol). Five derived units are designated: volume (liter, L, 10^{-3} m^3), force (newton, N, kg ms^{-2}), pressure (pascal, Pa, kg m^{-1} s^{-2}), energy (joule, J, kg m^2 s^{-2}), and power (watt, W, kg m^2 s^{-3}). However, it is difficult for clinicians to relate to molar concentrations (e.g., serum cholesterol 4.14 mmol•L^{-1} versus 160 mg/dL, or HbA1c mmol/mL versus 8%). In the United States, most laboratory results are reported in conventional units.

Rationale for Ordering Laboratory Tests

Laboratory tests are performed with the expectation that the results will

1. Discover occult disease
2. Confirm a suspected diagnosis
3. Differentiate among possible diagnoses
4. Determine the stage, activity, or severity of disease
5. Detect disease recurrence
6. Assess the effectiveness of therapy
7. Guide the course of therapy

Laboratory tests are categorized as screening or diagnostic tests. Screening tests, performed in individuals without signs or symptoms of disease, detect disease early when interventions (e.g., lifestyle modifications, drug therapy, and surgery) are likely to be effective. Screening tests are performed on healthy individuals and are generally inexpensive, quick and easy to perform, and reliable but do not provide a definitive answer. Screening tests require confirmation with other clinical tests. Diagnostic tests are performed on at-risk individuals, are typically more expensive, and are associated with some degree of risk but provide a definitive answer.[12]

Comparative features of screening tests are listed in Table 1-3. Examples of screening tests include the Papanicolaou smear, lipid profile, PSA, fecal occult blood, tuberculin skin test, sickle cell tests, blood coagulation tests, and serum chemistries. Screening tests may be performed on healthy outpatients (e.g., ordered by the patient's primary care provider or performed during public health fairs) or on admission to an acute care facility (e.g., prior to scheduled surgery). Abnormal screening tests are followed by more specific tests to confirm the abnormality.

Screening tests must be cost-effective and population-appropriate. The number needed to screen (NNS) is defined as "the number of people that need to be screened for a given duration to prevent one death or one adverse event."[14] For example, 465 women need to undergo mammographic screening every 24–33 months for 7 years to save one life from breast cancer.[15]

Diagnostic tests are performed in individuals with signs or symptoms of disease, a history suggestive of a specific disease or disorder, or an abnormal screening test. Diagnostic tests are used to confirm a suspected diagnosis, differentiate among possible diagnoses, determine the stage of activity of disease, detect disease recurrence, and assess and guide the therapeutic course. Diagnostic test features are listed in Table 1-3. Examples of diagnostic tests include blood cultures, serum cardiac-specific troponin I and T, kidney biopsy, and the cosyntropin test.

Many laboratories group a series of related tests (screening and/or diagnostic) into a set called a *profile*. For example, the basic metabolic panel (BMP) includes common serum electrolytes (sodium, potassium, and chloride), carbon dioxide content, blood urea nitrogen (BUN), calcium, creatinine, and glucose. The comprehensive metabolic panel (CMP) includes the BMP plus albumin, alanine aminotransferase (ALT), aspartate aminotransferase (AST), total bilirubin, and total protein. Grouped together for convenience, some profiles may be less costly to perform than the sum of the cost of each individual test. However, profiles may generate unnecessary patient data. Attention to cost is especially important in the current cost-conscious era. A test should not be done if it is unnecessary,

TABLE 1-3. Comparative Features of Screening and Diagnostic Laboratory Tests[a]

Feature	Screening Test	Diagnostic Test
Simplicity of test	Fairly simple	More complex
Target population	Individuals without signs or symptoms of the disease	Individuals with signs or symptoms of the disease
Performed by	Nonphysician providers and physicians	Physicians
Characteristic	High sensitivity	High specificity
Disease prevalence	Relatively common	Common or rare
Risks	Acceptable to population	Acceptable to individual

[a]Compiled from reference 13.

Figure 1-2. Contents of a typical Quickview chart.

QUICKVIEW	Contents of a typical Quickview chart		
PARAMETER	**DESCRIPTION**	**COMMENTS**
Common reference ranges		
Adults	Reference range in adults	Variability and factors affecting range
Pediatrics	Reference range in children	Variability, factors affecting range, age grouping
Critical value	Value beyond which immediate action usually needs to be taken	Disease-dependent factors; relative to reference range; value is a multiple of upper normal limit
Inherent activity	Does substance have any physiological activity?	Description of activity and factors affecting activity
Location		
Production	Is substance produced? If so, where?	Factors affecting production
Storage	Is substance stored? If so, where?	Factors affecting storage
Secretion/excretion	Is substance secreted/excreted? If so, where/how?	Factors affecting secretion or excretion
Causes of abnormal values		
High	Major causes	Modification of circumstances, other related causes or drugs that are commonly monitored with this test
Low	Major causes	
Signs and symptoms		
High level	Major signs and symptoms with a high or positive result	Modification of circumstances/other related signs and symptoms
Low level	Major signs and symptoms with a low result	Modification of circumstances/other related causes
After event, time to....		
Initial elevation	Minutes, hours, days, weeks	Assumes acute insult
Peak values	Minutes, hours, days, weeks	Assumes insult not yet removed
Normalization	Minutes, hours, days, weeks	Assumes insult removed and nonpermanent damage
Causes of spurious results	List of common causes	Modification of circumstances/assay specific
Additional information	Any other pertinent information regarding the lab value of assay	

redundant, or provides suboptimal clinical data (e.g., non-steady-state serum drug concentrations). Before ordering a test, the clinician should consider the following questions:

1. Was the test recently performed and in all probability the results have not changed at this time?
2. Were other tests performed that provide the same information?
3. Can the needed information be estimated with adequate reliability from existing data?

For example, creatinine clearance can be estimated using age, height, weight, and serum creatinine rather than measured from a 24-hour urine collection. Serum osmolality can be calculated from electrolytes and glucose rather than measured directly. Additionally, a clinician should ask, "What will I do if results are positive or negative (or absent or normal)?" If the test result will not aid in clinical decisions or change the diagnosis, prognosis, or treatment course, the benefits from the test are not worth the cost of the test.

Factors That Influence Laboratory Test Results

Laboratory results may be inconsistent with patient signs, symptoms, or clinical status. Before accepting reported laboratory values, clinicians should consider the numerous laboratory- and patient-specific factors that may influence the results (Table 1-4). For most of the major tests discussed in this book, a Quickview chart summarizes information helpful in interpreting results. Figure 1-2 depicts the format and content of a typical Quickview chart.

TABLE 1-4. Factors That Influence Assessment of Laboratory Results

Assay used and form of analyte
Free
Bound
Clinical situation
Acuity
Severity
Demographics
Age
Gender
Ethnicity
Height
Weight
Body surface area
Drugs
Drug–drug interactions
Drug–assay interactions
Food
Time of last meal
Type of food ingested
Nutritional status
Posture
Pregnancy
Specimen analyzed
Serum
Blood (venous or arterial)
Cerebrospinal fluid
Urine
Temporal relationships
Time of day
Time of last dose

Laboratory-Specific Factors

Laboratory errors are uncommon but may occur. Defined as a test result that is not the true result, laboratory error most appropriately refers to inaccurate results that occur because of an error made by laboratory personnel or equipment. However, laboratory error is sometimes used to refer to otherwise accurate results rendered inaccurate by specimen-related issues. Laboratory errors should be suspected for one or more of the following situations:

1. The result is inconsistent with trend in serial test results.
2. The magnitude of error is great.
3. The result is not in agreement with a confirmatory test result.
4. The result is inconsistent with clinical signs or symptoms or other patient-specific information.

True laboratory errors (inaccurate results) are caused by one or more laboratory processing or equipment errors, such as deteriorated reagents, calibration errors, calculation errors, misreading the results, computer entry or other documentation errors, or improper sample preparation. For example, incorrect entry of thromboplastin activity (International Sensitivity Index, [ISI]) when calculating the International Normalized Ratio (INR) results in accurately assayed but incorrectly reported INR results.

Accurate results may be rendered inaccurate by one or more specimen-related problems. Improper specimen handling prior to or during transport to the laboratory may alter analyte concentrations between the time the sample was obtained from the patient and the time the sample was analyzed in the laboratory.[16] For example, arterial blood withdrawn for blood gas analysis must be transported on ice to prevent continued in vitro changes in pH, $PaCO_2$, and PaO_2. Failure to remove the plasma or serum from the clot within 4 hours of obtaining blood for serum potassium analysis may elevate the reported serum potassium concentration. Red blood cell hemolysis elevates the serum potassium and phosphate concentrations. Failure to refrigerate samples may cause falsely low concentrations of serum enzymes (e.g., CK). Prolonged tourniquet time may hemoconcentrate analytes, especially those that are highly protein bound (e.g., calcium).

Patient-Specific Factors

Laboratory test values cannot be interpreted in isolation of the patient. Numerous age-related (e.g., age and renal function) and other patient-specific factors (e.g., time of day, posture) as well as disease-specific factors (e.g., time course) affect lab results. The astute clinician assesses laboratory data in context of all that is known about the patient.

Time course. Incorrectly timed laboratory tests produce misleading lab results. Disease states, normal physiologic patterns, pharmacodynamics, and pharmacokinetics time courses must be considered when interpreting lab values. For example, digoxin has a prolonged distribution phase. Digoxin serum concentrations obtained before tissue distribution is complete do not accurately reflect true tissue drug concentrations. Postmyocardial infarction enzyme patterns are an example of a more complex and prolonged postevent time course. Creatine kinase elevates about 6 hours following myocardial infarction (MI) and returns to baseline about 48–72 hours after the MI. Lactate dehydrogenase elevates about 12–24 hours following MI and returns to baseline about 10 days after the MI. Troponin elevates a few hours following MI and returns to baseline in about 5–7 days. Serial samples are used to assess myocardial damage.

Lab samples obtained too early or too late may miss critical changes and lead to incorrect assessments. For example, cosyntropin (synthetic ACTH) tests adrenal gland responsiveness. The baseline 8 a.m. plasma cortisol is compared to the stimulated plasma cortisol obtained 30 and 60 minutes following injection of the drug. Incorrect timing leads to incorrect results. The sputum acid-fast bacilli (AFB) smear may become

AFB-negative with just a few doses of antituberculous drugs, but the sputum culture may remain positive for several weeks. Expectations of a negative sputum culture too early in the time course may lead to the inappropriate addition of unnecessary antituberculous drugs.

Non-steady-state drug concentrations are difficult to interpret; inappropriate dosage adjustments (usually inappropriate dosage increases) may occur if the clinician fails to recognize that a drug has not reached steady-state concentrations. Although non-steady-state drug concentrations may be useful when assessing possible drug toxicity (e.g., overdose situations and new onset adverse drug events), all results need to be interpreted in the context of the drug's pharmacokinetics. Absorption, distribution, and elimination may change with changing physiology. For example, increased/decreased hepatic or renal perfusion may affect the clearance of a drug. Some drugs (e.g., phenytoin) have very long half-lives; constantly changing hemodynamics during an acute care hospitalization may prevent the drug from achieving steady-state while the patient is acutely ill.

Age. Age influences many physiologic systems. Age-related changes are well-described for neonates and young children, but less data are available for the elderly and the very elderly (usually described as ≥75 years of age). Age influences some but not all lab values; not all changes are clinically significant.

Pediatric reference ranges often reflect physiologic immaturity, with lab values approaching those of healthy adults with increasing age. For example, the complete blood count (CBC) (hemoglobin, hematocrit, RBC count, and RBC indices) ranges are greatly dependent on age with different values reported for premature neonates, term neonates, and young children. The fasting blood glucose reference range in premature neonates is approximately 20–65 mg/dL compared to 60–105 mg/dL for children 2 years of age and older and 70–110 mg/dL for adults. The serum creatinine reference range for children 1–5 years of age differs from the reference range for children 5–10 years of age (0.3–0.5 mg/dL versus 0.5–0.8 mg/dL). Reference ranges for children are well-described because it is relatively easy to identify age-differentiated populations of healthy children. Most laboratory reference texts provide age-specific reference values.

Geriatric reference ranges are more difficult to establish because of physiologic variability with increasing age and the presence of symptomatic and asymptomatic disease states that influence reference values. Diet (e.g., malnutrition) also influences some lab results. Some physiologic functions (e.g., cardiac, pulmonary, renal and metabolic functions) progressively decline with age, but each organ declines at a different rate.[17] Other physiologic changes associated with aging include decreased body weight, decreased height, decreased total body water, increased extracellular water, increased fat percentage, and decreased lean tissue percentage; cell membranes may leak.[17] Published studies sometimes lead to contradictory conclusions due to differences in study methodology (e.g., single point versus longitudinal evaluations) and populations assessed (e.g., nursing home residents versus general

population). Little data are available for the very elderly (≥90 years of age).[18] Most laboratory reference texts provide age-specific reference values.

Despite the paucity of data and difficulties imposed by different study designs and study populations, there is general consensus that some laboratory reference ranges are unchanged, some are different but of uncertain clinical significance, and some are significantly different in the elderly (Table 1-5). For example, decreased lean muscle mass with increased age results in decreased creatinine production. Decreased renal function is associated with decreased creatinine elimination. Taken together, the serum creatinine reference range in the elderly is not different from younger populations though creatinine clearance clearly declines with age.

Significant age-related changes are reported for the 2-hour postprandial glucose test, serum lipids, and arterial oxygen pressure (Table 1-5). The 2-hour postprandial glucose increases by about 5–10 mg/dL per decade. Progressive ventilation-perfusion mismatching from loss of elastic recoil with increasing age causes progressively decreased arterial oxygen pressure with increasing age. Cholesterol progressively increases from age 20 years reaching a plateau in the 5th to 6th decade in men and in the 6th to 7th decade in women followed by progressive decline. LDL and TG follow a similar pattern, though TG appears to progressively increase in women.

Genetics, ethnicity, and gender. Inherited ethnic and/or gender differences are identified for some laboratory tests. For example, the hereditary anemias (e.g., thalassemias and sickling disorders such as sickle cell anemia) are more common in individuals with African, Mediterranean, Middle Eastern, Indian, and southeast Asian ancestry.[24] Glucose-6-phosphate dehydrogenase (G6PD) deficiency is an example of an inherited sex-linked (X-chromosome) enzyme deficiency found primarily in men of African and Mediterranean ancestry.[25] The A-G6PD variant occurs mostly in Africans and affects about 13% of African-American males and 3% of African-American females in the United States. The Mediterranean G6PD variant, associated with a less common but more severe enzyme deficiency state, occurs mostly in individuals of Greek, Sardinian, Kurdish, Asian, and Sephardic Jewish ancestry.

Other enzyme polymorphisms influence drug metabolism. The genetically-linked absence of an enzyme may lead to drug toxicity secondary to drug accumulation or lack of drug effect if the parent compound is an inactive prodrug (e.g., codeine). The cytochrome P450 (CYP450) superfamily consists of greater than 100 isoenzymes with selective but overlapping substrate specificity. Some individuals are poor metabolizers while some are hyperextensive metabolizers. Several of the cytochrome P450 phenotypes vary by race. For example, the CYP2D6 poor metabolism phenotype occurs in 5% to 10% of Caucasians and the CYP2C19 poor metabolism phenotype occurs in 10% to 30% of Asians.[26,27]

Additional enzyme polymorphisms include pseudocholinesterase deficiency, phenytoin hydroxylation deficiency, inefficient N-acetyltransferase activity, inefficient or rapid debrisoquine hydroxylase activity, diminished thiopurine

TABLE 1-5. Laboratory Testing: Tests Affected by Aging[17-23]

No change

Amylase

Lipase

Hemoglobin

Hematocrit

Red blood cell count

Red blood cell indices

Platelet count

White blood cell count and differential

Serum electrolytes (sodium, potassium, chloride, bicarbonate, magnesium)

Coagulation

Total iron binding capacity

Thyroid function tests (thyroxine, T_3 resin uptake)

Liver function tests (AST, ALT, LDH)

Some change (unclear clinical significance)

Alkaline phosphatase

Erythrocyte sedimentation rate

Serum albumin

Serum calcium

Serum uric acid

Thyroid function tests (TSH, triiodothyronine)

Clinically significant change

Arterial oxygen pressure

2-hr postprandial glucose

Serum lipids (total cholesterol, low-density lipoprotein, triglycerides)

Serum testosterone (in men)

Serum estradiol (in women)

No change but clinically significant

Serum creatinine

ALT = alanine aminotransferase; AST = aspartate aminotransferase;
LDH = lactate dehydrogenase; TSH = thyroid-stimulating hormone.

methyltransferase activity, partial dihydropyrimidine dehydrogenase inactivity, and defective uridine diphosphate glucuronosyl transferase activity.[28] Other examples of genetic polymorphisms include variations in the beta-2 adrenoceptor gene that influence response to sympathomimetic amines and variations in drug transporters such as P-glycoprotein (P-gp), multidrug resistance gene associated proteins (MRP1, MRP2, MRP3), and organic anion transporting peptide (OATP1, OATP2).[28]

Biologic rhythms. Biologic rhythms are characterized as short (less than 30 minutes), intermediate (greater than 30 minutes but less than 6 days), and long (greater than 6 days).[29] The master clock, located in the suprachiasmatic nucleus of the hypothalamus, coordinates timing signals and multiple peripheral clocks.[30] A circadian rhythm is a 24-hour, endogenously generated cycle.[31] Well-described, human circadian rhythms include body temperature, cortisol production, melatonin production, and hormonal production (gonadotropin, testosterone, growth hormone, and thyrotropin). Platelet function, cardiac function, and cognition also follow a circadian rhythm.[32]

Other laboratory parameters follow circadian patterns. For example, statistically significant circadian rhythms have been reported for CK, ALT, gamma glutamyl transferase, LDH, and some serum lipids.[33,34] Glomerular filtration has a circadian rhythm.[35] Amikacin is almost completely excreted via glomerular filtration, and serum amikacin levels have been reported to have a diurnal variation.[36] Though the clinical significance of diurnally variable laboratory results is not well understood, diurnal variability should be considered when assessing laboratory values. Obtaining laboratory results at the same time of day (e.g., routine 7 a.m. blood draws) minimizes variability due to circadian rhythms. Different results obtained at different times of the day may be due to circadian variability rather than acute physiologic changes.

Other well-described biologic rhythms include the 8-hour rhythm for circulating endothelin, the approximately weekly (circaseptan) rhythm for urinary 17-ketosteroid excretion, the monthly rhythms of follicle-stimulating hormone, luteinizing hormone, progesterone production, and the seasonal rhythms for cholesterol and 25-hydroxycholecalciferol.[37]

Drugs. The four generally accepted categories of drug–laboratory interactions include methodological interference; drug-induced, end-organ damage; direct pharmacologic effect; and a miscellaneous category. Many drugs interfere with analytical methodology. Drugs that discolor the urine interfere with fluorometric, colorimetric, and photometric tests and mask abnormal urine colors. For example, amitriptyline turns the urine a blue–green color and phenazopyridine and rifampin turn the urine an orange–red color. Other drugs directly interfere with the laboratory assay. For example, high doses of ascorbic acid (greater than 500 mg/day) cause false-negative stool occult blood tests as well as false-negative urine glucose oxidative tests. Some drugs interfere with urinary fluorescence tests for urine catecholamines by producing urinary fluorescence themselves (e.g., ampicillin, chloral hydrate, and erythromycin).

Direct drug-induced, end-organ damage (e.g., kidney, liver, and bone marrow) change the expected lab results. For example, amphotericin B causes renal damage evidenced by increased serum creatinine; and bone marrow suppressants, such as doxorubicin and bleomycin, cause thrombocytopenia. Some drugs alter laboratory results as a consequence of a direct pharmacologic effect. For example, thiazide and loop diuretics increase serum uric acid by decreasing uric acid renal clearance or tubular secretion. Narcotics, such as codeine and morphine sulfate, increase serum lipase by inducing spasms of the sphincter of Oddi. Urinary specific gravity is increased in the presence of dextran. Other examples of drug–lab interactions include drugs that cause a positive direct Coombs test (e.g., isoniazid,

MINICASE 2

Interpretation of Hemoglobin and Hematocrit

ANNA W., A 72-YEAR-OLD FEMALE nursing home resident, suffered a minor stroke about 5 weeks ago. Her neurological deficits improved leaving her with residual weakness on her left side. She returned from an acute care hospital 12 days ago. Since that time, Anna W. has not been eating much and has been drinking even less. She has a history of chronic iron and folate deficiency anemia with her usual Hgb around 10 g/dL (reference range: 12–16 g/dL), Hct around 30% (reference range: 37% to 47%), iron concentration around 35 mcg/dL (reference range: 60–150 mcg/dL), and folate less than 1–3 ng/mL (reference range 4–15 ng/mL).

Anna W. takes daily iron and folate supplements as well as many other drugs. Her blood pressure has remained stable, but her heart rate has increased from 70s to 90s over the past 5–7 days. Her mucous membranes became dry, her skin turgor diminished, and her urine output decreased over that same time period. A complete blood count is ordered. Tests results indicate an Hgb of 13 g/dL and an Hct of 40%. Her BUN is 40 mg/dL (reference range: 8–20 mg/dL), creatinine is 0.8 mg/dL (reference range: 0.5–1.1 mg/dL), and sodium is 145 mEq/L (reference range: 136–145 mEq/L).

Question: Has the patient's anemia resolved? What is happening here?

Discussion: All the patient's laboratory values, including Hgb and Hct, have become temporarily hemoconcentrated because the patient is dehydrated. Thirst mechanisms are sometimes disrupted after a stroke. Her dry mucous membranes, decreased skin turgor, diminished urine output, and increased heart rate are all consistent with dehydration. As the patient is rehydrated, Hgb and Hct values should return to baseline.

If the patient is overhydrated, the opposite scenario can occur. Of course, assay interference by drugs, metabolites, and other foreign substances (as well as laboratory error) should always be kept in mind. If hemoconcentration had not been so apparent, laboratory error and interferences might be considered. In that case the test should be repeated.

---

sulfonamides, and quinidine), drugs that cause a positive anti-nuclear antibody test (e.g., penicillins, sulfonamides, and tetracyclines), and drugs that inhibit bacterial growth in blood or urine cultures (e.g., antibiotics).

Thyroid function tests are a good example of the complexity of potential drug-induced laboratory test changes. Thyroxine (T_4) and triiodothyronine (T_3) are displaced from binding proteins by salicylates, heparin, and high-doses of furosemide. Free T_4 levels initially increase, but chronic drug administration results in decreased T_4 levels with normal TSH levels. Phenytoin, phenobarbital, rifampin, and carbamazepine stimulate hepatic metabolism of thyroid hormone, resulting in decreased serum hormone concentration. Amiodarone, high-dose beta-adrenergic blocking drugs, glucocorticosteroids, and some iodine contrast dyes interfere with the conversion of T_4 to T_3. Ferrous sulfate, aluminum hydroxide, sucralfate, colestipol, and cholestyramine decrease T_4 absorption. Somatostatin, octreotide, and glucocorticosteroids suppress TSH production.

Pregnancy. Pregnancy is a normal physiologic condition that alters the reference range for many laboratory tests. Normal pregnancy increases serum hormone concentrations (e.g., estrogen, testosterone, progesterone, human chorionic gonadotropin, prolactin, corticotropin-releasing hormone, ACTH, cortisol, and atrial natriuretic hormone). The plasma volume increases by 30% to 50%, resulting in a relative hyponatremia (e.g., serum sodium decreased by about 5 mEq/L) and modest decreases in hematocrit. The metabolic adaptations to pregnancy include increased RBC mass and altered carbohydrate (e.g., 10% to 20% decrease in fasting blood glucose) and lipid (e.g., 300% increase in TGs and a 50% increase in total cholesterol) metabolism. Pregnancy changes the production and elimination of thyroid hormones, resulting in different reference values over the course of pregnancy.[38] For example, thyroxine-binding globulin increases during the first trimester, but pregnancy-associated accelerated thyroid hormone metabolism occurs later in the pregnancy. Other physiologic changes during pregnancy include an increased cardiac output (increases by 30% to 50%), decreased systemic vascular resistance, increased glomerular filtration rate (increases by 40% to 50%), shortened prothrombin and partial thromboplastin times, and hyperventilation resulting in compensated respiratory alkalosis and increased arterial oxygenation.[39]

Other Factors

Organ function, diet, fluid status, patient posture, and altitude affect some laboratory tests.

Organ function. Renal dysfunction may lead to hyperkalemia, decreased creatinine clearance, and hyperphosphatemia. Hepatic dysfunction may lead to reduced clotting factor production with prolonged partial thromboplastin times and prothrombin times. Bone marrow dysfunction may lead to pancytopenia.

Diet. Serum glucose and lipid profiles are best assessed in the fasting state. Unprocessed grapefruit juice down-regulates intestinal CYP3A4 and increases the bioavailability of some orally administered drugs.

Fluid status. Dehydration is associated with a decreased amount of fluid in the bloodstream; all blood constituents (e.g., sodium, potassium, creatinine, glucose, and BUN) become more concentrated. This effect is called *hemoconcentration*. Although the absolute amount of the substance in the body has not changed, the loss of fluid results in an abnormally high concentration of the measured analyte. The converse is true with hemodilution. Relativity must be applied or false impressions may arise (refer to Minicase 2).

Posture. Plasma renin release is stimulated by upright posture, diuretics, and low-sodium diets; plasma renin testing usually occurs after 2–4 weeks of normal sodium diets under fasting supine conditions.

Altitude. At high altitude, hemoglobin initially increases secondary to dehydration. However, hypoxia stimulates erythropoietin production, which in turn stimulates hemoglobin production resulting in increased hemoglobin concentration and increased blood viscosity. Serum hemoglobin reference ranges are adjusted progressively upward for individuals living above 1000 feet.[40]

NONCENTRALIZED LABORATORY TESTS

Point-of-Care Testing

Point-of-care (POC) testing (POCT), also known as *near patient testing, bedside testing,* or *extra-laboratory testing,* is clinician-directed diagnostic testing performed at or near the site of patient care rather than in a centralized laboratory.[41,42] Point-of-care test equipment ranges from small, hand-held devices to table-top analyzers. In vitro, in vivo, and ex vivo POC testing refer to tests performed near the patient (e.g., fingerstick blood glucose), in the patient (e.g., specialized intra-arterial catheter that measures lactate), and just outside the patient (e.g., intra-arterial catheter attached to an external analyzer), respectively. Although POC testing is not a new concept, recent technological advances (e.g., microcomputerization, miniaturization, biosensor development, and electrochemical advances) have rapidly expanded the variety of available POC tests beyond the traditional urinalysis dipsticks or fingerstick blood glucose monitors (Table 1-6).

The major advantages of POC testing include reduced turnaround time (TAT) and test portability. Reduced TAT is especially advantageous in settings where rapidly available laboratory test results may improve patient care (e.g., emergency departments, operating rooms, critical care units, accident scenes, and patient transport). Reduced TAT also enhances patient care in more traditional ambulatory settings by reducing patient and provider time and minimizing delays in initiating therapeutic interventions. Patient care sites

TABLE 1-6. Point-of-Care Tests

Arterial blood gases
Blood chemistries
Blood glucose
Cholesterol
Coagulation
Lactate, whole blood
Microbiological tests (influenza, RSV, group A streptococcus, *Clostridium difficile, Helicobacter pylori*)
Myocardial injury markers (creatine kinase MB, cardiac troponin T and troponin I)
Pregnancy tests
Urinalysis (glucose, red cells, leukocyte esterase, and nitrite)

RSV = respiratory syncytial virus.

without local access to centralized laboratories (e.g., nursing homes, rural physician practices, and military field operations) also benefit from POC testing. Other POC advantages include blood conservation (POC tests usually require drops of blood as opposed to the several milliliters required for traditional testing), less chance of preanalytical error from inappropriate transport, storage, or labeling of samples, and overall cost savings. Although the per test cost is usually higher with POC testing, cost analyses must consider the per unit cost of the test as well as other costs such as personnel time, length of stay, and quality of life.

The major disadvantages of POC testing include misuse or misinterpretation of results, loss of centrally-generated epidemiological data, documentation errors, inappropriate test material disposal, and quality assurance issues. All laboratory testing must meet the minimum standards established by the Clinical Laboratory Improvement Amendments of 1988 (CLIA-88).[43] Under CLIA-88, tests are categorized into one of three groups based on potential public health risk: waived tests, tests of moderate complexity, and tests of high complexity. Waived tests (e.g., fecal occult blood test) pose no risk of harm to the patient if used incorrectly or use such simple and accurate methodologies that inaccurate results are unlikely. Many POC tests meet the criteria for waived status but increasingly sophisticated POC tests may be subject to more stringent control. State-specific regulations may be more stringent than federal regulations.

Home Testing

Home testing refers to patient-directed diagnostic and monitoring testing usually performed by the patient or family member at home. More than 500 FDA-approved, home-use, nonprescription lab test kits are marketed; home glucose and pregnancy testing are among the most popular (Table 1-7). Many non-FDA-approved home-testing kits are marketed via the Internet. The FDA's Office of In Vitro Diagnostic Device and Evaluation and Safety maintains a searchable list of approved home-testing kits (www.fda.gov). Advantages of home testing include convenience, cost-savings (as compared to physician office visit), quickly available results, and privacy. Home monitoring of chronic drug therapy, such as blood glucose control with insulin therapy, may give the patient a better sense of control over the disease and improve patient outcomes. Disadvantages of home testing include misinterpretation of test results, delays in seeking medical advice, and lack of pre- and post-test counseling and psychological support. In addition, home test kits typically do not provide the consumer with information regarding sensitivity, specificity, precision, or accuracy. Home-use test kits are marketed as either complete test kits (the individual obtains their own sample, tests the sample and reads the results) or as collection kits (the individual obtains the sample, mails the sample to the laboratory, and receives the results by mail or telephone). Consumers should read and follow the test instructions to minimize testing error.

TABLE 1-7. Types of Nonprescription In Vitro Diagnostic Tests

TEST	BODY FLUID OR SPECIMEN TESTED
Alcohol	Breath
Blood, fecal occult	Feces
Drugs of abuse (amphetamines, barbiturates, benzodiazepines, cannabinoids, cocaine metabolites, methadone, methylenedioxymethamphetamine, morphine, phencyclidine)	Urine, hair
Fertility, male	Semen
Follicle-stimulating hormone (menopausal)	Urine
Glucose	Blood, urine
HDL cholesterol	Blood
Hemoglobin	Blood
HbA1c (glycosylated)	Blood
HIV-1	Blood
Human chorionic gonadotropin (pregnancy)	Urine, serum
Ketones	Blood, urine
Luteinizing hormone (ovulation)	Urine
Thyroid-stimulating hormone	Blood
Triglycerides	Blood

HbA1c = glycosylated hemoglobin; HDL = high-density lipoprotein; HIV = human immunodeficiency virus.

GUIDELINES FOR INTERPRETING LABORATORY RESULTS

Laboratory results must be interpreted in context of the patient and the limitations of the laboratory test. However, a laboratory result is only one piece of information; diagnostic and therapeutic decisions cannot be made on the basis of one piece of information. Clinicians typically give more weight to the presence or absence of signs and symptoms associated with the medical problem rather than to an isolated laboratory report. For example, an asymptomatic patient with a serum potassium concentration of 3 mEq/L (reference range: 3.5–5.0 mEq/L) should not cause as much concern as a patient who has a concentration of 3.3 mEq/L but is symptomatic. Tests for occult disease, such as colon cancer, cervical cancer, and hyperlipidemia, are exceptions to this logic because, by definition, the patients being tested are asymptomatic. Baseline results, rate of change, and patterns should be considered when interpreting laboratory results.

Baseline Results

Baseline studies establish relativity and are especially useful when reference ranges are wide or when reference values vary significantly among patients. For example, lovastatin and other HMG CoA (hydroxymethyl glutamyl coenzyme A) reductase inhibitors cause myopathy and liver dysfunction in a small percentage of patients. The myopathy is symptomatic (muscle pain or weakness) and elevates CK concentrations. The drug-induced liver dysfunction is asymptomatic and causes elevated AST and ALT. Some clinicians establish a pretreatment baseline

profile including CK, AST, and ALT and then conduct periodic testing thereafter to identify potential drug-induced toxicity. Creatine kinase has a wide reference range (55–170 units/L); establishment of a baseline allows the clinician to identify early changes, even within the reference range. The baseline value is also used to establish relative therapeutic goals. For example, the activated partial thromboplastin time (aPTT) is used to assess patient response to heparin anticoagulation. Therapeutic targets are expressed in terms of how much higher the patient's aPTT is compared to the baseline control.

Lab Value Compared to Reference Range

Not all lab values above the upper limit of normal (ULN) require intervention. Risk-to-benefit considerations may require that some evidence of drug-induced organ damage is acceptable given the ultimate benefit of the drug. For example, a 6-month course of combination drug therapy including isoniazid, a known hepatotoxin, is recommended for treatment of latent tuberculosis.[44] The potential benefit of at least 6 months of therapy (i.e., lifetime protection from tuberculosis in the absence of reinfection) means that clinicians are willing to accept some evidence of liver toxicity with continued drug therapy (e.g., isoniazid is continued until AST is greater than 5 times the ULN in asymptomatic individuals or greater than 3 times the ULN in symptomatic patients).[45]

Rate of Change

The *rate of change* of a laboratory value provides the clinician with a sense of risks associated with the particular signs and symptoms. For example, a patient whose RBC count falls from 5–3.5 million/mm^3 over several hours is more likely to be symptomatic and need immediate therapeutic intervention than if the decline took place over several months.

Isolated Results Versus Trends

An isolated abnormal test result is difficult to interpret. However, one of several values in a series of results or similar results from the same test performed at two different times suggests a pattern or trend. For example, a random serum glucose concentration of 300 mg/dL (reference range ≤200 mg/dL in adults) might cause concern unless it was known that the patient was admitted to the hospital the previous night for treatment of diabetic ketoacidosis with a random serum glucose of 960 mg/dL. A series of lab values adds perspective to an interpretation but may increase overall costs.

Spurious Results

A *spurious lab value* is a false lab value. The only way to differentiate between an actual and a spurious lab value is to interpret the value in context of what else is known about the patient. For example, a serum potassium concentration of 5.5 mEq/L (reference range: 3.5–5.0 mEq/L) in the absence of significant electrocardiographic changes (i.e., wide, flat P waves, wide QRS complexes, and peaked T waves) and risk factors for hyperkalemia (i.e., renal insufficiency) is most likely a spurious value. Possible causes of falsely elevated potassium, such as hemolysis, acidosis, and lab error, have to be ruled out before accepting that the elevated potassium accurately reflects the patient's actual serum potassium. Repeat testing of suspected spurious lab values increases the cost of patient care but may be necessary to rule out an actual abnormality.

FUTURE TRENDS

Point-of-care testing will progress and become more widely available as advances in miniaturization produce smaller and more portable analytical devices. Real-time, in vivo POC testing may become standard in many patient care areas. Laboratory test specificity and sensitivity will improve with more sophisticated testing. Genetic testing (laboratory analysis of human DNA, RNA, chromosomes, and proteins) will undergo rapid growth and development in the next few decades; genetic testing will be able to predict an individual's risk for disease, identify carriers of disease, establish diagnoses, and provide prognostic data. Genetic links for a diverse group of diseases including cystic fibrosis, Down syndrome, Huntington disease, breast cancer, Alzheimer disease, schizophrenia, PKU, and familial hypercholesterolemia are established; genetic links for many additional diseases will be established. Variations in DNA sequences will be well-described and linked to individualized disease management strategies.[46] Developments in nanotechnology will provide simple and inexpensive in vitro and in vivo assessments. Advances in array-based technologies (i.e., simultaneous evaluation of multiple analytes from one sample) will reduce sample volume and cost.[47]

PATIENT ASSESSMENT

Evaluation of patient laboratory data is an important component of designing, implementing, monitoring, evaluating, and modifying patient-specific medication therapy management plans. Depending on the setting, state laws, and collaborative practice agreements, some pharmacists have the authority to order and assess specific laboratory tests (e.g., drug serum concentrations, serum creatinine, liver function tests, serum electrolytes) or to perform POTC (e.g., lipid screening profiles, prothrombin time, HbA1c, rapid strep test). Pharmacists in ambulatory clinics and acute care inpatient settings have routine access to the same patient laboratory data as all other members of the healthcare team, but many community-based pharmacists do not have access to patient laboratory data. Though lack of access to laboratory data is currently a barrier, the increasing use of electronic patient charts and databases will improve pharmacist access to patient laboratory data.

SUMMARY

Clinical laboratory tests are convenient methods to investigate disease- and drug-related patient issues, especially since knowledge of pathophysiology and therapeutics alone is insufficient to provide high quality clinical considerations. This chapter should help clinicians appreciate general causes and mechanisms of abnormal test results. However, results within the reference range are not always associated with lack of signs and symptoms. Many factors influence the reference range. Knowing the sensitivity, specificity, and predictive value is important in selecting an assay and interpreting its results. Additionally, an understanding of the definitions, concepts, and strategies discussed should also facilitate mastering information in the following chapters.

Learning Points

1. **What factors should be considered when assessing a subtherapeutic INR?**

   Answer: Patient- and laboratory-related factors should be considered when assessing a subtherapeutic INR. Patient factors include adherence, anticoagulant dose, historical dose-related INRs, concomitant nonprescription and prescription medications, complementary and alternative medications, concurrent disease states, smoking status, and diet. Laboratory factors include analytical accuracy and precision, sample handling and processing procedures, and accuracy when calculating and reporting the INR.

2. **What factors should be considered when recommending PSA screening?**

   Answer: Sensitivity and specificity should be considered. Prostate specific antigen is specific for the prostate but has a low sensitivity for detecting prostate cancer. The PSA is elevated by urethral instrumentation, prostatitis, urinary retention, prostatic needle biopsy, and benign prostatic hyperplasia. Specificity for prostate cancer is lower in older men with benign prostatic hyperplasia than in younger men without prostatic hyperplasia. Thus, an elevated PSA level found during screening may result in unnecessary biopsies, treatment, and complications. Currently, there is not concurrence on the net benefit of PSA screening.[48]

3. **What factors should be considered when recommending at-home laboratory testing kits?**

   Answer: Advantages of patient-directed diagnostic and monitoring testing include convenience, cost-savings as compared to a physician office-visit, quickly available results, and privacy. Disadvantages include lack of information regarding sensitivity, specificity, precision, or accuracy; misinterpretation of the test results; the absence of pre- and post-test counseling; and delays in seeking medical advice. Patients who wish to purchase FDA-approved home-testing kits should be cautioned to seek advice before making treatment decisions based solely on home-testing laboratory results.

REFERENCES

1. Biomarkers and surrogate endpoints: preferred definitions and conceptual framework. *Clin Pharmacol Ther.* 2001;69:89-96.

2. Park KS, Baek KA, Kim DU, et al. Evaluation of a new immunochromatographic assay kit for the rapid detection of norovirus in fecal specimens. *Ann Lab Med.* 2012;32:79-81.

3. Solberg HE. Approved recommendation (1986) on the theory of reference values. Part 1. The concept of reference values. *J Clin Chem Clin Biochem.* 1987;25:337-342.

4. Expert Panel on Detection, Evaluation, and Treatment of High Blood Cholesterol in Adults. Executive summary of the third report of the National Cholesterol Education Program (NCEP) Expert Panel on detection, evaluation, and treatment of high blood cholesterol in adults (Adult Treatment Panel III). *JAMA.* 2001;285:2486-2497.

5. Wartofsky L, Dickey RA. The evidence for a narrower thyrotropin reference range is compelling. *J Clin Endocrinol Metab.* 2005;90:5483-5488.

6. Lalkhen AG, McCluskey A. Clinical tests: sensitivity and specificity. *Continuing Education in Anaesthesia, Critical Care & Pain.* 2008;8:221-223.

7. Weinstein S, Obuchowski NA, Lieber ML. Clinical Evaluation of diagnostic tests. *AJR.* 2005;184:14-19.

8. Hanley WB, Demshar H, Preston MA, et al. Newborn phenylketonuria (PKU) Guthrie (BIA) screening and early hospital discharge. *Early Human Development.* 1997;47:87-96.

9. Holmstrom B, Johansson M, Bergh A, et al. Prostate specific antigen for early detection of prostate cancer: longitudinal study. *BMJ.* 2009;339:b3537 doi:10.1136/bmj.b3537.

10. Kwon C, Farrell PM. The magnitude and challenge of false-positive newborn screening test results. *Arch Pediatr Adolesc Med.* 2000;154:714-718.

11. Council on Scientific Affairs. SI units for clinical laboratory data. *JAMA.* 1985;253:2553-2554.

12. Evans MI, Galen RS, Britt DW. Principles of screening. *Sem Perinatol.* 2005;29:364-366.

13. Boardman LA, Peipert JF. Screening and diagnostic testing. *Clin Obstet Gynecol.* 1998;41:267-274.

14. Rembold CM. Number needed to screen: development of a statistic for disease screening. *Br Med J.* 1998;317:307-312.

15. Tabar I, Vitak B, Yen MFA, et al. Number needed to screen: lives saved over 20 years of follow-up in mammographic screening. *J Med Screen.* 2004;11:126-129.

16. Lippi G, Giuseppe G, Cesare G. Preanalytic indicators of laboratory performances and quality improvement of laboratory testing. *Clinical Laboratory.* 2006;5:457-462.

17. Coodley EL, Coodley GO. Laboratory changes associated with aging. *Hospital Physician.* 1993;Jan:12-18, 25-31.

18. Tietz NW, Shuney DF, Wekstein DR. Laboratory values in fit aging individuals-sexagenarians through centenarians. *Clin Chem.* 1992;38:1167-1185.

19. Tietz NW, Wekstein DR, Shuey DF, et al. A two-year longitudinal reference range study for selected serum enzymes in a population more than 60 years of age. *J Am Geriatr Soc.* 1984;32:563-570.

20. Kelso T. Laboratory values in the elderly. Are they different? *Emerg Med Clinics North America.* 1990;8:241-254.

21. Duthie EH, Abbasi AA. Laboratory testing: current recommendations for older adults. *Geriatrics.* 1991;46:41-50.

22. Fraser CG. Age-related changes in laboratory test results. *Clin Pharmacol.* 1993;3:246-257.

23. Siest G. Study of reference values and biological variation: a necessity and a model for Preventive Medicine Centers. *Clin Chem Lab Med.* 2004;42:810-816.

24. Weatherall DJ, Clegg JB. Inherited haemoglobin disorders: an increasing global health problem. *Bull World Health Org.* 2001;79:704-712.

25. Frank JE. Diagnosis and management of G6PD deficiency. *Am Fam Physician.* 2005;72:1277-1282.

26. Caraco Y. Genes and the response to drugs. *N Engl J Med.* 2004;351:2867-2869.

27. Nguyen A, Desta Z, Flockhart DA. Enhancing race-based prescribing precision with pharmacogenomics. *Clin Pharmcol Ther.* 2007;81:323-325.

28. Prandota J. Advances of molecular clinical pharmacology in gastroenterology and hepatology. *Am J Ther.* 2010:17:e137-e162.

29. Smolensky MH, Peppas NA. Chronobiology, drug delivery, and chronotherapeutics. *Adv Drug Del Rev.* 2007;59:828-851.

30. Mendoza J, Challet E. Brain clocks: from the suprachiasmatic nuclei to a cerebral network. *The Neuroscientist.* 2009;15:477-488.

31. Edery I. Circadian rhythms in a nutshell. *Physiol Genomics.* 2000;3:59-74.

32. Rivkees SA. Mechanisms and clinical significance of circadian rhythms in children. *Curr Opinion Pediatr.* 2001;13:352-357.

33. Rivera-Coll A, Fuentes-Arderiu X, Diez-Noguera A. Circadian rhythms of serum concentrations of 12 enzymes of clinical interest. *Chronobiology International.* 1993;10:190-200.

34. Rivera-Coll A, Fuentes-Arderiu X, Diez-Noguera A. Circadian rhythmic variations in serum concentrations of clinically important lipids. *Clin Chemistry.* 1994;40:1549-1553.

35. Koopman MG, Koonen GCM, Krediet RT, et al. Circadian rhythm of glomerular filtration rate in normal individuals. *Clin Sci.* 1989;77:105-111.

36. Bleyzac N, Allard-Latour B, Laffont A, et al. Diurnal changes in the pharmacokinetic behavior of amikacin. *Ther Drug Monit.* 2000;22:307-312.

37. Otsuka K, Cornelissen G, Halberg F. Circadian rhythms and clinical chronobiology. *Biomed Pharmacother.* 2001;55:7-18.

38. Soldin OP. Thyroid function testing in pregnancy and thyroid disease. *Ther Drug Monit.* 2006;28:8-11.

39. Foley MR. Maternal cardiovascular and hemodynamic adaptation to pregnancy. In: UpToDate. Waltham, MA: UpToDate Version 19.3; 2011.

40. Sullivan KM, Mei Z, Grummer-Strawn L, et al. Haemoglobin adjustments to define anemia. *Trop Med International Health.* 2008;13:1267-1271.

41. Gutierres SL, Welty TE. Point-of-care testing: an introduction. *Ann Pharmacother.* 2004;38:119-125.

42. Gilbert HC, Szokol JW. Point-of-care technologies. *Int Anesthesiol Clin.* 2004;42:73-94.

43. Medicare, Medicaid, and CLIA Programs. Extension of Certain Effective Dates for Clinical Laboratory Requirements Under CLIA: final rule. *Federal Register.* 1998;63:55031-55034.

44. Mitchison DA. The diagnosis and therapy of tuberculosis during the past 100 years. *Am J Respir Crit Care Med.* 2005;171:699-706.

45. Saukkonen JJ, Cohn DL, Jasmer RM, et al. An official ATS statement: hepatotoxicity of antituberculosis therapy. *Am J Respir Crit Care Med.* 2006;174:935-952.

46. Pene F, Courtine E, Cariou A, et al. Toward theragnostics. *Crit Care Med.* 2009;37:S50-S58.

47. Hadd AG, Brown JT, Andruss BF, et al. Adoption of array technologies into the clinical laboratory. *Expert Rev Mol Diagn.* 2005;5:409-420.

48. Chou R, Croswell JM, Dana T, et al. Screening for prostate cancer: a review of the evidence for the US Preventive Services Task Force. *Ann Intern Med.* 2011;155:762-771.

BIBLIOGRAPHY

Bakerman S, Bakerman P, Strausbauch P. *Bakerman's ABC's of Interpretive Laboratory Data.* 4th ed. Scottsdale, AZ: Interpretive Laboratory Data Inc; 2002.

Fischbach FT, Dunning III, MB. *A Manual of Laboratory and Diagnostic Tests.* 8th ed. Philadelphia, PA: Lippincott Williams & Wilkins; 2008.

Jacobs DS, DeMott WR, Oxley DK. *Laboratory Test Handbook Concise with Disease Index.* 3rd ed. Hudson, OH: Lexi-Comp Inc; 2004.

Jacobs DS, Oxley DK, DeMott WR. *Laboratory Test Handbook with Key Word Index.* 5th ed. Hudson, OH: Lexi-Comp Inc; 2001.

Kraemer HC. *Evaluating Medical Tests.* Newbury Park, CA: Sage Publications; 1992.

Laposata M. *Laboratory Medicine: The Diagnosis of Disease in the Clinical Laboratory.* New York, NY: McGraw-Hill Companies Inc; 2010.

Sacher RA, McPherson RA, Campos JM. *Widmann's Clinical Interpretation of Laboratory Tests.* 11th ed. Philadelphia, PA: FA Davis Company; 2000.

Speicher CE. *The Right Test: A Physician's Guide to Laboratory Medicine.* Philadelphia, PA: WB Saunders; 1998.

Williamson MA, Snyder LM (eds.). *Wallach's Interpretation of Diagnostic Tests.* 9th ed. Philadelphia, PA: Lippincott Williams & Wilkins; 2011.

CHAPTER 2

INTRODUCTION TO COMMON LABORATORY ASSAYS AND TECHNOLOGY

PHILIP F. DUPONT

Objectives

After completing this chapter, the reader should be able to

- Describe the current and developing roles of laboratory testing in accurately diagnosing diseases

- Compare the fundamental elements of hospital-based laboratory testing procedures and automation with those of point-of-care testing

- Describe the basic elements of photometry and the major components of a spectrophotometer

- Explain the principles of turbidimetry and nephelometry as applied to laboratory testing

- Describe the analytic techniques of electrochemistry based on potentiometry, coulometry, voltammetry, and conductometry

- Describe the major electrophoresis techniques and their applications

- Describe the major analytic techniques of chromatography and compare gas- and high-performance liquid chromatography with respect to equipment and methodology

- Learn the basic principles of immunoassays; compare and contrast the underlying principles, methods, and tests performed involving
  - radioimmunoassay
  - enzyme-linked immunosorbent assay
  - enzyme-multiplied immunoassay technique
  - fluorescent polarization immunoassay
  - agglutination
  - enzyme-linked immunoassay tests

(continued on 18)

THE CHANGING ROLE OF THE LABORATORY IN THE DIAGNOSIS OF DISEASE

Traditionally, the physician bases a clinical diagnosis and patient management protocol on the patient's family and medical history, clinical signs/symptoms, and data derived from laboratory and imaging tests. An accurate history and physical examination of the patient are still considered among the most informative procedures in establishing accurate diagnoses of disease, with clinical laboratory test results playing important roles in confirming and/or ruling out certain diseases.

Consequently, pharmaceutical companies have developed drugs based on these collective empiric observations and known disease mechanisms. Some common examples include medications for high cholesterol, which modify the absorption, metabolism, and generation of cholesterol. Agents have been developed that are aimed at improving insulin release from the pancreas and sensitivity of the muscle and fat tissues to insulin action. Antibiotics are based on the observation that microbes produce substances, which inhibit other species. Hypotensive medications that lower blood pressure have typically been designed to act on certain pathways involved in hypertension (such as renal salt and water absorption, vascular contractility, and cardiac output. In a real sense this has often been a reactive approach with appropriate treatments and therapy starting after the signs and symptoms appear.

The past 30 years has seen remarkable progress in the role of laboratory in personalizing medicine, a consequence of the advances in human and medical genetics. These advances have enabled a more detailed understanding of the impact of genetics in disease and have led to new disciplines: genomics, epigenetics, and proteomics. It is anticipated that discoveries in these areas will change the practice of traditional clinical medicine into a more personalized medicine approach and will also impact pharmaceutical development.

Many of the traditional laboratory procedures and tests that are described in the following parts of this chapter will create the framework upon which these potential advances will be based—researchers are simplifying them, improving throughput, and running in real time. And as these tests are automated, they will take their place alongside current testing procedures. In the United States alone, each year clinicians order laboratory tests costing billions of dollars. Although these clinicians themselves do not usually perform laboratory tests, they still need an introduction to, and a basic understanding of, the more common methods and techniques (and newer methodologies) used to generate this information. This understanding is essential for the proper ordering of tests and the correct interpretation of results. This chapter provides an introduction to these methods and techniques.

Clinical laboratory tests represent a vast array of diverse procedures ranging from microscopic examination of tissue specimens (histopathology) to measurement of interactions of cellular and molecular components (typically clusters of atoms, molecules, and molecular fragments [nanotechnology]). A consideration of all of the diverse methodologies used in these procedures is beyond the scope of this chapter, but all share some of the common characteristics of automation and mechanization. These two often intertwine; automation commonly involves the mechanization of basic manual laboratory techniques or procedures such as

Objectives

- Describe the basic components of a mass spectrometry system

- Understand the basic principles of the commonly used cytometry systems

- Describe the impact of genomics, epigenetics, and proteomics on the personalization of medical practice and the newer roles that laboratory tests will play in the future

- Describe the basic principles of molecular diagnostics

- Describe the basic techniques of the polymerase chain reaction

- Discuss the laboratory testing implications for the emerging science of nanotechnology

those described throughout this chapter. The common goals of clinical laboratory mechanization and automation result in increased efficiency, reduced errors, and the ability to integrate various processes in the laboratory.

AUTOMATION IN THE HOSPITAL/CLINICAL LABORATORY

This trend toward automation in the hospital/clinical laboratory is, in part, motivated by the drive toward higher productivity and cost efficiency.[1] In its most comprehensive sense, total laboratory automation (TLA) encompasses all procedures from receipt of the specimen to the reporting of results. It can involve consolidated analyzers, individual or integrated, and automated devices that address specific tasks, coupled to specimen management and transportation systems, as well as process control software that automates each stage of the system. The centralized hospital/clinical laboratory of the future will consist mainly of automated laboratory systems capable of performing high volume and esoteric testing.[2]

Laboratory automation involves many varieties of steps and generally begins with processes that are manual in nature: obtaining the specimen, identification, transportation, and preparation of the sample. Once in the laboratory a quality control (QC) process begins with a check of the preordered specimen to ensure that specimens have correct identification labels and/or bar codes, correct cap colors on tubes, appropriate quality, and adequate quantity of material for the testing requested. Total laboratory automation systems are currently capable of performing only some of the above. Determining whether, for example, a specimen is hemolyzed or lipemic usually requires examination by a laboratory staff member.

In many divisions of the centralized laboratory, three major areas, for example, chemistry profile analyzers, complete blood count (CBC) instruments, and automated microbe identification systems, generate information in almost completely automated ways. Using the example of a chemistry analyzer, introduction of a specimen begins with aspiration of the

sample into a continuous-flow system. Each specimen passes through the same continuous stream and is subjected to the same various analytical reactions. The use of flushing systems prevents carryover between specimens. Many results generated by automated chemistry analyzers rely on reactions based on principles of photometry, which will be discussed later in this chapter. In addition to the more commonly requested serum chemistry levels, enzymes, therapeutic drugs, hormones, and other analytes are also measured using these techniques.

All modern automated analyzers rely on computers and sophisticated software to perform these processing functions. Calculations (statistics on patient or control values), monitoring (linearity and QC), and display (acquisition and collation of patient results and warning messages) functions are routinely performed by these instruments once the specimen has been processed. Automation does not end at this stage. While printed reports are almost always generated for placement on the patient's chart (and duplicated as electronic medical records used for long-term storage and retrieval), these instruments are also becoming interfaced with laboratory information systems, which can automatically order repeat and reflex testing, track samples and results through the system, and manage the storage and, when necessary, the retrieval of specimens.

Standardization within the laboratory automation arena is an essential means of assuring QC. The Clinical and Laboratory Standards Institute (CLSI) has developed a series of comprehensive automation standards that serves as the "gold standard" for laboratory automation: Clinical and Laboratory Standards Institute.[3]

The discipline of informatics is a parallel component of laboratory automation. As generators and collectors of information, large laboratories provide relevant clinical information to a wide network of physicians and other healthcare professionals in an efficient manner. Informatics in the laboratory involves the use of collected data for the purposes of problem solving and healthcare decision-making. Modern laboratory information systems have the capability of analyzing data in a variety of ways that enhance patient care. The ability to transmit and share such information via the Internet is becoming as indispensable a function of the laboratory as performing the tests themselves. The centralized clinical laboratory of the future will house automated laboratory systems capable of performing high volume and esoteric testing.[4] They will become centers of information management for hospital-based medicine practice as well as the community. In parallel with the development of the highly automated core laboratory, technological advances in miniaturization of analyzers will make point-of-care testing an essential and complementary tool for the diagnosis and treatment of disease.

POINT-OF-CARE TESTING

While TLA is well-suited for high volume laboratories, it is, at present, unaffordable for most small- or midsized hospital, reference laboratories, and professional offices. Currently, technological advances are being developed that involve

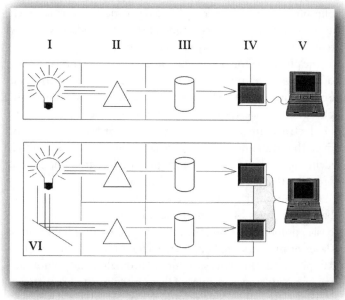

FIGURE 2-1. Schematic of single-beam (upper portion) and double-beam (lower portion) spectrophotometers. I = radiant light source; II = monochromator; III = analytical cuvette; IV = photomultiplier; V = recording device; VI = mirror.

miniaturization of analyzers, allowing for point-of-care testing, an essential and complementary facet of the centralized laboratory, in the diagnosis and treatment of disease.

Point-of-care testing may be thought of as any specimen testing that exists outside the walls of the large, central hospital laboratory. Community clinics, physician offices, emergency rooms, or patients' homes are common examples. Currently, hand-held analyzers exist that are capable of accurately measuring many common analytes such as electrolytes, blood gases, pH, blood urea nitrogen (BUN), creatinine, lactate, glucose, lipids, coagulation factors, hemoglobin, and hematocrit.[5] Wireless devices, such as PDAs, tablet PCs, and embedded computers are becoming commonplace at the patient's bedside.

The principle technology that underlies the function of these smaller instruments usually involves biosensor systems. *Biosensor systems* consist of two components: a bioreceptor and a transducer. The bioreceptor is a molecule such as an antibody, enzyme, receptor protein, or nucleic acid that recognizes a target analyte. The interaction between the bioreceptor and the target analyte generates either a specific molecular species or results in a physiochemical change that can be measured by electrochemical methods. The transducer detects this change and converts it into a measurable signal that is proportional to the concentration of the analyte. Common transducers used in these systems are based on amperometry, such as measurement of hydrogen peroxide and oxygen; potentiometry, measurement of pH and ions; and photometry, which uses optical fibers. In contrast to conventional assay methods that involve multiple steps and liquid reagents, both components are integrated into one sensor in these portable instruments. In the future, the centralized laboratory will provide highly specialized testing and will be a source of information storage and

retrieval, while point-of-care testing will likely continue to expand, providing clinicians with immediate results.[6,7]

Throughout the remainder of this text, many examples of the use of laboratory testing procedures are given as aids in diagnosing or confirming a diagnosis. These test procedures are based on one or more of the following methodologies.

PHOTOMETRY

Photometry is used to identify and/or quantify a given substance by measuring either the light absorbed or emitted on excitation by a specific narrow wavelength of light. In clinical laboratory instruments, the range of wavelengths measured is between 150 (the low ultraviolet) and 2500 nm (the near infrared region).[8] These instruments are classified by the source of light as well as whether the light is absorbed or emitted. Four types of photometric instruments are currently in use in laboratories: molecular absorption, molecular emission (fluorometers), atomic emission (flame photometers), and atomic absorption spectrophotometers.

Molecular Absorption Spectrophotometers

Molecular absorption spectrophotometers, usually referred to as *spectrophotometers,* are commonly employed in conjunction with other methodologies, such as nephelometry and enzyme immunoassay (EIA). Spectrophotometers are easy to use, have relatively high specificity, and the results are highly accurate. The high specificity and accuracy are obtained by isolated analytes reacting with various substances that produce colorimetric reactions.

The basic components of two types of spectrophotometers (single and double beam) are depicted in Figure 2–1. Single-beam instruments have a light source (I) (e.g., a tungsten bulb or laser), which passes through an entrance slit that minimizes stray light. Specific wavelengths of light are selected by the use of a monochromator (II). Light of a specific wavelength then passes through the exit slit and illuminates the contents of the analytical cell (cuvette) (III). After passing through the test solution the light strikes a detector, usually a photomultiplier tube (IV). This tube amplifies the electronic signal, which is then sent to a recording device (V). The result is then compared with a standard curve to yield a specific concentration of analyte.

The double-beam instrument, similar in design to single-beam instruments, is designed to compensate for changes in absorbance of the reagent blank and light source intensity. It utilizes a mirror (VI) to split the light from a single source into two beams, one passing through the test solution and one through the reagent blank. By doing so, it automatically corrects optical errors as the wavelength changes.

Most measurements are made in the visible range of the spectrum, although sometimes measurements in the ultraviolet and infrared ranges are employed. The greatest sensitivity is achieved by selecting the wavelength of light in the range of maximum absorption. If substances are known to interfere at this wavelength, measurements may be made at a different wavelength in the absorption spectrum. This modified procedure allows detection or measurement of the analyte with minimal interference from other substances.

Molecular Emission Spectrophotometers

Molecular emission spectrophotometry is usually referred to as *fluorometry*. The technology found in these instruments is based on the principle of luminescence, that is, an energy exchange process that occurs when electrons absorb electromagnetic radiation and then emit this excited energy level at a lower level. Three types of fluorescence phenomena—fluorescence, phosphorescence, and chemiluminescence—form the principle on which these sensitive clinical laboratory instruments operate.

Fluorescence results from a three-stage process that occurs in certain molecules known as *fluorophores*. The first stage involves the absorption of radiant energy by an electron in the ground state creating an excited singlet state. During the very short lifetime of this state (order of nanoseconds), energy from the electronic-vibrational excited state is partially dissipated through a radiationless transfer of energy that results from interactions with the molecular environment and leads to the formation of a relaxed excited singlet state. This is followed by relaxation to the electronic ground state by the emission of radiation (fluorescence). Because energy is dissipated, the energy of the emitted photon is lower and the wavelength is longer than the absorption photon. The difference between these two energies is known as *Stokes shift*. This principle is the basis for the sensitivity of the different fluorescence techniques since the emission photons can be detected at a different wavelength band than the excitation photons. Consequently, the background is lower than with absorption spectrophotometry where the transmitted light is detected against a background of incident light at the same wavelength.[9]

The phenomenon of *phosphorescence* is similar to fluorescence since it also results from the absorption of radiant energy by a molecule. However, it is also a competitive process. Unlike fluorescence, which results from a singlet-singlet transition, phosphorescence is the result of a triplet-singlet transition. When a pair of electrons occupies a molecular orbital in the ground or excited state, a singlet state is created. In this state, the electrons must have opposite spins (the Pauli exclusion principle), and only one magnetic moment is derived from this state. When the electrons are no longer paired, three different arrangements are possible, each with a different magnetic moment, the triplet state. The electronic energy of a triplet state is lower than a singlet state. Therefore, when the relaxed excited singlet state overlaps with a higher triplet state, energy may be transferred through a process called *intersystem crossing*. As in the case of an excited singlet state, energy may be dissipated through several radiationless mechanisms to the electronic ground state. However, when a triplet-singlet transition occurs, the result is phosphorescence. The probability of this type of transition is much lower than a singlet-singlet transition (fluorescence), and the emission wavelength and decay times are also longer than for fluorescence emission. Because the various forms of radiationless energy transfer compete so effectively, phosphorescence is generally limited to certain molecules, such as many aromatic and organometallic compounds, at very low temperatures, or in highly viscous solutions.[9,10]

The phenomenon of *chemiluminescence* is also similar to that of fluorescence in that it results from light emitted from an excited singlet state. However, unlike both fluorescence and phosphorescence, the excitation energy is caused by a chemical or electrochemical reaction. The energy is typically derived from the oxidation of an organic compound, such as luminol, luciferin, and acridinium ester. Light is derived from the excited products that are formed in the reaction.

Different instruments have been developed that use these basic principles of luminescence. These devices use similar basic components along the following pathway: a light source (laser or mercury arc lamp), an excitation monochromator, a sample cuvette, an emission monochromator, and a photodetector.[8] While the principles of these instruments are relatively straightforward, various modifications have been developed for specific applications.

An important example is fluorescent polarization in fluorometers. Fluorescent molecules (fluorophores) become excited by polarized light when the plane of polarization is parallel to their absorption transition vector, provided the molecule remains relatively stationary throughout the excited state. If the molecules rotate rapidly, light will be emitted in a different plane than the excitation plane. The intensity of light emitted by the molecules in the excitation polarization plane and at 90° permits the fluorescence polarization to be measured. The degree to which the emission intensity varies between the two planes of polarization is a function of the mobility of the fluorophore. Large molecules move slowly during the excited state and will remain highly polarized. Small molecules that rotate faster will emit light that is depolarized relative to the excitation plane.[10]

One of the most common applications of fluorescence polarization is competitive immunoassays, used to measure a wide range of analytes including therapeutic and illicit drugs, hormones, and enzymes. This important methodology involves the addition of a known quantity of fluorescent-labeled analyte molecules to a serum antibody (specific to the analyte) mixture. The labeled analyte will emit depolarized light because its motion is not constrained. However, when it binds to an antibody, its motion will decrease and the emitted light will be more polarized. When an unknown quantity of an unlabeled analyte is added to the mixture, competitive binding for the antibody will occur and reduce the polarization of the labeled analyte. By using standard curves of known drug concentrations versus polarization, the concentration of the unlabeled analyte can be determined.[10]

Another important application of fluorometry is flow cytometry, discussed later in this chapter. Like many modern laboratory instruments, flow cytometry involves the application of multiple physical, chemical, and biological principles and is, therefore, best considered as a separate category.

Atomic Emission and Atomic Absorption Spectrophotometers

Atomic emission (flame photometry) and *atomic absorption spectrophotometry* have limited use in modern laboratories. In the past, concentrations of metallic elements such as sodium, potassium, and lithium were commonly determined by flame photometry. The technique is based on the elementary quantum principle that electrons in an atom are excited to a higher energy level by heat. The electrons, being unstable in this state, return to a lower energy state. In doing so, the excess energy is liberated as photons in the visible light range. Usually, multiple energy levels are involved and the resulting spectral patterns are characteristic of each element. When conditions are held constant, the concentration of each ion is proportional to the light intensity at its characteristic wavelength.

Atomic absorption spectrophotometry procedures are currently associated mainly with toxicology laboratories where poisonous substances, such as lead and arsenic, need to be identified. Unlike flame photometry, the element that is analyzed by this technique is not appreciably excited. Rather, the element is dissociated from its chemical bonds. In this state, the element is in its lowest energy state and capable of absorbing energy in a narrow range that corresponds to its line spectrum.[11] Atomic absorption spectrophotometers are much more sensitive than flame photometers and more specific since the light sources used (hollow cathode lamps) emit at wavelengths that are specific for the element being measured.[2]

TURBIDIMETRY AND NEPHELOMETRY

When light passes through a solution, it can be either absorbed or scattered. *Turbidimetry* is the technique for measuring the percent light absorbed. A major advantage of turbidimetry is that measurements can be made with laboratory instruments, such as a spectrophotometer, used for other procedures in laboratory testing. Errors associated with this method usually involve sample and reagent preparation. For example, since the amount of light blocked depends on both the concentration and size of each particle, differences in particle size between the sample and the standard is one cause of error. The length of time between sample preparation and measurement, another cause of error, should be consistent since particles settle to varying degrees, allowing more or less light to pass. Large concentrations are necessary because this test measures small differences in large numbers.

Nephelometry, similar to turbidimetry, is the technique used for measuring the scatter of light by particles. The main differences are that (1) the light source is usually a laser, and (2) the detector, used to measure scattered light, is at a right angle to the incident light. Beam light scattered by particles is a function of the size and number of the particles. Nephelometric measurements are more precise than turbidimetric ones since the smaller signal generated for low analyte concentrations is more easily detected against a very low background.[12] Because antigen–antibody complexes are easily detected by this method, it is commonly employed in combination with EIAs.

REFRACTOMETRY

Refractometry measurements are based on the principle that light bends as it passes through different media. The ability of a liquid to bend light depends on several factors: wavelength of the incident light, temperature, physical characteristics of the medium, and the solute concentration in the medium. By keeping the first three parameters constant, refractometers can measure the total solute concentration of a liquid. This procedure is particularly useful, especially as a rapid screening test, since no chemical reagents and reactions are involved.[8]

Refractometers are commonly used to measure total dissolved plasma solids (mostly proteins) and urine specific gravity. In the refractometer, light is passed through the sample and then through a series of prisms. The refracted light is projected on an eyepiece scale. The scale is calibrated in grams per deciliter for serum protein, and in the case of urine, for specific gravity. In the eyepiece, a sharp line of demarcation is apparent and represents the boundary between the sample and distilled water. In the case of plasma samples, the refraction angle is proportional to the total dissolved solids. Although proteins are the predominant chemical species, other substances such as electrolytes, glucose, lipids, and urea contribute to the refraction angle. Therefore, measurements made on plasma do not correlate exactly to the true protein concentrations, but as the nonprotein solutes contribute to the total solutes in a predictable manner, accurate corrections are possible.[13]

OSMOMETRY

In the clinical laboratory, osmometer readings are interpreted as a measure of total concentration of solute particles and are used to measure the osmolality of biological fluids such as serum, plasma, and urine. When osmotically active particles are dissolved in a solvent (water, in the case of biological fluids), four physical properties of the water are affected: the osmotic pressure and the boiling point are increased, and the vapor pressure and the freezing point are decreased. Since each property is related, they can be expressed mathematically in terms of the others (colligative properties) and to osmolality. Consequently, several methods can be used to measure osmolality including freezing-point depression, colloid osmotic pressure (COP), and vapor pressure osmometry.[14]

The most commonly used devices to measure osmolality or other colligative properties of a solution are freezing-point depression osmometers. These are simple devices consisting of a sample chamber with a stirrer and a thermistor, a cooling chamber containing antifreeze, and a potentiometer with a direct readout. The sample is rapidly cooled several degrees below its freezing point in the cooling chamber. The sample is stirred to initiate freezing of the super-cooled solution. When the freezing point of the solution is reached (the point where the rate of the heat of fusion released by ice formation comes into equilibrium with the rate of heat removal by the cooling chamber), the osmolality can be calculated.[8]

In certain situations, it is important to measure the COP, a direct measure of the contribution of plasma proteins to the

TABLE 2-1. Common Laboratory Tests Performed with Various Assays

ASSAY	ANALYSIS TIME (MIN)	COMMON TESTS	USE
ISE	6–18	Electrolytes, (sodium potassium, chloride, calcium, lithium, total carbon dioxide)	Primary testing method
GC	30	Toxicologic screens, organic acids, drugs (e.g., benzodiazepines and TCAs)	Primary testing method
HPLC	30	Toxicologic screens, vanilmandelic acid, hydroxy-vanilmandelic acid, amino acids, drugs (e.g., indomethacin, anabolic steroids, cyclosporin)	Primary and secondary or confirmatory testing methods
ELISA	0.1–0.3	Serologic tests (e.g., ANA; rheumatoid factor; hepatitis B, cytomegalovirus, and human immunodeficiency virus antigens/antibodies)	Primary testing method
EMIT	0.1–0.3	General chemistries (e.g., albumin, BUN, creatine, glucose, cholesterol, bilirubin, total protein) and enzymes (e.g., acid and alkaline phosphatase, amylase, creatine kinase), coagulation factors (e.g., antithrombin III, fibrinogen, degradation products, heparin, plasminogen), drug levels for therapeutic drug monitoring (e.g., aminoglycosides, vancomycin, digoxin, antiepileptics, antiarrhythmics, theophylline), drug levels for toxicology (acetaminophen, salicylate, barbiturates, TCAs, amphetamines, cocaine, opiates)	Primary testing method
FPIA	0.1–0.2	Therapeutic drug monitoring (e.g., aminoglycosides, vancomycin, antiepileptics, antiarrhythmics, theophylline, methotrexate, digoxin, cyclosporine), general chemistries (e.g., thyroxine, triiodothyronine, cortisol, amylase, BUN, lactate dehydrogenase, creatinine, glucose, cholesterol, iron)	Primary testing method
PCR	0.1–0.2	Microbiologic and virologic markers of organisms and genetic markers	Primary testing method

ANA = antinuclear antibody; BUN = blood urea nitrogen; ELISA = enzyme-linked immunosorbent assay; EMIT = enzyme-multiplied immunoassay technique; FPIA = fluorescent polarization immunoassay; GC = gas chromatography; HPLC = high-performance liquid chromatography; ISEs = ion-selective electrodes; PCR = polymerase chain reaction; TCAs = tricyclic antidepressants.

osmolality. Because of the large molecular weight of plasma proteins, their contribution to the total osmolality is very small as measured by freezing-point depression and vapor pressure osmometers. Since a low COP favors a shift of fluid from the intravascular compartment to the interstitial compartment, measurement of the COP is particularly important in monitoring intravascular volume and useful in guiding fluid therapy in different circumstances to prevent peripheral and pulmonary edema.

The *COP osmometer*, also known as a *membrane osmometer*, consists of two fluid-filled chambers separated by a semipermeable membrane. One chamber is filled with a colloid-free physiologic saline solution that is in contact with a pressure transducer. When the plasma or serum is placed in the sample chamber, fluid moves by osmosis from the saline chamber to the sample chamber, thus causing a negative pressure to develop in the saline chamber. The resultant pressure is the colloidal osmotic pressure.[14]

ELECTROCHEMISTRY

In the clinical laboratory, analytic electrochemical techniques involve the measurement of current or voltage produced by the activity of different types of ions. These analytic techniques are based on the fundamental electrochemical phenomena of potentiometry, coulometry, voltammetry, and conductometry.

Potentiometry

Potentiometry involves the measurement of electrical potential differences between two electrodes in an electrochemical cell at zero current flow. This electrochemical method is based on the Nernst equation, which relates the potential to the concentration of an ion in solution, to measure analyte concentrations.[15] Each electrode or half-cell in an electrochemical cell consists of a metal conductor that is in contact with an electrolyte solution. One of the electrodes is a reference electrode with a constant electric potential; the other is the measuring or indicator electrode. The boundaries between the ion conductive phases in the cell determine the type of potential gradients that exist between the electrodes and are defined as redox (oxidation reduction), membrane, and diffusion potentials.

A redox potential occurs when the two electrolyte solutions in the electrochemical cell are brought into contact with each other by a salt bridge so that the two solutions can achieve equilibrium. A potentiometer may be used to measure the potential difference between the two electrodes. This is known as the *redox potential difference* since the reaction involves the transfer of electrons between substances that accept electrons (oxidant) and substances that donate electrons (reductant). Junctional potentials rather than redox potentials occur when either a solid state or liquid interface exists between the ion conductive phases. These produce membrane or diffusion potentials, respectively. In each case the concentration of an ion in solution can be measured using the Nernst equation, which relates the electrode potential to the activity of the measured ions in the test solution[8]:

$$E = E^0 - (0.059/z)\log (C_{red}/C_{ox})$$

where E = the total potential (in mV), E^0 = is the standard reduction potential, z = the number of electrons involved in the reduction reaction, C_{red} = the molar concentration of the ion in the oxidized form, and C_{ox} = the molar concentration of the ion in the reduced form.

Ion-selective electrodes (ISEs) consisting of a membrane that separates the reference and test electrolyte solutions are very selective and sensitive for the ions that they measure. For this reason further discussion on potentiometry will focus on these types of electrodes.

The ISE method, having comparable or better sensitivity than flame photometry, has become the principal test for determining urine and serum electrolytes in the clinical laboratory. Typically, ion concentrations such as sodium, potassium, chloride, calcium, and lithium, are measured using this method (Table 2-1).

The principle of ISE involves the generation of a small electrical current when a particular ion comes in contact with an electrode. The electrode selectively binds the ion to be measured. To measure the concentration, the circuit must be completed with a reference electrode. The three types of electrodes are

1. Ion-selective glass membranes
2. Solid-state electrodes
3. Liquid ion-exchange membranes

As shown in Figure 2-2, ion-selective glass membranes preferentially allow hydrogen (H^+), sodium (Na^+), and ammonium (NH_4^+) ions to cross a hydrated outer layer of glass. The H^+ glass electrode or pH electrode is the most common electrode for measuring H^+. Electrodes for Na^+, potassium (K^+), lithium (Li^+), and NH_4^+ are also available. An electrical potential is created when these ions diffuse across the membrane.

Solid-state electrodes consist of halide-containing crystals for measuring specific ions. An example is the silver–silver chloride electrode for measuring chloride.[8] Liquid ion-exchange membranes contain a water-insoluble, inert solvent that can dissolve an ion-selective carrier. Ions outside the membrane produce a concentration-related potential with the ions bound to the carrier inside the membrane.[8]

The electrodes are separated from the sample by a liquid junction or salt bridge. Since the liquid junction generates its own voltage at the sample interface, it is a source of error. This error is overcome by adjusting the composition of the liquid junction.[16] Another source of error is the selectivity of the electrode. Therefore, careful electrode selection is important. Overall, this method is simple to use and more accurate than flame photometry for samples having low plasma water due to conditions such as hyperlipoproteinemia.[17]

Ion-selective electrodes are relatively inexpensive and simple to use compared to other techniques and have an extremely wide range of applications and wide concentration range. They are also very useful in biomedical applications because they can measure the activity of the ion directly in addition to the concentration.

Coulometry

Coulometry is an analytical method for measuring an unknown concentration of an analyte in solution by completely converting the analyte from one oxidation state to another. This is

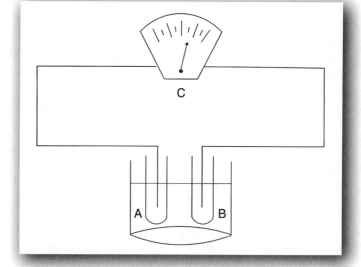

FIGURE 2-2. The pH meter is an example of a test that uses ISE to measure the concentration of hydrogen ions. An electric current is generated when hydrogen ions come in contact with the ISE (A). The circuit is completed through the use of a reference electrode (B) submerged in the same liquid as the ISE (also known as the *liquid junction*). The concentration can then be read on a potentiometer (C).

accomplished through a form of titration where a standardized concentration of the titrant is reacted with the unknown analyte, requiring no chemical standards or calibration. The point at which all of the analyte has been converted to the new oxidation state is called the *endpoint* and is determined by some type of indicator that is also present in the solution.

This technique is based on the Faraday law, which relates the quantity of electric charge generated by an amount of substance produced or consumed in the redox process and is expressed as

$$znF = It = Q$$

where z is the number of electrons involved in the reaction, n is the quantity of the analyte, F is the Faraday constant (96,487 C/mol), I is the current, t is time, and Q is the amount of charge that passes through the cell.

The chloridometer is a common instrument that employs this method. This instrument may be used to measure the chloride ion (Cl^-) concentration in sweat, urine, and CSF samples.[8] The device uses a constant current across two silver electrodes. The silver ions (Ag^+) that are generated at a constant rate react with the Cl^- ions in the sample. The reaction that produces insoluble AgCl ceases once excess Ag^+ ions are detected by an indicator and reference electrodes. Since the quantity of Ag^+ ions generated is known, the quantity of Cl^- ions may be calculated using the Faraday law.

Voltammetry

Voltammetry encompasses a group of electrochemical techniques in which a potential is applied to an electrochemical cell with the simultaneous measurement of the resulting current. By varying the potential of an electrode, it is possible to oxidize and reduce analytes in a solution. At more positive potentials, the electrons within the electrode become lower in energy and the oxidation of species in a solution becomes more likely. At lower potentials, the opposite occurs. By monitoring the current of an electrochemical cell at varying electrode potentials, it is possible to determine several parameters such as concentration, reaction kinetics, and thermodynamics of the analytes.[14]

This technique differs from potentiometry in a number of important ways. Voltammetric techniques use an externally applied force (potential) to generate a signal (current) in a way that would not normally occur, whereas in potentiometric techniques the analytical signal is produced internally through a redox reaction. The electrode arrangement is also quite different between the two techniques. In order to analyze both the potential and the resulting current, three electrodes are employed in voltammetric devices. The three electrodes include the working, auxiliary, and reference electrodes, which (when connected through a voltmeter) permit the application of specific potential functions. The measurement of the resulting current can yield results about ionic concentrations, conductivity, and diffusion. The ability to apply different types of potential functions or waveforms has led to the development of different voltammetric techniques: linear potential sweep polarography, pulse polarography, cyclic voltammetry, and anode stripping voltammetry.[8] These analytical methods, though not commonly used in clinical laboratories, are very sensitive (detection limits as low as the parts per billion range) and are capable of identifying trace elements in patient tissues such as hair and skin.

Conductometry

Conductometry is the measurement of current flow (proportional to conductivity) between two nonpolarized electrodes of which a known potential has been established. Clinical applications include urea estimation through the measurement of the rate-of-change of conductance that occurs with the urease-catalyzed formation of NH_4^+ and bicarbonate (HCO_3^-). The technique is limited at low concentrations because of the high conductance of biological fluids. Perhaps the most important application of impedance (inversely proportional to conductance) measurements in the clinical laboratory involves the Coulter principle for the electronic counting of blood cells. This method is discussed in detail in the cytometry section.

ELECTROPHORESIS

Routine diagnostic applications of *electrophoresis* technology exist for infectious diseases, malignancies, genetic diseases, paternity testing, forensic analysis, and tissue typing for transplantation. Electrophoresis tests, an important clinical laboratory method for molecular separations, involve the movement of charged molecules in a solution or on a support medium, associated with a direct current electrical field. The movement of molecules in this electrical field is dependent on molecular charge, shape, and size.[18] Since most molecules of biologic importance are both water-soluble and charged, this analytical tool is one of the most important techniques for molecular separation in the clinical laboratory. The main types of electrophoresis techniques used in both clinical and research laboratories include cellulose acetate, agarose gel, polyacrylamide gel, isoelectric focusing, two-dimensional, and capillary electrophoresis (CE). Because of a large number of clinical applications, electrophoresis apparatus, cellulose acetate and agarose gels, and reagents are available from commercial suppliers for each of these specific applications.

The primary application of electrophoresis is the analysis and purification of very large molecules such as proteins and nucleic acids. Electrophoresis also can be applied to the separation of smaller molecules, including charged sugars, amino acids, peptides, nucleotides, and simple ions. Through the proper selection of the medium for electrophoretic separations, extremely high resolution and sensitivity of separation can be achieved. Electrophoretic systems are usually combined with highly sensitive detection methods to monitor and analyze the separations that suit the specific application.[19]

The basic electrophoresis apparatus consists of a high voltage direct current supply, electrodes, a buffer, and a support for the buffer or a capillary tube. Supports for the buffer include filter paper, cellulose acetate membranes, agarose, and polyacrylamide gels. When an electrostatic force (EOF) is applied across the electrophoresis apparatus, the charged molecules will migrate to the anode or the cathode of the system depending on their charge. The force that acts on these molecules is proportional to the net charge on the molecular species and the applied voltage (electromotive force). This relationship is expressed as

$$F = qE/d$$

where F is the force exerted on the charged molecule, q is its net charge, E is the electromotive force, and d is the distance across the electrophoretic medium.[14]

While the basic principles are simple, procedures employed in the electrophoresis process are considerably more complex. Molecules to be separated must be dissolved in a buffer that contains electrolytes, which carry the applied current and fix the pH. The mobility of the molecules will be affected locally by the charge of the electrolytes, the viscosity of the medium, their size, and degree of asymmetry. These factors are related by the following equation:

$$\mu = q/6\eta r$$

where μ is the electrophoretic mobility of the charged molecule, q is its net charge, η is the viscosity of the medium, and r is the ionic radius.[20]

The conditions in which this process occurs are further complicated by the use of a support medium, necessary to minimize diffusion and convective mixing of the bands (caused by the heated current flowing through the buffer). Media used include polysaccharides (cellulose and agarose) and synthetic media such as polyacrylamide. The porosity of these media will, to a large extent, determine the resistance to movement for different ionic species. Therefore, the type of support medium used depends on the application. The above cited factors affecting the process of electrophoresis are controllable and provide optimal resolution for each specific application.

Gel Electrophoresis

Cellulose Acetate and Agarose Gel Electrophoresis

Cellulose acetate and *agarose gel electrophoresis* are commonly used for both serum protein and hemoglobin separations. Serum protein electrophoresis is often used as a screening procedure for the detection of disease states, such as inflammation, protein loss, monoclonal gammopathies, and other dysproteinemias. When the molecules have been separated into bands, specific stains are used to visualize them. Densitometry is typically used to quantify each band. When a monoclonal immunoglobulin pattern is identified, another technique, immunofixation electrophoresis, is used to quantify the immunoglobulins IgG, IgA, IgM, IgD, and IgE. Once these proteins are separated on an agarose gel, specific antibodies directed at the immunoglobulins are added. The sample is then fixed and stained to visualize and quantify the bands.[21] Separation of proteins may also be accomplished with isoelectric focusing where the proteins migrate through a stable pH gradient with the pH varying in the direction of migration. Each protein moves to its isoelectric point (i.e., the point where the protein's charge becomes zero and migration ceases). This technique is often used for separation of isoenzymes and hemoglobin variants.

Hemoglobin electrophoresis is the most common method for the screening of hemoglobin variants. Variant hemoglobins are separated on a cellulose acetate membrane at an alkaline pH (8.6) and on an agarose gel at an acid pH (6.2). Electrophoresis at both pH conditions is performed for optimal resolution of comigrating hemoglobin bands that occur at either of the pH conditions. For example, hemoglobin S, which comigrates with hemoglobins D and G at pH 8.6, can be separated at pH 6.2. The choice of support media is determined by the resolution of the hemoglobin bands that are achieved. Following electrophoresis, the bands are stained for visualization and the relative proportions of the hemoglobins are obtained by densitometry.[22]

Electrophoresis is also an important technique used in the laboratory where it is used to separate DNA, RNA, and protein fragments. Three common techniques used are Southern, Northern, and Western blots. These techniques differ in the target molecules that are separated. Southern blots separate DNA that is cut with restriction endonucleases and then identified with a labeled (usually radioactive) DNA probe. Northern blots separate fragments of RNA that are probed with labeled DNA or RNA. Western blots separate proteins that are probed with radioactive or enzymatically-tagged antibodies.

Each method involves a series of steps that leads to the detection of the various targets. Following electrophoresis, typically performed with an agarose or polyacrylamide gel, the molecules are transferred to a solid stationary support during the probe hybridization, washing, and detection stages of the assay. The DNA, RNA, or protein in the gel may be transferred onto nitrocellulose paper through electrophoresis or capillary blotting. In the former method the molecules, by virtue of their negative charge, are transferred by electrophoresis. The latter method involves layering the gel on wet filter paper with the nitrocellulose paper on top. Dry filter paper is placed on the nitrocellulose paper and the molecules are transferred with the flow of buffer from the wet to dry filter paper via capillary action. Following the transfer, the nitrocellulose paper is soaked in a blocking solution containing high concentrations of DNA, RNA, or protein. This prevents the probe from randomly sticking to the paper during hybridization. During the hybridization stage, the labeled DNA, RNA, or antibody is incubated with the blot where binding with the molecular target occurs. The probe-target hybrids are detected following a wash step to remove any unbound probe.

Two-Dimensional Electrophoresis

Two-dimensional electrophoresis (2-D electrophoresis) is a powerful and widely used method for the analysis of complex protein mixtures extracted from cells, tissues, or other biological samples. Proteins are sorted according to two independent properties: isoelectric focusing, which separates proteins according to their isoelectric points, and SDS-polyacrylamide gel electrophoresis, which separates proteins according to their molecular weights. Each spot on the resulting two-dimensional array corresponds to a single protein species in the sample.[23] Using this technique, thousands of different proteins can be separated, quantified, and characterized. This technology also has many research applications especially in the field of proteomics, which includes the large scale screening and cataloging of proteins in biological systems.

Capillary Electrophoresis

Capillary electrophoresis (CE) includes diversified analytical techniques, such as capillary zone electrophoresis (CZE), capillary gel electrophoresis (CGE), capillary chromatography, capillary isoelectric focusing, micelle electrokinetic capillary chromatography, and capillary isotachophoresis. Currently, only the first two in the above list have practical applications in the clinical laboratory. While historically a research tool, CE is being adapted for various applications in the clinical laboratory because of its rapid and high-efficiency separation power, diverse applications, and potential for automation. The possibility of CE becoming an important technology in the clinical laboratory is illustrated by its use in the separation and quantification of a wide spectrum of biological components ranging from macromolecules (proteins, lipoproteins, and nucleic acids) to small analytes (amino acids, organic acids, or drugs).

Capillary electrophoresis apparatus consists of a small-bore, silica-fused capillary (25–75 μm), approximately 50–100 cm in length, connected to a detector at one end and via buffer reservoirs to a high-voltage power supply (25–35 kV).[24] Because the small capillaries efficiently dissipate the heat, high voltages can be used to generate intense electric fields across the capillary to produce efficient separations with short separation times. In a CE separation, a very small amount of the sample (0.1–10 nL) is required. When the sample solution is injected into the apparatus, the molecules in the solution migrate through the capillary due to its charge in an electric field (electrophoretic mobility) or due to EOF. The negatively charged surface of the silica capillary attracts positively-charged ions in the buffer solution, which in turn migrate toward the cathode and carry solvent molecules in the same direction. The overall movement of the solvent is called *electroosmotic flow*. The separated proteins are eluted from the cathode end of the capillary. Quantitative detectors such as fluorescence, absorbance, electrochemical detectors, and mass spectrometry (MS) can be used to identify and quantify the proteins in the solution in amounts as little as 10–20 mol of substance in the injected volume.[24]

Capillary Zone Electrophoresis

Capillary zone electrophoresis (CZE) is the most widely-used type of CE and is used for the separation of both anionic and cationic solutes, usually in a single analysis. In CZE, the anions and cations migrate in different directions, but they both rapidly move toward the cathode due to EOF, which is usually significantly higher than the solute velocity. Therefore, all molecules, regardless of their charge, will migrate to the cathode. In this way the negative, neutral, and positive species can be detected and separated. Common clinical applications include high throughput separation of serum and urine protein and hemoglobin variants. In the future, other applications will become more commonplace. However, these systems are expensive, and currently conventional methods are used.

Capillary Gel Electrophoresis

Capillary gel electrophoresis (CGE) is the CE analog of traditional gel electrophoresis and is used for the size-based separation of biological macromolecules such as oligonucleotides, DNA restriction fragments, and proteins. The separation is performed by filling the capillary with a sieve-like matrix such as polyacrylamide or agarose to reduce the EOF. Therefore, larger molecules such as DNA will move more slowly resulting in better separation. Capillary gel electrophoresis is primarily used in research, but clinical applications are beginning to be developed.

DENSITOMETRY

Densitometry is a specialized form of spectrophotometry used to evaluate electrophoretic patterns. Densitometers can perform measurements in an absorbance optical mode and a fluorescence mode, depending on the type of staining of the electrophoretic pattern. An absorbance optical system consists of a light source, filter system, a movable carriage to scan the electrophoretic medium, an optical system, and a photodetector (silicon photocell) to detect light in the absorbance mode. When a densitometer is operated in the absorbance mode, an electrophoretic pattern located on the carriage system is moved across a focused beam of incident light. After the light passes through the pattern, it is converted to an electronic signal by the photocell to indicate the amount of light absorbed by the pattern. The absorbance is proportional to the sample concentration. The filter system provides a narrow band of visible light to provide better sensitivity and resolution of the different densities. This mode of operation is commonly used to evaluate hemoglobin and protein electrophoresis patterns

and applications of molecular diagnostics (MDx), including one- and two-dimensional, DNA, RNA, and polymerase chain reaction (PCR) gel electrophoresis bands; dot blots; slot blots; image analysis; and chromosome analysis.

The fluorescence method is used in the case of electrophoretic patterns that fluoresce when radiated by UV light (340 nm). Densitometers used in this mode include a UV light source and a photomultiplier tube instead of the silicon photocell. When the pattern located on the carriage moves across a focused beam of UV light, the pattern absorbs the light and emits visible light. The light is focused by a collection of lenses onto a UV blocking filter and then to a photomultiplier tube where the visible light is converted into an electronic signal that is proportional to the intensity of the light.

In each case, the electrophoretic patterns are evaluated by comparison of peak heights or peak areas of the sample and the standards. Current densitometry systems employ sophisticated software to provide analysis of the signal intensities with high resolution and sensitivity.[8]

CHROMATOGRAPHY

Chromatography is another method used primarily for separation and identification of various compounds. Three types of chromatography are currently and routinely used in the clinical laboratory: thin layer chromatography (TLC), gas chromatography (GC), and high-performance (or pressure) liquid chromatography (HPLC). Chromatographic assays require more time for specimen preparation and performance; they are usually performed only when another assay type is not available or when interferences are suspected with an immunoassay. Chromatographic assays do not require premanufactured antibodies and, therefore, afford better flexibility than an immunoassay.

Paper Chromatography

Paper chromatography, the original methodology, is simple and its principles apply to all other forms of chromatography. The procedure involves placing a drop of the sample near the bottom of a piece of chromatography paper and allowing it to dry. The paper is then hung in a chromatography jar so that the bottom edge contacts a solvent. Each component, having a different solubility and polarity, migrates toward the top of the paper as the solvent moves by capillary action. After separation is complete (usually 12–24 hours), the paper is sprayed with a developing solution. Various fractions are then identified by how far they migrated on the paper. Since quantification of a substance is not possible with this method, it is seldom employed today in the clinical laboratory

Thin Layer Chromatography

Thin layer chromatography (TLC) is commonly used for drug screening and analysis of clinically important substances such as oligosaccharides and glycosaminoglycans (e.g., dermatan sulfate, heparan sulfate, and chondroitin sulfate). In this method, a thin layer of gel (sorbent) is applied to glass or plastic, forming the stationary phase. The sorbent may be composed of silica, alumina, polyacrylamide, or starch. The choice of sorbent depends on the specific application since compounds have different relative affinities for the solvent (mobile phase) and the stationary phase. These factors affect the separation of a mixture into the different components. Silica gel is the most commonly used sorbent because it may be used to separate a broad range of compounds, including amino acids, alkaloids, sugars, fatty acids, lipids, and steroids.

Thin layer chromatography is used for identification and separation of multiple components of a sample in a single step, and initial component separation prior to analysis by another technique. Quantification of various substances is possible with TLC; each spot can be scraped off and analyzed individually.[8] While TLC is a useful screening technique, it has lower sensitivity and resolution than either gas or high-performance chromatography. Another disadvantage, as with gas and high-performance chromatography, is that someone with skill and expertise must interpret the results.

Gas Chromatography

Gas chromatography (GC) is used to identify and quantify volatile substances such as alcohols, steroids, and drugs in the picogram range (Table 2-1). This technique is also based on the principles of paper and TLC, but it has better sensitivity. Instead of a solvent, GC uses an inert gas (e.g., nitrogen or helium) as a carrier for the volatile substance. A column packed with inert material, coated with a thin layer of a liquid phase, is substituted for paper or gel.

The sample is injected into the column (contained in a heated compartment) where it is immediately volatilized and picked up by the carrier gas. Heating at precise temperature gradients is essential for good separation of the analytes. The gas carries the sample through the column where it contacts the liquid phase, which has a high boiling point. Analytes with lower boiling points migrate faster than those with higher boiling points, thus fractionating the sample components.

When the sample leaves the column, it is exposed to a detector. The most common detector consists of a hydrogen flame with a platinum loop mounted above it. When the sample is exposed to the flame, ions collect on the platinum loop and generate a small current. This current is amplified by an electrometer, and the signal is sent on to an integrator or recorder.

The recorder produces a chromatogram with various peaks being recorded at different times. Because each sample component is retained for a different length of time, the peak produced at a particular retention time is characteristic for a specific component (Figure 2-3). The amount of each component present is determined by the area of the characteristic peak or by the ratio of the peak heights calibrated against a standard curve.

This technique has many advantages, including high sensitivity and specificity. However, it requires sophisticated and expensive equipment. In addition, one or more compounds may produce peaks with the same retention time as the analyte of interest. In cases of such interference, the temperature and/

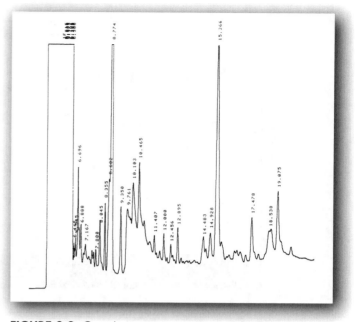

FIGURE 2-3. Gas chromatogram. Area under the curve or peak height of an analyte (e.g., drug or toxin) is compared to the area under the curve or peak height of an internal standard, and then the ratio is calculated. This ratio is compared to a standard curve of peak area ratios to give the concentration of the analyte.

or composition of the liquid phase can be adjusted for better peak resolution.

High-Performance Liquid Chromatography

High-performance liquid chromatography (HPLC) is widely used, especially in forensic laboratories, for toxicologic screening and to measure various drugs (Table 2-1). Its basic principles are similar to those of GC, but it is useful for nonvolatile or heat-sensitive substances. Instead of gas, HPLC utilizes a liquid solvent (mobile phase) and a column packed with a stationary phase, usually with a porous silica base. The mobile phase is pumped through the column under high pressure to decrease the assay time.

The sample is injected onto the column at one end and migrates to the other end in the mobile phase. Various components move at different rates, depending on their solubility characteristics and the amount of time spent in the solid versus liquid phases. As the mobile phase leaves the column, it passes through a detector that produces a peak proportional to the concentration of each sample component. The detector is usually a spectrophotometer with variable wavelength capability in the ultraviolet and visible ranges.

A signal from the detector is sent to a recorder or integrator, which plots peaks for each component as it elutes from the column (Figure 2-4). Once again, each component has its own characteristic retention time so each peak represents a specific component. As with GC, interferences may occur with compounds of similar structure or solubility characteristics; the peaks may fall on top of each other. Better resolution can be obtained by using a column packing with different

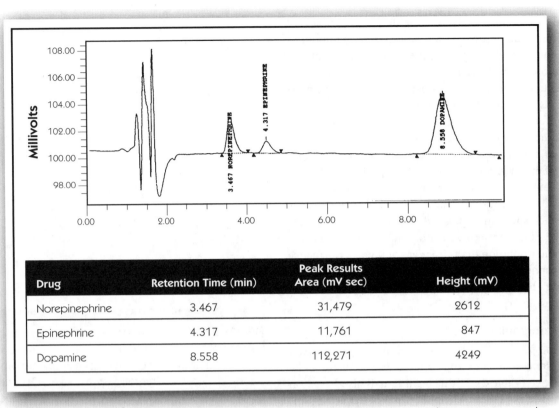

Drug	Retention Time (min)	Peak Results Area (mV sec)	Height (mV)
Norepinephrine	3.467	31,479	2612
Epinephrine	4.317	11,761	847
Dopamine	8.558	112,271	4249

FIGURE 2-4. HPLC chromatogram. Appearance of this chromatogram is similar to the gas chromatogram, and area or peak height ratio is used to quantify the analyte in a sample.

characteristics or by changing the composition and/or pH of the mobile phase.

Compounds are identified by their retention times and quantified either by computing the area of the peak or by comparing the peak height or area to an internal standard to obtain a peak height or peak area ratio. This ratio is then used to calculate a concentration by comparison to a predetermined standard curve.

Although HPLC offers both high sensitivity and specificity, it requires specialized equipment and personnel. Furthermore, since the substance being determined is usually in a body fluid (e.g., urine or serum), one or more extraction steps are needed to isolate it. Another concern is that since many assays require a mobile phase composed of volatile and possibly toxic solvents, Occupational Safety and Health Administration (OSHA) guidelines must be followed. In addition, assays developed for commercial use may be costly since modifications to published methods are almost always required.

IMMUNOASSAYS

Immunoassays are based on a reaction between an antigenic determinant or hapten and a labeled antibody.[25] The label may consist of a radioisotope, an enzyme, enzyme substrate, a fluorophore, or a chromophore. The reaction may be measured by several detection methods including liquid scintillation, ultraviolet absorbance, fluorescence, fluorescent polarization, and turbidimetry or nephelometry. The immunoassay method is commonly used for determination of drug concentrations in serum.

Immunoassays can be divided into two general categories: heterogeneous and homogeneous. In *heterogeneous* assays, the free and bound portions of the determinant must be separated before either or both portions can be assayed. This separation can be accomplished by various methods including protein precipitation, double antibody technique, adsorption of free drug, and removal by immobilized antibody on a solid phase support.

Homogeneous assays do not require a separation step and, therefore, can be easily automated. The binding of the labeled hapten to the antibody alters its signal in a way (color change or reduction in enzyme activity) that can then be used to measure the analyte concentration. Homogeneous assays are also suited to stat tests due to their rapid turnaround time.

Early immunoassays used polyclonal antibodies, generated as a result of an animal's natural immune response. Typically, an antigen is injected into an animal. The animal's immune system then recognizes the material as foreign and produces antibodies against it. These antibodies are then isolated from the blood. Many different antibodies may be generated in response to a single antigen. The numbers as well as the specificities of the antibodies depend on the size and number of antigenic sites on the antigen. In general, the larger and more complex the antigen (e.g., cell or protein), the more antigenic sites (epitopes) it has and the greater the variety of antibodies formed.

Although polyclonal antibodies have been used successfully, both specificity and response may vary greatly because of their heterogeneous nature. The result is a high degree of cross-reactivity with similar substances. This cross-reactivity difficulty was eliminated with the development of monoclonal antibodies (MoABs).

Prior to 1975, the only MoABs available were from patients suffering from multiple myeloma, a cancer of the blood and bone marrow in which uncontrolled numbers of malignant plasma cells are produced. Usually, these tumor cells produce a single (monoclonal) type of antibody. In 1975, a technique was developed to make MoABs in the laboratory.[26] The technique is based on the fusion of genetic material from plasma cells that produce antibody but cannot reproduce, and myeloma cells that do not produce antibody but can reproduce limitlessly. The plasma cells and myeloma cells are cultured together, resulting in a mixture of both parent cells and hybrid cells. This hybrid cell produces the specific antibody and reproduces indefinitely.

The mixture is incubated in a special medium, which kills the parent cells and leaves only the hybrid antibody-producing cells alive. The hybrid cells can then be grown using conventional cell culture techniques, resulting in large amounts of the MoAB. The development of MoABs has allowed for high sensitivity and specificity in immunoassay technology.

Radioimmunoassay

Today *radioimmunoassay (RIA)* is rarely used in the clinical laboratory and is discussed from a historical perspective. A heterogeneous immunoassay, RIA, was developed in the late 1950s and has been primarily used for endocrinology testing purposes.[27] This technique takes advantage of the fact that certain atoms can be either incorporated directly into the analyte's structure or attached to antibodies. The primary atoms used in the clinical laboratory fall into two classes: gamma emitters and beta emitters.

Gamma emitters (^{125}I and ^{57}Co) are generally incorporated into compounds such as thyroid hormone and cyanocobalamin (vitamin B_{12}).[12] These types of isotopes can be counted directly with standard gamma counters that utilize a sodium iodide–thallium crystal. When the gamma ray hits the crystal, it gives off a flash of light. This light, in turn, stimulates a photomultiplier tube to amplify the signal.

Beta emitters (^{14}C and ^{3}H) are primarily used to measure steroid concentrations.[5] Beta rays cannot be counted directly since endogenous substances tend to absorb the radiation. Therefore, this technique requires a scintillation cocktail with an organic compound capable of absorbing the beta radiation and reemitting it as a flash of light. This light is then amplified by a photomultiplier tube and counted.

Radioimmunoassay is extremely sensitive and has been made more specific with the introduction of MoABs. Unfortunately, this technique also has several significant disadvantages[12]:

- A short shelf-life for labeled reagents is a source of increased cost.
- Lead shielding is required, making the instrument heavy and bulky.
- Strict record keeping is required, resulting in a higher workload.
- Monitoring of personnel for radiation exposure is required.
- Special licensing is required.
- Waste disposal requires additional costs to comply with government regulations.

Since enzyme-linked immunoassays have none of these problems and can perform essentially the same tests as RIA, the clinical use of RIA has decreased in recent years.

Agglutination

The simplest immunoassay is *agglutination*. Typical tests that can be performed using this assay include human chorionic gonadotropin, rheumatoid factor, antigens from infectious agents such as bacteria and fungi, and antinuclear antibodies (ANAs). The agglutination reaction, used to detect either antigens or antibodies, results when multivalent antibodies bind to antigens with more than one binding site.

This reaction occurs through the formation of cross-linkages between antigen and antibody particles. When enough complexes form, clumping results, and a visible mass is formed (Figure 2-5). Since the reaction depends on the number of binding sites on the antibody, the greater the number, the better the reaction. For example, immunoglobulin M produces better agglutination than immunoglobulin G because the former has more binding sites.

The agglutination reaction is also affected by other factors[27]:

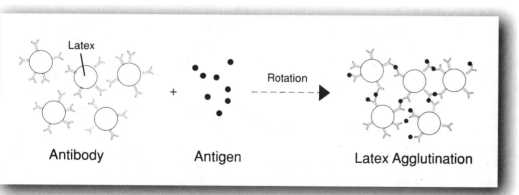

FIGURE 2-5. Schematic of latex agglutination immunoassay. The specimen (cerebrospinal fluid, serum, etc.) contains the analyte (in this case, antigens to bacteria) that causes an easily readable reaction (adapted, with permission, from Power DA, McCuen PJ, eds. *Manual of BBI Products and Laboratory Procedures.* Cockeysville, MD: Becton Dickinson Microbiology Systems; 1998:77).

- Avidity and affinity of the antibody
- Number of binding sites on the antigen as well as the antibody
- Relative concentrations of the antigen and antibody
- Z-potential (electrostatic interaction that causes particles in solution to repel each other)
- Viscosity of medium

The two types of agglutination reactions are direct and indirect. *Direct agglutination* occurs when the antigen and antibody are mixed together, resulting in visible clumping. An example of this reaction is the test for *Salmonella typhi* antibody. *Indirect agglutination* (also known as *passive* or *particle agglutination*) uses a carrier for either the antibody or antigen. Originally, erythrocytes were selected as the carrier (as described for hemolytic anemia tests). However, latex-coated particles are now commonly used, and the latex agglutination method is simpler and less expensive than the erythrocyte immunoassay. In addition, latex particles allow titration of the amount of antibody bound to the latex particle, thus reducing variability. Other advantages include a rapid performance time with no separation step, allowing full automation. Disadvantages include expensive equipment and lower sensitivity than either RIA or EIAs. The use of an automated particle counter increases the sensitivity of the test 10–1000 times.[28]

Enzyme Immunoassays

Enzyme immunoassays (EIAs) employ enzymes as labels for specific analytes. When antibodies bind to the antigen-enzyme complex, a defined reaction occurs (e.g., color change, fluorescence, radioactivity, or altered activity). This altered enzyme activity is used to quantitate the analyte. The advantages of EIAs include commercial availability at a relatively low cost, long shelf life, good sensitivity, automation, and none of the specific requirements mentioned for RIA.

Enzyme-Linked Immunosorbent Assay

Enzyme-linked immunosorbent assay (ELISA) is a heterogeneous EIA. This assay employs the same basic principles as RIA, except that enzyme activity rather than radioactivity is measured. This assay is commonly used to determine antibodies directed against a wide range of antigens such as rheumatoid factor, hepatitis B antigen, and bacterial and viral antigens in the serum (Table 2-1).

In a competitive ELISA assay, the specific antibody is adsorbed to a solid phase. Enzyme-labeled antigen is incubated together with the sample containing unlabeled antigen and the antibodies attached to the solid phase. After a specified time, equilibrium is reached between the binding of the enzyme-labeled and unlabeled antigens to the solid phase antibody, and the solid phase is washed with buffer. The remaining product is measured with a spectrophotometer or fluorometer. The amount of the reaction product will be inversely proportional to the amount of unlabeled antigen in the sample because an increasing amount of unlabeled antigen will displace enzyme-labeled antigen from antibody binding.

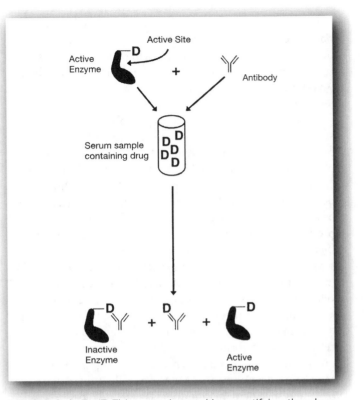

FIGURE 2-6. EMIT. This assay is used in quantifying the drug concentration in a serum sample, as described in the text.

Enzyme-Multiplied Immunoassay

Enzyme-multiplied immunoassay technique (EMIT) is a homogeneous EIA; the enzyme is used as a label for a specific analyte (e.g., a drug). Many drugs commonly assayed using EMIT are also measured by fluorescence polarization immunoassay (FPIA) (e.g., digoxin, quinidine, procainamide, *N*-acetylprocainamide, and aminoglycoside antibiotics) as are substances like BUN and creatinine (Table 2-1).

With the EMIT assay, the enzyme retains its activity after attaching to the analyte. For example, to determine a drug concentration, an enzyme is conjugated to the drug and incubated with antidrug antibody. As shown in Figure 2-6, the test drug (D) is covalently bound to an enzyme that retains its activity and acts as a label. When this complex is combined with antidrug antibody, the enzyme is inactivated. If the antibody and enzyme-bound drug are combined with serum that contains unbound drug, competition occurs. Since the amount of antidrug antibody is limited, the free drug in the sample and the enzyme-linked drug compete for binding to the antibody. When the antibody binds to the enzyme-linked drug, enzyme activity is inhibited. The result is that the serum drug concentration is proportional to the amount of active enzyme remaining. Since no separation step is required, this assay has been automated.

Fluorescent Polarization Immunoassay

Fluorescent polarization immunoassay (FPIA), the most common form of immunoassay, is used to measure concentrations of many serum analytes such as BUN and creatinine. It is also commonly employed for determining serum drug concentrations of aminoglycoside antibiotics, vancomycin, and theophylline (Table 2-1).

Molecules having a ring structure and a large number of double bonds, such as some aromatic compounds, can fluoresce when excited by a specific wavelength of light. These molecules must have a particular orientation with respect to the light source for electrons to be raised to an excited state. When the electrons return to their original lower energy state, some light is reemitted as a flash with a longer wavelength than the exciting light. Fluorescent immunoassays take advantage of this property by conjugating an antibody or analyte to a fluorescent molecule. The concentration can be determined by measuring either the degree of fluorescence or, more commonly, the decrease in the amount of fluorescence present.[12,28]

In FPIA, a polarizing filter is placed between the light source and the sample and between the sample and the detector. The first filter assures that the light exciting the molecules is in a particular orientation; the second filter assures that only fluorescent light of the appropriate orientation reaches the detector.

The fluorescent polarization of a small molecule is low because it rotates rapidly and is not in the proper orientation long enough to give off an easily detected signal. To decrease this molecular motion, the molecule is complexed with an antibody. Since this larger complex rotates at a slower rate, it stays in the proper orientation to be excited by the incident light.

When unlabeled analyte is mixed with a fixed amount of antibody and fluorescent-labeled analyte, a competitive binding reaction occurs between the labeled and unlabeled analytes. The result is a decrease in fluorescence. Thus, the concentration of unlabeled analyte is inversely proportional to the amount of fluorescence.[28]

Because of their simplicity, automation, and low cost, assays have been developed with relatively high sensitivity for many drugs (e.g., antiepileptics, antiarrhythmics, and antibiotics). The primary difficulty is interference from endogenous substances (lipids and bilirubin) or metabolites of the drugs.

MASS SPECTROMETRY

Mass spectrometry (MS) involves the fragmentation and ionization of molecules in the gas phase according to their mass to charge ratio (m/z). The resulting mass fragments are displayed on a mass spectrum, or a bar graph, that plots the relative abundance of an ion versus its m/z ratio. Since the mass spectrum is characteristic of the parent molecule, an unknown molecule can be identified by comparing its mass spectrum with a library of known spectra.

A wide array of MS systems has been developed to meet the increasing demands of the biomedical field. However, the basic principles and components of mass spectrometers are essentially the same. These include an inlet unit, an ion source, a mass analyzer, an ion detector, and a data/recording system. Compounds introduced into a mass spectrometer must first be isolated. This is accomplished with separation techniques such as GC, liquid chromatography (LC), and CE, which are used in tandem with mass spectrometers. In a GC/MS system, an interface between the GC and MS components, which restricts the gas flow from the GC column into the mass spectrometer, is required to prevent a mismatch in the operating pressures between the two instruments. The unit must also be heated to maintain the volatile compounds in the vapor state and remove most of the carrier gas from the GC effluent entering the ion source unit.[29]

Ionization Methods

The ionization of the molecules introduced into MS is accomplished by several methods. In each case, the ion sources are maintained at high temperatures and high vacuum conditions necessary for ionizing vaporized molecules. The *electron ionization (EI)* method, a form of gas-phase ionization, consists of a beam of high energy electrons that bombard the incoming gas molecules. The energy used is sufficiently high to not only ionize the gas molecules but also cause them to fragment through the breaking of their chemical bonds. This process yields ion fragments in addition to intact molecular ions that appear in the mass spectra. The EI method is most useful for low molecular weight compounds (<400 daltons) because of problems with excessive fragmentation and thermal decomposition of large molecules during vaporization.[30,31] Therefore, EI is typically used in GC/MS systems that are suitable for applications including the analysis of synthetic organic chemicals, hydrocarbons, pharmaceutical compounds, organic acids, and drugs of abuse.

Chemical ionization (CI) is another form of gas-phase ionization. This technique is a less energetic technique than EI because the sample molecule is ionized by a reagent such as methane or ammonia that is first ionized by an electron beam. Less fragmentation is produced by this method making it useful for determining the molecular weights of many organic compounds and for enhancing the abundance of intact molecular ions.

Electrospray ionization (ESI), a form of atmospheric pressure ionization, generates ions directly from solution permitting it to be used in combination with HPLC and CE systems. This method involves the creation of a fine spray in the presence of a strong electric field. As the droplets become declustered, the force of the surface tension of the droplet is overcome by the mutual repulsion of like charges, allowing the ions to leave the droplet and enter the mass analyzer. This technique will yield multiple ionic species especially for high molecular weight ions that have a large distribution of charge states, thus making this a very sensitive technique for small, large, and labile molecules.[32] This ionization method is well-suited for the analysis of peptides, proteins, carbohydrates, DNA fragments, and lipids.

Other common ionization techniques include *fast atom bombardment* (FAB), which uses high velocity atoms such as argon to ionize molecules in a liquid or solid, and *matrix-assisted laser desorption/ionization (MALDI)*, which uses high energy photons to ionize molecules embedded on a solid organic matrix.[32]

Mass Analyzers

Following ionization, the gas phase ions enter the mass analyzer. This component of the mass spectrometer separates the ions by their m/z ratios. Commonly used *mass analyzers* include the double-focusing magnetic sector analyzer, quadrupole, quadrupole ion trap mass spectrometers, and tandem mass spectrometers. The magnetic sector mass spectrometer uses a magnetic field perpendicular to the direction of the ion motion to deflect the ions into a circular path with a radius dependent on the m/z ratio and the velocity of the ion. The detector will then separate the ions by their m/z ratios. However, since the kinetic energy (or velocity) of the molecules leaving the ion source is not necessarily constant, the path radii will become dependent on the velocity and the m/z ratio. To enhance the resolution, an electrostatic analyzer or electric sector is used to allow molecules with only a specific kinetic energy to pass through its field. That is, for a particular kinetic energy, the radius of curvature is directly related to the m/z ratio. This type of analyzer is commonly used in combination with EI and FAB ionization systems.

Quadrupole mass spectrometers act as a filter for molecules or fragments with a specific m/z ratio. This is accomplished by using four equally spaced parallel rods with direct current (DC) and radio-frequency (RF) potentials on opposing rods of the quadrupole. The field produced is along the x- and y-axis. The radio frequency oscillation causes the ions to be attracted or repelled by the rods. Only ions with a specific m/z ratio will have a trajectory along the z-axis, allowing them to pass to the detector while others will be trapped by the rods of the quadrupole. By varying the RF field, other m/z ranges are selected, thus resulting in the mass spectrum.[31] The quadrupole mass spectrometer, commonly combined with the EI ionization system, is perhaps the most commonly used type of mass spectrometer because of its relatively low cost, ability to analyze m/z ratios up to 3000, and its compatibility with ESI ionization systems.

The ion trap analyzer is another form of a quadrupole mass spectrometer, consisting of a ring electrode to which an RF voltage is applied to two end caps at ground potential. This arrangement generates a quadrupole field trapping ions that are injected into the chamber or are generated within it. As the RF field is scanned, ions with specific and successive m/z ratios are ejected from the trap to the ion detector through holes in the caps.[31] The quadrupole ion trap mass spectrometer is notable for its high sensitivity and compact size.

Tandem MS is a technique that uses multiple stages of mass analysis on subsequent generations of ion fragments. This is accomplished by preselecting an ion from the first analysis and colliding it with an inert gas, such as argon or helium, to induce further fragmentation of the ion. The next stage involves analysis of the fragments generated by an earlier stage. The abbreviation MS[n] is applied to the stages, which analyze fragments beyond the initial ions (MS) to the first generation of ion fragments (MS[2]) and subsequent generations (MS[3], MS[4], and …). These techniques can be tandem in space (two or more instruments) or tandem in time. In the former case, many combinations have been used for this type of analysis. In the later cases, quadrupole ion trap devices are often used and can achieve multiple MS[n] measurements.[33] Tandem mass analysis is primarily used to obtain structural information such as peptides sequences, small DNA/RNA oligomers, fatty acids, and oligosaccharides. Other mass analyzers such as time-of-flight and Fourier transform mass spectrometers are not commonly used for clinical applications.

ION DETECTOR

The *ion detector* is the final element of the mass spectrometer. Once an ion passes through the mass analyzer, a signal is produced in the detector. The detector consists of an electron multiplier that converts the energy of the ion into a cascade of secondary electrons (similar to a photomultiplier tube), resulting in about a million-fold amplification of the signal. Due to the rapid rate at which data is generated, computerized data systems are indispensable components of all modern mass spectrometers. The introduction of rapid processors, large storage capacities, and spectra databases has lead to automated high throughput. Miniaturization of components has also led to the development of bench-top systems practical for routine clinical laboratory analysis. Clinical applications include newborn screening for metabolic disorders, hemoglobin analysis, and drug testing. Pharmaceutical applications include drug discovery, pharmacokinetics, and drug metabolism.

CYTOMETRY

Cytometry is defined as a process of measuring physical, chemical, or other characteristics of (usually) cells or other biological particles. While this definition encompasses the fields of flow cytometry and cellular image analysis, many additional methods are now used to study the vast spectrum of cellular properties. Consequently, the term *cytomics* has been introduced. Cytomics is defined as the science of cell-based analysis that integrates genomics and proteomics with dynamic functions of cells and tissues. The technology used includes techniques discussed in this chapter, such as flow cytometry and MS, and others that are beyond the scope of this chapter.

Flow Cytometry

Flow cytometry is the technology used to measure properties of cells as they move or flow in liquid suspension.[34] Instruments generally referred to as *flow cytometers* are based on the principles of laser-induced fluorometry and light scatter. The terminology can become confusing since various conventions have taken root over the years. However, regardless of the principles of detection or measurement, the term *flow cytometry* may in general be applied to technologies that rely on cells moving in a fluid stream for analysis.

The hematology analyzer, an instrument employing flow cytometry, also incorporates the principles of impedance, absorbance, and laser light scatter to measure cell properties, and generates a CBC laboratory report. The basis of cell counting and sizing in hematology analyzers is the Coulter principle, which relates counting and sizing of particles to changes in electrical impedance across an aperture in a conductive medium (which is created when a particle moves through it). The basic system consists of a smaller chamber within a larger chamber, both filled with a conductive medium and each with one electrode across in which a constant DC is applied. The fluids within each chamber communicate through a small aperture (100 μm) or sensing zone. When a nonconductive particle or cell passes through the aperture, it displaces an equivalent volume of conductive fluid. This increases the conductance and creates a voltage pulse for each cell counted, the intensity of which is proportional to the cell volume.[15]

In hematology analyzers, blood is separated into two volumes for measurement. One volume is mixed with a diluent and delivered to a chamber where platelet and erythrocyte counts are performed. Particles with volumes between 2 and 20 fL are counted as platelets, and particles with volumes >36 fL are counted as erythrocytes. The other volume is mixed with a diluent, and an erythrocyte lysing reagent is used to permit leukocyte (>36 fL) counts to be performed. The number of cells in this size range may be subtracted from the erythrocyte count performed in the other chamber.

Modern hematology analyzers employ additional technologies to enhance the resolution of blood cell analysis. Radio frequency energy is used to assess important information about the internal structure of cells such as nuclear volume. Laser light scatter is used to obtain information about cell shape and granularity. The combination of these and other technologies such as light absorbance (for hemoglobin measurements) provide accurate blood cell differentials, counts, and other important blood cell indices. These basic principles are common to many hematology analyzers used in clinical laboratories. However, each uses different proprietary detection, measurement and software systems, and ways of displaying this data.

Flow cytometers can also incorporate the principles of fluorometry and light scatter to the analysis of particles or cells that pass within a fluid stream. This technology provides multiparametric measurements of intrinsic and extrinsic properties of cells. Intrinsic properties, including cell size and cytoplasmic complexity, are properties that can be assessed directly by light scatter and do not require the use of any type of probe. Extrinsic cellular properties, such as cell surface or cytoplasmic antigens, enzymes or other proteins, and DNA/RNA, require the use of a fluorescent dye or probe to label the components of interest and a laser to induce the fluorescence (older systems used mercury arc lamps as a light source) to be detected.

The basic flow cytometer consists of four types of components: fluidics, optics, electronics, and data analysis. Fluidics refers to the apparatus that directs the cells in suspension to the flow cell where they will be interrogated by the laser light. Fluidics systems use a combination of air pressure and vacuum to create the conditions that allow the cells to pass through the flow chamber in single file. The optical components include the laser (or other light source), flow chamber, monochromatic filters, dichroic mirrors, and lenses. These are used to direct the scattered or fluorescent light to detectors, which measure the signals that are subsequently analyzed.[34]

The light scattered by the cell when it reaches the flow chamber is used to measure its intrinsic properties. Forward-angle light scattering (FALS) is detected by a diode and reflects the size of the passing cell. Right-angle light scattering (RALS) is detected by a photomultiplier tube and is a function of the cytoplasmic complexity of the cell. The analysis of extrinsic properties is more complicated. The measurement of DNA or RNA, for example, requires the use of intercalating nucleic acid dyes such as propidium iodide. The detection of antigenic determinants on cells can be performed with fluorescent-labeled MoABs directed at these antigens. In each case the principle of detection involves the use of laser light to excite the fluorescent dye and detect its emitted signal. Fluorescent dyes are characterized by their excitation (absorption) and emission wavelength spectra and by the difference between the maxima of these spectra or Stokes shift (discussed in the spectrophotometry section). These properties permit the use of multiple fluorescent probes on a single cell.

To illustrate the operation of a flow cytometer, consider a four-color, six-parameter (FALS and RALS) configuration (Figure 2-7).[35] An argon gas laser with a wavelength of 488 nm is commonly used because it simultaneously excites several different dyes that possess different emission wavelengths. Fluorochromes conjugated with MoABs that may be used include fluorescein isothiocyanate (FITC), phycoerythrin (PE), energy-coupled dye (ECD), and Cy5PE (tandem dye composed of the carbocyanine derivative Cy5 and PE) with peak emission wavelengths of approximately 520, 578, 613, and 670 nm, respectively. The emitted light at each of these wavelengths is detected at an angle of 90°. The array of optical filters selects light in each wavelength region and directs it to a different photomultiplier tube where it is detected, amplified, and converted into an electronic signal. This measurement can be made on thousands of cells in a matter of seconds. The result is a histogram that identifies distinct cell populations based on light scatter and extrinsic properties. In the case of blood, a histogram will distinguish lymphocytes, monocytes, and granulocytes by light scatter. The B cell, T cell, T cell subsets, and natural killer cell populations can all be distinguished.

This important method of cell analysis has found many applications in medicine making it a relatively common clinical laboratory instrument. Flow cytometry is routinely used to assist in the diagnosis of leukemia and lymphoma, derive prognostic information in these and other malignancies, monitor immunodeficiency disease states such as HIV/AIDS, enumerate stem cells by cluster differentiation (CD34), and assess various functional properties of cells.

Image Cytometry

Image cytometry is a form of cytometry that encompasses a class of instruments and techniques used to analyze tissue specimens or individual cells. The basic components of an image cytometry system include a microscope, camera, computer, and monitor. Variations and complexity of these systems exist, which are beyond the scope of this chapter. However, the essence of these instruments is the ability to acquire images in two or three (confocal microscopy) dimensions to study the distribution of various components within cells or tissues. The high optical resolution of these systems is an important determinant in obtaining morphometric information and precise data about cell and tissue constituents through the use of fluorescence/absorbance-based probes, as in flow cytometry.[36] Specific applications of image cytometry generally involve unique methods of cell or tissue preparation and other modifications. This lends to the versatility of this technology, which yields such applications as the measurement of DNA content in nuclei to assess prognosis in cancer and the detection of specific nucleic acid sequences to diagnose genetic disorders.

In Situ Hybridization

Among the methods of image cytometry, *in situ hybridization* is perhaps the most commonly used in the clinical laboratory, particularly in molecular cytogenetics laboratories. In situ hybridization is used to localize nucleic acid sequences (entire chromosomes or parts, including genes) in cells or tissues through the use of probes, which consist of a nucleic acid sequence that is complementary to the target sequence and labeled in some way that makes the hybridized sequence detectable. These principles are common to all methods of in situ hybridization, but they differ in the type of probe that is used. Fluorescent probes, which provide excellent spatial resolution, have become a preferred method of in situ hybridization for many applications. (Radioactive probes are also used for this application. However, because their spatial resolution is limited, detection and artifacts are often produced.)

Fluorescent in situ hybridization (FISH) is a powerful technique for detecting genes and genetic anomalies and monitoring different diseases at the genetic level. This technique involves the use of a system of coupled antibodies and fluorochromes similar to those used with flow cytometry. The probe, which is the complementary nucleic acid sequence, is incorporated with a fluorescent molecule or antigenic site to which fluorescently labeled antibodies may be directed (biotin-avidin system). When the two strands of DNA are separated through heating (denaturation), the labeled probe can hybridize the target sequence. Fluorescent microscopes are used to visualize the hybridized sequences. An appropriate arrangement of filters is used to direct the relevant

wavelength of light from the light source to excite the fluorescent molecule on the probe. All but the emission wavelength of light is blocked with a special filter permitting the signal from the probe to be visualized.[37]

MOLECULAR DIAGNOSTICS AND NANOTECHNOLOGY

Molecular diagnostics (MDx) have initially been introduced into the clinical laboratories as manual, labor intensive techniques. This discipline, still in its infancy, has experienced an overwhelming period of maturation in the past several years. Testing has moved quickly from highly complex, labor intensive procedures to more user friendly and semi-automated protocols. Nucleic acid amplification technologies are among the procedures that have most revolutionized MDx testing.

Nucleic Acid Amplification

Polymerase chain reaction (PCR) is the most frequently used of these technologies. Other techniques that are beginning to emerge in the clinical laboratory include ligase chain reaction (LCR), transcription mediated amplification (TMA), branched DNA amplification, and nucleic acid sequence-based amplification (NASBA).

Polymerase chain reaction is used principally for detecting microbiologic organisms and genetic diseases (Table 2-1). Microorganisms identified by this process include chlamydia, cytomegalovirus (CMV), Epstein-Barr virus, human immunodeficiency virus (HIV), mycobacteria, and herpes simplex virus. Although the number of organisms that can be identified is limited at present, this list is growing. Furthermore, PCR can

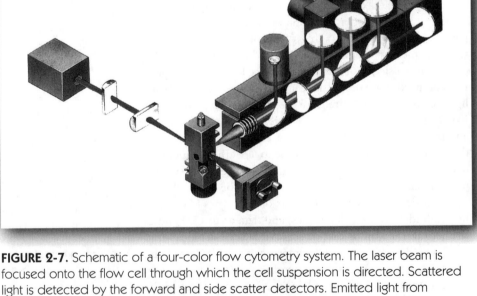

FIGURE 2-7. Schematic of a four-color flow cytometry system. The laser beam is focused onto the flow cell through which the cell suspension is directed. Scattered light is detected by the forward and side scatter detectors. Emitted light from specific MoAB labeled with fluorochromes are detected. Appropriate dichroic long pass filters direct the specific wavelength of light through a narrow band pass filter and then to the appropriate PMT (provided courtesy of Beckman Coulter, Inc.).

often identify organisms with greater rapidity and sensitivity than conventional methods.

Genetic diseases diagnosed using PCR include alpha-1 antitrypsin deficiency, cystic fibrosis, sickle cell anemia, fragile X syndrome, Tay–Sachs disease, drug-induced hemolytic anemia, and von Willebrand disease. In addition, cancer research has benefited from PCR through the diagnosis of various cancers (e.g., chronic myeloid leukemia and pancreatic and colon cancers) as well as through the detection of residual disease after treatment.[38] This technique is used to amplify specific DNA and RNA sequences enzymatically.

Polymerase chain reaction takes advantage of the normal DNA replication process. In vivo, DNA replicates when the double helix unwinds and the two strands separate. A new strand forms on each separate strand through the coupling of specific base pairs (e.g., adenosine with thymidine and cytosine with guanosine). The PCR cycle is similar and consists of three separate steps (Figure 2-8)[28]:

1. Denaturation—the two strands of DNA are thermally separated.
2. Primer annealing—sequence-specific primers are allowed to hybridize to opposite strands flanking the region of interest by decreasing the temperature.
3. Primer extension—DNA polymerase then extends the hybridized primers, generating a copy of the original DNA template.

The efficiency of the extension step can be increased by raising the temperature. Typical temperatures for the three steps are 201.2°F (94°C) for denaturation, 122°F to 149°F (50°C to 65°C) for annealing, and 161.6°F (72°C) for extension. Since the entire cycle is completed in only about 3 minutes, many cycles can occur within a short time, resulting in the exponential production of millions of copies of the target sequence.[39]

The genetic material is then identified by agarose gel electrophoresis. While not truly a chromatographic technique, gel electrophoresis utilizes principles similar to TLC in that the migration of bands is similar to the migration of spots. An electric current is applied to facilitate DNA migration, and the gene is identified by the distance it migrates through the gel.

One potential disadvantage of this method is contamination of the amplification reaction with products of a previous PCR (carryover), exogenous DNA, or other cellular material. Contamination can be reduced by prealiquoting reagents, using dedicated positive-displacement pipettes and physically separating the reaction preparation from the area where the product is analyzed. In addition, multiple negative controls are necessary to monitor for contamination. Several companies are currently developing instrumentation that can perform real-time (q)PCR as well as multiplex PCR, which allows amplification of two or more products in parallel in a singly reaction tube.[40]

GENOMICS, EPIGENETICS, AND PROTEOMICS

Newly developed techniques capable of examining the DNA, mRNA, and proteins of cells have provided a framework for detailed molecular classifications and treatments of diseases. Genetic analysis of cystic fibrosis, for example, has shown the disease to be the result of over 1500 different mutations in the gene cystic fibrosis transmembrane conductance regulator (CFTR).[41] The most common mutation accounts for two-thirds of cystic fibrosis cases. Most recently, a new pharmaceutical (Kalydeco) has been approved by the U.S. Food and Drug Administration, with orphan drug status, to treat

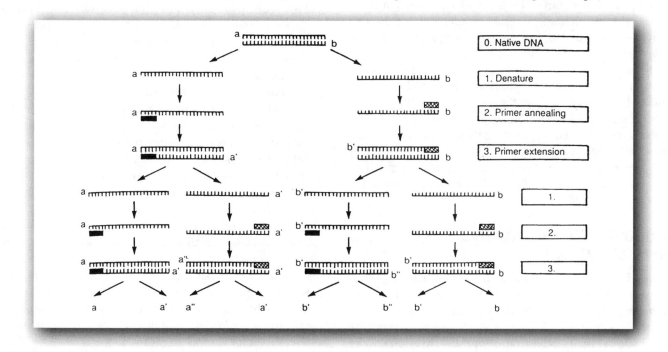

FIGURE 2-8. Schematic of the three steps in the PCR amplification of a specific DNA sequence, as described in the text (adapted from reference 39).

patients with one of the less common mutations. Several related developments, especially in the areas of tumor classifications, is based upon the fields of genomics, epigenetics, and proteomics. The most important laboratory procedures are array-based comparative hybridization and the data derived from these studies, bioinformatics.

Genomics

The study of all the genes of a cell, its DNA sequences, and the fine-scale mapping of genes is the science of *genomics*. A genome is the sum total of all genes of an individual organism. Knowledge of full genomes has created multiple possibilities, mainly concerned with patterns of gene expression associated with various diseases.[42]

Epigenetics

Epigenetics refers to modifications of the genome that are functionally relevant and do not involve a change in the nucleotide sequence. DNA methylation and histone deacetylation are examples of such changes, both of which serve to suppress gene expression without altering the sequence of the silenced genes. Such changes may continue to exist for many cell divisions, and even the remainder of the cell's life, as well as for future generations of cells. But since there is no change in the underlying DNA sequence of the organism, nongenetic factors cause the organism's genes to express themselves differently.[43]

Proteomics

The study of the full complement of proteins in a cell or tissue is called *proteomics* and includes the comprehensive analysis and characterization of all of the proteins encoded by the human genome. Protein-based assays were among the first assays to be approved by the FDA, mostly using immunohistochemistry techniques. Most important biological functions are controlled by signal transduction, processes governed by the enzyme activities of proteins. Diseases such as cancer, while fundamentally the result of genomic mutations, are functionally manifest as dysfunctional protein signal transduction. Many pharmaceuticals are now being developed to aim at modulating the aberrant protein activity, not the genetic defect.[44-46]

Proteomics will eventually have a great impact in the practice of medicine. Although the genome is the source of basic cellular information, the functional aspects of the cell are controlled by and through proteins, not genes. Currently, most of the FDA-approved targeted therapeutics are directed at proteins and not genes.

ARRAY-BASED COMPARATIVE HYBRIDIZATION

Molecular profiles of cells can now be determined using *array-based comparative hybridization*.[47] This technique is especially useful in profiling tumor cells. Until recently, changes occurring in cancer cells were studied one at a time or in small groups in small sets of tumors. New array comparative hybridization or microarray technology ("gene chips") has enabled investigators to simultaneously detect and quantify the expression of large numbers of genes (potentially all genes) in different tumors using mRNA levels. In this technique, samples are obtained from tissues embedded in paraffin blocks, and serve as the sources to prepare new blocks that may contain up to thousands of tissue fragments. These multiple samples are then used to test the expression of potential tumor markers by mRNA expression profiling. mRNA levels, however, do not always correspond to changes in tumor cell proteins. The quantity of protein within a cell depends not only on the amount and rate of transcription and translation, but also on protein breakdown and the rate of transport out of the cell. Whereas tissue used for mRNA profiling may include both tumor and stromal cells, by adding immunohistochemistry methods, specific proteins in tissue sections originating from both normal as well as tumor cells can be identified.

As a specific example, several types of breast cancer cells, which were previously identified only by morphology, are now being studied by array-based comparative hybridization techniques. Combined with immunohistochemistry staining and protein expression levels, new subtypes that were not previously well defined have been identified (e.g., the basal-like carcinomas).[48] As a consequence, new treatment modalities have been developed. Array-based comparative hybridization methods have also identified new subtypes of other tumors, such as lymphomas and prostate cancer with potential for susceptibility and prognosis.[49,50]

NANOTECHNOLOGY

Nanotechnology refers to the emerging science that studies interactions of cellular and molecular components at the most elemental level of biology, typically clusters of atoms, molecules, and molecular fragments. Nanoscale objects have dimensions smaller than 100 nm. At this dimension, smaller than human cells (which vary from 10,000–20,000 nm in diameter), small clusters of molecules and their interactions can be detected. Nanoscale devices smaller than 50 nm can easily enter most cells, while those smaller than 20 nm can move out of blood vessels, offering the possibility that these devices will be able to enter biological chambers, such as the blood–brain barrier or the gastrointestinal epithelium, and identify tumors, abnormalities, and deficiencies in enzymes and cellular receptor sites. Within these biological chambers, they will be able to interact with an individual cell in real time and in that cell's native environment.

Despite their small size, nanoscale devices can also hold tens of thousands of small molecules, such as a magnetic resonance imaging (MRI) contrast agent or a multicomponent diagnostic system capable of assaying a cell's metabolic state. A good example of this approach will capitalize on existing "lab-on-a-chip" and microarray technologies developed at the micron scale. Widely used in biomedical research and to a lesser extent for clinical diagnostic applications today, these technologies will find new uses when shrunk to nanoscale. (In some instances, nanotechnology has already taken advantage of previous clinically relevant technological developments on larger scales.)

Currently, innovative testing is available for many different viruses, mutation analysis, and hematological and solid tumors. With continuing advances and developments in nanotechnology, it is impossible to speculate as to what this new area of testing holds for the future of the clinical laboratory.

SUMMARY

This chapter presents a brief overview of the more common and emerging laboratory methodologies, including their potential advantages and problems. Flame photometry, paper chromatography, and RIA are discussed primarily to provide a historical basis and description of the simple principles on which the more complex methods are based. A summary of the most common assay methods performed for routine laboratory tests is provided in Table 2-1.

Due to its simplicity and improved sensitivity, ISE has replaced flame photometry as the principal method for measuring serum and urine electrolytes. Some methods, including turbidimetry, nephelometry, and spectrophotometry, are used in conjunction with other tests such as the immunoassay. With these methods, concentrations of substances such as immune complexes can be determined.

Chromatography remains one of the mainstays of the laboratory for drug detection. The two principal forms of chromatography are liquid and gas. Both types are similar in that they depend on differences in either solubilities or boiling points, respectively, to separate different analytes in a sample. Another group of important tests are the immunoassays: EIA, EMIT, ELISA, and FPIA. All of these methods depend on an immunologically mediated reaction that increases sensitivity and specificity over RIA. These assays are commonly used to determine routine clinical chemistries and drug concentrations. A relatively new technology, PCR is used to amplify specific DNA and RNA sequences, primarily in the areas of microbiology and detection of genetic diseases. Finally, with the potential advances envisioned in the area of nanotechnology, the laboratory will be able to provide clinicians with information and access to the patient's cellular and molecular environments, thus providing the ability to target therapies at the exact site of the pathologic process.

The rapid technological advancement of laboratory instrumentation has led to the implementation of new and enhanced clinical laboratory methodologies, including MS, cytometry, laboratory automation, and point-of-care testing. While laboratory medicine endeavors to keep pace with the burgeoning developments in biomedical sciences, especially with an increase in the sophistication of the tests, it is essential that today's clinicians have a basic understanding of the more common and esoteric tests in order to select the most appropriate one in each case. All of these developments will translate directly into improved patient care.

REFERENCES

1. Smith T. Quality automated. In: *Advance for Administrators of the Laboratory*. King of Prussia, PA: Merion Publications Inc; 2007:44–48.

2. Felder RA. Automation: survival tools for the hospital laboratory. The Second International Bayer Diagnostics Laboratory Testing Symposium; July 17, 1998; New York, NY. Available at http://marc.med.virginia.edu/pdfs/lib_automation.html.

3. Available at http://www.clsi.org/Content/NavigationMenu/Committees/AutomationandInformatics/Automation_Mission.htm. Accessed

4. Felder RA, Graves S, Mifflin T. Reading the future: increasing the relevance of laboratory medicine in the next century. *MLO Med Labs Obs*. 1999;31: 20–21, 24–26

5. Imants RL. Microfabricated biosensors and microanalytical systems for blood analysis. *Acc Chem Res*. 1998;31:317–324.

6. Ouellette J. Biosensors: microelectronics marries biology. *The Industrial Physicist*. 1998;September:11.

7. Wang J. Survey and summary from DNA biosensors to gene chips. *Nucleic Acids Research*. 2000;28:3011–3016.

8. Nguyen A. Principles of instrumentation. In: McPherson RA, Pinkus MR, eds. *Henry's Clinical Diagnosis and Management by Laboratory Method*. 21st ed. Philadelphia, PA: WB Saunders; 2006:60–79.

9. Wehry EA. Molecular fluorescence and phosphorescence spectrometry. In: Settle FA, ed. *Handbook of Instrumental Techniques for Analytical Chemistry*. Upper Saddle River, NJ: Prentice-Hall; 1997:507–539.

10. Tiffany TO. Fluorometry, nephelometry, and turbidimetry. In: Burtis CA, Ashwood ER, eds. *Tietz Fundamentals of Clinical Chemistry*. 5th ed. Philadelphia, PA: WB Saunders; 2001:74–90.

11. Evenson MA. Photometry. In: Burtis CA, Ashwood ER, eds. *Tietz Fundamentals of Clinical Chemistry*. 5th ed. Philadelphia, PA: WB Saunders; 2001:56–73.

12. Moore RE. Immunochemical methods. In: McClatchey KD, ed. *Clinical Laboratory Medicine*. 1st ed. Baltimore, MD: Williams & Wilkins; 1994:213–238.

13. George JW, O'Neill SL. Comparison of refractometer and biuret methods for total protein measurement in body cavity fluids. *Vet Clin Pathol*. 2001;30:16–18.

14. Freier ES. Osmometry. In: Burtis CA, Ashwood ER, eds. *Clinical Chemistry*. 2nd ed. Philadelphia, PA: WB Saunders; 1994:184–190.

15. Durst RA, Siggaard-Andersen. Electrochemistry In: Burtis CA, Ashwood ER, eds. *Tietz Fundamentals of Clinical Chemistry*. 5th ed. Philadelphia, PA: WB Saunders; 2001:104–120.

16. Burnett W, Lee-Lewandrowski E, Lewandrowski K. Electrolytes and acid base balance. In: McClatchey KD, ed. *Clinical Laboratory Medicine*. 1st ed. Baltimore, MD: Williams & Wilkins; 1994:331–354.

17. Ladenson JH, Apple FS, Koch DD. Misleading hyponatremia due to hyperlipemia: a method-dependent error. *Ann Intern Med*. 1981;95:707.

18. Southern EM. Detection of specific sequences among DNA fragments separated by gel electrophoresis. *J Mol Biol*. 1975;98:503–517.

19. Hoefer Scientific Instruments. *Protein Electrophoresis Applications Guide* (1994). Available at http://www.seas.upenn.edu /belab/ReferenceFiles/hofferelectrobook.pdf.

20. Chang R. *Physical Chemistry with Applications to Biological Systems*. New York, NY: MacMillan; 1977.

21. Christenson RH, Azzazy, HME. Amino acids and proteins. In: Burtis CA, Ashwood ER, eds. *Tietz Fundamentals of Clinical Chemistry*. 5th ed. Philadelphia, PA: WB Saunders; 2001:300–351.

22. Fairbanks VF, Klee GG. Biochemical aspects of hematology. In: Burtis CA, Ashwood ER, eds. *Clinical Chemistry*. 2nd ed. Philadelphia, PA: WB Saunders; 1994:1974–2072.

23. Görg A, Postel W, Günther S. The current state of two-dimensional electrophoresis with immobilized pH gradients. *Electrophoresis*. 1988;9:531–546.

24. Karcher RE, Nuttall KL. Electrophoresis. In: Burtis CA, Ashwood ER, eds. *Tietz Fundamentals of Clinical Chemistry*. 5th ed. Philadelphia, PA: WB Saunders; 2001:121–132.

25. Slagle, KM. Immunoassays: tools for sensitive, specific, and accurate test results. *Lab Med*. 1996:27:177.

26. Kohler G, Milstein C. Continuous cultures of fused cells secreting antibody of predefined specificity. *Nature*. 1975;256:445–497.

27. Berson SA, Yalow RS, Bauman A, et al. Insulin I131 metabolism in human subjects: demonstration of insulin binding globulin in the circulation of insulin treated subjects. *J Clin Invest*. 1956;35:170.

28. Ashihara Y, Kasahara Y, Nakamura RM. Immunoassays and Immunochemistry. In: McPherson RA, Pinkus MR, eds. *Henry's Clinical Diagnosis and Management by Laboratory Methods*. 21st ed. Philadelphia, PA: WB Saunders; 2001.

29. Kitson FG, Larsen BS, McEwen CN. *Gas Chromatography and Mass Spectrometry: a Practical Guide*. San Diego, CA: Academic Press; 1996.

30. Siuzdak G. *Mass Spectrometry for Biotechnology*. San Diego, CA: Academic Press; 1996.

31. Bowers LD, Ullman MD, Burtis CA. Chromatography. In: Burtis CA, Ashwood ER, eds. *Tietz Fundamentals of Clinical Chemistry*. 5th ed. Philadelphia, PA: WB Saunders; 2001:133–156.

32. Van Bramer SE. An introduction to mass spectrometry (1997). Available at http://science.widener.edu/svb/massspec/massspec.pdf.

33. Busch KL, Glish GL, McLuckey SA. *Mass Spectrometry/Mass Spectrometry: Techniques and Applications of Tandem Mass Spectrometry*. New York, NY: VCH Publishers Inc; 1988.

34. Melnick SJ. Acute lymphoblastic leukemia. *Clin Lab Med*. 1999;19:169–186.

35. Alamo AL, Melnick SJ. Clinical applications of four and five-color flow cytometry lymphocyte subset immunophenotyping. *Comm Clin Cytometry*. 2000;42:363–370.

36. Raap AK. Overview of fluorescent in situ hybridization techniques for molecular cytogenetics. *Current Protocols in Cytometry*. 1997;8.1.1–8.1.6.

37. Wilkinson DG. Chapter 1: The theory and practice of in situ hybridization. In: Wilkinson DG, ed. *In Situ Hybridization—A Practical Approach*. Oxford: Oxford University Press; 1992:1–13.

38. Erlich HA, Gelfand D, Sninsky JJ. Recent advances in the polymerase chain reaction. *Science*. 1991;252:1643–1651.

39. Remick DG. Clinical applications of molecular biology. In: McClatchey KD, ed. *Clinical Laboratory Medicine*. 1st ed. Baltimore, MD: Williams & Wilkins; 1994:165–174.

40. Biosearch Technologies, Inc. 81 Digital Dr., Novato, CA 94949-5728.

41. Ratjen F, Doring G. Cystic fibrosis. *Lancet*. 2003;361(9358):681–689.

42. Bloom, MV, Freyer GA, Micklos DA. *Laboratory DNA Science: An Introduction to Recombinant DNA Techniques and Methods of Genome Analysis*. Menlo Park, CA: Addison-Wesley; 1996.

43. Russo VEA, Martienssen RA, Riggs AD. *1996 Epigenetic Mechanisms of Gene Regulation*. Plainview, NY: Cold Spring Harbor Laboratory Press; 1996.

44. Anderson NL, Anderson NG. Proteome and proteomics: new technologies, new concepts, and new words. *Electrophoresis*. 1998;19:1853–1861.

45. Blackstock WP, Weir MP. Proteomics: quantitative and physical mapping of cellular proteins. *Trends Biotechnol*. 1999;17:121–127.

46. Wilkins MR, Pasquali C, Appel RD, et al. From proteins to proteomes: large scale protein identification by two-dimensional electrophoresis and amino acid analysis. *Biotechnology (NY)*. 1996;14:61–65.

47. Shinawi M, Cheung SW. The array CGH and its clinical applications. *Drug Discov Today*. 2008;13:760–770.

48. Peppercorn J, Perou CM, Carey LA. Molecular subtypes in breast cancer evaluation and management: divide and conquer. *Cancer Invest*. 2008;26:1–10.

49. Rosenwald A, Wright G, Chan WC, et al. The use of molecular profiling to predict survival after chemotherapy for diffuse large cell-B-cell lymphoma. *New Engl J Med*. 2002;346:1937–1947.

50. Eeles RA, Kote-Jarai Z, Giles GG, et al. Multiple newly identified loci associated with prostate cancer susceptibility. *Nat Genet*. 2008;40:316–321.

PRIMER ON DRUG INTERFERENCES WITH TEST RESULTS

MARY LEE

After completing this chapter, the reader should be able to

- Distinguish between in vivo and in vitro drug interferences with laboratory tests

- Identify suspected drug–laboratory test interference in a logical, systematic manner given a drug and a laboratory test

- Devise a stepwise process to confirm that a drug is causing a clinically significant drug–laboratory test interference

- Analyze differences among tertiary, secondary, and primary literature resources about drug–laboratory test interferences

- Apply a systematic method to search and identify medical literature relevant to a suspected drug–laboratory test interference situation

Through a variety of mechanisms, drugs can interfere with laboratory test results. If the clinician who has ordered the laboratory test is not aware that the drug has altered the results of the test, inappropriate management of the patient may follow including unnecessary hospitalization, extra office visits, or additional laboratory or clinical testing—all of which may increase the cost of healthcare. This chapter addresses this situation and provides resources that can be used by health professionals to better interpret laboratory tests when a drug is suspected to cause an interference with test results.

IN VIVO AND IN VITRO DRUG INTERFERENCES WITH LABORATORY TESTS[1]

When a drug interferes with a laboratory test result, it alters the lab value. Mechanisms for drug interference of clinical laboratory tests can be classified as either in vivo or in vitro. *In vivo drug interferences* can also be called biological and can be subclassified as pharmacological or toxicological. In vivo interferences account for most effects of drugs on laboratory tests.[2] In contrast, the term *in vitro interference* is used synonymously with analytical or methodological.

In Vivo Interference

An *in vivo interference* is an actual change in the analyte concentration or activity prior to specimen collection and analysis. The assay measurement is true and accurate and reflects a change in the measured substance that has occurred in the patient. Therefore, an in vivo interference will always change a laboratory test result, independent of the assay methodology. A drug can produce an in vivo interference in several ways. By a direct extension of its pharmacological effects, a drug can produce changes in some lab test results. For example, thiazide and loop diuretics will commonly cause increased renal elimination of potassium. Therefore, decreased serum potassium levels can occur in treated patients. In these patients, hypokalemia is true and accurate. Similarly, increased blood urea nitrogen (BUN) levels can occur as a result of excessive fluid loss during treatment with thiazide and loop diuretics.

Other drugs produce changes in lab test results by producing in vivo toxicological effects. As the drug damages a particular organ system, abnormal laboratory tests may be one of the first signs of the problem. For example, as isoniazid and rifampin produce hepatotoxicity, elevated hepatic transaminases will herald the onset of liver inflammation. Similarly, as a prolonged course of high-dose aminoglycoside antibiotic causes acute renal failure, serum creatinine and serum trough aminoglycoside levels will increase steadily. In the face of cyclophosphamide-induced bone marrow suppression, neutropenia will become evident 10–14 days after the dose has been administered.

In Vitro Interference

Drugs in a patient's body fluid or tissue can directly interfere with a clinical laboratory test during the in vitro analytical process. This type of drug–laboratory test interaction is highly dependent on the laboratory test methodology, as the reaction may occur with one specific assay method but not another. For example, serum digoxin levels are commonly determined using a radioimmunoassay, a fluorescent polarization immunoassay, or a TDx assay. However, these assays are based on the three-dimensional structure of the digoxin molecule, and many other drugs with a similar chemical structure to digoxin (e.g., spironolactone, estrogen replacement products, cortisol, or digoxin-like substances) can cross-react with the assay.[3] A falsely increased or decreased serum digoxin level can result.[3,4] To determine the true serum digoxin level in this situation, another assay technique (e.g., high pressure liquid chromatography) may be used. A similar problem occurs with fosphenytoin, which cross-reacts with phenytoin when measured with immunoassay methods.[5] In addition, substances that are prepackaged in or added to the in vitro system before or after sample collection can cause laboratory test interference in vitro. As an example, test tubes sometimes contain lithium heparin or sodium fluoride. Heparin can interfere with aminoglycoside assays, and fluoride can cause false increases in BUN when measured by the Ekatchem assay.

Alternatively, a drug may cause discoloration of the body fluid specimen, which may interfere with colorimetric, photometric, or fluorometric laboratory-based assay methods. For example, phenazopyridine causes an orange–red discoloration of urine that may be mistaken for blood. Nitrofurantoin may cause a brown discoloration of the urine that may cause alarm for the patient. These types of drug interference with lab testing can be detected visually and appropriate attribution of the abnormality should be made by knowledgeable clinicians.

Other common mechanisms by which drugs cause in vitro interferences with laboratory tests include the following:

1. A drug reacts with reagent to form a chromophore (e.g., cefoxitin or cephalothin) with the Jaffe-based creatinine assay.
2. A drug reacts with immunoassay's antibody that is intended to be specific for the analyte. For example, caffeine cross-reacts in the theophylline assay; digitoxin, digoxin metabolites, antigen-binding fragments derived from antidigoxin antibodies (used for treating digoxin intoxication), spironolactone, and canrenone (the major metabolite of spironolactone) cross-react with the digoxin immunoassays.[3]
3. A drug alters the specimen pH (usually urine) so that reagent reactions are inhibited or enhanced. For example, acetazolamide produces an alkaline urinary pH that causes false-positive proteinuria with reagent dip strips.
4. A drug has chemical properties similar to the analyte. For example, patients who receive radiographic contrast media, which contain iodine, may exhibit altered laboratory values for protein-bound iodine.
5. A drug chelates with an enzyme activator or reagent used in the in vitro laboratory analysis.
6. A drug absorbs at the same wavelength as the analyte. For example, methotrexate interferes with analytic methods using an absorbance range of 340–410 nm.

In addition to the parent drug, other drug-related components may cause significant interferences with laboratory tests. Metabolites can cross-react with the parent drug in an assay, such as in the case with cyclosporine. Its metabolites cross-react with the parent drug in high-pressure liquid chromatography

assays and can produce a falsely high measurement of the concentration of cyclosporine.[6] Inactive ingredients of some drug products may influence assay results. Inactive ingredients in dosage formulations include excipients such as lactose or starch, preservatives, colorants, or flavoring agents. Although most manufacturers do report the inactive ingredients in their products, little systematic research has been performed to assess the impact of these substances on laboratory tests. Compounding these factors, many laboratory test interferences are concentration-related, and many drug metabolites and their usual plasma concentrations have yet to be identified. Therefore, systematic study of all of these potential causes of interactions is difficult to conduct and is not available in many cases.[7]

Simultaneous In Vitro and In Vivo Effects

Some drugs can affect an analyte both in vivo and in vitro. In these rare situations, interpretation is extremely difficult because the degree of impact in each environment cannot be determined easily. The prototypic example involves reaction of aminoglycosides with penicillins, which leads to a loss of antibacterial activity in vivo and can decrease measured aminoglycoside concentrations and antibacterial activity in vitro. Although this inactivation mechanism is unclear, it seems to involve the formation of an adduct between the aminoglycoside and beta-lactam ring of the penicillins.

In vitro, carbenicillin is the most potent inactivator of aminoglycosides when compared to the other penicillins; tobramycin is the most susceptible when compared to the other aminoglycosides; and amikacin and netilmicin are degraded the least. Refrigeration does not significantly slow the reaction but centrifugation with freezing does. Unreasonably low aminoglycoside concentrations in patients receiving concomitant high-dose penicillins should alert the practitioner to this in vitro interaction.[8-10]

In vivo inactivation of aminoglycosides by a parenteral penicillin is a problem primarily in patients with renal failure. With normal renal function, these antibiotics are excreted at a rate faster than their interaction rate. In one study, the in vivo inactivation rate constant of gentamicin in patients with renal failure receiving carbenicillin was 0.025 hour^{-1}. The inactivation rate constant was defined as the difference between the elimination rate constant for gentamicin alone and that for its combination with carbenicillin. Thus, in renal failure patients, carbenicillin apparently eliminates gentamicin at the same rate as do the kidneys. The change corresponded to a shortening of the gentamicin half-life from 61.6–19.6 hours after carbenicillin was added. Fortunately, carbenicillin is no longer commercially available by the parenteral route. However, this drug–laboratory test interaction occurs with other penicillins.

The effect of penicillins on aminoglycosides can be minimized several ways[7]:

1. To eliminate in vitro problems, the sample can be centrifuged and frozen soon after it is drawn.
2. Antibiotics with less interaction potential (e.g., amikacin and piperacillin, or amikacin and a cephalosporin) can be used.

MINICASE 1

A Case of Polycythemia in an Elderly Patient Receiving Testosterone Replacement Therapy

SAMUEL M., A 68-YEAR-OLD, AFRICAN-AMERICAN MALE PATIENT, complains of decreased sexual drive and erectile dysfunction for 1 year. His wife, who is about 20 years younger, has sent him to the clinic for medical treatment. Samuel M. reports retiring from his job as a mailman about 3 years ago. Since then, he has kept active by volunteering at a nearby community center and babysitting his grandchildren. He reports no other problems.

Samuel M. also has well-controlled essential hypertension, which has been treated with hydrochlorothiazide and enalapril for the past 5 years. He is sickle cell trait positive. Pertinent findings on physical exam reveals mild gynecomastia, small testicles, and a normal penis.

Samuel M. is suspected of having late-onset hypogonadism, which is confirmed by two separate serum testosterone measurements of 200 ng/dL and 185 ng/dL. All other lab tests, including a complete blood count are normal. Samuel M. is prescribed testosterone enanthate 400 mg intramuscularly every 2–3 weeks for 3 months. At the end of the third month of treatment, hematocrit is 55%, BUN is 15 mg/dL, serum creatinine is 1.3 mg/dL, and serum testosterone is 1800 ng/dL.

Question: What is the cause of the hematocrit change in Samuel M.? Is this an in vivo or in vitro drug interference with a lab test? How should Samuel M. be managed?

Discussion: As men age, the testes decrease production of testosterone, the principal androgen in males. Whereas all men develop biochemical hypogonadism, when serum testosterone levels are below the normal range, only some men develop clinical symptoms that require medical intervention. This is similar to women who go through the menopause. In the short term, hypogonadism is associated with decreased libido, erectile dysfunction, and mood changes. In the long term, hypogonadism is associated with osteoporosis, weight gain, and decreased body muscle. For patients with confirmed hypogonadism-related decreased libido, erectile dysfunction, and mood changes, testosterone replacement therapy is effective in reducing these symptoms. The least expensive regimen is intramuscular injections of depot testosterone enanthate or testosterone cypionate, which are typically administered every 3 or 4 weeks. Serum testosterone levels should be obtained 2 or 3 months after the start of treatment, and the goal is to increase serum testosterone to the mid-normal physiologic range (300–1200 ng/dL). Excessive doses of testosterone are associated with adverse effects including mood swings and polycythemia. Polycythemia is a direct result of the anabolic effects of testosterone and its stimulatory effect on erythropoiesis. In elderly patients, polycythemia may clog small capillaries, which may predispose to the development of a cerebrovascular accident, myocardial infarction, or priapism. Therefore, testosterone supplementation should be discontinued when the hematocrit exceeds 50%.

In Samuel M., testosterone enanthate was likely the cause of polycythemia based on the temporal relationship of the adverse effect and the start of testosterone supplementation, and the high serum testosterone concentration indicates that Samuel M. is receiving an excessive dose. The elevated hematocrit is not due to dehydration, as Samuel M.'s BUN:creatinine ratio is less than 20:1. This is an in vivo, drug–laboratory test interference. Therefore, testosterone enanthate should be discontinued until the hematocrit and serum testosterone concentration return to the normal range. At that time, testosterone enanthate can be restarted at a lower dose of 200 mg intramuscularly every 3 weeks.

3. Administration times can be separated or blood can be drawn just before the next scheduled penicillin dose to decrease the penicillin concentration in the specimen tube, the concentration-exposure time (in vivo), and, thus, the degradation time.

This last maneuver would be less applicable in patients with renal failure, particularly if the penicillin dose was not adjusted. However, decreasing the daily penicillin dose according to renal function and target serum concentration would make testing more accurate even for these patients.

Simultaneous in vitro and in vivo effects also occur when drugs produce lipemia, hemolysis, or hyperbilirubinemia.[7] Drugs that increase cholesterol blood levels (e.g., protease inhibitors, estrogens, corticosteroids) do so by a variety of different mechanisms. The increase in lipids in the blood specimen produce a cloudy appearance, which interferes with light transmission, an essential component of nephelometric and turbidometric analytic procedures.[11] Similarly, drugs that produce hemolytic anemia cause in vivo toxic effects on red blood cells. As hemoglobin is released from lysed red blood cells into the circulation, in vitro interference with analytic methods results from a variety of mechanisms: (1) hemoglobin interferes with assay reactions directly; (2) cytoplasmic constituents of lysed red blood cells enter the bloodstream and produce elevations of plasma potassium and magnesium; and (3) hemoglobin interferes with optical absorbance measures on spectrophotometric assays.[12,13]

Some immunoassays use mouse monoclonal antibody as the reagent. Human antimouse antibody can interfere with the mouse monoclonal antibody reagent leading to incorrect assay results for creatine kinase and thyroid function.[13] Human antimouse antibody can be produced by patients who are regularly exposed to mice as pets, by people whose occupation is working with mice in a pet store, or by humans who are exposed to foods or other items contaminated by mice.[7] To avoid this lab test interference, another assay method should be chosen, or alternatively, employ an immunoassay that does not rely on mouse monoclonal antibody.[13]

IDENTIFYING DRUG INTERFERENCES

Incidence of Drug Interferences

The true incidence of drug interferences with laboratory tests is unknown. This is because many situations probably go undetected. However, as the number of laboratory tests and drugs on the U.S. commercial market increase, it is likely that the number of cases of in vivo interferences will also increase.

As a reflection of this, consider the number of drug–laboratory test interferences reported by D. S. Young, author of one of the classic literature references on this topic. In the first edition of *Effects of Drugs on Clinical Laboratory Tests,* published in the journal *Clinical Chemistry* in 1972, 9000 such interactions were included.[14] In the second edition of the same publication, which was published in 1975, 16,000 such interactions were reported.[15] In 2007, this resource, which had been converted to an online searchable database, included over 135,000 interactions.

As for in vitro interferences, the number of drug–laboratory test interferences may be moderated over time because of newer, more specific laboratory test methodologies that minimize cross-reactions with drug metabolites or drug effects on reagents or laboratory reactions.[12,16] In addition, manufacturers of commonly used laboratory equipment systematically study the effects of drugs on assay methods.[17] Therefore, this information is often available to clinicians who confront problematic laboratory test results in patients. This increased awareness reduces the number of patients who are believed to have experienced newly reported drug–laboratory test interferences.

Suspecting a Drug Interference

A clinician should suspect a drug–laboratory test interference when an inconsistency appears among related test results, or between test results and the clinical picture. Specifically, clinicians should become suspicious whenever

1. Test results do not correlate with the patient's signs, symptoms, or medical history.
2. Results of different tests—assessing the same organ anatomy or organ function or the drug's pharmacologic effects—conflict with each other.
3. Results from a series of the same test vary greatly over a short period of time.
4. Serial test results are inconsistent.

No Correlation with Patient's Signs, Symptoms, or Medical History

As emphasized elsewhere in this book, when an isolated test result does not correlate with signs, symptoms, or medical history of the patient, the signs and symptoms should be considered more strongly than the test result. This rule is particularly true when the test result is used to confirm suspicions raised by the signs and symptoms in the first place or when the test results are being used as surrogate markers or indirect indicators of underlying pathology.

For example, serum creatinine is used in various formulae to approximate the glomerular filtration rate, which is used to assess the kidney's ability to make urine. However, actual urine output and measurement of urinary creatinine excretion is a more accurate method of assessing overall renal function. If a patient's serum creatinine has increased from a baseline of 1–5 mg/dL over a 3-day period, but the patient has had no change

in urine output, urinary creatinine excretion, or serum electrolyte levels, then the serum creatinine level may be elevated because of a drug interference with the laboratory test. Similarly, if a patient has a total serum bilirubin of 6 mg/dL, but the patient is not jaundiced or does not have scleral icterus, then a drug interference with the laboratory test should be considered.

Conflicting Test Results

Occasionally, pharmacological or toxicological effects of a drug produce conflicting results of two tests that assess the same organ function. For example, a presurgical test screen shows a serum creatinine of 4.2 mg/dL in an otherwise healthy 20-year old patient with a BUN of 8 mg/dL. Usually, if a patient had true renal impairment, BUN and serum creatinine would likely be elevated in tandem. Thus, in this patient, a drug interference with the laboratory test is suspected. Further investigation revealed that the patient received cefoxitin shortly before blood was drawn for the lab test. Cefoxitin can falsely elevate serum creatinine concentrations. Thus, the elevated serum creatinine is likely due to drug interference with the laboratory test and not to renal failure. To confirm that this is the case, cefoxitin should be discontinued and the serum creatinine repeated after that. If due to the drug, the elevated serum creatinine should return to the normal range.[18]

Varying Serial Test Results Over a Short Time Period

Typically, the results of a specific laboratory test should follow a trend in a patient. However, in the absence of a new onset of medical illness or worsening of existing disease, a sudden change in the laboratory test result trend should cause examination of a possible drug interference with a laboratory test. For example, prostate specific antigen (PSA) is a tumor marker for prostate cancer. It is produced by glandular epithelial cells of the prostate. Whereas the normal serum level is less than 4 ng/mL in a patient without prostate cancer, the level is typically elevated in patients with prostate cancer. However, it is not specific for prostate cancer. Elevated PSA serum levels are also observed in patients with benign prostatic hyperplasia, prostatitis, or following instrumentation of the prostate. A 70-year-old male patient with stage T_3 (locally invasive) prostate cancer has a PSA of 20 ng/mL and has decided to undergo no treatment. Four serial PSA tests over the course of 1 year and done at 3-month intervals show no change. Despite the absence of any changes on pelvic computerized axial tomography, bone scan, or chest x-ray, his PSA is 10 ng/mL at his most recent office visit. After a careful interview of the patient, the urologist discovers that the patient has been treated for alopecia for the past 6 months with Propecia® (finasteride). The patient received the prescription from another physician. It is likely that his use of Propecia® caused the decrease in PSA.[19]

Changing Serial Test Results Which Are Inconsistent with Expected Results

Leuprolide, a luteinizing hormone-releasing hormone (LHRH) agonist, is useful in the management of prostate cancer, which is an androgen dependent tumor. Persistent use of leuprolide causes down-regulation of pituitary LHRH receptors, decreased secretion of luteinizing hormone, and decreased production of testicular androgens. A patient with prostate cancer, treated with leuprolide, should experience a sustained reduction in serum testosterone levels from normal (300–1200 ng/dL) to castration levels (less than 50 ng/dL) after 2–3 weeks. The serum testosterone level should remain below 50 ng/dL as long as the patient continues treatment with leuprolide, making sure that he makes visits to the clinic for repeated doses on schedule. However, one of the adverse effects of leuprolide is decreased libido and erectile dysfunction, which is a direct extension of the drug's testosterone-lowering effect. Such a patient may seek medical treatment of sexual dysfunction, and he may be inappropriately prescribed depot testosterone injections. Thus, in this case, depot testosterone injections will cause a change in serum testosterone levels in the wrong direction. If serum testosterone levels increase, this should be a signal that the patient has serial test results, which are inconsistent with expected results of leuprolide, and an investigation should be done as to the cause.[20]

MANAGING DRUG INTERFERENCES

When a drug is suspected to interfere with a laboratory test, the clinician should collect appropriate evidence to confirm the interaction. Important information includes
1. Establishing a temporal relationship between the change in the laboratory test and drug use and ensuring that the change in the laboratory test occurred after the drug was started or after the drug dose was changed
2. Ruling out other drugs as causes of the laboratory test change
3. Ruling out concurrent diseases as causes of the laboratory test change
4. If possible, discontinuing the causative agent and repeating the test to see if dechallenge results in correction of the abnormal laboratory test
5. Choosing another laboratory test that will provide assessment of the same organ's function but is unlikely to be affected by the drug (the clinician can conduct the lab test, compare the results against the original lab test result, and check for dissimilarity or similarity of results)[3]
6. Finding evidence in the medical literature that documents the suspected drug–laboratory test interference
7. Contacting the head of diagnostic labs who maintains or has access to computerized lists of drugs that interfere with laboratory tests (the person would also provide assistance in interpreting aberrant laboratory test results)[13]

For any particular patient case, it is often not possible to obtain information on all seven of the above items. However, the first four items are crucial in any suspected drug–laboratory test interference.

LITERATURE RESOURCES

A systematic search of the medical literature is essential for providing the appropriate background information to address steps 2–6. This search will ensure that a complete

and comprehensive review—necessary in making an accurate diagnosis—has been done. When searching the literature, it is recommended to use the method originally described by Watanabe et al. and, subsequently, modified by C. F. Kirkwood.[21,22] Using this technique, the clinician would search tertiary, secondary, and then primary literature.

Tertiary literature includes reference texts and monograph databases, which provide appropriate foundational content and background material essential for understanding basic concepts and historical data relevant to the topic. *Secondary literature*, functioning as a gateway to primary literature, includes indexing and abstracting services (i.e., PubMed and *International Pharmaceutical Abstracts*). *Primary literature* includes case reports, experimental studies, and other nonreview types of articles in journals about the topic. These represent the most current literature on the topic. By systematically scanning the literature in this order, the clinician can be sure to have identified and analyzed all relevant literature, which is crucial in developing appropriate conclusions for these types of situations.

Tertiary Literature

Tertiary literature, which contains useful information about drug–laboratory test interferences, includes the *Physicians' Desk Reference*. Each complete package insert included in this book contains a precautions section that includes information on drug–laboratory test interferences. However, it is important to note that the *Physicians' Desk Reference* does not include package inserts on all commercially available drugs, nor does it include complete package inserts for all of the products included in the text. Thus, additional resources will need to be checked. The drug monographs in the *AHFS Drug Information*, published by the American Society of Health-System Pharmacists, also include a section on lab test interferences. Although the information provided is brief, it can be used as an initial screen. *Meyler's Side Effects of Drugs*, although well-referenced, includes extensive information on adverse effects of medications that are associated with in vivo interference with laboratory test results. Information on various drug categories is subdivided among a number of texts that focus on antimicrobial agents, anesthetics, antineoplastic agents, immunobiologics, endocrine and metabolic drugs, psychiatric drugs, and cardiovascular agents. To do a complete search through *Meyler's Side Effects of Drugs*, the clinician may have to go through several texts. Also, unlike the other two texts, *Meyler's Side Effects of Drugs* is usually only available in drug information centers or medical libraries because of its expense.

One of the most comprehensive compilations of drug–laboratory test interactions is *Effects of Drugs on Clinical Laboratory Tests* by D. S. Young. Although originally published for many years as a special issue of the journal, *Clinical Chemistry*, it is available as a textbook, which can be purchased from the American Association of Clinical Chemistry. The last and fifth edition of the textbook was published in 2000. The content is searchable by the name of the laboratory test; specific drug, herb, or disease name; preanalytic variable; type of body fluid

MINICASE 2

Ciprofloxacin-Induced Hypoprothrombinemia

WILLIAM R., A 65-YEAR-OLD MALE PATIENT, is started on ciprofloxacin 500 mg by mouth twice daily for chronic prostatitis due to *E. coli*. Antibiotic treatment will continue for 6 months. William R. has atrial fibrillation and is also taking digoxin 0.125 mg by mouth daily and warfarin 2.5 mg by mouth daily. William R. has been on warfarin for years and says that he is fully aware of all the DOs and DON'Ts of taking warfarin. His international normalized ratio (INR) regularly and consistently is 2.5, which is therapeutic. William R. has no history of liver disease and appears healthy and well-nourished. Prior to the start of the antibiotic, William R.'s serum sodium was 137 mEq/L, potassium 4.0 mEq/L, BUN 10 mg/dL, creatinine 1 mg/dL, and INR is 2.5. After 3 days of antibiotics, a repeat INR is 5, and William R. complains of slight gum bleeding when he brushes his teeth.

Question: What do you think is causing the laboratory abnormality? How should William R. be managed?

Discussion: Ciprofloxacin inhibits cytochrome 1A2, the principal hepatic enzyme that catabolizes warfarin, and decreases vitamin K–producing bacteria in the gastrointestinal tract. A search of the medical literature documents multiple cases of enhanced warfarin effect when ciprofloxacin is taken concurrently.[23] Although some other antibiotics in the same pharmacologic class of quinolones may have less inhibitory effect on this enzyme, the interaction may still occur.

In William R., the drug interaction occurred after ciprofloxacin was started. William R. is not taking any other medications that could cause the drug–laboratory test interaction and has no history of vitamin K deficiency or liver disease, which could be causing hypoprothrombinemia. To confirm that ciprofloxacin is causing the drug interaction, the physician could discontinue the drug and then see if William R.'s INR returns to the range of 2–3. However, since the ciprofloxacin–warfarin interaction is well-known, a better approach might be to continue ciprofloxacin, hold warfarin until the INR has decreased to 2.5, and then resume warfarin at a reduced daily dose.

---

specimen; and specific laboratory test abnormality. Search results include a description of the drug–laboratory test interaction and a reference citation. No detail is provided on the dosage of drug that produced the interference. Hence, a clinician will need to obtain the original references and evaluate the data independently as a separate step.

A variety of other books about clinical laboratory tests are listed below. Some are comprehensive references while others are handbooks. All of them provide information about drug–laboratory test interferences. However, the reference texts are more complete than the handbooks. In addition, several comprehensive review articles include more current information about drug–laboratory test interferences.

DRUGDEX®, prepared by MICROMEDEX, is available electronically. For every drug included in the system, information is available in a drug monograph format, and any information about drug–laboratory test interferences is included in a unique section of the monograph. In addition, for some drugs, drug information questions and answers are included. To access relevant information, the clinician can search information using the name of the drug or the laboratory test.

Books and Handbooks

Anon. *AHFS Drug Information 2012*. Bethesda, MD: American Society of Health-System Pharmacists; 2012 (electronic reference, ISBN 9781585282609 158528260x).

Anon. *Physician's Desk Reference 2012*. Montvale, NJ: Thomson Publications; 2012.

Aronson JK, ed. *Meyler's Side Effects of Antimicrobial Drugs*. Amsterdam, Netherlands: Elsevier; 2009.

Aronson JK, ed. *Meyler's Side Effects of Cardiovascular Drugs*. Amsterdam, Netherlands: Elsevier; 2009.

Aronson JK, ed. *Meyler's Side Effects of Drugs: The International Encyclopedia of Adverse Drug Reactions and Interactions*. 15th ed. Amsterdam, Netherlands: Elsevier; 2006.

Aronson JK, ed. *Meyler's Side Effects of Drugs in Cancer and Immunology*. Amsterdam, Netherlands: Elsevier; 2009.

Aronson JK, ed. *Meyler's Side Effects of Drugs Used in Anesthesia*. Amsterdam, Netherlands: Elsevier; 2009.

Aronson JK, ed. *Meyler's Side Effects of Endocrine and Metabolic Drugs*. Amsterdam, Netherlands: Elsevier; 2009.

Aronson JK, ed. *Meyler's Side Effects of Psychiatric Drugs*. Amsterdam: Elsevier, Netherlands; 2009.

Chernecky CC, Berger BJ. *Laboratory Tests and Diagnostic Procedures*. 5th ed. St. Louis, MO: WB Saunders; 2007.

Dasgupta A, Hammett-Stabler CA, eds. *Herbal Supplements: Efficacy, Toxicity, Interactions with Western Drugs and Effects on Clinical Lab Tests*. Hoboken, NJ: Wiley; 2011.

Guder WG, Narayanan S, Wisser H, et al., eds. *Diagnostic Samples: from the Patient to the Laboratory*. 4th ed. Weinheim, Germany: Wiley-Blackwell; 2009.

Laposata M. *Laboratory Medicine. The Diagnosis of Disease in the Clinical Laboratory*. New York, New York: McGraw Hill Medical; 2010.

McPherson RA, Pincus MR, eds. *Henry's Clinical Diagnosis and Management by Laboratory Methods*. 22nd ed. Philadelphia, PA: Elsevier WB Saunders; 2011.

Schmidt J, Wieczorkiewicz J. *Interpreting Laboratory Data: A Point-of-Care Guide*. Bethesda, MD: American Society of Health-System Pharmacists; 2011.

Williamson MA, Snyder LM. *Wallach's Interpretation of Diagnostic Tests*. 9th ed. Philadelphia, PA: Wolters Kluwer Lippincott Williams & Wilkins; 2011.

Young DS. *Effects of Drugs on Clinical Laboratory Tests*. 5th ed. Washington, DC: American Association for Clinical Chemistry; 2000.

Young DS. *Effects of Preanalytic Variables on Clinical Laboratory Tests*. 3rd ed. Washington, DC: American Association for Clinical Chemistry; 2007.

Young DS, Friedman RB, Young DS. *Effects of Disease on Clinical Laboratory Tests*. 4th ed. Washington, DC: American Association for Clinical Chemistry; 2001.

Review Articles

- Sher PP. Drug interferences with clinical laboratory tests. *Drugs*. 1982;24:24-63.

  This useful reference provides many tables of drugs known to interfere with various laboratory tests. The data is arranged by laboratory test. For many common laboratory tests, summary tables of drugs known to interfere with the particular lab tests are provided. Also, mechanisms for the in vivo and in vitro interactions are described. Although this reference is dated and is not useful for newer drugs, it is an excellent resource for older drugs.

- Sonntag O, Scholer A. Drug interference in clinical chemistry: recommendation of drugs and their concentrations to be used in drug interference studies. *Ann Clin Biochem.* 2001;38:376-385.

  In 1995, 18 clinical laboratory test experts identified 24 commonly used drugs known to interfere with laboratory tests. Usual therapeutic and toxic drug concentrations were identified. Both concentrations of each drug were added in vitro to blood and urine specimens and then various laboratory tests were run on the specimens. Laboratory testing was duplicated in three different laboratories. This review article summarizes drug–laboratory test interactions for over 70 different laboratory tests.

- Kroll MH, Elin RJ. Interference with clinical laboratory analyses. *Clin Chem.* 1994;40(11 Part 1):1996-2005.

  This is an excellent overview of drug–laboratory test interactions. The article describes how drugs, metabolites, and additives (e.g., heparin, ethylenediamine tetra-acetic acid) can produce significant interactions and discrepancies during in vitro analytic procedures. It also provides a summary of useful references (although outdated) on the topic. In addition, a suggested approach to drug–laboratory test interactions is described.

- DasGupta A, Bernard DW. Herbal remedies: effects on clinical laboratory tests. *Arch Pathol Lab Med.* 2006;130:521-528.

  This review summarizes literature from 1980–2005 on herbal drug interactions with laboratory tests. Mechanisms include (1) herbal agent-induced in vivo toxic effects; (2) direct assay interference by the herbal agent; or (3) contaminant in the herbal agent produces in vivo or in vitro effects that produce changes in laboratory test results. The effect of Chan su on digoxin blood levels and St. John's wort on blood levels of cyclosporine, digoxin, theophylline, and protease inhibitors are just some of the herbal agent–laboratory test interactions discussed. This is a followup to the author's first article on the topic, which was published in the *American Journal of Clinical Pathology* in 2003.

Secondary and Primary Literature

For secondary literature, the main indexing or abstracting service that should be used is PubMed. This allows the clinician to check the literature from thousands of biomedical journals from 1950 to the present. Due to improvements in search capabilities, clinicians can search using text words (i.e., words as they might appear in the title or abstract of a journal article). The database will automatically convert that text word to official medical subject headings or accepted indexing terms. As a result, search output is optimized despite the lack of proficiency or experience of the searcher. If the search represents a combination of concepts, the concepts can be appropriately linked using Boolean logical operators, *or* or *and*. In addition, the database provides links enabling clinicians to locate related articles or order articles online, which enhance search capabilities and convenience in obtaining relevant primary literature articles.

This chapter does not allow a complete tutorial on search strategy development and conducting PubMed searches. However, the reader is encouraged to develop expertise in this area so that he or she can identify current, relevant literature efficiently.

SUMMARY

Although the number of drug–laboratory test interferences increases as the number of commercially available drugs increases, improved literature resources that compile information on this topic and improved assay methodologies have helped clinicians in dealing with suspected cases of this problem. Most drug–laboratory test interferences are due to in vivo effects of drugs; that is, the drug's pharmacological or toxic effects produce specific alterations in laboratory values. A drug–laboratory test interference should be suspected whenever a laboratory test result does not match the signs and symptoms in a patient, when the results of different tests—assessing the same organ function or drug effect—conflict with each other, or when serial laboratory test values vary greatly over a short period of time.

To determine if a drug is interfering with a drug–laboratory test, the clinician should, at a minimum, establish a temporal relationship between the change in the laboratory test and drug use; rule out other drugs and diseases as the cause; and discontinue the drug and repeat the lab test to see if dechallenge results in correction of the abnormal laboratory test. The literature should be checked to see if documentation of the drug–laboratory test interference can be found. The literature search should be systematic to ensure complete literature retrieval. Therefore, the clinician should proceed from the tertiary to the secondary and then to the primary literature. Many helpful literature resources provide relevant information on this topic.

Learning Points

1. **Distinguish an in vivo from an in vitro drug interference with a laboratory test.**

   Answer: An in vivo interaction is characterized by an actual change in measured analyte concentration or activity prior to specimen collection and analysis. That is, the change in the measured analyte occurred in the patient. An in vitro inter-action is characterized by a drug's physical presence in a body fluid or tissue specimen, which interferes with clinical laboratory testing during the analytical process. The interaction occurs outside the patient's body

2. **What clinical situations should signal a potential drug–laboratory test interaction?**

   Answer: A clinician should suspect a drug–laboratory test interaction when an inconsistency appears among related test results or between test results and the clinical presentation (i.e., the patient's signs and symptoms do not match). In addition, if test results vary greatly over a short period of time or if serial results of the same laboratory test are inconsistent, the clinician should evaluate the patient for this possibility.

3. **What key information should a clinician collect to confirm that a drug is causing a laboratory test interaction?**

   Answer: The key criteria in confirming the presence of a drug–laboratory test interaction include

   (1) Ensuring that the change in the laboratory test occurred after the drug was started

   (2) Ruling out other drugs as causes of the laboratory test change

   (3) Ruling out concurrent medical illness(es) as causes of the laboratory test change

   (4) Stopping the drug and seeing if the laboratory test result returns to the predrug value

REFERENCES

1. Sher PP. Drug interferences with clinical laboratory tests. *Drugs.* 1982;24:24-63.

2. Salway JG. Drug interference causing misinterpretation of laboratory results. *Ann Clin Biochem.* 1978;15:44-48.

3. Steimer W, Muller C, Eber B. Digoxin assays: frequent, substantial, and potentially dangerous interference by spironolactone, canrenone, and other steroids. *Clin Chem.* 2002;48:507-516.

4. Dasgupta A. Endogenous and exogenous digoxin-like immunoreactive substances. *Am J Clin Pathol.* 2002;118:132-140.

5. Datta P, Dasgupta A. Cross-reactivity of fosphenytoin in four phenytoin immunoassays. *Clin Chem.* 1998;44:696-697.

6. Steimer W. Performance and specificity of monoclonal immunoassays for cyclosporine monitoring: how specific is specific? *Clin Chem.* 1999;45:371-381.

7. Dimeski G. Interference testing. *Clin Biochem Rev.* 2008;29 (suppl 1):S43-S48.

8. Pickering LK, Rutherford I. Effect of concentration and time on inactivation of tobramycin, gentamicin, netilmicin, and amikacin by azlocillin, carbenicillin, mecillinam, mezlocillin, and piperacillin. *J Pharmacol Exp Ther.* 1981;217:345-349.

9. Chow MS, Quintiliani R, Nightingale CH. In vitro inactivation of tobramycin by ticarcillin. *JAMA.* 1982;247:658-659.

10. Thompson MI, Russo ME, Saxon BJ, et al. Gentamicin inactivation by piperacillin or carbenicillin in patients with end stage renal disease. *Antimicrob Agents Chemother.* 1982;21:268-273.

11. Kroll MH. Evaluating interference caused by lipemia. *Clin Chem.* 2004;50:1968-1969.

12. Lippi G, Salvagno GL, Montagnana M, et al. Influence of hemolysis on routine clinical chemistry testing. *Clin Chem Lab Med.* 2006;44:311-316.

13. Tate J, Ward G. Interferences in immunoassay. *Clin Biochem Rev.* 2004;25:105-119.

14. Young DS, Thomas DW, Friedman RB, et al. Effects of drugs on clinical laboratory tests. *Clin Chem.* 1972;18:1041-1303.

15. Young DS, Pestaner LC, Gibberman V. Effects of drugs on clinical laboratory tests. *Clin Chem.* 1975;21:1D-432D.

16. Young DS. Effects of drugs on clinical laboratory tests. *Ann Clin Biochem.* 1997;34:579-581.

17. Powers DM, Boyd JC, Glick MR, et al. *Interference Testing in Clinical Chemistry.* NCCLS Document. 1986; EP7–P:6(13).

18. Letellier G, Desjarlais F. Analytical interference of drugs in clinical chemistry: II—the interference of three cephalosporins with the determination of serum creatinine concentration by the Jaffe reaction. *Clin Biochem.* 1985;18:352-356.

19. D'Amico AV, Roehrborn CG. Effect of 1 mg/day finasteride on concentrations of serum prostate specific antigen in men with androgenic alopecia: a randomized controlled trial. *Lancet Oncol.* 2007;8:21-25.

20. deJong IJ, Eaton A, Bladou F. LHRH agonists in prostate cancer: frequency of treatment, serum testosterone measurement and castrate level: consensus opinion from a roundtable discussion. *Curr Med Res Opin.* 2007;23:1077-1080.

21. Watanabe AS, McCart G, Shimomura S, et al. Systematic approach to drug information requests. *Am J Hosp Pharm.* 1975;32:1282-1285.

22. Kirkwood CF. Modified systematic approach to answering questions. In: Malone PM, Mosdell KW, Kier KL, et al., eds. *Drug Information: A Guide for Pharmacists.* 2nd ed. Stamford, CT: Appleton & Lange; 2000:19-30.

23. Schelleman H, Bilker WB, Brensinger CM, et al. Warfarin with fluoroquinolones, sulfonamides, or azole antifungals: interactions and risk of hospitalization for gastrointestinal bleeding. *Clin Pharmacol Ther.* 2008;84:581-588.

CHAPTER 4

SUBSTANCE ABUSE AND TOXICOLOGICAL TESTS

PETER A. CHYKA

Objectives

After completing this chapter, the reader should be able to

- List the general analytical techniques used in substance abuse and toxicological screening and discuss their limitations

- Compare the uses of preliminary and confirmatory urine drug tests

- Discuss the considerations in interpreting a positive and negative drug screen result

- Discuss why interfering substances can cause false-negative and false-positive results of screening tests

- Recognize the uses of serum drug concentrations in the evaluation and treatment of a patient who has a suspected poisoning or overdose

- Describe how the pharmacokinetics of a drug in overdose may affect the interpretation of serum concentrations

- Discuss how toxicologic analyses may be helpful in medicolegal situations, postmortem applications, athletic competition and prescription drug abuse

When substance abuse, poisoning, or overdose is suspected, the testing of biological specimens is crucial for characterizing usage or exposure, monitoring therapy or abstinence, or aiding in diagnosis or treatment. Millions of Americans are potentially subject to these types of tests. According to the 2010 National Survey on Drug Use and Health, 22.6 million Americans aged 12 years and older (8.9% of the population) reported using an illicit drug in the past month and 38.8 million (15.3%) reported illicit drug use during the past year (Table 4-1).[1] During 2009 an estimated 4.6 million drug-related episodes were treated in emergency departments (EDs) with 49.8% due to adverse drug reactions, 45.1% from drug and substance misuse, and 2.1% from unintentional poisoning, primarily in preschool-age children.[2] Poison control centers document approximately 2.8 million unintentional and intentional poisonings each year with one-half occurring in children under 6 years of age and approximately 90% of cases occurring in homes (Table 4-2).[3]

Workplace illicit drug use has been estimated to involve 13.3 million part- and full-time workers between the ages of 18 and 65 years with another 12.3 million claiming heavy alcohol use (five or more drinks per occasion on five or more days).[1] Based on 6.4 million urine drug screens performed by a nationwide laboratory service in 2011 for the combined U.S. workforce, 3.5% had positive test results

TABLE 4-1. Americans Aged 12 Years or Older Reporting Use of Illicit Drugs During 2010[1]

PERCENTAGE OF THE TOTAL POPULATION

SUBSTANCE	PAST YEAR (%)	PAST MONTH (%)
Any illicit drug	15.3	8.9
Marijuana and hashish	11.5	6.9
Cocaine	1.8	0.6
Crack	0.3	0.1
Heroin	0.2	0.1
Hallucinogens	1.8	0.5
Lysergic acid diethylamide (LSD)	0.3	0.1
Phencyclidine (PCP)	0.0	0.0
3,4-methylenedioxy-N-methamphetamine (MDMA, Ecstasy)	1.0	0.3
Inhalants	0.8	0.3
Any illicit drug other than marijuana	8.1	3.6
Nonmedical use of any		
Psychotherapeutic drug	6.3	2.7
Pain reliever	4.8	2.0
Tranquilizer	2.2	0.9
Stimulant	1.1	0.4
Sedative	0.4	0.1

TABLE 4-2. Ranking of Twelve Most Frequent Poison Exposure Categories Reported to U.S. Poison Control Centers During 2010[a,b]

ALL EXPOSURES	CHILDREN (UNDER 6 YEARS)	ADULTS (OVER 19 YEARS)	FATALITIES
Analgesics	Cosmetics and personal care products	Analgesics	Analgesics
Cosmetics and personal care products	Analgesics	Sedative drugs	Sedative drugs
Cleaning substances	Cleaning substances	Antidepressant drugs	Cardiovascular drugs
Sedative drugs	Foreign bodies	Cleaning substances	Opioids
Foreign bodies	Topical drugs	Cardiovascular drugs	Alcohols
Topical drugs	Vitamins	Alcohols	Anticonvulsants
Antidepressant drugs	Antihistamines	Bites and envenomations	Stimulant and street drugs
Cardiovascular drugs	Pesticides	Pesticides	Antidepressant drugs
Antihistamines	Cough and cold drugs	Anticonvulsants	Muscle relaxant drugs
Pesticides	Gastrointestinal drugs	Cosmetics and personal care products	Antihistamines
Alcohols	Plants	Antihistamines	Gases and fumes
Cough and cold drugs	Antimicrobial drugs	Hormones and antagonists	Unknown drugs

[a]In decreasing order of frequency and based on 2,784,907 substances reported in 2,384,825 cases.
[b]Data from reference 3.

TABLE 4-3. Rate of Positive Urine Drug Screens for the Combined U.S. Workforce During 2011 As Reported by a Nationwide Laboratory Service for 6.4 Million Tests[4]

SUBSTANCE	PERCENTAGE OF POSITIVE URINE DRUG SCREENS[a]
Marijuana	1.60
Oxycodones	1.10
Amphetamines	0.69
Benzodiazepines	0.68
Opiates	0.36
Cocaine	0.28
Barbiturates	0.26
Methadone	0.20
Phencyclidine (PCP)	0.02
6-acetylmorphine (heroin)	0.01

[a]Some samples had multiple drugs identified.

(Table 4-3).[4] In 2010, 28.8 million persons (11.4% of Americans) reported driving under the influence of alcohol at least once during the past year with 10.6 million (4.2%) driving under the influence of illicit drugs.[1]

In 2010, 4.1 million Americans (1.6% of the population) received treatment for a problem with the use of alcohol or illicit drugs.[1] Of the 1.5 million people on parole and 5.4 million adults on probation in 2010, 27% to 30% were current illicit drug users and 37% to 38% were dependent or abusers of illicit drugs or alcohol.[1] In a 2010 study of 8,300 arrestees in 10 U.S. sites, there was a high percentage of congruence between self-reporting of drug use and positive urine drug screening (82% marijuana, 61% methamphetamine, 45% cocaine, and 37% heroin).[5]

For eighth-, tenth-, and twelfth-grade students, the lifetime prevalence of the use of illicit drugs during 2011 was 20.1%, 37.7%, and 49.9%, respectively (Table 4-4).[6] During 2009, 41,592 people died from poisoning or overdose with 99 deaths (0.2%) occurring in children under 5 years of age.[7] Poisoning became the leading cause of injury-related death in the United States in 2008 with 89% of these deaths caused by drugs. The number of drug-related poisoning deaths has increased sixfold during the past three decades.[8]

There is no comprehensive tabulation of all incidents of substance abuse or poisoning, and the available databases have strengths and weaknesses.[9,10] Nevertheless, substance abuse and poisoning are common problems facing healthcare professionals, law enforcement officials, employers, teachers, family members, and individuals throughout society. The detection and management of these incidents often involves laboratory testing and interpretation of the results. On a personal basis, healthcare professionals are asked by family members, acquaintances, and patients about drug testing and the potential impact on their lives. It is often prudent to refer the person to the testing laboratory or physician who ordered the test in question when pertinent facts are not available or when they are unable to be properly assessed. This chapter will focus on urine drug testing and serum drug concentration determinations as a means to aid in the management of substance abuse and poisoning.

URINE DRUG SCREENS

Objectives of Analysis

A *drug screen* provides a qualitative result based on the presence of a specific substance or group of substances. This determination is also called a *toxicology screen* or *tox screen*. Urine is the

TABLE 4-4. Categories of Substances Abused as Claimed by High School Seniors During 2011[6]

	PERCENTAGE OF SURVEY RESPONDENTS	
SUBSTANCE	**PAST YEAR (%)**	**EVER (%)**
Alcohol (to a drunken condition)	42.2	51.0
Any illicit drug	40.0	49.9
Marijuana and hashish	36.4	45.5
Opioids (excluding heroin)	8.7	13.0
Amphetamines	8.2	12.2
Tranquilizers	5.6	8.7
Inhalants	3.2	8.1
3,4-methylenedioxy-N-methamphetamine (MDMA, Ecstasy)	5.3	8.0
Sedatives	4.3	7.0
Cocaine	2.9	5.2
Lysergic acid diethylamide (LSD)	2.7	4.0
Phencyclidine (PCP)	1.3	2.3
Methamphetamine	1.4	2.1
Crack	1.0	1.9
Androgenic anabolic steroids	1.2	1.8
Heroin	0.8	1.4

TABLE 4-5. Federal Cutoff Concentrations for Urine Drug Tests[17,a]

DRUG	INITIAL TEST (ng/mL)	CONFIRMATORY TEST (ng/mL)
Amphetamines		
Methamphetamine	500	250[b]
Amphetamine		250
3,4-methylenedioxy-N-methamphetamine (MDMA, Ecstasy)	500	250[c]
Cocaine metabolites	150	100[d]
Marijuana metabolites	50	15[e]
Opiate metabolites		
Morphine	2000	2000
Codeine		2000
6-acetylmorphine[f]	10	10
Phencyclidine (PCP)	25	25

[a]Standards issued by Substance Abuse Mental Health Services Administration for urine specimens collected by federal agencies and by employers regulated by the Department of Transportation effective October 2010; check website for changes (http://workplace.samhsa.gov).
[b]Specimen must also contain amphetamine at a concentration of 100 ng/mL or more.
[c]Same cutoff for 3,4-methylenedioxyamphetamine (MDA) and 3,4-methylenedioxyethylamphetamine (MDEA).
[d]Metabolite as benzoylecgonine.
[e]Metabolite as delta-9-tetrahydrocannabinol-9-carboxylic acid.
[f]A metabolite specific to heroin.

specimen of choice, and it is widely used for most situations requiring a drug screen. The collection of urine is generally noninvasive and can be collected following urinary catheterization in unresponsive patients. Adequate urine samples of 20–100 mL are easily collected. Most drugs and their metabolites are excreted and concentrated in urine. They are also stable in frozen urine allowing long-term storage for batched analyses or reanalysis. Urine is a relatively clean matrix for analysis due to the usual absence of protein and cellular components, thereby eliminating preparatory steps for analysis.[11-16]

A urine drug screen result does not provide an exact determination of how much of the substance is present in the urine. The concentration of the substance is actually measured by urine drug screen assays in the process of determining whether the drug is present in a significant amount to render the test as positive. For each substance, the test has performance standards established by the intrinsic specificity and sensitivity of the analytical process that are linked to regulatory or clinical thresholds, commonly called *cutoff values*. These thresholds are a balance of the actual analytical performance, likelihood for interfering substances, and the potential for false positives, which together suggest that the substance is actually present in the urine. Cutoff values may be set by an individual laboratory to meet regulatory or clinical needs or by purchasing immunoassay kits with the desired cutoff values.

Regulatory cutoff values are typically used to monitor people in the workplace or patients undergoing substance abuse therapy. The Substance Abuse and Mental Health Services Administration (SAMHSA) in the Department of Health and Human Services specifies cutoff values and requires that five categories be routinely included in urine screens (Table 4-5).[17] In hospital and forensic settings, cutoff values are sometimes lowered relative to workplace values in order to detect more positive results, which can serve as an aid in verifying or detecting an overdose or poisoning.[13-15,18] Reports of urine drug screen results will often list the cutoff value for a substance and whether the substance was detected at the specified value.

General Analytical Techniques

There is no standardized urine drug screen that employs the same panel of tested drugs, analytical techniques, or turnaround times. Although there is some commonality among laboratories, tests differ by individual laboratory. Generally, urine drug screens are categorized by level of sensitivity of the analytical technique (preliminary versus confirmatory) and by the variety of drugs tested.[12,15,18] *Preliminary tests,* also known as *initial, provisional,* or *stat urine drug screens,* typically employ one of six currently available immunoassays (EMIT, KIMS, CEDIA, RIA, FPIA, or ELISA). (See Chapter 2: Introduction to Common Laboratory Assays and Technology.)

Immunoassays can readily be performed on autoanalyzers that are available in most hospitals. These assays are available for many substances of abuse, and results can be reported within 1–2 hours.[14,18] Many point-of-care tests (POCTs) also

MINICASE 1

Reliability of Amphetamine Results

KISHA T., A 21-YEAR-OLD COLLEGE STUDENT, is brought to the ED by her family because of bizarre behavior. She is having visual hallucinations and is paranoid and jittery. She is clinically dehydrated, tachycardic, and delirious. A stat preliminary urine drug screen is positive for amphetamines.

Question: Is Kisha T. abusing amphetamine?

Discussion: Amphetamine abuse is possible, but alternative causes should be considered. Her parents report that she has just completed a week of final exams, is taking a full course load, and is working two part-time jobs. She is described as studious and a compulsive achiever. After 6 hours of supportive therapy, rest, and IV fluids, she is lucid and confesses to drinking more than a dozen "energy drinks" to stay awake in the past 2 days and taking two loratadine and pseudoephedrine combination 12-hour tablets 6 hours ago for allergy symptoms. A targeted confirmatory assay for amphetamines was negative for amphetamines and methamphetamine. Urine drug screens by immunoassay for amphetamines are subject to cross-reactivity with several sympathomimetic amine-type drugs (e.g., ephedrine and pseudoephedrine and their vari-ants are often found in dietary supplements marketed for energy and weight loss and as decongestants), which would cause a false positive for amphetamines by immunoassay. Caffeine found in many energy drinks and dietary supplements for weight loss and energy is likely the principal cause of her symptoms. Caffeine was not detected in the urine screen because it was not on the testing panel of screened drugs.

The inclusion of a substance on a drug screen is also subject to individual laboratory discretion. Workplace and substance abuse monitoring programs are required to test for five categories of substances (marijuana metabolites, cocaine metabolites, opiate metabolites, PCP, and amphetamines) as specified by the "SAMHSA 5." Most immunoassay manufacturers design the range of assays to meet this need and offer additional categories that a laboratory may choose to include.[11,13] The expense of developing an immunoassay is balanced with the promise of economic recovery with widespread utilization. This economic reality precludes the development of a test for emerging substances of abuse, such as ketamine and gamma hydroxybutyrate, and life-threatening—albeit infrequent—overdoses, such as calcium channel antagonists and beta-adrenergic blockers.[18] Techniques used for confirmatory tests would be required to detect many of the substances not included in the panel of the preliminary drug screen.

use an immunoassay technique, and results can be available within 5–15 minutes. Unfortunately, the result of an immunoassay is preliminary due to compromises in specificity that lead to cross-reactivity, particularly with amphetamines and opiates. A preliminary urine drug screen result cannot stand alone for medicolegal purposes and must be confirmed with another type of analysis that is more specific.[11-13] For clinical purposes, some laboratories routinely confirm the results of preliminary drug screens, but others do so only on request of the physician. The need for confirming preliminary test results is based on several factors: whether the result would affect the patient's care; whether the patient is expected to be discharged by the time the results are known; whether any legal actions are anticipated; and whether the cost justifies the possible outcome.

Confirmatory techniques are more specific than preliminary tests and utilize another analytical technique.[12,15,18] These tests include high-performance liquid chromatography, gas chromatography, or mass spectrometry, depending on the substances being confirmed. The "gold standard" of confirmatory tests is the combination of *gas chromatography* and *mass spectrometry*, often referred to as *GC mass spec* or *GC-MS*. Compared to preliminary tests, these techniques are more time-consuming, more costly, require greater technical expertise, and require greater time for analysis—often several hours to days. Most hospital clinical laboratories do not have the capability to perform confirmatory tests and must send the specimen to a local reference laboratory or a regional laboratory. Transportation of the specimen will add to the delay in obtaining results. Confirmatory tests are routinely performed for workplace settings and forensic and medicolegal purposes, and the delay is often less critical than in clinical settings.[11,13] (See Minicase 1.)

Common Applications

The purpose of a urine drug screen depends on the circumstances for its use, the condition of the patient, and the setting of the test. In an ED where a patient is being evaluated for a poisoning or overdose, the primary purposes are to verify substances claimed to be taken by the patient and to identify other toxins that could be likely causes of the poisoning or symptoms.[14] This is particularly important when the patient has altered mental status and cannot give a clear history or is experiencing nondrug causes of coma, such as traumatic head injury or stroke. The value of routinely performing urine drug screens in the ED for patients who overdose has been questioned.[19] The benefits include having objective evidence of the toxin's presence to confirm the exposure; suggesting alternative toxins in the diagnosis; ruling out a toxin as a cause of symptoms of unknown etiology; and providing medicolegal documentation. The disadvantages include being misled by false-positive results; impractical delays in receiving the results that do not influence therapy; and limited practical value because many poisonings can be recognized by a collection of signs and symptoms.[20]

The American College of Emergency Physicians states in a clinical policy on the immediate treatment of poisonings that "qualitative toxicologic screening tests rarely assist the emergency physician in patient management."[21] Urine drug testing can be important with substances exhibiting delayed onset of toxic symptoms, such as sustained-release products, when patients ingest multiple agents, or when patients are found with multiple agents at the scene. Some trauma centers routinely perform urine drug screens on newly admitted patients, although the value of this practice has been questioned.[22]

MINICASE 2

Drug Screens and Emergent Care

BOB C., A 26-YEAR-OLD MALE, is dropped off at an ED in the late evening after he became progressively more unresponsive in a hotel room. His acquaintances do not know his medical history, but eventually admit that he had swallowed some drugs. They promptly leave the area. Bob C. is unconscious with some response to painful stimuli and exhibits pinpoint pupils and depressed respirations at 12 breaths/min. His other vital signs are satisfactory. Oxygen administration and intravenous fluids are started. A bedside stat glucose determination yields a result of 60 mg/dL. A 50-mL intravenous bolus of dextrose 50% is administered with no change in his level of consciousness. Naloxone 0.8 mg is given IV push, and within minutes Bob C. awakens, begins talking, and exhibits an improved respiratory rate. He admits to drinking some whiskey and taking a handful of several combination tablets of hydrocodone and acetaminophen shortly before he was dropped off at the ED. In addition to routine laboratory assessment, a serum acetaminophen concentration is determined. During the next 24 hours, he receives supportive care in the critical care unit and requires two additional doses of naloxone. He is scheduled for a psychiatric evaluation to assess treatment options for his substance abuse, but he walks out of the hospital against medical advice on the second day. A urine drug screen by immunoassay that was obtained in the ED is reported as positive for opiates and marijuana on the morning of his second day of hospitalization. The serum acetaminophen concentration reported 2 hours after ED arrival was 60 mcg/mL, which was obtained approximately 6 hours after drug ingestion. Ethanol was not included in the drug screen panel.

Question: Was a urine drug screen necessary for the immediate care of Bob C.? How is a urine drug screen helpful in this type of situation?

Discussion: In emergent situations like this one that involve an apparent acute opiate overdose, the results of a urine drug screen are not necessary for immediate evaluation and effective treatment. The symptoms and history clearly indicate that an opiate overdose is very likely. The response to naloxone confirms that an opiate is responsible for the central nervous system (CNS) depressant effects. Since immediate treatment was necessary, waiting for the results of the preliminary drug screen, even if it was reported within hours, would not change the use of supportive care, glucose, and naloxone. The urine drug screen may be helpful to confirm the diagnosis for the record and to assist in guiding substance abuse treatment. Obtaining a serum acetaminophen concentration is important in cases of intentional drug use (suicide attempt and substance abuse). This practice is particularly important in situations of a multiple drug exposure, an unknown drug exposure, or when acetaminophen may be contained in a multiple-ingredient oral drug product (e.g., analgesics, cough and cold medicines, sleep aids, and nonprescription allergy medicines). A serum specimen is needed because acetaminophen is not part of routine urine drug screens, and serum assays on acetaminophen generally have a quick turnaround time so they can be used clinically to assess the potential severity of the exposure. In Bob C.'s case, the serum acetaminophen concentration did not indicate a risk for hepatotoxicity. Another benefit of obtaining a serum acetaminophen concentration in this case is that it indirectly confirms that an opioid combination product was involved and is consistent with the Bob C.'s response to naloxone.

Suicidal and substance-abusing patients are poor or misleading historians, whereby the amounts, number of substances, and routes of exposure can be exaggerated or downplayed. A urine drug screen may assist in identifying potential substances involved in these cases and lead to specific monitoring or treatment. (See Minicase 2.)

In the workplace, the purpose of a urine drug screen may include pre-employment tests, monitoring during work, post-accident evaluation, and substance abuse treatment monitoring.[11,13] Employers who conduct pre-employment urine drug tests will generally make hiring contingent on a negative test result. Many positions in the healthcare industry require pre-employment drug tests, and some employers perform random tests for employees in positions requiring safety or security as a means to deter drug use and abuse that could affect performance. In addition to random tests, some employers test individuals based on a reasonable suspicion of substance abuse such as evidence of use or possession, unusual or erratic behavior, or arrests for drug-related crimes. For employees involved in a serious accident, employers may test for substances when there is suspicion of use—to determine whether substance abuse was a factor—or as a necessity for legal or insurance purposes. Employees who return to work following treatment for substance abuse are often randomly tested as one of their conditions for continued employment or licensure. In the workplace setting, specific procedures must be followed to ensure that the rights of employees and employers are observed.

The Division of Workplace Programs of SAMHSA specifies guidelines for procedures, due process and the appeals process, and lists certified laboratories.[11] Two critical elements of workplace drug testing include establishing a chain-of-custody and control for the specimen and involving a medical review officer (MRO) to interpret positive test results. The chain-of-custody starts with close observation of urine collection. Patients are required to empty their pockets, and they are placed in a collection room without running water and where blue dye has been added to the toilet water. These measures minimize the risk of adulteration or dilution of the urine sample. After the urine is placed in the container, the temperature is taken, the container is sealed, and the chain-of-custody documentation is completed. After the chain-of-custody form is completed by everyone in possession of the specimen, it reaches the laboratory where the seal is broken and further procedures are observed. Positive specimens are often frozen for 1 year or longer if requested by the client or if the results are contested by a court. Chain-of-custody procedures are time-consuming and are not typically considered in the clinical management of poisonings and overdoses, but they are important to sustain the validity of the sample and its result in a court of law.[11]

An MRO is typically a physician trained in this specialty who has responsibility to determine whether the result of the drug test is related to substance abuse.[11,13,23] Duties involve interviewing the donor; reviewing their therapeutic drug regimen; reviewing possible extraneous causes of a positive result, such as a false-positive result from a prescribed medication or substance interfering with the analytical test; rendering an opinion on the validity of the test result; considering a retest of the donor or the same specimen; reporting the result to the employer; and maintaining confidential records. This individualized interpretation is not only critical because people's careers, reputations, livelihood, and legal status can be affected, but also because it is a regulatory requirement.

Drug screening is also used in the criminal justice system for several purposes such as informing judges for bail-setting and sentencing, monitoring whether specified drug abstinence is being observed, and identifying individuals in need of treatment.[5] For example, a positive drug test at the time of arrest may identify substance abusers who need medical treatment prior to incarceration, which may result in a pretrial release condition that incorporates periodic drug testing. If a defendant is being monitored while on parole or work release, a drug screen can verify that he or she is remaining drug-free. Drug tests in prisons can also assist in monitoring substance use in jail.

The impact of a drug screen result can be profound if it affects decisions of medical care, employment, legal importance, and a person's reputation. In addition, several factors can affect the reliability and interpretation of drug screen results. These issues should be considered when evaluating a drug screen and are described in the following section.

Unique Considerations

When a urine drug screen is reported as negative, it does not mean that the drug was not present or not taken—it means that it was not detected. The drug in question may not be part of a testing panel of the particular drug screen (Table 4-6). For example, meperidine and pentazocine are not detected on current opioid immunoassays.[13,14,18] Likewise, the urine may be too dilute for detection of the substance. This may be due to renal disease, intentional dilution to avoid detection, or administration of large volumes of intravenous fluids as part of a critically ill patient's care. The urine may have been collected before the drug was excreted, but this is unlikely in symptomatic acute overdoses or poisonings. The time that an individual tests positive (i.e., the drug detection time) depends on pharmacologic factors including dose, route of administration, rates of metabolism and elimination, and analytical factors (e.g., sensitivity, specificity, and accuracy). In some cases, the urine sample may have been intentionally adulterated to mask or avoid detection.

Adulteration of a urine sample either intentionally or unintentionally can lead to negative or false-positive results through several means.[11,13,24] A freshly voided urine sample may be replaced with a drug-free sample when urine collection is not directly observed. The ingestion of large volumes of water with or without a diuretic may dilute a drug in the urine, thereby reducing the concentration of the urine below the assay

TABLE 4-6. Drugs and Chemicals Often Not Detected by Routine Drug Screens

Androgenic anabolic steroids
Angiotensin converting enzyme inhibitors
Animal venoms
Antidysrhythmic drugs
Anticoagulant drugs and rodenticides
Beta-adrenergic agonists
Beta-adrenergic antagonists
Calcium channel antagonists
Carbon monoxide
Chem-bioterrorism agents
Clonidine
Colchicine
Dietary supplements[a]
Ergot alkaloids
Ethylene glycol
Gamma-hydroxybutyrate
Heavy metals (lead, arsenic, and mercury)[b]
Hydrocarbon solvents and inhalants
Iron
Lithium
Methemoglobin producing agents
Methylphenidate
Pesticides
Plant toxins
Selective serotonin reuptake inhibitors

[a]Those without chemically similar drug counterparts are not detected on a drug screen.
[b]Heavy metals will require a special collection container, collection duration, and assay.

detection limit. Urine specimens for workplace testing will often be immediately tested for temperature and later tested for creatinine content and specific gravity in order to detect water dilution of the sample.

Adding a chemical to a urine sample may invalidate some test results. Adulteration products that are available through the Internet contain chemicals such as soaps, glutaraldehyde, nitrites, other oxidants, and hydrochloric acid. Depending on the assay method and test, these substances may interfere with absorbance rates or enzyme activity, produce false-positive or false-negative results, or oxidize metabolites that are measured in the immunoassay. For example, some chromate- and peroxidase-based oxidizers will degrade 9-carboxy-tetrahydrocannabinol, a principal metabolite of tetrahydrocannabinol, and lead to a negative result for marijuana.[13,24] Taking large amounts of sustained-release niacin (2.5–5.5 g over 36–48 hours) has been promoted on the Internet as a means to rid the body of cocaine and marijuana and interfere with urine drug screens. This practice is unlikely to produce the desired outcome, but

TABLE 4-7. Detection Times and Interfering Substances for Immunoassay Urine Drug Screens[a,b,c]

DRUG	DETECTION TIME	POTENTIAL FALSE-POSITIVE AGENTS AND COMMENTS
Amphetamines	2–5 days; up to 2 weeks with prolonged or heavy use	Ephedrine, pseudoephedrine, ephedra (ma huang), phenylephrine, selegiline, chlorpromazine, promethazine, trazodone, bupropion, desipramine, trimipramine, ritodrine, amantadine, ranitidine, phenylpropanolamine, brompheniramine, 3,4-methylenedioxy-N-methamphetamine (MDMA, Ecstacy), isometheptene, labetalol, phentermine, methylphenidate, isoxsuprine, trimethobenzamide
Barbiturates	Short-acting, 1–7 days; intermediate-acting, 1–3 weeks	Ibuprofen, naproxen; phenobarbital may be detected up to 4 weeks
Benzodiazepines	Up to 2 weeks; up to 6 weeks with chronic use of some agents	Oxaprozin, sertraline; benzodiazepines vary in cross-reactivity, persistence, and detectability; flunitrazepam may not be detected
Cocaine metabolite (benzoylecgonine)	12–72 hr; up to 1–3 weeks with prolonged or heavy use	Cross-reactivity with cocaethylene varies with the assay because assay is directed to benzoylecgonine; false positives from -caine anesthetics and other drugs are unlikely
Lysergic acid diethylamide (LSD)	1–2 days typically; up to 5 days possible	
Marijuana metabolite (delta 9-tetrahydrocannabinol-9-carboxylic acid)	7–10 days; 1 month or more with prolonged or heavy use	Ibuprofen, naproxen, tolmetin, efavirenz, pantoprazole; patients taking dronabinol will also have positive test results
Methadone	3–14 days	Diphenhydramine, doxylamine, clomipramine, chlorpromazine, thioridazine, quetiapine, verapamil
Opioids	2–3 days typically; up to 6 days with sustained-release formulations; up to 1 week with prolonged or heavy use	Rifampin, some fluoroquinolones, poppy seeds, quinine in tonic water; the assay is directed toward morphine with varying cross-reactivity for codeine, oxycodone, hydrocodone, and other semisynthetic opioids; synthetic opioids (e.g., fentanyl, meperidine, methadone, pentazocine, propoxyphene, and tramadol) have minimal cross-reactivity and may not be detected
Phencyclidine (PCP)	2–10 days; 1 month or more with prolonged or heavy use	Ketamine, dextromethorphan, diphenhydramine, imipramine, mesoridazine, thioridazine, venlafaxine, ibuprofen, meperidine, tramadol

[a]Time after which a drug screen remains positive after last use.
[b]Since performance characteristics may vary with the type of immunoassay, manufacturer, and lot, consult the laboratory technician and package insert for the particular test.
[c]Data from references 12, 16, 26, and 27.

it has produced niacin poisonings ranging from skin flushing to life-threatening symptoms that required hospitalization.[25] The effects of adulterants vary with the immunoassay technique and the specific test used by the laboratory; they are not reliable ways to mask drug use. Most adulterants do not affect the GC-MS analysis for drugs in urine, but such a confirmatory step would be ordered only if there was a high suspicion of adulteration. A positive immunoassay result is typically used to justify the use of a confirmatory GC-MS analysis.

A positive drug test can show the presence of specific drugs in urine at the detectable level of the test. It does not indicate the dosage, when the drug was administered, how it was administered, or the degree of impairment. Many drugs can be detected in urine for up to 3 days after being taken and some up to 2 weeks or more (Table 4-7).[12,14,26] It is possible for a legitimate substance in the urine to interact with the immunoassay and produce a false-positive result.[13,14,27,28]

Exposure to interfering substances can affect the results of an immunoassay urine drug screen (Table 4-7). A positive immunoassay result for opiates may result from the ingestion of

pastries containing poppy seeds because they contain codeine and morphine in small, but sufficient, amounts to render the test positive. The result is a true positive but not a positive indicator of drug abuse. The immunoassay for amphetamines is prone to false-positive results from drugs with similar structures such as ephedrine, pseudoephedrine, and buproprion.[13,14,27] Also, drugs seemingly dissimilar from the target of an immunoassay can cause false-positive results. For example, naproxen can produce false-positive results for marijuana and barbiturates and was found to do so in 1 in 14 volunteers tested.[29] Most fluoroquinolone antibiotics can produce false-positive opiate results, but this interference varies with the fluoroquinolone and immunoassay.[30] The immunoassay manufacturer's package insert should be consulted for information on known interfering substances. In workplace settings, the MRO is obligated to assess whether a person's legitimate drug therapy could interfere with the result. (See Minicase 3.)

The persistence of the substance in the urine is an important factor in the interpretation of the results (see Table 4-7).[23] For lab results reported as negative, it may indicate that the

MINICASE 3

Workplace Drug Screen Interpretations

JUAN G., A 45-YEAR-OLD PHARMACIST, applies for a position at a hospital pharmacy. As part of his pre-employment evaluation, he is asked to provide a urine specimen in a specially designed room for drug testing. His urine sample is positive for opiates and marijuana by immunoassay. His case is referred to the hospital's MRO for a review of the findings. The physician orders a confirmatory test on the same urine specimen. The human resources department of the hospital learns from his current employer that he is an above average worker with no history of substance abuse. A criminal background check is negative for any criminal record. The MRO contacts Juan G. and learns that he was taking acetaminophen and codeine prescribed for pain from suturing of a laceration of his hand for 2 days prior to drug testing. He also routinely takes naproxen for arthritis in his knees. He had forgotten to list the recent use of these drugs on his employment application because his injured hand began to ache while writing.

Question: Has Juan G. used any drugs or substances that should prevent him from being considered for employment?

Discussion: Consideration of several factors is important in interpreting the urine drug screen result in this case. Juan G. has no obvious symptoms of intoxication and has a good employment record. It is likely that the codeine prescribed for pain control produced the positive opiate result. This drug is being used for a legitimate purpose with a valid prescription. The positive test for marijuana is likely from Juan G.'s use of naproxen causing a false-positive result. The confirmatory test by GC-MS was negative for marijuana, but it was positive for codeine and morphine. Codeine is metabolized in part to morphine. The MRO reviewing Juan G.'s case would likely conclude that the test results are not indicative of opioid abuse and the marijuana immunoassay result was a false positive. If there were concerns about his suitability for employment, Juan G. may be subjected to an unannounced drug test during his probationary employment period. Acetaminophen and naproxen were not reported as a result, because they were not on the routine assay panel.

specimen was obtained too early or too late after exposure to a chemical, thereby producing a urine specimen with insufficient concentration of the drug to lead to a positive result. Drugs with short half-lives, such as amphetamines, may not be detectable several hours after use. A common concern for individuals undergoing workplace testing is the length of time after use that the drug will still be detectable. This will vary with the sensitivity of the assay; whether the assay is directed to the parent drug or the metabolite; whether the drug or its metabolites exhibits extensive distribution to tissues that will affect its half-life; the dose of the drug taken; and whether the drug was used chronically or only once. For example, cocaine is rarely detected in a urine specimen because of its rapid metabolism. Immunoassays are directed to cocaine metabolites, such as benzoylecgonine, which are detected for up to 2–3 days after use and up to 8 days with heavy use. The major active component of marijuana, delta-9-tetrahydrocannabinol, is converted to several metabolites of which delta-9-tetrahydrocannabinol-9-carboxylic acid is the agent to which antibodies are directed in many immunoassays. This metabolite is distributed to tissues and can be detected for days to weeks after use.[13,14] Chronic or heavy use can lead to detection up to a month or more after stopping use. (See Minicase 4.)

For clinical applications, the time it takes for the test result to be reported to the clinician after specimen collection, also known as *turnaround time*, can affect the utility of the drug screen.[18] Many hospital laboratories can perform preliminary immunoassay urine drug screens using mechanized analytical technology, which is used for common clinical tests or using dedicated desktop analyzers. Results from in-hospital laboratories can often be returned within 2 hours of collection. For many urgent situations such as an acute overdose or poisoning, this delay is unlikely to influence the immediate therapy of the victim. The results may lead to later consideration of alternative or additional diagnoses. Most clinics, small hospitals, or specimen collection sites do not possess such capability and must rely on making the specimen a *send out* that is performed at a nearby or regional reference laboratory. The turnaround time from a reference laboratory varies with the laboratory and the need for urgency. Most results for clinical applications are reported within 24–48 hours. However, some results may take up to 3–7 days. In some situations, such as pre-employment workplace testing, this delay is acceptable. The turnaround time for confirmatory testing depends on the laboratory, transportation time from the collection site to the laboratory, the tests being performed or requested, and the need for urgency. The delay could be as short as 24 hours or as long as a month or more, particularly for postmortem samples. (See Minicase 5.)

SERUM CONCENTRATIONS

Objectives of Analysis

Quantitative assays determine the concentration of a substance in a biological specimen, typically this involves serum. The availability of serum concentrations for toxins is based on considerations of whether the concentration correlates with an effect; the outcome or need for therapy; the existing use of the assay for another application such as therapeutic drug monitoring; and technical ease of performing the assay. Serum is typically not used for drug screening purposes in clinical or workplace settings.

Many poisonings and overdoses can be adequately managed without quantitative analysis.[10,13] A history of the exposure, signs and symptoms, and routinely available clinical tests—such as full blood count, electrolytes, glucose, international normalized ratio (INR), liver function tests, blood urea nitrogen, serum creatinine, anion gap, serum osmolality and osmolal gap, arterial blood gases, and creatinine kinase—can guide patient management decisions.

MINICASE 4

Differences Involving Opioids

DANNY W., A 23-YEAR-OLD ASSEMBLY LINE WORKER at a computer manufacturing facility, is examined by the company's physician within an hour of being involved in a workplace accident. She observes a laceration on his left arm, pupil size of 1–2 mm, bilateral ptosis, and recent punctate lesions on the left antecubital fossa. The rest of the physical exam is unremarkable. Danny W. denies eating poppy seeds, taking any medication or dietary supplement, or having a neurological condition. He has no history of substance abuse in his files. The physician suspects heroin use and orders a focused urine drug test for opiates. Several days later, the laboratory report indicates positive results for morphine, codeine, and 6-acetylmorphine.

Question: Has Danny W. used a drug or substance that would impair his ability to work? What, if any, substance is likely?

Discussion: Danny W. has likely used heroin several hours before the accident and several symptoms are consistent with opiate intoxication. Heroin may not be present in sufficient amounts to be detected, in part, because it is metabolized to several compounds such as morphine and 6-acetylmorphine, which can be detected in the urine of heroin users. Since 6-acetylmorphine is only found in urine following heroin use, its presence confirms heroin but other opioids could also contribute to Danny W.'s symptoms. The presence of small amounts of codeine in heroin abusers is likely from contamination of the heroin with codeine and is not a metabolic byproduct (or he had consumed codeine).

MINICASE 5

Interpreting Cocaine Results

SHELLY N., A 56-YEAR-OLD SUPERVISOR for a large utility company, had recently conducted an inspection at a nuclear power plant. She then left for a 2-week vacation with a friend. After returning to work, she is asked to submit a urine sample for drug testing because the company performs random drug tests for compliance with regulatory, insurance, and contractual requirements. A week later, the results of the immunoassay are reported as positive for the cocaine metabolite, benzoylecognine. A confirmatory test by GC-MS confirms the immunoassay result. Shelly N. is asked to report to the company's medical office. During the interview with the physician, she denies illicit drug use but states that she had dental work performed immediately before returning to work from her vacation and that she had received procaine hydrochloride (Novocain) for local anesthesia.

Question: What caused the positive test result for cocaine?

Discussion: Shelly N. apparently believed that any substance with a name ending in -caine must share chemical similarity with cocaine and could be a probable cause of a false-positive result. While interference with immunoassays is possible, a false positive for cocaine with local anesthetics is not likely unless the anesthetic preparation contains cocaine. The positive result was confirmed by a confirmatory test that is not subject to this type of interference. In Shelly N.'s case, use of cocaine is the most likely explanation for the positive result.

Serum concentrations of potential toxins can be complementary to clinical tests or become essential in several situations (Table 4-8).[18,32] A serum concentration can confirm the diagnosis of a poisoning when in doubt or when a quantitative assessment in the serum is important to interpret a qualitative urine drug screen. When there is a relationship between serum concentration and toxicity, a serum concentration can assist in patient evaluation or for medicolegal purposes. When sustained-release drug formulations have been ingested, serial serum concentrations can indicate when peak serum concentrations have occurred and whether efforts to decontaminate the gastrointestinal tract with activated charcoal or whole bowel irrigation have been achieved. A serum concentration can also be useful in determining when to reinitiate drug therapy after the drug has caused toxicity. For some agents, serum concentrations can guide the decision to use therapies that are often risky, invasive, or expensive such as antidotes (e.g., acetylcysteine, digoxin immune antibody, and fomepizole) or special treatments (e.g., hemodialysis and hyperbaric oxygen).

General Analytical Techniques

There is no standardized panel of quantitative serum assays for toxicologic use. Tests differ by individual laboratory, but a set of essential tests has been proposed (Table 4-8).[18,32] Generally, serum concentrations utilize existing technologies (e.g., immunoassay, spectrophotometry, gas chromatography,

high-performance liquid chromatography, and atomic absorption spectrometry) that are commonly used for therapeutic drug monitoring (see Chapter 2: Introduction to Common Laboratory Assays and Technology). Assays for carboxyhemoglobin, methemoglobinemia, and serum cholinesterase activity are available in many hospitals.[18] In most toxicological applications, the specimen is usually 5–10 mL of blood in adults (1–5 mL in children depending on the assay) that has been allowed to clot for several minutes. It is then centrifuged and the clear serum, which is devoid of red blood cells and coagulants, is aspirated and subjected to analysis or frozen for later analysis. The type of test tube, test tube additive, and quantity of blood necessary should be verified with the laboratory prior to blood collection.

Common Applications

Serum concentrations of several drugs and chemicals can be helpful in the assessment of patients who may be poisoned or overdosed and arrive at a hospital for evaluation and treatment. Although general treatment approaches—such as supportive care, resuscitation, symptomatic care, and decontamination—are performed without the need of serum concentrations, the severity of several toxicities are related to serum concentrations (Table 4-8). A more detailed discussion of the toxicity relationships can be found in toxicology references.[10,32] The examples of ethanol, salicylates, acetaminophen, and digoxin demonstrate

TABLE 4-8. Toxicologically Important Serum Concentrations for Selected Agents[a]

ASSAY	INDICATION	TIMING OF SAMPLE	REPEAT SAMPLING	EXPOSURE
Acetaminophen	Suspected acetaminophen overdose; every intentional overdose where acetaminophen poisoning has not been reliably excluded	At least 4 hr after ingestion	Rarely required unless timing of overdose is uncertain or for sustained-release formulations	Refer to nomogram to assess toxicity and need for acetylcysteine; toxic concentrations depend on patient's individual risk factors
Carboxyhemoglobin	Suspected carbon monoxide poisoning or smoke inhalation	Immediate	No	Greater than 20% to 25% indicates significant exposure, but there is a poor relationship with severity and outcome
Digoxin	Severe digoxin toxicity and prior to use of digoxin antibodies	Immediate	No	Greater than 2.0 ng/L associated with toxicity but may be lower with patient risk factors
Ethanol	Undiagnosed coma with widened osmolal gap; prior to anesthesia when ethanol abuse is suspected; assessment for hemodialysis with severe intoxication; monitor ethanol therapy when used as an antidote	Immediate	Every 2–4 hr monitoring when used as an antidote; repeat following hemodialysis; used as treatment for methanol or ethylene glycol poisoning	Target of 100–150 mg/dL when used as an antidote for ethylene glycol or methanol poisoning; greater than 180–200 mg/dL associated with systemic ethanol toxicity in the absence of other agents and in patients without tolerance to ethanol
Iron	Ingestion of greater than 40 mg/kg elemental iron and obtained within 6 hr; symptoms suggesting acute iron toxicity at any time after poisoning	At least 4 hr after overdose	No	Greater than 450–500 mcg/dL may be associated with systemic toxicity; greater than 500 mcg/dL usually treated with deferoxamine
Lithium	Suspected acute or chronic lithium poisoning	Immediate for suspected chronic or acute-on-chronic poisoning, or for patients with symptoms suggesting lithium intoxication; after 6 hr for asymptomatic acute overdose	Every 6–12 hr in severe poisoning or following use of a sustained-release formulation until concentrations are decreasing after hemodialysis when used as treatment for lithium toxicity	Usual therapeutic range 0.6–1.2 mEq/L (mmol/L); varies with the laboratory and patient factors; acute ingestions may achieve high concentrations that may not lead to serious toxicity
Methemoglobin	Exposure to relevant toxins or sources (e.g., well water) that produce methemoglobinemia	Immediate	Worsening symptoms	Values greater than 20% are associated with hypoxic symptoms, but there is poor correlation with clinical severity
Salicylate	Salicylate overdose (acute aspirin dose over 150 mg/kg); ingestion of concentrated methyl salicylate; unidentified poisoning with clinical features suggesting salicylate toxicity (e.g., altered mental status with acid–base disorder)	At least 2 hr if symptomatic; at least 4 hr if asymptomatic	Repeat in 2–4 hr in patients with suspected severe toxicity or if enteric-coated aspirin; measurements should be repeated until concentrations are falling	Systemic toxicity usually associated with concentrations greater than 30 mg/dL; severe toxicity usually associated with concentrations greater than 90–100 mg/dL following acute overdose

[a]These concentrations are given for general guidance only. Drug/toxin concentrations may not correlate closely with the severity of poisoning in individual patients and values may vary between laboratories.

Source: Reprinted, with permission, from reference 32 with adaptations from reference 31.

important principles in the application of serum concentrations to toxicity and therapy.

One of the most widely studied and used toxicologic tests involves blood, serum, or breath ethanol concentrations. Due to the absence of protein binding and small volume of ethanol distribution, the serum concentration generally correlates with many of the acute toxic effects of ethanol as shown in Table 4-9.[33] Regular ethanol use can lead to tolerance, and ethanol concentrations in excess of 0.4% (400 mg/dL) can easily be tolerated by some patients (e.g., they can converse and exhibit stable vital signs).[34,35] Conversely, uninitiated drinkers, such as small children who ingest household products containing ethanol (e.g., cologne and mouthwash) and those who concurrently ingest other CNS depressants, may have an exaggerated effect. Most acute poisonings can be managed with supportive and symptomatic care; an unstable patient with exceedingly high ethanol concentrations may be the rare candidate for hemodialysis.[31]

Ethanol concentrations also have medicolegal applications involving driving or work performance and ethanol intake. In 2005, the minimum legal threshold for driving under the influence of ethanol intoxication was set by all states of the United States at blood ethanol concentrations of 0.08% (equivalent to 0.08 g/dL or 80 mg/dL).[34] This value can be determined at the scene or at bedside by a breath alcohol test.[36] The breath alcohol test is based on the assumption that equilibrium exists between ethanol in the blood supply of the lung and the alveolar air at a relatively uniform partition ratio. A number of variables can affect this relationship such as temperature, hematocrit, and sampling technique. The National Highway Traffic and Safety Administration publishes a list of breath alcohol testing devices that conform to their standards (www.nhtsa.gov).

Since ethanol concentrations are reported in several different units for either serum or blood, verification of the unit of measure is important.[18,37] Further, many hospital-based laboratories perform ethanol determinations on serum and use the units of mg/dL versus forensic situations that typically use blood and report the value as %, g%, or g/dL (all of which are equivalent expressions except mg/dL). Serum concentrations of ethanol are greater than blood concentrations by a median factor of 1.2, which varies with the hematocrit value because of the greater water content of serum compared to whole blood.[14,18] Although legal standards are written in terms of whole blood concentrations, this difference is without clinical significance.

Ethanol is also used as a drug to treat poisonings by methanol (blindness, acidosis, and death) and ethylene glycol (acidosis, renal failure, and death). In order to achieve a consistent concentration near 100 mg/dL, serial serum ethanol concentrations are obtained to ensure that sufficient quantities have been administered to prevent severe toxicities of methanol and ethylene glycol (during therapy, hemodialysis removes ethanol while also removing methanol and ethylene glycol).[31]

An early attempt to correlate serum drug concentrations with acute toxicity over time involved the Done nomogram for salicylate poisoning.[38] Categories of toxicity (mild, moderate, and severe) were demarcated on a semilogarithmic plot of serum salicylate versus time after ingestion as an aid to interpreting serum concentrations. Given the limited knowledge available at the time, the nomogram was based on several assumptions (zero-order kinetics and back extrapolation of single concentrations to time zero) that were later proven to be false. The nomogram did not guide therapy to any great extent and was not confirmed to be clinically useful in subsequent studies.[39]

Clinical findings such as vital signs, electrolytes, anion gap, and arterial blood gases, which have quick turnaround times in most hospitals, are more direct indicators of salicylate toxicity and are now preferred to the Done nomogram. A patient, with exceedingly high serum salicylate concentrations (in excess of 100–120 mg/dL) who is unresponsive to supportive and symptomatic therapy, may benefit from hemodialysis to remove salicylate from the body. Elderly and very young patients with unexplained changes in consciousness, acid–base balance, and respiratory rate who present to an ED could be suffering from unrecognized acute or chronic salicylate poisoning.[40,41] A routine serum salicylate concentration in such patients could determine the contribution of excessive salicylate to their symptoms.

Serum acetaminophen concentrations following acute overdoses are essential in assessing the potential severity of poisoning and determining the need for antidotal therapy with acetylcysteine. Acetaminophen toxicity differs from many other poisonings in that there is delay of significant symptoms by 1–3 days after ingestion, whereas most other poisonings have definite symptoms within 6 hours of exposure.[10,31] This delay in onset makes it difficult to use signs, symptoms, and

TABLE 4-9. Relationship of Blood Ethanol Concentration and Toxic Effects[33]

BLOOD ETHANOL CONCENTRATION	TOXIC EFFECT OR CONSEQUENCE
0.08% (80 mg/dL)	Legal definition for driving impairment
0.15% (150 mg/dL)	Euphoria, loss of critical judgment, slurred speech, incoordination, drowsiness
0.2% (200 mg/dL)	Increased incoordination, staggering gait, slurred speech, lethargy, disorientation, visual disturbances (diplopia, reduced acuity and perception)
0.3% (300 mg/dL)	Loss of motor functions, marked decreased response to stimuli, impaired consciousness, marked incoordination and inability to stand or walk, vomiting and incontinence, possible amnesia of the event
0.4% (400 mg/dL) and higher	Comatose, unresponsive to physical stimuli, absent reflexes, unstable vital signs, shallow and decreased respirations, hypotension, hypothermia, potentially lethal

clinical diagnostic tests (such as serum transaminase, bilirubin, or INR) as an early means to assess the risk of acetaminophen toxicity.[10] A serum concentration of acetaminophen obtained at least 4 hours after an acute ingestion (Figure 4-1) can be used to assess whether a patient is at risk of developing acetaminophen hepatotoxicity. The acetaminophen nomogram is intended to be used only for an acute, single-episode ingestion of immediate-release acetaminophen and not in situations when acetaminophen is ingested in supratherapeutic doses over several hours or days.

The semilogarithmic plot of serum acetaminophen concentration versus time (also called the *Rumack-Matthew nomogram* or *acetaminophen nomogram*) is also used to determine whether there is a need to administer acetylcysteine to reduce the risk of toxicity.[42] If the results are not expected to be available within 10 hours of ingestion, acetylcysteine is typically administered provisionally and then continued or discontinued based on the serum acetaminophen concentration. In situations when the specimen is sent to a reference laboratory, the results may take several days to be reported, and, consequently, the patient may receive the entire course of therapy that may last for 72 hours with the oral regimen or 21 hours with the intravenous regimen. Due to the widespread availability of acetaminophen, it is commonly ingested in suicide attempts. Several professional groups have advocated that all patients who are suspected of intentionally taking drugs should have a serum acetaminophen concentration determined as part of their evaluation in the ED.[18,21,32] In the case of acetaminophen poisoning, the serum concentration becomes a valuable determinant of recognition, therapy, and disposition. (See Minicase 6.)

A serum concentration can also guide the utilization or dosage determination of antidotes that are in short supply or are expensive, such as digoxin immune fragment antibody

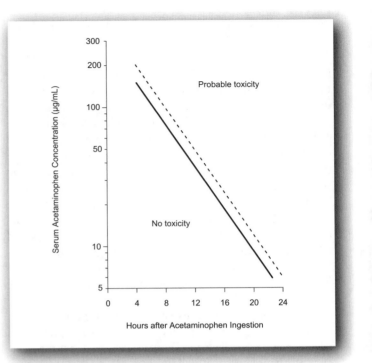

FIGURE 4-1. Nomogram for prediction of acetaminophen hepatoxicity following acute overdose from nonextended-release oral dosage forms. The lower line (starting at 150 mcg/mL at 4 hours) allows a margin for error and should be used as a guide as to whether treatment with acetylcysteine is necessary. (Reprinted, with permission, from reference 42.)

(Digibind and Digifab). Life-threatening acute or chronic digoxin toxicity may require the administration of digoxin immune fragment antibody to quickly reverse the toxic effects of digoxin. The dose of digoxin immune fragment antibody can be determined empirically, based on the amount ingested, or by a steady-state serum concentration (consult current prescribing

---

MINICASE 6

Value of Acetaminophen Concentrations

A MOTHER CALLS A POISON CONTROL CENTER about her 16-year-old daughter, Kelly, who has acutely ingested approximately 30 acetaminophen 500-mg tablets 1 hour ago. She thinks that her daughter was "trying to hurt herself." The pharmacist at the poison center refers Kelly to the nearest hospital for evaluation due to the amount of acetaminophen and the intent of the ingestion. The mother is asked to bring any medicine to which Kelly may have had access. At the ED, Kelly vomits several times but has no other physical complaints or symptoms. A physical exam is unremarkable except for the vomiting. Baseline electrolytes, complete blood count, liver function tests, urine drug screen, and a pregnancy test are ordered. An intravenous line is placed and maintenance intravenous fluids are started. At 4 hours after the acetaminophen ingestion, a blood specimen is drawn to determine the serum acetaminophen concentration. Ninety minutes later, the result is reported as 234 mcg/mL.

Question: Is Kelly at risk for acetaminophen hepatotoxicity? Should she be treated with acetylcysteine?

Discussion: When the serum acetaminophen concentration of 234 mcg/mL is plotted on the acetaminophen nomogram at 4 hours, it is clearly above the treatment line. This indicates that Kelly is at risk for developing hepatotoxicity and that treatment with acetylcysteine should be initiated immediately. The dose of acetaminophen that Kelly ingested is also associated with a risk of developing hepatotoxicity, but patients with intentional overdoses (substance abuse or attempted suicide) do not always provide accurate histories. If the results of the acetaminophen assay would not be available within 2 hours of sampling or within 8–10 hours of ingestion, acetylcysteine therapy would be started provisionally. After learning the acetaminophen concentration, the decision to continue or stop therapy with acetylcysteine could be determined. Since most patients do not exhibit signs and symptoms of acute hepatic injury until 1–3 days after acute acetaminophen overdose, serum transaminase and bilirubin values would not be expected to be abnormal at the time of Kelly's assessment in the ED.

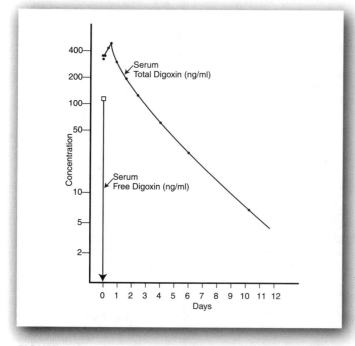

FIGURE 4-2. Serum digoxin concentrations changed dramatically after administration of digoxin immune fragment antibodies at time zero. Serum free digoxin was greater than 100 ng/mL at the time of administration and decreased to undetectable amounts (<0.3 ng/mL) by 1 hour after antibody administration was complete. Serum total digoxin concentration (including that bound to the antibody) increased to >400 ng/mL during the first 12 hours and then fell rapidly. (Reprinted, with permission, from reference 43.)

information).[43,44] Number of vials of digoxin immune fragment antibody = serum concentration of digoxin (ng/mL) × patient weight (kg)/100.

Once the digoxin immune fragment antibody is administered, the serum concentration of digoxin precipitously rises and has no correlation to the degree of toxicity (Figure 4-2).[43] This sharp increase of digoxin reflects total digoxin (protein-bound and unbound) in the serum that has been redistributed

from tissue sites. The digoxin bound to digoxin immune fragment antibody is not toxicologically active, and it is eventually excreted in the urine.

Unique Considerations

The timing of sample collection for poisoned or overdosed patients is variable due to the varying times of arrival at an ED after the exposure and the delay in the recognition of poisoning (unless it is obvious from the history or symptoms).[45] Most specimens are collected at the time of admission to the ED except when specified times are important, such as acetaminophen or when adequate absorption has yet to occur (Table 4-8). This variability makes comparison of serum concentrations among patients difficult to clearly establish a relationship with the concentration and toxicity.

The pharmacokinetics of drugs and chemicals on overdose, sometimes termed *toxicokinetics*, can affect interpretation of a serum concentration.[10] Few studies have compared the pharmacokinetics of drugs in therapeutic and toxic doses since toxic doses cannot be administered to human volunteers and overdosed patients are too heterogeneous to make clear assessments. Nevertheless, there are several examples where the absorption, distribution, metabolism, and elimination of drugs are different on overdose (Table 4-10). It is difficult to apply pharmacokinetic parameters derived from therapeutic doses to situations when massive overdoses are involved. Many patients who are poisoned or have overdosed are critically ill, and multiple samples of blood have been obtained for a variety of tests to monitor their condition. When the toxic agent is recognized late in the course of therapy or when serial determinations could be helpful in understanding some aspect of therapy or toxicity, scavenging aliquots of existing serum samples may be helpful for retrospective toxicological analysis. Laboratories often retain serum samples for several days in case a retest is needed so immediate consultation with the clinical laboratory technician is essential in order to save the specimen for testing. Another sample collection technique involves collecting a blood or urine specimen at presentation to the ED but not performing the assay. This approach, sometimes called

TABLE 4-10. Influence of Toxicokinetic Changes in Poisoned and Overdosed Patients

EFFECT OF OVERDOSAGE[a]	EXAMPLES
Slowed absorption due to formation of poorly soluble semisolid tablet masses in the gastrointestinal tract	Aspirin, lithium, phenytoin, sustained-release theophylline
Slowed absorption due to slowed gastrointestinal motility	Benztropine, nortriptyline
Slowed absorption due to toxin-induced hypoperfusion	Procainamide
Decreased serum protein binding	Lidocaine, salicylates, valproic acid
Increased volume of distribution associated with toxin-induced acidemia	Salicylates
Slowed elimination due to saturation of biotransformation pathways	Ethanol, phenytoin, salicylates, theophylline
Slowed elimination due to toxin-induced hypothermia (<35°C)	Ethanol, propranolol
Prolonged toxicity due to formation of longer-acting metabolites	Carbamazepine, dapsone, glutethimide, meperidine

[a]Compared to characteristics following therapeutic doses or resolution of toxicity.

Source: Reprinted, with permission, from reference 10.

TABLE 4-11. Characteristics of Selected Specimens for Toxicological Analysis[13,46]

SPECIMEN	STRENGTHS	WEAKNESSES	DETECTION TIMES
Urine	• Available in sufficient quantities • Higher concentrations of drugs or metabolites in urine than in blood • Well-researched testing techniques • Availability of POCTs	• Specimen can be adulterated, substituted, or diluted • May require observed collection • Some individuals experience "shy bladder" syndrome and cannot produce a specimen • Biological hazard for specimen handling and shipping to lab	• Limited window of detection after drug use • Typically 1–5 days
Hair	• Observed and noninvasive specimen collection • Good specimen stability (does not deteriorate) • Convenient shipping and storage (no need to refrigerate) • Difficult to adulterate or substitute	• Few labs perform testing • Costly and time consuming to prepare specimen for testing • Difficult to interpret results • Cannot detect alcohol use • Will not detect very recent drug use (7–10 days prior to test) • Difficult to detect low-level use (e.g., single-episode)	• Longest window of detection; best suited for chronic drug use • Depends on hair length in the sample • 1½ inch specimen reflects a 3-month history; hair grows about ½ inch per month
Oral fluids (saliva)	• Observed and noninvasive specimen collection • Minimal risk of tampering • Samples can be collected easily in virtually any setting • Availability of POCTs	• Drugs and metabolites do not remain in oral fluids as long as they do in urine • Limited specimen volume • Requires supervision for 10–30 min before sampling • Oral fluids contaminated by cannabinoids do not reflect presence in saliva and blood	• Reflects recent drug use • Approximately 10–24 hr
Sweat	• Observed and noninvasive specimen collection • Simple application and removal of skin patch • Variable application time (generally 1–14 days) • Difficult to adulterate	• Few labs perform testing • Risk of accidental or deliberate removal of patch • External contamination of the patch may affect results • Requires two visits (application and removal of patch)	• Patch retains evidence of drug use for at least 7 days • Detects low levels of some drugs 2–5 hr after last use

POCTs = point-of-care tests.

toxicology hold, allows collection of a specimen at a time when concentrations may be highest even if the need for the assay may not be clear.[14] The blood specimen can be refrigerated or the serum or urine can be frozen and assayed on request.

SPECIAL SITUATIONS

Other Biological Specimens

There is great interest in utilizing other biological specimen, such as hair, saliva, perspiration, and expired breath and the application of POCTs for quantitative or qualitative analysis.[13,46] These are typically less invasive than venipuncture and some provide unique markers of long-term exposure or use (Table 4-11). Once a technology has been fully validated and sampling techniques refined to minimize interference, POCTs can be useful for drug screens at the bedside and worksite or longitudinal evaluation of chronic use (e.g., cocaine and marijuana in hair samples).[47] To date, SAMHSA has not accepted these alternative specimen nor POCTs for federal regulatory requirements,

but the FDA has approved several types of POCTs for clinical use. The most common and accepted application of POCTs is breath alcohol determination to assess driving impairment from ethanol use at the scene of an accident or arrest.[36]

Forensic and Legal Issues

In addition to clinical and regulatory applications for urine drug screens and serum drug concentrations, toxicological analysis has an important role in providing evidence for suspected cases of homicide, suicide, child abuse, drug-aided sexual assault ("drugged date rape"), environmental contamination, malpractice, workers' compensation, insurance claims, and product liability litigation. Chemical exposure monitoring of workers or the work environment requires specialized approaches such as long-term, on-site monitoring by an industrial hygiene specialist. Toxicological tests are also important in establishing brain death in patients being considered for organ donation or to remove life support. It is essential to establish that the apparent vegetative or unresponsive state is not due to drugs. Whenever legal action is anticipated, it is necessary to maintain a specimen chain-of-custody that can be documented as part of the evidence presentation.[14]

Postmortem analysis of biological specimens, such as gastric contents, organs, vitreous humor, bile, blood, and urine, can assist in the cause of death. These specimens are often collected at the time of autopsy, which may be weeks after death. The study of the changes that occur in drug distribution and metabolism after death has been called *postmortem toxicology* or *necrokinetics*. In addition to diffusion of some drugs to or from tissues and blood after death, the effects of putrefaction, fluid shifts on drug concentrations, and chemical stability need to be considered. This is an evolving field of study, which has already demonstrated that postmortem drug concentrations from various biological specimens may not always be appropriately referenced to drug concentration results derived from living humans.[48-50]

Pediatrics

The toxicological testing of newborn babies, preschool-age poisoning victims, and adolescents involves several unique ethical, technical, and societal concerns. Intrauterine drug exposure can lead to medical complications of newborns and such abuse may be confirmed by drug screens. When mothers do not admit to prepartal drug use, the routine screening of a newborn's urine or meconium poses economic and practical challenges, such as the cost of a generalized screening policy, difficulty in obtaining an adequate urine sample from a neonate and the preanalytical processing of meconium to make it suitable for analysis. Guidelines for newborn urine drug testing involve consideration of maternal and neonatal risk factors.[51]

The use of urine drug screens in the pediatric ED provides minimally useful information because the offending agent is typically known and attempts at concealment are infrequent.[52] However, a broad or focused drug screen may be helpful for cases of suspected child abuse by poisoning or when the history of the poisoning is unclear.[50]

Prerequisite drug testing of adolescents for participation in school activities and routine screening by school officials, concerned parents, and pediatricians, presents several ethical dilemmas. Parents and school officials want assurance that substance abuse is not occurring, but the confidentiality and consent of the adolescent should be recognized. The American Academy of Pediatrics states that it "has strong reservations about testing adolescents at school or at home and believes that more research is needed on both safety and efficacy before school-based testing programs are implemented."[53] This policy statement is at odds with the desire of some parent groups to perform such tests without the adolescent's consent and with court rulings upholding a school's ability to perform mass or random drug tests of its students.[54] Drug use in school-age children has been associated with a variety of risk taking behaviors, such as carrying a gun, engaging in unprotected sexual intercourse with multiple partners, and suffering injury from a physical fight.[55] These behaviors may indicate the need for monitoring drug abuse with appropriate behavioral and

TABLE 4-12. Some Purported Athletic Performance-Enhancing Substances

Amino acids (e.g., arginine, ornithine, lysine, aspartate, glutamine, leucine, tryptophan, carnitine)

Amphetamines[a]

Androgenic anabolic steroids

Androstenedione

Antiestrogenic agents (e.g., anastrozole, tamoxifen, clomiphene, fulvestrant)

Antioxidants (e.g., megadoses of ascorbic acid [vitamin C], tocopherol [vitamin E], beta-carotene)

Beta-adrenergic blockers

Beta-2 agonists

Caffeine

Clenbuterol

Cocaine[a]

Corticotropin (ACTH)

Creatine

Dihydroepiandrostenedione (DHEA)

Diuretics

Erythropoietin

Ethanol

Gamma-hydroxybutyrate (GHB)

Human chorionic gonadotropin

Human growth hormone

Selective androgen receptor modulators

Theophylline

[a]Can be detected on most routine immunoassay urine drug screens; the others are not typically detected on routine drug screens.

health counseling. Many drug testing products are promoted for home use on the Internet, but their reliability and benefits are questionable.[56]

Sports and Drugs

Drugs have been used by amateur and professional athletes in hopes of enhancing athletic performance and by nonathletes to improve physical appearance. An estimated 2% to 7% of high school students (approximate ratio of 2:1 for boys to girls) have used androgenic anabolic steroids; of these students, nearly one-third do not participate in sports but use steroids to change their appearance.[6,55,57] The types and variety of substances are typically different from those encountered in poisonings or substance abuse. Most workplace or clinical drug screens will not detect athletic performance enhancing drugs such as anabolic androgenic steroids, growth hormone, and erythroid-stimulating agents (Table 4-12).[58] The international term for drug use in sports is *doping* and efforts to combat this practice are referred to as *doping control* or *antidoping*.

Governing athletic organizations, such as the International Olympic Committee, the United States Olympic Committee, and the National Collegiate Athletic Association, have established policies and analytical procedures for testing athletes as well as lists of banned substances. Most organized sports observe the World Antidoping Agency's guidelines for analytical tests, banned substances, and screening procedures.[59] The technical and scientific challenges in detecting many of these substances are unique to this field.[62] Using banned drugs can result in an unfair, artificial advantage for competitive athletes and physical injury or permanent disability from the drug's effects, such as those from anabolic steroids.[57,58]

Prescription Drug Abuse

During the past decade the abuse of prescription drugs has risen dramatically and has increased in all age groups.[8] Nationwide 20% of Americans aged 12 years and older reported taking prescription drugs for nonmedical purposes during their lifetime.[1,55] For the first time the number of poisoning deaths exceeded the number of motor vehicle traffic deaths in 2008. Drugs were the cause of 89% of these deaths with opioid analgesics involved in 41% of the cases.[8] Since 2003, deaths from opioid analgesics have exceeded the number from heroin and cocaine combined.[8,60] These trends have been recognized as a national epidemic.[60,61] In evaluating patients who may be abusing prescription drugs, a careful history, physical examination, and use of behavioral screening tools are important elements, which can be supported by drug screens.[62-64] A urine drug screen can assist in the detection of inappropriate use when there is sufficient suspicion. If a patient is on a methadone treatment program or is regularly receiving opioids for the relief of chronic pain, the urine drug screen should produce positive results. A negative finding could suggest poor adherence and possible diversion. Characteristics of the drug (e.g., short duration of action) and the assay (e.g., ability to detect some synthetic opioids) should be considered before discussing the issue with the patient. In a national sample of pediatricians and family physicians, a survey indicated that 48% followed no defined procedures to ensure proper collection of the urine sample and most had poor responses on knowledge of drugs that are detected and those that could cause false-positive results. The authors concluded that primary care physicians are not prepared to assist with drug testing programs.[65] Knowledge and training at primary care settings on urine drug screening would enhance the ability to detect and help patients who are abusing prescription drugs and help stem the rise in drug abuse, diversion, and deaths. Differences in federal workplace testing and the clinical setting, such as specimen type, collection procedures, drug testing panel, cutoff concentrations, and MRO involvement, should be recognized.[11,46,66]

SUMMARY

Testing for substance abuse, poisonings, and overdose affects society at several levels. Knowledge of assay limitations, sampling procedures, interfering substances, patient factors, and regulatory requirements will aid in the interpretation of the value of the test and its clinical relevance. In this chapter, several approaches and applications are discussed, but other situations

---

MINICASE 7

Monitoring Chronic Therapy with Opioid Analgesics

ALEX P., A 32-YEAR-OLD DAY LABORER, developed chronic pain after a lower back injury. He currently has a prescription for a long-acting morphine preparation. Alex P. has had a history of anxiety and substance abuse of a variety of illicit and prescription drugs. He is otherwise healthy. During the past 24 months on this medication he has lost his prescription twice and asked for a replacement. His physician has also written additional prescriptions at times when he complained that the dosage was inadequate to provide pain relief. His current daily total dose of morphine is 120 mg. He was recently arrested for forging a prescription to obtain additional opioid medication. Alex P. has had several random urine drug screens during the past 18 months that have been positive for morphine. On one occasion the test result was positive for oxycodone for which he had a prescription from another physician.

Question: How can urine drug screens be helpful in assessing adherence to an opioid analgesic regimen and identifying potential abuse of opioids?

Discussion: The opioid drug treatment of noncancer-related chronic pain can be complicated by many factors such as need for escalating doses for adequate pain relief, potential for diversion of the drugs by selling or giving the drugs to others, abuse of the drugs to get high or satisfy a drug craving, and the risks of overdose and death. One of the approaches to monitor chronic therapy with opioids is to perform random drug screens. A positive drug screen can support that the person is taking the drug, while a negative result should raise the question of whether the person is diverting it to others or has stopped taking it for some reason. A drug screen that shows illicit, nonprescribed drugs or prescriptions from multiple or other prescribers, such as oxycodone in this case, strongly suggests that abuse of other medications is taking place which all raise the risks for overdose and death. The physician is faced with several significant signals in this case that need attention to provide safe and effective care. If the physician is not a pain specialist, referral to one for Alex P.'s chronic pain care should be considered.

---

that involve potential toxins—such as environmental contamination, chemical terrorism, and product safety testing—call for different approaches and pose unique challenges.

Sources of Information

Since test characteristics vary with the type of test, manufacturer, assay kit, setting, and application, information about a specific test is critical for proper utilization and interpretation. Good communication with laboratory technicians is an important first step in ensuring proper testing. Laboratory technicians can provide guidance on sample collection, cutoff values, interfering substances, and other technical aspects. The package insert for immunoassays or other commercial assay kits is an important and specific guide to assay performance and known interfering substances with the specific assay. There are several textbooks that can be helpful in understanding techniques, values, and interfering substances.[13,67,68] Clinical toxicologists in poison control centers (list at www.aapcc.org or contact the local program at 1-800-222-1222 nationwide) can also provide useful information on laboratory tests particularly as they relate to poisonings. Several relevant publications are available at Internet websites of governmental agencies such as the SAMHSA (www.samhsa.gov), Office of Drug Policy Control (www. whitehouse.gov/ondcp), and the U.S. Drug Enforcement Administration (www.justice.gov/dea). These websites can also increase awareness of persistent or emerging drugs of abuse. Quickviews of eight common urine drug screens by immunoassay include information on the signs and symptoms of these agents following abuse and overdose.[10,12,26-28,69] (See Minicase 7.)

Learning Points

1. **How long does it take for a drug to clear the body and result in a negative urine drug screen?**

   Answer: It depends on a number of factors. Length of time for detection will vary with the sensitivity of the assay, whether the assay is directed to the parent drug or the metabolite, whether the drug or its metabolites exhibit extensive distribution to tissues, the dose of the drug taken, and whether the drug was used chronically or only once.

2. **What does a negative result from a drug screen mean?**

   Answer: A *negative* result does not mean that the drug was not present or not taken; it means that it was not detected. Some reasons include that the drug may not have been part of the testing panel; the urine may have been too dilute for detection; the urine may have been collected before the drug was excreted in the urine; the urine sample may have been adulterated after collection to mask or avoid detection; or the specimen was obtained too late after the exposure.

3. **How can serum concentrations be useful in the treatment of poisoned patients?**

   Answer: When a poisoning or overdose is suspected, a serum concentration is obtained when it can confirm the diagnosis of a poisoning when in doubt, aid the interpretation of a qualitative urine drug screen, determine whether antidotal therapy is indicated, or determine the effectiveness of a therapy. For assays not primarily intended for overdoses or poisonings (e.g., acetaminophen), drug concentrations occasionally are measured when the assay is used for another application such as therapeutic drug monitoring. In clinical settings, serum is typically not used for drug screening.

4. **What should you do if the results do not make sense?**

   Answer: Consider actions that include checking the report and units of measure, talking with the laboratory technician, checking the package insert of the assay, searching the literature, seeking alternative causes of symptoms, and repeating the assay at the same or different laboratory.

REFERENCES

1. Substance Abuse and Mental Health Services Administration. *Results from the 2010 National Survey on Drug Use and Health: summary of national findings* (NSDUH Series H-41, HHS Publication No. SMA 11-4658); Rockville, MD: Substance Abuse and Mental Health Services Administration; 2011. Available at http://oas.samhsa.gov/NSDUH/2k10NSDUH/2k10Results.pdf. Accessed January 9, 2012.

2. Substance Abuse and Mental Health Services Administration. *Drug Abuse Warning Network, 2009: national estimates of drug-related emergency department visits.* (HHS Publication No. SMA 11-4659, DAWN Series D-35); Rockville, MD: Substance Abuse and Mental Health Services Administration; 2011. Available at http://www.samhsa.gov/data/2k11/DAWN/2k9DAWNED/PDF/DAWN2k9ED.pdf. Accessed January 9, 2012.

3. Bronstein AC, Spyker DA, Cantelina LR, et al. 2010 Annual Report of the American Association of Poison Control Centers' National Poison Data System (NCDS) 28th Annual Report. *Clin Toxicol*. 2010;49:910-941. Available at http://www.aapcc.org/dnn/Portals/0/2010%20NPDS%20Annual%20Report.pdf. Accessed December 22, 2011.

4. Anon. Drug Testing Index 2011 Report. Lyndhurst, NJ: Quest Diagnostics Inc; March 12, 2012. Available at http://www.questdiagnostics.com/home/physicians/health-trends/drug-testing. Accessed July 21, 2012.

5. Executive Office of The President of the United States. ADAM II 2010 annual report: Arrestee Drug Abuse Monitoring Program II. Washington, DC: Office of National Drug Control Policy; 2011. Available at http://www.whitehouse.gov/sites/default/files/ondcp/policy-and-research/adam2010.pdf. Accessed February 2, 2012.

6. Johnston LD, O'Malley PM, Bachman JG, Schulenberg JE. *Monitoring the Future national results on adolescent drug use: overview of key findings, 2011*. Ann Arbor: Institute for Social Research, The University of Michigan; 2012. Available at http://monitoringthefuture.org/pubs/monographs/mtf-overview2011.pdf. Accessed February 4, 2012.

7. Centers for Disease Control and Prevention. *Web-Based Injury Statistics Query and Reporting System (WISQARS) [Online]*. Atlanta, GA: Centers for Disease Control and Prevention. Available at http://www.cdc.gov/injury/wisqars/fatal.html. Accessed February 4, 2012.

8. Warner M, Li Hui C, Makuc DM, Anderson RN, Minino AM. Drug poisoning deaths in the United States, 1980-2008. NCHS Data Brief No. 81. Hyattsville, MD: National Center for Health Statistics; 2011. Available at http://www.cdc.gov/nchs/data/databriefs/db81.pdf. Accessed February 4, 2012.

9. Executive Office of The President of the United States. Research and data; federal drug data sources. Washington, DC: Office of National Drug Control Policy. Available at http://www.whitehouse.gov/ondcp/research-and-data. Accessed February 4, 2012.

10. Chyka PA. Clinical toxicology. In: DiPiro JT, Talbert RL, Yee GC, et al., eds. *Pharmacotherapy: A Pathophysiologic Approach*. 8th ed. New York, NY: McGraw-Hill; 2011:27-49.

11. Division of Workplace programs. *Drug Testing*. Rockville, MD: Substance Abuse and Mental Health Services Administration, Department of Health and Human Services. Available at http://workplace.samhsa.gov/Dtesting.html. Accessed February 4, 2012.

12. Anon. Tests for drugs of abuse. *Med Lett Drugs Ther*. 2002;44:71-73.

13. Ropero-Miller JD, Goldberger BA, eds. *Handbook of Workplace Drug Testing*. 2nd ed. Washington, DC: American Association of Clinical Chemistry Press Press; 2009.

14. Rainey PM. Laboratory principles. In: Nelson LS, Lewin NA, Howland MA, et al., eds. *Goldfrank's Toxicologic Emergencies*. 9th ed. New York, NY: McGraw-Hill; 2011:70-89.

15. Rosenfeld W, Wingert WE. Scientific issues in drug testing and use of the laboratory. In: Schydlower M (ed). *Substance Abuse: A Guide for Health Professionals*. 2nd ed. Elk Grove, IL: American Academy of Pediatrics; 2002:105-121.

16. Hammertt-Stabler CA, Pesce AJ, Cannon DJ. Urine drug screening in the medical setting. *Clinica Chimicia Acta*. 2002;315:125-135.

17. Department of Health and Human Services, Substance Abuse and Mental Health Services Administration. Mandatory guidelines for federal workplace drug testing programs. *Fed Regist*. 2008;73:71858-1907 and 2010;75:22809-22810. Available at http://edocket.access.gpo.gov/2008/pdf/e8-26726.pdf. Accessed February 4, 2012.

18. Wu AB, McKay C, Broussard LA, et al. National Academy of Clinical Biochemistry laboratory medicine practice guidelines: recommendations for the use of laboratory tests to support poisoned patients who present to the emergency department. *Clin Chem*. 2003;49:357-379.

19. Tenenbein M. Do you really need that emergency drug screen? *Clin Toxicol*. 2009;47:286-291.

20. Nice A, Leikin JB, Maturen A, et al. Toxidrome recognition to improve efficiency of emergency urine drug screens. *Ann Emerg Med*. 1988;17:676-680.

21. American College of Emergency Physicians. Clinical policy for the initial approach to patients presenting with acute toxic ingestion or dermal or inhalation exposure. *Ann Emerg Med*. 1999;33:735-761.

22. Carrigan TD, Field H, Illingworth RN, et al. Toxicological screening in trauma. *J Accid Emerg Med*. 2000;17:33-37.

23. Substance Abuse and Mental Health Services Administration. *Medical review officer manual for federal workplace drug testing programs, 2010*. Rockville, MD: Department of Health and Human Services. Available at http://workplace.samhsa.gov/DrugTesting/pdf/MRO_Manual_2010_100908.pdf. Accessed February 4, 2012.

24. Wu AH. Urine adulteration before testing for drugs of abuse. In: Shaw LM, Kwong TC, Rosana TG, et al., eds. *The Clinical Toxicology Laboratory: Contemporary Practice of Poisoning Evaluation*. Washington, DC: American Association of Clinical Chemistry Press; 2001:157-171.

25. Mittal MK, Florin T, Perrone J, et al. Toxicity from the use of niacin to beat urine drug screening. *Ann Emerg Med*. 2007; 50:587-590.

26. Anon. Urine drug detection. In: *Poisindex System* (Internet database). Greenwood Village, CO: Thomson Healthcare; 2010. Accessed February 4, 2012.

27. Moeller KE, Lee KC, Kissack JC. Urine drug screening: practical guide for clinicians. *Mayo Clin Proc*. 2008;83:66-76.

28. Brahm NC, Yeager LL, Fox MD, et al. Commonly prescribed medications and potential false-positive urine drug screens. *Am J Health Syst Pharm*. 2010;67:1344-1350.

29. Rollins DE, Jennison TA, Jones G. Investigation of interference by nonsteroidal anti-inflammatory drugs in urine tests for abused drugs. *Clin Chem*. 1990;36:602-606.

30. Zacher JL, Givone DM. False-positive urine opiate screening associated with fluoroquinolone use. *Ann Pharmacother*. 2004;38:1525-1528.

31. Olson KR, ed. *Poisoning & Drug Overdose*. 6th ed. New York, NY: Lange/McGraw-Hill; 2012.

32. National Poisons Information Service and Association of Clinical Biochemists. Laboratory analyses for poisoned patients: joint position paper. *Ann Clin Biochem*. 2002;39:328-339.

33. National Highway Traffic Safety Administration. The ABCs of BAC: a guide to understanding blood alcohol concentration and alcohol impairment. Washington, DC: Department of Transportation; 2005. Available at http://www.stopimpaireddriving.org/ABCsBACWeb/images/ABCBACscr.pdf. Accessed February 4, 2012.

34. Hammond KB, Rumack BH, Rodgerson DO. Blood ethanol: a report of unusually high levels in a living patient. *JAMA*. 1973;226:63-64.

35. Van Heyningen C, Watson ID. Survival after very high blood alcohol concentrations (letter). *Ann Clin Biochem*. 2002;39:416-417.

36. Kwong TC. Point-of-care testing for alcohol. In: Shaw LM, Kwong TC, Rosana TG, et al., eds. *The Clinical Toxicology Laboratory: Contemporary Practice of Poisoning Evaluation*. Washington, DC: American Association of Clinical Chemistry Press; 2001:190-196.

37. Orsay E, Doan-Wiggins L. Serum alcohol is not the same as blood alcohol concentration. *Ann Emerg Med*. 1995;25:430-431.

38. Done AK. Salicylate intoxication: significance of measurements of salicylate in blood in cases of acute ingestion. *Pediatrics*. 1960;26:800-807.

39. Dugandzic RM, Tierney MG, Dickinson GE, et al. Evaluation of the validity of the Done nomogram in the management of acute salicylate intoxication. *Ann Emerg Med*. 1989;18:1186-1190.

40. Gabow PA, Anderson RJ, Potts DE, et al. Acid-base disturbances in the salicylate-intoxicated adult. *Arch Intern Med*. 1978;38:1481-1484.

41. Sporer KA, Khayam-Bashi H. Acetaminophen and salicylate serum levels in patients with suicidal ingestion or altered mental status. *Am J Emerg Med.* 1996;14:443-446.

42. Smilkstein MJ, Knapp GL, Kulig KW, et al. Efficacy of oral *N*-acetylcysteine in the treatment of acetaminophen overdose: analysis of the national multicenter study (1976 to 1985). *N Engl J Med.* 1988;319:1557-1562.

43. Zucker AR, Lacina SJ, DasGupta DS, et al. Fab fragments of digoxin-specific antibodies used to reverse ventricular fibrillation induced by digoxin ingestion in a child. *Pediatrics.* 1982;70:468-471.

44. Antman EM, Wenger TL, Butler VP, et al. Treatment of 150 cases of life-threatening digitalis intoxication with digoxin-specific Fab antibody fragments: final report of a multicenter study. *Circulation.* 1990;81:1744-1752.

45. Bosse GM, Matyunas NJ. Delayed toxidromes. *J Emerg Med.* 1999;17:679-690.

46. Substance Abuse and Mental Health Services Administration. *Clinical drug testing in primary care.* Technical Assistance Publication (TAP) 32. HHS Publication No. SMA 12-4668. Rockville, MD: Substance Abuse and Mental Health Services Administration, 2012. Available at http://www.kap.samhsa.gov/products/manuals/pdfs/TAP32.pdf. Accessed August 17, 2012.

47. George S, Braithwaite RA. Use of on-site testing for drugs of abuse. *Clin Chem.* 2002;48:1639-1646.

48. Leikin JB, Watson WA. Postmortem toxicology: what the dead can and cannot tell us. *J Toxicol Clin Toxicol.* 2003;41:47-56.

49. Ferner RE. Post-mortem clinical pharmacology. *Br J Clin Pharmacol* 2008;66:430-443.

50. Rao RB, Flomenbaum M. Postmortem toxicology. In: Nelson LS, Lewin NA, Howland MA, et al., eds. *Goldfrank's Toxicologic Emergencies.* 9th ed. New York, NY: McGraw-Hill; 2011:471-478.

51. Kwong TC, Ryan RM. Detection of intrauterine illicit drug exposure by newborn drug testing. *Clin Chem.* 1997;43:235-242.

52. Belson MG, Simon HK, Sullivan K, et al. The utility of toxicologic analysis in children with suspected ingestions. *Pediatr Emerg Care.* 1999;15:383-387.

53. American Academy of Pediatrics. Testing for drugs of abuse in children and adolescents: addendum – testing in schools and at home. *Pediatrics.* 2007;119:627-630. Available at http://aappolicy.aappublications.org/cgi/reprint/pediatrics;119/3/627.pdf. Accessed February 4, 2012.

54. Schwartz RH, Silber TJ, Heyman RB, et al. Urine testing for drugs of abuse. *Arch Pediatr Adolesc Med.* 2003;157:158-161.

55. Eaton DK, Kann L, Kinchen S, et al. Youth risk behavior surveillance—United States, 2009. In: *Surveillance Summaries MMWR.* 2010;59(SS-5):1-148. Available at http://www.cdc.gov/mmwr/pdf/ss/ss5905.pdf. Accessed February 4, 2012.

56. Levy S, Van Hook S, Knight JR. A review of internet-based home drug testing products for parents. *Pediatrics.* 2004;113:720-726.

57. Calfee R, Fadale P. Popular ergogenic drugs and supplements in young athletes. *Pediatrics.* 2006;117;577-589.

58. De Rose EH. Doping in athletes—an update. *Clin Sports Med.* 2008;27:107-130.

59. World Antidoping Agency. *The world anti-doping code. The 2012 prohibited list: international standard.* Available at http://www.cdc.gov/mmwr/pdf/ss/ss5905.pdf. Accessed February 4, 2012.

60. Paulozzi L, Baldwin G, Franklin G, Kerlikowske RG, et al. CDC Grand Rounds: prescription drug overdoses—a U.S. epidemic. *MMWR.* 2012;61:10-13.

61. Executive Office of the President of the United States. *Epidemic: responding to America's prescription drug abuse crisis.* Washington, DC: Office of National Drug Control Policy; 2011. Available at http://www.whitehouse.gov/sites/default/files/ondcp/policy-and-research/rx_abuse_plan.pdf. Accessed February 4, 2012.

62. Substance Abuse and Mental Health Services Administration. *Clinical drug testing in primary care. Technical Assistance Publication (TAP) 32.* (HHS Publication No. SMA 12-4668). Rockville, MD: Substance Abuse and Mental Health Services Administration; 2012. Available at http://www.kap.samhsa.gov/products/manuals/pdfs/TAP32.pdf. Accessed August 17, 2012.

63. Christo PJ, Manchikanti L, Ruan X, et al. Urine drug testing in chronic pain. *Pain Physician.* 2011;14:123-143

64. Passik SD. Issues in long-term opioid therapy: unmet needs, risks, and solutions. *Mayo Clin Proc.* 2009;84:593-601.

65. Levy S, Harris SK, Sherritt L, et al. Drug testing of adolescents in ambulatory medicine. *Arch Pediatr Adolesc Med.* 2006;160:146-150.

66. Phan HM, Yoshizuka K, Murry DJ, et al. Drug testing in the workplace. *Pharmacotherapy* 2012;32:649-656.

67. Baselt RC. *Disposition of Toxic Drugs and Chemicals in Man.* 9th ed. Foster City, CA: Biomedical Publications; 2011.

68. Shaw LM, Kwong TC, Rosana TG, et al., eds. *The Clinical Toxicology Laboratory: Contemporary Practice of Poisoning Evaluation.* Washington, DC: American Association of Clinical Chemistry Press; 2001.

69. National Institute on Drug Abuse. *InfoFacts.* Washington, DC: National Institutes of Health. Available at http://www.drugabuse.gov/publications/term/160/InfoFacts. Accessed February 4, 2012.

Quickview | Urine Drug Screen, Amphetamines, and Methamphetamine

PARAMETER	DESCRIPTION	COMMENTS
Critical Value	Positive	Check for possible interferents; confirm result with confirmatory test such as GC-MS
Major causes of...		
Positive results	Following ingestion, intranasal application, injection, smoking (methamphetamine)	
Associated signs and symptoms	None may be evident at time of specimen collection; may involve exposure to illicit substances; may be used for legitimate purposes or abuse may involve exposure to illicit forms	Typical symptoms include CNS stimulation, euphoria, irritability, insomnia, tremors, seizures, paranoia, and aggressiveness; overdoses cause hypertension, tachycardia, stroke, arrhythmias, cardiovascular collapse, rhabdomyolysis, and hyperthermia
After use, time to...		
Negative result from light, sporadic use	2–5 days; clearance is faster in acidic urine	Methylphenidate typically will not be detected
Negative result from chronic use	Up to 2 weeks	
Possible spurious positive results with immunoassays	Ephedrine, pseudoephedrine, ephedra (ma huang), phenylephrine, selegiline, chlorpromazine, promethazine, trazodone, bupropion, desipramine, trimipramine, ritodrine, amantadine, ranitidine, phenylpropanolamine, brompheniramine, isometheptene, labetalol, phentermine, methylphenidate, isoxsuprine, trimethobenzamide, 3,4-methylenedioxy-N-methamphetamine (MDMA, Ecstasy)	A false-positive result may be caused by patient's use of drugs and dietary supplements; verify possible false positive with laboratory and assay package insert

CNS = central nervous system; GC-MS = gas chromatography/mass spectrometry; MDMA = 3,4-methylenedioxy-N-methamphetamine.

Quickview | Urine Drug Screen, Barbiturates

PARAMETER	DESCRIPTION	COMMENTS
Critical Value	Positive	Check for possible interferents; confirm result with confirmatory test such as GC-MS
Major causes of...		
Positive results	Following ingestion; rarely injected or used as a suppository	
Associated signs and symptoms	None may be evident at time of specimen collection; may involve exposure to medicines used for legitimate purposes or abuse	Typical symptoms include sedation; overdoses cause coma, ataxia, nystagmus, depressed reflexes, hypotension, and respiratory depression; consider coingestion of ethanol; primidone is metabolized to phenobarbital
After use, time to...		
Negative result from light, sporadic use	1–7 days	Depends on drug and extent and duration of use
Negative result from chronic use	1–3 weeks	Phenobarbital may be detected up to 4 weeks after stopping use
Possible spurious positive results with immunoassays	Ibuprofen, naproxen	Verify possible false positive with laboratory and assay package insert

GC-MS = gas chromatography/mass spectrometry.

Quickview | Urine Drug Screen, Benzodiazepines

PARAMETER	DESCRIPTION	COMMENTS
Critical Value	Positive	Check for possible interferents; confirm result with confirmatory test such as GC-MS
Major causes of...		
Positive results	Following ingestion or injection	Benzodiazepines vary in cross-reactivity and detectability
Associated signs and symptoms	None may be evident at time of specimen collection; may involve exposure to medicines used for legitimate purposes or abuse; may involve exposure to illicit forms	Typical symptoms include drowsiness, ataxia, slurred speech, sedation; oral overdoses can cause tachycardia and coma with rare severe respiratory or cardiovascular depression; rapid IV use can cause severe respiratory depression; consider coingestion of ethanol
After use, time to...		
Negative result	Typically up to 2 weeks; up to 6 weeks with chronic use of some agents	Some benzodiazepines may persist for a longer period of time and some have an active metabolite that may or may not be detected; flunitrazepam may not be detected; not all benzodiazepines will be detected by all immunoassays
Possible spurious positive results with immunoassays	Oxaprozin, sertraline	Verify possible false positive with laboratory and assay package insert

GC-MS = gas chromatography/mass spectrometry; IV = intravenous.

Quickview | Urine Drug Screen, Benzoylecgonine (cocaine metabolite)

PARAMETER	DESCRIPTION	COMMENTS
Critical Value	Positive	Check for possible interferents; confirm result with confirmatory test such as GC-MS
Major causes of...		
Positive results	Following snorting, smoking, injection, topical application (vagina, penis) or rectal insertion; possible passive inhalation; ingestion	
Associated signs and symptoms	None may be evident at time of specimen collection with heavy or chronic use; may involve exposure to medicines used for legitimate purposes or abuse; may involve exposure to illicit forms	Typical symptoms include CNS stimulation that produces euphoric effects and hyperstimulation such as dilated pupils, increased temperature, tachycardia and hypertension; overdoses cause stroke, acute myocardial infarction, seizures, coma, respiratory depression, arrhythmias
After use, time to...		
Negative result from light, sporadic use	12–72 hr	Cross-reactivity with cocaethylene (metabolic product of concurrent cocaine and ethanol abuse) varies with the assay
Negative result from chronic use	Up to 1–3 weeks	
Possible spurious positive results with immunoassays	Topical anesthetics containing cocaine; coca leaf tea	False finding for abuse
		False positives from caine anesthetics (e.g., lidocaine, procaine, benzocaine) are unlikely; verify possible false positive with laboratory and assay package insert

CNS = central nervous system; GC-MS = gas chromatography/mass spectrometry.

Quickview | Urine Drug Screen, Delta-9-tetrahydrocannabinol-9-carboxylic Acid

PARAMETER	DESCRIPTION	COMMENTS
Critical Value	Positive	Check for possible interferents; confirm result with confirmatory test such as GC-MS
Major causes of...		
Positive results	Following smoking, ingestion, possible passive inhalation	May be caused by sodium phosphate used as drug screen adulterant; patients taking dronabinol will also have positive test results
Associated signs and symptoms	None may be evident at time of specimen collection with heavy or chronic use; may involve exposure to illicit substances; may involve exposure to medicine used for legitimate purposes or abuse	Typical symptoms include delirium, conjunctivitis, food craving; other effects include problems with memory and learning, distorted perception, difficulty in thinking and problem solving, loss of coordination, sedation, and tachycardia
After use, time to...		
Negative result from light, sporadic use	7–10 days	
Negative result from chronic use	6–8 weeks typically, up to 3 months possible	May persist for a longer period of time with heavy, long-term use
Possible spurious positive results with immunoassays	Ibuprofen, naproxen, tolmetin, efavirenz, pantoprazole	False-positive result
		False positive for abuse; verify possible false positive with laboratory and assay package insert

GC-MS = gas chromatography/mass spectrometry.

Quickview | Urine Drug Screen, LSD

PARAMETER	DESCRIPTION	COMMENTS
Critical Value	Positive	Check for possible interferents; confirm result with confirmatory test such as GC-MS
Major causes of...		
Positive results	Following ingestion, placement in buccal cavity or ocular instillation	Not well-absorbed topically
Associated signs and symptoms	May involve exposure to illicit substances	Typical symptoms include unpredictable hallucinogenic effects; physical effects include mydriasis, elevated temperature, tachycardia, hypertension, sweating, loss of appetite, sleeplessness, dry mouth, and tremors; flash-backs months later are possible
After use, time to...		
Negative result	24–48 hr typically, up to 120 hr possible	
Possible spurious positive results with immunoassays		LSD is a schedule I drug with no legitimate routine medical use; verify possible false positive with laboratory and assay package insert

GC-MS = gas chromatography/mass spectrometry; LSD = lysergic acid diethylamide.

Quickview | Urine Drug Screen, Opiates

PARAMETER	DESCRIPTION	COMMENTS
Critical Value	Positive	Check for possible interferents; confirm result with confirmatory test such as GC-MS
Major causes of...		
Positive results	Following ingestion, injection, dermal application of drug-containing patches, rectal insertion	Synthetic opioids (e.g., fentanyl, fentanyl derivatives, meperidine, methadone, pentazocine, propoxyphene, and tramadol) have minimal cross-reactivity and may not be detected
Associated signs and symptoms	None may be evident at time of specimen collection; may involve exposure to illicit substances; may involve exposure to medicines used for legitimate purposes or abuse; ingestion of large amounts of food products made with poppy seeds	Typical symptoms include CNS depression, drowsiness, miosis, constipation; overdoses cause coma, hypotension, respiratory depression, pulmonary edema, and seizures Heroin use is confirmed by the presence of 6-acetylmorphine (6-AM)
After use, time to...		
Negative result	2–3 days typically, up to 6 days with sustained-release formulations, up to 1 week with prolonged or heavy use	
Possible spurious positive results with immunoassays	Poppy seeds	False positive for drug abuse
	Rifampin, some fluoroquinolones, quinine	False-positive result; consider patient's legitimate use of opioid analgesics including long-term pain management and opioid withdrawal treatment with methadone, or buprenorphine; verify possible false positive with laboratory and assay package insert

CNS = central nervous system; GC-MS = gas chromatography/mass spectrometry.

Quickview | Urine Drug Screen, PCP

PARAMETER	DESCRIPTION	COMMENTS
Critical Value	Positive	Check for possible interferents; confirm result with confirmatory test such as GC-MS
Major causes of...		
Positive results	Following ingestion, smoking, snorting, or injection	
Associated signs and symptoms	None may be evident at time of specimen collection; may involve exposure to illicit substances; may involve exposure to medicines containing dextromethorphan or diphenhydramine used for legitimate purposes or abuse	Typical symptoms include hallucinations, schizophrenia-like behavior, hypertension, elevated temperature, diaphoresis, tachycardia; high doses cause nystagmus, ataxia, hypotension, bradycardia, depressed respirations, seizures, and coma
After use, time to...		
Negative result from light, sporadic use	2–10 days	May persist for a longer period of time with heavy, long-term use or massive overdose preceded by chronic use
Negative result from chronic use	Weeks or months	
Possible spurious positive results with immunoassays	Ketamine, dextromethorphan, diphenhydramine, imipramine, mesoridazine, thioridazine, venlafaxine, ibuprofen, meperidine, tramadol	False-positive result; verify possible false positive with laboratory and assay package insert

GC-MS = gas chromatography/mass spectrometry; PCP = phencyclidine.

CHAPTER 5

INTERPRETATION OF SERUM DRUG CONCENTRATIONS

JANIS J. MACKICHAN

Special thanks to Jaclyn Kruse, BS, MS, PharmD for her invaluable contributions to this chapter.

Objectives

After completing this chapter, the reader should be able to

- Justify the need for concentration monitoring of a drug based on its characteristics and the clinical situation

- Identify and justify information needed when requesting and reporting drug concentrations

- Describe and categorize factors that may contribute to interpatient variation in a therapeutic range of drug concentrations

- Explain the importance of documenting the time a sample is obtained relative to the last dose, as well as factors that can affect interpretation of a drug concentration, depending on when it was obtained

- Compare the types of specimens that may be obtained (serum, plasma, whole blood, and saliva), and the types of artifacts that may be caused by collection methods and assay choice

- Compare linear to nonlinear pharmacokinetic behavior with respect to how drug concentration measurements are used to make dosage regimen adjustments

- Describe how altered serum binding, active metabolites, or stereoselective pharmacokinetics can impact the interpretation of drug concentration measurements

The pharmacist is a key member in the therapeutic drug monitoring process. This chapter is designed to review the indications for drug concentration monitoring and to discuss how drug concentrations obtained from the clinical laboratory, specialized reference laboratory, or physician's office should be interpreted. General considerations for interpretation will be described, as well as unique considerations for drugs that commonly undergo therapeutic drug monitoring. Future directions of therapeutic drug monitoring will also be discussed.

This chapter is not intended to provide an in-depth review of pharmacokinetic dosing methods; nevertheless, knowledge of certain basic pharmacokinetic terms and concepts is expected. The general phrase *drug concentration* will be used throughout the chapter unless specific references to serum, plasma, whole blood, saliva, or tears are more appropriate. The bibliography lists numerous texts about therapeutic drug monitoring and clinical pharmacokinetic principles with applications to clinical practice.

THERAPEUTIC DRUG MONITORING

Therapeutic drug monitoring is broadly defined as the use of drug concentrations to optimize drug therapy for individual patients.[1] Prior to the use of drug concentrations to guide therapy, physicians adjusted drug doses based on their interpretation of clinical response. In many cases, drug doses were increased until obvious signs of toxicity were observed (e.g., nystagmus for phenytoin or tinnitus for salicylates). The idea that intensity and duration of pharmacologic response depended on serum drug concentration was first reported by Marshall and then tested for the screening of antimalarials during World War II.[2,3] Koch-Weser, in a hallmark paper, described how steady-state serum levels of commonly used drugs can vary 10-fold among patients receiving the same dosage schedule.[4] He further described how serum concentrations predict intensity of therapeutic or toxic effects more accurately than dosage.

Starting in the 1960s, there was rapid improvement in analytical methods used for drug concentration measurements; extensive research correlating serum or plasma drug concentrations with clinical efficacy and toxicity quickly followed. In the 1970s, physicians, pharmacists, and laboratory technologists began forming specialized therapeutic drug monitoring or clinical pharmacokinetics services in hospitals. Today, with the emergence of immunoassays that require no specialized equipment, drug concentration measurements can be easily performed in physician offices.[5]

The drug concentration assays most widely available in hospital laboratories are for antiepileptics (carbamazepine, ethosuximide, primidone/phenobarbital, phenytoin, and valproic acid), cardiac drugs (digoxin, procainamide/N-acetylprocainamide [NAPA], and quinidine), antibiotics (aminoglycosides and vancomycin), theophylline, and lithium. But there is new research showing correlations between drug concentration and response for additional groups of drugs such as the psychotropics, immunosuppressants, and antimycobacterial, anticancer, and antiretroviral drugs. Drugs in these groups are currently monitored only in certain circumstances, in special treatment centers, or in research settings, but they may become more routinely monitored as the relationships between drug concentration and response become clearer.

The increased availability and convenience of drug assay methods has led to a number of concerns. Is therapeutic drug monitoring being done simply because it is available, rather than because it is clinically necessary? There are numerous reports of suboptimal therapeutic drug monitoring practices that contribute to inappropriate decision-making as well as wasted resources.[6-8] Questions are also being raised about whether therapeutic drug monitoring actually improves patient outcomes.[9,10] However, many clinicians claim that therapeutic drug monitoring is greatly underused and could, if appropriately used, further improve patient care and save healthcare dollars.[11,12] Clearly, there is a need for more education of all healthcare professionals involved in the therapeutic drug monitoring process in order to make its use more appropriate and cost-effective. Such education efforts have been shown to effectively reduce the numbers of inappropriate drug concentration requests.[13]

Goal and Indications for Drug Concentration Monitoring

The primary goal of therapeutic drug monitoring is to maximize the benefit of a drug to a patient in the shortest possible time with minimal risk of toxicity. The number of hospitalizations or office visits used to adjust therapies or manage and diagnose adverse drug reactions may therefore be reduced, resulting in cost savings.

Drug concentration measurements should not be performed unless the result will affect some future action or decision. Monitoring should not be done simply because the opportunity presents itself; it should be used discriminatingly to answer clinically relevant questions and resolve or anticipate problems in drug therapy management.[14] The clinician should always ask, "Will this drug concentration value provide more information to me than sound clinical judgment alone?"[9] The following are examples of clinical situations and the clinical questions that drug concentration measurements might be able to answer:

- **Therapeutic confirmation:** A patient is on a regimen that appears to offer maximum benefit with acceptable side effects. *Question: What is the drug concentration associated with a therapeutic effect in this patient for future reference?*
- **Dosage optimization:** A patient has a condition in which clinical response is not easily measured, and has been initiated on a standard regimen of a drug. There is modest improvement and no symptoms of toxicity are evident. *Question: Can I increase the dose rate to further enhance effect? If so, by how much?*
- **Confirmation of suspected toxicity:** A patient is experiencing certain signs and symptoms that could be related to the drug. *Question: Are these signs and symptoms most likely related to a dose rate that is too high? Can I reduce the daily dose, and if so, by how much?*
- **Avoidance of inefficacy or toxicity:** A patient is initiated on a standard regimen of an antibiotic that is known to be poorly absorbed in a small percentage of patients. Sustained subtherapeutic concentrations of

this drug can lead to drug-resistance. *Question: Will a higher daily dose be needed in this patient?* A patient has been satisfactorily treated on a dosage regimen of Drug A. The patient experiences a change in health or physiologic status or a second drug, suspected to interact with Drug A, is added. *Question: Will a dosage regimen adjustment be needed to avoid inefficacy or toxicity?*
- **Distinguishing nonadherence from treatment failure:** A patient has not responded to usual doses and noncompliance is a possibility. *Question: Is this a treatment failure or does the patient need counseling on adherence?*

Characteristics of Ideal Drugs for Therapeutic Drug Monitoring

Not all drugs are good candidates for therapeutic drug monitoring, no matter how appropriate the indication seems to be. Those for which drug concentration monitoring will be most useful have the following characteristics[15]:

- **Readily available assays:** Methods for drug concentration measurement must be available to the clinician at a cost to justify the information to be gained. Analytical methods for some drugs are routinely available in hospitals or in physician offices. Methods for newer drugs or drugs used in specialized treatment centers are not as widely available but, nevertheless, are essential for that patient population.
- **Lack of easily observable, safe, or desirable clinical endpoint:** Clinically, there is no immediate, easily monitored, and/or predictable clinical parameter to guide dosage titration. For example, waiting for arrhythmias or seizures to occur or resume may be an unsafe and undesirable approach to dosing antiarrhythmics and antiepileptics.
- **Dangerous toxicity or lack of effectiveness:** Toxicity or lack of effectiveness of the drug presents a danger to the patient. For example, serum drug concentrations of the antifungal drug, flucytosine, are not routinely monitored. However, specialized monitoring may be done to ensure that levels are below 100 mg/L to avoid gastrointestinal side effects, blood dyscrasias, and hepatotoxicity. As another example, specialized monitoring of the protease inhibitors (PIs) may be done to ensure adequate levels since rapid emergence of antiviral resistance is observed with sustained exposure to subtherapeutic levels.
- **Unpredictable dose–response relationship:** There is an unpredictable dose–response relationship, such that a dose producing therapeutic benefit in one patient may cause toxicity in another patient. This would be true for drugs that have significant interpatient variation in pharmacokinetic parameters, drugs with nonlinear behavior, and drugs whose pharmacokinetic parameters are affected by concomitant administration of other drugs. For example, patients given the same daily dose of phenytoin can demonstrate a wide range of serum concentrations and responses.
- **Narrow therapeutic range:** The drug concentrations

associated with therapeutic effect overlap considerably with the concentrations associated with toxic effects, such that the zone for therapeutic benefit without toxicity is very narrow. For example, the therapeutic range of phenytoin is widely accepted to be 10–20 mg/L for most patients; the upper limit of the range is only twice the lower limit.

- **Good correlation between drug concentration and efficacy or toxicity:** This criterion must apply if we are using drug concentrations to adjust the dosage regimen of a drug. For example, a patient showing unsatisfactory asthma control with a serum theophylline concentration of 5 mg/L is likely to show improved control with a doubling of the daily dose to attain a serum concentration of 10 mg/L.

TABLE 5-1. Information Needed on Laboratory Request Form

TYPE OF DATA	SPECIFIC DATA	WHY NECESSARY
Patient identification	• Name, address, identification number, and physician name	All blood samples look alike and could easily be switched among patients without appropriate identification
Patient demographics and characteristics	• Age, gender, ethnicity, height, weight, and pregnancy	The therapeutic range for a given drug may depend on the specific indication being treated (e.g., digoxin for atrial arrhythmias versus heart failure); if there is no history of prior drug concentration measurements, information about concurrent disease states, physiologic status, and social habits may help with initial determination of population pharmacokinetic parameters, in order to determine if the resulting level is expected or not; information about renal function and albumin is important if a total drug level is being measured for a drug normally highly bound to serum proteins; it is also important to know if any endogenous substances due to diseases will interfere with the assay; electrolyte abnormalities may affect interpretation of a given concentration (e.g., digoxin)
History and physical examination	• Condition being treated • Organ involvement (renal, hepatic, cardiac, gastrointestinal, and endocrine) • Fluid balance and nutritional status • Labs (albumin, total protein, liver function enzymes, INR, bilirubin, serum creatinine or creatinine clearance, thyroid status, and electrolyte abnormalities) • Smoking and alcohol history	
Specimen information	• Time of collection • Nature of specimen: blood, urine, or other body fluid site of collection • Order of sample, if part of a series • Type of collection tube • Time of receipt by laboratory	Laboratories often retain samples for several days and detailed information will help to find a sample if important pre-post or random samples are needed; the time of collection relative to the dose is extremely important for proper interpretation; (Close to a trough? Closer to a peak?) knowing the type of collection tube is important because of the many interferences that may occur; it is important to know the collection site relative to the administration site, if intravenous route is used; if a series of samples is to be drawn, the labeled timing of the collection tubes can get mixed up
Drug information	• Name of drug to be assayed • Current dosage regimen, including route • Type of formulation (sustained-release, delayed-release, or prompt-release) • Length of time on current regimen • Time of last dose • Concurrent drug therapy • Duration of intravenous infusion	It is important to know if the concentration was drawn at a steady-state and when the level was drawn relative to the last dose; it is also important to know if there are any potential drug interferences with the assay to be used
Drug concentration history	• Dates and times of prior concentration measurements • Response and drug regimen schedules associated with prior concentrations	It is important to know what drug concentrations have been documented as effective or associated with toxicity; it is also important to know how drug concentrations have changed as a consequence of dosage regimen
Purpose of assay and urgency of request	• Therapeutic confirmation • Suspected toxicity • Anticipated inefficacy or toxicity due to change in physiologic/health status or drug–drug interaction • Identification of drug failure • Suspected overdose	This forces the clinician to have a specific clinical question in mind before ordering a sample; it also aids in the interpretation of results

Source: Adapted with permission from references 15 and 16.

TABLE 5-2. Common Reasons Why Drug Concentration Results Do Not Make Sense

CATEGORY OF FACTOR	SPECIFIC EXAMPLES
Related to drug administration or blood sampling logistics	• Wrong dose or infusion rate administered • Dose skipped or infusion held for a period of time • Dose given at time other than recorded; blood drawn as ordered • Dose given at right time; blood drawn at time other than recorded • Sample taken through an administration line, which was improperly flushed prior to sample withdrawal • Sample taken from the wrong patient • Improper or prolonged storage prior to delivery to laboratory • Wrong collection tube/device used • Patient was dialyzed between doses
Related to pharmacokinetics	• Sample is drawn prior to a steady-state • Orders for digoxin samples are not clearly specified to be drawn at least 6 hr postdistribution • Samples are ordered for the wrong times relative to last dose to reflect specific needs (e.g., peaks and/or troughs) • Concentrations of active metabolites are not ordered when appropriate • Concentrations for total drug are ordered for a drug with unusual serum protein binding without recognition that the usual therapeutic range of total drug will not apply • Samples following intravenous administration are drawn prior to completion of distribution phase (e.g., vancomycin, aminoglycosides)
Related to the laboratory	• The wrong drug is assayed • Critical active metabolites are not assayed • Interferences or artifacts caused by endogenous substances (bilirubin, lipids, and hemolysis) or concurrent drugs • Improper or prolonged storage prior to assay • Technical errors with the assay
Related to the patient	Patient is not adherent with therapy

Source: Adapted with permission from references 16 and 20.

Other than availability of an assay, it may not be necessary for a drug to fulfill all of the above characteristics for drug concentration monitoring to help guide clinical decision-making. Newer drugs that do not yet have clearly defined therapeutic ranges may be monitored only under special circumstances (e.g., to ensure adherence). Other drugs may not have a clearly defined upper or lower limit to the therapeutic range but are monitored under special circumstances to ensure efficacy or avoid toxicity. This goes back to the importance of the drug concentration for answering a specific clinical question: Will the information provided by this measurement help to improve the patient's drug therapy?

Information Needed for Planning and Evaluating Drug Concentrations

Drug concentrations should be interpreted in light of full information about the patient, including clinical status. Information about the timing of the sample relative to the last dose is especially critical and is one of the biggest factors making drug concentrations unusable or cost-ineffective.[6,17–19] Table 5-1 provides a list of the essential information needed for a drug concentration request. Laboratory request forms or computer entry forms must be designed to encourage entry of the most important information. All relevant information should be included on both the request form and the report form to facilitate accurate interpretation. It is particularly important to verify the time of sample draw because phlebotomists or computer-generated labels commonly identify samples with the time of the intended draw instead of the actual draw time. Some hospital laboratories have minimized the number of inappropriate samples by refusing to run any samples that are not accompanied by critical information, such as the timing of the sample relative to the last dose.[6] The laboratory report form should also include the assay used; active metabolite concentration (if measured); and parameters reflecting the sensitivity, specificity, and precision of the method.

Accuracy and completeness of the information provided on a laboratory request form is particularly important in light of the many problems that can occur during the therapeutic drug monitoring process. A drug concentration that seems to be illogical, given the information provided on the form, may be explained by a variety of factors as shown in Table 5-2. (See Minicase 1.)

Considerations for Appropriate Interpretation of Drug Concentrations

To appropriately interpret a drug concentration, it is important to have as many answers as possible to the following questions:

- **Therapeutic range:** What do the studies show to be the usual therapeutic range? How frequently will patients show response at a concentration below the lower limit of the usual range? How frequently will patients show toxicity at a level below the upper limit of the usual range? What are the usual signs and symptoms indicating toxicity?

MINICASE 1

Bouncing Theophylline Levels

CHARLES W., A 65-YEAR-OLD MALE patient with COPD, had been taking sustained-release oral theophylline at home, 300 mg q 12 hr. Previous testing showed Charles W.'s bronchospasm was relieved at this dose rate with serum theophylline levels between 12 and 13 mg/L. The theophylline half-life was documented as 12 hours.

Charles W. now arrives at the local emergency room experiencing bronchospasm; he admits that he stopped taking his theophylline 3 days ago. He is started on an aminophylline infusion of 30 mg/hr at 6 p.m. on Monday. His physician orders a theophylline level for Tuesday morning; the level is drawn then at 6 a.m. A concentration of 6 mg/L is reported Tuesday afternoon at 3 p.m., and the physician immediately increases the aminophylline infusion rate to 60 mg/hr because of poor clinical response. He assumed that doubling the infusion rate would double the serum theophylline concentration.

At 6 p.m. on Wednesday, Charles W. complains of nausea, palpitations, and jitteriness; his heart rate is 110. The physician orders a stat theophylline level; the laboratory calls 2 hours later with a critical value of 21 mg/L. The physician decreases the infusion rate back to 30 mg/hr; a level drawn 48 hours later is 13 mg/L. Charles W.'s bronchospasm is relieved.

Question: Why did the original rate of 30 mg/hr not yield a serum theophylline concentration of 12 mg/L as it did at the end of the case?

What could have been done to avoid the bouncing concentrations and side effects?

Discussion: This case shows how drug toxicity and unnecessary costs can result when practitioners fail to consider the concept of a steady-state when interpreting drug concentrations. It also illustrates practical issues when this type of patient comes to the emergency room. The outpatient theophylline dose rate of 300 mg q 12 hr had previously been shown to result in a serum level between 12 and 13 mg/L. By converting this to a similar dose rate of theophylline, given in the salt form of aminophylline, we would predict a serum theophylline level close to 12 mg/L once at a steady-state. The physician failed to understand that the level of 6 mg/L (in the blood sample drawn after only one half-life) represented only 50% of the eventual steady-state concentration. By doubling the infusion rate, serum theophylline concentrations would have doubled to a steady-state level of 24 mg/L if a steady-state had been attained. Charles W. exhibited signs and symptoms of theophylline toxicity after three half-lives (36 hours) and the serum level of 18 mg/L at that time represented 88% of the eventual steady-state level. By returning to the original infusion rate of 30 mg/hr and waiting four half-lives before sampling, it was confirmed that this is an appropriate infusion rate for Charles W., who is responding.

Minicase 1 is adapted from the second edition chapter titled "Interpretation of Serum Drug Concentrations," which was written by Scott L. Traub.

- **Sample timing:** Was the sample drawn at a steady-state? Was the sample drawn at a time during the dosing interval (if intermittent therapy) that reflects the intended indication for monitoring (a peak, a trough, a so-called "random" level, or an average level)? During the dosing interval, when is a peak level most likely to occur for the formulation administered? Does the formulation exhibit a lag-time for release or absorption, such that the lowest level will occur into the next dosing interval?
- **Specimen, collection method, and assay:** Was the collected specimen (serum, plasma, whole blood, and saliva) appropriate for the assay that was used? Was the blood collection method artifact-free or interference-free? Is saliva (or some other fluid) an appropriate non-invasive alternative to blood collection? Was the saliva collected according to a standardized protocol? Was the storage method appropriate based on studies of stability in the specimen used? Was the assay suitably sensitive and precise for concentrations being measured? Is there any reason to believe, based on the assay, that there might be interferences (over-reading, under-reading) from endogenous substances in the specimen, concurrent drugs, or metabolites?
- **Use of levels for dosage adjustment:** Does the drug display first-order (linear) pharmacokinetic behavior such that an increase in daily dose will produce a proportional increase in the drug concentration? Is the dosage adjustment method focused on attaining specific peaks and/or trough, or specific average levels?
- **Protein binding, active metabolites, and enantiomers:** How are total drug concentrations in serum interpreted in cases of altered serum protein binding? How are concentrations or contributions of active metabolite considered along with parent drug? Is the drug administered as a racemic mixture and if so, do the enantiomers differ in activity and pharmacokinetic behavior? Do certain physiologic or pathologic conditions affect a patient's response to the drug at a given concentration?

Each of these categories will be described in general below and, more specifically, for each drug or drug class in the Applications section.

THE THERAPEUTIC RANGE

A *therapeutic range* (also referred to as a *therapeutic reference range*[21,22]) is best defined as a "range of drug concentrations within which the probability of the desired clinical response is relatively high and the probability of unacceptable toxicity is relatively low."[1] This means that the reference range reported by a laboratory is actually a population-based average for which the majority of patients are expected to respond with acceptable side effects. Thus, there will always be some patients who exhibit therapeutic effect at drug concentrations below the lower limit, while others will experience unacceptable toxicity at levels below the upper limit. Therefore, a patient's therapy is always best guided by that patient's individual therapeutic concentration.[21,22]

Figure 5-1 illustrates how the probability of response and toxicity increases with drug concentration for a hypothetical drug and how a therapeutic range might be determined based on these relative probabilities. Figure 5-2 shows how patterns for response and toxicity can differ in two different patients receiving the same drug. If the hypothetical drug in question has an active metabolite that accumulates more than the parent drug in renal impairment, and if that metabolite contributes more to toxicity than to efficacy, then the individual therapeutic range in the patient with renal impairment will be narrower with lower concentrations. Concentration monitoring of the active metabolite would be especially important in that situation.

Drug concentration monitoring is often criticized by claims that therapeutic ranges are not sufficiently well defined.[11,12] The lack of clearly-defined therapeutic ranges for older drugs is partially attributable to how these ranges were originally determined. Eadie describes the process that was typically used for determination of the therapeutic ranges of the antiepileptic drugs: "These ranges do not appear to have been determined by rigorous statistical procedures applied to large patient populations. Rather, workers seem to have set the lower limits for each drug at the concentration at which they perceived a reasonable (though usually unspecified) proportion of patients achieved seizure control, and the upper limit at the concentration above which overdosage-type adverse effects appear to trouble appreciable numbers of patients, the values then being rounded off to provide a pair of numbers, which are reasonably easy to remember."[14] In an ideal world, studies to define therapeutic ranges for drugs should use reliable methods for measurement of response and should be restricted to patients with the same diseases, age range, and concurrent medications.[1] In recent years, the Food and Drug Administration (FDA) has recognized the importance of determining concentration versus response relationships early during clinical trials.[23]

What factors can affect a therapeutic range for a given patient? Anything that affects the pharmacodynamics of a drug, meaning the response at a given drug concentration, will affect the therapeutic range. These factors include

- **Indication:** Drugs that are used for more than one indication are likely to be interacting with different receptors. Thus, a different concentration versus response profile might be expected depending on the disease being treated. For example, higher serum concentrations of digoxin are needed for treatment of atrial fibrillation as compared to congestive heart failure. Higher antibiotic drug concentrations may be needed for resistant organisms or to penetrate certain infected tissues.
- **Active metabolites:** As shown in Figure 5-2, variable presence of an active metabolite can shift the therapeutic range for that individual patient up or down. These

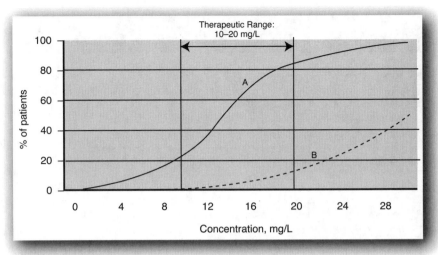

FIGURE 5-1. The therapeutic range for a hypothetical drug. Line A is the percentage of patients displaying a therapeutic effect; line B is the percentage of patients displaying toxicity.

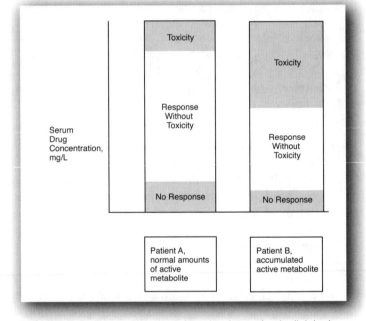

FIGURE 5-2. Representation showing how the individual therapeutic range of a hypothetical drug can differ in a patient with renal impairment because of accumulated active metabolite.

metabolites may behave in a manner similar to the parent drug or may interact with different receptors altogether. In either case, the relationship between parent drug concentration and response will be altered.
- **Concurrent drug treatment:** In a manner similar to active metabolites, the presence of other drugs that have similar pharmacodynamic activities will contribute to efficacy or toxicity but not to measurement of the drug concentration. The therapeutic range will be shifted.
- **Patient's age:** While there is not much information concerning developmental changes in pharmacodynamics, it is believed that the numbers and affinities of pharma-

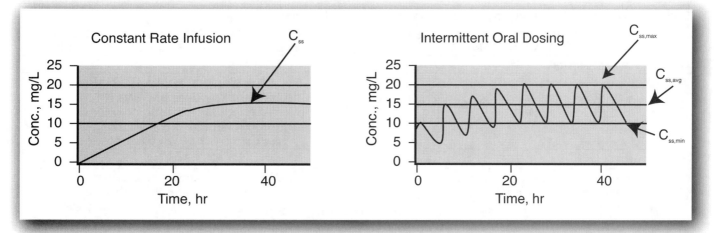

FIGURE 5-3. Concentration versus time plots for a constant infusion and intermittent therapy after initiation of therapy, without a loading dose. The half-life for this hypothetical drug is 8 hours. Thus, 88% of the eventual average steady-state concentration ($C_{ss,avg}$) is attained in 24 hours.

cologic receptors change with progression of age from newborns to advanced age.[24] This would be expected to result in a shift of the therapeutic range.

- **Electrolyte status:** As an example, hypokalemia, hypomagnesemia, and hypercalcemia are all known to increase the cardiac effects of digitalis glycosides and enhance the potential for digoxin toxicity at a given serum concentration.[25]
- **Concurrent disease:** As an example, patients with underlying heart disease (cor pulmonale or coronary, atherosclerotic heart disease) have increased sensitivity to digoxin.[25] There is also evidence that thyroid disease alters the usual response patterns of digoxin.[22]
- **Variable ratios of enantiomers:** Some drugs are administered as racemic mixtures of enantiomers, which may have different response/toxicity profiles as well as pharmacokinetic behaviors. Thus, a given level of the summed enantiomers (using an achiral assay method) will be associated with different levels of response or toxicity in patients with different proportions of the enantiomers. This has been extensively studied for disopyramide.[26]
- **Variable genotype:** There is growing evidence that response to certain drugs is genetically determined. For selected drugs, patients may be genotyped before starting drug treatment in order to identify them as nonresponders, responders, or toxic responders (see Chapter 7: Pharmacogenomics and Molecular Testing).[27-29]
- **Variable serum protein binding:** Theoretically, only the unbound concentration of drug in blood is capable of establishing equilibrium with pharmacologic receptors, thus making it a better predictor of response than total drug concentration. Most drug concentrations in serum, plasma, or blood, however, are measured as the summed concentration of bound and unbound drug. It is very likely that some of the patients who show toxicity within the conventional therapeutic range have abnormally low protein binding and high concentrations of

unbound drug in blood.[30] Low protein binding of a drug in blood can be the result of either reduced protein concentrations or the presence of other substances in blood that displace the drug from protein binding sites.

In summary, the therapeutic range reported by the laboratory is only an initial guide and is not a guarantee of desired clinical response in any individual patient. Every effort must be made to consider other signs of clinical response and toxicity in addition to the drug concentration measurement. Therapeutic ranges for the most commonly monitored drugs discussed in the Applications section of this chapter are reported in Table 5-3.

SAMPLE TIMING

Incorrect timing of sample collection is the most frequent source of error when therapeutic drug monitoring results do not agree with the clinical picture.[19,31] Warner reviewed five studies in which 70% to 86% of the samples obtained for therapeutic drug monitoring purposes were not usable. In most cases, this was the result of inappropriate sample timing, including lack of attention to the time required to reach a steady-state. There are two primary considerations for sample timing: (1) how long to wait after initiation or adjustment of a dosage regimen, and (2) when to obtain the sample during a dosing interval.

At steady-state. When a drug dosage regimen (a fixed dose given at a regularly repeated interval) is initiated, concentrations are initially low and gradually increase until a steady-state is reached. Pharmacokinetically, *steady-state* is defined as the condition in which the rate of drug entering the body is equal to the rate of its elimination. For the purpose of therapeutic drug monitoring, a steady-state means that drug concentrations have leveled off at their highest and, when given as the same dose at a fixed interval, the concentration versus time profiles are constant from interval to interval. This is illustrated in Figure 5-3 for a constant infusion and a chronic intermittent dosage regimen.

TABLE 5-3. Data to Aid Interpretation of Concentrations of Drugs That Are Commonly Monitored

	RECOMMENDED CONCENTRATIONS	RECOMMENDED TIMING	CONSIDERATIONS FOR INTERPRETATION: PROTEIN BINDING, ACTIVE METABOLITES, OTHER FACTORS
Analgesic/Anti-Inflammatory			
Salicylate	20–100 mg/L (analgesic/antipyretic 100–250 mg/L (anti-inflammatory)	Trough or $C_{ss,avg}$ Steady-state occurs after 1 week	Salicylic acid binding to albumin is concentration-dependent; unbound fractions increase in pregnancy and in patients with liver disease, nephrotic syndrome, and uremia; lower total levels might be more appropriate in these patients with decreased serum binding
Antiasthmatics			
Theophylline	Adult: 5–15 mg/L Neonate: 5–10 mg/L	Trough or $C_{ss,avg}$ Steady-state occurs in 24 hr for an average adult nonsmoker receiving a maintenance infusion but may take longer for sustained-release products	Levels up to 20 mg/L may be necessary in some patients; the caffeine metabolite is of minor significance in adults but may contribute to effect in neonates
Caffeine	Neonate: 10–20 mg/L	At least 2-hr postdose Steady-state not necessary	
Antiepileptics			
Carbamazepine	4–12 mg/L	Trough or $C_{ss,avg}$ Steady-state may require up to 2–3 weeks after initiation of full dose rate	Lower total concentrations may be more appropriate in patients with decreased protein binding—liver disease, hypoalbuminemia, and hyperbilirubinemia
Ethosuximide	40–100 mg/L	Anytime during interval; steady-state may require up to 12 days	
Phenobarbital	10–40 mg/L	Anytime during interval; steady-state may require up to 3 weeks	
Phenytoin	Adult: 10–20 mg/L (total) Infant: 6–11 mg/L (total)	Trough or $C_{ss,avg}$ Steady-state may require up to 3 weeks	Measurement of unbound phenytoin levels (therapeutic range of 1–2 mg/L) may be preferred in most patients; lower total phenytoin levels may be more appropriate in patients with decreased protein binding due to hypoalbuminemia (e.g., liver disease, nephrotic syndrome, pregnancy, cystic fibrosis, burns, trauma, malnutrition, AIDS, and advanced age), end-stage renal disease, concurrent salicylic acid or valproic acid
Primidone	5–12 mg/L	Steady-state may require up to 3 weeks	Phenobarbital is a metabolite of primidone and may be a primary determinant of primidone effect; it must always be measured when primidone is administered
Valproic acid	50–120 mg/L	Trough or $C_{ss,avg}$ Steady-state may require up to 5 days	Lower total valproic acid levels may be more appropriate in patients with hypoalbuminemia, (liver disease, cystic fibrosis, burns, trauma, malnutrition, and advanced age), hyperbilirubinemia, end-stage renal disease, and concurrent salicylic acid; valproic acid shows interpatient variability in unbound fraction because of nonlinear protein binding; total concentrations will increase less than proportionately with increases in daily dose, while unbound concentrations will increase proportionately
Antimicrobial Drugs			
Amikacin	Traditional dosing: Peaks: 20–30 mg/L Troughs: 1–8 mg/L	Traditional dosing: steady-state should be based on estimated half-life, particularly in patients with renal impairment Pulse dosing: per protocol	
Gentamicin, netilmicin, tobramycin	Traditional dosing: Peaks: 6–10 mg/L Troughs: 0.5–2 mg/L	Traditional dosing: steady-state should be based on estimated half-life, particularly in patients with renal impairment Pulse dosing: per protocol	

TABLE 5-3. Data to Aid Interpretation of Concentrations of Drugs That Are Commonly Monitored, cont'd

	RECOMMENDED CONCENTRATIONS	RECOMMENDED TIMING	CONSIDERATIONS FOR INTERPRETATION: PROTEIN BINDING, ACTIVE METABOLITES, OTHER FACTORS
Vancomycin	Peaks: 30–50 mg/L Troughs: 5–15 mg/L	Trough, within 1 hr of next dose; steady-state may require up to 2–3 days in patients with normal renal function	Desired trough levels may be as high as 20 mg/L in some institutions for certain resistant strains
Cardiac Drugs			
Digoxin	0.5–2.0 mcg/L	NEVER sooner than 6 hr after an oral dose; steady-state may require up to 7 days with normal renal function	Lower end of range used for heart failure; higher end for atrial arrhythmias; toxicity more likely within therapeutic range in patients with hypokalemia, hypomagnesemia, hypercalcemia, underlying heart disease, and hypothyroidism; patients with hyperthyroidism may be resistant at a given digoxin level
Lidocaine	1.5–5 mg/L	Anytime during infusion once steady-state is reached; steady-state may require up to 24 hr	High lidocaine levels in postmyocardial infarction patients may not be associated with toxicity because of increased serum binding; higher total levels may be acceptable in other conditions associated with increased binding—rheumatoid arthritis, cancer, morbid obesity, or any kind of physiologic trauma
Procainamide/ N-acetyl-procainamide (NAPA)	Procainamide: 4–8 mg/L, up to 12 mg/L in some NAPA: 5–30 mg/L	May require up to 18 hr with normal renal function for steady-state of both parent and NAPA	NAPA levels will accumulate more than procainamide in patients with renal impairment; NAPA should always be measured along with procainamide in these patients. Levels of procainamide and NAPA should be separately compared to their own therapeutic ranges, rather than to a therapeutic range of summed concentrations
Quinidine	2–8 mg/L	Trough, within 1 hr of next oral dose; steady-state may require up to 3 days	Higher total levels may be acceptable in conditions associated with increased binding—myocardial infarction, cardiac surgery, atrial arrhythmias, heart failure, or any other kind of physiologic trauma
Cytotoxic Drugs			
Methotrexate	0.01–0.1 μM (per protocol)	Per protocol for determination of leucovorin rescue regimen	Decreased protein binding is observed in some situations, but implications for interpretation of total levels are unclear
Immunosuppressives			
Cyclosporine	100–500 mcg/L (whole blood, using specific assay)	Trough or 2-hr postdose; steady-state may require up to 5 days	Highly variable unbound fraction in blood; higher total levels may be acceptable in patients with hypercholesterolemia or prior to acute rejection episodes (increased serum binding); lower total levels might be acceptable in patients with decreased binding in serum (low cholesterol)
Psychotropics			
Amitriptyline	Amitriptyline + nortriptyline: 120–250 mcg/L	12–14 hr after the bedtime dose for once-daily dosing; steady-state may require up to 11 days	
Nortriptyline	50–150 mcg/L		
Imipramine	Imipramine + desipramine: 180–350 mcg/L	12–14 hr after the bedtime dose for once-daily dosing; steady-state may require up to 6 days for steady-state	Unbound fractions are decreased in alcoholics and cardiac patients; higher total concentrations may be acceptable in patients suspected to have higher binding; active metabolites (desipramine of imipramine and nortriptyline of amitriptyline) must always be determined in addition to the parent drug, as they contributed significantly to therapeutic effect
Desipramine	115–250 mcg/L		
Lithium	0.5–1.2 mEq/L (acute management) 0.6–0.8 mEq/L (maintenance)	12 hr after the evening dose on BID or TID schedule; steady-state may require up to 1 week	

AIDS = acquired immune deficiency syndrome.

Drug concentration measurements should not be made until the drug is sufficiently close to a steady-state, so that the maximum benefit of the drug is ensured. (See Minicase 2.) The time required to reach a steady-state can be predicted if the drug's half-life is known, as follows:

Number of Half-Lives	Percentage of Steady-State Attained
2	75%
3	88%
4	94%
5	97%

This means the clinician should wait three half-lives at a minimum before obtaining a sample for monitoring purposes. The clinician should also anticipate that the "usual" half-life in a given patient may be actually longer due to impaired elimination processes, and it may be prudent to wait longer if possible. The half-lives of drugs that are typically monitored are reported in the Applications section, and typical times to steady-state are reported in Table 5-3.

Sometimes drugs are not given as a fixed dose at a fixed interval, or they may undergo diurnal variations in pharmacokinetic handling.[32,33] While the concentration versus time profiles may differ from each other within a given day, the patterns from day-to-day will be the same if a steady-state has been attained. In cases of irregular dosing or diurnal variations, it is important that drug concentration measurements on different visits be obtained at similar times of the day for comparative purposes.

An unusual situation is caused by autoinduction, as exemplified by carbamazepine. The half-life of carbamazepine is longer after the first dose but progressively shortens as the enzymes that metabolize carbamazepine are induced by exposure to itself.[34] The half-life of carbamazepine during chronic therapy cannot be used to predict the time required to reach a steady-state. The actual time to reach a steady-state is somewhere between the time based on the first-dose half-life and that based on the chronic-dosing half-life.

It is a common misconception that a steady-state is reached faster when a loading dose is given. While a carefully chosen loading dose will provide desired target levels following that first dose, the resulting level is only an approximation of the true steady-state level, and it will still require at least three half-lives to attain a true steady-state. Whenever possible, it is best to allow more time for a steady-state to be attained than less. This is also important because the average half-life for the population may not apply to a specific patient.

There are some exceptions to the rule of waiting until a steady-state is reached before sampling. If there is suspected toxicity early during therapy, a drug concentration measurement is warranted and may necessitate immediate reduction of the dose rate. Dosing methods designed to predict maintenance dosage regimens using pre-steady-state drug levels are useful when rapid individualization of the dosage regimen is needed.[35-40]

Within the dosing interval. Figure 5-3 shows typical concentration versus time profiles for a drug given by constant infusion and a drug given by oral intermittent dosing. Once a

---

MINICASE 2

Importance of Documenting Drug Administration Times

ANGELA M. IS A 35-YEAR-OLD FEMALE who is receiving aminoglycoside monotherapy for treatment of a gram-negative infection. According to the medical chart, she has received 5 doses of tobramycin as 100 mg infused over 30 minutes, q 8 hr on a 6 a.m./2 p.m./10 p.m. schedule. The estimated half-life of tobramycin, based on Angela M.'s creatinine clearance, is 4.5 hours. Two serum tobramycin levels are ordered in order to determine if peak and trough serum levels are within the desired ranges of 6–10 mg/L and 0.5–2 mg/L, respectively. A trough serum level drawn at 1:50 p.m., just before the start of infusion of the 6th dose is 0.8 mg/L. A second level, drawn 30 minutes after the end of infusion of the 6th dose, is used to calculate a peak serum tobramycin level of 7.8 mg/L. Based on this information, the current regimen is continued. Repeat levels drawn 2 days later, however, reveal a peak tobramycin level of 10.1 mg/L and trough of 2.9 mg/L. Renal function, as indicated by creatinine clearance, has not changed in this patient. If this second set of serum concentrations is accurate, a dosage adjustment is critical to avoid aminoglycoside toxicity.

Question: What are the possible explanations for the apparent change in serum tobramycin level results? Which set of tobramycin levels accurately reflects the current dosage regimen?

Discussion: In a situation such as this, one should always consider whether the first levels were drawn at a steady-state. With an estimated tobramycin half-life of 4.5 hours, a steady-state was most certainly attained after 5 doses or 40 hours. A second consideration would be changing renal function. Since the aminoglycoside antibiotics are handled almost exclusively by the kidney, a decrease in renal function would explain the increase in serum tobramycin levels. In this case, however, renal function has not changed. A third consideration would be laboratory error or assay interference/artifact. Artifactually low serum tobramycin concentrations might have resulted if beta-lactam antibiotics had been coadministered during the time that the first set of samples was drawn; no other antibiotics were being coadministered, however. Assuming that laboratory error is ruled out, one must finally investigate the possibility of inaccurate documentation of either blood sample or drug administration times. Further scrutiny revealed that the 5th dose of tobramycin was held. Consequently, an extra 8 hours of washout occurred prior to blood sampling and the levels drawn before and after the 6th dose where lower than would be expected. These levels did not reflect the 100 mg, q-8-hr tobramycin regimen. After ensuring that all subsequent doses were appropriately administered and that the second set of blood samples was appropriately timed and documented, an adjusted dosage regimen of 80 mg q 12 hr was ordered.

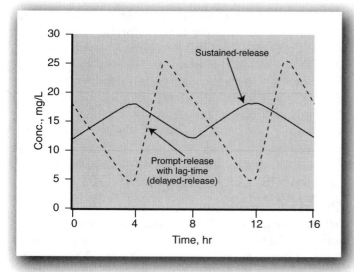

FIGURE 5-4. Concentration versus time profiles for a prompt-release formulation that exhibits a lag-time in its release or absorption (delayed-release) as compared to a sustained-release formulation without lag-time. Note that the lowest concentration during the dosing interval for the delayed-release product occurs at a time that is typically expected for the peak to occur.

(Interval-Peak Time)/ Half-Life	Peak:Trough Ratio
2.00	4.0
1.50	2.8
1.00	2.0
0.50	1.4
0.25	1.2

Using the information above, concentrations during the interval fluctuate very little (peaks are only 1.2 times troughs) if the difference between the dosing interval and peak time is one-quarter of the drug's half-life. In that case, it may be assumed that concentrations obtained anytime during the interval are almost equivalent; the peak, trough, and average concentrations are roughly equal.

The choice of timing for samples within the dosing interval should be based on the clinical question to be addressed. Troughs are usually recommended for therapeutic confirmation, especially if the therapeutic range was formulated based on trough levels as for most of the antiepileptic drugs.[14] Trough concentrations are also recommended if the indication for concentration monitoring is avoidance of inefficacy or distinguishing nonadherence from therapeutic failure. Trough concentrations should also be monitored if the patient tends to experience symptoms of inefficacy before the next dose (in which case a shortening of the dosing interval might be all that is needed). While it is logical to assume that the lowest concentration during the interval will occur immediately before the next dose, this is not always the case. Some products are formulated as delayed-release products (e.g., enteric-coated valproic acid) that are designed to be absorbed from the intestine rather than the stomach. As such, they may not begin to be absorbed for several hours after administration, and the level of drug from the previous dose continues to decline for several hours into the next interval. It is important to recognize that the predose level for those formulations is not the lowest level during the interval (Figure 5-4).

Peak concentrations are monitored less often for drugs given orally because the time at which peak concentrations occur is difficult to predict. If a peak concentration is indicated, the package insert should be consulted for peak times of individual products. Peak concentration monitoring would be appropriate if the patient complains of symptoms of toxicity at a time believed to correspond with a peak concentration. Peaks may also be used for intravenous drugs (aminoglycosides and chloramphenicol) because the time of the peak is known to correspond to the end of the infusion. For the aminoglycosides, the peak level is believed to be a predictor of efficacy, while for chloramphenicol the peak concentration predicts both efficacy and adverse effects.[42]

Sometimes the clinician wishes to get an idea of the average level of drug during the day or dosing interval. This is particularly useful when the level is to be used for a dosage adjustment. Pharmacokinetically, the average level equals the area-under-the-curve (AUC) during the dosing interval (requiring multiple samples) divided by the interval. (Note: The AUC during an

steady-state is attained, drug concentrations during a constant infusion remain constant, and samples for drug concentration measurements can be obtained at any time. When a drug is given intermittently, however, there is fluctuation in the drug concentration profile. The lowest concentration during the interval is known as the *steady-state minimum concentration*, or the *trough*. The highest concentration is known as the *steady-state maximum concentration*, or the *peak*. Also shown in Figure 5-3 is the *steady-state average concentration* ($C_{ss,avg}$), which represents the time-averaged concentration during the dosage interval. An important principle of dosing for drugs that show first-order behavior is that the average concentration during the interval or day will change in direct proportion to the change in the daily dose. This is covered in more detail in the Use of Levels for Dosage Adjustment section.

The degree of fluctuation within a dosing interval will depend on three factors: the half-life of the drug in that patient; how quickly the drug is absorbed (as reflected by the time at which a peak concentration occurs for that particular formulation); and the dosing interval. The least fluctuation (lowest peak:trough ratio) will occur for drugs with relatively long half-lives that are slowly absorbed or given as sustained-release formulations (prolonged peak time) and are given in divided doses (short dosing interval). However, drugs with relatively short half-lives that are quickly absorbed (or given as prompt-release products) and given only once daily will show the greatest amount of fluctuation within the interval.

The estimated degree of fluctuation (peak:trough ratio) for a given dosage regimen can be estimated by comparing the drug's half-life in a patient to the difference between the dosing interval and the estimated time required to reach a peak concentration.[41] The following guidelines may be used:

interval or portion of an interval is used as the monitoring parameter in place of single drug concentration measurements for certain drugs, such as some immunosuppressant and cytotoxic drugs, because it provides a better indication of overall drug exposure.) However, determination of the AUC, or $C_{ss,avg}$, by multiple sampling is not cost-effective for the most commonly monitored drugs. The following are alternatives to estimating the $C_{ss,avg}$ without multiple samples:

- Look up the expected time to reach a peak concentration for the particular formulation and obtain a sample midway between that time and the end of the dosing interval.[20]
- Measure the trough level (as close to the time of administration of the next dose as possible) and use that along with the population value for the drug's volume of distribution (Vd) to estimate the peak level as follows:

$$\text{Peak}_{\text{steady-state}} = (\text{Dose/Vd}) + \text{measured trough}$$

Then take the simple average of the trough and the peak to get an estimate of the average steady-state level.

- If you have reason to believe that there is very little fluctuation during the dosing interval, then a sample drawn anytime during the interval will provide a reasonable reflection of the average concentration.

There are special and extremely important timing considerations for some drugs, such as digoxin. It must reach specific receptors, presumably in the myocardium, to exhibit its therapeutic effect, but this takes a number of hours after the dose is administered. Early after a digoxin dose, levels in serum are relatively high, but response is not yet evident because digoxin has not yet equilibrated at its site of action. Thus, only digoxin levels that are in the postdistribution phase should be monitored and compared to the reported therapeutic range.

The timing of samples for other drugs may be based on the requirements for certain dosing methods. This is true for the aminoglycosides and certain lithium dosing methods. Sample timing for drugs like methotrexate will be specified in protocols because concentrations are used to determine the need for rescue therapy with leucovorin to minimize methotrexate toxicity.

While samples for drug concentration measurements may be preferred at certain times during a dosing interval, visits to physician offices often do not coincide with desired times for blood draws. One is then faced with the matter of how to interpret a level that is drawn at a time that happens to be more convenient to the patient's appointment. The most critical pieces of information to obtain in this situation are (1) when the last drug dose was taken; (2) how compliant the patient has been; (3) timing of the sample relative to the last dose; and (4) the expected time of peak concentration. Some drugs are available as a wide variety of formulations (solutions, suspensions, prompt-release, and sustained- or extended-release solid dosage forms), and the package insert may be the best source of information for the expected peak time. Once again, drugs with relatively long half-lives given as sustained-release or slowly absorbed products in divided doses will have the flattest concentration versus time profiles, and levels drawn anytime during the interval are going to be similar. However, prompt-release drugs with short half-lives given less frequently will show more fluctuation. Knowing the expected peak time for the formulation in question is especially important for drugs that show more fluctuation during that interval. In that case, one can at least judge if the reported concentration is closer to a peak, an average (if midway between the peak and trough), or a trough.

SPECIMENS, COLLECTION METHODS, AND ASSAYS

Whole blood, plasma, and serum. Whole blood, plasma, serum, and ultrafiltrate of serum are commonly used specimens for drug concentration measurements. Unbound drug molecules in blood distribute themselves among red blood cells, binding proteins (albumin, alpha-1-acid glycoprotein [AAG], and lipoproteins) and plasma water based on how avidly they partition into red blood cells; the concentrations of binding proteins in blood; and the affinities of the binding proteins for the drug.[30]

Samples for plasma or whole blood analysis are collected in tubes that contain an anticoagulant. Plasma is created by centrifugation of the anticoagulated whole blood sample and collection of the upper layer containing plasma water, protein, unbound drug, and protein-bound drug. Samples for serum are collected in tubes without an anticoagulant and allowed to clot followed by centrifugation, while samples for unbound drug measurements, preferably serum, are ultrafiltered (as described below) to create serum water that contains only unbound drug. Concentrations of drug in ultrafiltrate of serum are always lower than the corresponding total (bound plus unbound) concentrations, especially for drugs that are highly bound to serum proteins. Because the only difference between plasma and serum is that the clotting factors have been consumed when serum is created, drug concentrations in plasma and serum are generally regarded to be equivalent. Concentrations of drug in whole blood are higher than the corresponding serum or plasma concentrations if the drug happens to concentrate within red blood cells.

The choice of serum, plasma, or whole blood for a drug concentration measurement depends in part on the requirements of the assay to be used. Serum or plasma would be preferred if hemoglobin interferes with the assay. An assay with marginal sensitivity might be more useful if whole blood is used for a drug such as cyclosporine that concentrates in the red blood cell. Some of the newer point-of-care methods have the advantage of using capillary whole blood from fingersticks, thus obviating the need for centrifugation or other sample preparation steps.

The choice of blood collection method is extremely important. For plasma analyses, it is important to know if the particular anticoagulant interferes with the assay, affects the stability or protein binding of the drug, or even dilutes the sample.[43] There have been numerous reports that polymer-based gels, designed to form a barrier between serum and the clot during centrifugation, may also absorb drugs from the serum to varying extents. Technical improvements in these devices (known as *serum separator tubes*) have been made, but, nevertheless, several groups have categorically recommended that separation gels not be used for blood collection unless rigorous testing has first been done.[44,45] Finally, there were a number of reports in the 1970s and 1980s of artifacts caused by contact of serum or plasma with rubber stoppers of evacuated blood collection tubes.[46,47] Tris-(2-butoxyethyl)phosphate (TBEP) in the rubber stoppers leached into the serum or plasma and displaced basic drugs from AAG, thus causing redistribution of unbound drug into the red blood cells. When the samples were centrifuged, the total plasma or serum drug concentration was decreased to varying extents. Although recent studies of reformulated stoppers for these tubes show no artifacts, each laboratory must perform their own tests to ensure that similar artifacts are not observed.[47]

Specific recommendations for blood collection methods and collection tubes will be presented in the appropriate sections that follow for each drug or drug category.

Alternatives to blood sampling. Saliva has been proposed as a noninvasive alternative to blood sampling, particularly for children, for a number of drugs.[48-50] Collection at home and mailing of samples may further offer convenience and cost savings.[51] Saliva is a natural ultrafiltrate of plasma and, thus, may provide a closer reflection of the therapeutically active unbound drug concentration in serum as compared to the total drug concentration.[52] Concentrations of drug in saliva are much lower than total concentrations in serum of highly bound drugs, and assay sensitivity should be considered if saliva samples are used for drug concentration monitoring.

Use of saliva drug concentration as a substitute for total or unbound drug concentration in serum or plasma requires that the saliva:plasma (S:P) drug concentration ratio be stable, at least within a patient. The S:P ratio, however, can be influenced by salivary flow rate, saliva pH, and contamination by residual drug in the mouth. With the exception of saliva pH, these factors can be controlled by careful selection of the collection method. The degree of a drug's ionization affects the extent to which it passively diffuses from blood into saliva. Blood pH is relatively constant, but saliva pH varies widely during the day within a patient, and the S:P ratio may, therefore, change considerably during the day. Neutral drugs are not expected to show variable S:P ratios within patients, while acids or bases with pKa values similar to blood pH are most likely to be sensitive to variations in saliva pH. Correction of the S:P ratio may be possible, however, if the saliva pH is measured.[52,53]

Whole saliva is most often collected, and it can be either *stimulated* or *unstimulated*. Stimulated saliva is preferred: it produces a larger volume, minimizes the pH gradient between saliva and blood, and provides more stable S:P ratios. Methods for stimulating whole saliva production include the chewing or rolling of inert materials (paraffin, wax, and glass marble) in the mouth or applying a small amount of citric acid to the tongue.[54] Novel methods have been proposed for collection of saliva for home monitoring purposes in children. One involves placing a gauze-wrapped cotton ball, with attached string, in the child's mouth for a period of time and squeezing saliva from the retrieved cotton using a plastic syringe.[55] Special devices that collect saliva from specific salivary glands are commercially available. While they offer the advantage of reduced viscosity, they must be checked to ensure stability and recovery of any absorbed drug.[48,56] Regardless of the method used, contamination of saliva from residual drug in the mouth must be avoided by collecting saliva no earlier than 2–3 hours after a dose and rinsing the mouth with deionized water prior to collection.

Lacrimal fluid has been proposed as an ideal medium for monitoring unbound drug, since it does not have the problem with pH changes.[57-59] Tears may be stimulated by exposing the eye to cigarette smoke or having the patient sniff formaldehyde fumes. In another method, tears are collected by hooking small strips of blotting paper over the lower lid of the eye for a few minutes.[58] The major limitation for assay of drug in tears is the sensitivity of the assay, since large volumes cannot be collected.

Storage. The following factors can affect drug concentrations in serum, serum ultrafiltrate, plasma, whole blood, saliva, and lacrimal fluid: exposure to light, temperature, storage container, and presence of other drugs or endogenous substances.

Assays. Interpretation of any drug concentration measurement requires full knowledge of the strengths and limitations of the analytical method that was used. Laboratories should readily supply clinicians with all details of assay performance, including linearity, coefficients of variation at high and low concentrations, minimum detection limit, and potential interferences. While the laboratory must consistently conform to accepted standards for accuracy and reproducibility, requirements for assay sensitivity and specificity will depend on the intended use, the therapeutic range, the volume to be analyzed, and the nature of the specimen (serum/plasma, whole blood, serum ultrafiltrate, or saliva).

Knowledge of the sensitivity of a method (the ability to quantitate drug when drug is present) is helpful to interpret a laboratory report of *nondetectable*. If the method is highly sensitive, nondetectable may actually mean there is no drug in the sample. If the method is less sensitive, however, there could be drug in the sample but just not enough to register.[60] The minimum detection limit will be of greatest concern for drugs with lower therapeutic ranges (i.e., in the mcg/L range) such as digoxin and the PIs. More sensitive assays are also required when there are small sample volumes, such as in neonates. Drug concentrations in saliva or in ultrafiltrates of serum may require more sensitive assays if the drugs are highly bound to serum proteins. In some cases, assays may be based on blood concentrations for drugs that concentrate in red blood cells in order to overcome limitations of sensitivity.[61]

Knowledge of the specificity (the ability to detect nothing when nothing is there) of a method is equally important. If the drug concentration report from the laboratory is higher than would be expected with no attendant toxicity, the clinician might suspect an interference with the assay. Substances that may interfere with assays include drug metabolites, other drugs, and endogenous substances (e.g., lipids, bilirubin, hemoglobin, or uremic byproducts that accumulate in renal impairment). As an example, endogenous digoxin-like immunoreactive substances accumulate in the serum of neonates, pregnant patients, and patients with liver or renal disease and are reported to cause falsely elevated digoxin concentration readings.[62] Some assays are purposely developed to be nonspecific for purposes of drug abuse screens. Examples are the immunoassays used for detection of *benzodiazepines*, *tricyclics*, or *barbiturates*.

Knowledge of the condition or appearance of the sample at the time of assay may be important. A sample with a milky appearance may indicate lipemia; one with a dark yellow to gold appearance may mean high bilirubin levels; one with a pinkish tinge may mean hemolysis. All of these conditions can result in either overreading (positive bias) or underreading (negative bias) of a drug concentration, depending on the analytical method. Drugs that are more concentrated in red blood cells than in serum will have artifactually high-serum concentration readings in a hemolyzed sample, while drugs that are less concentrated in the red blood cell will dilute the serum or plasma resulting in artifactually low readings.

High-performance liquid chromatography (HPLC) and gas-liquid chromatography (GLC) are still used in clinical laboratories and are considered in many cases to be the reference methods. Homogenous immunoassays (fluorescence polarization immunoassay [FPIA], enzyme-multiplied immunoassay [EMIT], and cloned enzyme-donor immunoassay [CEDIA]) have become the methods of choice, however, because of ease of use, ability to automate, and rapid turnaround time. These immunologic methods are generally specific for the parent drug, but in some cases metabolites or other drug-like substances are recognized by the antibody.[63] Certain drugs are not suitable for immunologic assays. Lithium, an electrolyte, is an example of this and must be analyzed using ion-selective electrode (ISE) technology, atomic absorption spectroscopy, or flame emission photometry.

The increased interest in drug assay methods for use in ambulatory settings, such as physician offices, has led to the development of immunoassay systems purported to be fast, reliable, and cost-effective.[5,64-67] Most of these point-of-care testing methods have the capacity to produce results within 1–5 minutes; some use whole blood. Prior to 1988, less than 10% of all clinical laboratories were required to meet quality standards. Growing concern about lack of quality control in settings such as physician offices led to adoption of the 1988 Clinical Laboratory Improvement Amendments (CLIA) in which three levels of testing complexity were defined: waived, moderately complex, and highly complex. All drug concentration measurement testing is currently classified either as moderate or high complexity, and laboratories that perform these assays must maintain a quality control program, participate in proficiency testing programs, and be periodically inspected.[5] These point-of-care testing methods vary in their reliability as compared to reference methods.[68-71]

USE OF LEVELS FOR DOSAGE ADJUSTMENT

A chronic intermittent dosage regimen has three components: the dose rate, the dosing interval, and the dose. For the dosage regimen of 240 mg q 8 hr, the dose is 240 mg, the interval is 8 hours, and the dose rate can be expressed as 720 mg/day or 30 mg/hr. The dose rate is important because it determines the average concentration ($C_{ss,avg}$) during the day. The degree of fluctuation within a dosing interval is highly influenced by the dosing interval.

Dosage adjustments for linear behavior. If a drug is known to have first-order bioavailability and elimination behavior after therapeutic doses, one can use simple proportionality to make an adjustment in the daily dose:

- If average levels are being monitored or estimated, one can predict that the average, steady-state drug concentration will increase in proportion to the increase in daily dose, regardless of any changes that were made in the dosing interval.

- If trough levels are monitored and the dosing interval will be held constant, the trough level will increase in proportion to the increase in daily dose.

- If trough levels are monitored for a drug that exhibits considerable fluctuation during the interval, and both the dose rate and dosing interval will be adjusted, the trough concentration will not be as easy to predict at a new steady-state and is beyond the scope of this chapter. If the trough concentration can be used to estimate the $C_{ss,avg}$, as described above, the $C_{ss,avg}$ can be predicted with certainty to change in proportion to the change in daily dose.

Sampling after a dosage regimen adjustment, if appropriate, should not be done until a new steady-state has been reached. For a drug with first-order behavior, this should take the same period of time (three half-lives at a minimum) that it did after initiation of therapy with this drug.

Dosage adjustments for drugs with nonlinear behavior. All drugs will show nonlinear elimination behavior if sufficiently high doses are given. Some drugs, however, show pronounced nonlinear (Michaelis-Menten) behavior following doses that produce therapeutic drug concentrations. This means that an increase in the dose rate of the drug will result in a greater-than-proportional increase in the drug concentration. Phenytoin is an example of a drug with this behavior. Theophylline, procainamide, and salicylate also show some degree of nonlinear behavior but only at the higher end of their therapeutic ranges (and not enough to require special dosing methods).

Methods have been described to permit predictions of the effect of dose rate increases for phenytoin using population averages or actual measurements of the parameters that define nonlinearity, namely Vmax (maximum rate of metabolism) and Km (the "Michaelis constant"), but they are beyond the scope of this chapter.[72] The most important rule to remember for dosage adjustments of drugs like phenytoin is to be conservative; small increases in the dose rate will produce unpredictably large increases in the serum drug concentration. It must also be remembered that the half-life of a drug like phenytoin will be progressively prolonged at higher dose rates. Increases in dose rate will require a longer period of time to reach a steady-state as compared to when the drug was first initiated.

Population pharmacokinetic or Bayesian dosage adjustment methods, which involve the use of statistical probabilities, are preferred by many for individualization of therapy.[40,73] They are useful for drugs with both linear and nonlinear behavior.

PROTEIN BINDING, ACTIVE METABOLITES, AND OTHER CONSIDERATIONS

Altered serum binding. Total (unbound plus protein-bound) drug concentrations measured in blood, serum, or plasma are almost always used for therapeutic drug monitoring, despite the fact that unbound drug concentrations are more closely correlated to drug effect.[30] This is because it is easier to measure the total concentration and because the ratio of unbound to total drug concentration in serum is usually constant within and between individuals. For some drugs, however, the relationship between unbound and total drug concentration is extremely variable among patients, or it may be altered by disease or drug interactions. For drugs that undergo concentration-dependent serum binding, the relationship between

unbound and total concentration varies within patients. In all of these situations, total drug concentration does not reflect the same level of activity as with normal binding and must be cautiously interpreted because the usual therapeutic range will not apply. (See Minicase 3.)

The direct measurement of unbound drug concentration would seem to be appropriate in these situations. Drugs for which total concentration monitoring is routinely performed (but for which unbound concentration monitoring has been proposed) include carbamazepine, disopyramide, lidocaine, phenytoin, quinidine, and valproic acid. Of these, correlations between unbound drug concentration and response have been only weakly established for carbamazepine and disopyramide but more firmly established for phenytoin.[26,30,74]

Unbound drug concentration measurements involve an extra step prior to analysis—separation of the unbound from the bound drug. Equilibrium dialysis and ultracentrifugation may be used in a research setting, but ultrafiltration is the method of choice for a clinical laboratory.[30,75] Commercial systems for unbound drug concentration measurements involve centrifugation of serum in tubes containing a semipermeable membrane (e.g., Millipore Centrifree® UF device). The ultrafiltrate, containing unbound drug, is collected in a small

---

MINICASE 3

Value of Unbound Antiepileptic Drug Serum Levels

FRANK S., A 66–YEAR-OLD CAUCASIAN MALE, was admitted to the emergency department (ED) with a chief complaint of vomiting, diarrhea, blurred vision and unsteady gait. He was diagnosed with epilepsy 3 years ago and was taking the following oral antiepileptic drugs at home: valproic acid 1000 mg BID; sodium phenytoin 200 mg TID; carbamazepine 300 mg BID; and levetiracetam 400 mg at bedtime. The patient also had a past medical history of hypertension and hyperlipidemia and was taking aspirin 81 mg every day, simvastatin 40 mg at bedtime, and metoprolol 100 mg BID. Physical examination in the ED revealed bilateral nystagmus and significant ataxia. The clinical picture was deemed consistent with antiepileptic drug toxicity and total serum concentrations of three of the antiepileptic drugs were ordered:

Carbamazepine:	6.4 mg/L (reference range: 4–12 mg/L)
Phenytoin:	9.3 mg/L (reference range 10–20 mg/L)
Valproic acid:	72 mg/L (reference range 50–100 mg/L)

Free levels of the same three drugs were subsequently determined:

Carbamazepine:	1.9 mg/L (reference range: 1–3 mg/L)
Phenytoin:	1.3 mg/L (reference range 1–2 mg/L)
Valproic acid:	13.4 mg/L (reference range 2.5–10 mg/L)

The valproic acid was held for 24 hours and then reintroduced at a dose rate of 250 mg TID. His symptoms resolved within 24 hours. A repeat unbound serum valproic acid level 1 week later was 5.2 mg/L.

Questions: How were total levels of antiepileptic drug misleading in this patient? How might sole reliance on total antiepileptic serum concentrations have led to a different clinical decision and outcome? How did

free serum concentration monitoring aid in understanding the cause of the patient's signs and symptoms?

Discussion: Frank S. had total serum concentrations of carbamazepine and valproic acid within the reference ranges for total concentrations of these drugs, while the total level of phenytoin was slightly below the lower limit of the laboratory's reference range. Based solely on these total drug concentrations, the unaware clinician would be tempted to seek alternative explanations and likely delay the resolution of the patient's signs and symptoms. Even worse, the clinician might be tempted to increase the daily dose of sodium phenytoin in an attempt to get the total phenytoin level to within the usual reference range for phenytoin. Measurement of free levels of these anticonvulsants revealed that the patient was probably getting appropriate daily doses of carbamazepine and phenytoin but was clearly receiving too much valproic acid. This was confirmed when the signs and symptoms resolved after reduction of the valproic acid dose rate and a repeat unbound serum valproic acid level at a new steady-state was within the laboratory's reference range for free valproic acid.

Explanations for the "supratherapeutic" free valproic acid level in face of a "therapeutic" total level in this patient may include one or more of the following: (1) saturable (nonlinear) protein binding of valproic acid to albumin at higher dose rates of valproic acid; (2) inhibition of valproic acid metabolism by salicylic acid; and (3) displacement of valproic acid from albumin by phenytoin and/or salicylic acid. As a result, total valproic acid concentrations no longer reflect what is happening to the free, active valproic acid moiety, and the usual therapeutic reference range of total concentrations cannot be used.

Minicase 3 is adapted from reference 142.

cup and assayed. The method used for analysis of the ultrafiltrate must be sufficiently sensitive since lower drug concentrations will be observed for highly bound drugs. Specificity of the assay may also be especially important. The ratio of metabolite to parent drug is likely to be greater in the ultrafiltrate since most metabolites are not as highly bound to protein as the parent. Thus, an immunoassay that shows acceptable specificity using total serum might show unacceptable specificity using ultrafiltrate.[76]

If unbound drug concentration measurements are unavailable, too costly, or considered impractical, the following alternative approaches to interpreting total drug concentrations in situations of altered serum protein binding may be used:

- **Use of equations to normalize the measured total concentration:** Sheiner and Tozer were the first to propose equations that can be used to convert a measured total concentration of drug (phenytoin in this case) to an approximation of what the total level would be if the patient had normal binding.[77] Equations to normalize total phenytoin concentrations have been used for patients with hypoalbuminemia, impaired renal function, and concurrent valproic acid therapy.[78] Once the total level has been normalized, it may be compared to the conventional therapeutic range. It must be noted that this normalization method may not be a reliable substitute for measurement of the unbound phenytoin level.

- **Normalize the measured total concentration using literature estimates of the abnormal unbound drug fraction:** An alternative method for normalizing the total concentration can be used if reasonable estimates of the abnormal and normal unbound reactions of the drug can be ascertained (i.e., from the literature). The normalized total concentration ($C_{normalized}$) can be estimated as

$$C_{normalized} = C_{measured} \times \frac{\text{abnormal unbound fraction}}{\text{normal unbound fraction}}$$

where $C_{measured}$ is the measured total concentration reported by the laboratory.

- **Predictive linear regression equations:** Some studies have reported the ability to predict unbound drug concentrations in the presence of displacing drugs if the total concentrations of both drugs are known. This has been done to predict unbound concentrations of phenytoin and carbamazepine, both in the presence of valproic acid.[79,80] These unbound drug concentrations should be compared to corresponding therapeutic ranges of unbound drug, which can be estimated for any drug if the normal unbound fraction and the usual therapeutic range of total concentrations (TR) are known:

$$TR_u = TR \times \text{normal unbound fraction}$$

- **Use of saliva or tears as a substitute for unbound drug concentration:** This may be a reasonable alternative so long as studies have shown a strong correlation between unbound concentrations in serum and concentrations in saliva or lacrimal fluid. The concentration of drug in saliva or tears may not be equal to the concentration in serum ultrafiltrate. Therefore, the laboratory should have determined a reliable conversion factor for this. The calculated unbound concentration may then be compared to the estimated therapeutic range for unbound concentrations as described above.

Active metabolites. Interpretation of parent drug concentration alone, for drugs with active metabolites that are present to varying extents, is difficult at best. Active metabolites may contribute to therapeutic response, to toxicity, or to both. Since metabolites will likely have different pharmacokinetic characteristics, they will be affected differently than the parent drug under different physiologic and pathologic conditions.

For drugs like primidone (metabolized to phenobarbital) and procainamide (metabolized to NAPA), the laboratory will typically report both the parent drug and the metabolite as well as a therapeutic range for both. While a therapeutic range for the sum of procainamide and NAPA may be reported by some laboratories, this practice is discouraged since the parent and metabolites have different types of pharmacologic activities.

Enantiomeric pairs. Some drugs exist as an equal mixture (racemic mixture) of enantiomers, which are chemically identical but are mirror images of each other. Because they can interact differently with receptors, they may have very different pharmacodynamic and pharmacokinetic properties. The relative proportions of the enantiomers can differ widely among and within patients. Thus, a given concentration of the summed enantiomers (what is routinely measured using achiral methods) can represent very different activities.

Table 5-3 provides relevant information about protein binding, active metabolites, enantiomers, and other influences on serum concentration interpretation for drugs discussed in the Applications sections that follow.

APPLICATIONS

Analgesic/Anti-inflammatory Drugs

Salicylic Acid

Therapeutic range. Salicylic acid is used to reduce fever and relieve pain and inflammation associated with a variety of conditions. The therapeutic range for the analgesic and antipyretic effects of salicylic acid is commonly reported as 20–100 mg/L.[81,82] Salicylate is more commonly monitored, however, for its anti-inflammatory effect: while the commonly reported therapeutic range is 100–250 mg/L, effective concentrations may be as low as 70 mg/L and as high as 300 mg/L.[81,82] The concentrations associated with toxicity can overlap considerably with those associated with efficacy. Tinnitus, for example, may be experienced at concentrations as low as 200 mg/L. Indications for monitoring salicylate concentrations, other than suspected overdose or chronic salicylate abuse, include suspected toxicity; suspected nonadherence; change in renal function, mental status, acid–base balance, or pulmonary status; and anticipated drug–drug interactions.

Sample timing. Salicylic acid undergoes nonlinear elimination, and, thus, the half-life progressively increases from 3–20 hours as drug accumulates to within the range of 100–300 mg/L.[83] Because of the progressive prolongation of half-life during initiation of therapy, samples for salicylate monitoring should not be obtained earlier than after 1 week of therapy.[84] The rate of salicylate absorption, while usually fast, is slowed during food intake or when enteric-coated formulations are administered.[84] Trough samples are generally advised for purposes of therapeutic drug monitoring, as they are the most reproducible.[84] Timing of the sample within the interval was not deemed critical in patients with juvenile rheumatoid arthritis who are dosed using an interval of 8 hours or less.[85]

Specimens, collection methods, and assays. Blood samples for determination of salicylate concentration should be collected in tubes without additives or in tubes containing heparin or ethylenediaminetetraacetic acid (EDTA).[81] Recent studies of certain evacuated serum separator tubes show they are also acceptable for blood collection for salicylate monitoring.[44,86] Saliva concentrations are extremely variable when compared to unbound salicylate concentrations, and the variability is not explained by pH alone.[50] Salicylate in serum may be stored refrigerated for up to 2 weeks.[81]

Colorimetric methods are used for salicylate determination as well as GLC, HPLC, and FPIA. The FPIA method performs exceptionally well and is recommended over colorimetric methods especially for icteric serum or plasma.[87,88] Saliva is proposed to be a reasonable alternative to icteric serum, however, if a colorimetric method must be used.[81] An immunoassay-based point-of-care method has been developed to simultaneously screen for salicylate and acetaminophen overdose.[89]

Use of levels for dosage adjustment. Two of the metabolic pathways for salicylate are capacity-limited, such that increases in dose rate produce greater-than-proportional increases in unbound serum drug concentrations and response. Because there is also concentration-dependent serum protein binding, total concentrations may mask this nonlinear relationship between dose rate and unbound drug concentration. Droomgoole and Furst provide an algorithm for adjustment of salicylate doses based on total serum salicylate levels.[82]

Protein binding, active metabolites, and other considerations. The binding of salicylate to albumin is concentration-dependent. Specifically, it is approximately 90% bound at total concentrations of 100 mg/L and decreases to 76% bound at levels as high as 400 mg/L.[82] The unbound fraction of salicylate is known to increase during pregnancy and in patients with nephrotic syndrome, liver disease, and uremia.[82] While salicylate would seem to be an ideal candidate for unbound concentration monitoring, a therapeutic range for unbound salicylate has not been established. Nevertheless, the clinician should be cautious that total concentrations within the usual therapeutic range may be associated with toxic responses in patients who are suspected to have abnormally low serum binding. No significant differences in the unbound percentage of salicylate in serum were observed among patients with

juvenile rheumatoid arthritis, despite widely variable albumin concentrations, suggesting that total concentration monitoring is more appropriate in this group.[90]

Antiasthmatics

Theophylline

Therapeutic range. Some clinicians still use 10–20 mg/L as the accepted therapeutic range for theophylline for management of acute bronchospasm associated with asthma and chronic obstructive pulmonary disease.[91] The 2007 NIH Expert Panel Report, Guidelines for the Diagnosis and Management of Asthma, stipulates, however, a more conservative range of 5–15 mg/L.[92] Most patients will respond at serum concentrations within this range, but levels as low as 2 mg/L may provide anti-inflammatory effects in some patients, while levels up to 20 mg/L may be necessary in others.[91,93] There is an 85% probability of adverse effects with levels above 25 mg/L, and levels above 30–40 mg/L can be associated with dangerous adverse events.[94] Adverse effects typically experienced by adults include nausea, vomiting, diarrhea, irritability, and insomnia at levels above 15 mg/L; supraventricular tachycardia, hypotension, and ventricular arrhythmias at levels above 40 mg/L; and seizures, brain damage, and even death at higher levels. It must also be noted that side effects such as nausea and vomiting, while common, do not occur in all patients and should never be considered prodromal to the occurrence of the more serious side effects.[95]

Theophylline is also indicated for treatment of neonatal apnea, although caffeine is usually preferred.[96] The therapeutic range in neonates is generally considered to be 5–10 mg/L but may be as low as 3 mg/L on the low end to 14 mg/L on the high end.[91,97-99] Adverse effects in neonates include lack of weight-gain, sleeplessness, irritability, diuresis, dehydration, hyperflexia, jitteriness, and serious cardiovascular and neurologic events.[94] Tachycardia has been reported in neonates with levels as low as 13 mg/L.[100]

In summary, there is considerable overlap of therapeutic and toxic effects within the usual therapeutic ranges reported for theophylline in neonates, children, and adults. Therefore, serum concentrations should never be interpreted in the absence of information about the patient's clinical status. Indications for theophylline monitoring include therapeutic confirmation of effective levels after initiation of therapy or a dosage regimen adjustment, anticipated drug–drug interactions, change in smoking habits, and/or changes in health status that might affect the metabolism of theophylline.

Sample timing. The half-life of theophylline is greatly affected by age, disease, concurrent drugs, smoking, and any physiologic condition that affects its metabolism. The half-life of theophylline can range anywhere from 3–5 hours in children or adult smokers to as long as 50 hours in nonsmoking adults with severe heart failure or liver disease.[91] Steady-state will be reached in 24 hours for the average patient with an elimination half-life of 8 hours but will require much longer for patients with heart failure or liver disease (or for patients who are taking drugs known to inhibit theophylline metabolism). The time to steady-state in premature neonates may be as long as 9 days.[97]

The fluctuation of theophylline concentrations within a steady-state dosing interval can be quite variable—depending not only on the frequency of administration, type of formulation (sustained- or prompt-release), and half-life—but also on whether or not the dose was taken with a meal.[94] There are many theophylline formulations available. Thus, it is important to consult the product information to determine the anticipated peak times. For prompt-release formulations, peak times are 1–2 hours; peak times for sustained-release formulations occur later and are difficult to predict.[95]

Trough concentrations of theophylline are most reproducible and should always be obtained if at all possible. Comparisons of trough levels from visit to visit will also be facilitated if samples are obtained at the same time of day on each visit. This is because of diurnal variations in the rate of theophylline absorption.[94]

Specimens, collection methods, and assays. Plasma or serum is used for most assays; whole blood may be used in some of the point-of-care systems.[94] There are no particular concerns about blood collection tubes. Prolonged storage in red-top evacuated tubes or serum separator tubes had no effect on theophylline concentrations in serum.[44]

Many studies suggest saliva theophylline concentrations to be reliable predictors of total or unbound theophylline concentrations in serum or plasma.[56,101,102] Both unstimulated and stimulated saliva were equally good predictors of theophylline concentrations in serum in one study.[101] Either citric acid or the chewing of Parafilm® may be used for stimulation of whole saliva production.[102] A study of an oral mucosal transudate collection device showed that once the S:P ratio was established for a given patient, saliva samples collected at home by the patient are reliable predictors of serum theophylline concentrations.[56]

While theophylline is often measured using HPLC, the most common assays for point-of-care methods and in clinical laboratories are based on FPIA or EMIT. The immunoassay methods offer acceptable sensitivity but may not be suitable for patients with renal failure who have accumulated theophylline metabolites.[103,104] Caffeine and theobromine have been reported to interfere with theophylline measurements by some point-of-care methods. The Abbott Vision® system showed no interferences by bilirubin and triglycerides, but hemolyzed samples gave lower readings.[68,105]

Use of levels for dosage adjustment. Theophylline is usually assumed to undergo first-order elimination, but some of its metabolic pathways are nonlinear at concentrations at the higher end of the therapeutic range.[94] The clearance of theophylline decreases by 20% as daily doses are increased from 210 mg to 1260 mg.[94] While the magnitude of this nonlinear behavior does not require special methods for dosing, the clinician should expect somewhat greater-than-proportional increases in serum theophylline concentration with increases in dose rate, particularly as concentrations get into the upper end of the therapeutic range.

Protein binding, active metabolites, and other considerations. Theophylline is 35% bound to serum proteins in neonates and 40% to 50% bound to serum proteins in adults. Therefore, significant alterations in serum protein binding are unlikely.[94] Theophylline is metabolized to the active metabolite caffeine, which is of minor consequence in adults. Caffeine concentrations in the serum of neonates who are receiving theophylline, however, are approximately 30% of theophylline concentrations and therefore contribute to the effect of theophylline during treatment of neonatal apnea. This may account for the slightly lower therapeutic range of theophylline in neonates as compared to adults. There are many other metabolites of theophylline, none of which possess significant activity.

Caffeine

Therapeutic range. Caffeine is indicated for neonatal apnea (apnea of prematurity) and is recommended over theophylline because it can be given once daily and is considered to have a wider therapeutic range.[96] Concentrations as low as 5 mg/L may be effective, but most pediatric textbooks consider 10 mg/L to be the lower limit of the therapeutic range.[99,106] Most clinicians consider 20 mg/L to be the upper limit of the range, and serious toxicity is associated with serum concentrations above 50 mg/L. Signs of toxicity include jitteriness, vomiting, irritability, tremor of the extremities, tachypnea, and tonic-clonic movements. Serum concentration measurements of caffeine may not be routinely necessary for apnea of prematurity in neonates.[107] Neonates who do not respond as expected or in whom there is recurrence of apnea after a favorable response may benefit, however.

Sample timing. The half-life of caffeine in preterm infants at birth is 65–103 hours.[106] Thus, a loading dose is always administered to attain effective levels as soon as possible. The long half-life means that caffeine concentrations will not fluctuate much during the interval, even when caffeine is administered once daily. Sampling in the postdistribution phase is recommended, but at least 2 hours postdose.

Baseline levels of caffeine must be obtained prior to the first caffeine dose in the following situations: (1) if the infant had been previously treated with theophylline, since caffeine is a metabolite of theophylline; and (2) if the infant was born to a mother who consumed caffeine prior to delivery. Reductions in the usual caffeine dose will be necessary if predose caffeine levels are present.

Specimens, collection methods, and assays. Because of the limited blood volume in neonates, it is generally recommended that blood samples of 75 µL or less be used.[99] Caffeine from blood samples is measured as either serum or plasma. Recommendations for collection tubes include evacuated tubes without additives or tubes containing EDTA. Refrigeration at 4°C for up to 24 hours is acceptable.[106] Common assays for caffeine include HPLC, GLC, and EMIT. The immunoassay method was demonstrated to be unaffected by hemolysis, hyperbilirubinemia, and lipemia.[108]

Saliva concentrations have been recommended as a noninvasive alternative to blood sampling, which would be particularly helpful in this population.[106] The reported S:P concentration ratio can vary depending on the methods used. Therefore, it is important that collection and assay methods be consistently used within a given institution. De Wildt et al. developed a novel saliva collection method in which a cotton swab with attached gauze was placed in the mouth of the neonate 5–10 minutes after a drop of 1% citric acid solution had been placed in the cheek pouch.[106] Saliva concentrations measured by HPLC predicted plasma concentrations reliably. Other collection methods (no stimulation or citric acid placed on the gauze) did not predict plasma concentrations as well.[106]

Use of levels for dosage adjustment. There is no data to suggest that caffeine undergoes nonlinear elimination. Thus, dosage adjustments by proportionality are acceptable. Dosage adjustments for caffeine are complicated by the fact that a true steady-state is not reached for at least 4 days, so any adjustments should be conservative.

Protein binding, active metabolites, and other considerations. Caffeine is only 31% bound to serum proteins and has no active metabolites.[106]

Antiepileptics

The antiepileptics that have clearly defined therapeutic ranges should be routinely monitored. Because they are used as prophylaxis for seizures that may not occur frequently, it is particularly important that effective serum concentrations of these drugs be ensured early in therapy. Indications for monitoring antiepileptic drugs include[14,109] (1) documentation of an effective steady-state concentration after initiation of therapy; (2) after dosage regimen adjustments; (3) after adding a drug that has potential for interaction; (4) changes in disease state or physiologic status that may affect the pharmacokinetics of the drug; (5) within hours of a seizure recurrence; (6) after an unexplained change in seizure frequency; (7) suspected dose-related drug toxicity; and (8) suspected nonadherence.

Carbamazepine

Therapeutic range. Carbamazepine is indicated for the prevention of partial seizures and generalized tonic-clonic seizures, and the treatment of pain associated with trigeminal neuralgia.[91,110] Most textbooks report a therapeutic range of 4–12 mg/L. Concentrations above 12 mg/L are most often associated with nausea and vomiting, unsteadiness, blurred vision, drowsiness, dizziness, and headaches in patients who are taking carbamazepine alone.[34] Patients taking other antiepileptic drugs such as primidone, phenobarbital, valproic acid, or phenytoin, however, may show these adverse effects at levels as low as 9 mg/L. For this reason, many clinicians use a more conservative target therapeutic range of 4–8 mg/L.[110] Serious adverse reactions are seen at levels greater than 50 mg/L.[109]

Carbamazepine 10,11-epoxide is an active metabolite that can be present in concentrations containing 12% to 25% carbamazepine, but it is not routinely monitored along with the parent drug. A suggested therapeutic range for this metabolite, used at some research centers, is 0.4–4 mg/L.[91]

In addition to the usual indications for monitoring, it is important to monitor carbamazepine concentrations if the patient is switched to another formulation (e.g., generic), since the bioavailability may be different.[109]

Sample timing. Because carbamazepine induces its own metabolism, it is recommended that initial dose rates of carbamazepine be relatively low and gradually increased over a 3- to 4-week period.[34] For maximal induction or deinduction to occur, 2–3 weeks may be required after the maximum dose rate has been attained. Thus, a total of 6–7 weeks may be required for a true steady-state to be reached after initiation of therapy. After any dose rate changes or addition/discontinuation of enzyme-inducing or inhibiting drugs, 2–3 weeks will be required to reach a new steady-state.[91]

A trough level is generally preferred if there is a choice. The absorption of immediate-release carbamazepine tablets from the gastrointestinal tract is relatively slow and erratic, reaching a peak between 3 and 8 hours after a dose.[111] Extended-release formulations are even more slowly absorbed. If carbamazepine is administered every 6 or 8 hours, serum levels during the dosing interval will remain fairly flat, and all levels will be fairly representative of a trough concentration. Less frequent dosing will result in more fluctuation in which case the time of the level relative to the last dose should be documented for appropriate interpretation. Use of the extended-release formulation of carbamazepine will minimize fluctuations caused by diurnal variations.[112] Nevertheless, it is recommended that samples on repeated visits always be obtained at the same time of the day for purposes of comparison.[109]

Specimens, collection methods, and assays. Either serum or plasma collected in EDTA-treated tubes is acceptable for total carbamazepine measurements. Oxalate and citrate were shown to cause significant negative interferences in the measurement of carbamazepine by an EMIT method and a GLC method.[113] Studies of a new serum separator tube (SST II®, Becton-Dickinson) showed that serum carbamazepine concentrations were stable for 24 hours at room temperature.[44] Saliva has been proposed as a convenient noninvasive alternative, especially for children and for home monitoring.[48,52,114] If saliva is used, a standardized protocol for obtaining the specimen must be approved by the laboratory. Both the chewing of Parafilm® and stimulation by citric acid have been used successfully.[52,115] Saliva collected within 2 hours of oral administration may be contaminated by residual drug in the mouth.[34]

The most common assays for total carbamazepine include a wide variety of immunoassays.[111] Some of the immunoassays cross-react with the 10,11-epoxide metabolite.[116] This can be a particular problem if saliva is measured, as the ratio of epoxide to parent drug is higher in saliva.[115] The active carbamazepine 10,11-epoxide is generally not routinely measured separately, even though it has been shown to exhibit anticonvulsant activity. Assays for unbound carbamazepine, monitored rarely, are done by ultrafiltration followed by one of the other assay methods.[30] Severe hemolysis may result in inaccurate measurement by the immunologic methods in which case one of the chromatographic methods is suggested.[117]

Use of levels for dosage adjustment. Carbamazepine exhibits first-order behavior following therapeutic doses. Thus, increases in dose rate will result in a proportional increase in the average steady-state level of carbamazepine. If the dose is adjusted without a change in the interval, a level drawn at the same time within the interval will increase in proportion to the increase in dose.

Protein binding, active metabolites, and other considerations. In most patients, carbamazepine is 70% to 80% bound to serum proteins, including albumin and AAG.[118] In some patients, however, unbound percentages as low as 10% have been reported.[91] Measurements of unbound carbamazepine concentrations are not generally recommended or necessary. Rather, total carbamazepine concentrations should be carefully interpreted in situations of suspected altered protein binding. Decreased binding might be anticipated in liver disease, hypoalbuminemia, or hyperbilirubinemia.[91] Increased binding might be expected in cases of physiologic trauma due to elevated AAG concentrations, but this would be a rare occurrence. Valproic acid has been shown to displace carbamazepine from albumin; an equation was proposed to predict unbound carbamazepine concentrations in this situation.[80] Correlations between saliva and unbound carbamazepine concentrations are strong.[52] Thus, saliva sampling might be considered in situations of suspected alterations in carbamazepine binding.

Drug–drug interactions that are expected to result in a higher proportion of active 10,11-epoxide metabolite relative to the parent drug (e.g., concurrent phenytoin, phenobarbital, or valproic acid) may alter the activity associated with a given carbamazepine concentration. It is suggested that a lower therapeutic range of 4–8 mg/L be used when those drugs are given concurrently.[14]

Ethosuximide

Therapeutic range. Ethosuximide is indicated for the management of absence seizures. The therapeutic range is generally considered to be 40–100 mg/L.[119] Eighty percent of patients will achieve partial control within that range, and 60% will be seizure-free. Some patients will require levels up to 150 mg/L.[91] Side effects are usually seen at concentrations above 70 mg/L and include drowsiness, fatigue, ataxia, and lethargy.[91] Ethosuximide does not require as much monitoring as some of the other antiepileptics, but it is important to ensure effective levels after initiation of therapy or a change in dosage regimen.

Sample timing. The half-life of ethosuximide is quite long—60 hours in adults and 30 hours in children.[111] Thus, it is advised to wait as long as 1 week to 12 days before obtaining ethosuximide levels for monitoring purposes.[14,119] While it is generally advised that trough concentrations be obtained, levels drawn anytime during the dosing interval should be acceptable because there will be very little fluctuation if ethosuximide is given in divided doses. Peak concentrations of ethosuximide administered as a capsule are attained in 3–7 hours.[111,119]

Specimens, collection methods, and assays. Ethosuximide is usually measured by immunoassay.[111] Serum or plasma may be used for determination of ethosuximide concentrations. A variety of blood collection tubes have been tested, and none have interfered with measurement of ethosuximide.[47] Ethosuximide does not bind to serum proteins. Therefore, measurement of unbound levels is never necessary. Studies have shown saliva ethosuximide concentrations to be equal to serum or plasma

concentrations, thus making saliva a convenient alternative, especially in children.[48,115]

Use of levels for dosage adjustment. Ethosuximide is reported to display nonlinear elimination, but primarily at concentrations near the upper end of its therapeutic range. Somewhat greater-than-proportional increases in drug concentration with increases in doses can therefore be expected when higher dose rates are use.

Protein binding, active metabolites, and other considerations. Ethosuximide is negligibly bound to serum proteins and its metabolites have insignificant activity. While ethosuximide is administered as a racemic mixture, the enantiomers have the same pharmacokinetic properties. Thus, measurement of the summed enantiomers is acceptable.[120]

Phenobarbital/Primidone

Primidone and phenobarbital are both used for management of generalized tonic-clonic and partial seizures.[91] Phenobarbital is used for febrile convulsions and hypoxic ischemic seizures in neonates and infants.[107] Primidone is used for treatment of essential tremor in the elderly.[109] Although primidone has activity of its own, most clinicians believe that phenobarbital—a metabolite of primidone—is predominantly responsible for primidone's therapeutic effects. These two drugs will, therefore, be considered together.

Therapeutic ranges. The therapeutic range of phenobarbital for treatment of tonic-clonic, febrile, and hypoxic ischemic seizures is generally regarded as 10–40 mg/L, while concentrations as high as 70 mg/L may be required for refractory status epilepticus.[109,121] Eighty-four percent of patients are likely to respond with concentrations between 10 and 40 mg/L.[121] Management of partial seizures seems to require higher phenobarbital concentrations than management of bilateral tonic-clonic seizures.[14] Concentrations of phenobarbital are always reported when primidone levels are ordered. The therapeutic range of primidone reported by most laboratories is 5–12 mg/L.[14,109] Fifteen to 20% of a primidone dose is metabolized to the active phenobarbital; the side effects of primidone are mostly related to phenobarbital.[91] Central nervous system side effects such as sedation and ataxia generally occur in chronically treated patients at phenobarbital levels between 35 and 80 mg/L. Stupor and coma have been reported at phenobarbital concentrations above 65 mg/L.[111,121]

Sample timing. The half-life of phenobarbital is the rate-limiting step for determining the time to reach steady-state after primidone administration. The half-life of phenobarbital averages 5 days for neonates and 4 days for adults.[121] Since phenobarbital or primidone dosage may be initiated gradually, steady-state is not attained until 2–3 weeks after full dosage has been implemented. Because phenobarbital has such a long half-life, levels obtained anytime during the day would provide reasonable estimates of a trough concentration. Ideally, levels should be obtained from visit to visit at similar times of the day.[121]

Specimens, collection methods, and assays. Serum or plasma is acceptable for measurements of phenobarbital and primidone; whole blood is generally used for point-of-care methods. Use of a new serum separator tube (SST II®, Becton-Dickinson) did not cause a problem with phenobarbital determinations.[44] The partitioning of phenobarbital into saliva is pH-sensitive. However, some studies have shown acceptable correlations with or without pH correction.[48] Saliva concentrations of primidone are particularly sensitive to saliva flow rate changes but show strong correlations with serum concentrations of primidone when standardized collection methods are used.[48] The clinical utility of just measuring primidone concentration in saliva is questionable.

Chromatographic methods (GLC, HPLC) may permit simultaneous determination of both primidone and phenobarbital, but immunoassays are most commonly used.[111] There is potential for cross-reactivity of the immunoassay methods with coadministered barbiturates.[111] No interferences from endogenous substances or blood collection tube components were observed with one immunoassay method for phenobarbital.[122,123]

Use of levels for dosage adjustment. Phenobarbital and primidone exhibit first-order elimination behavior, thus, a change in the dose rate of either drug will result in a proportional change in the average, steady-state serum concentrations.[111,121]

Protein binding, active metabolites, and other considerations. Phenobarbital is approximately 50% bound to serum proteins (albumin) in adults; primidone is not bound to serum proteins.[109,124] Thus, total concentrations of both drugs are reliable indicators of the active, unbound concentrations of these drugs. While primidone has an active metabolite, phenylethylmalonamide (PEMA), the contribution to activity is unlikely to be significant.

Phenytoin

Therapeutic range. Phenytoin is primarily used for treatment of generalized tonic-clonic and complex partial seizures.[125] It may also be used in the treatment of trigeminal neuralgia and for seizure prophylaxis following neurosurgery.[91,125] Studies have shown that serum or plasma concentrations of phenytoin between 10 and 20 mg/L will result in maximum protection from primary or secondary generalized tonic-clonic seizures in most adult patients with normal serum binding. Ten percent of patients with controlled seizures have phenytoin levels less than 3 mg/L, 50% have levels less than 7 mg/L, and 90% have levels less than 15 mg/L.[14] Levels at the lower end of the range are effective for bilateral seizures, while higher concentrations appear to be necessary for partial seizures.[14] The therapeutic range of total concentrations in infants is lower due to lower serum protein binding: 6–11 mg/L.[109] Concentration-related side effects include nystagmus, central nervous system depression (ataxia, inability to concentrate, confusion, and drowsiness), and changes in mental status, coma, or seizures at levels above 40 mg/L.[109] While mild side effects may be observed at concentrations as low as 5 mg/L, there have been cases in which concentrations as high as 50 mg/L have been required for effective treatment without negative consequences.[126]

Some clinicians have proposed that monitoring of phenytoin be limited to unbound concentrations, particularly in patients who are critically ill or likely to have unusual protein

binding.[74,127,128] Unbound phenytoin concentrations are more predictive of clinical toxicity than are total phenytoin concentrations in these individuals.[129] The therapeutic range of unbound phenytoin levels is presumed to be 1–2 mg/L for laboratories that determine the unbound phenytoin fraction at 25°C and 1.5–3 mg/L if done at 37°C.[109]

Sample timing. The time required to attain a steady-state after initiation of phenytoin therapy is difficult to predict due to phenytoin's nonlinear elimination behavior. While the $T_{50\%}$ is approximately 24 hours (considering the average population Vmax and Km values when levels are between 10 and 20 mg/L), there can be extreme variations in these population values. Half-lives between 6 and 60 hours have been reported in adults.[109] Thus, a steady-state might not be attained for as long as 3 weeks. Some clinicians advise that samples be obtained prior to steady-state (after 3–4 days) in order to make sure that levels are not climbing too rapidly.[125] Equations have been developed to predict the time required to reach a steady-state once Vmax and Km values are known.[72] It is important to recognize that the time required to reach a steady-state in a given patient will be longer each time the dose rate is further increased.

Most clinicians advise that trough phenytoin concentrations be monitored.[109] Phenytoin is quite slowly absorbed so that the concentration versus time profile is fairly flat. This is especially true when oral phenytoin is administered 2 or 3 times per day. In this case, a serum phenytoin sample drawn any time during the dosage interval is likely to be close to a trough concentration. The greatest fluctuation would be seen for the more quickly absorbed products (chewable tablets and suspension) in children (who have a higher clearance of phenytoin) given once daily. In this case, it is particularly important to document the time of sample relative to the dose—to identify if the level is closer to a peak, a trough, or a $C_{ss,avg}$.

Specimens, collection methods, and assays. Serum or plasma is generally recommended for total phenytoin measurements. Blood collected for plasma should not be anticoagulated with citrate or oxalate because these anticoagulants have been reported to cause negative interferences with measurements of phenytoin using the EMIT method.[109,113] Anticoagulation with heparin is also of concern since activation of lipoprotein lipases may increase free fatty acid concentrations and displace phenytoin from albumin.[109] While serum separator tubes are generally not recommended, more recent studies with a serum separator tube, the SST II (Becton Dickinson) tubes, showed that serum phenytoin concentrations were stable for 24 hours at room temperature.[44,109]

Saliva has been proposed as a viable alternative to monitoring plasma phenytoin concentrations, especially for children.[48,51,54,115] It has also been proposed as a useful specimen for monitoring unbound phenytoin concentrations, particularly in patients taking valproic acid concurrently.[48] Successful results in infants and children have been shown when saliva is stimulated using a small amount of citric acid on the tongue.[50] Since the S:P ratio is affected by salivary flow rate, it is particularly important that the saliva collection procedure be carefully standardized.[48]

Immunoassays are the most common methods for measurement of total phenytoin concentrations in serum or plasma.[72] The metabolites of phenytoin do not contribute to antiepileptic activity, but certain immunologic methods may measure accumulated phenytoin metabolites in patients with renal impairment. Immunoassays that use monoclonal antibodies or HPLC would be appropriate alternative methods for samples from patients with renal impairment.[76] Fosphenytoin, the phenytoin prodrug, interferes with commonly used immunoassay methods.[72] For this reason, serum for phenytoin monitoring should not be obtained earlier than 4 hours after administration of fosphenytoin, at which time it has been maximally converted to phenytoin.[130] Assays for unbound phenytoin are usually done using ultrafiltered serum followed by one of the other assay methods.[76] The unbound phenytoin fraction is affected by temperature. Therefore, this variable must be controlled.[109] Hemolysis and lipemia do not interfere with phenytoin measurements using an FPIA method.[131]

Use of levels for dosage adjustment. Phenytoin exhibits pronounced nonlinear behavior following therapeutic doses. Thus, increases in dose rate will produce greater-than-proportional increases in the average serum concentration during the dosing interval. Several methods, described elsewhere, use population and/or patient-specific Vmax and Km values to predict the most appropriate dose rate adjustment.[72] The clinician must be aware that the size of phenytoin daily dose increases should typically not be greater than 30 or 60 mg using sodium phenytoin or 25 or 50 mg using the chewable tablets.

Protein binding, active metabolites, and other considerations. The metabolites of phenytoin have insignificant activity. Phenytoin binds primarily to albumin in plasma and the normal unbound fraction of drug in plasma of adults is 0.1.[109,125] Lower serum binding of phenytoin is observed in neonates and infants and in patients with hypoalbuminemia, liver disease, nephrotic syndrome, pregnancy, cystic fibrosis, burns, trauma, malnourishment, AIDS, and advanced age.[91,132] Concurrent drugs (valproic acid, salicylate, and other nonsteroidal anti-inflammatory drugs [NSAIDs]) are known to displace phenytoin.[91] Thus, a total level of phenytoin that is within the range of 10–20 mg/L in these patients might represent an unbound level that is higher than 1–2 mg/L (the therapeutic range of unbound levels). A total concentration of phenytoin in this situation can be misleading. Several approaches can be used in these situations: (1) an unbound phenytoin level can be ordered, if available; (2) the patient's unbound phenytoin level can be calculated by estimating the unbound fraction in the patient (using the literature) and multiplying that by the patient's measured phenytoin level (the resulting unbound level should then be compared to 1–2 mg/L); or (3) special equations may be used to convert the total phenytoin level to what it would be if the patient had normal serum protein binding.

The following equation was developed to normalize phenytoin (PHT) levels in patients with hypoalbuminemia and/or renal failure[91,125,133]:

$$\frac{\text{normalized}}{\text{PHT level}} = \frac{\text{measured PHT level}}{(X \times \text{albumin concentration, gm\%}) + 0.1}$$

The value "X" is 0.2 for patients with low albumin and creatinine clearances equal to or above 25 mL/min and 0.1 mL/min for patients with normal or low albumin who are receiving dialysis. Total levels of phenytoin in patients with creatinine clearance values between 10 and 25 mL/min cannot be as accurately normalized; the clinical status of such patients should be carefully considered since total levels can be misleading. This equation for normalizing total phenytoin concentrations has been tested by groups of investigators in different groups of patients with mixed reviews; it is emphasized that it should be used only as a guide.

Valproic acid is known to increase the unbound fraction of phenytoin in serum.[134] It has also been variably reported to inhibit the metabolism of phenytoin. These two occurrences together could mean that a level within the range of 10–20 mg/L is associated with adverse effects and an unbound phenytoin level greater than 2 mg/L. If unbound phenytoin concentrations are not available, the following equation—modified from its original form—may be useful to normalize the total phenytoin (PHT) level if the level of valproic acid (VPA) in that same sample has been measured[78,125]:

$$\text{normalized PHT level} = \text{measured PHT level} + (0.01 \times \text{VPA level} \times \text{measured PHT level})$$

Other equations have been used for estimating the unbound phenytoin concentration in the presence of valproic acid.[135]

Valproic Acid

Therapeutic range. Valproic acid is used for management of absence seizures, in addition to partial and generalized tonic-clonic and myoclonic seizures. It is also used for a variety of other conditions, including prophylaxis against migraine headaches and bipolar disorder.[109] Most laboratories use 50–100 mg/L as the therapeutic range for trough total valproic acid concentrations. Some patients are effectively treated at lower levels, and others may require trough levels as high as 120 mg/L.[136] Levels at the upper end of the therapeutic range appear to be necessary for treatment of complex partial seizures.[136] The same therapeutic range has been used for patients with migraines or bipolar disorder, although the value of routine serum concentration monitoring for bipolar disorder has been questioned.[137] The following concentration-related side effects may be seen: ataxia, sedation, lethargy, and fatigue at levels above 75 mg/L; tremor at levels above 100 mg/L; and stupor and coma at levels greater than 175 mg/L.[81] The therapeutic range of total valproic acid concentrations is confounded by the nonlinear serum protein binding of this drug, which might explain some of the variable response among and within patients at a given total serum concentration.[97]

Sample timing. The half-life of valproic acid ranges between 7 and 18 hours in children and adults and 17 and 40 hours in infants.[109] Thus, as long as 5 days may be required to attain a steady-state. The pattern of change in valproic acid concentrations varies from interval to interval during the day because of considerable diurnal variation.[109,136] It is, therefore, recommended that samples always be obtained prior to the morning dose as this has been shown to be most consistent from day to day.[136] Considerable fluctuation within the interval will be seen with the immediate-release capsule and syrup, which are rapidly absorbed. The enteric-coated, delayed-release Depakote® tablet displays a shift-to-the-right with respect to its concentration versus time profile, such that the lowest concentration during the interval may not be observed until 4–6 hours into the next dosing interval.[111] It is important to know, however, that concentrations during the interval following administration of the enteric-coated tablet will show considerable fluctuation. The extended-release formulations (Depakote®ER and Sprinkle® capsules), if given in divided doses, provide less fluctuation in concentrations, and samples may be drawn at any time.

Specimens, collection methods, and assays. Serum or heparinized plasma are recommended; other anticoagulants may cross-react if immunoassay methods are used.[109,113] Concentrations of valproic acid in saliva are very low and do not correlate well with plasma concentrations.[48,54] Concentrations of valproic acid measured in tears collected using absorbent paper strips were shown to correlate well with unbound, valproic acid concentrations.[58]

Immunoassays are the most common methods for routine valproic acid serum concentration determinations.[111] Unbound concentrations of valproic acid in ultrafiltrates of serum have been measured by immunoassay or HPLC.[138]

Use of levels for dosage adjustment. The metabolism of unbound valproic acid is linear following therapeutic doses. Thus, unbound valproic acid levels will increase in proportion to increases in dose rate.[109,111] Because valproic acid shows nonlinear, saturable protein binding in serum over the therapeutic range, however, total concentrations will increase less than proportionally. This is important to keep in mind when interpreting total valproic acid levels.

Protein binding, active metabolites, and other considerations. Valproic acid is 90% to 95% bound to albumin and lipoproteins in serum. The unbound fraction of valproic acid shows considerable interpatient variability. It is increased in neonates, in conditions in adults associated with hypoalbuminemia (e.g., liver disease, nephrotic syndrome, cystic fibrosis, burns, trauma, malnutrition, and advanced age) and as a result of displacement by endogenous substances (e.g., bilirubin, free fatty acids, and uremic substances in end-stage renal disease) and other drugs (e.g., salicylate and other NSAIDs).[91,139,140] The increase in the unbound fraction of valproic acid during labor is believed to be the result of displacement by higher concentrations of free fatty acids.[141] Valproic acid also shows intrapatient variability in the unbound fraction due to nonlinear binding. The unbound fraction of valproic acid is fairly constant at lower concentrations but progressively increases as total concentrations rise above 75 mg/L.[109] Thus, total concentrations do not reflect unbound concentrations at the upper end of the therapeutic range. A therapeutic range for unbound valproic acid concentrations can be only approximated; assuming unbound

fractions of 0.05–0.1 and a therapeutic range of total valproic acid concentrations of 50–100 mg/L, an unbound therapeutic range of 2.5–10 mg/L can be deduced.

Other Antiepileptic Drugs

Routine serum concentration monitoring is not recommended for most of the newer antiepileptic drugs.[143,144] Lamotrigine, levetiracetam, felbamate, oxcarbazepine, tiagabine, topiramate, and zonisamide, however, have characteristics that might make concentration monitoring helpful for guiding therapy in certain situations or in special populations.[22,145] While seizure control is associated with a wide range of gabapentin serum concentrations, some feel that its dose-dependent bioavailability may make serum concentration monitoring justified in some cases. Vigabatrin serum levels do not correlate with clinical effect because of its unusual mechanism of action—irreversible binding to an enzyme. Because severe adverse reactions observed in the postmarketing period have resulted in severe restrictions of felbamate use, it will not be discussed here.

Lamotrigine. The considerable pharmacokinetic variability among patients taking lamotrigine, due in part to significant drug–drug interactions, makes it a good candidate for therapeutic drug monitoring.[143,146] The therapeutic range of lamotrigine was originally defined as 1–4 mg/L, but more recently 2.5–15 mg/L has been proposed.[22,144,147] Some patients may tolerate concentrations above 20 mg/L.[148] It has been suggested that concomitant therapy with other antiepileptics may alter the response to lamotrigine or its side effect profile at a given lamotrigine serum concentration.[146] The half-life of lamotrigine can range from 15–30 hours on monotherapy.[143] Thus, one should wait at least 1 week before obtaining samples after initiating or adjusting lamotrigine therapy.[146] This drug exhibits linear pharmacokinetics; therefore, dose rate adjustments will result in proportionate changes in average serum concentrations. Because it is only 55% bound to serum proteins, measurements of unbound lamotrigine levels in serum are not necessary. Saliva concentrations of lamotrigine may be a useful alternative to blood sampling.[143,149] There are HPLC assays currently available for lamotrigine.[147] Routine lamotrigine monitoring is generally not recommended, but serum concentrations might be helpful in special populations or to determine if lack of response is related to unusually low levels or nonadherence.[145,147]

Levetiracetam. Serum concentration monitoring of levetiracetam is more important in pregnancy and in infants and children because of the higher clearances in these patients.[22,145] The half-life ranges from 6–8 hours in adults and a steady-state should be attained within a week.[144] Serum concentrations between 6 and 20 mg/L appear to be associated with response in most patients. Serum protein binding of levetiracetam is less than 10%, obviating the need for measurement of unbound levetiracetam concentrations.[144]

Oxcarbazepine. The pharmacologic effect of oxcarbazepine is primarily related to serum concentrations of its active monohydroxy metabolite (MHD). A therapeutic range of 13 to 35 mg/L for MHD may be used as a rough guide.[22,144] The elimination half-life of MHD is quite variable, ranging from

7–20 hours, and is prolonged in renal impairment. The serum protein binding of MHD is low at 40%; therefore, unbound concentration monitoring of MHD is unnecessary. Routine monitoring of MHD is not warranted, but may be useful in patients with extremes of age or renal impairment, during pregnancy, or to rule out medication nonadherence.[150]

Tiagabine. Tiagabine shows pronounced interpatient pharmacokinetic variability. Trough levels between 20 and 100 mcg/L are associated with improved seizure control, but there is wide variation in response at any given total concentration.[22,143,144] This could, in part, be due to variable serum binding (96% bound in serum on average). Valproic acid, salicylate, and naproxen have been shown to displace tiagabine from serum proteins.[143,144] Tiagabine half-life ranges from 5–13 hours and may be even shorter in the presence of enzyme-inducing drugs.[144,146] Tiagabine shows linear elimination behavior following therapeutic doses.

Topiramate. Topiramate levels are particularly influenced by interactions with other drugs, with levels as much as twofold lower when enzyme-inducing drugs are administered concurrently.[151] The half-life ranges from 18–23 hours, and it has linear elimination behavior.[143,144,146] Topiramate is less than 40% bound to serum proteins but shows saturable binding to red blood cells, thus suggesting that whole blood might be a preferable specimen for monitoring.[144,146] Effective serum levels are generally reported to be between 5 and 20 mg/L with most patients responding at levels below 20 mg/L.[22,143,144] No active metabolites have been identified. An FPIA assay method has been developed.[146]

Zonisamide. The pharmacokinetics of zonisamide are variable among patients and also highly influenced by interactions with other drugs.[143] Zonisamide is approximately 40% bound to serum albumin, and, like topiramate, shows saturable binding to red blood cells, suggesting that whole blood monitoring might be preferable.[144,146] The half-life is 50–70 hours but may be as short as 25 hours when enzyme inducers are coadministered.[143] There are some reports suggesting nonlinear behavior at higher doses. The serum concentration range associated with response is 10–38 mg/L; cognitive dysfunction is reported at levels above 30 mg/L.[22,144,146] No active metabolites have been identified.[143] Both HPLC and immunoassays are available.

Antimicrobials

Aminoglycosides
Therapeutic ranges. Amikacin, gentamicin, and tobramycin are administered intravenously to treat infections of gram-negative bacilli that are resistant to less toxic antibiotics.[42] They are bactericidal, and, thus, their efficacy is highly related to peak concentration after an infusion.[152] They also exhibit a postantibiotic effect in which bacterial killing continues even after the serum concentration is below the minimum inhibitory concentration (MIC).[91] The concentration-dependent killing and postantibiotic effects of the aminoglycosides explain why extended-interval (pulse) dosing of the aminoglycosides is shown to be safe and effective in many patients. Nephrotoxicity

and ototoxicity are the most frequently reported adverse effects of the aminoglycoside antibiotics. Ototoxicity seems to be associated with a prolonged course of treatment (for greater than 7–10 days) with peaks above 12–14 mg/L for gentamicin and tobramycin and 35–40 mg/L for amikacin.[91] Patients with trough levels above 2–3 mg/L (gentamicin, and tobramycin) or 10 mg/L (amikacin) for sustained periods of time are predisposed to increased risk of nephrotoxicity.[91]

Therapeutic ranges for peaks and troughs are reported for the aminoglycosides and pertain only to dosing approaches that involve multiple doses during the day. For gentamicin and tobramycin, peaks between 6 and 10 mg/L and troughs between 0.5 and 2 mg/L are recommended.[153] The approximately fourfold higher MIC for amikacin explains why peaks between 20 and 30 mg/L and troughs between 1 and 8 mg/L are recommended.[153] There is no therapeutic range when the pulse-dosing method is used; doses are given to attain peaks that are approximately 10 times the MIC, and troughs are intended to be nondetectable within 4 hours of administration of the next dose.[152,153] A serum level drawn sometime after infusion of the dose is used only for adjustment of the dosing interval, not to check for efficacy or toxicity.

There has been some concern over the years that aminoglycosides are overmonitored. Uncomplicated patients with normal renal function, who do not have life-threatening infections and will be treated for less than 5 days, may not need to have serum aminoglycoside levels measured.[154] At the other extreme, dosage individualization using serum levels of aminoglycosides are absolutely necessary in patients with serious infections who are on prolonged treatment courses, especially if unusual pharmacokinetic parameters are expected (e.g., renal impairment, burns, cystic fibrosis, extremes of age, sepsis, and pregnancy) and if risk of toxicity is high (such as in patients taking concomitant loop diuretics or nephrotoxic drugs [e.g., amphotericin, cyclosporine, or vancomycin]).[153,154]

Sample timing. For pulse dosing in patients with normal renal function, a steady-state is never reached since each dose is washed out prior to the next dose. The method developed by Nicolau et al. (the so-called *Hartford method*) requires that a single blood sample be obtained between 6 and 14 hours after the end of the first infusion.[155] This sample is referred to as a *random sample*, but the time of the collection must be documented. The level is used with a nomogram in order to determine if a different dosing interval should be used.[42,155] Levels that are too high, according to this nomogram, will indicate that the drug is not being cleared as well as originally predicted, suggesting the need for a longer interval. For traditional dosing, it is important to wait until a steady-state is reached before obtaining blood samples. The half-lives of the aminoglycosides are 1.5–3 hours for adults with normal renal function but as long as 72 hours in patients with severe renal impairment.[91] Since the dosing interval for aminoglycosides is usually adjusted to be 2–3 times the drug's half-life, then a conservative rule of thumb is that steady-state is reached after the third or fourth dose.[42] Some patients may have blood samples drawn immediately after the first dose ("off the load") in order to determine their pharmacokinetic parameters for purposes of dosage regimen individualization. These would most likely be patients who are anticipated to have unpredictable or changing pharmacokinetic parameters, such as those in a critical care unit, and who require immediate effective treatment because of life-threatening infections.

Two blood samples are sufficient for purposes of individualizing traditional aminoglycoside therapy, and will provide reasonable estimates of aminoglycoside pharmacokinetic parameters.[156] It is crucial that the times of the sample collections be accurately recorded.[42,152] The two samples should be spaced sufficiently apart from each other so that an accurate determination of the log-linear slope can be made in order to determine the elimination rate constant. One sample (sometimes referred to as the *measured peak*) should be drawn no earlier than 1 hour after the end of a 30-minute, at minimum, infusion.[156] A second sample may be drawn any time later but is usually drawn within 30 minutes of the start of infusion of the next dose (assumed to be the trough).[42,152,154] If it is expected that the trough level will be close to the limit of the assay sensitivity, the second sample may be drawn earlier.[154,156] Once the elimination rate constant has been calculated using these two levels, the true peak and true trough can be calculated and their values compared to desired target peaks and troughs.

Specimens, collection methods, and assays. Serum or EDTA-treated plasma is recommended. Blood collection tubes using gel barriers are acceptable for serum.[157,158] Heparin has been shown to interfere with some assays and is not recommended unless the laboratory has ruled out any problems.[42] A study showed that gentamicin concentrations in citric acid-stimulated saliva of pediatric patients were good predictors of trough plasma gentamicin concentrations, but only when pulse dosing was used (24-hour dosing interval).[159] It was suggested that gentamicin may require a long period of time to fully equilibrate between plasma and saliva, thus explaining the lack of correlation in measured levels when divided doses were used.[159] Aminoglycoside concentrations in cerebrospinal fluid are between 10% and 50% of serum concentrations; no therapeutic ranges for cerebrospinal fluid concentrations have been established.[42]

Serum or plasma should either be assayed within 2 hours of collection, or frozen at 0°C to 5°C.[42] This is particularly important for samples that contain beta-lactam antibiotics such as penicillin G, ampicillin, carbenicillin, nafcillin, or ticarcillin.[91] The beta-lactam antibiotics, commonly administered with aminoglycosides, physically bind aminoglycoside antibiotics in blood resulting in their inactivation.[42,91,152] In vivo, this means the aminoglycoside is cleared more rapidly than usual. The primary concern, however, is continued inactivation of the aminoglycoside that can occur after a blood sample has been collected. A serum concentration that is 7 mg/L at the time of collection might become 6 mg/L after a period of time at room temperature. Use of the artifactually low serum concentration would lead to errors in determination of the aminoglycoside pharmacokinetic parameters. If immediate assay is not possible, the serum or plasma sample should be immediately frozen.

Use of levels for dosage adjustment. Various pulse-dosing methods are used to take advantage of the concentration-related killing and postantibiotic effects of the aminoglycosides.[154] The original Hartford method involves giving a mg/kg dose that is administered in order to attain a peak concentration that is approximately 10 times the MIC. Then a sample is obtained between 6 and 14 hours after the end of the infusion and compared to a nomogram, which indicates the appropriate maintenance dosing interval—usually 24, 36, or 48 hours.[155] Pulse-dosing methods are not routinely recommended for certain patients, including those with enterococcal endocarditis, renal failure, meningitis, osteomyelitis, or burns.[154] However, studies are ongoing to show safety and efficacy in more subpopulations of patients. The results of clinical trials do not consistently show a reduction in nephrotoxicity, and it has been proposed that pulse doses be lowered to provide daily AUC similar to those measured following traditional daily doses.[152,160]

Serum concentrations of aminoglycosides obtained during traditional dosing are used to determine an individual patient's pharmacokinetic parameters, as well as the true peak and true trough in order to compare these to desired target levels. Equations that account for time of drug infusion are used to determine an appropriate dosing interval and dose.[161] Other dosage adjustment methods include nomograms and population pharmacokinetic (Bayesian) methods.[153,161]

Protein binding, active metabolites, and other considerations. The aminoglycosides are less than 10% bound to serum proteins, and unbound concentrations will always reflect total concentrations in serum.[153] The metabolites of the aminoglycosides are inactive.

Chloramphenicol

Therapeutic range. Chloramphenicol is a broad spectrum antibiotic reserved for treatment of serious infections, including treatment of meningitis caused by ampicillin-resistant *Haemophilus influenzae* type b.[42,162] The therapeutic range for peak levels is generally considered to be 10–20 mg/L. A dose-related reversible type of bone marrow depression may occur and is associated with sustained peak serum levels above 25 mg/L. Irreversible aplastic anemia occurs rarely and is not believed to be related to the serum concentration of chloramphenicol. A somewhat lower therapeutic range may be used for neonates (7.5–14 mg/L) because of the lower serum binding of chloramphenicol in this group—32% versus 53% in adults.[99,162] Toxic reactions, including fatalities, have occurred in premature infants and newborns who have had sustained chloramphenicol serum levels above 40–50 mg/L.[42,162] These reactions, known as the *Gray syndrome,* are likely caused by the immature conjugation and renal clearance pathways in these patients.

Chloramphenicol should be monitored closely in patients to guide dosing and avoid toxicity in patients with liver or renal disease or in whom drug–drug interactions are anticipated.[42] One study in children, ages 1–66 months, showed progressive decreases in chloramphenicol levels during treatment, suggesting that this group should be frequently monitored.[163] It is important that baseline blood counts and hepatic and renal function tests be done before initiation of therapy and repeated during treatment.

Sample timing. The half-life of chloramphenicol is 2–5 hours in adults; steady-state is usually assumed to occur within 12–24 hours.[162] The half-life in neonates and infants may range from 8–22 hours.[164] Thus, a steady-state should not be assumed in these groups for at least 3 days.

Because both efficacy and toxicity to chloramphenicol are related to peak levels, it is necessary to anticipate when the peak level will occur. Chloramphenicol is available orally as either chloramphenicol base or the chloramphenicol palmitate, which is hydrolyzed to active chloramphenicol in the intestine. Chloramphenicol succinate is the only available intravenous product and is hydrolyzed to chloramphenicol by esterases in the liver, kidneys, and lungs. The peak times for chloramphenicol, therefore, depend not only on the rate of absorption or infusion but also on the rate of hydrolysis in the case of these prodrugs.[162] Times associated with peak serum concentrations of chloramphenicol are approximately 1 hour for the orally administered base, 1.5–3 hours for the orally administered palmitate suspension, and between 0.5 and 1 hour after the end of a 30-minute succinate infusion.[42] Times of peak chloramphenicol levels following intravenous infusion of the succinate to infants are highly affected by infusion rate, injection site, volume of fluid in the tubing, and type of infusion system.[165] It is important that specific guidelines be established at individual institutions to best estimate the times at which peak chloramphenicol levels will occur.

Specimens, collection methods, and assays. Both serum and plasma are acceptable for analysis of chloramphenicol. Gel barrier serum separator tubes have not caused a problem with chloramphenicol.[42] There is some suggestion that serum or plasma should be protected from light.[42] Also, in vitro hydrolysis of the succinate has been reported, and samples are not stable when stored at –20°C for longer than 1 week.[166] The most commonly used assays for chloramphenicol are HPLC and immunoassay (EMIT). The immunoassay method has the necessary sensitivity and specificity but does not permit measurements of palmitate or succinate concentrations.[167] High-performance liquid chromatography is sufficiently sensitive and may also permit simultaneous determination of both prodrug and active drug. This ability to determine concentrations of prodrug would be useful only for explaining the reason for a particular chloramphenicol level. For example, low concentrations of chloramphenicol along with high concentrations of the succinate would indicate limited capacity for hydrolysis of the prodrug.[162]

Cerebrospinal fluid concentrations of chloramphenicol are sometimes measured (in which case the assay must ensure the necessary sensitivity). Concentrations in cerebrospinal fluid need to be above the MIC of the organism, usually between 1 and 6 mg/L.[42] Saliva concentrations of chloramphenicol are not reliable predictors of serum chloramphenicol concentrations.[168]

Use of levels for dosage adjustment. Chloramphenicol has linear elimination characteristics. Therefore, serum chloramphenicol concentrations should change in proportion to the change in daily dose.

Protein binding, active metabolites, and other considerations. Chloramphenicol is 53% to 60% bound in the serum of adults, with lower binding in neonates (32%) and adults with cirrhosis (42%).[162] Unbound chloramphenicol concentrations in neonates who have total concentrations between 7.5 and 14 mg/L are similar to unbound concentrations in adults who have total levels between 10 and 20 mg/L.[99] None of the metabolites of chloramphenicol show significant activity, and, therefore, do not need to be considered when interpreting chloramphenicol serum concentrations.

Vancomycin

Therapeutic range. Vancomycin, a glycopeptide antibiotic with a narrow spectrum of activity, is used intravenously to treat gram-positive organisms resistant to other antibiotics.[42,91] Emergence of vancomycin-resistant enterococci has led to the need to restrict its use. The major toxicities associated with vancomycin are nephrotoxicity and ototoxicity (likely aggravated by concurrent administration of other nephro- and ototoxic drugs). Another adverse effect known as *red man syndrome* (intense flushing, tachycardia, and hypotension) is usually associated with infusion times shorter than 1 hour.[91,169]

While many institutions monitor both peaks and troughs of vancomycin, this practice has been questioned, in part because of a lack of standardization of when a sample should be drawn to appropriately reflect a "peak." In contrast to the aminoglycosides, it is more important to maintain vancomycin levels above the MIC during the dosing interval (to ensure efficacy) than it is to have high peaks and low troughs. It is usually assumed that trough concentrations for vancomycin should be between 5 and 15 mg/L, and greater than 10 mg/L for deep seated infections such as endocarditis.[169,170] A range of 15–20 mg/L for troughs is recommended for treatment of pneumonia or other nafcillin- or methicillin-resistant *Staphylococcus aureus* infections.[169,170] While it is sometimes recommended that peak concentrations must be kept below 50 mg/L to avoid ototoxicity, this recommendation is based on only two cases.[152] It is more likely that ototoxicity is the result of all levels being too high during the dosing interval (an excessively high total vancomycin exposure).[152] Some pharmacokinetic dosing methods are, therefore, based on targeting peak vancomycin serum concentrations (those drawn 2 hours after the end of the infusion) between 30 and 50 mg/L.[169]

Vancomycin is routinely monitored in all patients in some hospitals, but many question the need for this in uncomplicated patients with normal renal function.[42,152] Indications for monitoring include decreased or changing renal function, especially in patients receiving other nephrotoxic or ototoxic drugs; patients expected to have unusual pharmacokinetics (burns, malignancies, and intravenous drug abusers); patients on therapy for longer than 10 days; patients showing poor response; and patients with unusually high MICs.[42,170,171]

Sample timing. The half-life of vancomycin is 7–9 hours in adults with normal renal function but can be as long as 120–140 hours in patients with renal failure. Vancomycin half-life is approximately 7 hours in full-term neonates, 6 hours in children, and 12 hours in patients older than 65.[170] Half-lives are 3–4 hours in obese patients and 4 hours in burn patients.[91] Samples should be obtained as troughs, within 0.5–1 hour of the start of the next infusion.

Specimens, collection methods, and assays. Serum or plasma, using EDTA-treated tubes, may be used. Heparinized tubes should be avoided based on reports of instability of vancomycin in the presence of heparin. There are no reports or problems using serum separator tubes.[42]

Immunoassays (EMIT and FPIA) are the most common assays used for routine measurements of serum or plasma vancomycin concentration measurements. High-performance liquid chromatography or radioimmunoassay may also be used.[170] Serum vancomycin concentrations in patients with renal failure were overestimated by one FPIA method because of cross-reactivity of the polyclonal antibody with a vancomycin crystalline degradation product which accumulates in renal failure patients.[172] This same method underestimated serum vancomycin concentrations in patients with hyperbilirubinemia.[173] An EMIT method and a modified FPIA method, which both used monoclonal antibodies, did not significantly overestimate vancomycin serum concentrations in these patients.[174]

Use of levels for dosage adjustment. Vancomycin elimination is linear, and an increase in the dose (without a change in the dosing interval) can be expected to provide a proportional change in the trough serum concentration. It must be cautioned that vancomycin has a very pronounced distribution phase, making the standardization of any so-called peak sample to be especially important. More sophisticated prediction methods for dosing adjustments must be used if the dosing interval is adjusted with or without a change in dose.

Many methods have been proposed for vancomycin dosage regimen adjustment.[91,169,175,176] A relatively simple method proposed by Ambrose and Winter permits the use of a single trough level (drawn within 1 hour of the start of the next infusion) along with an assumption of the population distribution volume to predict the necessary pharmacokinetic parameters needed for individualization.[169] Once those parameters are determined, the aminoglycoside individualization equations can be used to target desired peak and trough vancomycin concentrations.

Protein binding, active metabolites, and other considerations. Vancomycin is 30% to 55% bound to serum proteins in adults with normal renal function. The binding is lower (19%) in patients with end-stage renal disease.[176] With binding this low, total concentrations of vancomycin will always provide reliable indications of the unbound concentrations in serum. Vancomycin metabolites are inactive, and, thus, do not contribute to antibacterial effect or toxicity.

Amphotericin B

While amphotericin B continues to be considered the drug of choice for most systemic fungal infections, serum concentration

monitoring is not recommended.[177] The nephrotoxic effects of amphotericin B do not appear to be related to serum concentration, and the range of concentrations associated with beneficial effect is, likewise, unclear.[177]

Flucytosine

Therapeutic range. Flucytosine is a synthetic antifungal agent that is often used in combination with amphotericin B for treatment of systemic fungal infections.[178] It is also used increasingly in combination with the azole antifungal agents and is part of a new therapeutic approach in the treatment of certain tumors, such as colorectal carcinoma.[179] Most clinicians agree that peak serum concentrations of flucytosine should be kept below 100 mg/L to avoid dose-related hepatotoxicity, bone marrow depression, and gastrointestinal disturbances.[152,179,180] Some clinicians also advise that trough concentrations of flucytosine be kept between 25 and 50 mg/L (or kept above 25 mg/L) in order to avoid rapid development of resistance.[152,178,179] If a constant infusion is used, steady-state serum concentrations of 50 mg/L should be targeted.[152] The hepatotoxicity and bone marrow suppression are both usually reversible with discontinuation. Indications for monitoring flucytosine include avoidance of toxicity—particularly in patients with impaired renal function or those receiving concomitant amphotericin B—and avoidance of resistance due to sustained low levels.[152,178-180]

Sample timing. The half-life of flucytosine is approximately 3–4 hours in patients with normal renal function; it is usually advised to wait 24 hours before a steady-state is assumed.[179,180] The half-life can be as long as 85 hours in patients with renal failure in which case steady-state would not be reached for approximately 10 days.[178] Peak concentrations should be obtained 1–2 hours after an oral dose or 30 minutes after the end of an infusion.[152,177-179] The peak time occurs later after an oral dose of flucytosine in patients with poor renal function because of either slowed absorption or a shift in peak time related to the drug's longer half-life.[179] Trough concentrations, if indicated, should be drawn within 30 minutes of the next dose.

Specimens, collection methods, and assays. Serum is the most common specimen reported for analysis. There do not appear to be special precautions for blood collection devices. The most common assays include microbiological, GLC, HPLC, and an automated enzymatic method.[178,180,181] The enzymatic method compares well to HPLC but shows some degree of nonspecificity with icteric and lipemic samples.[181]

Use of levels for dosage adjustment. Because there are no reports of nonlinear elimination behavior, a given increase in dose rate or infusion rate should produce a proportional increase in serum flucytosine concentration.

Protein binding, active metabolites, and other considerations. Flucytosine does not exist as enantiomers, has no active metabolites, and is minimally bound to serum proteins.

Azole Antifungals

Therapeutic ranges. While serum concentrations of the azoles have been measured and documented following successful therapy, serum concentrations associated with toxicity have not been clearly documented. Serum concentrations of ketoconazole between 1.5 and 6 mg/L, and of fluconazole between 30 and 90 mg/L have been associated with effective chronic therapy.[177,180] Efficacy has been associated with the following serum concentration ranges of the triazole antifungals, as measured by HPLC methods: 0.5–2 mg/L for itraconazole, 0.5–1.5 mg/L for posaconazole, and 0.5–2 mg/L for voriconazole.[182,183]

The primary reason for monitoring the azole antifungal drugs is to ensure efficacy. Itraconazole levels are known to be relatively low in patients with AIDS or acute leukemia, most likely due to malabsorption and concurrent administration of enzyme-inducing drugs.[184] For this reason, some consider the serum concentration monitoring of itraconazole to be essential in patients with life-threatening fungal infections.[177] Ketoconazole is recommended for monitoring only in patients with treatment failure or relapse, or if drug–drug interactions or malabsorption are suspected.[177,180] Fluconazole is the least likely to require monitoring, as its absorption is predictable and it is less affected by drug–drug interactions.[177]

Sample timing. The half-lives of fluconazole, itraconazole, and posaconazole range between 24 and 31 hours.[182] Thus, steady-state will not be attained for at least 1 week after initiation of therapy or adjustment of the dosage regimen. The half-lives of ketoconazole and voriconazole are shorter (3–6 hours) and steady-state can therefore be expected after 24–48 hours.[180,182] Since the purpose of monitoring the azoles is to ensure that minimum levels of drug are present, trough levels should be obtained when possible.

Specimens, collection methods, and assays. Serum is the most common specimen reported for analysis of the azole drugs. There do not appear to be any reported problems associated with blood collection methods. The most common assays for the azoles include microbiological (bioassay), GLC, and HPLC.[177,180,184] Because itraconazole has an active metabolite that may be present at concentrations that are 2–3 times higher than the parent drug, concentration readings using microbiologic assays will be higher than those reported using the chromatographic methods.[183,184] An HPLC method that measures both the parent and hydroxylated metabolite is preferred for itraconazole. Although concentrations of fluconazole in stimulated saliva were highly correlated with concentrations in plasma, the accuracy of plasma concentration prediction was not adequate.[185]

Use of levels for dosage adjustment. Although azole levels are not used for the purpose of dosage adjustment, fluconazole, ketoconazole, fluconazole, and posaconazole exhibit first-order elimination behavior, and increases in dose rate or infusion rate can be expected to produce proportional increases in drug concentrations.[177] Itraconazole and voriconazole are reported to have nonlinear elimination behavior, such that greater-than-proportional increases in serum drug concentration should be expected with increases in dose rate.[152,183]

Protein binding, active metabolites, and other considerations. Itraconazole, ketoconazole, and posaconazole are 98% to 99% bound to serum proteins, primarily albumin, For these drugs, it is possible that some of the inability to correlate total concentrations with response and toxicity is complicated by variable serum protein binding among patients. Voriconazole is 60% bound, while fluconazole is only 12% bound.[183] Itraconazole concentrations in the presence of variable quantities of the active metabolite may also complicate the correlation of itraconazole serum concentrations with effect and toxicity.[183]

Antimycobacterials

The optimal use of therapeutic drug monitoring for mycobacterial infections is currently under study. Drugs that are FDA-approved and considered first line as part of an initial four-drug regimen are isoniazid, rifampin, pyrazinamide, and either ethambutol or streptomycin. Of these, isoniazid and rifampin are the most important based on their relatively high potency and favorable side-effect profiles. Second-line agents that are more toxic must be used if drug resistance emerges and include ethionamide, cycloserine, capreomycin, para-aminosalicylic acid, and dapsone.[186]

It is essential that adequate levels of these antimycobacterial drugs be present in serum for effective treatment. This does not always occur, even in patients in whom adherence has been documented.[186] Lower-than-expected levels of antimycobacterial drugs have been reported in patients with diabetes and in those with HIV infections, which in some cases was associated with malabsorption.[187-189] There is also considerable potential for drug–drug interactions among the antimycobacterial drugs, given the effects of rifampin, isoniazid, and the fluoroquinolones in either inducing or inhibiting cytochrome P450 isozymes.[190] Drugs used to treat HIV patients may also contribute to this drug–drug interaction quagmire.

A study in non-HIV infected tuberculosis patients who were not responding to treatment as expected showed that 29% to 68% of them had serum antimycobacterial drug levels below target ranges.[191] In another study, a small percentage of nonresponding patients all showed suboptimal levels of rifampin.[192] After dosage adjustments were made, all patients responded to treatment. The authors recommended that low serum rifampin levels be suspected in patients who do not respond after 3 months of supervised drug administration, or earlier in patients with HIV infection, malnutrition, known gastrointestinal or malabsorptive disease, or hepatic or renal disease.

Specialized laboratories have been developed that offer sensitive and specific assays for serum concentrations for the most commonly used antimycobacterial drugs.[186] As more specific information about the efficacy of therapeutic drug monitoring of these drugs becomes available, more laboratories and services of this type will likely be available.[193]

Antiretrovirals

Therapeutic ranges. There is some evidence that favors limited serum concentration monitoring of drugs used in the treatment of HIV-1 infection, in particular the PIs and the nonnucleoside reverse-transcriptase inhibitors (NNRTIs).[194,195] These drugs, particularly the PIs, show marked interpatient variability in their pharmacokinetics, and retrospective studies show strong relationships between drug concentrations and virologic response.[196] In addition, suboptimal levels of the antiretroviral drugs are associated with acquired drug resistance and virologic failure.[197] A substudy of the randomized, prospective clinical trial, ATHENA, showed that patients who underwent serum drug concentration monitoring for the antiretroviral drugs had a significantly higher likelihood of virological response as compared to those who did not undergo monitoring.[196]

Minimum effective concentrations have been determined for the most common PIs based on in vitro determinations of drug concentrations (corrected for serum binding) required for 50% or 90% inhibition of replication in the patient's virus isolate (IC_{50} or IC_{90}). Attention has turned more recently, however, to the use of a new parameter that may be a better predictor of response. The inhibitory quotient (IQ) is the ratio of the patient's trough plasma concentration to the IC_{50} or IC_{90}.[196] A high IQ would indicate more drug is present in the patient than is needed for virologic response, while a low IQ would indicate inadequate drug levels or a resistant virus. Recent studies show virologic response may be better related to IQ than to trough levels alone.[196] Future studies may focus on the definition of therapeutic ranges of IQ rather than minimum concentrations.

The most commonly used PIs are fosamprenavir (a prodrug of amprenavir), darunavir, atazanavir, indinavir, lopinavir, nelfinavir, ritonavir, saquinavir and tipranavir. The most commonly used NNRTIs are efavirenz, nevirapine and etravirine. Serum concentrations of newer agents (enfuvirtide, a fusion inhibitor, and raltegravir, an integrase inhibitor) may also be monitored in select situations.[194,195] Some clinicians advocate the monitoring of these drugs in all patients on initiation of therapy to ensure adequate levels; others reserve use for selected situations including patients with renal or liver disease, pregnancy, children, patients at risk for drug interactions, and suspected toxicity.[196,198]

Sample timing. Half-lives of the NNRTIs average 25–50 hours, and steady-state will be reached after a week in most patients.[199] However, a steady-state will be reached within 2 days for the PIs, which have half-lives ranging from 2–12 hours.[199] Predose samples are recommended as the minimum effective concentrations and the IQs are based on the lowest drug concentration during the dosing interval. There may be logistic problems with this timing, however, in cases when the drug is administered once daily in the evening. Some drugs, such as nelfinavir, exhibit a lag in their absorption, such that the lowest concentration actually occurs about an hour after administration of the next dose.

Specimen, collection methods, and assays. Serum or plasma has been used as the specimen for analysis. It is important that the possible influence of gel barrier or serum separator tubes be determined by the laboratory prior to use. Given the high binding of these drugs to AAG, tubes with stoppers possibly formulated with TBEP must be avoided. Nevirapine concentrations in citric-acid simulated saliva strongly correlated with concentrations in plasma and plasma ultrafiltrate.[200] Indinavir concentrations in saliva also show promise as noninvasive alternatives to plasma concentrations.[201] Concentration monitoring in saliva for the other antiretroviral drugs is not

likely to be as promising because they are highly protein bound (>90%), and assay sensitivity would be limiting.

High-performance liquid chromatography is most commonly used to determine serum concentrations of the antiretroviral drugs, and HPLC methods have been developed to measure as many as seven PIs and two NNRTIs in a single run using ultraviolet absorption.[202,203]

Use of levels for dosage adjustment. Dosage adjustments of the antiretroviral drugs, for the most part, should result in proportional changes in the trough serum drug concentration, provided the dosing interval is not altered. Reports showing serum drug concentrations to be unpredictable after dosage adjustments in some patients suggest that nonadherence with antiretroviral regimens is a major concern.[196] Serum concentrations of amprenavir, lopinavir, nelfinavir, and saquinavir may be difficult to maintain above their minimum effective concentrations because of rapid clearances and large first-pass effects. Rather than increasing their dose rate, ritonavir, a potent inhibitor of CYP3A4-mediated metabolism in the gut wall and liver, may be coadministered as a *pharmacoenhancer*. This results in decreased gastrointestinal enzyme metabolism of the PI, higher trough levels, and, in most cases, prolonged elimination half-lives.[204]

Protein binding, active metabolites, and other considerations. The serum protein binding of nevirapine and indinavir is 50% to 60%, while the protein binding of the other antiretrovirals is greater than 90%.[196,199] Alpha-1-acid glycoprotein and albumin are the primary binding proteins for these drugs in serum.[196] As would be expected, there is considerable variability in the unbound fraction of these drugs in serum. In addition, AAG concentrations are elevated in patients with HIV-1 infection and can return to normal with treatment. Thus, the same total level of the drug would be expected to reflect a lower level of response early in treatment as compared to later. Clearly, total concentrations of the PIs and NNRTIs should be cautiously interpreted if unusual serum binding is anticipated, but no clear guidelines are yet available. Only nelfinavir has a metabolite that is known to be active.[196] While studies indicate the measurement of the metabolite is probably not crucial, there is likely to be considerable variability among and within patients in the presence of this metabolite.

Cardiac Drugs

Digoxin

Therapeutic ranges. There has been a dramatic reduction in digoxin toxicity since the advent of therapeutic drug monitoring for digoxin.[62] Digoxin's inotropic effect is the basis for its use for treatment of congestive heart failure, while its chronotropic effects are the basis for treatment of atrial arrhythmias such as atrial fibrillation, atrial flutter, and paroxysmal atrial tachycardia. The commonly reported therapeutic range is 0.5–2.0 mcg/L in adults and 1–2.6 mcg/L in neonates.[62,99,205] The lower end of the range (0.5–1 mcg/L) is generally used for treatment of heart failure, with levels up to 1.5 mcg/L possibly leading to additional benefit.[81] Higher serum digoxin concentrations are required for treatment of atrial arrhythmias (0.8–1.5 mcg/L), with additional benefit gained in some patients with levels up to 2 mcg/L.[91]

Fifty percent of patients with serum digoxin concentrations above 2.5 mcg/L show some form of digoxin toxicity.[91] Symptoms of toxicity include muscle weakness; gastrointestinal complaints (anorexia, nausea, vomiting, abdominal pain, and constipation); CNS effects (headache, insomnia, confusion, vertigo, and changes in color vision); and serious cardiovascular effects (second- or third-degree atrioventricular [AV] bradycardia, premature ventricular contractions, and ventricular tachycardia).[91,205] In fact, many of the cardiac arrhythmias observed with high digoxin concentrations resemble the clinical condition being treated, hence the need to monitor serum digoxin concentrations to distinguish toxicity from inadequate therapy.

There are several physiologic or pathologic conditions that can shift the therapeutic range of digoxin. Its toxicity may be more likely within the therapeutic range if the patient has hypokalemia, hypomagnesemia, hypercalcemia, or underlying heart disease (e.g., coronary atherosclerotic heart disease or an old myocardial infarction).[25,62] Patients with hyperthyroidism are believed to be more resistant to digoxin.[25]

The primary indications for digoxin monitoring include (1) suspected digoxin toxicity in order to determine the appropriate amount of antidote (digoxin-immune Fab fragments; Digibind®) needed; (2) suspected poisoning from ingestion of plants or herbal medications that contain structurally similar glycosides; (3) impaired renal function to adjust the dose rate; and (4) suspected interactions with drugs such as antacids, amiodarone, oral antibiotics, cholestyramine, cyclosporine kaolin-pectin, metoclopramide, neomycin, quinidine, spironolactone, sulfasalazine, verapamil, and St. John's wort.[25,206]

Sample timing. The average digoxin half-life in adults with normal renal function is approximately 2 days; at least 7 days are recommended to attain a steady-state.[205] In the case of treatment of digoxin overdose with digoxin-immune Fab fragments (a fragment of an antibody that is very specific for digoxin), blood samples for serum digoxin measurements should not be obtained sooner than 10 days after administration of the fragments.[62,205] Since most immunoassays measure both the free and Fab-bound digoxin, premature sampling would lead to artifactually high digoxin concentration readings.

Samples drawn during the absorption and distribution phases after administration of digoxin cannot be appropriately interpreted by comparison to the usual therapeutic range. Digoxin levels in blood do not reflect the more important levels in myocardial tissue until at least 6 hours after the dose (some say at least 12 hours).[205-207] Blood samples should, therefore, be drawn anytime between 6 hours after the dose and right before the next dose (Figure 5-5).

Inappropriate timing of samples for digoxin determinations is a major problem in hospitals. One study showed that 55% of the samples submitted to the laboratory for digoxin analysis lacked clinical value because of inappropriate timing.[208] In another study, standardization of digoxin administration times for 1700 and blood sample times for 0700 resulted in a dramatic reduction in inappropriately timed samples.[209] Another recommendation is that the laboratory immediately contact the clinician if digoxin levels are above 3.5 mcg/L.[205] If it is confirmed that the sample was drawn too early after the dose, another sample should be requested. Alternatively, the laboratory should collect sample timing information as part of the laboratory request form and refuse to assay any samples that are inappropriately timed.

Specimens, collection methods, and assays. Serum or plasma, anticoagulated with heparin or EDTA, may be used. In general, serum separator tubes should be avoided.[205] Serum is recommended if ultrafiltration is to be done for purposes of determining unbound concentrations of digoxin in patients treated with Fab fragments (Digibind®). Samples are stable for 24 hours at 2°C to 8°C and 1–2 weeks at –20°C.[205] Saliva concentrations of digoxin have been measured in a number of studies, but none show a sufficiently strong correlation with either total or unbound levels in serum. Part of the poor correlation was proposed to be related to active secretion of digoxin into saliva or interferences from endogenous digoxin-like immunoreactive substances (DLIS).[159]

Digoxin serum concentrations are measured almost exclusively using commercial immunoassay methods.[62,205] The digoxin antibodies used in these immunoassays cross-react to varying extents with digoxin metabolites, endogenous DLIS, and other drugs and their metabolites (spironolactone and its active metabolite canrenone, digitoxin, and digitoxin metabolites). In fact, immunoassays for digoxin may cross-react with structurally similar substances in Chinese medicines (e.g., dried venom of Chinese toad) or plants (oleander) and, therefore, may be used to detect the presence of these substances, which cause digoxin-like toxicity.[205] It is important to note that these interferences can result in overreading or underreading of digoxin. One study comparing nine different commercial immunoassay methods showed that three of the nine methods underreported potentially toxic digoxin concentrations because of negative interferences caused by spironolactone and canrenone.[71] Potentially interfering digoxin metabolites will accumulate in renal impairment; DLIS are predominant in the blood of patients with renal and liver disease, those who are pregnant, and in neonates.[62] The high potential for interferences reinforces the importance of monitoring signs and symptoms in addition to serum levels.

One major cause of interference with digoxin serum concentration determinations by immunoassay is the presence of Fab fragments (Digibind®) used as an antidote to digoxin toxicity. The digoxin antibodies from the immunoassay cause this interference by competing with the Fab fragments for digoxin in the same samples. In patients with renal failure, this source of interference persists for more than 10 days after administration of the antidote. Ultrafiltration of the serum sample removes the digoxin-bound Fab fragments and permits a fairly reliable measurement of the unbound digoxin concentration.[210] Newer assays have been developed to directly measure unbound digoxin in the presence of Digibind® without ultrafiltration.[211]

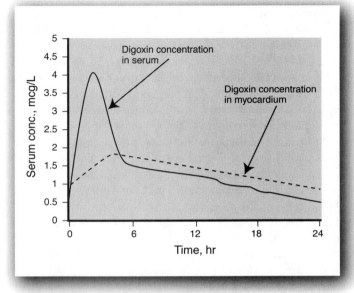

FIGURE 5-5. Simulated plot showing concentrations of digoxin in serum (mcg/L) and concentrations in myocardial tissue (units not provided) after a dose of digoxin at steady-state. Tissue concentrations do not parallel concentrations in serum until at least 6 hours after the dose.

Use of levels for dosage adjustment. Dose rate adjustments of digoxin based on serum digoxin concentrations are straightforward. Because of linear elimination behavior, a given increase in the daily digoxin dose will produce a proportional increase in the serum concentration at that time during the dosing interval. Again, it is extremely important that a serum level used for dose rate adjustment be obtained no earlier than 6–8 hours after the last dose.

Protein binding, active metabolites, and other considerations. Digoxin is only 20% to 30% bound to serum proteins.[25] Therefore, total concentrations in serum will reflect the pharmacologically active unbound concentration. The biologic activity of digoxin metabolites is modest compared to the parent drug, and variable presence of metabolites should not affect the interpretation of a digoxin serum concentration.

Lidocaine

Therapeutic range. Lidocaine is a Type 1B antiarrhythmic used as second-line therapy for the acute treatment for ventricular tachycardia and fibrillation. The therapeutic range is generally considered to be 1.5–5 mg/L with concentrations greater than 6 mg/L considered to be toxic.[91,205,212] Minor side effects—drowsiness, dizziness, euphoria, and paresthesias—may be observed at serum concentrations above 3 mg/L. More serious side effects observed at concentrations above 6 mg/L include muscle twitching, confusion, agitation, and psychoses, while cardiovascular depression, AV block, hypotension, seizures, and coma may be observed at concentrations above 8 mg/L.[91,205,213]

Lidocaine is not monitored as commonly as some of the other cardiac drugs because its effect (abolishment of the ECG-monitored arrhythmia) is easy to directly observe.

Indications should be restricted to situations in which the expected response is not evident (inefficacy or toxicity) or when decreased hepatic clearance is suspected or anticipated: liver disease, congestive heart failure, advanced age, severe trauma, and/or concurrent drugs such as beta-adrenergic blockers, fluvoxamine, or cimetidine.[62,205,212]

Sample timing. The half-life of lidocaine ranges from 1.5 hours to as long as 5 hours in patients with liver disease.[91,213] Thus, steady-state may not be attained for 18–24 hours even if a loading dose is administered. Because lidocaine is administered as a continuous infusion, there are no fluctuations in levels, and blood for lidocaine serum concentration determinations can be drawn anytime at steady-state.

Specimens, collection methods, and assays. Blood collected in serum separator tubes and tubes using TBEP-containing rubber stoppers have resulted in artifactually low lidocaine levels. A new formulation of the Becton-Dickinson serum separator tube, SST II®, was shown to be acceptable, however, with complete recovery of lidocaine from serum stored for as long as 7 days.[44] Plasma is also acceptable as a specimen if heparin or EDTA is used as the anticoagulant.[175] Lidocaine is stable in serum or plasma stored 24 hours at 2°C to 8°C or 1–2 weeks at –20°C.[175]

Immunoassays for determination of lidocaine are commercially available and show little cross-reactivity with lidocaine metabolites.[62] They do not permit separate determination of the primary active metabolite, monoethylglycinexylidide (MEGX), which has 80% to 90% of the activity of lidocaine.[91,205] Chromatographic methods (HPLC and GLC) are preferred if monitoring of the active metabolite is deemed necessary.

Use of levels for dosage adjustment. Adjustments of lidocaine infusion rate should result in a proportional increase in lidocaine serum concentration.

Protein binding, active metabolites, and other considerations. The unbound percentage of lidocaine is normally 30% but can range from 10% to 40% due to variations in AAG concentrations.[91,205] The AAG concentrations are decreased in patients with nephrotic syndrome and increased in conditions of trauma, after surgery, and in patients with rheumatoid arthritis, cancer, and morbid obesity.[205] Thus, higher total concentrations may be considered therapeutic for patients with higher AAG concentrations.

The AAG concentrations are also increased after a myocardial infarction, resulting in a lower unbound lidocaine fraction during prolonged infusions of lidocaine in these patients.[214] The combination of higher total levels of lidocaine during prolonged infusions (believed to be due to competition between lidocaine and its accumulated metabolites) and a lower unbound fraction mean that unbound lidocaine concentrations during prolonged infusions are probably therapeutic.[215] It is important to be aware that total lidocaine levels at the higher end of the therapeutic range may not present a danger of toxicity in patients receiving prolonged infusions of lidocaine after a myocardial infarction.

The MEGX metabolite of lidocaine has 80% to 90% of the antiarrhythmic potency of lidocaine, and its concentration accumulates in renal failure. Thus, MEGX may contribute to the pharmacologic effects of lidocaine in patients with renal impairment.[91,212]

Procainamide

Therapeutic range. Procainamide is not used much anymore in the oral form, but may be used intravenously for select indications, such as patients with atrial fibrillation or flutter who require acute conversion to normal sinus rhythm.[216] The therapeutic range of procainamide is complicated by the presence of an active metabolite, NAPA, which has different electrophysiologic properties. Procainamide is a Type 1A antiarrhythmic, while NAPA is a Type III antiarrhythmic.[62,91,205] The enzyme that acetylates procainamide is bimodally distributed, such that patients are either slow or fast acetylators. In addition, NAPA is more dependent on the kidneys for elimination than is procainamide, and its levels accumulate more than procainamide for a given level of renal impairment.[205,214] Thus, the ratio of NAPA to procainamide in serum can be quite variable, necessitating the use of separate therapeutic ranges for the parent and metabolite.

Most patients respond when serum procainamide concentrations are between 4 and 8 mg/L; some receive additional benefit with levels up to 12 mg/L.[216] There have been reports of patients requiring levels between 15 and 20 mg/L without adverse effects.[216] Serum concentrations of NAPA associated with efficacy are reported to be as low as 5 mg/L and as high as 30 mg/L. Most clinicians consider toxic NAPA levels to be above 30–40 mg/L.[205] Some clinicians feel that NAPA does not need to be monitored except in patients with renal impairment.[216] Most laboratories, however, automatically measure both procainamide and NAPA concentrations in the same sample. The practice of summing the two concentrations and comparing to a therapeutic range for summed procainamide and NAPA (often reported as 10–30 mg/L) is to be discouraged.[91,205,216] To do this validly, the molar units of the two chemicals would need to be used.[62] More importantly, however, is the fact that procainamide and NAPA have completely different electrophysiologic behaviors. The best practice is to independently compare each chemical to its own reference range.[62,91,205]

Side effects to procainamide and NAPA are similar. Anorexia, nausea, vomiting, diarrhea, weakness, and hypotension may be seen with procainamide levels above 8 mg/L, while levels above 12 mg/L may be associated with more serious adverse effects: heart block, ventricular conduction disturbances, new ventricular arrhythmias, and even cardiac arrest.[91] A syndrome known as *torsades de pointes* may also be seen after procainamide administration, although this is more commonly seen after quinidine or disopyramide administration.[91]

Indications for procainamide and NAPA serum level monitoring include recurrence of arrhythmias that were previously controlled, suspected toxicity or overdose, anticipated pharmacokinetic alterations caused by drug–drug interactions (including amiodarone, cimetidine, ethanol, ofloxacin, quinidine, ranitidine, and trimethoprim), and disease state changes (renal failure or congestive heart failure, in particular).[91,205,214,216]

Sample timing. The half-life of procainamide in adults without renal impairment or congestive heart failure ranges from 2.5 hours (fast acetylator) to 5 hours (slow acetylator).[91,205] The half-life of NAPA is longer, averaging 6 hours in patients with normal renal function, and 30 hours or longer in patients with renal impairment.[91,216] Thus, a steady-state of both chemicals is not observed until at least 18 hours in patients with good renal function or as long as 4 days in renal impairment.

Specimens, collection methods, and assays. Serum or plasma, anticoagulated with heparin, EDTA, or oxalate, may be used.[205] Recovery of procainamide and NAPA are not affected by use of serum separator tubes, but the influence of any special blood collection devices should always be confirmed by individual laboratories.[205] Serum and plasma are stable for 24 hours at 2°C to 8°C, and for 1–2 weeks at –20°C.[205] Saliva levels of procainamide and NAPA have been shown to correlate strongly with plasma levels and are proposed as acceptable, noninvasive alternatives to blood sampling.[217]

The most commonly used commercial, automated assays for procainamide and NAPA are FPIA and EMIT. These methods require separate determinations of procainamide and NAPA on the same serum sample. Samples that are hemolyzed, lipemic, or icteric may affect the reading of these immunoassay methods.[205] Chromatographic methods (HPLC and GLC) allow the simultaneous measurement of procainamide and NAPA and are not subject to interferences from hemoglobin, lipids, or bilirubin.[205]

Use of levels for dosage adjustment. The 24% lower clearance of procainamide at higher dose rates has been attributed to nonlinear hepatic clearance.[218] The clinician should be aware that increases in infusion rate may produce somewhat greater-than-proportional increases in serum procainamide concentration in some patients, particularly those with serum levels at the upper end of the therapeutic range.

Protein binding, active metabolites, and other considerations. Procainamide is only 10% to 20% bound to serum proteins.[62,205] Thus, total procainamide and NAPA levels always reflect the pharmacologically active unbound concentrations of these drugs.

Quinidine

Therapeutic range. The therapeutic range of quinidine for treatment of severe malaria due to *P. falciparum* is reported as 3–8 mg/L.[219] When used in combination with verapamil for prevention of atrial fibrillation, the therapeutic range of quinidine is reported to be 2–6 mg/L.[220] Common side effects are gastrointestinal in nature (anorexia, nausea, and diarrhea) and more serious side effects include cinchonism (blurred vision, lightheadedness, tremor, giddiness, and tinnitus), hypotension, and ventricular arrhythmias.[91,205] Torsades de pointes is more likely to occur at concentrations at the lower end of the therapeutic range, thus complicating the interpretation of quinidine concentrations.[62]

Indications for monitoring of quinidine concentrations include therapeutic confirmation; suspected toxicity; recurrence of arrhythmias after initial suppression; suspected drug–drug interactions or other conditions known to alter quinidine pharmacokinetics; suspected nonadherence; and changes in administered formulation.[91,205,220]

Sample timing. The half-life of quinidine is reported to range from 4–8 hours in adults and up to 10 hours in patients with liver disease. Steady-state should be attained within 2 or 3 days, and most clinicians agree that samples should be drawn as a trough within 1 hour of the next dose.[62,91,205,220]

Specimens, collection methods, and assays. Serum or plasma may be used. Plasma should be collected in EDTA-treated tubes. Serum separator tubes should generally be avoided.[205] Quinidine in serum or plasma is stable for 1–2 weeks at −20°C.[205]

Quinidine in serum or plasma is most frequently assayed using immunoassay, but HPLC may also be used. Dihydroquinidine (an impurity in quinidine dosage forms), quinine, and the quinidine metabolite, 3-hydroxyquinidine, may all interfere to varying extents with immunoassay methods.[205] Moderate (20%) cross-reactivity with the 3-hydroxy metabolite was reported with an FPIA method.[62]

Use of levels for dosage adjustment. Quinidine displays linear elimination behavior for most patients; a change in daily quinidine dose will cause a proportional change in the average steady-state serum quinidine concentration. Nonlinear elimination may be evident in some patients, due either to saturable first-pass metabolism or saturable renal tubular secretion.[220] Thus, a greater-than-proportional increase in average quinidine concentration with increase in daily quinidine dose may be evident in some patients.

Protein binding, active metabolites, and other considerations. Quinidine is a weak base that is normally between 70% and 80% bound to albumin and AAG in the serum of healthy patients.[205] These protein levels are known to increase in trauma, myocardial infarction, cardiac surgery, atrial fibrillation/flutter, and congestive heart failure, and the percentage binding of quinidine can increase to as high as 92% in these patients.[91] The unbound fraction of quinidine was shown to be decreased in patients with atrial fibrillation or atrial flutter, and the unbound quinidine concentration was shown to correlate better with ECG interval changes than total quinidine.[221,222] All of this suggests that total serum concentrations of quinidine must be cautiously interpreted in patients with suspected elevations in AAG concentrations. A total quinidine level that is above 5 mg/L could be therapeutic with respect to unbound quinidine concentration.

The dihydroquinidine impurity may be present in amounts that are between 10% and 15% of the labeled amount of quinidine and is believed to have similar electrophysiologic properties as quinidine.[205] The 3-hydroxyquinidine metabolite has activity that is less than the parent (anywhere between 20% and 80% have been reported) and is not as highly bound to serum proteins.[214] Although not reported, this leads one to wonder about possible accumulation of these substances in renal failure patients with a resultant shift in the quinidine therapeutic range.

Other Cardiac Drugs

Amiodarone. Amiodarone is used for the treatment of life-threatening recurrent ventricular arrhythmias that do not respond to adequate doses of other antiarrhythmics. The primary metabolite, desethylamidarone, has similar electrophysiologic properties as amiodarone and accumulates to levels similar to or higher than the parent drug, especially in renal failure patients.[62] The concentration versus effect relationship for amiodarone is poorly defined; some say that serum concentrations between 0.5 and 2.5 mg/L are associated with effectiveness with minimal toxicity.[62] The occurrence of toxicity, however, appears to be more reliably related to the total amount of drug administered rather than serum concentration. Laboratories that measure serum amiodarone concentrations report only the parent drug, despite high levels of the active metabolite. In general, therapeutic drug monitoring of amiodarone is of limited benefit because activity of the drug is mostly associated with concentrations in the tissue.[62] Serum concentrations might be most useful in cases of suspected nonadherence.

Disopyramide. Disopyramide is used to treat life-threatening ventricular arrhythmias in selected patients.[205] Disopyramide has several characteristics that confound the use of serum disopyramide concentration monitoring. It is administered as a racemic mixture, and only the S(+) enantiomer is believed to significantly contribute to the drug's antiarrhythmic effect.[26] Both enantiomers demonstrate concentration-dependent binding, such that increases in dose rate produce proportional increases in unbound (pharmacologically active) enantiomer but less-than-proportional increases in total summed enantiomer concentration.[26,62,205] The primary metabolite of disopyramide, mono-N-dealkyldisopyramide, has 50% of the antiarrhythmic activity of the parent but 2–4 times the anticholinergic activity, which is responsible for many of the side effects.[205] The metabolite accumulates more than disopyramide in renal failure patients. Despite all of these confounding factors, most laboratories monitor summed enantiomer levels of total parent drug only (no metabolite) and, in most cases, rely on a therapeutic range between 2 and 5 mg/L with levels greater than 7 mg/L considered toxic.[205] The use of serum disopyramide concentrations as a guide to dosage adjustments is, understandably, on the decline. Indications that might be appropriate include suspected toxicity or nonadherence and drug–drug interactions or diseases that are anticipated to affect the pharmacokinetics of the enantiomers.[205]

Flecainide. Flecainide is used for prevention of paroxysmal atrial fibrillation/flutter or paroxysmal supraventricular tachycardias.[205] It is administered as a racemic mixture, but unlike disopyramide, there is little difference in the pharmacologic effects of these enantiomers.[62] The commonly used therapeutic range for trough concentrations, based on the flecainide acetate salt, is 0.2–1 mg/L; the range based on the flecainide base is 0.175–0.870 mg/L.[62,205] Toxicity is likely observed at acetate concentrations greater than 1.6 mg/L.[62] Although this is a fairly wide therapeutic range, the pharmacokinetics of flecainide are quite variable among patients, suggesting that serum concentration monitoring might be helpful. Indications for monitoring may include patients who have a recent myocardial infarction, impaired renal function, or in whom drug–drug interactions are suspected.[205] The serum binding of flecainide is low (32% to 58%) so that total flecainide concentrations provide a reliable reflection of the active, unbound concentration. Flecainide is assayed by FPIA or HPLC.[205]

Mexiletine. Mexiletine is structurally similar to lidocaine but has the advantage that it can be given orally. It is used for the treatment of life-threatening ventricular arrhythmias in select patients and may also be used for treatment of chronic pain syndromes.[62] It is given as a racemic mixture—with the S(+) enantiomer showing greater activity than the R(–) enantiomer—and is only 50% to 60% bound to serum proteins. Mexiletine is usually assayed by achiral methods (GLC or HPLC); no studies have yet been done to relate effect to individual enantiomers.[62] The therapeutic range for the summed total enantiomers is most commonly reported to be 0.5–2.0 mg/L.[62,214] Toxicity may occur, however, at concentrations within the range of effective concentrations.[214] Mild side effects may be seen between 0.8 and 3 mg/L, and severe side effects between 1 and 4.4 mg/L.[214] Because the extent of mexiletine absorption can be significantly affected by changes in the rate of gastric emptying, patients receiving narcotics and those who have had a recent myocardial infarction might benefit from serum concentration monitoring.[214] Higher serum levels of mexiletine may be seen in patients with liver disease and patients with congestive heart failure.[223]

Cytotoxic Drugs

While cytotoxic drugs have some characteristics that make them ideal candidates for therapeutic drug monitoring (narrow therapeutic indices and variable pharmacokinetics) they have many more characteristics that make therapeutic drug monitoring difficult or unsuitable.[224,225] They lack a simple, immediate indication of pharmacologic effect in order to aid definition of a therapeutic range (the ultimate outcome of cure could be years). They are given in combination with other cytotoxic drugs, such that concentration versus effect relationships for any single drug is difficult to isolate. They are used to treat cancer, which is a highly heterogeneous group of diseases, each possibly having its own concentration versus effect relationships. Finally, many of these drugs require tedious assay techniques. In summary, cytotoxic drugs are not routinely monitored because they are in need of more clearly defined therapeutic ranges. If ranges are established, they are usually more helpful to avoid toxicity than to define zones for efficacy.

Methotrexate

Therapeutic range. Methotrexate is the only antimetabolite drug for which serum concentrations are routinely monitored.[224] It acts by blocking the conversion of intracellular folate to reduced folate cofactors necessary for cell replication. While cancer cells are more susceptible to the toxic effects of methotrexate, healthy host cells are also affected by prolonged exposure to methotrexate. It is for this reason that leucovorin, a folate analogue that prevents further cell damage, is administered following high-dose methotrexate treatments.[224]

Measurements of serum methotrexate concentrations at critical times following high-dose methotrexate regimens are imperative to guide the amount and duration of leucovorin rescue treatments, thus preventing methotrexate toxicity. Institution of protocols for methotrexate serum concentration monitoring for this purpose has resulted in dramatic reductions in high-dose methotrexate-related toxicity and mortality.[226]

While it is known that methotrexate levels must be sufficiently high in order to prevent relapse of the malignancy, the specific range of levels defining efficacy has been difficult to define.[226] However, the relationship between methotrexate levels and toxicity has been much more clearly defined. Depending on the protocol, methotrexate levels that remain above 0.1 µM for longer than 48 hours are associated with a high risk of cytotoxicity.[227] Prolonged levels of methotrexate can lead to nephrotoxicity, myelosuppression, gastrointestinal mucositis, and liver cirrhosis.[224,226]

Serum concentration monitoring is not generally indicated when relatively low doses of methotrexate are given for chronic diseases such as rheumatoid arthritis, asthma, psoriasis, and maintenance for certain cancers.

Sample timing. The timing of samples for determination of methotrexate concentrations is highly dependent on the administration schedule. As one example of such a protocol, a methotrexate dose may be administered by intravenous infusion over 36 hours followed by a regimen of leucovorin doses administered over the next 72 hours.[227] Additional or larger leucovorin doses might be given depending on the methotrexate levels in samples drawn at various times after the start of the methotrexate infusion. It is important that methotrexate levels continue to be monitored until they are below the critical levels (usually between 0.05 and 0.1 µM).[224,227]

Specimen, collection methods, and assays. Serum or plasma concentrations are generally used. Saliva concentrations correlate poorly with total and unbound methotrexate concentrations, precluding the clinical use of saliva as a noninvasive alternative for blood samples.[228] Rapid reporting of methotrexate levels is important, and the immunoassay methods are preferred for determination of methotrexate levels. All immunoassays have different specificities and sensitivity limits and none stand out as clearly superior.[226] The most widely used method, FPIA, offers a sensitivity limit as low as 0.02 µM, and minimal cross-reactivity with the major metabolite, 7-hydroxymethotrexate.[226] Chromatographic methods such as HPLC must be used if quantitation of methotrexate metabolites is desired, most likely for research purposes.

Use of levels for dosage adjustment. Methotrexate and leucovorin doses are based on protocols.

Protein binding, active metabolites, and other considerations. Methotrexate binds to albumin in serum ranges from 20% to 57%.[224] While studies have shown the unbound fraction of methotrexate to be increased by concomitant administration of NSAIDs, salicylate, sulfonamides, and probenecid, the implications for interpretation of methotrexate levels are probably not important.[227] The methotrexate metabolite, 7-hydroxymethotrexate, has only 1/100th the activity of methotrexate but may cause nephrotoxicity due to precipitation in the renal tubules.[226]

Other Cytotoxic Drugs

Petros and Evans provide an excellent summary of cytotoxic drugs and the types of measurements that have been used to predict their toxicity and/or response.[226] Correlations between response or toxicity and serum concentration or area under the serum concentration (AUC) versus time curve for total drug have been shown for bisacetamide, busulfan, carboplatin, cisplatin, cyclophosphamide, docetaxel, etoposide, 5-fluorouracil hexamethylene, irinotecan, paclitaxel, teniposide, topotecan, and vincristine.[226,229,230] The strong correlation between busulfan AUC and bone marrow transplant outcome led the FDA to include instructions for AUC monitoring in the package insert for intravenous busulfan. Unbound AUC values for etoposide and teniposide, which demonstrate concentration-dependent binding, correlate more strongly with toxicity than corresponding total plasma AUC values.[231] Systemic drug clearance has been predictive of response/toxicity for amsacrine, fluorouracil, methotrexate, and teniposide.[226,232] Steady-state average serum concentrations or concentrations at designated postdose times have also been predictive of response/toxicity for cisplatin, etoposide, and methotrexate.[226] Finally, concentrations of cytosine-arabinoside metabolite in leukemic blasts and concentrations of mercaptopurine metabolite in red blood cells have been predictive of response or toxicity for these drugs. Correlations between systemic exposure and response/toxicity for cyclophosphamide, carmustine, and thiotepa have also been reported.[233]

Other than methotrexate, none of the assays for these drugs (often done by HPLC) is available commercially as an immunoassay.[226] While most studies up to this point have focused on use of cytotoxic drug concentration measurements to minimize toxicity, future studies will be increasingly focused on use of drug concentrations to maximize efficacy.

Immunosuppressants

Cyclosporine

Therapeutic range. Cyclosporine is a potent cyclic polypeptide used for prevention of organ rejection in patients who have received kidney, liver, or heart transplants. It is also used for the management of psoriasis, rheumatoid arthritis, and other autoimmune diseases. The therapeutic range of cyclosporine is highly dependent on the specimen (whole blood or serum/plasma) and assay. Most transplant centers use whole blood with one of the more specific assays—HPLC or immunoassays that use monoclonal antibodies (monoclonal radioimmunoassay or monoclonal fluorescence polarization immunoassay).[91,234,235] The commonly cited therapeutic range for whole blood troughs using one of these specific methods is 100–500 mcg/L.[91,236] Troughs at the higher end of this range may be desired initially after transplantation and in patients at high risk for rejection.[236] Therapeutic ranges are lower if serum or plasma is used and higher if a less specific assay is used, such as an immunoassay based on polyclonal antibodies. The

therapeutic range also depends on the specific organ transplantation procedure and the stage of treatment after surgery (higher concentrations during induction and lower concentrations during maintenance to minimize side effects).[61,91,235-237] Thus, it is important that the therapeutic range guidelines established by each center be used. While most centers still use single trough levels to adjust cyclosporine doses, the area under the blood concentration versus time curve is believed to be a more sensitive predictor of clinical outcome.[238] Studies that have investigated the use of single cyclosporine concentrations measured 2 hours after the dose, as a surrogate for the AUC value, suggest a better clinical outcome as compared to the use of single trough levels.[234,238,239]

Cyclosporine has a narrow therapeutic index and extremely variable pharmacokinetics among and within patients. The implications of ineffective therapy and adverse reactions are serious. Thus, it is imperative that cyclosporine concentrations be monitored in all patients starting immediately after transplant surgery. The primary side effects associated with high cyclosporine blood concentrations are nephrotoxicity, neurotoxicity, hypertension, hyperlipidemia, hirsutism, and gingival hyperplasia.[61,91,236] Blood cyclosporine concentrations should also be monitored when there is a dosage adjustment, signs of rejection or adverse reactions, suspected nonadherence, or initiation or discontinuation of drugs known to induce or inhibit cyclosporine metabolism.[61,236]

Sample timing. Monitoring is often done immediately after surgery before a steady-state is reached. Initially, levels may be obtained daily or every other day, then every 3–5 days, then monthly. Changes in dose rate or initiation or discontinuation of potential enzyme inducers or inhibitors will require resampling once a new steady-state is reached. The half-life of cyclosporine ranges from 5–27 hours and is dependent on the particular formulation. Thus, 3–5 days is generally adequate in most patients for attainment of a new steady-state. Most centers continue to sample predose (trough) cyclosporine levels, while some are using 2-hour postdose levels, which appear to more closely predict total exposure to cyclosporine as measured by AUC.[234,239] Multiple samples to determine the AUC are generally unnecessary.

Specimens, collection methods, and assays. Blood concentrations of cyclosporine are 2–5 times the concentration in serum because of extensive partitioning into red blood cells. Whole blood is the preferred specimen and should be collected in tubes with EDTA.[61] Samples are stable for 7 days in plastic tubes at 4°C.[240] Capillary blood by skin puncture is also acceptable.[61] While the popular monoclonal immunoassays offer improved specificity over the older polyclonal versions, they continue to measure varying amounts of cross-reactive metabolites.[61,234] The reference method of HPLC offers optimal specificity but takes longer; it might be considered in selected cases where significant interferences from metabolites are suspected.

Use of levels for dosage adjustment. In most cases, simple proportionality may be used for dosage adjustments. Trough or 2-hour postdose levels will change in proportion to the change in dose rate so long as the dosing interval remains the same.

Protein binding, active metabolites, and other considerations. Cyclosporine is 90% bound to albumin and lipoproteins in blood.[237] Unbound fractions in blood vary widely among patients and are weakly correlated to lipoprotein concentrations in blood.[237] For example, lower unbound fractions of cyclosporine have been reported in patients with hypercholesterolemia.[61] Lindholm and Henricsson reported a significant drop in the unbound fraction of cyclosporine in plasma immediately prior to acute rejection episodes.[241] An association between low cholesterol levels (and presumably high unbound fractions of cyclosporine) and increased incidence of neurotoxicity has also been reported.[61] These studies suggest that efforts to maintain all patients within a certain range of total concentrations may be misleading. Routine monitoring of unbound cyclosporine levels is not yet feasible, given the many technical difficulties with this measurement. Instead, the clinician should cautiously interpret total levels of cyclosporine in situations where altered protein binding of cyclosporine has been reported.

Other Immunosuppressants

Tacrolimus. Tacrolimus is a macrolide antibiotic with immunosuppressant activity and is generally used in combination with other immunosuppressant drugs. Like cyclosporine, whole blood is the preferred specimen.[242] Trough blood concentrations of tacrolimus as high as 20 mcg/L are targeted during initial treatment and gradually decrease to between 5 and 10 mcg/L during maintenance therapy, often after 12 months.[55] Toxicities to tacrolimus are very similar to those with cyclosporine, including nephrotoxicity and neurotoxicity.[236,242] The unpredictable and variable extent of tacrolimus bioavailability (5% to 67%) contribute to the need for monitoring of this drug.[242] Monitoring should always be done after changes in dose rate or initiation/discontinuation of enzyme-inducing or inhibiting agents. The half-life of tacrolimus ranges from 4–41 hours, and a new steady-state will be attained after approximately 3–5 days.[61,236] While trough concentrations are still the method of choice for monitoring, a second level might be needed if Bayesian approaches to dosage individualization are used.[239,243] The majority of centers use immunoassay methods, either a microparticle enzyme immunoassay (MEIA) or EMIT, which show some cross-reactivity with tacrolimus metabolites. More specific methods, such as HPLC, may be required in patients with liver disease who are anticipated to have high levels of metabolites.[61] Bilirubin and alkaline phosphatase do not interfere with measurements of tacrolimus using MEIA, but abnormally high hematocrit levels have caused underreading of tacrolimus.[244] Tacrolimus appears to exhibit linear elimination behavior. Thus, an increase in the daily dose is expected to result in a proportional increase in the steady-state trough level. Tacrolimus is 75% to 99% bound to plasma proteins (albumin, alpha-1-glycoprotein, lipoproteins and globulins).[61,242] Reports of lower unbound serum concentrations of tacrolimus during episodes of rejection lead one to be cautious with interpretation of total tacrolimus concentrations in patients with suspected alterations in protein binding.[245]

Mycophenolic acid. Mycophenolate mofetil, the prodrug of mycophenolic acid, is often used in combination with cyclosporine or tacrolimus with or without corticosteroids.[61] While troughs of mycophenolic acid may be monitored (plasma levels between 2.5 and 4 mg/L are targeted with good success), AUC values appear to be better predictors of postoperative efficacy (avoidance of acute rejection).[239,246,247] Reliable measurements of AUC may be determined with as few as three samples (trough, 30 minutes, and 120 minutes postdose) with a desired target AUC range of 30–60 mg x hr/L.[246] The half-life of mycophenolic acid is approximately 17 hours. Thus, a new steady-state will be attained approximately 3 days after a dose rate change or the addition/discontinuation of drugs that affect the metabolism of mycophenolic acid. In contrast to cyclosporine, tacrolimus, and sirolimus, plasma anticoagulated with EDTA is the preferred specimen for mycophenolic acid concentration measurements.[61,246] The acyl glucuronide metabolite of mycophenolic acid is active, but its clinical significance for the interpretation of mycophenolic acid levels is not yet clear. This metabolite cross-reacts with immunoassay using the EMIT method, giving higher readings as compared to HPLC.[61] Mycophenolic acid is 98% bound to plasma proteins, and the unbound fraction is greatly influenced by changes in albumin concentration, displacement by metabolites, renal failure, and hyperbilirubinemia.[234,246] Several groups of investigators suggest that unbound mycophenolic acid concentrations should be monitored when altered binding is suspected.[61,246-249] There is evidence that unbound mycophenolic acid concentration may be a better predictor of adverse effects.[245,248]

Sirolimus. Sirolimus is a macrolide antibiotic with potent immunosuppressant activity. When used in combination with cyclosporine and corticosteroids, trough blood concentrations of 5–15 mcg/L are generally targeted.[236] It has a relatively long half-life (62 hours), and a new steady-state will not be attained in many patients until at least 6 days after dose rate adjustments or the addition/discontinuation of interacting drugs.[236] At present, trough concentrations are used for monitoring as they correlate well with AUC.[234] Whole blood is the preferred specimen and should be collected using EDTA as the anticoagulant.[250] Samples are not stable at temperatures above 35°C but may be stored at room temperature for up to 24 hours, between 2°C and 8°C for up to 7 days, and at 20°C for up to 3 months.[250] An MEIA method is under development, but it overestimates sirolimus concentrations measured by HPLC because of cross-reactivities with sirolimus metabolites.[61]

Psychotropics

Amitriptyline, Nortriptyline, Imipramine, Desipramine

Therapeutic ranges. Although tricyclic antidepressants (TCAs) continue to be used for treatment of depression, their use has significantly declined in favor of the newer antidepressants which have more favorable side effect profiles.[251] The therapeutic ranges of amitriptyline, imipramine, desipramine, and nortriptyline are well-defined.[21,252,253] Desipramine and nortriptyline, while drugs in their own right, are also active metabolites of imipramine and amitriptyline, respectively. Thus, amitriptyline is included as a fourth TCA for serum concentration monitoring.

When imipramine is administered, combined serum concentrations of imipramine and desipramine that are considered therapeutic but not toxic are between 180 and 350 mcg/L.[252,253] Combined levels above 500 mcg/L are extremely toxic.[253] When desipramine is administered, levels between 115 and 250 mcg/L are frequently associated with therapeutic effect.[252,253] When amitriptyline is administered, combined serum concentrations of amitriptyline and nortriptyline should be between 120 and 250 mcg/L.[252] Combined levels above 450 mcg/L are not likely to produce additional response and are associated with cardiotoxicity anticholinergic delirium.[253] The therapeutic range of nortriptyline is the most firmly established of these four drugs; target serum concentrations after nortriptyline administration are between 50 and 150 mcg/L.[252-254]

The most common side effects of the TCAs are anticholinergic in nature—dry mouth, constipation, urinary retention, and blurred vision.[252] Toxicities seen at higher concentrations include cardiac conduction disturbances (with prolonged QRS interval evident on EKG), seizures, and coma.[252] For all of the TCAs, these toxic effects occur at serum concentrations that are approximately 5 times those needed for antidepressant efficacy.[12]

Since it takes 3 or more weeks beyond the final dose rate adjustment to fully assess clinical response to a TCA, routine monitoring once a steady-state has been attained would shorten the overall dosage titration period as compared to a trial-and-error dose rate adjustment method. A dosage individualization method, using serum nortriptyline levels drawn following the first dose, resulted in patients being discharged 6 days earlier and returning to work 55 days earlier as compared to a control group.[37] Response rates to TCAs are reported to increase from 30% to 40% to as high as 80% by use of serum TCA concentration monitoring.[255] Other indications for monitoring include suspected nonadherence or inadequate response, suspected toxicity, and suspected unusual or altered pharmacokinetics (children, elderly, and drug interactions).

Sample timing. While the half-lives of amitriptyline and nortriptyline range from 9–56 hours with a steady-state attained within 4–11 days in most patients, the half-lives of imipramine and desipramine range from 6–28 hours with a steady-state attained in 6 days.[253,254] As a general rule, the clinician should wait at least a week before drawing any blood samples for serum concentration monitoring. Trough levels are ideal for monitoring purposes because they are the most reproducible. Troughs are inconvenient, however, since patients usually take the drug once daily at bedtime. Therefore, a standardized sampling time is commonly used—12 to 14 hours after the bedtime dose.[253,254] Since this sample is taken midway through the dosing interval, it provides a fairly good approximation of the average steady-state level of TCA. If the TCA happens to be given in divided doses, a 4- to 6-hour postdose sample time is recommended.[252,254]

Specimens, collection methods, and assays. Serum or plasma collected using EDTA as the anticoagulant is preferred. There is some suggestion that heparin lowers the concentrations of TCAs, and there were numerous reports in the literature about TCAs having spuriously low serum levels due to displacement from AAG by TBEP in the rubber stopper.[252] Although the stopper has since been reformulated, it is a good idea to avoid blood collection materials that have not been tested by the laboratory, as well as special serum separator tubes with gel barriers.[252] Serum or plasma should be immediately separated from red blood cells to avoid the possibility of hemolysis.[252] Serum or plasma can be stored for 24 hours at room temperature, for 4 weeks at 4°C, or for more than 1 year at –20°C.

Chromatographic and immunoassay methods are most commonly used for measurements of serum TCA concentrations with immunoassay being most common.[253,254] Of the two available immunoassay methods, only the EMIT system uses a monoclonal antibody to determine individual concentrations of these four TCAs. An FPIA method measures for the presence of all tricyclic drugs (*total tricyclics*) using a less specific polyclonal antibody and is, therefore, useful for toxicology screenings.[252] False positives may result from such screenings, however, if carbamazepine is present.[256] One limitation of the EMIT method is that the tertiary amines (imipramine, amitriptyline, and others) cross-react with one another, while the secondary amines (desipramine and nortriptyline) also cross-react with one another.[252] This becomes a problem if the patient is receiving more than one TCA or is being switched from one to another.

Use of levels for dosage adjustment. Some mild nonlinearity has been described for desipramine, in which case, increases in the daily dose will be expected to produce somewhat greater-than-proportional increases in the standardized 12-hour sample. The other TCAs, however, exhibit proportionality. A method proposed by Browne et al. for the dosing of nortriptyline involves the use of a serum level drawn following a first dose to predict an appropriate maintenance dosage regimen.[37] This method, very similar to methods used for initiation of lithium therapy, is not commonly used, but has demonstrated great promise in speeding up the dose-titration period.

Protein binding, active metabolites, and other considerations. The TCAs in general are highly bound to serum proteins, including albumin, AAG, and lipoproteins.[251] Based on this, one would expect unbound TCA serum concentrations to be much better predictors of response than total concentrations, particularly in populations suspected to have unusually high or low serum binding. Until now, studies that have attempted to examine this have not been able to clarify relationships between response and total serum concentrations based on variable protein binding. Assays for accurate and direct measurement of unbound TCA concentrations in serum need to be sufficiently sensitive for these kinds of studies.

The TCAs are extensively metabolized and undergo significant first-pass metabolism. While the primary active metabolites have been identified and are separately measured, other active metabolites can accumulate in some circumstances and affect the response at a given parent drug concentration. In one study, levels of conjugated and unconjugated hydroxylated metabolites of the TCAs were markedly elevated in patients with renal failure and believed to contribute to the hypersensitivity of these patients to TCA side effects.[257]

Lithium

Therapeutic range. Lithium is a monovalent cation used for the treatment of bipolar disorder and the manic phase of affective disorders. The concentration units for lithium are expressed as mEq/L, which is the same as mmol/L. While the overall therapeutic range for treatment of manic depression is commonly cited as 0.5–1.2 mEq/L,[21] there appear to be two distinct ranges used in practice, depending on the stage of therapy.[252] For acute management of manic depressive episodes, the therapeutic range of 0.5–1.2 mEq/L is desired, going up to 1.5 mEq/L if necessary.[91,258,259] For maintenance treatment, the therapeutic range of 0.6–0.8 mEq/L is usually recommended.[91,258,259] Serum concentrations above 1.5 mEq/L are associated with fine tremors of the extremities, gastrointestinal disturbances, muscle weakness, fatigue, polyuria, and polydipsia. Concentrations above 2.5 mEq/L are associated with coarse tremors, confusion, delirium, slurred speech, and vomiting. Concentrations above 2.5–3.5 mEq/L are associated with seizures, coma, and death.[252] It is important to point out that the values for the therapeutic ranges are based on samples obtained at a specific time during the day—just before the morning dose and at least 12 hours after the evening dose for patients on a BID or TID regimen.[259,260]

Most clinicians require that every patient taking lithium be regularly monitored, which is cost-effective considering the potential avoidance of toxicity.[91,254] Specific indications for lithium concentration monitoring include evaluation of nonadherence; suspicion of toxicity; confirmation of the level associated with efficacy; and any situation in which altered pharmacokinetics of the drug is anticipated (drug–drug interactions, pregnancy, children, geriatric patients, and fluid and electrolyte imbalance). Despite the strong indication for lithium monitoring in all patients, 37% of lithium users on Medicaid did not have serum drug concentrations monitored.[261]

Sample timing. The half-life of lithium ranges from 18–24 hours, and steady-state will be reached within a week of therapy.[259] However, 2–3 weeks of treatment may be required after that before the full response to the drug can be assessed.[259] When initiating lithium therapy, it is recommended that serum levels be measured every 2–3 days (before a steady-state is reached) to ensure that levels do not exceed 1.2 mEq/L during that time.[91] Because of the extreme variability of serum lithium levels during the absorption and distribution periods, the current standard of practice is to draw all samples for lithium serum concentration determination 12 hours after the evening dose, regardless of whether a twice or thrice daily dosing schedule is used. For example, the time for blood sampling for a patient on a 0900/1500/2100 schedule would be right before the 0900 dose.[91] The timing of blood samples for a patient taking once daily lithium is less clear, given the greater degree of serum lithium concentration fluctuation with this dosing method.[259]

Specimens, collection methods, and assays. While plasma is acceptable, it must be collected using sodium heparin as the anticoagulant, not lithium heparin. Serum is the preferred specimen, therefore, just to avoid any possible confusion.[215] The serum sample should be rejected if there is any evidence of hemolysis since release of high concentrations of lithium from the red blood cells will artifactually raise the serum concentration.[252] To minimize the chance of hemolysis, serum should be separated from the red blood cells within 1 hour of collection.[254] Other than one exception, involving an interference from a silica clot activator, blood collection tubes generally have not introduced any artifacts for lithium assays.[262] Lithium in serum or plasma is stable at room temperature or refrigeration temperature for extended periods of time.[252]

Lithium erythrocyte concentration has been proposed to correlate better with response and toxicity since it represents intracellular lithium.[252] This method, however, has never been routinely adopted for monitoring. Saliva concentrations of lithium have been proposed as noninvasive substitutes for serum or plasma lithium concentrations. However, the S:P ratio is quite variable, even within some patients. The average S:P ratio ranges from two to four and is affected by many variables. If the S:P ratio is shown to be stable for an individual patient over time, saliva monitoring might prove to be useful for some patients.[263] Based on an audit of clinical laboratories in Europe and the United Kingdom, flame emission photometry and atomic absorption spectroscopy are still the most commonly used methods for lithium quantitation and offer excellent precision, accuracy, and few interferences.[264] Ion-selective electrode methods are more rapid and less costly but may have problems with interferences. Carbamazepine, quinidine, procainamide, NAPA, lidocaine, and valproic acid can all produce biases in lithium measurements by ISE.[252] High calcium levels may also produce a positive bias with some ISE methods.[252] A new colorimetric dry slide-based serum lithium assay is concluded to offer an acceptable alternative to currently available methods for monitoring lithium.[265]

Use of levels for dosage adjustment. Lithium exhibits linear elimination behavior and proportionality can be assumed when dosage adjustments are made. The assumption of linearity is the basis for several dosing methods that are used for initiating lithium therapy in patients. The Cooper method involves drawing a sample for lithium analysis 24 hours after a first dose of 600 mg.[38] The resulting level, believed to provide a reflection of the drug's half-life, is used with a nomogram that indicates the optimal maintenance regimen. The Perry method requires that two levels be drawn during the postabsorption-postdistribution phase after a first dose of lithium.[39] These two levels are used to determine the first-order elimination rate constant, which can then be used to determine the expected extent of lithium accumulation in the patient. The maintenance regimen required to attain a desired target lithium concentration in that patient can then be determined. Population-pharmacokinetic dosing-initiation methods (Bayesian) can also be used.[91]

Protein binding, active metabolites, and other considerations. Lithium is not bound to serum proteins, nor is it metabolized.

Other Psychotropics

Other antidepressants. Assays have been developed to document the serum concentrations observed following administration of other cyclic antidepressants as well as the selective serotonin reuptake inhibitors, serotonin and norepinephrine reuptake inhibitors, and norepinephrine reuptake inhibitors.[12,253,258,266-268] While reference ranges have been established, there does not appear to be any compelling reason for routine monitoring of these drugs given their relatively wide therapeutic indices and more favorable side effect profiles. Because 50% of patients do not achieve optimal relief from symptoms of depression, some clinicians advocate the use of serum concentration monitoring in patients who do not initially respond to identify nonadherence or to identify unusually low serum concentrations.[12,21,252,253]

Antipsychotics. The existence of well-defined therapeutic ranges for most antipsychotic drugs remains controversial.[255,269,270] There is some justification, however, for serum concentration monitoring of clozapine, fluphenazine, haloperidol, olanzapine, perphenazine, risperidone, and thioridazine in special circumstances.[21,270,271] Reference ranges for other antipsychotic drugs are primarily based on average serum concentrations observed during chronic therapy.[254,255,272] One difficulty in establishing clear therapeutic range guidelines is that chronicity of illness and duration of antipsychotic drug exposure can shift the therapeutic range; separate therapeutic ranges may need to be developed depending on duration of illness.[272]

FUTURE OF TDM

Drug assays are rapidly improving with regard to specificity, sensitivity, speed, and convenience. Methods that separate drug enantiomers may help to elucidate therapeutic ranges for compounds administered as racemic mixtures.[273] Capillary electrophoresis-based assays will be increasingly used in clinical laboratories because of their low cost, specificity, utility for small sample volumes, and speed.[274] Methods for measurement of drugs in hair samples are being proposed for assessment of long-term drug adherence.[275] Implanted amperometric biosensors, currently used for glucose monitoring, may be useful for continuous monitoring of drug concentrations.[276] Subcutaneous microdialysis probes may also be useful for continuous drug monitoring, particularly since they monitor pharmacologically active unbound drug concentrations.[277] Point-of-care assay methods, currently used in private physician offices, group practices, clinics, and emergency rooms, could eventually be used in community pharmacies in the future.[278,279]

The therapeutic drug monitoring of the near future may also involve determination of genotypes, characterization of proteins produced in particular diseases (proteomics), and analysis of drug metabolite profiles (metabonomics).[280,281] These sciences may help to identify those subsets of patients who will be *nonresponders* or *toxic responders,* and help to determine appropriate initial doses. Such testing would not require special sample timing, might be possible using noninvasive methods (e.g., hair, saliva, and buccal swabs), and would need to be done only once as the results would apply over a lifetime. These types of testing may help patients to receive the best drug for the indication and rapid individualization of drug dosage to achieve desired target concentrations.[28,29,280,282] This will likely result in increased demand for new types of tests from clinical laboratories currently involved in routine therapeutic drug monitoring.

There is a movement to change the terminology and practice of therapeutic drug monitoring to *target concentration strategy, target concentration intervention,* or *therapeutic drug management.*[40,283] Critics of the therapeutic drug monitoring terminology claim that it suggests a passive process that is concerned only with after-the-fact monitoring to ensure that levels are within an ill-defined range without proper regard to evaluation of the response to the drug in an individual patient.[283] Target concentration intervention is essentially a new name for a process used by clinical pharmacokinetics services for years and involves the following steps: (1) choosing a target concentration (usually within the commonly accepted therapeutic range) for a patient; (2) initiating therapy to attain that target concentration using best-guess population pharmacokinetic parameters; (3) fully evaluating response at the resulting steady-state concentration; and (4) adjusting the regimen as needed using pharmacokinetic parameters that have been further refined by use of the drug concentration measurement(s).

Methods to improve the therapeutic drug monitoring process itself are needed. Every effort should be made to focus on patients who are most likely to benefit from therapeutic drug monitoring, and minimize time and money spent on monitoring that provides no value.[9] The biggest problems with the process continue to be lack of education, communication, and documentation.[6,19] Approaches to changing physician behavior with regard to appropriate sampling and interpretation include educational sessions; formation of formal therapeutic drug monitoring services; multidisciplinary quality improvement efforts; and computerization of requests for drug concentration measurement samples.[284] Pharmacists will continue to have a pivotal role in the education of physicians and others involved in the therapeutic drug monitoring process. Future studies that evaluate the effect of therapeutic drug monitoring on patient outcomes will likely use quality management approaches.[285]

Learning Points

1. **A patient who was diagnosed with generalized tonic-clonic seizures was initiated on phenytoin sodium, 300 mg/day. She returns to the clinic after 4 weeks and reports that she has not had any seizures since taking the phenytoin. There are no signs or symptoms consistent with phenytoin toxicity. Why should a serum phenytoin level be measured in this patient?**

   Answer: Because the endpoint of therapy is the absence of something (seizures in this case), there is no way to ensure that the patient is taking enough phenytoin. Some types of seizures occur infrequently, and it is possible that the patient's serum phenytoin level is low and she simply hasn't had a seizure yet. It is important to ensure that the level is within the therapeutic range of 10–20 mg/L (for patients with normal serum albumin levels) before assuming the patient is adequately protected from future seizure activity

2. **A patient with hypoalbuminemia has been initiated on valproic acid for treatment of absence seizures. A serum valproic acid level is measured and reported as 75 mg/L. The patient reports that she has not experienced any seizures since starting the drug, but she's been feeling drowsy every day. The laboratory reports a serum albumin level of 2.8 g/dL (normal is 3.5–5 g/dL). How do you interpret the valproic acid level?**

   Answer: The target therapeutic range for total valproic acid concentrations is reported as 50–100 mg/L. This range, however, assumes an albumin concentration that is within the normal range. A patient with abnormally low albumin concentrations is likely to show toxicity when total valproic acid levels are between 50–100 mg/L. This is because the unbound level of valproic acid is too high. It is likely in this case that the dose of valproic acid is too high, thus accounting for the drowsiness. A total valproic acid concentration at the low end of the usual therapeutic range would be a more appropriate goal.

3. **A 60-year-old patient with normal renal function was initiated on oral digoxin, 0.25 mg every morning, for treatment of supraventricular arrhythmias. He returned to his primary care physician 1 month later for an 8 a.m. appointment. A blood sample, drawn at 8:30 a.m., revealed a digoxin serum concentration of 2.9 mcg/L. There are no signs or symptoms of digoxin toxicity. On further inquiry, the patient reveals that he took his digoxin dose at 7:30 a.m. that morning. A repeat sample drawn right before the next digoxin dose is 1.2 mcg/L.**

   Answer: This illustrates the importance of blood sample timing relative to intake of the last drug dose. The serum digoxin level in this case is above the upper limit generally defined for patients with atrial arrhythmias (2 mcg/L), and might lead to the conclusion that the daily digoxin dose is excessively high. However, the sample should have been drawn sometime between 6 hours after the dose and right before the next dose, when the digoxin in blood will have equilibrated with digoxin in myocardial tissue. Significant resources are wasted by inappropriate timing of blood samples for digoxin measurements, and/or incomplete documentation of dose or blood sample timing.

REFERENCES

1. Evans WE. General principles of clinical pharmacokinetics. In: Burton ME, Shaw LM, Schentag JJ, et al., eds. *Applied Pharmacokinetics and Pharmacodynamics: Principles of Therapeutic Drug Monitoring.* 4th ed. Baltimore, MD: Lippincott Williams & Wilkins; 2006:3-7.
2. Marshall EK. Experimental basis of chemotherapy in the treatment of bacterial infections. *Bull N Y Acad Med.* 1940;16:722-731.
3. Shannon JA. The study of antimalarials and antimalarial activity in the human malarias. *Harvey Lect.* 1946;41:43-89.
4. Koch-Weser J. Drug therapy. Serum drug concentrations as therapeutic guides. *N Engl J Med.* 1972;287:227-231.
5. Oles KS. Therapeutic drug monitoring analysis systems for the physician office laboratory: a review of the literature. *DICP.* 1990;24:1070-1077.
6. Carroll DJ, Austin GE, Stajich GV, et al. Effect of education on the appropriateness of serum drug concentration determination. *Ther Drug Monit.* 1992;14:81-84.
7. Mason GD, Winter ME. Appropriateness of sampling times for therapeutic drug monitoring. *Am J Hosp Pharm.* 1984;41:1796-801.
8. Travers EM. Misuse of therapeutic drug monitoring: an analysis of causes and methods for improvement. *Clin Lab Med.* 1987;7:453-472.
9. Ensom MH, Davis GA, Cropp CD, et al. Clinical pharmacokinetics in the 21st century. Does the evidence support definitive outcomes? *Clin Pharmacokinet.* 1998;34:265-279.
10. Touw DJ, Neef C, Thomson AH, et al. Cost-effectiveness of therapeutic drug monitoring: a systematic review. *Ther Drug Monit.* 2005;27:10-17.
11. Walson PD. Therapeutic drug monitoring in special populations. *Clin Chem.* 1998;44:415-419.
12. Burke MJ, Preskorn SH. Therapeutic drug monitoring of antidepressants: cost implications and relevance to clinical practice. *Clin Pharmacokinet.* 1999;37:147-165.
13. Bates DW. Improving the use of therapeutic drug monitoring. *Ther Drug Monit.* 1998;20:550-555.
14. Eadie MJ. Therapeutic drug monitoring—antiepileptic drugs. *Br J Clin Pharmacol.* 2001;52(suppl 1):S11-S20.
15. Robinson JD, Taylor W.J. Interpretation of serum drug concentrations. In: Taylor WJ, Caviness MHD, eds. *A Textbook for the Application of Therapeutic Drug Monitoring.* Irving, TX: Abbott Laboratories, Diagnostics Division; 1986:31-45.
16. Traub SL. Interpretation of serum drug concentrations. In: Traub SL, ed. *Basic Skills in Interpreting Laboratory Data.* 2nd ed. Bethesda, MD: American Society of Health-System Pharmacists; 1996:61-92.
17. D'Angio RG, Stevenson JG, Lively BT, et al. Therapeutic drug monitoring: improved performance through educational intervention. *Ther Drug Monit.* 1990;12:173-181.
18. Sieradzan R, Fuller AV. A multidisciplinary approach to enhance documentation of antibiotic serum sampling. *Hosp Pharm.* 1995;30:872-877.
19. Warner A. Setting standards of practice in therapeutic drug monitoring and clinical toxicology: a North American view. *Ther Drug Monit.* 2000;22:93-97.
20. Murphy JE. Introduction. In: Murphy JE, ed. *Clinical Pharmacokinetics.* 5th ed. Bethesda, MD: American Society of Health-System Pharmacists; 2012:xxix-xxxvii.

21. Hiemke C, Baumann P, Bergemann N, et al. AGNP consensus guidelines for therapeutic drug monitoring in psychiatry: Update 2011. *Pharmacopsychiatry.* 2011;44:195-235.

22. Johannessen SIJ Landmark. Value of therapeutic drug monitoring in epilepsy. *Expert Rev Neurother.* 2008;8:929-39.

23. Food and Drug Administration. *Guidance for Industry: Exposure-Reponses Relationships—Study Design, Data Analysis, and Regulatory Applications: 2003.* Silver Spring, MD: US Department of Health & Human Services; 2003.

24. Reed MD, Blumer JL. Therapeutic drug monitoring in the pediatric intensive care unit. *Pediatr Clin North Am.* 1994;41:1227-1243.

25. Schentag JJ, Bang AJ, Kozinski-Tober JL. Digoxin. In: Burton ME, Shaw LM, Schentag JJ, et al., eds. *Applied Pharmacokinetics and Pharmacodynamics: Principles of Therapeutic Drug Monitoring.* 4th ed. Baltimore, MD: Lippincott Williams & Wilkins; 2006:410-439.

26. Lima JJ, Wenzke SC, Boudoulas H, et al. Antiarrhythmic activity and unbound concentrations of disopyramide enantiomers in patients. *Ther Drug Monit.* 1990;12:23-28.

27. Ensom MH, Chang TK, Patel P. Pharmacogenetics: the therapeutic drug monitoring of the future? *Clin Pharmacokinet.* 2001;40:783-802.

28. McLeod HL, Evans WE. Pharmacogenomics: Unlocking the human genome for better drug therapy. *Annu Rev Pharmacol Toxicol.* 2001;41:101-121.

29. MacKichan JJ, Lee M. Factors contributing to drug-induced diseases. In: Tisdale JE, Miller DA, eds. *Drug-Induced Diseases: Prevention, Detection and Management.* Bethesda, MD: American Society of Health-System Pharmacists; 2010:23-30.

30. MacKichan JJ. Influence of protein binding and use of unbound (free) drug concentrations. In: Burton ME, Shaw LM, Schentag JJ, et al., eds. *Applied Pharmacokinetics and Pharmacodynamics: Principles of Therapeutic Drug Monitoring.* 4th ed. Baltimore, MD: Lippincott Williams & Wilkins; 2006:82-120.

31. Traugott KA, Maxwell PR, Green K, et al. Effects of therapeutic drug monitoring criteria in a computerized prescriber-order-entry system on the appropriateness of vancomycin level orders. *Am J Hosp Pharm.* 2011;68:347-352.

32. Bruguerolle B. Chronopharmacokinetics. Current status. *Clin Pharmacokinet.* 1998;35:83-94.

33. Baraldo M. The influence of circadian rhythms on the kinetics of drugs in humans. *Expert Opin Drug Metab Toxicol.* 2008;4:175-192.

34. MacKichan JJ, Kutt H. Carbamazepine. In: Taylor WJ, Finn AL, eds. *Individualizing Drug Therapy: Practical Applications of Drug Monitoring.* Vol. 2. New York, NY: Gross, Townsend Frank Inc; 1981:1-25.

35. Rodvold KA, Paloucek FP, Zell M. Accuracy of 11 methods for predicting theophylline dose. *Clin Pharm.* 1986;5:403-408.

36. Slattery JT, Gibaldi M, Koup JR. Prediction of maintenance dose required to attain a desired drug concentration at steady-state from a single determination of concentration after an initial dose. *Clin Pharmacokinet.* 1980;5:377-385.

37. Browne JL, Perry PJ, Alexander B, et al. Pharmacokinetic protocol for predicting plasma nortriptyline levels. *J Clin Psychopharmacol.* 1983;3:351-356.

38. Cooper TB, Simpson GM. The 24-hr lithium level as a prognosticator of dosage requirements: a 2-year follow-up study. *Am J Psychiatry.* 1976;133:440-443.

39. Perry PJ, Alexander B, Dunner FJ, et al. Pharmacokinetic protocol for predicting serum lithium levels. *J Clin Psychopharmacol.* 1982;2:114-118.

40. Neely M, Jelliffe R. Practical, individualized dosing: 21st century therapeutics and the clinical pharmacometrician. *J Clin Pharmacol.* 2010;50:842-847.

41. Winter ME. *Basic Clinical Pharmacokinetics.* 4th ed. Baltimore, MD: Lippincott Williams & Wilkins; 2004.

42. Hammett-Stabler C, Johns T. Laboratory guidelines for monitoring of antimicrobial drugs. *Clin Chem.* 1998;44:1129-1140.

43. Uges DR. Plasma or serum in therapeutic drug monitoring and clinical toxicology. *Pharm Weekbl Sci.* 1988;10:185-188.

44. Bush V, Blennerhasset J, Wells A, et al. Stability of therapeutic drugs in serum collected in vacutainer serum separator tubes containing a new gel (SST II). *Ther Drug Monit.* 2001;23:259-262.

45. Kaplan LA. Standards of laboratory practice: guidelines for the maintaining of a modern therapeutic drug monitoring service. *Clin Chem.* 1998;44:1072.

46. Devine JE. Drug-protein binding interferences caused by the plasticizer TBEP. *Clin Biochem.* 1984;17:345-347.

47. Janknegt R, Lohman JJ, Hooymans PM, et al. Do evacuated blood collection tubes interfere with therapeutic drug monitoring? *Pharm Weekbl Sci.* 1983;5:287-290.

48. Drummer OH. Introduction and review of collection techniques and applications of drug testing of oral fluid. *Ther Drug Monit.* 2008;30:203-206.

49. Liu H, Delgado MR. Therapeutic drug concentration monitoring using saliva samples. Focus on anticonvulsants. *Clin Pharmacokinet.* 1999;36:453-470.

50. Gorodischer R, Koren G. Salivary excretion of drugs in children: theoretical and practical issues in therapeutic drug monitoring. *Dev Pharmacol Ther.* 1992;19:161-177.

51. Tennison M, Ali I, Miles MV, et al. Feasibility and acceptance of salivary monitoring of antiepileptic drugs via the US Postal Service. *Ther Drug Monit.* 2004;26:295-299.

52. MacKichan JJ, Duffner PK, Cohen ME. Salivary concentrations and plasma protein binding of carbamazepine and carbamazepine 10,11-epoxide in epileptic patients. *Br J Clin Pharmacol.* 1981;12:31-37.

53. Nishihara K, Uchino K, Saitoh Y, et al. Estimation of plasma unbound phenobarbital concentration by using mixed saliva. *Epilepsia.* 1979;20:37-45.

54. Gorodischer R, Burtin P, Verjee Z, et al. Is saliva suitable for therapeutic monitoring of anticonvulsants in children: an evaluation in the routine clinical setting. *Ther Drug Monit.* 1997;19:637-642.

55. Chee KY, Lee D, Byron D, et al. A simple collection method for saliva in children: potential for home monitoring of carbamazepine therapy. *Br J Clin Pharmacol.* 1993;35:311-313.

56. Holden WE, Bartos F, Theime T, et al. Theophylline in oral mucosal transudate. A practical method for monitoring outpatient therapy. *Am Rev Respir Dis.* 1993;147:739-743.

57. Barre J, Didey F, Delion F, et al. Problems in therapeutic drug monitoring: free drug level monitoring. *Ther Drug Monit.* 1988;10:133-143.

58. Nakajima M, Yamato S, Shimada K, et al. Assessment of drug concentrations in tears in therapeutic drug monitoring: I. Determination of valproic acid in tears by gas chromatography/mass spectrometry with EC/NCI mode. *Ther Drug Monit.* 2000;22:716-722.

59. Monaco F, Piredda S, Mutani R, et al. The free fraction of valproic acid in tears, saliva, and cerebrospinal fluid. *Epilepsia.* 1982;23:23-26.

60. Friedman H, Greenblatt DJ. Rational therapeutic drug monitoring. *JAMA.* 1986;256:2227-2233.

61. Wong SH. Therapeutic drug monitoring for immunosuppressants. *Clin Chim Acta.* 2001;313:241-253.

62. Campbell TJ, Williams KM. Therapeutic drug monitoring: antiarrhythmic drugs. *Br J Clin Pharmacol.* 2001;52(suppl 1):S21-S34.

63. Dasgupta A. Therapeutic drug monitoring: recognizing the sources of interferences in immunoassays. *Clinical Laboratory News* [serial online]. 2008 April; 34. http://www.aacc.org/publications/cln/2008/april/Pages/series_0408.aspx. Accessed December 19, 2011.

64. Nierenberg DW. Measuring drug levels in the office: rationale, possible advantages, and potential problems. *Med Clin North Am.* 1987;71:653-664.

65. Blecka LJ, Jackson GJ. Immunoassays in therapeutic drug monitoring. *Clin Lab Med.* 1987;7:357-370.

66. Taylor AT. Office therapeutic drug monitoring. *Prim Care.* 1986; 13:743-760.

67. Tachi T, Hase T, Okamoto Y, et al. A clinical trial for therapeutic drug monitoring using microchip-based fluorescence polarization immunoassay. *Anal Bioanal Chem.* 2011;401:2301-2305.

68. Cook JD, Platoff GE, Koch TR, et al. Accuracy and precision of methods for theophylline measurement in physicians' offices. *Clin Chem.* 1990;36:780-783.

69. Wallinder H, Gustafsson LL, Angback K, et al. Assay of theophylline: in vivo and in vitro evaluation of dry chemistry and immunoassay versus high-performance liquid chromatography. *Ther Drug Monit.* 1991;13:233-239.

70. Iosefsohn M, Soldin SJ, Hicks JM. A dry-strip immunometric assay for digoxin on the Ames Seralyzer. *Ther Drug Monit.* 1990;12:201-205.

71. Steimer W, Muller C, Eber B. Digoxin assays: frequent, substantial, and potentially dangerous interference by spironolactone, canrenone, and other steroids. *Clin Chem.* 2002;48:507-516.

72. Winter ME, Tozer TN. Phenytoin. In: Burton ME, Shaw LM, Schentag JJ, et al., eds. *Applied Pharmacokinetics and Pharmacodynamics: Principles of Therapeutic Drug Monitoring.* 4th ed. Baltimore, MD: Lippincott Williams & Wilkins; 2006:463-490.

73. Jelliffe RW, Schumitzky A, Van Guilder M, et al. Individualizing drug dosage regimens: roles of population pharmacokinetic and dynamic models, Bayesian fitting, and adaptive control. *Ther Drug Monit.* 1993;15:380-393.

74. Burt M, Anderson DC, Kloss J, et al. Evidence-based implementation of free phenytoin therapeutic drug monitoring. *Clin Chem.* 2000; 46:1132-1135.

75. Musteata FM. Monitoring free drug concentrations: challenges. *Bioanalysis.* 2011;3:1753-1768.

76. Roberts WL, Annesley TM, De BK, et al. Performance characteristics of four free phenytoin immunoassays. *Ther Drug Monit.* 2001;23:148-154.

77. Sheiner LB, Tozer TN, Winter ME. Clinical pharmacokinetics: the use of plasma concentrations of drugs. In: Melmon KL, Morelli HF, eds. *Clinical Pharmacology: Basic Principles in Therapeutics.* New York, NY: MacMillan; 1978:71-109.

78. Kerrick JM, Wolff DL, Graves NM. Predicting unbound phenytoin concentrations in patients receiving valproic acid: a comparison of two prediction methods. *Ann Pharmacother.* 1995;29:470-474.

79. Haidukewych D, Rodin EA, Zielinski JJ. Derivation and evaluation of an equation for prediction of free phenytoin concentration in patients comedicated with valproic acid. *Ther Drug Monit.* 1989;11:134-139.

80. Haidukewych D, Zielinski JJ, Rodin EA. Derivation and evaluation of an equation for prediction of free carbamazepine concentrations in patients comedicated with valproic acid. *Ther Drug Monit.* 1989;11:528-532.

81. White S, Wong SH. Standards of laboratory practice: analgesic drug monitoring. National Academy of Clinical Biochemistry. *Clin Chem.* 1998;44:1110-1123.

82. Dromgoole SH, Furst DE. Salicylates. In: Evans WE, Schentag JJ, Jusko WJ, eds. *Applied Pharmacokinetics: Principles of Therapeutic Drug Monitoring.* 3rd ed. Vancouver, WA: Applied Therapeutics; 1992:32.1-32.34.

83. Levy G. Pharmacokinetics of salicylate in man. *Drug Metab Rev.* 1979;9:3-19.

84. Levy G, Tsuchiya T. Salicylate accumulation kinetics in man. *N Engl J Med.* 1972;287:430-432.

85. Pachman LM, Olufs R, Procknal JA, et al. Pharmacokinetic monitoring of salicylate therapy in children with juvenile rheumatoid arthritis. *Arthritis Rheum.* 1979;22:826-831.

86. Dasgupta A, Yared MA, Wells A. Time-dependent absorption of therapeutic drugs by the gel of the Greiner Vacuette blood collection tube. *Ther Drug Monit.* 2000;22:427-431.

87. Berkovitch M, Uziel Y, Greenberg R, et al. False-high blood salicylate levels in neonates with hyperbilirubinemia. *Ther Drug Monit.* 2000;22:757-761.

88. Dasgupta A, Zaidi S, Johnson M, et al. Use of fluorescence polarization immunoassay for salicylate to avoid positive/negative interference by bilirubin in the Trinder salicylate assay. *Ann Clin Biochem* 2003;40:684-688.

89. Dale C, Aulawi AAM, Baker J, et al. Assessment of point-of-care test for paracetamol and salicylate in blood. *Q J Med.* 2005;98:113-118.

90. Poe TE, Mutchie KD, Saunders GH, et al. Total and free salicylate concentrations in juvenile rheumatoid arthritis. *J Rheumatol.* 1980;7:717-723.

91. Bauer LA. *Applied Clinical Pharmacokinetics.* 2nd ed. New York, NY: McGraw-Hill; 2008.

92. National Heart, Lung and Blood Institute, National Asthma Education and Prevention Program. Expert panel report 3: Guidelines for the diagnosis and management of asthma. August 2007. http://www.nhlbi.nih.gov/guidelines/asthma/asthgdln.pdf. Accessed December 16, 2011.

93. Tilley SL. Methylxanthines in asthma. *Handb Exp Pharmacol.* 2011;200:439-456.

94. Edwards DJ, Zarowitz BJ, Slaughter RL. Theophylline. In: Evans WE, Schentag JJ, Jusko WJ, eds. *Applied Pharmacokinetics: Principles of Therapeutic Drug Monitoring.* 3rd ed. Vancouver, WA: Applied Therapeutics Inc; 1992:13.1-13.38.

95. Murphy JE, Winter ME. Theophylline. In: Winter ME, ed. *Basic Clinical Pharmacokinetics.* 5th ed. Baltimore, MD: Lippincott Williams & Wilkins;1020:403-441.

96. Scanlon JE, Chin KC, Morgan ME, et al. Caffeine or theophylline for neonatal apnea? *Arch Dis Child.* 1992;67:425-428.

97. Murphy JE, Phan H. Theophylline. In: Murphy JE, ed. *Clinical Pharmacokinetics.* 5th ed. Bethesda, MD: American Society of Health System Pharmacists; 2012:315-325.

98. Juarez-Olguin H, Flores-Perez J, Perez-Guille G, et al. Therapeutic monitoring of theophylline in newborns with apnea. *P&T* 2004;29:322-324.

99. Koren G. Therapeutic drug monitoring principles in the neonate. National Academy of Clinical Biochemistry. *Clin Chem.* 1997;43:222-227.

100. Aranda JV, Chemtob S, Laudignon N, et al. Pharmacologic effects of theophylline in the newborn. *J Allergy Clin Immunol.* 1986;78:773-780.

101. Blanchard J, Harvey S, Morgan WJ. Relationship between serum and saliva theophylline levels in patients with cystic fibrosis. *Ther Drug Monit.* 1992;14:48-54.

102. Kirk JK, Dupuis RE, Miles MV, Gaddy GD, Miranda-Massari JR, Williams DM. Salivary theophylline monitoring: reassessment and clinical considerations. *Ther Drug Monit.* 1994;16:58-66.

103. Patel JA, Clayton LT, LeBel CP, et al. Abnormal theophylline levels in plasma by fluorescence polarization immunoassay in patients with renal disease. *Ther Drug Monit.* 1984;6:458-460.

104. Jenny RW, Jackson KY. Two types of error found with the Seralyzer ARIS assay of theophylline. *Clin Chem.* 1986;32:2122-2123.

105. Chan KM, Koenig J, Walton KG, et al. The theophylline method of the Abbott "Vision" analyzer evaluated. *Clin Chem.*1987;33:130-132.

106. de Wildt SN, Kerkvliet KT, Wezenberg MG, et al. Use of saliva in therapeutic drug monitoring of caffeine in preterm infants. *Ther Drug Monit.* 2001;23:250-254.

107. Natarajan G, Botica ML, Aranda JV. Therapeutic drug monitoring for caffeine in preterm neonates: an unnecessary exercise? *Pediatrics.* 2007:119;936-940.

108. Aranda JV, Beharry K, Rex J, et al. Caffeine enzyme immunoassay in neonatal and pediatric drug monitoring. *Ther Drug Monit.* 1987;9:97-103.

109. Warner A, Privitera M, Bates D. Standards of laboratory practice: antiepileptic drug monitoring. National Academy of Clinical Biochemistry. *Clin Chem.* 1998;44:1085-1095.

110. Van Tyle JH, Winter ME. Carbamazepine. In: Winter ME, ed. *Basic Clinical Pharmacokinetics.* 5th ed. Baltimore, MD: Lippincott Williams & Wilkins; 2010:182-197.

111. Garnett WR, Anderson GD, Collins RJ. Antiepileptic drugs. In: Burton ME, Shaw LM, Schentag JJ, et al., eds. *Applied Pharmacokinetics and Pharmacodynamics: Principles of Therapeutic Drug Monitoring.* 4th ed. Baltimore, MD: Lippincott Williams & Wilkins; 2006:491-511.

112. Bonneton J, Iliadis A, Genton P, et al. Steady state pharmacokinetics of conventional versus controlled-release carbamazepine in patients with epilepsy. *Epilepsy Res.* 1993;14:257-263.

113. Godolphin W, Trepanier J, Farrell K. Serum and plasma for total and free anticonvulsant drug analyses: effects on EMIT assays and ultrafiltration devices. *Ther Drug Monit.* 1983;5:319-323.

114. Rosenthal E, Hoffer E, Ben-Aryeh H, et al. Use of saliva in home monitoring of carbamazepine levels. *Epilepsia.* 1995;36:72-74.

115. Drobitch RK, Svensson CK. Therapeutic drug monitoring in saliva. An update. *Clin Pharmacokinet.* 1992;23:365-379.

116. Contin M, Riva R, Albani F, et al. Determination of total and free plasma carbamazepine concentrations by enzyme multiplied immunoassay: interference with the 10,11-epoxide metabolite. *Ther Drug Monit.* 1985;7:46-50.

117. Lacher DA, Valdes R Jr, Savory J. Enzyme immunoassay of carbamazepine with a centrifugal analyzer. *Clin Chem.* 1979;25:295-28.

118. MacKichan JJ, Zola EM. Determinants of carbamazepine and carbamazepine 10,11-epoxide binding to serum protein, albumin and alpha 1-acid glycoprotein. *Br J Clin Pharmacol.* 1984;18:487-493.

119. Garnett WR, Bainbridge JL, Johnson SL. Ethosuximide. In: Murphy JE, ed. *Clinical Pharmacokinetics.* 5th ed. Bethesda, MD: American Society of Health-System Pharmacists; 2012:197-201.

120. Villen T, Bertilsson L, Sjoqvist F. Nonstereoselective disposition of ethosuximide in humans. *Ther Drug Monit.* 1990;12:514-516.

121. Tallian KB, Anderson DM. Phenobarbital. In: Murphy JE, ed. *Clinical Pharmacokinetics.* 5th ed. Bethesda, MD: American Society of Health-System Pharmacists; 2012:263-272.

122. Fairchild L, Wong E, Li TM, et al. Phenobarbital monitoring in whole blood with a quantitative noninstrumented test. *Ther Drug Monit.* 1991;13:425-427.

123. Nielsen IM, Gram L, Dam M. Comparison of AccuLevel and TDx: evaluation of on-site monitoring of antiepileptic drugs. *Epilepsia.* 1992;33:558-563.

124. Eadie MJ. Therapeutic drug monitoring—antiepileptic drugs. *Br J Clin Pharmacol.* 1998;46:185-193.

125. Winter ME. Phenytoin and fosphenytoin. In: Murphy JE, ed. *Clinical Pharmacokinetics.* 5th ed. Bethesda, MD: American Society of Health-System Pharmacists; 2012:273-287.

126. Kozer E, Parvez S, Minassian BA, et al. How high can we go with phenytoin? *Ther Drug Monit.* 2002;24:386-389.

127. Banh HL, Burton ME, Sperling MR. Interpatient and intrapatient variability in phenytoin protein binding. *Ther Drug Monit.* 2002;24:379-385.

128. Brodtkorb E, Reimers A. Seizure control and pharmacokinetics of antiepileptic drugs in pregnant women with epilepsy. *Seizure.* 2008;17:160-165.

129. Von Winckelmann SL, Spriet I, Willems L. Therapeutic drug monitoring of phenytoin in critically ill patients. *Pharmacotherapy.* 2008;28:1391-400.

130. Kugler AR, Annesley TM, Nordblom GD, et al. Cross-reactivity of fosphenytoin in two human plasma phenytoin immunoassays. *Clin Chem.* 1998;44:1474-1480.

131. Oeltgen PR, Shank WA Jr, Blouin RA, et al. Clinical evaluation of the Abbott TDx fluorescence polarization immunoassay analyzer. *Ther Drug Monit.* 1984; 6:360-367.

132. Toler SM, Wilkerson MA, Porter WH, et al. Severe phenytoin intoxication as a result of altered protein binding in AIDS. *DICP.* 1990;24:698-700.

133. Anderson GD, Pak C, Doane KW, et al. Revised Winter-Tozer equation for normalized phenytoin concentrations in trauma and elderly patients with hypoalbuminemia. *Ann Pharmacother.* 1997;31:279-284.

134. MacKichan JJ. Protein binding drug displacement interactions fact or fiction? *Clin Pharmacokinet.* 1989;16:65-73.

135. May TW, Rambeck B, Jurges U, et al. Comparison of total and free phenytoin serum concentrations measured by high-performance liquid chromatography and standard TDx assay: implications for the prediction of free phenytoin serum concentrations. *Ther Drug Monit.* 1998;20:619-623.

136. Gidal BE. Valproic acid. *Clinical Pharmacokinetics.* 5th ed. Bethesda, MD: American Society of Health-System Pharmacists; 2012:327-236.

137. Haymond J, Ensom MH. Does valproic acid warrant therapeutic drug monitoring in bipolar affective disorder? *Ther Drug Monit.* 2010;32:19-29.

138. Liu H, Montoya JL, Forman LJ, et al. Determination of free valproic acid: evaluation of the Centrifree system and comparison between high-performance liquid chromatography and enzyme immunoassay. *Ther Drug Monit.* 1992;14:513-521.

139. Ueshima S, Aiba T, Ishikawa N, et al. Poor applicability of estimation method for adults to calculate unbound serum concentrations of valproic acid in epileptic neonates and infants. *J Clin Pharm Ther.* 2009;34:415-322.

140. Dasgupta A, Volk A. Displacement of valproic acid and carbamazepine from protein binding in normal and uremic sera by tolmetin, ibuprofen, and naproxen: presence of inhibitor in uremic serum that blocks valproic acid-naproxen interactions. *Ther Drug Monit.* 1996;18:284-287.

141. Bardy AH, Hiilesmaa VK, Teramo K, et al. Protein binding of antiepileptic drugs during pregnancy, labor, and puerperium. *Ther Drug Monit.* 1990;12:40-46.

142. Chan K, Beran RG. Value of therapeutic drug level monitoring and unbound (free) levels. *Seizure.* 2008;17:572-575.

143. Johannessen SI, Tomson T. Pharmacokinetic variability of newer antiepileptic drugs: when is monitoring needed? *Clin Pharmacokinet.* 2006;45:1061-1075.

144. Garnett WR, Bainbridge JL, Egeberg MD, et al. Newer antiepileptic drugs. In: Murphy JE, ed. *Clinical Pharmacokinetics.* 5th ed. Bethesda, MD: American Society of Health-System Pharmacists; 2012:135-157.

145. Tomson T, Battino D. Pharmacokinetics and therapeutic drug monitoring of newer antiepileptic drugs during pregnancy and the puerperium. *Clin Pharmacokinet.* 2007;46:209-219.

146. Perucca E. Is there a role for therapeutic drug monitoring of new anticonvulsants? *Clin Pharmacokinet.* 2000;38:191-204.

147. Chong E, Dupuis LL. Therapeutic drug monitoring of lamotrigine. *Ann Pharmacother.* 2002;36:917-920.

148. Perucca E, Dulac O, Shorvon S, et al. Harnessing the clinical potential of antiepileptic drug therapy: dosage optimization. *CNS Drugs.* 2001;15:609-621.

149. Malone SA, Eadie MJ, Addison RS, et al. Monitoring salivary lamotrigine concentrations. *J Clin Neurosci.* 2006;13:902-907.

150. Bring P, Ensom MHH. Does oxcarbazepine warrant therapeutic drug monitoring? A critical review. *Clin Pharmacokinet.* 2008;47:767-778.

151. Contin M, Riva R, Albani F, et al. Topiramate therapeutic monitoring in patients with epilepsy: effect of concomitant antiepileptic drugs. *Ther Drug Monit.* 2002;24:332-337.

152. Begg EJ, Barclay ML, Kirkpatrick CM. The therapeutic monitoring of antimicrobial agents. *Br J Clin Pharmacol.* 2001;52(suppl 1):S35-S43.

153. Schentag JJ, Meagher AK, Jelliffe RW. Aminoglycosides. In: Burton ME, Shaw LM, Schentag JJ, et al., eds. *Applied Pharmacokinetics and Pharmacodynamics: Principles of Therapeutic Drug Monitoring.* 4th ed. Baltimore, MD: Lippincott Williams & Wilkins; 2006:285-327.

154. Murphy JE, Matthias KR. Aminoglycosides. In: Murphy JE, ed. *Clinical Pharmacokinetics.* 5th ed. Bethesda, MD: American Society of Health-System Pharmacists; 2012:91-118.

155. Nicolau DP, Freeman CD, Belliveau PP, et al. Experience with once-daily aminoglycoside program administered to 2,184 adult patients. *Antimicrob Agents Chemother.* 1995;39:650-655.

156. Beringer P, Winter ME. Aminoglycoside antibiotics. In: Winter ME, ed. *Basic Clinical Pharmacokinetics.* 5th ed. Baltimore, MD: Lippincott Williams & Wilkins; 2010:134-181.

157. Landt M, Smith CH, Hortin GL. Evaluation of evacuated blood-collection tubes: effects of three types of polymeric separators on therapeutic drug-monitoring specimens. *Clin Chem.* 1993;39:1712-1717.

158. Koch TR, Platoff G. Suitability of collection tubes with separator gels for therapeutic drug monitoring. *Ther Drug Monit.* 1990;12:277-280.

159. Berkovitch M, Bistritzer T, Aladjem M, et al. Clinical relevance of therapeutic drug monitoring of digoxin and gentamicin in the saliva of children. *Ther Drug Monit.* 1998;20:253-256.

160. Barclay ML, Kirkpatrick CM, Begg EJ. Once daily aminoglycoside therapy. Is it less toxic than multiple daily doses and how should it be monitored? *Clin Pharmacokinet.* 1999;36:89-98.

161. Tod MM, Padoin C, Petitjean O. Individualizing aminoglycoside dosage regimens after therapeutic drug monitoring: simple or complex pharmacokinetic methods? *Clin Pharmacokinet.* 2001;40:803-814.

162. Nahata MC. Chloramphenicol. In: Evans WE, Schentag JJ, Jusko WJ, eds. *Applied Pharmacokinetics: Principles of Therapeutic Drug Monitoring.* 3rd ed. Vancouver, WA: Applied Therapeutics; 1992:16.1-16.24.

163. Coakley JC, Hudson I, Shann F, et al. A review of therapeutic monitoring of chloramphenicol in patients with *Haemophilus influenzae* meningitis. *J Paediatr Child Health.* 1992;28:249-253.

164. Soldin OP, Soldin SJ. Review: therapeutic drug monitoring in pediatrics. *Ther Drug Monit.* 2002;24:1-8.

165. Nahata MC. Intravenous infusion conditions. Implications for pharmacokinetic monitoring. *Clin Pharmacokinet.* 1993;24:221-229.

166. Nahata MC, Powell DA. Bioavailability and clearance of chloramphenicol after intravenous chloramphenicol succinate. *Clin Pharmacol Ther.* 1981;30:368-372.

167. Schwartz JG, Casto DT, Ayo S, et al. A commercial enzyme immunoassay method (EMIT) compared with liquid chromatography and bioassay methods for measurement of chloramphenicol. *Clin Chem.* 1988;34:1872-1875.

168. Koup JR, Lau AH, Brodsky B, et al. Relationship between serum and saliva chloramphenicol concentrations. *Antimicrob Agents Chemother.* 1979;15:658-661.

169. Ambrose PJ, Winter ME. In: Winter ME, ed. *Basic Clinical Pharmacokinetics.* 5th ed. Baltimore, MD: Lippincott Williams & Wilkins; 2010:459-487.

170. Matzke GR, Duby JJ. Vancomycin. In: Murphy JE, ed. *Clinical Pharmacokinetics.* 5th ed. Bethesda, MD: American Society of Health-System Pharmacists; 2012:337-350.

171. Pou L, Rosell M, Lopez R, et al. Changes in vancomycin pharmacokinetics during treatment. *Ther Drug Monit.* 1996;18:149-153.

172. Somerville AL, Wright DH, Rotschafer JC. Implications of vancomycin degradation products on therapeutic drug monitoring in patients with end-stage renal disease. *Pharmacotherapy.* 1999;19:702-707.

173. Wood FL, Earl JW, Nath C, et al. Falsely low vancomycin results using the Abbott TDx. *Ann Clin Biochem.* 2000;37(part 3):411-413.

174. Trujillo TN, Sowinski KM, Venezia RA, et al. Vancomycin assay performance in patients with acute renal failure. *Intensive Care Med.* 1999;25:1291-1296.

175. Matze GR, McGory R, Halstenson CE, et al. Pharmacokinetics of vancomycin in patients with various degrees of renal function. *Antimicrob Agents Chemother.* 1984;25:433-437.

176. Moise-Broder PA. Vancomycin. In: Burton ME, Shaw LM, Schentag JJ, et al., eds. *Applied Pharmacokinetics and Pharmacodynamics: Principles of Therapeutic Drug Monitoring.* 4th ed. Baltimore, MD: Lippincott Williams & Wilkins; 2006:328-340.

177. British Society for Antimicrobial Chemotherapy Working Part. Laboratory monitoring of antifungal chemotherapy. *Lancet.* 1991;337:1577-1580.

178. Petersen D, Demertzis S, Freund M, et al. Individualization of 5-fluorocytosine therapy. *Chemotherapy.* 1994;40:149-156.

179. Vermes A, Guchelaar HJ, Dankert J. Flucytosine: a review of its pharmacology, clinical indications, pharmacokinetics, toxicity and drug interactions. *J Antimicrob Chemother.* 2000;46:171-179.

180. Summers KK, Hardin TC, Gore SJ, et al. Therapeutic drug monitoring of systemic antifungal therapy. *J Antimicrob Chemother.* 1997;40:753-764.

181. Huang CM, Kroll MH, Ruddel M, et al. An enzymatic method for 5-fluorocytosine. *Clin Chem.* 1988;34:59-62.

182. Lewis RE. Current concepts in antifungal pharmacology. *Mayo Clin Proc* 2011;86:805-817.

183. Haria M, Bryson HM, Goa KL. Itraconazole. A reappraisal of its pharmacological properties and therapeutic use in the management of superficial fungal infections. *Drugs.* 1996;51:585-620.

184. Al-Rawithi S, Hussein R, Al-Moshen I, et al. Expedient microdetermination of itraconazole and hydroxyitraconazole in plasma by high-performance liquid chromatography with fluorescence detection. *Ther Drug Monit.* 2001;23:445-448.

185. Koks CH, Crommentuyn KM, Hoetelmans RM, et al. Can fluconazole concentrations in saliva be used for therapeutic drug monitoring? *Ther Drug Monit.* 2001;23:449-453.

186. Peloquin CA. Therapeutic drug monitoring in the treatment of tuberculosis. *Drugs* 2002;62:2169-2183.

187. Holland DP, Hamilton CD, Weintrob AC, et al. Therapeutic drug monitoring of antimycobacterial drugs in patients with both tuberculosis and advanced human immunodeficiency virus infection. *Pharmacotherapy.* 2009;39:503-510.

188. Sahai J, Gallicano K, Swick L, et al. Reduced plasma concentrations of antituberculosis drugs in patients with HIV infection. *Ann Intern Med.* 1997;127:289-293.

189. Heysell SK, Moore JL, Keller SJ, et al. Therapeutic drug monitoring for slow response to tuberculosis treatment in a state control program, Virginia, USA. *Emerg Infect Dis.* 2010;16:1546-1553.

190. Yew W. Clinically significant interactions with drugs used in the treatment of tuberculosis. *Drug Saf.* 2002;25:111-133.

191. Kimerling ME, Phillips P, Patterson P, et al. Low serum antimycobacterial drug levels in non-HIV-infected tuberculosis patients. *Chest.* 1998;113:1178-1183.

192. Mehta JB, Shantaveerapa H, Byrd RP Jr, et al. Utility of rifampin blood levels in the treatment and follow-up of active pulmonary tuberculosis in patients who were slow to respond to routine directly observed therapy. *Chest.* 2001;120:1520–1524.

193. Yew WW. Therapeutic drug monitoring in antituberculosis chemotherapy: clinical perspectives. *Clin Chim Acta.* 2001;313:31-316.

194. Pretorius E, Klinker H, Rosenkranz B. The role of therapeutic drug monitoring in the management of patients with human immunodeficiency virus infection. *Ther Drug Monit.* 2011;33:265-274.

195. Panel on Antiretroviral Guidelines for Adults and Adolescents. Guidelines for the use of antiretrovirals in HIV-1-infected adults and adolescents. Washington DC: Department of Health and Human Services; October 13, 2011:1-67. http://www.aidsinfo.nih.gov/ContentFiles/AdultandAdolescentGL.pdf. Accessed December 28, 2011.

196. Rayner CR, Dooley JM, Nation RL. Antivirals for HIV. In: Burton ME, Shaw LM, Schentag JJ, et al., eds. *Applied Pharmacokinetics and Pharmacodynamics: Principles of Therapeutic Drug Monitoring.* 4th ed. Baltimore, MD: Lippincott Williams & Wilkins; 2006:354-409.

197. Back DJ, Khoo SH, Gibbons SE, Merry C. The role of therapeutic drug monitoring in treatment of HIV infection. *Br J Clin Pharmacol.* 2001;52(suppl 1):S89-S96.

198. Khoo SH, Gibbons SE, Back DJ. Therapeutic drug monitoring as a tool in treating HIV infection. *Aids.* 2001;15(suppl 5):S171-S181.

199. Dasgupta A, Okhuysen PC. Pharmacokinetic and other drug interactions in patients with AIDS. *Ther Drug Monit.* 2001;23:591-605.

200. van Heeswijk RP, Veldkamp AI, Mulder JW, et al. Saliva as an alternative body fluid for therapeutic drug monitoring of the nonnucleoside reverse transcription inhibitor nevirapine. *Ther Drug Monit.* 2001;23:255-258.

201. Wintergerst U, Kurowski M, Rolinski B, et al. Use of saliva specimens for monitoring indinavir therapy in human immunodeficiency virus-infected patients. *Antimicrob Agents Chemother.* 2000;44:2572-2574.

202. Titier K, Lagrange F, Pehourcq F, et al. High-performance liquid chromatographic method for the simultaneous determination of the six HIV-protease inhibitors and two non-nucleoside reverse transcriptase inhibitors in human plasma. *Ther Drug Monit.* 2002;24:417-424.

203. Dailly E, Raffi F, Jolliet P. Determination of atazanavir and other antiretroviral drugs (indinavir, amprenavir, nelfinavir and its active metabolite M8, Saquinavir, ritonavir, lopinavir, nevirapine, and efavirenz) plasma levels by high performance liquid chromatography with UV detection. *J Chromatogr Analyt Technol Biomed Life Sci.* 2004;813:353-358.

204. Moyle GJ, Back D. Principles and practice of HIV-protease inhibitor pharmacoenhancement. *HIV Med.* 2001;2:105-113.

205. Valdes R Jr, Jortani SA, Gheorghiade M. Standards of laboratory practice: cardiac drug monitoring. National Academy of Clinical Biochemistry. *Clin Chem.* 1998;44:1096-1109.

206. Boro MS, Winter ME. Digoxin. In: Winter ME, ed. *Basic Clinical Pharmacokinetics.* 5th ed. Baltimore, MD: Lippincott Williams & Wilkins; 2010:198-239.

207. Page RL. Digoxin. In: Murphy JE, ed. *Clinical Pharmacokinetics.* 5th ed. Bethesda, MD: American Society of Health-System Pharmacists; 2012:185-195.

208. Bernard DW, Bowman RL, Grimm FA, et al. Nighttime dosing assures postdistribution sampling for therapeutic drug monitoring of digoxin. *Clin Chem.* 1996;42:45-49.

209. Matzuk MM, Shlomchik M, Shaw LM. Making digoxin therapeutic drug monitoring more effective. *Ther Drug Monit.* 1991;13:215-219.

210. Ujhelyi MR, Green PJ, Cummings DM, et al. Determination of free serum digoxin concentrations in digoxin toxic patients after administration of digoxin Fab antibodies. *Ther Drug Monit.* 1992;14:147-154.

211. Ocal IT, Green TR. Serum digoxin in the presence of digibind: determination of digoxin by the Abbott AxSYM and Baxter Stratus II immunoassays by direct analysis without pretreatment of serum samples. *Clin Chem.* 1998;44:1947-1950.

212. Nolan PE, Trujillo TC. Lidocaine. In: Murphy JE, ed. *Clinical Pharmacokinetics.* 5th ed. Bethesda, MD: American Society of Health-System Pharmacists; 2012:229-242.

213. Ohara KY, Winter ME. Lidocaine. In: Winter ME, ed. *Basic Clinical Pharmacokinetics.* 5th ed. Baltimore, MD: Lippincott Williams & Wilkins; 2010:277-293.

214. Brown JE, Shand DG. Therapeutic drug monitoring of antiarrhythmic agents. *Clin Pharmacokinet.* 1982;7:125-148.

215. Bauer LA, Brown T, Gibaldi M, et al. Influence of long-term infusions on lidocaine kinetics. *Clin Pharmacol Ther.* 1982;31:433-437.

216. Page RL, Murphy JE. Procainamide. In: Murphy JE, ed. *Clinical Pharmacokinetics.* 5th ed. Bethesda, MD: American Society of Health-System Pharmacists; 2012:289-298.

217. Koike Y, Mineshita S, Uchiyama Y, et al. Monitoring of procainamide and N-acetyl-procainamide concentration in saliva after oral administration of procainamide. *Am J Ther.* 1996;3:708-714.

218. Coyle JD, Lima JJ. Procainamide. In: Evans WE, Schentag JJ, Jusko WJ, eds. *Applied Pharmacokinetics: Principles of Therapeutic Drug Monitoring.* 3rd ed. Vancouver, WA: Applied Therapeutics; 1992:22.1-22.33.

219. Griffith KS, Lewis LS, Mali S, et al. Treatment of malaria in the United Stated: A systematic review. *JAMA.* 2007;297:2264-2275.

220. Nolan PE, Trujillo TC, Yeaman CM. Quinidine. In: Murphy JE, ed. *Clinical Pharmacokinetics.* 5th ed. Bethesda, MD: American Society of Health-System Pharmacists; 2012:299-313.

221. McCollam PL, Crouch MA, Watson JE. Altered protein binding of quinidine in patients with atrial fibrillation and flutter. *Pharmacotherapy.* 1997;17:753-759.

222. Ochs HR, Grube E, Greenblatt DJ, et al. Intravenous quinidine: pharmacokinetic properties and effects on left ventricular performance in humans. *Am Heart J.* 1980;99:468-475.

223. Bauman J. Mexiletine. In: Taylor W, Caviness MHD, eds. *A Textbook for Clinical Application of Therapeutic Drug Monitoring.* Irving, TX: Abbott Laboratories, Diagnostics Division; 1986:125-131.

224. Lennard L. Therapeutic drug monitoring of cytotoxic drugs. *Br J Clin Pharmacol.* 2001;52(suppl 1):S75-S87.

225. Hon YY, Evans WE. Making TDM work to optimize cancer chemotherapy: a multidisciplinary team approach. *Clin Chem.* 1998;44:388-400.

226. Petros WP, Evans WE. Anticancer Agents. In: Burton ME, Shaw LM, Schentag JJ, et al., eds. *Applied Pharmacokinetics and Pharmacodynamics: Principles of Therapeutic Drug Monitoring.* 4th ed. Baltimore, MD: Lippincott Williams & Wilkins; 2006:617-636.

227. Yuen CW, Winter ME. Methotrexate. In: Winter ME, ed. *Basic Clinical Pharmacokinetics.* 5th ed. Lippincott Williams & Wilkins; 2010:304-325.

228. Press J, Berkovitch M, Laxer R, et al. Evaluation of therapeutic drug monitoring of methotrexate in saliva of children with rheumatic diseases. *Ther Drug Monit.* 1995;17:247-250.

229. McCune JS, Gibbs JP, Slattery JT. Plasma concentration monitoring of busulfan: does it improve clinical outcome? *Clin Pharmacokinet.* 2000;39:155-165.

230. Tabak A, Hoffer E, Rowe JM, et al. Monitoring of busulfan area under the curve: estimation by a single measurement. *Ther Drug Monit.* 2001;23:526-528.

231. Sparreboom A, Nooter K, Loos WJ, et al. The (ir)relevance of plasma protein binding of anticancer drugs. *Neth J Me.* 2001;59:196-207.

232. Gusella M, Ferrazzi E, Ferrari M, et al. New limited sampling strategy for determining 5-fluorouracil area under the concentration-time curve after rapid intravenous bolus. *Ther Drug Monit*. 2002;24:425-431.

233. Petros WP, Colvin OM. Metabolic jeopardy with high-dose cyclophosphamide?—not so fast. *Clin Cancer Res*. 1999;5:723-724.

234. Holt DW, Armstrong VW, Griesmacher A, et al. International Federation of Clinical Chemistry/International Association of Therapeutic Drug Monitoring and Clinical Toxicology working group on immunosuppressive drug monitoring. *Ther Drug Monit*. 2002;24:59-67.

235. Oellerich M, Armstrong VW, Kahan B, et al. Lake Louise Consensus Conference on cyclosporin monitoring in organ transplantation: report of the consensus panel. *Ther Drug Monit*. 1995;17:642-654.

236. Formea CM, Karlix JL. Antirejection agents. In: Murphy JE, ed. *Clinical Pharmacokinetics*. 5th ed. Bethesda, MD: American Society of Health-System Pharmacists; 2012:159-166.

237. Johnston A, Holt DW. Cyclosporine. In: Burton ME, Shaw LM, Schentag JJ, et al., eds. *Applied Pharmacokinetics and Pharmacodynamics: Principles of Therapeutic Drug Monitoring*. 4th ed. Baltimore, MD: Lippincott Williams & Wilkins; 2006:512-528.

238. Quan DJ, Winter ME. Immunosuppressants: cyclosporine, tacrolimus, and sirolimus. In: Winter ME, ed. *Basic Clinical Pharmacokinetics*. 5th ed. Lippincott Williams & Wilkins; 2010:250-276.

239. Johnston A, Holt DW. Immunosuppressant drugs—the role of therapeutic drug monitoring. *Br J Clin Pharmacol*. 2001;52(suppl 1):S61-S73.

240. Faynor SM, Robinson R. Suitability of plastic collection tubes for cyclosporine measurements. *Clin Chem*. 1998 44:2220-2221.

241. Lindholm A, Henricsson S. Intra- and interindividual variability in the free fraction of cyclosporine in plasma in recipients of renal transplants. *Ther Drug Monit*.1989;11:623-630.

242. Christians U, Pokaiyavanichkul T, Chan L. Tacrolimus. In: Burton ME, Shaw LM, Schentag JJ, et al., eds. *Applied Pharmacokinetics and Pharmacodynamics: Principles of Therapeutic Drug Monitoring*. 4th ed. Baltimore, MD: Lippincott Williams & Wilkins; 2006:529-562.

243. Macchi-Andanson M, Charpiat B, Jelliffe RW, et al. Failure of traditional trough levels to predict tacrolimus concentrations. *Ther Drug Monit*. 2001;23:129-133.

244. Kuzuya T, Ogura Y, Motegi Y, et al. Interference of hematocrit in the tacrolimus II microparticle enzyme immunoassay. *Ther Drug Monit*. 2002;24:507-511.

245. Dasgupta A. Usefulness of monitoring free (unbound) concentrations of therapeutic drugs in patient management. *Clin Chim Acta*. 2007;277:1-13.

246. Nawrocki A, Korecka M, Solari S, et al. Mycophenolic acid. In: Burton ME, Shaw LM, Schentag JJ, et al., eds. *Applied Pharmacokinetics and Pharmacodynamics: Principles of Therapeutic Drug Monitoring*. 4th ed. Baltimore, MD: Lippincott Williams & Wilkins; 2006:563-594.

247. Kuypers DRJ, Le Meur Y, Cantarovich M, et al. Consensus report on therapeutic drug monitoring of mycophenolic acid in solid organ transplantation. *Clin J Am Soc Nephrol*. 2010;5:341-358.

248. Weber LT, Shipkova M, Armstrong VW, et al. The pharmacokinetic-pharmacodynamic relationship for total and free mycophenolic Acid in pediatric renal transplant recipients: a report of the German study group on mycophenolate mofetil therapy. *J Am Soc Nephrol*. 2002;13:759-768.

249. Ensom MH, Partovi N, Decarie D, et al. Pharmacokinetics and protein binding of mycophenolic acid in stable lung transplant recipients. *Ther Drug Monit*. 2002;24:310-314.

250. Yatscoff RW, Boeckx R, Holt DW, et al. Consensus guidelines for therapeutic drug monitoring of rapamycin: report of the consensus panel. *Ther Drug Monit*. 1995;17:676-680.

251. DeVane CL. Cyclic antidepressants. In: Burton ME, Shaw LM, Schentag JJ, et al., eds. *Applied Pharmacokinetics and Pharmacodynamics: Principles of Therapeutic Drug Monitoring*. 4th ed. Baltimore, MD: Lippincott Williams & Wilkins; 2006:781-797.

252. Linder MW, Keck PE Jr. Standards of laboratory practice: antidepressant drug monitoring. National Academy of Clinical Biochemistry. *Clin Chem*. 1998;44:1073-1084.

253. Finley PR. Antidepressants. In: Murphy JE, ed. *Clinical Pharmacokinetics*. 5th ed. Bethesda, MD: American Society of Health-System Pharmacists; 2012:119-134.

254. Mitchell PB. Therapeutic drug monitoring of psychotropic medications. *Br J Clin Pharmacol*. 2001;52(suppl 1):S45-S54.

255. Eilers R. Therapeutic drug monitoring for the treatment of psychiatric disorders. Clinical use and cost effectiveness. *Clin Pharmacokinet*. 1995;29:442-450.

256. Chattergoon DS, Verjee Z, Anderson M, et al. Carbamazepine interference with an immune assay for tricyclic antidepressants in plasma. *J Toxicol Clin Toxicol*. 1998;36:109-113.

257. Lieberman JA, Cooper TB, Suckow RF, et al. Tricyclic antidepressant and metabolite levels in chronic renal failure. *Clin Pharmacol Ther*. 1985;37:301-307.

258. Ghibellini G, Carson SW. Lithium. In: Murphy JE, ed. *Clinical Pharmacokinetics*. 5th ed. Bethesda, MD: American Society of Health-System Pharmacists; 2012:243-262.

259. Finley PR, Winter ME. Lithium. In: Winter ME, ed. *Basic Clinical Pharmacokinetics*. 5th ed. Baltimore, MD: Lippincott Williams & Wilkins; 2010:294-303.

260. Bettinger TL, Crismon ML. Lithium. In: Burton ME, Shaw LM, Schentag JJ, et al., eds. *Applied Pharmacokinetics and Pharmacodynamics: Principles of Therapeutic Drug Monitoring*. 4th ed. Baltimore, MD: Lippincott Williams & Wilkins; 2006:798-812.

261. Marcus SC, Olfson M, Pincus HA, et al. Therapeutic drug monitoring of mood stabilizers in Medicaid patients with bipolar disorder. *Am J Psychiatry*. 1999;156:1014-1018.

262. Sampson M, Ruddel M, Albright S, et al. Positive interference in lithium determinations from clot activator in collection container. *Clin Chem*. 1997;43:675-679.

263. Perry R, Campbell M, Grega DM, et al. Saliva lithium levels in children: their use in monitoring serum lithium levels and lithium side effects. *J Clin Psychopharmacol*. 1984;4:199-202.

264. Thomson AH, Watson ID, Wilson JF, et al. An audit of therapeutic drug monitoring service provision by laboratories participating in an external quality assessment scheme. *Ther Drug Monit*. 1998;20:248-252.

265. Frezzotti A, Margarucci AM, Coppa G, et al. An evaluation of the Ektachem serum lithium method and comparison with flame emission spectrometry. *Scand J Clin Lab Invest*. 1996;56:591-596.

266. Burke MD. Principles of therapeutic drug monitoring. *Postgrad Med*. 1981;70:57-63.

267. Leucht S, Steimer W, Kreuz S, et al. Doxepin plasma concentrations: is there really a therapeutic range? *J Clin Psychopharmacol*. 2001;21:432-439.

268. DeVane CL. Metabolism and pharmacokinetics of selective serotonin reuptake inhibitors. *Cell Mol Neurobiol*. 1999;19:443-466.

269. Perel JM, Jann MW. Antipsychotics. In: Burton ME, Shaw LM, Schentag JJ, et al., eds. *Applied Pharmacokinetics and Pharmacodynamics: Principles of Therapeutic Drug Monitoring*. 4th ed. Baltimore, MD: Lippincott Williams & Wilkins; 2006:813-838.

270. Mauri MC, Volonteri LS, Colasanti AF, et al. Clinical pharmacokinetics of atypical antipsychotics. A critical review of the relationship between plasma concentrations and clinical response. *Clin Pharmacokinet*. 2007;46:359-388.

271. Nielsen J, Damkier P, Taylor LH. Optimizing clozapine treatment. *Acta Psychiatr Scand*. 2011;123:411-422.

272. Preskorn SH, Burke MJ, Fast GA. Therapeutic drug monitoring. Principles and practice. *Psychiatr Clin North Am*. 1993;16:611-645.

273. Williams ML, Wainer IW. Role of chiral chromatography in therapeutic drug monitoring and in clinical and forensic toxicology. *Ther Drug Monit*. 2002;24:290-296.

274. Thormann W, Theurillat R, Wind M, et al. Therapeutic drug monitoring of antiepileptics by capillary electrophoresis. Characterization of assays via analysis of quality control sera containing 14 analytes. *J Chromatogr A*. 2001; 924:429-437.

275. Williams J, Patsalos PN, Mei Z, et al. Relation between dosage of carbamazepine and concentration in hair and plasma samples from a compliant inpatient epileptic population. *Ther Drug Monit*. 2001;23:15-20.

276. Wang J. Amperometric biosensors for clinical and therapeutic drug monitoring: a review. *J Pharm Biomed Anal*. 1999;19:47-53.

277. Stahle L, Alm C, Ekquist B, et al. Monitoring free extracellular valproic acid by microdialysis in epileptic patients. *Ther Drug Monit*. 1996;18:14-18.

278. Campbell M. Community-based therapeutic drug monitoring. Useful development or unnecessary distraction? *Clin Pharmacokinet*. 1995;28:271-274.

279. Hawksworth GM, Chrystyn H. Therapeutic drug and biochemical monitoring in a community pharmacy: Part 1. *Int J Pharm Pract*. 1995;3:133-138.

280. Nebert DW, Vessell ES. Can personalized drug therapy be achieved? A closer look at pharmaco-metabonomics. *Trends in Pharmacol Sci*. 2006;27:580-586.

281. Ferraldeschi R, Newman WG. Pharmacogenetics and pharmacogenomics: a clinical reality. *Ann Clin Biochem*. 2011;48:410-417.

282. Innocenti F, Ratain MJ. Update on pharmacogenetics in cancer chemotherapy. *Eur J Cancer*. 2002;38:639-644.

283. Holford NH. Target concentration intervention: beyond Y2K. *Br J Clin Pharmacol*. 2001;52(suppl 1):S55-S59.

284. Bates DW, Soldin SJ, Rainey PM, et al. Strategies for physician education in therapeutic drug monitoring. *Clin Chem*. 1998;44:401-407.

285. Schumacher GE, Barr JT. Total testing process applied to therapeutic drug monitoring: impact on patients' outcomes and economics. *Clin Chem*. 1998;44:370-374.

BIBLIOGRAPHY

Bauer LA. *Applied Clinical Pharmacokinetics*. 2nd ed. New York, NY: McGraw-Hill; 2008.

Burton ME, Shaw LM, Schentag JJ, et al., eds. *Applied Pharmacokinetics and Pharmacodynamics: Principles of Therapeutic Drug Monitoring*. 4th ed. Baltimore, MD: Lippincott Williams & Wilkins; 2006.

Murphy JE, ed. *Clinical Pharmacokinetics*. 5th ed. Bethesda, MD: American Society of Health-System Pharmacists; 2012.

Taylor WJ, Caviness MHD, eds. *A Textbook for the Application of Therapeutic Drug Monitoring*. Irving, TX: Abbot Laboratories, Diagnostics Division; 1986.

Winter ME, ed. *Basic Clinical Pharmacokinetics*. 5th ed. Baltimore, MD: Lippincott Williams & Wilkins; 2010.

CHAPTER 6

ELECTROLYTES, OTHER MINERALS, AND TRACE ELEMENTS

ALAN LAU, LINGTAK-NEANDER CHAN

Serum or plasma electrolyte concentrations are among the most commonly used laboratory tests by clinicians for assessment of a patient's clinical conditions and disease states. The purpose of this chapter is to present the physiological basis of the need to assess serum concentrations of common electrolytes and minerals. The interpretation of these laboratory results and the clinical significance are addressed.

Sodium, potassium, and chloride are among the most commonly monitored electrolytes in clinical practice. Magnesium, calcium, and phosphate are also monitored as determined by the patient's disease states and/or clinical indication. The homeostasis of calcium and phosphate is frequently discussed in the context of the endocrine system because of the effects of vitamin D and parathyroid hormone (PTH) on the regulation of these minerals. Serum total carbon dioxide content, often measured in conjunction with electrolytes, is discussed in Chapter 9: Arterial Blood Gases and Acid–Base Balance, because of its significance for the evaluation of acid–base disorders. Listed in Table 6-1 are the average daily dietary intakes of electrolytes, minerals, and trace elements.

ELECTROLYTES

The traditional units, International System (SI) units as well as their conversion factors for electrolytes, minerals, and trace elements discussed in this chapter, are listed in Table 6-2. Although the normal ranges of serum concentrations for each of the electrolytes are listed below, clinicians should always confirm with the institutional clinical laboratory department for their institutional reference range due to the variance introduced by equipments, analytical technique, and quality assurance data.

Sodium

Normal range: 136–142 mEq/L or 136–142 mmol/L

TABLE 6-1. Normal Dietary Intake of Electrolytes, Other Minerals, and Trace Elements for Healthy Adults

NUTRIENT	NORMAL DAILY DIETARY INTAKE[a]
Sodium	Variable; average 3.4 g (148 mEq)
Potassium	50–100 mEq
Chloride	Varies with potassium and sodium intakes
Magnesium	300–400 mg
Calcium	~1000 mg
Phosphate	800–1500 mg
Copper	2–5 mg
Zinc	4–14 mg
Manganese	3–4 mg
Chromium	50–100 mcg

[a]According to recommendations in 2010 from the National Academy of Sciences; Institute of Medicine; Food and Nutrition Board.

TABLE 6-2. Conversion Factors to SI Units

NUTRIENT	TRADITIONAL UNITS	CONVERSION FACTORS TO SI UNITS	SI UNITS
Sodium	mEq/L	1	mmol/L
Potassium	mEq/L	1	mmol/L
Chloride	mEq/L	1	mmol/L
Magnesium	mEq/L	0.5	mmol/L
Calcium	mg/dL	0.25	mmol/L
Phosphate	mg/dL	0.3229	mmol/L
Copper	mcg/dL	0.1574	µmol/L
Zinc	mcg/dL	0.1530	µmol/L
Manganese	mcg/L	18.2	µmol/L
Chromium	mcg/L	19.2	nmol/L

Sodium is the most abundant cation in the extracellular fluid and is the major regulating factor for bodily water balance. Extracellular (i.e., intravascular and interstitial) and intracellular sodium contents are closely affected by the body fluid status. Thus, an accurate interpretation of serum sodium concentration must include an understanding of body water homeostasis and the inter-relationship between the regulation of sodium and water.[1]

Physiology

While sodium is essential for maintaining the optimal transmembrane electric potential for action potential and neuromuscular functioning, the principal role of sodium is to regulate serum osmolality as well as water balance. Serum osmolality is an estimate of the water-solute ratio in the vascular fluid. It is useful in determining volume status, especially the intravascular volume.[2] Figure 6-1 summarizes the inter-relationship and regulation between water and sodium. Normal serum osmolality is usually between 280–295 mOsm/kg H$_2$O. The presence of a significant amount of other extracellular solutes (e.g., alcohol, glucose, and organic solvents) can further elevate serum osmolality, thus affecting body water and sodium status.

Changes in body water and plasma volume can directly or indirectly affect the serum sodium concentration. For example, as the result of changes in effective circulating volume, baroreceptors and osmoreceptors will respond accordingly in an attempt to restore an isovolemic state of the body. Baroreceptors are located in the carotid sinus, aortic arch, cardiac atria, hypothalamus, and the juxtaglomerular apparatus in the kidney. Stimulation of these receptors will promote urinary loss of water and sodium. Osmoreceptors are present primarily in the hypothalamus. The three major effectors in response to the stimulation of the osmoreceptors include vasopressin or antidiuretic hormone (ADH), the renin-angiotensin-aldosterone system (RAAS), and natriuretic peptides. The resultant renal effects from these three distinct pathways will alter the homeostasis of water and sodium.

The kidneys are the primary organ responsible for the retention and excretion of body sodium and water. The glomeruli

receive and filter about 180 L of plasma and 600 g (nearly 26,000 mEq) of sodium per day. On average, less than 2 L of water and between 0.1–40 g of sodium are excreted in the urine, depending on the fluid status of the individual. While almost 100% of the plasma sodium is filtered by the glomeruli, less than 1% is excreted in the urine under normal circumstances. The proximal tubule and the loop of Henle each account for approximately 45% of sodium reabsorption.

The homeostatic mechanism for water and sodium also involves the equilibrium among intravascular, interstitial, and intracellular fluids.[3] Net movement of water occurs from areas of low osmolality to areas of high osmolality. This effect can be readily observed in patients with a low serum osmolality due to a deficit of serum sodium or excess of plasma water. Water then moves from the plasma compartment to the higher osmolality in the interstitial space to minimize the osmolar gap.[3] In the presence of high hydrostatic and oncotic pressure gaps across capillary walls, the net effect is excessive interstitial water accumulation and edema formation.[3,4]

Antidiuretic hormone (vasopressin). *Antidiuretic hormone (ADH)*, also known as *arginine vasopressin*, is a nonapeptide hormone that regulates renal handling of free water exclusively. By altering the amount of water reabsorbed by the kidney, ADH has a pivotal effect in changing or maintaining serum sodium concentration, and it is secreted by the magnocellular neurons in the supraoptic and paraventricular nuclei of the hypothalamus, where both osmoreceptors and baroreceptors are present to detect vascular fluid changes. Its release is stimulated by (1) hypovolemia (detected by baroreceptors), (2) thirst, (3) increased serum osmolality, and (4) angiotensin II. The plasma half-life of ADH is 10–20 minutes, and it is rapidly deactivated and eliminated by the liver, kidneys, and a plasma enzyme called *vasopressinase*.

Antidiuretic hormone decreases urine output by augmenting the permeability of the collecting tubules to increase the net reabsorption of water. Circulating serum ADH binds to type 2 vasopressin (V2) receptors in the collecting tubule, which in turn stimulates the formation of a water channel, known as *aquaporin-2*. Aquaporin-2 facilitates the reabsorption of water from the lumen back into the renal blood supply in the systemic circulation, causing a decrease in diuresis. However, if serum sodium is high but blood volume is normal (e.g., normovolemia with hyperosmolality), the effect from the baroreceptors overrides the further release of ADH, thus preventing volume overload (i.e., hypervolemia).[3]

In patients with the syndrome of inappropriate ADH (SIADH) secretion, an abnormally high quantity of ADH is present in the systemic circulation. This condition results in increased water reabsorption, which could cause a dilutional effect in serum sodium. In conjunction with an increased free water intake, a low serum sodium concentration is commonly observed in these patients. Urine osmolality and urine electrolyte concentrations are often increased due to the decreased urinary excretion of free water. Conversely, central diabetes insipidus (DI) occurs when hypothalamic ADH synthesis or release is impaired. Patients with DI commonly present with

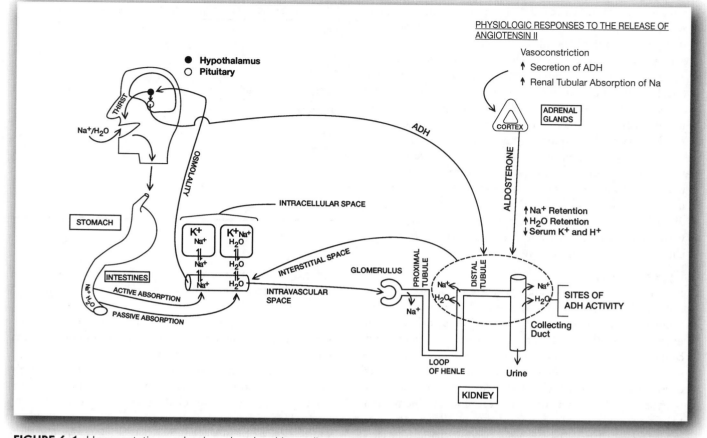

FIGURE 6-1. Homeostatic mechanisms involved in sodium, potassium, and water balance.

hypernatremia due to the increased renal wasting of free water. In some cases, the kidneys fail to respond to normal or high quantities of circulating ADH. This condition is called *nephrogenic diabetes insipidus*. In central or nephrogenic DI, little water reabsorption occurs, resulting in a large urine output with low urine osmolality.[3] (Chapter 8: The Kidneys offers an in-depth discussion of the effects of other diseases on urine composition.)

Drugs may affect ADH release or action, which may exacerbate SIADH or DI. Increased ADH release has been reported with chlorpropamide, tolbutamide, cyclophosphamide, carbamazepine, oxcarbazepine, some opiate derivatives, clofibrate, oxytocin, vincristine, phenothiazines, some tricyclic antidepressants, and a number of serotonin reuptake inhibitors. Because of their ability to increase ADH release, some of these drugs are used in the treatment of central DI. In contrast, other drugs that decrease ADH release (e.g., demeclocycline or lithium carbonate) have been used to treat SIADH. Selective type-2 vasopressin receptor (V2) antagonists (e.g., tolvaptan, conivaptan) modulate the renal handling of water and have a direct effect on sodium homeostasis.

Renin-angiotensin-aldosterone system. Renin is a glycoprotein that catalyzes the conversion of angiotensinogen to angiotensin I, which is further converted to angiotensin II primarily in the lungs. However, angiotensin II can also be formed locally in the kidneys. Angiotensin II, a potent vasoconstrictor, is important in maintaining optimal perfusion

pressure to end organs especially when plasma volume is decreased. In addition, it induces the release of aldosterone, ADH, and, to a lesser extent, cortisol.

Aldosterone is a hormone with potent mineralocorticoidal actions. It affects the distal tubular reabsorption of sodium rather than water.[4] This hormone is released from the adrenal cortex. Besides angiotensin II, various dietary and neurohormonal factors including low serum sodium, high serum potassium, and low blood volume can also stimulate its release. Aldosterone acts on renal Na-K-ATPase to increase urinary excretion of potassium from the distal tubules in exchange for sodium reabsorption. Because of its effect on renal Na/K exchange, aldosterone has a profound effect on serum potassium, while its effect on serum sodium is relatively modest. As serum sodium increases, so does water reabsorption, which follows the osmotic gradient.[3] Renal arteriolar blood pressure (BP) then increases, which helps maintain the glomerular filtration rate (GFR). Ultimately, more water and sodium pass through the distal tubules, overriding the initial effect of aldosterone.[3,4]

Natriuretic peptides. *Atrial natriuretic factor (ANF),* also known as *atrial natriuretic peptide,* is a vasodilatory hormone synthesized and primarily released by the right atrium. It is secreted in response to plasma volume expansion, as a result of increased atrial stretch. Atrial natriuretic factor inhibits the juxtaglomerular apparatus, zona glomerulosa cells of the adrenal gland, and the hypothalamus-posterior pituitary. As a result, a global down regulation of renin, aldosterone, and ADH, respectively, is achieved. Atrial natriuretic factor directly induces glomerular hyperfiltration and reduces sodium reabsorption in the collecting tubule. A net increase in sodium excretion is achieved. Therefore, ANF can decrease serum and total body sodium. Brain natriuretic peptide (BNP) is produced and secreted primarily by the ventricles in the brain, and to a much smaller extent, the atrium. Similar to ANP, BNP also regulates natriuretic, endocrine, and hemodynamic responses and may affect sodium homeostasis. An increase in blood volume or pressure, such as chronic heart failure and hypertension, enhances BNP secretion, which induces a significant increase in natriuresis and to a lesser extent, urinary flow (i.e., diuresis). Plasma BNP concentrations are found to correlate with the magnitude of left ventricular heart failure and the clinical prognosis of these patients.

Hyponatremia

Hyponatremia is loosely defined as a serum sodium concentration less than 136 mEq/L (<136 mmol/L). Hyponatremia may occur when total body water status is low (i.e., dehydration), normal, or high (i.e., fluid overload). Therefore, natremic status cannot be assessed without first assessing the fluid and water status of the patient. Fluid status should be evaluated based on vital signs; other supportive laboratory findings if available (e.g., serum, blood urea nitrogen–creatinine ratio, hematocrit to hemoglobin concentration ratio, or urine electrolyte assessment); recent changes in body weight; recent medical, surgical, and nutrition history; and findings from the physical examination. More importantly, the patient's renal function, hydration status, and fluid intake and output must be carefully assessed and closely monitored. The most common causes of hyponatremia can be broken down into two types: sodium depletion in excess of total body water loss (e.g., severe dehydration with true depletion of total body sodium) and dilutional hyponatremia (i.e., water intake greater than water output). Dilutional hyponatremia can be further categorized into five subtypes: (1) primary dilutional hyponatremia (e.g., SIADH and renal failure); (2) neuroendocrine (e.g., adrenal insufficiency and myxedema); (3) psychiatric disorder (e.g., psychogenic polydipsia); (4) osmotic hyponatremia (e.g., severe hyperglycemia); and (5) thiazide diuretic-induced.

Most patients with hyponatremia remain asymptomatic until serum sodium approaches 120 mEq/L. Infusion of hypertonic saline (e.g., 3% NaCl solution) is usually not necessary unless serum sodium concentration is less than 120 mEq/L, altered mental status is present, and if the patient is fluid restricted (e.g., heart failure, chronic renal failure). As with most electrolyte disorders, the chronicity of the imbalance is a major determinant of the severity of signs and symptoms. For example, hyponatremia in patients with congestive heart failure (CHF) secondary to chronic, progressive volume overload and decreased renal perfusion is less likely to be symptomatic than a patient who is hyponatremic due to rapid infusion of a hypotonic solution. The most commonly reported symptom associated with hyponatremia is altered mental status (List 6-1). If serum sodium continues to fall, cerebral edema can worsen

LIST 6-1. Signs and Symptoms of Hyponatremia

Agitation

Anorexia

Apathy

Depressed deep-tendon reflexes

Disorientation

Hypothermia

Lethargy

Muscle cramps

Nausea

Seizures

and intracranial pressure will continue to rise. More severe symptoms such as seizure, coma, and, subsequently, death may result.[3–6]

Hyponatremia associated with total body sodium depletion. Hyponatremia associated with low total body sodium reflects a reduction in total body water, with an even larger reduction in total body sodium. This condition is primarily caused by depletion of extracellular fluid, which stimulates ADH release to increase renal water reabsorption even at the expense of causing a transient hypo-osmotic state. Some common causes include vomiting; diarrhea; intravascular fluid losses due to burn injury and pancreatitis; Addison disease; and certain forms of renal failure (e.g., salt-wasting nephropathy).[3] This type of hyponatremia may also occur in patients treated too aggressively with diuretics who receive sodium-free solutions as replacement fluid.

Low serum sodium can also result when a large quantity of an osmotically active substance enters the bloodstream, resulting in a dilutional hyponatremia.[3] This situation can occur with the use of mannitol, an osmotic diuretic agent, as well as in the presence of hyperglycemia. In hyperglycemia, the elevated serum glucose concentration results in high serum osmolarity, thus creating an osmolar gradient between the plasma compartment and the extracellular fluid leading to a shift of water into the intravascular space. The net effect is a dilution of the serum sodium concentration resulting in hyponatremia.[3,5] In the absence of other causes impairing sodium homeostasis, the effect should be transient and should be reversed once serum glucose is normalized. However, hyperglycemia also leads to fluid loss through an osmotic diuretic effect. Hence, dilutional hyponatremia occurs as long as the rate of water moving from the cells into the blood is greater than the volume of water excreted through the urine. As cellular water diminishes and diuresis continues, plasma sodium may increase progressively.[3,5]

Patients with hyponatremia associated with low total body sodium often exhibit signs and symptoms of dehydration. These manifestations include thirst, dry mucous membranes, weight loss, sunken eyes, diminished urine output, and diminished skin turgor.[3]

Causes of SIADH

CNS Disorders
- Head trauma
- Subdural hematoma
- Subarachnoid hemorrhage
- Menengitis/encephalitis
- Hydrocephalus
- Brian mass or abscess
- Stroke/TIAs

Guillain-Barré Syndrome
Neoplasms (especially in lung cancer, lymphoma)

Pulmonary Diseases
- Tuberculolsis
- Aspergillosis
- Cystic fibrosis
- Bronchiectasis

Positive Pressure Ventilation
Surgery
Pain
Psychosis
Drug-induced →

DRUGS THAT ↑ ADA RELEASE
- Carbamazepine
- Oxcarbazepine
- Chlorpropamide
- clofibrate
- Nicotine

DRUGS THAT ↑ RENAL ADH RESPONSE OR MAY MIMIC ADH'S ACTION
- ADH analogs
- Carbamazepine
- Chlorpropamide
- Cyclophosphamide
- Fluoxetine
- Ifosfamide
- Indomethacin
- Lamotrigine
- MDMA
- Oxcarbazepine
- Vinca alkaloids

FIGURE 6-2. Etiology of SIADH.

Hyponatremia associated with normal total body sodium. Also called *euvolemic* or *dilutional hyponatremia*, this condition refers to impaired water excretion without any alteration in sodium excretion. Etiologies include any mechanism that enhances ADH secretion or potentiates its action at the collecting tubules. This condition can occur as a result of glucocorticoid deficiency, severe hypothyroidism, and administration of water to a patient with impaired water excretion capacity.[3,5] Syndrome of inappropriate ADH commonly results in hyponatremia, secondary to continued ADH secretion despite low serum osmolality.

Impaired ADH response can be precipitated by many factors, including medications (Figure 6-2). Syndrome of inappropriate ADH has been reported in patients with certain tumors, such as lung cancer, pancreatic carcinoma, thymoma, and lymphoma. Antidiuretic hormone release from the parvicellular and magnocellular neurons may be stimulated by cytokines such as interleukin (IL-2, IL-6, IL-1 beta), and tumor necrosis factor (TNF-a). Likewise, head trauma, subarachnoid hemorrhage, hydrocephalus, Guillain-Barré syndrome, pulmonary aspergillosis, and occasionally tuberculosis may increase hypothalamic ADH production and release. Patients with SIADH produce concentrated urine with high urine osmolality (usually >200 mOsm/kg H_2O) and urine sodium excretion (as reflected in a urine sodium concentration that is usually >20 mEq/L). They have normal renal, adrenal, and thyroid function and have no evidence of volume abnormalities.[3,5]

Hyponatremia may also be associated with an increase of total body sodium. This condition implies an increase in total body sodium with an even larger increase in total body water. It is frequently observed in edematous states such as CHF, cirrhosis, nephrotic syndrome, and chronic kidney disease (CKD). In these patients, renal handling of water and sodium is usually impaired.[3,5]

Tests for Assessing Fluid Status

Fractional Excretion of Sodium (FENa)

Normal range: 1% to 2%

In most cases, natremic disorders cannot be effectively managed without first optimizing the overall fluid status. Therefore, when a serum sodium value is abnormal, the clinician should first evaluate whether vascular volume is optimal. In addition to physical examinations and history, FE_{Na} may help validate these findings, especially in patients whose physical examination results may be limited by other confounders (e.g., the use of antihypertensive drugs, heart failure). The FE_{Na} may be determined by the use of a random urine sample to determine renal handling of sodium. FE_{Na}, the measure of the percentage of filtered sodium excreted in the urine, can be calculated using the following equation:

$$FE_{Na}(\%) = \frac{Urine_{Na}/Serum_{Na}}{Urine_{cr}/Serum_{cr}} \times 100\%$$

Values greater than 2% usually suggest that the kidneys are excreting a higher than normal fraction of the filtered sodium, implying likely renal tubular damage. Conversely, FE_{Na} values less than 1% generally imply preservation of intravascular fluid through renal sodium retention, suggesting prerenal causes of renal dysfunction (e.g., hypovolemia and cardiac failure). Since acute diuretic therapy can increase the FE_{Na} to 20% or more, urine samples should be obtained at least 24 hours after diuretics have been discontinued.[3] Minicase 1 demonstrates how to calculate FE_{Na}.

Blood Urea Nitrogen (BUN): Serum Creatinine (SCr) Ratio

Normal range: <20:1

The BUN: SCr ratio can provide useful information to assess fluid status. When this ratio is higher than 20:1, dehydration

MINICASE 1

A Case of Hyponatremia

JANE W., A 74-YEAR-OLD WOMAN, had a history of coronary artery disease, CHF, and type 2 diabetes mellitus. She was brought to the emergency department by her daughter, who complained about her mother's increasing disorientation over the past week. Medications (all taken orally) at the time of admission were benazepril 10 mg daily, digoxin 0.125 mg daily, furosemide 40 mg twice a day, metformin extended-released 2 g daily, sitagliptin 100 mg daily, and acetaminophen 650 mg PRN. She last took these medications the morning before presentation to the hospital. A review of systems revealed lethargy and apathy with no apparent distress. Vital signs showed a BP of 110/75 mm Hg at supine position (standing BP 105/70 mm Hg), a regular heart rate at 96 beats per minute (standing 100 beats per minute), and a rapid and shallow respiratory rate of 36 breaths per minute. Her laboratory findings were unremarkable, except for serum sodium of 120 mEq/L (136–142 mEq/L) and serum glucose of 185 mg/dL (70–110 mg/dL).

Question: What subjective and objective findings in Jane W. are consistent with the presentation of hyponatremia? What are the potential etiologies of hyponatremia in Jane W.?

Discussion: Aside from her low serum sodium concentration, her other major symptoms consistent with hyponatremia are mostly CNS-related symptoms, such as lethargy and apathy. Rapid shallow breathing (Cheyne-Stokes respiration) may be related to severe heart failure or an altered vascular fluid status. A clinician must determine volume status when assessing a patient with sodium abnormality. To further determine possible etiologies, the clinician should assess Jane W.'s body fluid status. The fact that she had normal blood pressure and a lack of orthostatic hypotension with essentially no change in heart rate suggests that hypovolemia is unlikely. Therefore, the primary cause of her symptoms at presentation is most likely associated with hyponatremia. Furosemide should be held as it is known to cause increased renal sodium loss which would worsen her current condition. Renal handling of sodium using other laboratory or diagnostic tests such as urine sodium excretion, and urine osmolality and FE_{Na} should be considered 24 hours after the discontinuation of furosemide, as the natriuretic action of loop diuretics could limit the accuracy in interpreting these test results.

is usually present. As extracellular fluid volume is diminished, the kidneys increase their reabsorption of urea but not creatinine. Therefore, BUN increases by a larger magnitude than the SCr concentration in dehydrated individuals, leading to a rise in the BUN: SCr ratio.

Hypernatremia

Hypernatremia is defined as a serum sodium concentration greater than 142 mEq/L (>142 mmol/L). High serum sodium concentrations are common in patients with either an impaired thirst mechanism (e.g., neurohypophyseal lesion, especially after suffering from a stroke) or an inability to replete water deficit through normal insensible losses (i.e., uncontrollable water loss through respiration or skin) or from renal or GI losses. All hypernatremic states increase serum osmolality. Similar to hyponatremia, hypernatremia may occur in the presence of high, normal, or low total body sodium content.[3,4,6]

The clinical manifestations of hypernatremia primarily involve the neurological system (List 6-2). These manifestations are the consequence of cellular dehydration, particularly

LIST 6-2. Signs and Symptoms of Hypernatremia

Thirst

Restlessness

Irritability

Lethargy

Muscle twitching

Seizures

Hyperreflexia

Coma

Death

in the brain. In adults, acute elevation in serum sodium above 160 mEq/L (>160 mmol/L) is associated with 75% mortality rate. Unfortunately, neurological sequelae are common even in survivors. In order to assess the etiology of hypernatremia, it is important to determine (1) urine production; (2) sodium intake; and (3) renal solute concentrating ability, which reflects ADH activity.

Hypernatremia associated with low total body sodium occurs when the loss of water exceeds the loss of sodium.[3] The thirst mechanism generally increases water intake, but this adjustment is not always possible (e.g., institutionalized elderly patients). This condition may also be iatrogenic when hypotonic fluid losses (e.g., profuse sweating and diarrhea) are replaced with an inadequate quantity of water and salt. In these circumstances, fluid loss should be replaced with intravenous (IV) dextrose solutions or hypotonic saline solutions.[3,5] In hypernatremic patients presenting with high urine osmolality (>800 mOsm/L, roughly equivalent to a specific gravity of 1.023) and low urine sodium concentrations (<10 mEq/L), these laboratory results reflect an intact renal concentrating mechanism. Signs and symptoms of dehydration should be carefully examined. These include orthostatic hypotension, flat neck veins, tachycardia, poor skin turgor, and dry mucous membranes. In addition, the BUN: SCr ratio may be greater than 20 secondary to dehydration.[3,5]

Hypernatremia may be associated with normal total body sodium, also known as *euvolemic hypernatremia*. This condition refers to a general water loss without concurrent sodium loss.[3] Because of water redistribution between the intracellular and extracellular fluid, no plasma volume contraction is usually evident unless water loss is substantial (Minicase 2). Etiologies include increased insensible water loss (e.g., fever,

LIST 6-3. Drugs That Can Cause Nephrogenic Diabetes Insipidus

Acetohexamide

Amphotericin B

Angiographic dyes

Cisplatin

Clozapine

Colchicine

Demeclocycline

Foscarnet

Gentamicin

Glyburide

Lithium

Loop diuretics

Methicillin

Methoxyflurane

Norepinephrine

Osmotic diuretics

Phenytoin

Propoxyphene

Thiazide diuretics

Tolazamide

Tolvaptan

Vinblastine

extensive burns, and mechanical ventilation) and central and nephrogenic DI. The clinician should be aware of drugs that may cause nephrogenic DI (List 6-3).[3,5]

Free water supplementation by mouth or IV fluid administration with dextrose 5% is necessary for correcting hypernatremia and preventing hypovolemia. If the diagnosis of DI is subsequently established, vasopressin or desmopressin, a synthetic analog of vasopressin, will be reasonable option for long-term maintenance therapy. Hypernatremia may be associated with high total body sodium. This form of hypernatremia is the least common, since sodium homeostasis is maintained indirectly through the control of water, and defects in the system usually affect total body water more than total body sodium.[3] This form of hypernatremia usually results from exogenous administration of solutions containing large amounts of sodium:

- Resuscitative efforts using hypertonic sodium bicarbonate
- Inadvertent IV infusion of hypertonic saline (i.e., solutions >0.9% sodium chloride)
- Inadvertent dialysis against high sodium-containing solution
- Sea water, near drowning

Primary hyperaldosteronism and Cushing syndrome may also cause this form of hypernatremia. Large quantities of sodium can be found in the urine of these patients. Signs and symptoms include diminished skin turgor and elevated plasma proteins.[3,5]

MINICASE 2

A Case of Hypernatremia After a Complete Hypophysectomy

RYAN L., A 21-YEAR-OLD MAN, was admitted to the neurosurgical service for a complete hypophysectomy to remove a pituitary tumor. He was otherwise in good health and was on no chronic medication. His postoperative medications included morphine (administered in a patient-controlled analgesia pump) and IV cefazolin 1 g intravenously every 8 hours.

On the day after surgery, Ryan L.'s urine output reached 4.5 L in 24 hours. His physical exam was unremarkable, and his vital signs were stable. Clinical laboratory tests included serum sodium 152 mEq/L (136–142 mEq/L), potassium 3.8 mEq/L (3.8–5.0 mEq/L), chloride 102 mEq/L (95–103 mEq/L), total carbon dioxide content 24 mmol/L (24–30 mmol/L), glucose 98 mg/dL (70–110 mg/dL), serum phosphate 2.9 mg/dL (2.3–4.7 mg/dL), BUN 18 mg/dL (8–23 mg/dL), and SCr 0.9 mg/dL (0.6–1.2 mg/dL). Urine specific gravity was 1.003 (1.016–1.022). On the following day, his daily urine volume reached 8 L, and he complained of being persistently thirsty despite drinking 14 glasses of water in the past 24 hour period.

Question: What is the primary cause of the sodium disorder in Ryan L.?

Discussion: Surgical procedures that could potentially affect pituitary gland functions are a major risk factor for sodium disorders since the release and regulation of ADH may be affected. Postoperatively, this patient presented with severely elevated urine output with persistent thirst. This suggests that an ADH-related disorder, DI, is likely present with a serious concern for altered sodium homeostasis. His relatively normal vital signs were maintained by his ability to dramatically increase his water intake; otherwise, he likely would have developed hypotension. This is an acute medical problem and the diagnosis should be established quickly with the help of several laboratory tests such as urine sodium, serum sodium, and urine osmolality. The diagnosis of DI can be confirmed with low urine osmolality, low urine sodium. These results, together with his elevated serum sodium and low urine specific gravity, as well as his clinical manifestation of polyuria and polydipsia, are consistent with the diagnosis of DI.

Potassium

Normal range: 3.8–5.0 mEq/L or 3.8–5.0 mmol/L

Potassium is the primary cation in the intracellular space, with an average intracellular fluid concentration of about 140 mEq/L (140 mmol/L). The major physiological role of potassium is in the regulation of muscle and nerve excitability. It may also play important roles in the control of intracellular volume (similar to the ability of sodium in controlling extracellular volume), protein synthesis, enzymatic reactions, and carbohydrate metabolism.[7,8]

Physiology

The most important aspect of potassium physiology is its effect on action potential, especially on muscle and nervous tissue excitability.[2] During periods of potassium imbalance, the cardiovascular system is of principal concern. Cardiac muscle cells depend on their ability to change their electrical potentials, with accompanying potassium flux when exposed to the proper stimulus, to result in muscle contraction and nerve conduction.[7,8]

One important aspect of potassium homeostasis is its distribution equilibrium. In a 70-kg man, the total body potassium content is about 4000 mEq. Of that amount, only 60 mEq is located in the extracellular fluid with the remainder residing within cells. The average daily Western diet contains 50–100 mEq of potassium, which is completely and passively absorbed in the upper gastrointestinal (GI) tract. To enter cells, potassium must first pass through the extracellular compartment. If the serum potassium concentrations rise above 6 mEq/L (>6 mmol/L), symptomatic hyperkalemia may occur. Potassium homeostasis is altered by insulin, aldosterone, changes in acid–base balance, renal function, or GI and skin losses. These conditions can be modulated by various pathological states as well as pharmacotherapy. Although potassium may affect different bodily functions, its effect on cardiac muscle is the most important due to the potential life-threatening effect of arrhythmias, as a result of either high or low serum potassium concentrations.[4,6-10]

Renal Homeostasis

When the serum potassium concentration is high, the body has two different mechanisms to restore potassium balance. One quick way is to shift the plasma potassium into cells, while the other slower mechanism is renal elimination.[10] The kidneys are the primary organs involved in the control and elimination of potassium. Potassium is freely filtered at the glomeruli and almost completely reabsorbed before the filtrate reaches the collecting tubules. However, an amount equal to about 10% of the filtered potassium is secreted into the urine at the distal and collecting tubules. Virtually all the potassium recovered in urine is, therefore, delivered via tubular secretion rather than glomerular filtration.[7]

In the distal tubule, potassium is being secreted into the tubule while sodium is reabsorbed. There are several mechanisms that can modulate this sodium-potassium exchange. Aldosterone plays an important role since it increases potassium secretion into the urine (Figures 6-1 and 6-3).[10] The hormone is secreted by the adrenal glands in response to high serum potassium concentrations. The delivery of large quantities of sodium and fluid to the distal tubules may also cause potassium secretion and its subsequent elimination, as seen in diuretic-induced hypokalemia.[11] As the delivery of sodium and fluid is decreased, potassium secretion declines.

The presence of anions in the distal tubules, which are relatively permeable to reabsorption, can increase renal potassium loss because the negatively charged anions attract positively charged potassium ions. This mechanism is responsible for hypokalemia caused by renal tubular acidosis and the administration of high doses of drugs with sodium salts (e.g., penicillin and its derivatives).[10] Potassium secretion is also influenced by the potassium concentration in distal tubular cells. When the intracellular potassium concentration is high, such as during dehydration, potassium secretion into the urine is increased.

In addition to the mechanisms addressed above, there are several additional points that we should consider regarding the maintenance of potassium homeostasis:

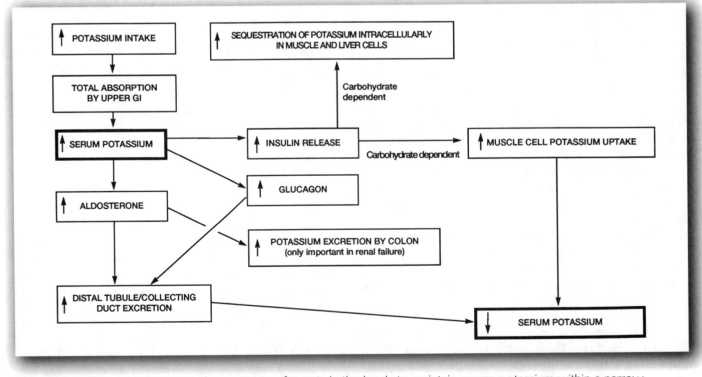

FIGURE 6-3. The acute homeostatic sequence of events in the body to maintain serum potassium within a narrow concentration range.

MINICASE 3

A Case of Hyperkalemia

JAMES D., A 65-YEAR-OLD, 150-LB MAN, was admitted to University Hospital for surgical management of acute urinary retention due to bladder outlet obstruction. His past medical history was significant for hypertension and diet-controlled type 2 diabetes mellitus. His medications (all orally) included atenolol 100 mg daily, hydrochlorothiazide 25 mg daily, and enalapril 10 mg every morning.

Vital signs upon presentation included a respiratory rate 25 breaths per minute, pulse 60 beats per minute with regular rhythm, and BP 160/95 mm Hg. Remarkable findings from physical examination included an audible S_4 heart sound and decreased deep-tendon reflexes bilaterally. The only other abnormal clinical finding was an indurated, fixed prostate gland. Abnormal clinical laboratory tests included serum potassium 5.6 mEq/L (3.8–5.0 mEq/L), serum total carbon dioxide 16 mmol/L (24–30 mmol/L), glucose 237 mg/dL (70–110 mg/dL), phosphate 6.4 mg/dL (2.3–4.7 mg/dL), BUN 56 mg/dL (8–23 mg/dL), and SCr 3.3 mg/dL (0.6–1.2 mg/dL). A presurgery arterial blood gas showed pH 7.30 (7.36–7.44), partial pressure of arterial carbon dioxide ($PaCO_2$) 17 mm Hg (35–40 mm Hg), and partial pressure of arterial oxygen (PaO_2) 99 mm Hg (95–100 mm Hg) on room air.

Twenty-four hours after surgery, he complained of muscle weakness and developed anuria. His pulse was around 40 beats per minute and with irregular rhythms, and his BP was 130/70 mm Hg. His EKG showed flat P waves, tall T waves, and widened QRS intervals. Repeat serum chemistry test revealed serum potassium concentration of 7.1 mEq/L (3.8–5.0 mEq/L).

Question: What are the potential causes of symptomatic hyperkalemia in James D.?

Discussion: James D. is exhibiting signs and symptoms of hyperkalemia (e.g., muscle weakness, rhythm disturbances, worsening of bradycardia, and reduced BP). He has several predisposing factors that may have contributed to his hyperkalemia. Acute renal failure is the most significant cause. If his underlying metabolic acidosis has not yet been corrected, extracellular shifting of potassium could occur leading to an elevated serum potassium concentration. Although clinically insignificant, his serum potassium value may be corrected for his acidosis to more accurately reflect his extracellular potassium status. The corrected serum potassium value is

$$K_{corr} = ([7.4 - pH]/0.1 \times 0.6 \text{ mEq/L}) + K_{uncorr}$$

$$K_{corr} = ([7.4 - 7.3]/0.1 \times 0.6 \text{ mEq/L}) + 7.1 = 7.7 \text{ mEq/L}$$

This correction implies that if the acidemia is treated to restore plasma pH to 7.4, the serum potassium concentration will increase by 0.6 mEq/L without any addition of potassium to the body. Such correction becomes more significant when the metabolic acid–base disorder is more severe.

Medications such as ACE-inhibitors can also contribute to hyperkalemia, although in this case, the impact is likely to be limited because (1) the dose used is small; (2) it is a chronic medication; and (3) the presence of acute renal failure would have a much more immediate and profound impact in elevating serum potassium.

1. Although the kidneys are the primary route of elimination, potassium secretion into the colon becomes important in patients with advanced renal failure.[10]
2. Unlike sodium, the kidneys are not fully able to arrest potassium's secretion into the urine. During hypokalemia, the urinary potassium concentration may decrease to as low as 5 mEq/L, however, potassium excretion does not cease completely.

The modulation of renal potassium excretion by these mechanisms may take hours to cause significant changes in serum potassium concentration, even during drastic, acute changes. Extrarenal mechanisms, therefore, often play important roles in keeping the serum potassium concentration within the narrow acceptable range.

Acid–Base Homeostasis

Another potentially relevant factor influencing renal potassium secretion is serum pH. When arterial pH increases due to metabolic, but not respiratory, alkalosis, a compensatory efflux of hydrogen ions from the cells into the extracellular fluid (bloodstream) takes place with a concurrent influx of potassium ions into the cells in order to maintain an electropotential gradient.[7] During the early phase of metabolic alkalosis, the serum potassium concentration is reduced due to a pH-dependent intracellular influx of serum potassium from the serum without altering the total body amount. Thus, although there is no immediate change in the amount of total body potassium,

this movement of ions increases the cellular potassium content and results in hypokalemia.

However, a shift in potassium and hydrogen ions also takes place in the renal distal tubular cells. In the presence of persistent alkalemia, renal potassium secretion into the urine is increased. Over time, the serum potassium concentration declines through increased renal loss, resulting in a reduced body store.

Metabolic acidosis has the opposite effect. Decreased pH results in an extracellular shift of potassium as a result of an intracellular shift of hydrogen ions, causing an elevated serum potassium concentration.[7] Since the intracellular potassium content of the distal tubular cell is decreased, secretion of potassium in the urine is diminished. Chronically, however, renal potassium loss gradually increases due to unknown mechanisms.

When a severe metabolic acid–base abnormality exists, adjustment of the measured serum potassium concentration may be necessary to more accurately assess the body potassium status. For every 0.1-unit reduction in arterial pH less than 7.4, roughly 0.6 mEq/L (range: 0.2–1.7 mEq/L) could be added to the serum potassium value:

$$K_{corr} = ([7.4 - pH]/0.1 \times 0.6 \text{ mEq/L}) + K_{uncorr}$$

where K_{corr} is the corrected serum potassium concentration and K_{uncorr} is the uncorrected or measured serum potassium concentration (Minicase 3).[7] It is important to note that K_{corr}

is a hypothetical value and only reflects what the serum potassium concentration would be if the serum pH is normalized and in the absence of other factors affecting potassium homeostasis. As long as the serum pH remains abnormal, the measured serum potassium concentration (K_{uncorr}) is the true reflection of actual serum potassium concentration. The K_{corr} value should always be assessed together with the actual serum potassium concentration and the patient's clinical presentation. The clinical value of calculating K_{corr} is mostly to avoid overcorrection of potassium based solely on K_{uncorr}, as well as to provide a more complete picture that reflects total potassium stores in the body. Clinicians should remember that regardless of the value of K_{corr}, a patient with a significantly abnormal measured (uncorrected) serum potassium concentration is still at risk for developing cardiac arrhythmias.

Acute Homeostasis

Figure 6-3 summarizes the acute homeostatic mechanism involved in potassium distribution. During hyperkalemia, along with the release of aldosterone, increased glucagon and insulin release also contribute to reducing the serum potassium concentration. Glucagon stimulates potassium secretion into the distal tubules and collecting ducts, while insulin promotes intracellular potassium uptake. Although insulin is not a major controlling factor in potassium homeostasis, it is useful for the emergency treatment of hyperkalemia.[7,12]

Pharmacological stimulation of beta-2 adrenergic receptors may also affect the transcellular equilibrium of potassium. It leads to the movement of potassium from extracellular fluid to the intracellular fluid compartment. Beta-2 adrenergic agonists (e.g., albuterol) can, therefore, be used short term to treat certain hyperkalemic patients.[7-9]

Hypokalemia

Hypokalemia is defined as a serum potassium concentration less than 3.8 mEq/L (<3.8 mmol/L).[10] To interpret the significance of low potassium values, clinicians should determine whether hypokalemia is due to intracellular shifting of potassium (apparent deficit) or increased loss from the body (true deficit) (List 6-4).

Intracellular shifting occurs as a result of metabolic alkalosis or after administration of insulin, or large doses of beta-2 adrenergic agonists (e.g., continuous or hourly use of albuterol in ICU patients receiving mechanical ventilation).[9,13] Increased elimination of potassium can occur in the kidneys or GI tract. There may be decreased potassium reabsorption in the proximal tubules or increased secretion in the distal tubules and collecting ducts.[10]

Amphotericin B. Proximal tubular damage can occur with amphotericin B therapy, resulting in renal tubular acidosis. Impaired reabsorption of potassium, magnesium, and bicarbonate may lead to hypokalemia, hypomagnesemia, and metabolic acidosis.[7,13] A concurrent deficiency in magnesium may affect the ability to restore potassium balance. Magnesium maintains the sodium–potassium adenosine triphosphate (ATP) pump activity and facilitates renal preservation of potassium. A hypokalemic patient who is also hypomagnesemic

LIST 6-4. Etiologies of Hypokalemia

Apparent deficit—intracellular shifting of potassium

Alkalosis

Beta-2 adrenergic stimulation

Insulin

True deficit

Decreased intake

"Tea and toast" diet

Alcoholism

Indigence

Potassium-free IV fluids

Anorexia nervosa

Bulimia

Increased output (extrarenal)

Vomiting

Diarrhea

Laxative abuse

Intestinal fistulas

Renal loss

Corticosteroids

Amphotericin B

Diuretics

Hyperaldosteronism

Cushing syndrome

Licorice abuse

may not, therefore, respond to potassium replacement therapy unless the magnesium balance is restored.[7,8,12] It appears that the lipid formulations of amphotericin B may still affect potassium homeostasis, although the magnitude may be less severe and the presentation is less acute.

Diuretics. Nonpotassium-sparing diuretic agents are drugs most commonly associated with renal potassium wasting. Although their mechanisms of natriuretic action differ, diuretic-induced hypokalemia is primarily caused by increased secretion of potassium at the distal sites in the nephron in response to an increased load of exchangeable sodium. Diuretics increase the distal urinary flow by inhibiting sodium reabsorption. This increased delivery of fluid and sodium in the distal segment of the nephron results in an increase in sodium reabsorption at that site. To maintain a neutral electropotential gradient in the lumen, potassium is excreted as sodium is reabsorbed. Therefore, any inhibition of sodium absorption by diuretics proximal to or at the distal tubules can increase potassium loss. Renal potassium excretion is further enhanced when nonabsorbable anions are present in the urine.

Use of loop diuretics (e.g., furosemide) and thiazides (e.g., hydrochlorothiazide) may both result in hypokalemia and the effect is dose-dependent. Serum potassium concentrations should be monitored regularly, especially in patients

LIST 6-5. Signs, Symptoms, and Effects of Hypokalemia on Various Organ Systems

Cardiovascular

Decrease in T-wave amplitude

Development of U waves

Hypotension

Increased risk of digoxin toxicity

PR prolongation (with severe hypokalemia)

Rhythm disturbances

ST segment depression

QRS widening (with severe hypokalemia)

Metabolic/endocrine (mostly serve as compensatory mechanisms)

Decreased aldosterone release

Decreased insulin release

Decreased renal responsiveness to antidiuretic hormone

Neuromuscular

Areflexia (with severe hypokalemia)

Cramps

Loss of smooth muscle function (ileus and urinary retention with severe hypokalemia)

Weakness

Renal

Inability to concentrate urine

Nephropathy

---

receiving high doses of loop diuretics, to avoid the increased risk of cardiovascular events secondary to hypokalemia and other electrolyte imbalances. In addition, elderly patients with ischemic heart disease and patients receiving digoxin are more susceptible to the adverse consequences of hypokalemia.[15-17] Other drugs commonly used in managing hypertension and other cardiac diseases such as spironolactone, triamterene, amiloride, eplerenone, angiotensin-converting enzyme (ACE) inhibitors, and angiotensin receptor antagonists are not expected to cause potassium loss due to their mode of action. On the contrary, they cause retention of potassium due to their effects related to aldosterone-dependent exchange sites in the collecting tubules.[11,18]

Other causes. Conditions that cause hyperaldosteronism, either primary (e.g., adrenal tumor) or secondary (e.g., renovascular hypertension), can produce hypokalemia.[13] Cushing syndrome leads to increased circulation of mineralocorticoids such as aldosterone. Corticosteroids with strong mineralocorticoid activity (e.g., cortisone) also can cause hypokalemia.[10]

GI loss of potassium can be important. Aldosterone influences both renal and intestinal potassium handling.[10] A decrease in extracellular volume increases aldosterone secretion, resulting in renal and colonic potassium wasting. Diarrheal fluid can contain 20–120 mEq/L (20–120 mmol/L) of

potassium; consequently, profuse diarrhea can rapidly result in potassium imbalance. In contrast, vomitus contains only 0–32 mEq/L (0–32 mmol/L) of potassium, and loss secondary to vomiting is unlikely to be significant. However, with severe vomiting, the resultant metabolic alkalosis may lead to hypokalemia due to intracellular shifting of potassium. Finally, patients receiving potassium-free parenteral fluids can become hypokalemic if not monitored properly.[7,10]

Clinical diagnosis. Signs and symptoms of hypokalemia involve many physiological systems. Abnormalities in the cardiovascular system may result in serious consequences (i.e., disturbances in cardiac rhythm). Hypokalemia-induced arrhythmias are of particular concern in patients receiving digoxin. Both digitalis glycosides and hypokalemia inhibit the sodium-potassium ATP pump in the cardiac cells. Together, they can deplete intracellular potassium, which may result in fatal arrhythmias. The signs and symptoms of hypokalemia are listed in List 6-5. Skeletal muscle weakness is often seen; severe depletion may lead to decreased reflexes and paralysis. Death can occur from respiratory muscle paralysis.[7,9,19]

Hyperkalemia

Hyperkalemia is defined as a serum potassium concentration greater than 5.0 mEq/L (>5.0 mmol/L). As with hypokalemia, hyperkalemia may indicate a true or apparent potassium imbalance, although the signs and symptoms are indistinguishable.[10] To interpret a high serum potassium value, the clinician should determine whether hyperkalemia is due to apparent excess caused by extracellular shifting of potassium or true potassium excess in the body caused by increased intake with diminished excretion (List 6-6).[4,6,9,11]

Causes. Since renal excretion is the major route of potassium elimination, renal failure is the most common cause of hyperkalemia. However, potassium handling by the nephrons is relatively well-preserved until the GFR falls to less than 10% of normal. Many patients with renal impairment can, therefore, maintain a near normal, serum potassium concentration. They are still prone to developing hyperkalemia if excessive potassium is consumed and when renal function deteriorates.[9,12]

Increased potassium intake rarely causes any problem in subjects in the absence of significant renal impairment. With normal renal function, increased potassium intake will lead to increased renal excretion and redistribution to the intracellular space through the action of aldosterone and insulin, respectively. Interference with either mechanism may result in hyperkalemia. Decreased aldosterone secretion can occur with Addison disease or other defects affecting the hormone's adrenal output.[7,12] Pathological changes affecting the proximal or distal renal tubules can also lead to hyperkalemia.[7,12]

Use of potassium-sparing diuretics (e.g., spironolactone) is a common cause of hyperkalemia, especially in patients with renal function impairment. Concurrent use of potassium supplements (including potassium-rich salt substitutes) will also increase the risk.

Similar to hypokalemia, hyperkalemia can result from transcellular shifting of potassium. In the presence of severe acidemia, potassium shifts from the intracellular to the

LIST 6-6. Etiologies of Hyperkalemia

Apparent excess—extracellular shifting of potassium

Metabolic acidosis

True excess

Increased intake

   Endogenous causes

   • Hemolysis

   • Rhabdomyolysis

   • Muscle crush injuries

   • Burns

   Exogenous causes

   • Salt substitutes

   • Drugs (e.g., penicillin potassium)

Decreased output

   Chronic or acute renal failure

   Drugs

   • Potassium-sparing diuretics

   • Angiotensin-converting enzyme inhibitors

   • Nonsteroidal anti-inflammatory agents

   • Angiotensin II receptor antagonists

   • Heparin

   • Trimethoprim

   Deficiency of adrenal steroids

   Addison disease

extracellular space, which may result in a clinically significant increase in the serum potassium concentration.[10]

Clinical diagnosis. The cardiovascular manifestations of hyperkalemia are of major concern. They include cardiac rhythm disturbances, bradycardia, hypotension, and, in severe cases, cardiac arrest. At times, muscle weakness may occur before these cardiac signs and symptoms. To appreciate the potent effect of potassium on the heart, one has to realize that potassium is the principal component of cardioplegic solutions commonly used to arrest the rhythm of the heart during cardiac surgeries.[7,9,12]

Causes of spurious laboratory results. There are several conditions that will result in fictitious hyperkalemia in which the high serum concentration reported is not expected to have any significant clinical sequelae. Erythrocytes, similar to other cells, have high potassium content. When there is substantial hemolysis in the specimen collection tube, the red cells will release potassium in quantities large enough to produce misleading results. Hemolysis may occur when a very small needle is used for blood draw, the tourniquet is too tight, or when the specimen stands too long or is mishandled. When a high serum potassium concentration is reported in a patient without pertinent signs and symptoms, the test needs to be repeated to rule out hemolysis.[6,7,10]

A similar phenomenon can occur when the specimen is allowed to clot (when nonheparinized tubes are used) because

platelets and white cells are also rich in potassium. In patients with leukemia or thrombocytosis, the potassium concentration should be obtained from plasma rather than serum samples. However, the normal plasma potassium concentration is 0.3–0.4 mEq/L lower than the serum values.

Chloride

   Normal range: 95–103 mEq/L or 95–103 mmol/L

Physiology

Chloride is the most abundant extracellular anion. However, its intracellular concentration is small (about 4 mEq/L). Chloride is passively absorbed from the upper small intestine. In the distal ileum and large intestine, its absorption is coupled with bicarbonate ion secretion. Chloride is primarily regulated by the renal proximal tubules, where it is exchanged for bicarbonate ions. Throughout the rest of the nephron, chloride passively follows sodium and water.

Chloride is influenced by the extracellular fluid balance and acid–base balance.[19,20] Although homeostatic mechanisms do not directly regulate chloride, they indirectly regulate it through changes in sodium and bicarbonate. The physiological role of chloride is primarily passive. It balances out positive charges in the extracellular fluid and, by passively following sodium, helps to maintain extracellular osmolality.

Hypochloremia and Hyperchloremia

Serum chloride values are used as confirmatory tests to identify fluid balance and acid–base abnormalities.[21] Like sodium, a change in the serum chloride concentration does not necessarily reflect a change in total body content. Rather, it indicates an alteration in fluid status and/or acid–base balance. One of the most common causes of hyperchloremia in hospitalized patients results from saline infusion. Chloride has the added feature of being influenced by bicarbonate. Therefore, it would be expected to decrease to the same proportion as sodium when serum is diluted with fluid and to increase to the same proportion as sodium during dehydration. However, when a patient is on acid-suppressive therapy (e.g., high-dose H2-blockers or proton pump inhibitors), has been receiving continuous or frequent nasogastric suction, or has profuse vomiting, a greater loss of chloride than sodium can occur because gastric fluid contains 1.5–3 times more chloride than sodium. Gastric outlet obstruction, protracted vomiting and self-induced vomiting can also lead to hypochloremia.

Drug and parenteral nutrition causes. Even though drugs can influence serum chloride concentrations, they rarely do so directly. For example, although loop diuretics (e.g., furosemide) and thiazide diuretics (e.g., hydrochlorothiazide) inhibit chloride uptake at the loop of Henle and distal nephron, respectively, the hypochloremia that may result is due to the concurrent loss of sodium and contraction alkalosis.[18,21] Since chloride passively follows sodium, salt and water retention can transiently raise serum chloride concentrations. This effect occurs with corticosteroids, guanethidine, and nonsteroidal anti-inflammatory agents (NSAIDs) such as ibuprofen. Also, parenteral nutrition solutions with high chloride concentrations are associated with an increased risk of hyperchloremia.

Acetate or phosphate salts used in place of chloride salts (e.g., potassium chloride) reduce this risk. Acetazolamide also can cause hyperchloremia.

Acid–base status and other causes. The acid–base balance is partly regulated by renal production and excretion of bicarbonate ions. The proximal tubules are the primary regulators of bicarbonate. These cells exchange bicarbonate with chloride to maintain the intracellular electropotential gradient. Renal excretion of chloride increases during metabolic alkalosis, resulting in a reduced serum chloride concentration.

The opposite situation also may be true: metabolic or respiratory acidosis results in an elevated serum chloride concentration. Hyperchloremic metabolic acidosis is not common but may occur when the kidneys are unable to conserve bicarbonate, as in interstitial renal disease (e.g., obstruction, pyelonephritis, and analgesic nephropathy), GI bicarbonate loss (e.g., cholera and staphylococcal infections of the intestines), and acetazolamide-induced carbonic anhydrase inhibition. Falsely elevated chloride rarely occurs from bromide toxicity due to a lack of distinction between these two halogens by the laboratory's chemical analyzer.

Since the signs and symptoms associated with hyperchloremia and hypochloremia are related to fluid status or the acid–base balance and underlying causes, rather than to chloride itself, the reader is referred to discussions in Chapter 9: Arterial Blood Gases and Acid–Base Balance.

OTHER MINERALS

Magnesium

Normal range: 1.3–2.1 mEq/L or 0.65–1.05 mmol/L

Physiology

Magnesium has a widespread physiological role in maintaining neuromuscular functions and enzymatic functions. Magnesium acts as a cofactor for phosphorylation of ATPs from adenosine phosphates (ADPs). Magnesium is also vital for binding macromolecules to organelles (e.g., messenger ribonucleic acid [mRNA] to ribosomes).

The average adult body contains 21–28 g (1750–2400 mEq) of magnesium with the following distribution:

- About 50% in bone (about 30% or less of this pool is slowly exchangeable with extracellular fluid)
- 20% in muscle
- Around 10% in nonmuscle soft tissues
- 1% to 2% in extracellular fluid (for plasma magnesium, about 50% is free; approximately 15% is complexed to anions; and 30% is bound to protein, primarily albumin)

The average daily magnesium intake is 20–40 mEq/day. Approximately 30% to 40% of the ingested magnesium is absorbed from the jejunum and ileum through intercellular and intracellular pathways. Both passive diffusion down an electrochemical gradient and active transport process are involved. The extent of magnesium absorption may be affected by dietary magnesium intake, calcium intake, vitamin D, and PTH. However, conflicting data are available and the extent of these parameters in affecting absorption is unresolved. Certain medications (e.g., cyclosporine, tacrolimus, cisplatin, amphotericin B) can significantly increase renal magnesium loss, predisposing the patient to hypomagnesemia.

Urinary magnesium accounts for one-third of the total daily magnesium output while the other two-thirds are in the GI tract (e.g., stool). Magnesium is excreted in the kidneys, where unbound serum magnesium is freely filtered at the glomerulus. All but about 3% to 5% of filtered magnesium is normally reabsorbed (100 mg/day). In other words, 97% of the filtered magnesium is reabsorbed under normal circumstances. Reabsorption is primarily through the ascending limb of the loop of Henle (50% to 60%). About 30% is reabsorbed in the proximal tubule and 7% from the distal tubule. This explains why loop diuretics have a more profound effect on renal magnesium wasting. The drive of magnesium reabsorption is mediated by the charge difference generated by the sodium-potassium-chloride cotransport system in the lumen.

The regulation of magnesium is primarily driven by the plasma magnesium concentration. Changes in plasma magnesium concentrations have potent effects on renal reabsorption and stool losses. These effects are seen over 3–5 days and may persist for a long time. Hormonal regulation of magnesium seems to be much less critical for its homeostasis.

Factors affecting calcium homeostasis also affect magnesium homeostasis.[22] A decline in serum magnesium concentration stimulates the release of PTH, which increases serum magnesium by increasing its release from the bone store and renal reabsorption. Hyperaldosteronism causes increased magnesium renal excretion. Insulin by itself does not alter the serum magnesium concentration. But in a hyperglycemic state, insulin causes a rapid intracellular uptake of glucose. This process causes an increase in the phosphorylation by sodium-potassium ATPase on the cell membrane. Since magnesium is a cofactor for sodium potassium ATPase, magnesium is consumed, which subsequently decreases the serum magnesium concentration. Excretion of magnesium is influenced by serum calcium and phosphate concentrations. Magnesium movement generally follows that of phosphate (i.e., if phosphate declines, magnesium also declines) and is the opposite of calcium.[21,22] Other factors that increase magnesium reabsorption include acute metabolic acidosis, hyperthyroidism, and chronic alcohol use.

Hypomagnesemia

Hypomagnesemia is defined as a serum magnesium concentration less than 1.3 mEq/L (<0.65 mmol/L). The common causes of hypomagnesemia include renal wasting, chronic alcohol use, diabetes mellitus, protein-calorie malnutrition, refeeding syndrome, and postparathyroidectomy. Since serum magnesium deficiency can be offset by magnesium release from bone, muscle, and the heart, the serum value may not be a useful indicator of cellular depletion and complications (e.g., arrhythmias). However, low serum magnesium usually indicates low cellular magnesium as long as the patient has a normal extracellular fluid volume.[22,23]

Causes. Magnesium deficiency is more common than magnesium excess. Depletion usually results from excessive loss from the GI tract or kidneys (e.g., use of loop diuretics). Magnesium depletion is not commonly the result of decreased intake because the kidneys can cease magnesium elimination in 4–7 days to conserve the ion. However, with chronic alcohol consumption, deficiency can occur from a combination of poor intake, poor GI absorption (e.g., vomiting or diarrhea), and increased renal elimination. Depletion can also occur from poor intestinal absorption (e.g., small-bowel resection). Diarrhea can be a source of magnesium loss because diarrhea stools may contain as much as 14 mEq/L (7 mmol/L) of magnesium.

Urinary magnesium loss may result from diuresis or tubular defects, such as the diuretic phase of acute tubular necrosis. Some patients with hypoparathyroidism may exhibit low magnesium serum concentrations from renal loss and, possibly, decreased intestinal absorption. Other conditions associated with magnesium deficiency include hyperthyroidism, primary aldosteronism, diabetic ketoacidosis, and pancreatitis. Magnesium deficiency associated with these conditions may be particularly dangerous because often there are concurrent potassium and calcium deficiencies. Although loop diuretics lead to significant magnesium depletion, thiazide diuretics do not cause hypomagnesemia, especially at lower doses (50 mg/day). Furthermore, potassium-sparing diuretics (e.g., spironolactone, triamterene, and amiloride), are also magnesium-sparing and have some limited clinical role in diuretic-induced hypokalemia and hypomagnesemia.[22,24]

Clinical diagnosis. Magnesium depletion is usually associated with neuromuscular symptoms such as weakness, muscle fasciculation with tremor, tetany, and increased reflexes.[22] They occur because the release of acetylcholine to motor endplates is affected by the presence or absence of magnesium. Motor endplate sensitivity to acetylcholine is also affected. When serum magnesium decreases, acetylcholine release increases, resulting in increased muscle excitation.

Magnesium also affects the central nervous system (CNS). Magnesium depletion can cause personality changes, disorientation, convulsions, psychosis, stupor, and coma.[22,25] Severe hypomagnesemia may result in hypocalcemia due to intracellular cationic shifts. Many symptoms of magnesium deficiency result from concurrent hypocalcemia.

Perhaps the most important effects of magnesium imbalance are on the heart. Decreased magnesium in cardiac cells may manifest as a prolonged QT interval (increased risk of arrhythmias, especially torsades de pointes).[25] Moderately decreased concentrations can cause electrocardiogram (EKG) abnormalities similar to those observed with hypokalemia. In addition, vasodilation may occur by a direct effect on blood vessels and ganglionic blockade.

A 24-hour urine magnesium excretion test may be helpful in determining the magnitude of a total body magnesium deficiency. If the value is normal, the patient is not considered deficient as long as serum magnesium is also normal. The diagnosis of total body magnesium deficiency is established when the 24-hour urinary magnesium excretion is low even in the presence of normal serum magnesium concentration.

TABLE 6-3. Signs and Symptoms of Hypermagnesemia

5–7 mEq/L	Bradycardia, flushing, sweating, sensation of warmth, fatigue, drowsiness
7–10 mEq/L	Lower blood pressure, decreased deep-tendon reflexes, altered mental status possible
10–15 mEq/L	Flaccid paralysis and increased PR and QRS intervals, severe mental confusion, coma
>15 mEq/L	Respiratory distress and asystole

Hypermagnesemia

Hypermagnesemia is defined as a serum magnesium concentration greater than 2.1 mEq/L (>1.05 mmol/L).

Causes. Besides magnesium overload (e.g., over-replacement of magnesium, treatment for preeclampsia, and antacid/laxative overuse), the most important risk factor for hypermagnesemia is renal dysfunction. Rapid infusions of IV solutions containing large amounts of magnesium, such as those given for myocardial infarction, preeclampsia, and status asthmaticus, may result in hypermagnesemia.

Clinical diagnosis. Plasma magnesium concentrations below 5 mEq/L (<2.5 mmol/L) rarely cause serious symptoms. No specific symptoms, such as muscle weakness, decrease in deep tendon reflexes or fatigue, may be present. As magnesium concentration rises above 5 mEq/L, more notable symptoms such as lethargy, mental confusion, and hypotension may be observed (Table 6-3).[22,24,27] In severe hypermagnesemia (>10 mEq/L), life-threatening symptoms, including coma, paralysis, or cardiac arrest, can be observed and urgent therapy is indicated.

Treatment for severe or symptomatic hypermagnesemia may include IV calcium gluconate 1–2 g over 30 minutes to reverse the neuromuscular and cardiovascular blockade of magnesium. Increased renal elimination of magnesium can be achieved by forced diuresis with IV saline hydration and a loop diuretic agent. Hemodialysis should be reserved as a last resort.

Calcium

Normal range: 9.2–11.0 mg/dL or 2.3–2.8 mmol/L for adults

Physiology

Calcium plays an important role in the propagation of neuromuscular activity; regulation of endocrine functions (e.g., pancreatic insulin release and gastric hydrogen secretion), blood coagulation including platelet aggregation, and bone and tooth metabolism.[2,28]

The serum calcium concentration is closely regulated by complex interaction among PTH, serum phosphate, vitamin D system, and the target organ (Figure 6-4). About one-third of the ingested calcium is actively absorbed from the proximal area of the small intestine, facilitated by 1,25-dihydroxycholecalciferol (1,25-DHCC or calcitriol, the most active form of vitamin D). Passive intestinal absorption is negligible with intake of less than 2 g/day. The average daily calcium intake is 2–2.5 g/day.

The normal adult body contains about 1000 g of calcium, with only 0.5% found in the extracellular fluid; 99.5% is

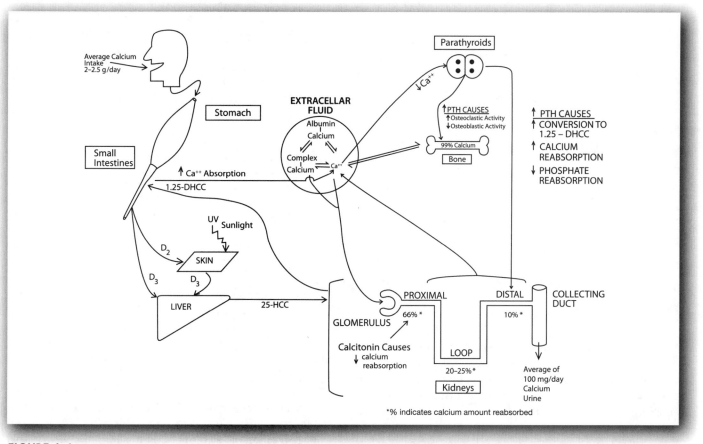

FIGURE 6-4. Calcium physiology: relationship with vitamin D, calcitonin, PTH, and albumin.

integrated into bones. Therefore, the tissue concentration of calcium is small. Since bone is constantly remodeled by osteoblasts and osteoclasts, a small quantity of bone calcium is in equilibrium with the extracellular fluid. Extracellular calcium exists in three forms:

1. Complexed to bicarbonate, citrates, and phosphates (6%)
2. Protein bound, mostly to albumin (40%)
3. Ionized or free fraction (54%)

Intracellular calcium. Imbalance of body calcium results in disturbances in muscle contraction and nerve action.[28] Within the cells, calcium maintains a low concentration. The calcium that is attracted into the negatively charged cell is either actively pumped out or sequestered by mitochondria or the endoplasmic reticulum. Such differences in concentrations allow calcium to be used for transmembrane signaling. In response to stimuli, calcium is allowed either to enter a cell or released from internal cellular stores where it interacts with specific intracellular proteins to regulate cellular functions or metabolic processes.[2,26,27] Calcium enters cells through one of the three types of calcium channels that have been identified: T (transient or fast), N (neuronal), and L (long lasting or slow). Subsets of these channels may exist. Calcium channel-blockers are likely to affect the L channels.[29]

In muscle, calcium is released from the intracellular sarcoplasmic reticulum. The released calcium binds to troponin and stops troponin from inhibiting the interaction of actin and myosin. This interaction results in muscle contraction. Muscle

relaxation occurs when calcium is pumped back into the sarcoplasmic reticulum. In cardiac tissue, calcium becomes important during phase 2 of the action potential. During this phase, fast entry of sodium stops and calcium entry through the slow channels begins (Figure 6-5), resulting in contraction. During repolarization, calcium is actively pumped out of the cell.[2]

Calcium channel-blocking drugs (e.g., nifedipine, diltiazem, and verapamil) inhibit the movement of calcium into muscle cells, thus decreasing the strength of contraction. The areas most sensitive to these effects appear to be the sinoatrial and atrioventricular nodes and vascular smooth muscles, which explains the hypotensive effects of nifedipine.

Extracellular calcium. Complex-bound calcium usually accounts for less than 1 mg/dL (<0.25 mmol/L) of blood calcium. The complex usually is formed with bicarbonate, citrate, or phosphate. In patients with CKD, calcium may also be bound with sulfate because the anion is retained. Phosphate plays an important role in calcium homeostasis. Under normal physiological conditions, the product of calcium concentration times phosphate concentration (the so-called calcium–phosphate product) is relatively constant: an increase in one ion necessitates a corresponding decline in the other. In addition, many homeostatic mechanisms that control calcium also regulate phosphate. This relationship is particularly important in renal failure; the decreased phosphate excretion may ultimately lead, through a complex mechanism, to hypocalcemia, especially if the hyperphosphatemia is untreated.[30,31]

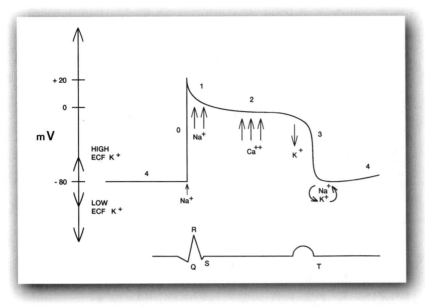

FIGURE 6-5. Cardiac intracellular potential and its relationship to the ECG.

Calcium is bound primarily to serum albumin (80%) and globulins (20%). Protein-bound calcium is in equilibrium with ionized calcium, which is affected by the serum anion concentration and blood pH. This equilibrium is important since ionized calcium is the physiologically active moiety. Alkalosis increases protein binding of calcium, resulting in a lower free fraction, whereas acidosis has the opposite effect. In patients with respiratory or metabolic alkalosis, the signs and symptoms of hypocalcemia may become more pronounced due to increased binding. Conversely, signs and symptoms of hypercalcemia become more apparent in patients with metabolic or respiratory acidosis. Therefore, total serum calcium concentration, which is commonly reported by clinical laboratories, is not as clinically significant as the quantity of available ionized calcium. In fact, it is the free calcium concentration that is closely regulated by the different homeostatic mechanisms.

Clinically, serum protein concentrations, especially albumin, have an important influence on regulating the amount of physiologically active calcium in the serum. The normal serum calcium range is 9.2–11.0 mg/dL (2.3–2.8 mmol/L) for a patient with a serum albumin of approximately 4 g/dL. In normal healthy adults, only 40% to 50% of the total serum calcium is free from protein-binding and thus considered as physiologically active. In patients with hypoalbuminemia (due to acute illnesses, severe malnutrition), the free concentration of calcium is elevated despite a "normal" total serum calcium concentration. Therefore, it is a common practice to either measure ionized calcium or to correct the total serum calcium concentration based on the measured albumin concentration. The following formula is commonly used in an attempt to "correct" total serum calcium concentration:

$$Ca_{corr} = ([4.0 - albumin] \times 0.8 \text{ mg/dL}) + Ca_{uncorr}$$

where Ca_{corr} is the corrected serum calcium concentration, and Ca_{uncorr} is the uncorrected (or measured total) serum calcium concentration. For example, a clinician may be asked to write parenteral nutrition orders for an emaciated cancer patient. The serum albumin is 1.9 g/dL (19 g/L), and the total serum calcium concentration is 7.7 mg/dL (1.9 mmol/L). At first glance, one might consider the calcium to be low. But with the reduced serum albumin concentration, more ionized calcium is available to cells.

$$Ca_{corr} = ([4.0 - 1.9] \times 0.8) + 7.7 = 9.4 \text{ mg/dL}$$
$$(2.34 \text{ mmol/L})$$

The corrected serum calcium concentration is, thus, within the normal range. More importantly, the patient does not exhibit any signs and symptoms of hypocalcemia. Calcium supplementation is not therefore indicated. In the presence of severe hypoalbuminemia, as in nutritionally deprived patients, an apparently low total serum calcium may in fact be sufficient or in some instances, excessive. If such a patient were given IV albumin, the free concentration of calcium would acutely decline due to the resultant increased binding. The measured total calcium concentration will need to be corrected with the new albumin concentration.

Although this serum calcium correction method may be useful, the clinician must be aware of its limitations and potential for inaccuracy. The correction factor of 0.8 represents an average fraction of calcium bound to albumin under normal physiology. To have an accurate determination of the free concentration, a direct measurement of serum ionized calcium concentration should be available in most clinical laboratories (normal range: 4.0–4.8 mg/dL or 1.00–1.20 mmol/L). Ultimately, the patient's clinical presentation is the most important factor to determine if immediate treatment for a calcium disorder is indicated.

Although calcium absorption takes place throughout the entire small intestine, the proximal region of the small intestine (jejunum and proximal ileum) are the most active and regulated areas. Calcium absorption from the human GI tract is mediated by two processes: (1) transcellular active transport, a saturable, vitamin D–responsive process mediated by specific calcium binding proteins primarily in the upper GI tract, particularly in the distal duodenum and upper jejunum; and (2) paracellular processes, a nonsaturable linear transfer via diffusion that occurs throughout the entire length of the intestine. Under normal physiology, the total calcium absorptive capacity is the highest in the ileum because of the longer residence time. The rate of paracellular calcium absorption is fairly stable regardless of calcium intake. However, when dietary calcium intake is relatively limited, the efficiency of transcellular calcium transport becomes higher and accounts for a significant fraction of the absorbed calcium. Transcellular calcium transport is closely regulated by vitamin D, although other mechanisms may also be involved. Specifically, 1,25-DHCC induces the intestinal expressions of transcellular calcium transporters through its binding with the vitamin D receptors (VDR) in the intestinal epithelial cells.

Effect of vitamin D. A small amount of calcium is excreted daily into the GI tract through saliva, bile, and pancreatic and intestinal secretions. However, the primary route of elimination is filtration by the kidneys. Calcium is freely filtered at the glomeruli, where approximately 65% is reabsorbed at the proximal tubules under partial control by calcitonin and 1,25-DHCC. Roughly 25% is reabsorbed in the loop of Henle, and another 10% is reabsorbed at the distal tubules under the influence of PTH.

Despite being classified as a vitamin, the physiological functions of vitamin D more closely resemble a hormone. Vitamin D is important for

- Intestinal absorption of calcium
- PTH-induced mobilization of calcium from bone
- Calcium reabsorption in the proximal renal tubules

Vitamin D must undergo several conversion steps before the active form, calcitriol or 1,25-DHCC, is formed. It is absorbed by the intestines in two forms, 7-dehydrocholesterol and cholecalciferol (vitamin D_3). 7-dehydrocholesterol is converted into cholecalciferol in the skin by the sun's ultraviolet radiation. Rickets, one of the causes of childhood hypocalcemia, is caused by reduced exposure to sunlight, resulting in diminished conversion of 7-dehydrocholesterol to cholecalciferol.

Hepatic and intestinal enzymes, including CYP27A1, CYP2J2 and CYP3A4, convert cholecalciferol to 25-hydroxycholecalciferol (25-HCC), which is then further activated by CYP27B1 in the kidneys to form the active 1,25-DHCC. This last conversion step is regulated by PTH. When PTH is increased during hypocalcemia, renal production of 1,25-DHCC increases, which increases intestinal absorption of calcium. 1,25-DHCC may in turn regulate PTH synthesis and secretion.[30,32]

Influence of calcitonin. Calcitonin is a hormone secreted by specialized C cells of the thyroid gland in response to a high level of circulating ionized calcium. Calcitonin inhibits osteoclastic activity, thereby inhibiting bone resorption. It also decreases calcium reabsorption in the renal proximal tubules to result in increased renal calcium clearance.[28] Calcitonin is used for the treatment of acute hypercalcemia and several different forms of the hormone are available.

Influence of parathyroid hormone. Parathyroid hormone is the most important hormone involved in calcium homeostasis. It is secreted by the parathyroid glands, which are embedded in the thyroid, in direct response to low circulating ionized calcium. Parathyroid hormone closely regulates, and is also regulated by, the vitamin D system to maintain the serum ionized calcium concentration within a narrow range. Generally, PTH increases the serum calcium concentration and stimulates the enzymatic activity of CYP27B1 to promote renal conversion of 25-HCC to 1,25-DHCC, which enhances intestinal calcium absorption. Conversely, 1,25-DHCC is a potent suppressor of PTH synthesis via a direct mechanism that is independent of the serum calcium concentration.[28,31] The normal reference range for serum PTH concentrations is 10–65 pg/mL.

Tubular reabsorption of calcium and phosphate at the distal nephron is controlled by PTH; it increases renal reabsorption of calcium and decreases the reabsorption of phosphate, resulting in lower serum phosphate and higher serum calcium concentrations. Perhaps the most important effect of PTH is on the bone. In the presence of PTH, osteoblastic activity is diminished and bone-resorption processes of osteoclasts are increased. These effects increase serum ionized calcium, which feeds back to the parathyroid glands to decrease PTH output.[30]

The suppressive effect of 1,25-DHCC (calcitriol) on PTH secretion is used clinically in patients with CKD who have excessively high serum PTH concentrations due to secondary hyperparathyroidism. Parathyroid hormone is a known uremic toxin, and its presence in supraphysiological concentrations has many adverse effects (e.g., suppression of bone marrow erythropoiesis and increased osteoclastic bone resorption with replacement by fibrous tissue).[33] Figure 6-6 depicts the relationship between serum PTH and serum calcium concentrations.

Abnormalities. True abnormal serum concentrations of calcium may result from an abnormality in any of the previously mentioned mechanisms, including

- Altered intestinal absorption[8,30,31,34]
- Altered number or activity of osteoclast and osteoblast cells in bone[8,30,31,34]
- Changes in renal reabsorption of calcium[8,30,31,34]
- Calcium or phosphate IV infusions

Patients with CKD have increased serum phosphate and decreased serum calcium concentrations as a result of the following factors that interact via a complex mechanism: decreased phosphate clearance by the kidneys, decreased renal production of 1,25-DHCC, and skeletal resistance to the calcemic action of PTH. This interaction is further complicated by the metabolic acidosis of renal failure, which can increase bone resorption to result in decreased bone integrity.

Hypocalcemia

Hypocalcemia indicates a total serum calcium concentration of less than 9.2 mg/dL (<2.3 mmol/L). The most common cause of hypocalcemia is low serum proteins. As discussed previously, decreased serum protein leads to an increased free fraction of ionized calcium. If there is no other coexisting factor that could impair or alter calcium homeostasis, this should not be associated with a functional calcium deficit and clinical symptoms. Therefore, serum protein concentration should always be taken into consideration when interpreting serum total calcium concentration. Even in the case of true, mild hypocalcemia, the patient may remain asymptomatic and often no treatment is required.

The most common causes of a true reduction in total serum calcium are disorders of vitamin D metabolism or impaired PTH production (List 6-7). Osteomalacia (in adults) and rickets (in children) can result from severe deficiency in dietary calcium or vitamin D, diminished synthesis of vitamin D_3 from insufficient sunlight exposure, or resistance of the intestinal wall to the action of vitamin D. The reduction in serum calcium leads to secondary hyperparathyroidism, which increases bone resorption. Over a long period to time, bones lose their

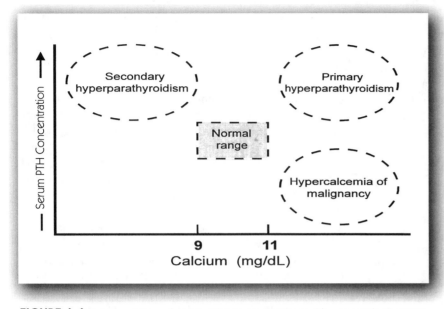

FIGURE 6-6. Interpretation of serum PTH concentrations with concomitant serum calcium concentrations.

structural integrity and become more susceptible to fracture. The diminished serum calcium concentration, if significant, may result in tetany.

Diminished intake. Although uncommon, diminished intake of calcium is an important cause of hypocalcemia, especially in patients receiving long-term total parental nutrition solutions.[37,38]

Medications. Excessive use of certain drugs to lower serum calcium by either increasing bone deposition or decreasing renal reabsorption of calcium may lead to hypocalcemia. These drugs include plicamycin, calcitonin, glucocorticoids, loop diuretics, etidronate, pamidronate, and alendronate.

Intravenous bicarbonate administration and hyperventilation can cause systemic alkalosis, resulting in decreased ionized serum calcium. This decrease is usually important only in patients who already have low serum calcium concentrations. Other drugs that may cause hypocalcemia include phenytoin, phenobarbital, aluminum-containing antacids, cisplatin, theophylline, sodium fluoride, and magnesium sulfate.

Another cause is rapid IV administration of phosphate salts, especially at high doses. Phosphate can bind calcium and form an insoluble complex that can deposit into soft tissues and clog the microcirculation, causing metastatic calcification, hardening of normally pliable tissues, or blockage of capillary blood flow.[37,38] Soft-tissue deposition of the calcium–phosphate complex in lungs and blood vessels occurs when the serum solubility product of calcium times phosphate is high. The product of serum calcium and phosphate concentrations (both expressed in mg/dL) is often calculated, especially in patients with CKD, to minimize the risk for tissue calcification. The risk of deposition is higher in patients with a calcium–phosphate product that exceeds 50 or in patients with alkalosis. Other than the IV route, a large amount of phosphate may be absorbed from the GI tract with the use of certain enema and laxative preparations (e.g., Fleet's enema or Fleet's Phospho-Soda).[33]

Hypoparathyroidism. Hypoparathyroidism can reduce serum calcium concentrations. The most common cause of hypoparathyroidism is thyroidectomy, when the parathyroid glands are removed along with the thyroid glands. Since PTH is the major hormone regulating calcium balance, its absence significantly reduces serum calcium.[38]

Hyperparathyroidism. Hypocalcemia is commonly seen in patients with secondary hyperparathyroidism resulting from CKD (see Figure 6-6). The mechanism is complex and involves elevated serum phosphate concentrations and reduced activation of vitamin D. Parathyroid hormone acts on bone to increase calcium and phosphate resorption. Since renal phosphate elimination is reduced because of renal failure, the serum phosphate concentration is often high and depresses the serum calcium level. Because of the high phosphate concentrations in the intestinal lumen, dietary calcium is bound and absorption is impaired while phosphate absorption continues.

Metabolic acidosis. Common in CKD, metabolic acidosis further enhances bone resorption. With prolonged severe hyperparathyroidism, excessive osteoclastic resorption of bones results in replacement of bone material with fibrous tissues. This condition is termed *osteitis fibrosa cystica*.[31,34,35] Such diminution of bone density may result in pathological fractures. Although the serum total calcium concentrations are low, patients may not show symptoms of hypocalcemia because the accompanying acidosis helps to maintain ionized serum calcium through the reduction in protein binding.

LIST 6-7. Common Etiologies of Hypocalcemia

Diminished intake
Medications
Calcitonin
Ethylenediaminetetraacetic acid (EDTA)
Glucocorticoids
Loop diuretics
Phosphate salts
Plicamycin
Hyperphosphatemia
Hypoalbuminemia
Hypomagnesemia
Hypoparathyroidism (common)
Pancreatitis
Renal failure
Secondary hyperparathyroidism
Vitamin D deficiency (common)

Magnesium. Similar to potassium, calcium balance depends strongly on magnesium homeostasis. Therefore, if a hypocalcemic patient is also hypomagnesemic, as a result of loop diuretic therapy, calcium replacement therapy may not be effective unless magnesium balance is restored.

Clinical diagnosis. As with any electrolyte disorder, the severity of the clinical manifestations of hypocalcemia depends on the acuteness of onset. Hypocalcemia can at times be a medical emergency with symptoms primarily in the neuromuscular system.[37,38] They include fatigue, depression, memory loss, hallucinations, and, in severe cases, seizures, and tetany. The early signs of hypocalcemia are finger numbness, tingling and burning of extremities, and paresthesia. Mental instability and confusion may be seen in some patients as the primary manifestation.

Tetany is the hallmark of severe hypocalcemia. The mechanism of muscle fasciculation during tetany is the loss of the inhibitory effect of ionized calcium on muscle proteins. In extreme cases, this loss leads to increased neuromuscular excitability that can progress to laryngospasm and tonic-clonic seizures. Chvostek and Trousseau signs are hallmarks of hypocalcemia. *Chvostek sign* is a unilateral spasm induced by a slight tap over the facial nerve. *Trousseau sign* is a carpal spasm elicited when the upper arm is compressed by a blood pressure cuff.[31,38,40]

As hypocalcemia worsens, the cardiovascular system may be affected, as evidenced by myocardial failure, cardiac arrhythmias, and hypotension.[37,38] Special attention should be given to serum calcium concentrations in patients receiving diuretics, corticosteroids, digoxin, antacids, lithium, and parenteral nutrition and in patients with renal disease.

Hypercalcemia

Hypercalcemia indicates a total serum calcium concentration greater than 11.0 mg/dL (>2.8 mmol/L).

Causes. The most common causes of hypercalcemia are malignancy and primary hyperparathyroidism (see Figure 6-6). Malignancies can increase serum calcium by several mechanisms. Osteolytic metastases can arise from breast, lung, thyroid, kidney, or bladder cancer. These tumor cells invade bone and produce substances that directly dissolve bone matrix and mineral content. Some malignancies, such as multiple myeloma, can produce factors that stimulate osteoclast proliferation and activity. Another mechanism is the ectopic production of PTH or PTH-like substances by tumor cells, resulting in a pseudohyperparathyroid state.[39,41]

In primary hyperparathyroidism, inappropriate secretion of PTH from the parathyroid gland, usually due to adenoma, increases serum calcium concentrations. The other major cause of hypercalcemia in hyperparathyroidism is the increased renal conversion of 25-HCC to active 1,25-DHCC. As the serum calcium concentration rises, the renal ability to reabsorb calcium may be exceeded, leading to an increased urinary calcium concentration and the subsequent formation of calcium–phosphate and calcium–oxalate renal stones. Typically, this condition results from parathyroid adenomas but

may also be caused by primary parathyroid hyperplasia of chief cells or parathyroid carcinomas.[31,41]

Approximately 2% of patients treated with thiazide diuretics may develop hypercalcemia. Patients at risk are those with hyperparathyroidism. The mechanism appears to be multifactorial and includes enhanced renal reabsorption of calcium and decreased plasma volume.

The milk-alkali syndrome (Burnett syndrome), rarely observed today, is another drug-related cause of hypercalcemia.[33] This syndrome occurs from a chronic high intake of milk or calcium products combined with an absorbable antacid (e.g., calcium carbonate, sodium bicarbonate, or magnesium hydroxide). This syndrome was more common in the past when milk or cream was used to treat gastric ulcers and before the advent of nonabsorbable antacids. Renal failure can occur as a result of calcium deposition in soft tissues.[33,42]

Hypercalcemia can also result from the following[28,40,41,43]:

- Excessive administration of IV calcium salts
- Calcium supplements
- Chronic immobilization
- Paget disease
- Sarcoidosis
- Hyperthyroidism
- Acute adrenal insufficiency
- Some respiratory diseases
- Lithium-induced renal calcium reabsorption
- Excessive vitamin D, vitamin A, or thyroid hormone, which increases intestinal absorption
- Tamoxifen
- Androgenic hormones
- Estrogen
- Progesterone

Clinical diagnosis. Similar to hypocalcemia and other electrolyte disorders, the severity of the clinical manifestations of hypercalcemia depends on the acuteness of onset. Hypercalcemia can be a medical emergency, especially when serum concentrations rise above 14 mg/dL (>3.5 mmol/L). Symptoms associated with this condition often consist of vague GI complaints such as nausea, vomiting, abdominal pain, dyspepsia, and anorexia. More severe GI complications include peptic ulcer disease, possibly due to increased gastrin release, and acute pancreatitis.[43,44]

Severe hypercalcemic symptoms primarily involve the neuromuscular system (e.g., lethargy, obtundation, psychosis, cerebellar ataxia, and, in severe cases, coma and death). However, EKG changes and spontaneous ventricular arrhythmias may also be seen. It may also enhance the inotropic effects of digoxin, increasing the likelihood of cardiac arrhythmias.[35-38]

Renal function may be affected by hypercalcemia through the ability of calcium to inhibit the adenyl cyclase–cyclic adenosine monophosphate system that mediates the ADH effects on the collecting ducts. This inhibition results in diminished conservation of water by the kidneys. The renal effect is further compounded by diminished solute transport in the loop of Henle, leading to polyuria, nocturia, and polydipsia.[28] Other chronic renal manifestations include nephrolithiasis, nephrocalcinosis, chronic interstitial nephritis, and renal tubular acidosis.

In addition, hypercalcemia can cause vasoconstriction of the renal vasculature, resulting in a decrease in renal blood flow and GFR. If hypercalcemia is allowed to progress, oliguric acute renal failure may ensue.[28] In the presence of high calcium–phosphate product, soft-tissue calcification by the calcium–phosphate complex may occur.

The signs and symptoms described above are mostly seen in patients with severe hypercalcemia. With serum concentrations less than 13 mg/dL (3.2 mmol/L), most patients should be asymptomatic.

Causes of spurious laboratory results. False hypercalcemia can occur if the tourniquet is left in place too long when the blood specimen is drawn. This results from increased plasma-protein pooling in the phlebotomized arm. Falsely elevated calcium should be suspected if serum albumin is greater than 5 g/dL (>50 g/L). Table 6-4 contains the normal range values for tests related to calcium metabolism.

Phosphate

Normal range: 2.3–4.7 mg/dL or 0.74–1.52 mmol/L for adults
Many of the factors that influence serum calcium concentrations also affect serum phosphate, either directly or indirectly. Laboratory values for calcium and phosphate should, therefore, be interpreted together. Since phosphate exists as several organic and inorganic moieties in the body, some clinical laboratories simply report the phosphate value as phosphorus.

Physiology

Phosphate is a major intracellular anion with several functions. It is important for intracellular metabolism of proteins, lipids, and carbohydrates, and it is a major component in phospholipid membranes, RNAs, nicotinamide diphosphate (an enzyme cofactor), cyclic adenine and guanine nucleotides (second messengers), and phosphoproteins. Another important function of phosphate is in the formation of high-energy bonds for the production of ATP, which is a source of energy for many cellular reactions. Phosphate is a component of 2,3-diphosphoglycerate (2,3-DPG), which regulates the release of oxygen from hemoglobin (Hgb) to tissues. In addition, phosphate has a regulatory role in the glycolysis and hydroxylation of cholecalciferol. It is also an important acid–base buffer.[35,40]

TABLE 6-4. Normal Ranges for Tests Related to Calcium Metabolism in Adults

Calcium (free)	4.0–4.8 mg/dL
Calcium (total)	9.2–11.0 mg/dL
1,25-DHCC	15–60 pg/mL
Phosphate	2.3–4.7 mg/dL
PTH	10–65 pg/mL
Urine calcium	0–300 mg/day
Urine hydroxyproline	10–50 mg/day (adults)
Urine phosphate	1 g/day (average)

A balanced diet for adults usually contains about 800–1500 mg/day of phosphate. About two-thirds is actively absorbed from the small intestine. Some of the phosphate is absorbed passively with calcium and some is absorbed under the influence of 1,25-DHCC, which also increases the intestinal absorption of calcium. However, phosphate is the first of the two to be absorbed.[40]

Phosphate absorption is diminished when a large amount of calcium or aluminum is present in the intestine due to the formation of insoluble phosphate compounds. Such large amounts of calcium and aluminum may result from the consumption of antacids. In fact, for patients with CKD who have high serum phosphate concentrations, calcium- and aluminum-containing antacids may be given with meals as phosphate binders to reduce intestinal phosphate absorption.[45] It should be noted that due to concerns of detrimental accumulation of aluminum in the CNS as well as the ability to worsen anemia and bone disease, chronic use of aluminum-containing antacids should be avoided.

Phosphate is widely distributed in the body throughout the plasma, extracellular fluid, cell membrane structures, intracellular fluid, collagen, and bone. Bone contains 85% of the phosphate in the body. About 90% of plasma phosphate is filtered at the glomeruli, and the majority is actively reabsorbed at the proximal tubule. Some reabsorption also takes place in the loop of Henle, distal tubules, and possibly the collecting ducts.[31] The amount of renal phosphate excretion is, therefore, the amount filtered minus the amount reabsorbed. Increased urinary phosphate excretion can result from an increase in plasma volume and the action of PTH, which can block phosphate reabsorption throughout the nephron. In contrast, vitamin D_3 and its metabolites can directly stimulate proximal tubular phosphate reabsorption. In all, 90% of eliminated phosphate is excreted renally while the remainder is secreted into the intestine.[31,35,46] Renal handling of phosphate, especially the proximal tubules, therefore, plays an important role in maintaining the homeostatic balance of phosphate. Renal phosphate transport is active, saturable, and dependent on pH and sodium ion. However, fluctuation in serum phosphate mostly results from changes in either the GFR or the rate of tubular reabsorption.[2,31,35]

Serum phosphate and calcium concentrations as well as PTH and vitamin D levels are intimately related with each other. Serum phosphate indirectly controls PTH secretion via a negative feedback mechanism. With a decrease in the serum phosphate concentration, the conversion of vitamin D_3 to 1,25-DHCC increases (which increases serum concentrations of both phosphate and calcium). Both the intestinal absorption and renal reabsorption of phosphate are increased. The concomitant increase in serum calcium then directly decreases PTH secretion. This decrease in serum PTH concentration permits a further increase in renal phosphate reabsorption.[30,31]

A true phosphate imbalance may result from an abnormality in any of the previously discussed mechanisms and hormones for maintaining calcium and phosphate homeostasis. They may include altered intestinal absorption, altered number or activity of osteoclast and osteoblast cells in bone, changes in renal calcium and phosphate reabsorption, and IV infusions of calcium or phosphate salts.[35,40]

Hypophosphatemia

Hypophosphatemia indicates a serum phosphate concentration of less than 2.3 mg/dL (<0.74 mmol/L). The following three clinical conditions are common causes of decreased serum phosphate concentrations:

1. Increased renal excretion[40,47,48]
2. Intracellular shifting
3. Decreased phosphate or vitamin D intake[41,47,48]

To identify the etiology of hypophosphatemia, the serum and urine phosphate concentrations should be evaluated simultaneously. Low urine and serum phosphates indicate either a diminished phosphate intake or excessive use of phosphate-binders. An increased urine phosphate suggests either hyperparathyroidism or renal tubular dysfunction. If the increased urine phosphate is accompanied by elevated serum calcium, the presence of primary hyperparathyroidism or decreased vitamin D metabolism must be considered.

Common causes. Hypophosphatemia commonly results from decreased renal reabsorption or increased GFR, shift of phosphate from extracellular to intracellular fluid, alcoholism, or malnutrition. Phosphate is added to total parenteral nutrition solutions for muscle growth and replenishment of hepatic glycogen storage in malnourished patients. The infusion of concentrated glucose solution increases insulin secretion from the pancreas, which facilitates glucose and phosphate cell entry. Phosphate is used to form phosphorylated hexose intermediates during cellular utilization of glucose. An inadequate phosphate content in these nutritional fluids can decrease anabolism, glycolysis, and ATP and 2,3-DPG production.[48]

Infusion of concentrated glucose solutions, especially when accompanied by insulin, can produce hypophosphatemia through intracellular phosphate shifting. This condition, known as *refeeding syndrome*, can occur when an inadequate amount of phosphate is given during total parenteral nutrition (i.e., when a large amount of phosphate is taken up by the newly produced cells during anabolism).

Hypophosphatemia can also occur during treatment of hyperkalemia with insulin and dextrose. In addition, aluminum- and calcium-containing antacids, as well as magnesium hydroxide, are potent binders of intestinal phosphate.[45] Overuse of these agents can severely reduce serum phosphate concentrations in patients with normal renal function. Moreover, calcitonin, glucagon, and beta-adrenergic stimulants can decrease serum phosphate concentrations. Thiazide and loop diuretics can increase renal phosphate excretion. However, this effect is often insignificant clinically in otherwise healthy individuals.

Other conditions known to cause hypophosphatemia include nutritional recovery after starvation, treatment of diabetic ketoacidosis, decreased absorption or increased intestinal loss, alcohol withdrawal, the diuretic phase of acute tubular necrosis, and prolonged respiratory alkalosis. To compensate for respiratory alkalosis, carbon dioxide shifts from intracellular to extracellular fluid. This shift increases the intracellular fluid pH, which activates glycolysis and intracellular phosphate trapping. Metabolic acidosis, in contrast, produces a minimal change in serum phosphate.

Uncommon causes. Burn patients often retain a great amount of sodium and water. During wound healing, diuresis often ensues, which results in a substantial loss of phosphate. Since anabolism also occurs during recovery, hypophosphatemia may be inevitable without proper replacement. A moderate reduction in serum phosphate can occur from prolonged nasogastric suctioning, gastrectomy, small bowel or pancreatic disease resulting in malabsorption, and impaired renal phosphate reabsorption in patients with multiple myeloma, Fanconi syndrome, heavy-metal poisoning, amyloidosis, and nephrotic syndrome.[47,48]

Severe hypophosphatemia. Severe phosphate depletion (<1 mg/dL or <0.32 mmol/L) can occur during diabetic ketoacidosis. The resultant acidosis mobilizes bone, promotes intracellular organic substrate metabolism, and releases phosphate into the extracellular fluid. The glycosuria and ketonuria caused by diabetic ketoacidosis results in an osmotic diuresis that increases urinary phosphate excretion. The combined effects of these events may produce a normal serum phosphate concentration with severe intracellular deficiency. When diabetic ketoacidosis is corrected with insulin, phosphate accompanies glucose to move intracellularly. Serum phosphate is usually reduced within 24 hours of treatment. As the acidosis is corrected, there is further intracellular shifting of phosphate to result in profound hypophosphatemia. The accompanying volume repletion may exacerbate the hypophosphatemia further.

Clinical diagnosis. Patients with a moderate reduction in serum phosphate (2–2.3 mg/dL or 0.64–0.74 mmol/L) are often asymptomatic. Neurological irritability may occur as the serum phosphate concentration drops below 2 mg/dL (<0.64 mmol/L). Severe hypophosphatemia is often associated with muscle weakness, rhabdomyolysis, paresthesia, hemolysis, platelet dysfunction, and cardiac and respiratory failure.

Central nervous system effects often include encephalopathy, confusion, obtundation, seizures, and ultimately, coma. The mechanism for these effects may involve decreased glucose utilization by the brain, decreased brain cell ATP, or cerebral hypoxia from increased oxygen-Hgb affinity, secondary to diminished erythrocyte 2,3-DPG content. This decreased content results in decreased glycolysis, which leads to decreased 2,3-DPG and ATP production. The decreased contents of 2,3-DPG and ATP result in an increased affinity of Hgb for oxygen, eventually leading to decreased tissue oxygenation. The ensuing cerebral hypoxia may explain the persistent coma often seen in patients with diabetic ketoacidosis. Hemolysis may occur, but it is rarely seen at serum phosphate concentrations greater than 0.5 mg/dL (>0.16 mmol/L).

Hyperphosphatemia

Hyperphosphatemia indicates a serum phosphate concentration greater than 4.7 mg/dL (>1.52 mmol/L). There are three basic causes for elevated serum phosphate concentrations:

1. Decreased renal phosphate excretion

2. Shift of phosphate from intracellular to extracellular fluid

3. Increased intake of vitamin D or phosphate-containing products (orally, rectally, or intravenously)

Elevated phosphate concentrations may also result from reduced PTH secretion, increased body catabolism, and certain malignant conditions (e.g., leukemias and lymphomas).[4,47,48]

Causes. The most common cause of hyperphosphatemia is renal dysfunction, which commonly occurs as the GFR falls below 25 mL/min. Chronic kidney disease results in secondary hyperparathyroidism, which can further reduce renal phosphate elimination. The increase in serum phosphate concentration increases the risk for deposition of insoluble calcium–phosphate complex in soft tissues (i.e., metastatic calcification). This deposition may further reduce the serum concentration of ionized calcium and lead to increased PTH production and release. A sustained period of high PTH level leads to excessive bone resorption, which will severely weaken its structural integrity.[36,40]

Hyperphosphatemia can be caused by a shift of phosphate from intracellular to extracellular fluid. This shift of phosphate can result from massive cell break down after administering chemotherapy for leukemia or lymphoma, and during rhabdomyolysis and septic shock. In addition, hyperthyroidism can elevate serum phosphate by directly increasing renal tubular phosphate reabsorption.

Clinical diagnosis. Signs and symptoms of hyperphosphatemia commonly result from the accompanying hypocalcemia and hyperparathyroidism (see Hypocalcemia section). Renal function may diminish if hyperphosphatemia is left untreated. In the presence of renal dysfunction, phosphate excretion is further reduced to cause an even greater increase of serum phosphate concentration and a further decline in serum calcium concentration (Minicase 4).[36,40,45]

Causes of Spurious Laboratory Results

Hemolysis can occur during phlebotomy, which may lead to a falsely elevated serum phosphate concentration. If the serum is not separated soon after phlebotomy, phosphate may be falsely decreased as it is taken up by the cellular components of blood.

Similar to what may occur to specimens for potassium concentration determination, when the blood is allowed to clot with the use of nonheparinized tubes, phosphate may leach out of platelets to result in a falsely elevated concentration. In patients with thrombocytosis, phosphate concentrations should, therefore, be obtained from plasma rather than serum samples.

Serum phosphate may vary by 1–2 mg/dL (0.32–0.64 mmol/L) after meals. Meals rich in carbohydrate can reduce serum phosphate; and meals with high phosphate contents, such as dairy products, can increase serum phosphate. If accurate assessment of the phosphate concentration is necessary, the blood specimen should be obtained from the patient after fasting.

TRACE ELEMENTS

Copper

Normal range: 70–140 mcg/dL (11–22 µmol/L) (males); 80–155 mcg/dL (12–24 µmol/L) (females) for serum copper, 23–50 mg/dL for ceruloplasmin, 0.47 ± 0.06 mg/g for erythrocyte superoxide dismutase (SOD)

Physiology

The relationship between copper homeostasis and human diseases was uncovered in 1912 shortly after Wilson disease was described. In the early 1930s, a link between copper deficiency and anemia was suspected, although the hypothesis was not proven at that time. In the 1970s, the physiological functions of copper were better understood and its link to various disease states was better appreciated. An official dietary copper recommendation and adequate daily dietary intake was introduced for the first time in 1979.

Copper plays an integral part in the synthesis and functions of many circulating proteins and enzymes. In addition, copper is an essential factor for the formation of connective tissues, such as the cross-linking of collagen and elastin. Copper also shares similar physiological functions with iron.[49] In the CNS, copper is required for the formation or maintenance of myelin and other phospholipids. Cuproenzymes (copper-dependent enzymes) are crucial in the metabolism of catecholamines. For example, the functions of dopamine hydroxylase and monoamine oxidase are impaired by copper deficiency. Copper also affects the function of tyrosinase in melanin synthesis, which is responsible for the pigmentation of skin, hair, and eyes. Deficiency of tyrosinase results in albinism. Other physiological functions of copper include thermal regulation, glucose metabolism, blood clotting (e.g., factor V function), and protection of cells against oxidative damage.[50,51]

The normal adult daily intake of copper, from both animal and plant sources, is 2–3 mg. Plant copper is in the inorganic (free ionic) form, while meat (animal) copper is in the form of cuproproteins (copper–protein complex). Inorganic copper is absorbed in the upper portion of the GI tract (stomach and proximal duodenum) under acidic conditions. Cuproprotein copper is absorbed below the pancreatic duct after digestion. The absorption of copper from the GI tract is saturable. The oral bioavailability of copper ranges from 15% to 97% and shows a negative correlation with the amount of copper present in the diet.

Once absorbed, copper is bound to a mucosal copper-binding protein called *metallothionein* (a sulfur-rich, metal-binding protein present in intestinal mucosa). From this protein, copper is slowly released into the circulation, where it is taken up by the liver and other tissues.[50] Animal data suggest that the liver serves as the ultimate depot for copper storage. Copper absorption may be reduced by a high intake of zinc (>20 mg/day), ascorbic acid, and dietary fiber. Zinc may induce the synthesis of intestinal metallothionein and form a barrier to copper ion absorption.[50,51]

The normal adult body contains 75–150 mg of copper, which is significantly lower when compared with other trace

MINICASE 4

Calcium and Phosphate Disorders in a Patient with Chronic Renal Failure

MICHAEL S., A 65-YEAR-OLD MAN, had a 1-week history of nausea, vomiting, and general malaise. His appetite had severely decreased over the past 2 months. He had a longstanding history of uncontrolled hypertension and type 2 diabetes mellitus as well as diabetic nephropathy, retinopathy, and neuropathy.

His current medications include levothyroxine 0.1 mg orally daily, metoclopramide 10 mg orally 3 times a day, and a subcutaneous insulin regimen given twice a day. His physical examination revealed a BP of 160/99 mm Hg, diabetic retinopathic changes with laser scars bilaterally, and diminished sensation bilaterally below the knees.

His laboratory values were serum sodium 146 mEq/L (136–142 mEq/L), potassium 4.7 mEq/L (3.8–5.0 mEq/L), chloride 104 mEq/L (95–103 mEq/L), total carbon dioxide content 15 mmol/L (24–30 mmol/L), SCr 3.2 mg/dL (0.6–1.2 mg/dL), BUN 92 mg/dL (8–23 mg/dL), and random blood glucose of 181 mg/dL (70–110 mg/dL). Because of his renal failure, additional laboratory tests were obtained: calcium 7.5 mg/dL (9.2–11.0 mg/dL), phosphate 9.1 mg/dL (2.3–4.7 mg/dL), albumin 3.3 g/dL (3.5–5 g/dL), and uric acid 8.9 mg/dL (4.0–8.5 mg/dL).

Over the next several days, he complained of finger numbness, tingling, and burning of extremities. He also experienced increasing confusion and fatigue. A neurological examination was positive for both Chvostek and Trousseau signs. Repeated laboratory tests showed substantial changes in serum calcium (6.1 mg/dL) and phosphate (10.4 mg/dL). The patient's intact serum PTH was 280 pg/mL (10–65 pg/mL).

Question: What calcium and phosphate disorders does Michael S. have?

Discussion: Michael S. has three laboratory abnormalities that are related specifically to calcium–phosphate metabolism: (1) hypocalcemia, (2) hyperphosphatemia, and (3) hyperparathyroidism. He is exhibiting classic signs and symptoms of hypocalcemia, such as finger numbness, tingling, burning of extremities, confusion, fatigue, and positive Chvostek and Trousseau signs.

Chronic kidney disease, as seen in Michael S., is commonly associated with hypocalcemia, hyperphosphatemia, hyperparathyroidism, and vitamin D deficiency. These calcium–phosphate abnormalities are responsible for the development of renal osteodystrophy. During the early stages of renal failure, renal phosphate excretion began to decrease. His serum phosphate concentration was thus increased and the ionized calcium concentration became reduced, which stimulated the release of PTH, resulting in secondary hyperparathyroidism. The higher concentration of PTH reduced his renal tubular phosphate reabsorption, thereby increasing its excretion. The hyperparathyroidism thus helped to maintain his serum phosphate and calcium concentrations within normal ranges during the early stage of renal failure (Figure 6-3).

As renal function continues to deteriorate (GFR below 30 mL/min), renal tubules ceased to respond adequately to the high serum PTH concentration, resulting in hyperphosphatemia. In response to the hypocalcemia that followed, calcium was mobilized from the bone through the action of PTH. However, such compensatory response is not sufficient as hypocalcemia and hyperphosphatemia continued. The persistent hyperphosphatemia may contribute to the diminished renal conversion of 25-HCC to its biologically active metabolite 1,25-DHCC. As a result, the gut absorption of dietary calcium was diminished. Deficiency in active vitamin D can therefore aggravate his hypocalcemia, which subsequently can stimulate PTH secretion increasing mobilization of calcium from bone. The metabolic acidosis that is common in renal failure may also contribute to the negative calcium balance in the bone.

Michael S. was relatively asymptomatic up to this point, primarily because these laboratory abnormalities were developed over a long period of time and therefore allowed the body to compensate. In the presence of nausea and vomiting and the lack of appetite, his oral calcium intake was probably reduced substantially, which might have enhanced his malaise. Since calcium is commonly reported as total calcium and not as the free or ionized fraction, his total serum calcium concentration must be corrected for his low serum albumin value. For every 1 g/dL reduction in serum albumin below 4 g/dL, 0.8 mg/dL should be added to his serum calcium concentration. Therefore, with his serum albumin concentration of 3.3 g/dL, his initial serum calcium value of 7.5 mg/dL is equivalent to a total calcium concentration of about 8.1 mg/dL. Therefore, he does have true hypocalcemia, although the deficit is mild.

---

elements such as zinc and iron. Approximately one-third of the total body copper is found in the liver and brain at high tissue concentrations.[52] Another one-third is located in the muscles at low tissue concentrations. The rest is found in the heart, spleen, kidneys, and blood (erythrocytes and neutrophils).[50,52]

In the plasma, copper is highly bound (95%) to ceruloplasmin (also known as ferroxidase I), a blue copper protein.[49] This protein contains six to seven copper atoms per molecule. The fraction of plasma copper associated with ceruloplasmin seems to be relatively constant for the same individual. However, a significant interindividual variation exists. The remainder of the plasma copper is bound to albumin and amino acids or is free.[50,52] Copper is eliminated mainly by biliary excretion (average 25 mcg/kg/day), with only 0.5% to 3% of the daily intake in the urine.[50]

Ceruloplasmin is considered the most reliable indicator of copper status because of its large and relatively stable binding capacity with plasma copper. Therefore, when evaluating copper status in the body, ceruloplasmin concentration should be assessed together with plasma copper concentration.

Hypocupremia

Copper deficiency is relatively uncommon in humans.[51] *Hypocupremia* usually occurs in infants with chronic diarrhea or malabsorption syndrome or in low-birth-weight infants fed with milk (rather than formulas).[49,51,53] Premature infants, who typically have low copper stores, are at a higher risk for developing copper deficiency under these circumstances.[50]

Copper deficiency may occur in patients receiving long-term parenteral nutrition. Chronic malabsorption syndromes (e.g., celiac disease and ulcerative colitis), protein-wasting enteropathies, short bowel syndrome, and the presence of significant bowel resection or bypass (e.g., malabsorptive bariatric surgical procedures such as long-limb Roux-en-Y, or jejunoileal bypass) are all potential risk factors resulting in copper deficiency. However, symptomatic deficiency is rare.[49,53] Individuals on a vegetarian diet may be at risk because (1) meat is a major food source of copper, and (2) plant sources often have high-fiber content that may interfere with copper absorption.[49]

Prolonged hypocupremia leads to a syndrome of neutropenia and iron-deficiency anemia, which are correctable with copper.[53] The anemia is normocytic or microcytic and hypochromic. It results mainly from poor iron absorption and ineffective heme incorporation of iron.[45,52] Copper deficiency can affect any system or organ whose enzymes require copper for proper functioning. As such, copper deficiency may lead to abnormal glucose tolerance, arrhythmias, hypercholesterolemia, atherosclerosis, depressed immune function, defective connective tissue formation, demineralization of bones, and pathological fractures.[51]

There are two well-known genetic defects associated with impaired copper metabolism in humans. *Menkes syndrome* (also called *kinky-* or *steely-hair syndrome*) is an X-linked disorder that occurs in 1 out of every 50,000 to 100,000 live births. These patients have defective copper absorption, and are commonly deceased by the age of 3. They have reduced copper concentrations in the blood, liver, and brain.[49,51] Most of them are children suffering from slow growth and retardation, defective keratinization and pigmentation of hair, hypothermia, and degenerative changes in the aortic elastin and neurons. Progressive nerve degeneration in the brain results in intellectual deterioration, hypotonia, and seizures. However, anemia and neutropenia, hallmark symptoms of nutritional copper deficiency, are not found in Menkes syndrome. Administration of parenteral copper increases serum copper and ceruloplasmin concentrations but does not have any apparent effect on slowing disease progression.

Wilson disease is an autosomal recessive disease of copper storage. Its frequency is uncertain, but it is believed to be not as common as Menkes syndrome. Wilson disease appears to be associated with altered copper catabolism and excretion of ceruloplasmin copper into the bile. It is associated with elevated urinary copper loss and low plasma ceruloplasmin and low plasma copper concentrations. However, copper deposition occurs in the liver, brain, and cornea. If untreated, significant copper accumulation in these organs will eventually lead to irreversible damage such as cirrhosis and neurological impairment. Interestingly, treatment with dietary adjustment of copper intake does not seem to be effective. Chelation therapy using D-penicillamine is much more effective in preventing copper deposition. Oral zinc supplementation has also been used to reduce copper accumulation.

Hypercupremia

Copper excess is not common in humans and usually occurs with a deliberate attempt to ingest large quantities of copper. The exact amount of copper that results in toxicity is unknown.

Acute or long-term ingestion of greater than 15 mg of elemental copper may lead to symptomatic copper poisoning.[52] It has also been reported that drinking water with 2–3 mg/L of copper is associated with hepatotoxicity in infants. Similar to other metallic poisonings, acute copper poisoning leads to nausea, vomiting, intestinal cramps, and diarrhea.[52] A larger ingestion can result in shock, hepatic necrosis, intravascular hemolysis, renal impairment, coma, and death.[53] Elevated intrahepatic copper concentrations may be present in patients with primary biliary cirrhosis and biliary atresia.[49,50,53] Long-term parenteral nutrition use is also a risk factor for hepatic copper overload. The mechanism is not well-established. Chronic cholestasis secondary to parenteral nutrition-associated liver disease has been suggested as the primary cause. Since copper plays an important role in the neurological system, it has been suggested that copper-induced free radical-induced neurodegeneration may be a contributing factor for Alzheimer disease. At present, there is no known treatment for *hypercupremia*.

Zinc

Normal range: 50–150 mcg/dL or 7.6–23 μmol/L

Physiology

Next to iron, zinc is the most abundant trace element in the body. It is an essential nutrient that is a constituent of, or a cofactor to, many enzymes. These metalloenzymes participate in the metabolism of carbohydrates, proteins, lipids, and nucleic acids.[50] As such, zinc influences[50,53]

- Tissue growth and repair
- Cell membrane stabilization
- Bone collagenase activity and collagen turnover
- Immune response, especially T cell mediated response
- Sensory control of food intake
- Spermatogenesis and gonadal maturation
- Normal testicular function

The normal adult body contains 1.5–2.5 g of zinc.[51] Aside from supplementation with zinc capsules, dietary intake is the only source of zinc for humans. Food sources of zinc include meat products, oysters, and legumes.[50] Food zinc is largely bound to proteins and released below the common duct for absorption by the ileum. Ionic zinc found in zinc supplements is absorbed in the duodenum due to a lower pH in that region.[50] Body zinc stores determine, to some extent, the percentage of zinc that is absorbed from food and mineral supplements. Foods rich in calcium, dietary fiber, or phytate may interfere with zinc absorption, as can folic acid supplements.[50]

After absorption, zinc is transported from the small intestine to the portal circulation where it binds to proteins such as albumin, transferrin, and other globulins.[50] Circulating zinc is bound mostly to serum proteins; two-thirds are loosely bound to albumin and transthyretin while one-third is bound tightly to beta-2 macroglobulin.[53] Only 2% to 3% (3 mg) of zinc is either in free ionic form or bound to amino acids.[50]

Zinc can be found in many organs. Tissues high in zinc include liver, pancreas, spleen, lungs, eyes (retina, iris, cornea, and lens), prostate, skeletal muscle, and bone. Because of their mass, skeletal muscle (60% to 62%) and bone (20% to 28%) have the highest zinc contents among the body tissues.[50] Only 2% to 4% of total body zinc is found in the liver. In blood, 85% is in erythrocytes, although each leukocyte contains 25 times the zinc content of an erythrocyte.[51]

Plasma zinc concentration is a poor indicator of total body zinc store. Since 98% of the total body zinc is present in tissues and end organs, the plasma zinc concentration tends to be maintained by continuous shifting from intracellular sources. Additionally, metabolic stress, such as infection, acute myocardial infarction, and critical illnesses increase intracellular shifting of zinc to the liver and lower serum zinc concentrations, even when total body zinc is normal. Conversely, serum zinc concentrations may be normal during starvation or wasting syndromes due to release of zinc from tissues and cells.[50] Therefore, serum/plasma zinc concentration alone has little meaning clinically. It has been suggested that the rate of zinc turnover in the plasma provides better assessment of the body zinc status. This may be achieved by measuring 24-hour zinc loss in body fluids (e.g., urine and stool). However, this approach is rarely practical for critically ill patients as renal failure is often present. Alternatively, zinc turnover and mobilization may be determined by adjusting plasma zinc concentrations with serum beta-2 macroglobulin and albumin concentrations.[56,57] To more accurately assess the body zinc status, others have suggested monitoring the functional indices of zinc, such as erythrocyte alkaline phosphatase, serum superoxide dismutase, and lymphocyte 5' nucleotidase. However, the clinical validity of these tests remains to be substantiated, especially in patients who are acutely ill.

Zinc undergoes substantial enteropancreatic recirculation and is excreted primarily in pancreatic and intestinal secretions. Zinc is also lost dermally through sweat, hair and nail growth, and skin shedding. Except in certain disease states, only 2% of zinc is lost in the urine.[50]

Hypozincemia

In Western countries, zinc deficiency is rare from inadequate intake. Individuals with serum zinc concentrations below 50 mcg/dL (<7.6 μmol/L) are at an increased risk for developing symptomatic zinc deficiency. It must also be emphasized that serum zinc exhibits a negative acute phase response. The presence of proinflammatory cytokines causes an intracellular and intrahepatic influx of zinc from the serum which would lead to transient hypozincemia. Therefore, serum or plasma zinc concentration alone should not be used to assess zinc status in patients with acute illnesses or any acute inflammatory response. Given the caveats of measuring serum zinc concentrations in certain disease states, response to zinc supplements may be the only way of diagnosing this deficiency. In the presence of chronic diseases, it is difficult to determine if zinc deficiency is clinical or subclinical because of the reduced protein binding.[53] Conditions leading to deficiency may be divided into five classes (List 6-8)[50,53]:

1. Low intake
2. Decreased absorption
3. Increased utilization
4. Increased loss
5. Unknown causes

The most likely candidates for zinc deficiency are infants; rapidly growing adolescents; menstruating, lactating, or pregnant women; individuals with low meat intake; chronically ill patients who have been institutionalized for extended periods; patients with chronic uncontrolled diarrhea or ostomy output, and those who have been receiving zinc-deficient parenteral nutrition solutions.[53] Acrodermatitis enteropathica is an autosomal, recessive disorder involving zinc malabsorption that occurs in infants of Italian, Armenian, and Iranian heritage. It is characterized by severe dermatitis, chronic diarrhea, emotional disturbances, and growth retardation.[50] Examples of malabsorption syndromes that may lead to zinc deficiency include Crohn disease, celiac disease, and short-bowel syndrome.

Excessive zinc may be lost in the urine (hyperzincuria), as occurs in alcoholism, beta-thalassemia, diabetes mellitus, diuretic therapy, nephrotic syndrome, sickle cell anemia, and treatment with parenteral nutrition. Severe or prolonged diarrhea (e.g., inflammatory bowel diseases and graft versus host disease) may lead to significant zinc loss in the stool.[50,53] Patients with end-stage liver disease frequently have depleted zinc storage due to decreased functional hepatic cell mass.

Because zinc is involved in a diverse group of enzymes, its deficiency manifests in numerous organs and physiological systems (List 6-9).[50] Dysgeusia (lack of taste) and hyposmia (diminished smell acuity) are common. Pica is a pathological craving for specific food or nonfood substances (e.g., geophagia). Chronic zinc deficiency, as occurs in acrodermatitis enteropathica, leads to growth retardation, anemia, hypogonadism, hepatosplenomegaly, and impaired wound healing. Additional signs and symptoms of acrodermatitis enteropathica include diarrhea; vomiting; alopecia; skin lesions in oral, anal, and genital areas; paronychia; nail deformity; emotional lability; photophobia; blepharitis; conjunctivitis; and corneal opacities.[50,53]

Hyperzincemia

Zinc is one of the least toxic trace elements.[53] Clinical manifestations of excess zinc occur with chronic, high doses of a zinc supplement. However, patients with Wilson disease who commonly take high doses of zinc rarely show signs of toxicity. This may be explained by the stabilization of serum zinc concentrations during high-dose administration.[50] As much as 12 g of zinc sulfate (>2700 mg of elemental zinc) taken over 2 days has caused drowsiness, lethargy, and increased serum lipase and amylase concentrations. Nausea, vomiting, and diarrhea also may occur.[50]

Serum zinc concentrations must be measured using nonhemolyzed samples. Erythrocytes and leukocytes, like many other cells, are rich in zinc. When they undergo hemolysis in the tube (e.g., too small a needle is used to draw the sample, tourniquet is too tight, or specimen left standing for too long or is mishandled), these cells release zinc into the specimen in quantities large enough to produce misleading results. This phenomenon

LIST 6-8. Etiologies of Zinc Deficiency

Low intake

Anorexia

Nutritional deficiencies

  Alcoholism

  Chronic kidney disease

  Premature infants

  Certain vegetarian diets

  Use of hyperalimentation solutions

Decreased absorption

  Acrodermatitis enteropathica

  Malabsorption syndromes

Increased utilization

  Adolescence

  Lactation

  Menstruation

  Pregnancy

Increased loss

  Alcoholism

  β-thalassemia

  Cirrhosis

  Diabetes mellitus

  Diarrhea

  Diuretic therapy

  Enterocutaneous fistula drainage

  Exercise (long term, strenuous)

  Glucagon

  Loss of enteropancreatic recycling

  Nephrotic syndrome

  Protein-losing enteropathies

  Sickle cell anemia

  Therapy with hyperalimentation solutions

Unknown causes

  Arthritis and other inflammatory diseases

  Down syndrome

can also occur when the specimen is allowed to clot, with the use of nonheparinized tubes.[50]

Manganese

Normal range: unknown

Physiology

Manganese is an essential trace element that serves as a cofactor for numerous diverse enzymes involved in carbohydrate, protein, and lipid metabolism; protection of cells from free radicals; steroid biosynthesis; and metabolism of biogenic amines.[54] Interestingly, manganese deficiency does not affect the functions of most of these enzymes, presumably because magnesium may substitute for manganese in most instances.[53] In animals, manganese is required for normal bone growth, lipid metabolism, reproduction, and CNS regulation.[51]

Manganese has an important role in the normal function of the brain, primarily through its effect on biogenic amine metabolism. This effect may be responsible for the relationship between brain concentrations of manganese and catecholamines.[54]

The manganese content of the adult body is 10–20 mg. Manganese homeostasis is regulated through control of its absorption and excretion.[54] Plants are the primary source of food manganese since animal tissues have low contents.[54] Manganese is absorbed from the small intestine by a mechanism similar to that of iron.[51] However, only 3% to 4% of the ingested manganese is absorbed. Dietary iron and phytate may affect manganese absorption.[49]

Human and animal tissues have low manganese content.[54] Tissues relatively high in manganese are the bone, liver, pancreas, and pituitary gland.[49,54] Most circulating manganese is loosely bound to the beta-1 globulin transmanganin, a transport protein similar to transferrin.[51,53] With overexposure, excess manganese accumulates in the liver and brain, causing severe neuromuscular signs and symptoms.[49]

Manganese is excreted primarily in biliary and pancreatic secretions. In manganese overload, other GI routes of elimination may also be used. Little manganese is lost in urine.[53,54]

Manganese Deficiency

Due to its relative abundance in plant sources, manganese deficiency is rare among the general population.[49] Deficiency normally occurs after several months of deliberate manganese omission from the diet.[53,54] Little is known regarding serum manganese concentrations and the accompanying disease states in humans.[53]

Information from the signs and symptoms of manganese deficiency comes from experimental subjects who intentionally followed low manganese diets for many months. Their signs and symptoms included weight loss, slow hair and nail growth, color change in hair and beard, transient dermatitis, hypocholesterolemia, and hypotriglyceridemia.[54]

Adults and children with convulsive disorders have lower mean serum manganese concentrations than normal subjects, although a cause-and-effect relationship has not been established. However, serum manganese concentrations correlate with seizure frequency.[54] Animals deficient in manganese show defective growth, skeletal malformation, ataxia, reproductive abnormalities, and disturbances in lipid metabolism.[49,53]

Manganese Excess

Manganese is one of the least toxic trace elements.[53] Overexposure primarily occurs from inhalation of manganese compounds (e.g., manganese mines).[54] The excess amount accumulates in the liver and brain resulting in severe neuromuscular manifestations. Symptoms include encephalopathy and profound neurological disturbances mimicking Parkinson disease.[49,53,54] These manifestations are not surprising since

LIST 6-9. Signs and Symptoms of Zinc Deficiency

Signs

Acrodermatitis enteropathica

Anemia

Anergy to skin test antigens

Complicated pregnancy

- Excessive bleeding
- Maternal infection
- Premature or stillborn birth
- Spontaneous abortion
- Toxemia

Decreased basal metabolic rate

Decreased circulating thyroxine (T$_4$) concentration

Decreased lymphocyte count and function

Effect on fetus, infant, or child

- Congenital defects of skeleton, lungs, and CNS
- Fetal disturbances
- Growth retardation
- Hypogonadism

Impaired neutrophil function

Impairment and delaying of platelet aggregation

Increased susceptibility to dental caries

Increased susceptibility to infections

Mental disturbance

Pica

Poor wound healing

Short stature in children

Skeletal deformities

Symptoms

Acne and recurrent furunculosis

Ataxia

Decreased appetite

Defective night vision

Hypogeusia

Hyposmia

Erectile dysfunction

Mouth ulcers

---

metabolism of biogenic amines is altered in both manganese excess and Parkinson disease. Other signs and symptoms include anorexia, apathy, headache, erectile dysfunction, and speech disturbances.[53] Inhalation of manganese products may cause manganese pneumonitis.[54]

Chromium

Normal range: 0.12–2.1 mcg/L (6–109 nmol/L)

Physiology

The main physiological role of chromium is as a cofactor for insulin.[55] In its organic form, chromium potentiates the action of endogenous and exogenous insulin, presumably by augmenting its adherence to cell membranes.[49] The organic form is in the dinicotinic acid–glutathione complex or glucose tolerance factor (GTF).[51] Chromium is the metal portion of GTF; with insulin, GTF affects the metabolism of glucose, cholesterol, and triglycerides.[53] Therefore, chromium is important for glucose tolerance, glycogen synthesis, amino acid transport, and protein synthesis. Chromium is also involved in the activation of several enzymes.[51]

The adult body contains an average of 5 mg of chromium.[53] Food sources of chromium include brewer's yeast, spices, vegetable oils, unrefined sugar, liver, kidneys, beer, meat, dairy products, and wheat germ.[50,51] Glucose tolerance factor is present in the diet and can be synthesized from inorganic trivalent chromium (Cr^{+3}) available in food and dietary supplements.[50] Chromium is absorbed via a common pathway with zinc; its degree of absorption is inversely related to dietary intake, varying from 0.5% to 2%.[49,50] Absorption of Cr^{+3} from GTF is 10% to 25%, but the absorption is only 1% for inorganic chromium.[51]

Chromium circulates as free Cr^{3+}, bound to transferrin and other proteins, and as the GTF complex.[50,53] Glucose tolerance factor is the biologically active moiety and is more important than total serum chromium concentration.[53] Trivalent chromium accumulates in the hair, kidneys, skeleton, liver, spleen, lungs, testes, and large intestine. Glucose tolerance factor concentrates in insulin-responsive tissues such as the liver.[50,51]

The metabolism of chromium is not well-understood for several reasons[51]:

- Low concentrations in tissues
- Difficulty in analyzing chromium in biological fluids and tissue samples
- Presence of different chromium forms in food

Homeostasis is controlled by release of chromium from GTF and by dietary absorption.[50] The kidneys are the main site of elimination where urinary excretion is constant despite variability in the fraction absorbed.[53] However, excretion increases after glucose or insulin administration.[50,53] Insulin, or a stimulus for insulin release, can therefore mobilize chromium from its stores. The chromium that is released will then be excreted in the urine. The amount of insulin in the circulation can thus affect the elimination and daily requirement of chromium.[55]

Chromium Deficiency

It is important to stress that the body store of chromium cannot be reliably assessed.[50] Serum or plasma chromium may not be in equilibrium with other pools. As with other trace elements, the risk for developing deficiency may be increased in patients receiving prescribed nourishment low in chromium content (e.g., parenteral nutrition solutions).[55] Marginal deficiencies or defects in utilization of chromium may be present in the elderly, patients with diabetes, or patients with atherosclerotic coronary artery disease.[50] The hepatic store of chromium decreases 10-fold in the elderly, suggesting a predisposition to deficiency. Since chromium is involved in lipid and cholesterol metabolism, its deficiency is a suspected risk factor for the development of atherosclerosis.[50,55]

Hyperglycemia increases the urinary losses of chromium. Coupled with marginal intake, a type II diabetic patient is predisposed to chromium deficiency, which can further impair glucose tolerance.[50,55] Finally, multiparous women are at a higher risk than nulliparous women for becoming chromium deficient because, over time, chromium intake may not be adequate to meet fetal needs and to maintain the mother's body store.[55]

The manifestations of chromium deficiency may involve insulin resistance and impaired glucose metabolism. Such manifestations may present clinically in three stages as the deficiency progresses:

1. Glucose intolerance is present but is masked by a compensatory increase in insulin release.
2. Impaired glucose tolerance and lipid metabolism are clinically evident.
3. Marked insulin resistance and symptoms associated with hyperglycemia are evident.[55]

Chromium supplementation has been shown in diabetic patients to increase insulin sensitivity, improve glucose control, and shorten EKG QTc interval, suggesting a potential favorable effect on cardiovascular risk. However, there is at present no conclusive support demonstrating the benefit of chromium supplementation in diabetic patients or in those with impaired glucose metabolism.

Chromium deficiency may lead to hypercholesterolemia and become a risk factor for developing atherosclerotic disease.[50] Low chromium tissue concentrations have been associated with increased risk for myocardial infarction and coronary artery disease in both healthy subjects and diabetic patients, although a cause-and-effect relationship has not been established.[55,58]

Chromium Excess

Chromium has very low toxicity. The clinical significance of a high body store of chromium is unknown.

SUMMARY

Hyponatremia and hypernatremia may be associated with high, normal, or low total body sodium. Hyponatremia may result from abnormal water accumulation in the intravascular space (dilutional hyponatremia), a decline in both extracellular water and sodium, or a reduction in total body sodium with normal water balance. Hypernatremia is most common in patients with either an impaired thirst mechanism (e.g., neurohypophyseal lesion) or an inability to replace water depleted through normal insensible loss or from renal or GI loss. Neurological manifestations are signs and symptoms often associated with sodium and water imbalance. The most common symptom of hyponatremia is confusion. However, if sodium continues to fall, seizures, coma, and death may result. Thirst is a major symptom of hypernatremia; elevated urine specific gravity, indicating concentrated urine, is uniformly observed.

Hypokalemia and hyperkalemia may indicate either a true or an apparent (due to transcellular shifting) potassium imbalance. Hypokalemia can occur due to excessive loss from the kidneys (diuretics) or GI tract (vomiting). The most serious manifestation involves the cardiovascular system (i.e., cardiac arrhythmias). Renal impairment, usually in the presence of high intake, commonly causes hyperkalemia. Like hypokalemia, the most serious clinical manifestations of hyperkalemia involve the cardiovascular system.

Serum chloride concentration may be used as a confirmatory test to identify abnormalities in fluid and acid–base balance. Hypochloremia may be diuretic-induced and results from the concurrent loss of sodium and also contraction alkalosis. Hyperchloremia may develop with the use of parenteral nutrition solutions that have a chloride:sodium ratio greater than 1. Signs and symptoms associated with these conditions are related to the abnormalities in fluid or acid–base balance and underlying causes rather than to chloride itself.

Hypomagnesemia usually results from excessive loss from the GI tract (e.g., nasogastric suction, biliary loss, or fecal fistula) or from the kidneys (e.g., diuresis). Magnesium depletion is usually associated with neuromuscular symptoms such as weakness, muscle fasciculation with tremor, tetany, and increased reflexes. Increased magnesium intake in the presence of renal dysfunction commonly causes hypermagnesemia. Neuromuscular signs and symptoms that are opposite to those caused by hypomagnesemia may be observed.

The most common causes of true hypocalcemia are disorders of vitamin D metabolism and PTH production. Severe hypocalcemia can be a medical emergency and lead to cardiac arrhythmias and tetany, with symptoms primarily involving the neuromuscular system.

The most common causes of hypercalcemia are malignancy and primary hyperparathyroidism. Symptoms often consist of vague GI complaints such as nausea, vomiting, abdominal pain, anorexia, constipation, and diarrhea. Severe hypercalcemia can cause cardiac arrhythmias, which can be a medical emergency.

The most common causes of hypophosphatemia are decreased intake and increased renal loss. Although mild hypophosphatemia is usually asymptomatic, severe depletion (<1 mg/dL or <0.32 mmol/L) is typically associated with muscle weakness, rhabdomyolysis, paresthesia, hemolysis, platelet dysfunction, and cardiac and respiratory failure. The most common cause of hyperphosphatemia is renal dysfunction, often with a GFR below 25 mL/min. Signs and symptoms, if present, primarily result from the ensuing hypocalcemia and hyperparathyroidism.

Hypocupremia is uncommon in adults but can occur in infants, especially those born prematurely. Also susceptible are infants who have chronic diarrhea, malabsorption syndrome, or those whose diet consists mostly of milk. Prolonged hypocupremia results in neutropenia and iron-deficiency anemia that is correctable with copper.

Copper excess is not common and may result from a deliberate attempt to ingest large quantities. Similar to other metallic poisonings, acute copper poisoning leads to nausea and vomiting, intestinal cramps, and diarrhea.

Likely candidates for zinc deficiency are infants; rapidly growing adolescents; menstruating, lactating, or pregnant women; persons with low meat intake; institutionalized patients; and patients receiving parenteral nutrition solutions. Because zinc is involved with a diverse group of enzymes, its deficiency manifests in different organs and physiological systems. Zinc excess develops from chronic, high-dose zinc supplementation. Signs and symptoms include nausea, vomiting, diarrhea, drowsiness, lethargy, and increases in serum lipase and amylase concentrations.

Manganese deficiency can occur after several months of deliberate omission from the diet. Signs and symptoms include weight loss, slow hair and nail growth, color change in hair and beard, transient dermatitis, hypocholesterolemia, and hypotriglyceridemia. Manganese excess primarily occurs through inhalation of manganese compounds (e.g., manganese mines). As a result of manganese accumulation, severe neuromuscular manifestations occur, including encephalopathy and profound neurological disturbances, which mimic Parkinson disease. Inhalation of manganese products may cause manganese pneumonitis.

Chromium deficiency may be found in patients receiving prescribed chronic nutrition regimens that are low in chromium content (e.g., parenteral nutrition solutions). Insulin resistance and impaired glucose metabolism are the main manifestations.

Learning Points

1. What does an abnormal serum electrolyte concentration mean?

Answer: An isolated abnormal serum electrolyte concentration may not always necessitate immediate treatment because it can be the result of a poor sample (hemolyzed blood sample), wrong timing (immediately after hemodialysis), or other confounding factors. Careful assessment of the patient's existing risk factors, history of illness, and clinical symptoms should be made to confirm the accuracy of the specific laboratory result. Patients with abnormal serum electrolyte concentrations who are also symptomatic, especially with potentially life-threatening clinical presentations such as EKG changes, should be treated promptly. The cause or precipitating factor of the electrolyte abnormality should be identified and corrected, if possible.

2. How should we approach a patient who has an abnormal serum sodium concentration?

Answer: Alteration of serum sodium concentration can be precipitated by sodium alone (either excess or deficiency), or abnormal water regulation. It is important to fully assess the patient's sodium and fluid status, symptoms, physical exam findings, and medical and surgical history for factors that may precipitate sodium disorders. Since the homeostasis of sodium and water is closely regulated by the kidney, it is useful to check urine electrolytes and osmolality to help establish the diagnosis and guide clinical management.

3. What is the clinical significance of abnormal serum calcium and phosphorus concentrations?

Answer: Severe hypocalcemia and hypercalcemia can result in neuromuscular problems. In addition, significant hypercalcemia may cause EKG changes and arrhythmias. While hyperphosphatemia is not expected to cause any acute problems, severe hypophosphatemia can result in neurologic and CNS manifestations.

In the presence of chronic hyperphosphatemia, especially in patients with CKD, the risk is increased for phosphorus to bind with calcium to form insoluble complexes which will result in soft tissue and vascular calcification. There is an increasing amount of evidence to show that such vascular calcification can increase the mortality and morbidity of CKD patients. Concurrent hypercalcemia will further increase the serum calcium–phosphorus product and exacerbate the calcification process.

REFERENCES

1. Sterns RH, Spital A, Clark EC. Disorders of water balance. In: Kokko JP, Tannen RL, eds. *Fluids and Electrolytes*. 3rd ed. Philadelphia, PA: WB Saunders; 1996:63-109.

2. Guyton AC, Hall JE. *Textbook of Medical Physiology*. 10th ed. Philadelphia, PA: WB Saunders; 2001.

3. Berl T, Schrier RW. Disorders of water metabolism. In: Schrier RW, ed. *Renal and Electrolyte Disorders*. 6th ed. Philadelphia, PA: Lippincott Williams & Wilkins; 2003:1-63.

4. Rose BD. *Clinical Physiology of Acid–Base and Electrolyte Disorders*. 5th ed. New York, NY: McGraw-Hill; 2001.

5. Briggs JP, Singh IIJ, Sawaya BE, et al. Disorders of salt balance. In: Kokko JP, Tannen RL, eds. *Fluids and Electrolytes*. 3rd ed. Philadelphia, PA: WB Saunders; 1996:3-62.

6. Halperin ML, Goldstein MB, eds. *Fluid, Electrolyte, and Acid–Base Physiology: A Problem-Based Approach*. 2nd ed. Philadelphia, PA: WB Saunders; 1994.

7. Zull DN. Disorders of potassium metabolism. *Emerg Med Clin North Am*. 1989;7:771-794.

8. Oh MS, Carroll HJ. Electrolyte and acid–base disorders. In: Chernow B, ed. *The Pharmacologic Approach to the Critically Ill Patient*. 3rd ed. Baltimore, MD: Williams & Wilkins; 1994:957-968.

9. Peterson LN, Levi M. Disorders of potassium metabolism. In: Schrier RW, ed. *Renal and Electrolyte Disorders*. 6th ed. Philadelphia, PA: Lippincott Williams & Wilkins; 2003:171-215.

10. Tannen RL. Potassium disorders. In: Kokko JP, Tannen RL, eds. *Fluids and Electrolytes*. 3rd ed. WB Saunders; 1996:111-199.

11. Rose BD. Diuretics. *Kidney Int*. 1991;39:336-352.

12. Williams ME. Endocrine crises. Hyperkalemia. *Crit Care Clin*. 1991;7:155-174.

13. Freedman BI, Burkart JM. Endocrine crises: hypokalemia. *Crit Care Clin*. 1991;7:143-153.

14. The seventh report of the Joint National Committee on Prevention, Detection, Evaluation, and Treatment of High Blood Pressure: The JNC 7 Report. *JAMA*. 2003;289:2560-2572.

15. Siegel D, Hulley SB, Black DM, et al. Diuretics, serum and intracellular electrolyte levels, and ventricular arrhythmias in hypertensive men. *JAMA*. 1992;267:1083-1089.

16. Moser M. Current hypertension management: separating fact from fiction. *Cleve Clin J Med*. 1993;60:27-37.

17. Papademetriou V, Burris JF, Notargiacomo A, et al. Thiazide therapy is not a cause of arrhythmia in patients with systemic hypertension. *Arch Intern Med*. 1988;148:1272-1276.

18. Ellison DH. Diuretic drugs and the treatment of edema: from clinic to bench and back again. *Am J Kidney Dis*. 1994;23:623-643.

19. Shapiro JI, Kaehny WD. Pathogenesis and management of metabolic acidosis and alkalosis. In: Schrier RW, ed. *Renal and Electrolyte Disorders*. 6th ed. Philadelphia, PA: Lippincott Williams & Wilkins; 2003:115-153.

20. Kaehny WD. Pathogenesis and management of respiratory and mixed acid–base disorders. In: Schrier RW, ed. *Renal and Electrolyte Disorders*. 6th ed. Philadelphia, PA: Lippincott Williams & Wilkins; 2003:154-170.

21. Koch SM, Taylor RW. Chloride ion in intensive care medicine. *Crit Care Med*. 1992;20:227-240.

22. Alfrey AC. Normal and abnormal magnesium metabolism. In: Schrier RW, ed. *Renal and Electrolyte Disorders*. 6th ed. Philadelphia, PA: Lippincott Williams & Wilkins; 2003:278-302.

23. Salem M, Munoz R, Chernow B. Hypomagnesemia in critical illness: a common and clinically important problem. *Crit Care Clin*. 1991;7:225-252.

24. Rude RK. Magnesium disorders. In: Kokko JP, Tannen RL, eds. *Fluids and Electrolytes*. 3rd ed. Philadelphia, PA: WB Saunders; 1996:421-445.

25. Ghamdi SM, Cameron EC, Sutton RA. Magnesium deficiency: pathophysiologic and clinical overview. *Am J Kidney Dis*. 1994;24:737-752.

26. Berkelhammer C, Bear RA. A clinical approach to common electrolyte problems: hypomagnesemia. *Can Med Assoc J*. 1985;132:360-368.

27. Van-Hook JW. Endocrine crises: hypermagnesemia. *Crit Care Clin*. 1991;7:215-223.

28. Kumar R. Calcium disorders. In: Kokko JP, Tannen RL, eds. *Fluids and Electrolytes*. 3rd ed. Philadelphia, PA: WB Saunders; 1996:391-419.

29. Zelis R, Moore R. Recent insights into the calcium channels. *Circulation*. 1989;80(suppl IV):14-16.

30. Brown AJ, Dusso AS, Slatopolsky E. Vitamin D analogues for secondary hyperparathyroidism. *Nephrol Dial Transplant*. 2002;17 (suppl)10:10-19.

31. Hruska KA, Slatopolsky E. Disorders of phosphorus, calcium, and magnesium metabolism. In: Schrier RW, Gottschalk CW, eds. *Diseases of the Kidney*. 7th ed. Philadelphia, PA: Lippincott Williams & Wilkins; 2001:2607-2660.

32. Slatopolsky E, Lopez-Hilker S, Delmez J, et al. The parathyroid-calcitriol axis in health and chronic renal failure. *Kidney Int*. 1990; 29(suppl):S41-S47.

33. Hudson JQ, Johnson CA. Chronic renal failure. In: Young LY, Koda-Kimble MA, eds. *Applied Therapeutics: The Clinical Use of Drugs*. 7th ed. Philadelphia, PA: Lippincott Williams & Wilkins; 2001:30.1-30.38.

34. Malluche HH, Mawad H, Koszewski NJ. Update on vitamin D and its newer analogues: actions and rationale for treatment in chronic renal failure. *Kidney Int*. 2002;62(2):367-374.

35. Zaloga GP, Chernow B. Divalent ions: calcium, magnesium, and phosphorus. In: Chernow B, ed. *The Pharmacologic Approach to the Critically Ill Patient*. 3rd ed. Baltimore, MD: Williams & Wilkins; 1994:777-804.

36. Ritz E, Matthias S, Seidel A, et al. Disturbed calcium metabolism in renal failure—pathogenesis and therapeutic strategies. *Kidney Int*. 1992;42(suppl 38):S37-S42.

37. Zaloga GP. Hypocalcemic crisis. *Crit Care Clin*. 1991;7:191-200.

38. Zaloga GP. Hypocalcemia in critically ill patients. *Crit Care Med*. 1992;20: 251-262.

39. Mundy GR. Hypercalcemia of malignancy. *Kidney Int*. 1987;31:142-155.

40. Popovtzer MM. Disorders of calcium, phosphorus, vitamin D, and parathyroid hormone activity. In: Schrier RW, ed. *Renal and Electrolyte Disorders*. 6th ed. Philadelphia, PA: Lippincott Williams & Wilkins; 2003:216-277.

41. Hall TG, Schaiff RA. Update on the medical treatment of hypercalcemia of malignancy. *Clin Pharm*. 1993;12:117-125.

42. Randall RE, Straus MB, McNeely WF, et al. The milk-alkali syndrome. *Arch Intern Med*. 1961;107:63-81.

43. Bilezikian JP. Management of acute hypercalcemia. *N Engl J Med*. 1992;326:1196-1203.

44. Davis KD, Attie MF. Management of severe hypercalcemia. *Crit Care Clin*. 1991;7:175-190.

45. Delmez JA, Slatopolsky E. Hyperphosphatemia: its consequences and treatment in patients with chronic renal disease. *Am J Kidney Dis*. 1992;19:303-317.

46. Dennis VW. Phosphate disorders. In: Kokko JP, Tannen RL, eds. *Fluids and Electrolytes*. 3rd ed. Philadelphia, PA: WB Saunders; 1996:359-390.

47. Peppers MP, Geheb M, Desai T. Endocrine crises: hypophosphatemia and hyperphosphatemia. *Crit Care Clin*. 1991;7:201-214.

48. Halevy J, Bulvik S. Severe hypophosphatemia in hospitalized patients. *Arch Intern Med*. 1988;148:153-155.

49. Williams SR, ed. *Nutrition and Diet Therapy*. St. Louis, MO: CV Mosby; 1993.

50. Flodin N, ed. *Pharmacology of Micronutrients.* New York, NY: Alan R Liss; 1988.

51. Robinson CH, Lawler MR, Chenoweth WL, et al., eds. *Normal and Therapeutic Nutrition.* 7th ed. New York, NY: Macmillan; 1990.

52. Grant JP, Ross LH. Parenteral nutrition. In: Chernow B, ed. *The Pharmacologic Approach to the Critically Ill Patient.* 3rd ed. Baltimore, MD: Williams & Wilkins; 1994:1009-1033.

53. Lindeman RD. Minerals in medical practice. In: Halpern SL, ed. *Quick Reference to Clinical Nutrition.* 2nd ed. Philadelphia, PA: JB Lippincott; 1987:295-323.

54. Hurley LS. Clinical and experimental aspect of manganese in nutrition. In: Prasad AR, ed. *Clinical, Biochemical, and Nutritional Aspects of Trace Elements.* 1st ed. New York, NY: Alan R Liss; 1982:369-378.

55. Mertz W. Clinical and public health significance of chromium. In: Prasad AS, ed. *Clinical, Biochemical, and Nutritional Aspects of Trace Elements.* 1st ed. New York, NY: Alan R Liss; 1982:315-323.

56. De Haan KE, De Goeij JJ, Van Den Hamer CJ, et al. Changes in zinc metabolism after burns: observations, explanations, clinical implications. *J Trace Elem Electrolytes Health Dis.* 1992;6:195-201.

57. Foote JW, Delves HT. Albumin bound and alpha-2-macroglobumin bound zinc concentrations in the sera of healthy adults. *J Clin Pathol.* 1984;37:1050-1054.

58. Cefalu WT, Hu FB. Role of chromium in human health and in diabetes. *Diabetes Care.* 2004;27:2741-2751.

QUICKVIEW | Sodium

PARAMETER	DESCRIPTION	COMMENTS
Common reference ranges		
Adults	136–142 mEq/L (136–145 mmol/L)	Useful for assessment of fluid status
Pediatrics: premature infants	130–140 mEq/L (130–140 mmol/L)	
Pediatrics: older children	135–142 mEq/L (135–145 mmol/L)	
Critical value	>160 or <120 mEq/L (>160 or <120 mmol/L)	Acute changes more dangerous than chronic abnormalities
Natural substance?	Yes	Most abundant cation in extracellular fluid
Inherent activity?	Yes	Maintenance of transmembrane electric potential
Location		
Storage	Mostly in extracellular fluid	
Secretion/excretion	Filtered by kidneys, mostly reabsorbed; some secretion in distal nephron	Closely related to water homeostasis
Major causes of...		
High results	Multiple (discussed in text)	Can occur with low, normal, or high total body sodium
Associated signs and symptoms	Mostly neurological	List 6-2
Low results	Multiple (discussed in text)	Can occur with low, normal, or high total body sodium
Associated signs and symptoms	Mostly neurological	List 6-1
After insult, time to...		
Initial elevation or positive result	Hours to years, depending on chronicity	The faster the change, the more dangerous the consequences
Peak values	Hours to years, depending on chronicity	
Normalization	Days, if renal function is normal	Faster with appropriate treatment
Drugs often monitored with test	Diuretics, ACE inhibitors, aldosterone antagonists, angiotensin II antagonists, ADH analogs	Any drug that affects water homeostasis
Causes of spurious results	None	

ACE = angiotensin-converting enzyme; ADH = antidiuretic hormone.

QUICKVIEW | Potassium

PARAMETER	DESCRIPTION	COMMENTS
Common reference ranges		
Adults and pediatrics	3.8–5.0 mEq/L (3.8–5.0 mmol/L)	Age: >10 days old
Critical value	>7 or <2.5 mEq/L (>7 or <2.5 mmol/L)	Acute changes more dangerous than chronic abnormalities
Natural substance?	Yes	Most abundant cation; 98% in intracellular fluid
Inherent activity?	Yes	Control of muscle and nervous tissue excitability, acid–base balance, intracellular fluid balance
Location		
Storage	98% in intracellular fluid	
Secretion/excretion	Mostly secreted by distal nephron	Some via GI tract secretion
Major causes of...		
High results	Renal failure (GFR <10 mL/min)	Especially with increased intake
Associated signs and symptoms	Mostly cardiac	EKG changes, bradycardia, hypotension, cardiac arrest
Low results	Decreased intake or increased loss	Usually combination of the two
Associated signs and symptoms	Involves many physiological systems	List 6-5
After insult, time to...		
Initial elevation or positive result	Hours to years, depending on chronicity	The faster the change, the more dangerous the consequences
Peak values	Hours to years, depending on chronicity	
Normalization	Days, if renal function is normal	Faster with appropriate treatment
Drugs often monitored with test	Diuretics, ACE inhibitors, amphotericin B, angiotensin receptor antagonists, cisplatin	Potassium-containing preparations if renal failure present
Causes of spurious results	Hemolyzed samples (falsely elevated)	High potassium content in erythrocytes

ACE = angiotensin-converting enzyme; GFR = glomerular filtration rate; GI = gastrointestinal.

QUICKVIEW | Chloride

PARAMETER	DESCRIPTION	COMMENTS
Common reference ranges		
Adults and pediatrics	95–103 mEq/L (95–103 mmol/L)	
Critical value		Depends on underlying disorder
Natural substance?	Yes	
Inherent activity?	Yes	Primary anion in extracellular fluid and gastric juice, cardiac function, acid–base balance
Location		
Storage	Extracellular fluid	Most abundant extracellular anion
Secretion/excretion	Passively follows sodium and water	Also influenced by acid–base balance
Major causes of...		
High results	Dehydration	
	Acidemia	
Associated signs and symptoms	Associated with underlying disorder	
Low results	Nasogastric suction	
	Vomiting	
	Serum dilution	
	Alkalemia	
Associated signs and symptoms	Associated with underlying disorder	
After insult, time to...		
Initial elevation or positive result	Hours to years, depending on chronicity	The faster the change, the more dangerous the consequences
Peak values	Hours to years, depending on chronicity	
Normalization	Days, if renal function is normal	Faster with appropriate treatment of underlying disorder
Drugs often monitored with test	Same as with sodium	
Causes of spurious results	Bromides; iodides (falsely elevated)	

QUICKVIEW | Magnesium

PARAMETER	DESCRIPTION	COMMENTS
Common reference ranges		
Adults and pediatrics	1.3–2.1 mEq/L (0.65–1.05 mmol/L)	
Critical value	>5 or <1 mEq/L (>2.5 or <0.5 mmol/L)	Acute changes more dangerous than chronic abnormalities
Natural substance?	Yes	
Inherent activity?	Yes	Enzyme cofactor, thermoregulation, muscle contraction, nerve conduction, calcium and potassium homeostasis
Location		
Storage	50% bone, 45% intracellular fluid, 5% extracellular fluid	
Secretion/excretion	Filtration by kidneys	3% to 5% reabsorbed
Major causes of...		
High results	Renal failure	Usually in presence of increased intake
Associated signs and symptoms	Neuromuscular manifestations	Table 6-3
Low results	Excessive loss from GI tract or kidneys	Alcoholism and diuretics
	Decreased intake	
Associated signs and symptoms	Neuromuscular and cardiovascular manifestations including weakness, muscle fasciculations, tremor, tetany, increased reflexes, and EKG abnormalities	More severe with acute changes
After insult, time to...		
Initial elevation or positive result	Hours to years, depending on chronicity	The faster the change, the more dangerous the consequences
Peak values	Hours to years, depending on chronicity	
Normalization	Days, if renal function is normal	Faster with appropriate treatment
Drugs often monitored with test	Diuretics	
Causes of spurious results	Hemolyzed samples (falsely elevated)	

EKG = electrocardiogram; GI = gastrointestinal.

QUICKVIEW | Calcium

PARAMETER	DESCRIPTION	COMMENTS
Common reference ranges		
Adults	9.2–11.0 mg/dL (2.3–2.8 mmol/L)	Approximately half is bound to serum proteins; only ionized (free) calcium is physiologically active
Pediatrics	8–10.5 mg/dL (2–2.6 mmol/L)	
Critical value	>14 or <7 mg/dL (>3.5 or <1.8 mmol/L)	Also depends on serum albumin and pH values
Natural substance?	Yes	
Inherent activity?	Yes	Preservation of cellular membranes, propagation of neuromuscular activity, regulation of endocrine functions, blood coagulation, bone metabolism, phosphate homeostasis
Location		
Storage	99.5% in bone and teeth	Very closely regulated
Secretion/excretion	Filtration by kidneys	Small amounts excreted into GI tract from saliva, bile, and pancreatic and intestinal secretions
Major causes of…		
High results	Malignancy	Also thiazide diuretics, lithium, vitamin D, and calcium supplements
	Hyperparathyroidism	More severe with acute onset
Associated signs and symptoms	Vague GI complaints neurological and cardiovascular symptoms, and renal dysfunction	
Low results	Vitamin D deficiency	Hypocalcemia due to hypoalbuminemia is asymptomatic (ionized calcium concentration unaffected)
	Chronic kidney disease	
	Hypoparathyroidism	
	Hyperphosphatemia	
	Pancreatitis	
	Loop diuretics	
	Calcitonin	
	Hypoalbuminemia	
Associated signs and symptoms	Primarily neuromuscular (e.g., fatigue, depression, memory loss, hallucinations, seizures, tetany)	More severe with acute onset
After insult, time to…		
Initial elevation or positive result	Hours to years, depending on chronicity	The faster the change, the more dangerous the consequences
Peak values	Hours to years, depending on chronicity	
Normalization	Days, if renal function is normal	Faster with appropriate treatment
Drugs often monitored with test	Loop diuretics, calcitonin, vitamin D, calcium supplements, phosphate binders	
Causes of spurious results	Hypoalbuminemia	Ionized calcium concentration usually unaffected

GI = gastrointestinal.

QUICKVIEW | Phosphate

PARAMETER	DESCRIPTION	COMMENTS
Common reference ranges		
Adults	2.3–4.7 mg/dL (0.74–1.52 mmol/L)	
Pediatrics	4–7.1 mg/dL (1.3–2.3 mmol/L)	
Critical value	>8 or <1 mg/dL (>2.6 or <0.3 mmol/L)	Acute changes more dangerous than chronic abnormalities
Natural substance?	Yes	Most abundant intracellular anion
Inherent activity?	Yes	Bone and tooth integrity, cellular membrane integrity, phospholipid synthesis, acid–base balance, calcium homeostasis, enzyme activation, formation of high-energy bonds
Location		
Storage	Extracellular fluid, cell membrane structure, intracellular fluid, collagen, bone	85% in bone
Secretion/excretion	Filtration by kidneys	Mostly reabsorbed
Major causes of...		
High results	Decreased renal excretion	Renal failure the most common cause
	Extracellular shifting	
	Increased intake of phosphate or vitamin D	
Associated signs and symptoms	Due primarily to hypocalcemia and hyperparathyroidism	See Quickview for calcium (hypocalcemia)
Low results	Increased renal excretion	Also can occur in renal failure
	Intracellular shifting	
	Decreased intake of phosphate or vitamin D	
Associated signs and symptoms	Bone pain, weakness, malaise, hypocalcemia, cardiac failure, respiratory failure	Usually due to diminished intracellular ATP and erythrocyte 2,3-DPG concentrations
After insult, time to...		
Initial elevation or positive result	Usually over months to years	
Peak values	Usually over months to years	
Normalization	Over days with renal transplantation	
Drugs often monitored with test	Vitamin D, phosphate binders	
Causes of spurious results	Hemolyzed samples (falsely elevated) and methotrexate (falsely elevated)	

ATP = adenosine triphosphate.

QUICKVIEW | Copper

PARAMETER	DESCRIPTION	COMMENTS
Common reference ranges		
Adults	70–140 mcg/dL (11–22 μmol/L) (males); 80–155 mcg/dL (12–24 μmol/L) (females)	
Pediatrics	20–70 mcg/dL (3.1–11 μmol/L)	0–6 months
	90–190 mcg/dL (14.2–29.9 μmol/L)	6 years
	80–160 mcg/dL (12.6–25.2 μmol/L)	12 years
Critical value	Not applicable	
Natural substance?	Yes	
Inherent activity?	Yes	Companion to iron enzyme cofactor, hemoglobin synthesis, collagen and elastin synthesis, metabolism of many neurotransmitters, energy generation, regulation of plasma lipid levels, cell protection against oxidative damage
Location		
Storage	One-third in liver and brain; one-third in muscles; the rest in heart, spleen, kidneys, and blood (erythrocytes and neutrophils)	95% of circulating copper is protein bound as ceruloplasmin
Secretion/excretion	Mainly by biliary excretion; only 0.5% to 3% of daily intake found in urine	
Major causes of...		
High results	Deliberate ingestion of large amounts (>15 mg of elemental copper) Wilson disease	Uncommon in humans
Associated signs and symptoms	Nausea, vomiting, intestinal cramps, diarrhea	Larger ingestions lead to shock, hepatic necrosis, intravascular hemolysis, renal impairment, coma, and death
Low results	Infants with chronic diarrhea	
	Malabsorption syndromes	
	Decreased intake over months	
	Menkes syndrome	
Associated signs and symptoms	Neutropenia, iron-deficiency anemia, abnormal glucose tolerance, arrhythmias, hypercholesterolemia, atherosclerosis, depressed immune function, defective connective tissue formation, demineralization of bones	Can affect any system or organ whose enzymes require copper for proper functioning
Drugs often monitored with test	Copper supplements, possibly during chronic total parenteral nutrition	Serum copper concentrations not routinely monitored

QUICKVIEW | Zinc

PARAMETER	DESCRIPTION	COMMENTS
Common reference ranges		
Adults and pediatrics	50–150 mcg/dL (7.6–23 μmol/L)	Increased risk for developing symptomatic zinc deficiency
Critical value	<50 mcg/dL (<7.6 μmol/L)	
Natural substance?	Yes	
Inherent activity?	Yes	Enzyme constituent and cofactor; carbohydrate, protein, lipid, and nucleic acid metabolism; tissue growth; tissue repair; cell membrane stabilization; bone collagenase activity and collagen turnover; immune response; food intake control; spermatogenesis and gonadal maturation; normal testicular function
Location		
Storage	Liver, pancreas, spleen, lungs, eyes (retina, iris, cornea, lens), prostate, skeletal muscle, bone, erythrocytes, neutrophils	60% to 62% in skeletal muscle, 20% to 28% in bone, 2% to 4% in liver
Secretion/excretion	Primarily in pancreatic and intestinal secretions; also lost dermally through sweat, hair and nail growth, and skin shedding	Except in certain disease states, only 2% lost in urine
Major causes of...		
High results	Large intake	Uncommon in humans
Associated signs and symptoms	Drowsiness, lethargy, nausea, vomiting, diarrhea, increases in serum lipase and amylase concentrations	
Low results	Low intake (infants)	Rare from inadequate dietary intake
	Decreased absorption (acrodermatitis enteropathica)	
	Increased utilization (rapidly growing adolescents and menstruating, lactating, or pregnant women)	
	Increased loss (hyperzincuria)	
Associated signs and symptoms	Manifests in numerous organs and physiological systems	List 6-9
Drugs often monitored with test	Zinc supplements, possibly during chronic total parenteral nutrition	Serum zinc concentrations not routinely monitored
Causes of spurious results	Hemolyzed samples; 24-hr intrapatient variability	High zinc content in erythrocytes and neutrophils

QUICKVIEW | Manganese

PARAMETER	DESCRIPTION	COMMENTS
Common reference ranges		
Adults	Unknown normal range	
Pediatrics	2–3 mcg/L (36–55 μmol/L)	
	2.4–9.6 mcg/L (44–175 μmol/L)	Newborn
	0.8–2.1 mcg/L (15–38 μmol/L)	2–18 years
Critical value	Not applicable	
Natural substance?	Yes	
Inherent activity?	Yes	Enzyme cofactor; carbohydrate, protein, and lipid metabolism; protection of cells from free radicals; steroid biosynthesis; metabolism of biogenic amines; normal brain function
		Magnesium may substitute for manganese in most instances
Location		
Storage	Bone, liver, pancreas, pituitary gland	Circulating manganese loosely bound to transmanganin
Secretion/excretion	Primarily in biliary and pancreatic secretions; limited excretion in urine	Other GI routes also may be used in manganese overload
Major causes of...		
High results	Primarily through inhalation of manganese compounds, such as in manganese mines	One of least toxic trace elements
Associated signs and symptoms	Encephalopathy and profound neurological disturbances mimicking Parkinson disease	Accumulates in liver and brain
Low results	After several months of deliberate omission from diet	Rare from inadequate dietary intake
Associated signs and symptoms	Weight loss, slow hair and nail growth, hair color change, transient dermatitis, hypocholesterolemia, hypotriglyceridemia	Seen mostly in experimental subjects
Drugs often monitored with test	Manganese supplements, possibly during chronic total parenteral nutrition	Serum manganese concentration not routinely monitored

GI = gastrointestinal.

QUICKVIEW | Chromium

PARAMETER	DESCRIPTION	COMMENTS
Common reference ranges		
Adults	0.12–2.1 mcg/L (6–109 nmol/L)	Analysis of chromium in biological fluids and tissues is difficult
Pediatrics	Unknown	Analysis of chromium in biological fluids and tissues is difficult
Critical value	Unknown	
Natural substance?	Yes	
Inherent activity?	Yes	Cofactor for insulin and metabolism of glucose, cholesterol, and triglycerides
Location		
Storage	Hair, kidneys, skeleton, liver, spleen, lungs, testes, large intestines	Chromium circulates as free Cr3+, bound to transferrin and other proteins, and as organic complex
Secretion/excretion	Excretion in urine	Circulating insulin may affect excretion
Major causes of...		
Low results	Decreased intake	
Associated signs and symptoms	Glucose intolerance; hyperinsulinemia; hypercholesterolemia; possibly, risk of cardiovascular disease	Mainly due to its role as insulin cofactor
Drugs often monitored with test	Chromium supplement, possibly during chronic total parenteral nutrition	Serum chromium concentration not routinely monitored

CHAPTER 7

Pharmacogenomics and Molecular Testing

AMBER L. BEITELSHEES, ROSANE CHARLAB*

*The views expressed in this article are those of the author and may not necessarily represent FDA policy. No official endorsement is intended nor should be inferred.

Objectives

After completing this chapter, the reader should be able to

- Define pharmacogenetics

- Differentiate germline and somatic mutations

- Understand the use of molecular testing in pharmacogenetics/ genomics as tools for personalizing therapy

- Describe the difference between empirical pharmacotherapy and genotype-enhanced pharmacotherapy

- Understand how pharmacogenetics can enhance therapeutic drug monitoring

- Assess the utility of genotype in addition to other patient-specific factors for specific medications in the provision of pharmaceutical care

- Discuss the role of laboratory medicine in pharmacogenetics in terms of turnaround time, interpretative reporting, and assay performance

PHARMACOGENETICS

As early as the 1950s, the heritable nature of drug response was noted for agents such as succinylcholine, isoniazid, and primaquine.[1-3] Later, twin studies confirmed this heritability by showing that the half-lives of some drugs were tightly correlated in monozygotic twins and had little correlation in dizygotic twins.[4] Since that time, the fields of pharmacogenetics and pharmacogenomics have taken off ,and the genetic basis for variability in drug metabolism, transport, and pharmacodynamic effect is increasingly being appreciated. In fact, pharmacogenetic and molecular tests are routinely used in therapeutic areas such as hematology/oncology, and their usefulness is being explored in every major therapeutic drug class.[5]

Pharmacogenetics/pharmacogenomics is the translational science of correlating inter-individual genetic variation with variability in drug response. Historically and practically, the terms *pharmacogenetics* and *pharmacogenomics* have been used interchangeably (as in this chapter). However, definitions may vary depending on the context. For example, pharmacogenetics can be seen as the study of variants in a handful of candidate genes. Contrarily, because of our expanding technological ability to simultaneously investigate millions of variants across the human genome using either genomewide genotyping arrays or high-throughput sequencing, pharmacogenomics may refer to genomewide investigation of drug response variability.

Pharmacogenetics has the potential to provide personalized medicine to patients, much the same way therapeutic drug monitoring by serum drug concentrations customizes certain medication regimens for individual patients. One goal of pharmacogenetics is to refine the current empirical approach to drug therapy management so that it is less "trial-and-error" in nature. There are often many drug classes available to treat a given condition, and several drugs within each of those classes that a clinician may opt to use. This large armamentarium of drug therapy choices can lead to an inefficient, time-consuming management strategy in which the therapeutic decision is based on little more than clinician preference. Another goal of pharmacogenetics is to provide the appropriate dose to individual patients so that the "one dose fits all" strategy is avoided. Incorporating the results of genetic tests along with nongenetic factors (e.g., age, sex, smoking status, interacting drugs, and others) into the pharmacotherapy decision-making may help streamline this process such that the likelihood for response is maximized while the chance of toxicity is minimized.[6]

Understanding the results of molecular tests that are used in the application of pharmacogenetics is of critical importance to healthcare providers if this form of personalized medicine is going to improve patient care. Many institutions are attempting to implement preemptive genotyping so that results will be in the electronic medical record before a particular drug with a useful genetic test is prescribed. Furthermore, direct-to-consumer genetic tests are already available to patients, regardless of whether or not they have been proven to improve care. Despite the great promise of personalized medicine, the field is changing very rapidly and exactly how and when tests should be applied clinically is still very much a work in progress. Therefore, this chapter will focus on pharmacogenetic laboratory tests which are FDA-approved, used commonly in clinical practice, or are most likely to be incorporated into clinical practice in the near future.

Presently, organizations such as the National Academy of Clinical Biochemistry (NACB) have established practice guidelines for the application of pharmacogenetics in the practice of laboratory medicine.[7] Coordinately, clinical pharmacology groups such as the Clinical Pharmacogenetics Implementation Consortium (CPIC) have published practice guidelines for specific drug/gene pairs with clinical importance as data become available.[8] Taken together, guidelines from these organizations and others will likely be useful in bringing together the fields of laboratory medicine and clinical pharmacology in the application of pharmacogenetics. An overview of such guidelines and their implications will be discussed.

Pharmacogenetics Testing Versus Genetic Testing

While laboratory testing for pharmacogenetic and genetic polymorphisms/mutations will yield the same general types of results, the target populations and how the test results are used may be quite different. Clinically used pharmacogenetic tests provide information that may aid in selection or dosing of medications. Therefore, individuals receiving pharmacogenetic tests will typically be candidates for a particular therapeutic agent. Individuals receiving genetic tests, on the other hand, will usually be those who are at risk of developing or are suspected of having a particular disease or condition.

Historically, pharmacogenetic testing has been considered to have fewer ethical issues surrounding it than disease genetic testing.[9] However, while this is still generally considered to be the case, the risks of pharmacogenetic testing have also been outlined and a framework created to ensure appropriate delivery of pharmacogenetic information in the healthcare system.[10] This framework outlines three major considerations regarding whether a particular pharmacogenetic test raises ethical issues: whether the genetic variant is inherited or acquired, whether the goal of testing is to address a specific clinical question or to provide information for future clinical care, and whether the test reveals ancillary clinical information (e.g., disease risk).[10]

Pharmacogenetics and Personalized Medicine

Pharmacogenetics offers one piece to the puzzle of personalized medicine. Personalized medicine seeks to tailor medical therapy to individual characteristics of patients. It can include genetics information, as in pharmacogenetics, or any other molecular analyses (such as metabolomics, proteomics, etc.). This chapter will focus on pharmacogenetics as a means of providing personalized medicine.

DRUG DISPOSITION-RELATED MOLECULAR TESTS

Pharmacokinetics is concerned with the fate of drugs or other substances once administered and studies the rate and extent of **a**bsorption, **d**istribution, **m**etabolism, and **e**xcretion (ADME). As early as the 1950s, it was noted that a great deal of interpatient variability existed in the pharmacokinetics of many drugs. One common source of interpatient variability occurs in drug metabolism. Drug metabolism reactions can be

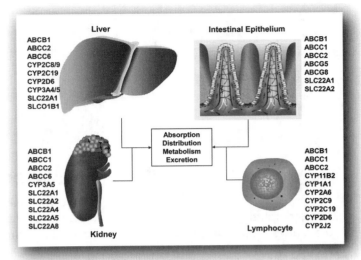

FIGURE 7-1. Sample polymorphic genes involved in drug pharmacokinetics. Polymorphic genes involved in drug pharmacokinetics are listed next to organs involved in drug absorption, distribution, metabolism, and excretion. VisiScience, Inc. software was used in the creation of the image.

divided into phase I, phase II, and phase III reactions. Phase I reactions typically involve processes such as oxidation, reduction, and hydrolysis of compounds and are typified by hepatic cytochrome P450 (CYP) drug metabolism. Phase II reactions include conjugation or synthetic reactions such as glucuronidation, sulfation, methylation, acetylation, and others. The purpose of phase II metabolism is to make compounds more water-soluble and facilitate excretion. Finally, phase III reactions are characterized by transport protein-mediated cellular efflux of drugs usually at the level of the gut, liver, kidney, and highly sequestered tissues. Genetic variability occurs in each of the above phases of drug disposition (Figure 7-1).

Cytochrome P450 System

While many of the genes encoding CYP enzymes are highly polymorphic, *CYP2D6*, *CYP2C9*, and *CYP2C19* have genetic variations (polymorphisms), which can describe fairly predictable distributions of drug concentrations, making them clinically relevant for some pharmacogenetic tests. Metabolizer status can be described as extensive (i.e., "normal"), intermediate, poor, or ultra-rapid based on the presence or absence of gene variations. The specific polymorphisms leading to these phenotypes are typically described using star (*) nomenclature as defined by the Cytochrome P450 Nomenclature Committee (http://www.cypalleles.ki.se), whereby the *1/*1 genotype is considered the common or normal, fully-functioning form of the gene. This genotype–phenotype relationship could help identify poor metabolizers likely to experience side effects (or therapeutic failure in the case of prodrugs requiring activation) to usual doses of CYP450-metabolized drugs or ultra-rapid metabolizers more prone to therapeutic failure (or toxicity in the case of prodrugs). The doses of these individuals with altered metabolism could then be increased or decreased as appropriate or alternative drugs chosen. This ability of genotype to predict drug metabolizing phenotype may be especially important for drugs with narrow therapeutic indices and less important for wide therapeutic index drugs.[11]

CYP2D6

The *CYP2D6* gene contains over 80 alleles, which can lead to normal-functioning, reduced- or nonfunctional protein, or even multiple copies of the gene. The most common nonfunctional alleles are *3, *4, *5, and *6. One of the most reproducible associations between *CYP2D6* genotype and a drug response occurs with codeine. Codeine is a prodrug requiring metabolism by CYP2D6 into its active form, morphine, for its analgesic effect. Therefore, individuals who are *CYP2D6* poor metabolizers are at risk of therapeutic failure and those who are ultra-rapid metabolizers are at risk of toxicity. Alternative analgesic therapy is recommended in both of these groups of patients. Guidelines have been published with recommendations for *CYP2D6* genetic testing interpretation and suggested clinical action for the test results.[12]

CYP2C19

The *CYP2C19* gene contains over 25 alleles leading to normal-, reduced-, non-, or over-functioning protein. The most common nonfunctional alleles are *2 and *3, which account for 85% of reduced function alleles in Caucasians and Africans and 99% of reduced function alleles in Asians. The other reduced or nonfunctional alleles, *4 to *8, are less common. The *17 allele is a gain-of-function allele and has a frequency of 3% to 20% depending on ethnicity.

One of the most clinically actionable associations between *CYP2C19* polymorphisms and a drug response is with clopidogrel. Clopidogrel is a prodrug requiring activation by two CYP450-dependent steps, both of which involve CYP2C19. Individuals carrying reduced function *CYP2C19* alleles have been shown to have lower active metabolite concentrations, reduced inhibition of platelet aggregation, and increased risk of adverse cardiovascular outcomes when treated with clopidogrel at standard doses compared to those without reduced function alleles.[13-17] Based on these data, the FDA updated the clopidogrel label to indicate that individuals with two reduced function *CYP2C19* alleles should receive alternative treatment or treatment strategies. Guidelines have been published with treatment recommendations based on *CYP2C19* genotype.[18]

CYP2C9

CYP2C9 contains over 30 alleles that lead to decreased or nonfunctional protein. The most common variants in *CYP2C9* are the *2 and *3 alleles. The *2 allele has a frequency of approximately 13% in whites, 0% in Asians, and 3% in blacks. The *3 allele has a frequency of approximately 7% in whites, 4% in Asians, and 2% in blacks. The most well-documented association with *CYP2C9* is with warfarin dose requirements (discussed below).

Other CYP450s

CYP3A4 contains over 30 reported polymorphisms, but these variations result in a unimodal distribution of drug clearance, lending themselves less well to use in the clinic setting. None of the discovered *CYP3A4* variants, with the exception of one rare variant—*20 (which has a frequency of less than 0.6% in Europeans)—result in nonfunctional protein.[19] This unimodal distribution likely results from the small contribution each individual polymorphism in the gene makes to phenotypic variation and the fact that environmental factors may play a bigger role in CYP3A4 activity than with other enzymes. *CYP3A5* has proved to have more predictable associations between polymorphisms and expression of CYP3A5 enzyme. Roughly 10% to 20% of whites, 85% of blacks, 60% of Hispanics, and 50% of east Asians have genetic variants in *CYP3A5* that cause them to express CYP3A5 hepatically and intestinally.[20] Consequently, this proportion of individuals may require dose modifications of CYP3A5-metabolized drugs, and in fact *CYP3A5* genetic variants have been implicated in variable drug responses for many drugs.

Thiopurine Methyltransferase

Thiopurine methyltransferase (TPMT) is the enzyme responsible for the conversion of azathioprine and 6-mercaptopurine into inactive metabolites (Figure 7-2). Genetic variants in the *TPMT* gene can result in deficient or absent TPMT activity leading to severe hematological adverse effects with azathioprine or 6-mercaptopurine (6-MP) treatment. The wild-type (common) allele in *TPMT* is designated *TPMT*1. The most common variants in *TPMT* are referred to as *TPMT*2, *3A, and *3C and are derived based on the presence or absence of any of three single nucleotide variants in the gene (G238→C; G460→A; and A719→G). Approximately one in 300 individuals possess two copies of these variant alleles and therefore lack TPMT activity. These individuals require dose reductions of thioguanines like 6-MP on the magnitude of 90% to avoid hematological toxicity. Individuals with one copy of a variant allele make up about 10% of the Caucasian population and require dose reductions of approximately 50%.

Azathioprine and 6-MP are used in the treatment of childhood acute lymphoblastic leukemia (ALL), rheumatoid arthritis, prevention of renal allograft rejection, and in the management of autoimmune disorders. In 2004, the FDA added language to the package insert of 6-MP indicating that *TPMT* genotyping or phenotyping should be considered prior to treatment.[21] Many major academic cancer hospitals routinely perform TPMT activity testing prior to 6-MP dosing for this indication and practice guidelines have been published.[22] Individuals with two deficient *TPMT* alleles (or deficient activity) require 10-fold starting dose reductions in order to avoid severe myelosuppression (recommendation classification strong).[22] Individuals with one deficient allele (or intermediate activity) have more variable dose requirements, with 30% to 60% of heterozygotes being unable to tolerate full doses. Starting dose reductions of 30% to 50% are recommended in heterozygotes (recommendation classification moderate).[22] Thiopurine methyltransferase activity can be determined either by enzymatic testing of red blood cell lysate or by genotyping. A study addressed the prevalence of TPMT enzyme and

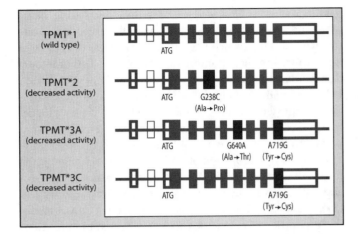

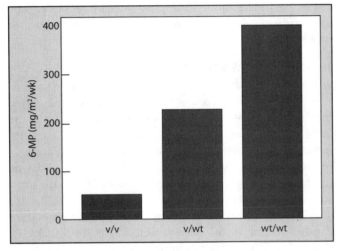

FIGURE 7-2. *TPMT* polymorphisms and 6-mercaptopurine dose requirements. (**A; top**) The *TPMT* gene structure is shown with exons indicated by boxes and introns as the horizontal line. The thin line box indicates exon 2, which is rarely expressed in the general population. Four major *TPMT* alleles are shown. The wild-type allele encodes a fully active enzyme, whereas the variant alleles *TPMT*2, *TPMT*3A, and *TPMT*3C, which together account for >95% of intermediate- and low-activity variants, encode proteins with decreased enzymatic activity. (**B; bottom**) Variable 6-MP dosage requirements for individuals with homozygous variant (v/v), heterozygous (v/wt), and homozygous wild-type (wt/wt) alleles. (Source: Reprinted from reference 70.)

genotype testing across a national survey of dermatologists, gastroenterologist, and rheumatologists in England.[23] Overall, TPMT enzyme testing was reportedly used by 67% of respondents. This testing was most frequently used by dermatologists (94%), followed by gastroenterologists (60%), and rheumatologists (47%). Genotype testing was not routinely available to practitioners participating in this survey and, hence, was only used by 5% of respondents.

It is important to note that the measurement of TPMT enzyme activity can be impacted by concurrent drugs such as salicylates and by recent blood transfusions. There has been some debate regarding whether genotyping or measurement of enzyme activity is superior.[24] Genotyping may be more useful at the start of therapy to minimize the likelihood of life-threatening toxicity, in the setting of blood transfusion (as phenotyping is inaccurate), and in bowel disease or rheumatoid arthritis where, unlike in leukemia, serial blood draws are not routinely performed. Phenotyping may be more useful after a disease flare (as a compliance measure), after several months of therapy (TPMT induction effect has been described), or at the time of an adverse event.

Dihydropyrimidine Dehydrogenase

Dihydropyrimidine dehydrogenase (DPD) metabolizes 5-fluorouracil, an agent commonly used in the treatment of solid organ tumors. In the mid-1980s, it was recognized that deficiencies in DPD were heritable and associated with severe 5-fluorouracil toxicity.[25,26] Many polymorphisms in the gene encoding DPD, *DPYD*, have been identified, although very few of them have any effect on enzyme activity. An intronic polymorphism, IVS14 +1 G>A (*DPYD*2A) has been the most widely studied and has been found in approximately half of cases of DPD deficiency. Other common polymorphisms, which have been assessed and found in cases of DPD deficiency, are 2846 A>T and 1679 T>G.

As with TPMT testing, DPD deficiency can be tested for genetically or with enzymatic testing. The analytical performance of using genetic testing to predict toxicity has ranged from 6.3% to 83% for sensitivity, 82% to 100% for specificity (although specificity was not determinable in most studies evaluated), 62% to 100% for positive predictive value, and 86% to 94% for negative predictive value (again, not determinable for most studies).[27] Fewer studies have evaluated the test performance characteristics of enzymatic testing, but two that did had a sensitivity of 60%.[27]

Clinical Significance

When deciding whether drug metabolism polymorphisms might be clinically significant for particular drugs, three main factors should be considered. First, is the drug metabolism enzyme of interest an important route of elimination for the drug in question? If not, even functional polymorphisms in this gene are not going to have a great impact on the pharmacokinetics of the drug. Second, does the medication of interest have a narrow therapeutic index or steep exposure/response curve? If not, changes in plasma concentrations may not be great enough to influence the dose-response relationship. Last, are other therapeutic alternatives available to the medication in question? If so, these alternatives may have other routes of metabolism that are not polymorphic, and the variability in pharmacokinetics could be avoided altogether.

DRUG-TARGET-RELATED MOLECULAR TESTS

While pharmacokinetics is concerned with ADME, pharmacodynamics is concerned with drug effects on target molecules, tissues, and physiological processes. There are abundant examples of pharmacogenetic studies in the literature, where the candidate gene of interest was one related to drug target physiology (vis-à-vis drug metabolism).[5] Furthermore, there are illustrative examples in cardiology and oncology where consideration of genetic variation may improve drug therapy. In oncology, in addition to germline (inherited) variations, tumor cells can also exhibit acquired or noninherited (somatic) variations only present in the tumor tissue. This adds a layer of complexity to molecular testing, involving the acquisition and processing of tumor tissue with adequate quality and quantity to accommodate the test of interest. Moreover, laboratories performing specialized testing should have demonstrated proficiency in the specific technology being used. This section deals with five such drugs: the anticoagulant warfarin, the breast cancer drug trastuzumab, the lung and pancreatic cancer drug erlotinib, the lung cancer drug crizotinib, and the melanoma drug vemurafenib.

Warfarin

Warfarin is the most commonly prescribed anticoagulant for the treatment and prevention of thrombosis. Despite its widespread use, warfarin has a narrow therapeutic range (as measured by the international normalized ratio [INR]) below which thrombosis risk is increased and above which bleeding risk is increased. While patient-specific factors such as age, sex, race, and diet partially explain variability in warfarin response, these factors don't reliably predict the likelihood for efficacy or bleeding risk. As such, investigators have studied the role of genetic variants in an enzyme responsible for warfarin's metabolism *(CYP2C9)* and target gene *(VKORC1)* on warfarin responses. These studies have investigated the impact of genetic and nongenetic factors on endpoints related to INR, bleeding, and clinical efficacy.

CYP2C9 is the major metabolic route for the more potent warfarin enantiomer. The *CYP2C9*1* allele is associated with full metabolic capacity, while the well-studied *2 and *3 alleles are associated with decreased activity, diminished warfarin clearance, and lower warfarin dose requirements.[28-33] By extension, these variant carriers exhibit longer than normal time to achieve target INR and are at increased risk for bleeding.[34] More recently, pharmacogenetic studies have also included analysis of *VKORC1* polymorphisms. Taken in sum, *CYP2C9* and *VKORC1* polymorphisms when considered with clinical correlates of warfarin dose explain approximately 50% of the variability in warfarin dose requirements.[35,36] Dosing algorithms including *CYP2C9*, *VKORC1*, and clinical information are continually being developed and tested, and the FDA updated the warfarin label with estimated doses by genotype.[37-39] The Couma-Gen study demonstrated the feasibility of performing prospective comparisons of pharmacogenetic-guided versus traditional dosing of warfarin, and the National Institutes of Health has a large prospective analysis of warfarin pharmacogenetics that is underway.[40] Guidelines have also been published with recommendations for clinical interpretation of warfarin pharmacogenetics data.[39]

Trastuzumab

Trastuzumab is a monoclonal antibody against the human epidermal growth factor receptor 2 (HER2), encoded by the *ERBB2* gene and represents a modality for the treatment of breast cancer. It was noted in the early drug development process that trastuzumab was only effective in a subset of patients. It was subsequently elucidated that trastuzumab is only effective in breast cancers that overexpress the HER2 protein, representing approximately 25% of breast cancer tumors. Consequently, treatment with trastuzumab is predicated on this molecular diagnostic and accurate classification of HER2 tumor status is necessary for optimum treatment of HER2-positive tumors. While not a test for genetic polymorphisms per se, HER2 testing is performed by methods including immunohistochemistry (IHC) and fluorescence in situ hybridization (FISH) to determine the HER2 overexpression and gene amplification, respectively.[41] Both IHC and FISH assays have been approved by the FDA for HER2 testing.[42]

Clinically, tumor biopsies are obtained from individuals with breast cancer in which trastuzumab may be an option. Immunohistochemistry is often used as initial screening for HER2/neu overexpression because of its more routine availability in clinical laboratories and lower cost than FISH. Guidelines regarding HER2 testing have recently been updated.[42,43] In one algorithm, a semiquantitative IHC test is performed on the tissue sample to determine the extent of HER2 overexpression. Samples with scores of 0/1+ are considered negative; those with scores of 2+ are borderline/equivocal; 3+ tissues are considered positive.[42,44] In cases of borderline specimens, FISH is recommended for subsequent evaluation with a FISH ratio greater than 2.0 generally considered a positive test.

The test performance characteristics of IHC and FISH have been well described. For example, in analysis of approximately 3,000 breast cancer specimens, the positive predictive value of IHC (3+) was 92%, and the negative predictive value (0 or 1+) was 97%.[45] These molecular tests are widely available and used clinically in the setting of breast cancer treatment with trastuzumab. Furthermore, the techniques are not limited to breast tumors and are likely to be extended to other disease states and drug therapies in which gene product expression is a determinant of clinical responsiveness.

More recently, trastuzumab has been approved in combination with chemotherapy as an option for the treatment of patients with HER2-overexpressing metastatic gastric cancer, or gastroesophageal junction (GEJ) adenocarcinoma. Due to differences in tumor histopathology (breast or gastric/GEJ adenocarcinoma), tests developed for the specific tumor type to assess HER2 protein overexpression and HER2 gene amplification should be used.[46]

Erlotinib

Erlotinib is an epidermal growth factor receptor tyrosine kinase inhibitor (EGFR-TKI). Much like HER2 discussed above, EGFR aberrant signaling is associated with development and prognosis of certain cancers, and EGFR inhibition with drugs such as erlotinib results in blockage of important processes in the pathogenesis of these cancers. Erlotinib is currently used for the treatment of non-small cell lung cancer (NSCLC) and pancreatic cancer.

Increased sensitivity to EGFR-TKIs in NSCLC has been linked to the presence of EGFR activating mutations in the tumor (mostly in exons 18 to 21 of the *EGFR* gene). These mutations are most common in women, Asian individuals, never-smokers, and patients with adenocarcinoma histology.[47] In a 2004 landmark study, Lynch and colleagues identified mutations in the *EGFR* gene in tumors of patients with NSCLC who were responsive to gefitinib, another EGFR-TKI.[48] Sensitivity and specificity were 89% and 100%, respectively; positive and negative predictive values were 100% and 88%. Since this publication, several clinical trials have prospectively tested the impact of somatic *EGFR*-activating mutations on clinical response to TKIs (e.g., gefitinib and erlotinib) among lung cancer patients. Results from these studies have underscored the importance of *EGFR* mutation testing in guiding therapy choices for advanced NSCLC.[49,50] Approximately 20% of lung adenocarcinomas harbor an *EGFR* activation mutation (this frequency can be higher in East Asians), and several methods are being used to detect these mutations in tumor tissues with different performance characteristics.[51]

Crizotinib

Crizotinib is a multitargeted receptor tyrosine kinase inhibitor of anaplastic lymphoma kinase (ALK) and potentially other kinases. Different lung cancer subsets can be molecularly defined by the presence of specific "driver" mutations (e.g., EGFR-activating mutations), which are key in tumor pathogenesis. These driver molecular alterations are being targeted for therapy, and the prospective genotyping of lung cancers is becoming a new standard of care.[52] One of these unique molecular subsets is characterized by rearrangements involving the *ALK* gene. In NSCLC, the *EML4-ALK* is the most commonly reported *ALK* rearrangement. The resulting fusion gene encodes a cytoplasmic chimeric protein with constitutive kinase activity and tumor promoting potential. *EML4-ALK* occurs in approximately 5% of unselected NSCLC, and is more common in never- or light-smokers, in young adult patients, and in patients with adenocarcinomas. Multiple distinct *EML4-ALK* chimeric variants, as well as other ALK fusion partners have been reported.[53]

Crizotinib was developed along with a companion diagnostic and is indicated for locally advanced or metastatic NSCLC with *ALK* rearrangements, as detected by an FDA-approved test. Therefore, the detection of *ALK*-positive NSCLC is necessary for selection of patients for treatment with crizotinib. The companion diagnostic test currently available is a FISH Break Apart assay. This assay employs one probe 5' of the *ALK* locus and one probe within the *ALK* gene. When the probe set is hybridized against normal nuclei, it generates a merged (green–red fluorescent) signal that can be visualized microscopically. However, the signal is split when the probe set is hybridized against nuclei with a rearrangement involving the 5' portion of the *ALK* locus. To be considered positive

for *ALK* rearrangements and eligible for treatment with crizotinib, at least 15% of the tumor cells analyzed have to harbor either the break-apart signals or have a single 3' *ALK* (red) signal, 50 cells or more have to be counted, and the separation between the 5' and 3' *ALK* probes has to be at least two signal diameter.[54,55] Other tests are being developed as alternatives to FISH, including IHC and reverse transcription polymerase chain reaction (RT-PCR), which has the potential of identifying fusion variants missed by FISH.[56,57]

Vemurafenib

Vemurafenib is a BRAF serine-threonine kinase inhibitor indicated for patients with advanced melanoma harboring a somatic V600E mutation in the *BRAF* gene. Mutated BRAF proteins often have elevated kinase activity leading to aberrant activation of survival and anti-apoptotic signaling pathways in the tumor cells.[58] As with crizotinib, vemurafenib was also developed along with a companion diagnostic.[59] The assay is a PCR-based system that detects *BRAF* V600E mutations in paraffin-embedded, formalin-fixed tumor samples. Approximately 40% to 60% of cutaneous melanomas are positive for *BRAF* V600 mutations. Among these, the V600E mutations constitute 80% to 90% of reported V600 *BRAF* mutations, but other mutations such as V600K and V600D can also occur in this disease setting. During vemurafenib's phase III pivotal trial, 10 *BRAF* V600 positive patients (as identified by the Cobas test) were subsequently found to harbor the V600K mutation using DNA sequencing. Four of these patients still had partial responses to the drug.[59] These results suggest that melanoma patients with V600 mutations other than V600E such as V600K may still be sensitive to vemurafenib and highlight the importance of understanding the performance of tests used to determine eligibility to therapy. Vemurafenib has not been studied in patients with wild-type *BRAF* melanoma, and is not recommended for this population.

Resistance to Targeted Therapy

Only a percentage of patients respond to targeted therapies. Moreover, responders often develop resistance. Elucidating underlying mechanisms of primary or acquired resistance at a molecular level is an intense area of research in oncology. For example, somatic point mutations in the *KRAS* gene, most commonly found in codons 12 and 13, have been strongly associated with primary resistance to the anti-EGFR monoclonal antibodies panitumumab and cetuximab in colorectal cancer. Therefore, these antibodies are not indicated for colorectal cancer patients with tumors positive for these mutations. Of note, different *KRAS* mutations may not predict in the same extent resistance to anti-EGFR antibodies.[60] Point mutations, gene amplifications, changes in protein expression and activation of alternate pathways are among the mechanisms implicated in resistance.[61] Molecular assays are being developed to identify these alterations and evaluate their clinical significance.

IMMUNE-RELATED MOLECULAR TESTS

Variants in immune-related genes are increasingly being associated with drug-induced adverse events. One of the most

Clopidogrel Pharmacogenetics

CHARLES B. IS A 59-YEAR-OLD African-American male who presents to the emergency department with chest pain. His cardiac enzymes and electrocardiogram are consistent with an acute coronary syndrome (ACS) and a percutaneous coronary intervention (PCI) with stent implantation is immediately planned. A decision is made to start Charles B. on clopidogrel per the hospital's standard ACS protocol.

PMH

Hypertension x 20 years
Hyperlipidemia x 10 years

Social history

Smoked 1.5 packs per day x 38 years; quit 10 years ago

Medications

HCTZ 25 mg daily
Verapamil SR 240 mg daily
Atorvastatin 40 mg daily

Weight: 77 kg

Height: 68"

BP: 138/88

HR: 90

Question: Variations in which candidate genes could be expected to impact clopidogrel effectiveness?

Answer: Clopidogrel is a prodrug that needs to be biotransformed to an active metabolite to exert its antiplatelet activity. The metabolism of clopidogrel to its active metabolite is a two-step process that involves the following cytochrome P450s: CYP1A2, CYP2B6, CYP2C9, CYP2C19, and CYP3A4/5. Variations in any of these genes could conceivably be associated with variable formation of the active metabolite with consequent variability in antiplatelet effects and clinical efficacy. In fact, several of these genes have been studied from a pharmacogenetic perspective, with *CYP2C19* being the most widely studied and consistently associated. In addition to drug metabolism enzymes, the p-glycoprotein transporter, encoded by the *ABCB1* gene has also been found in some studies to influence clopidogrel response and the paraoxonase I, encoded by *PON1*, has been identified in one study but not replicated in others. From a pharmacodynamic perspective, the P2Y12 platelet receptor (encoded by *P2RY12*) is the target of clopidogrel activity and has been associated with clopidogrel efficacy in some studies, although with no robust associations that currently influence treatment recommendations.

Charles B. had been previously seen in a progressive cardiovascular clinic for the management of his hypertension and dyslipidemia. As part of routine practice, preemptive genotyping for "VIPs" (Very Important Pharmacogenes) was performed several months ago. Charles B.'s *CYP2C19* genotype status according to his electronic medical record is as follows: *CYP2C19 *2/*2* (homozygous for loss-of-function allele).

Question: How would this genotype be expected to impact clopidogrel effectiveness in Charles B.?

Answer: CYP2C19 is involved in both steps of clopidogrel's two-step transformation to its active metabolite. *CYP2C19* is polymorphic with common alleles including *1 (normal activity), *2 and *3 (loss of activity), and *17 (increased activity). Patients are assigned the following likely drug metabolism phenotypes based on their genotypes: ultra-rapid metabolizer (UM): *1/*17, *17/*17; extensive metabolizer (EM): *1/*1; intermediate metabolizer (IM): *1/*2, *1/*3, *2/*17, *3/*17; poor metabolizer (PM): *2/*2, *2/*3, *3/*3. Charles B. is a PM, and PMs are prevalent in about 2% to 15% of the population and have the lowest levels of clopidogrel active metabolite, antiplatelet activity, and worse cardiovascular outcomes compared with EMs. Because of a growing body of evidence suggesting that PMs are at significant risk for not experiencing a treatment benefit when given clopidogrel, the FDA updated the clopidogrel label with a boxed warning in 2010. Specifically, the label notes that "[PMs] treated with [clopidogrel] at recommended doses exhibit higher cardiovascular event rates following ACS or PCI than patients with normal CYP2C19 function" and that one should "consider alternative treatment or treatment strategies in patients identified as CYP2C19 [PMs]."

Question: What possible courses of action are there for people with Charles B.'s genotype in his clinical context?

Answer: The FDA recommends alternative treatments or treatment strategies for known CYP2C19 PMs in the ACS or PCI contexts. Alternative treatments may include antiplatelet agents that are not susceptible to polymorphic metabolism in a clinically significant way (e.g., prasugrel or ticagrelor). Alternative treatment strategies might include increased clopidogrel doses beyond the standard 75 mg daily dose. Pharmacodynamic studies suggest that increased clopidogrel doses of 225 mg per day in IMs achieve platelet inhibition comparable to the standard 75mg dose in EMs, but that increased doses up to 300 mg per day cannot achieve comparable platelet inhibition in PMs.[62] Currently, the CPIC recommends PMs and IMs receive prasugrel or alternative therapy if no contraindications exist (classification of recommendation: strong for PMs, moderate for IMs). The guidelines recommend UMs and EMs receive clopidogrel at the standard label-recommended doses.

noted examples is that of abacavir. Immune-mediated hypersensitivity reactions occur in 5% to 8% of abacavir-treated patients, usually within the first 6 weeks of treatment. Retrospective case-control studies identified the major histocompatibility complex (MHC) Class I region as being associated with this hypersensitivity reaction.[63] Subsequent, prospective randomized-controlled trials demonstrated that screening for the *HLA-B**5701 allele eliminated immunologically-confirmed hypersensitivity reaction with a negative predictive value of 100% and a positive predictive value of 47.9%.[64] Current HIV treatment guidelines recommend screening for *HLA-B**5701 prior to the initiation of an abacavir-containing treatment regimen.[65]

Since the association between HLA genotype and abacavir hypersensitivity reaction was identified, severe adverse effects with many other drugs have been noted to be associated with MHC regions as well. Some examples of these associations are phenytoin-induced cutaneous reactions and *HLA-B**1502,

HER2 Testing

RACHEL K., DIAGNOSED WITH METASTATIC GASTRIC ADENOCARCI-NOMA, has not received prior treatment for metastatic disease. She had a tumor sample (resection specimen) tested for HER2 overexpression by IHC to determine eligibility for treatment with trastuzumab. Although the laboratory had available the FDA-approved test for HER2 testing in gastric cancer, it used breast cancer scoring criteria to determine HER2 positivity on the gastric cancer sample because it was more familiar with its use. Rachel K.'s tumor sample had strong basolateral membranous reactivity in 10% of cells. For breast cancer, the cutoff has been increased from 10% to 30%, and the completeness of membrane staining (circumferential staining) is a condition for positivity. The gastric sample was classified as HER2-negative and was not retested by FISH. Rachel K. was not offered trastuzumab therapy.

Question: Do you agree on using breast scoring system for HER2 testing in Rachel K.?

Answer: As in breast cancer, patients with HER2-positive metastatic disease whose tumors are IHC 3+ or IHC 2+/FISH-positive are eligible for trastuzumab therapy. However, the HER2 testing scoring criteria are significantly different due to higher intratumor heterogeneity in gastric cancer (compared to breast cancer) and to variations in the pattern of membrane staining. In gastric tumor cells, the HER2 receptors are predominantly expressed at the basolateral surface, and due to the biology of the tumor, the circularity (IHC membrane staining pattern) is mostly missing (often only lateral in IHC 2+/3+) but is a must in IHC

2+/3+ breast cancer sample.[68] The number of stained cells needed to consider a case HER2 positive is also different. The required percent of membrane staining in resections is 10% for positive HER2 status in gastric cancer (versus the accepted 30% in breast). Moreover, different criteria are also applied for gastric biopsy specimens versus resected (surgical) specimens. Due to the potential heterogeneity of HER2 positivity in gastric tumors, not all biopsies may appear HER2-positive and approximately six to eight biopsies are needed for accurate testing compared to usually only one in breast cancer. Therefore, scoring systems for breast cancer must not be used on gastric samples. Of note, also due to gastric cancer histological heterogeneity, bright-field methodologies (such as chromogenic in situ hybridization [CISH] or silver in situ hybridization [SISH]) may be useful in identifying HER2-positive tumor foci within a heterogeneous sample.[68] Studies are required to compare the results obtained with various methodologies in gastric cancer.

Rachel K. was incorrectly diagnosed as HER2-negative because breast criteria were used rather than gastric criteria for HER2 testing. Applying the breast cancer testing principles (including biospecimen considerations) and scoring criteria to determine HER2 status in gastric cancer patients may result in the underscoring and impact treatment choices.[68] When considering molecular tests for personalizing therapies, it is imperative to follow established guidelines and use appropriate technologies from laboratories with expertise in performing and interpreting the results in order to provide accurate test results. It is also important to keep in mind that test result interpretation must be made within the context of the patient's clinical history by a qualified professional.

carbamazepine-induced cutaneous reactions and *HLA-B**1502 as well as *HLA-A**3101, flucloxacillin (not currently available in the United States)-induced liver injury and *HLA-B**5701, amoxicillin-clavulanate-induced liver injury and *HLA-A**0201 and *HLA-DRB1**1501-*DQB1**0602, lumiracoxib (not currently available in the United States)-induced liver injury and *HLA-DQA1**0102, and allopurinol-induced cutaneous reactions and *HLA-B**5801.[66,67]

GENOTYPING PLATFORMS AND TEST PERFORMANCE AND DECISION-MAKING

Genotyping Platforms

Commercial genetic tests are available for several pharmacogenetic-related panels. The AmpliChip® (Roche Molecular Diagnostics, Basel, Switzerland) microarray provides analysis for *CYP2D6* and *CYP2C19* genotypes in order to predict enzymatic activities. The assay tests for up to 33 *CYP2D6* alleles, including gene duplications, and three *CYP2C19* variants and includes software to predict the drug metabolism phenotype based on the combination of alleles present (e.g., extensive, intermediate, poor, and ultra-rapid metabolizers). Another such product is the DMET (Drug Metabolizing Enzymes and Transporters) Plus® (Affymetrix, Santa Clara, CA) Micro-Array that assesses over 1,900 drug metabolism-related

polymorphisms in approximately 230 genes. The platform also includes software that translates genotypes into standardized star allele nomenclature.

These prototypical drug metabolism genotyping arrays do have two limitations with which the clinician should be familiar: (1) new alleles that alter metabolic function are constantly being discovered, so there are patients who will not be perfectly assigned to a drug metabolism group or could be inappropriately assigned the *1/*1 genotype by default because these alleles are untested; and (2) since these chips are not directly measuring metabolic activity or drug concentrations, the effect of drug interactions on the drug metabolizing phenotype are not captured by the test. In other words, a person may genotypically be an extensive metabolizer but phenotypically be a poor metabolizer because they are taking a drug that inhibits the particular CYP450 enzyme. This limitation highlights the importance of proper patient-specific interpretation of CYP genotyping results in clinical practice.

The cost of pharmacogenetic testing varies depending on the number of alleles being tested. The turnaround time also varies but is usually 24–96 hours. In institutions where the clinical laboratory is on site, turnaround could be as fast as 4 hours depending on the assay being run. Generally, clinicians have increased confidence in genotyping results that are generated from certified labs (such as those approved or certified by the

Clinical Laboratory Improvements Amendments (CLIA) or the College of Pathologists (CAP).

Test Performance and Decision-Making

Laboratory testing and clinical decision-making using pharmacogenetics can be incorporated into the total testing process (TTP) as outlined by Shumacher and Barr.[69] The TTP is divided into the preanalytical, analytical, and postanalytical phases and is designed to systematically improve patient care by asking a patient-oriented question, determining and ordering the appropriate test to answer the question, collecting and processing the sample, performing the test, reporting and interpreting the results, and taking clinical action to positively impact the patient.

Total testing process is well established in therapeutic drug monitoring using serum drug concentrations, where the appropriate test (e.g., free or total drug concentration) is ordered, the phlebotomist draws the appropriate sample (e.g., steady-state peak or trough), the results are reported and interpreted in the context of the patient's status (e.g., exhibiting signs of toxicity), and a clinical decision is made (e.g., dosage change or drug discontinuation). The TTP applied to pharmacogenetics is somewhat more complex. Firstly, with the exception of a few cases as described above, the relationship between genotype and clinical phenotype (e.g., toxicity or effectiveness) is not strong enough for any one test to be the "best" test. In fact, since variations exist in genes that encode for transport proteins involved in absorption, drug metabolizing enzymes, receptors, and intracellular proteins, a multiple-gene approach (i.e., a battery of pharmacogenetic tests) may be most appropriate. Secondly, because of potential associations with diseases and prognoses independent of drug effects, informed consent will in all likelihood be required for genotyping.

Perhaps the biggest barrier to application of pharmacogenetics is the inability to apply genotype results. This would require an adequate knowledge of the literature with respect to genetic associations and clinical outcomes. In this regard, the TTP as applied to pharmacogenetics could be interdisciplinary, involving physicians, translational scientists, clinical pharmacists, and others. Additionally, accreditation standards such as those put forth by The Joint Commission (TJC), CLIA, CAP and others will have to be addressed when formally incorporating pharmacogenetic testing into institution-based practice.

As mentioned elsewhere in the chapter, organizations including the NACB and CPIC are working in a multidisciplinary fashion to address issues related to pharmacogenetic test methodology; standardization and quality control/assurance of tests; selection of appropriate test panels; reporting and interpretation of results; and other issues related to testing applied in clinical practice.[7,8] While expansive in its scope, the NACB guidelines specifically highlight the role of the clinical laboratory in development of genotyping strategies that maximize test performance (i.e., sensitivity and specificity) for clinical application. Furthermore, the guideline recommendations develop criteria for a pharmacogenetic test to be clinically useful. These criteria include *analytical reliability* (consistent measurement of the genotype/allele tested), *operational implementation* (operational characteristics should not be beyond the complexity level certified by CLIA for reference laboratories); *clinical predictive power* (specificity and sensitivity consistent with other diagnostics in use); and *compatibility with therapeutic management* (interpretation of genotype results should inform clinical decision-making). Interestingly, model examples outlined by the guidelines for drugs in which pharmacogenetics can be implemented include warfarin (*CYP2C9* and *VKORC1*) and irinotecan (*UGT1A1*). The CPIC has taken the approach of publishing clinical practice guidelines for specific drug/gene pairs as enough data become available to warrant clinical action based on genotype. A sample of drug products that contain pharmacogenetic information in their labeling is shown in Table 7-1.

SUMMARY

Pharmacogenetics is currently being used most widely in hematology/oncology and holds the promise of improving patient care by adding another dimension to therapeutic drug monitoring in other diseases. The use of genetic information will likely be applied to chronic drug therapy for agents with narrow therapeutic indices such as warfarin. The field of pharmacogenetics is evolving rapidly. Consequently, specific information regarding molecular tests and labeling information are likely to constantly change. Basic skills in interpreting genetic information will serve as an important foundation for laboratory medicine and drug therapy as more clinical applications of pharmacogenetics emerge.

In order for pharmacogenetics to translate to practice, the research and clinical communities jointly must create a meaningful level of evidence in support of pharmacogenetics-enhanced therapeutic decision-making. Because of their unique training and position in the healthcare sector, pharmacists can foresee the forefront of pharmacogenetics research and application. Pharmacists will likely be called upon to synthesize evidence-based practices for incorporating genetic information into treatment algorithms. Once a genetic biomarker is validated (e.g., warfarin pharmacogenetics), clinicians (including pharmacists) will be responsible for appropriate use and interpretation of the genetic test. The pharmacist's drug and disease expertise, coupled with an understanding of pharmacogenetic principles, may lead to a revolutionary treatment paradigm with enhanced patient outcomes as the ultimate goal.

TABLE 7-1. Sample Package Inserts with Pharmacogenetic Information Included[a,b]

DRUG	EXAMPLES OF OTHER DRUGS ASSOCIATED WITH BIOMARKER	BIOMARKER	LABEL SECTIONS[a]
Abacavir		HLA-B* 5701	Boxed warning, contraindications, warnings and precautions, patient counseling information
Atomoxetine	Venlafaxine, risperidone, tiotroprium bromide, tamoxifen, timolol maleate	CYP2D6	Dosage and administration, warnings and precautions, drug interactions, clinical pharmacology
Azathioprine	6-mercaptopurine, thioguanine	TPMT	Precautions, drug interactions, adverse reactions, clinical pharmacology
Boceprevir		IL28B	Clinical pharmacology
Busulfan		Philadelphia chromosome deficiency	Clinical studies
Capecitabine	Fluorouracil cream, fluorouracil topical solution and cream	DPD deficiency	Contraindications, precautions, patient information
Carbamazepine		HLA-B* 1502	Boxed warning, warnings and precautions
Cetuximab		KRAS and EGFR	Indications and usage, warnings and precautions, description, clinical pharmacology, clinical studies
Clopidogrel		CYP2C19	Boxed warning, dosage and administration, warnings and precautions, drug interactions, clinical pharmacology
Crizotinib		ALK	Indications and usage, warnings and precautions, adverse reactions, clinical pharmacology, clinical studies
Fluoxetine	Codeine, olanzapine, cevimeline hydrochloride, tolterodine, terbinafine, tramadol + acetaminophen, clozapine, aripiprazole, metoprolol, propranolol, carvedilol, propafenone	CYP2D6	Warnings, precautions, clinical pharmacology
Imatinib mesylate		C-KIT	Indications and usage, dosage and administration, clinical pharmacology, clinical studies
Imatinib mesylate		Ph chromosome	Indications and usage, dosage and administration, clinical pharmacology, clinical studies
Imatinib mesylate		PDGFR	Indications and usage, dosage and administration, clinical studies
Imatinib mesylate		FIP1L1-PDGFRa	Indications and usage, dosage and administration, clinical studies
Irinotecan		UGT1A1	Dosage and administration, warnings, clinical pharmacology
Rifampin, isoniazid, and pyrazinamide	Isosorbide dinitrate and hydralazine hydrochloride	NAT1; NAT2	Adverse reactions, clinical pharmacology
Trastuzumab		HER2/neu	Indications and usage, precautions, clinical pharmacology
Tretinoin	Arsenic oxide	PML/RAR alpha gene expression	Boxed warning, dosage and administration, precautions
Vemurafenib		BRAF V600E	Indications and usage, warning and precautions, clinical pharmacology, clinical studies, patient counseling information
Voriconazole	Omeprazole, pantoprazole, esomeprazole, diazepam, nelfinavir, rabeprazole	CYP2C19	Clinical pharmacology, drug interactions
Warfarin		CYP2C9 and VKORC1	Dosage and administration, precautions, clinical pharmacology

[a]For primary drug listed.
[a]Not a comprehensive listing. Based on http://www.fda.gov/drugs/scienceresearch/researchareas/pharmacogenetics/ucm083378.htm.

Learning Points

1. How might pharmacogenomics enhance therapeutic drug monitoring?

Answer: Traditional patient-specific factors such as age, sex, renal function, hepatic function, and body weight are frequently used to determine appropriateness of a particular drug or dose for an individual. However, these factors only partially account for the likelihood of efficacy or toxicity. As our knowledge of how genetic variability impacts drug response is solidified, we can begin to incorporate pharmacogenetic information into algorithms for optimizing pharmacotherapy for individual patients and move toward personalized medicine.

2. Who is best equipped to incorporate pharmacogenomics into clinical decision-making?

Answer: The incorporation of pharmacogenomics will require an interdisciplinary team of healthcare providers with knowledge of the specific pharmacological properties of individual drugs, molecular biology, genetics, laboratory medicine, clinical medicine, genetic counseling, and economics. In addition, patients/consumers will likely be active participants and drivers of the use of genetic tests in clinical practice.

3. Where can pharmacogenomics information be obtained?

Answer: The majority of pharmacogenomics information is in the primary literature. Relevant pharmacogenomics information can also be communicated through product labeling, although this information may not be sufficient by itself to guide clinical decision-making, as patient-specific factors will also have to be taken into account. For example, the clopidogrel label has incorporated pharmacogenomics information on *CYP2C19* in a boxed warning that states, "…poor metabolizers treated with Plavix at recommended doses exhibit higher cardiovascular event rates following ACS or PCI than patients with normal *CYP2C19* function. Tests are available to identify a patient's *CYP2C19* genotype and can be used as an aid in determining therapeutic strategy. Consider alternative treatment or treatment strategies in patients identified as *CYP2C19* poor metabolizers." However, practical recommendations for when genotyping should occur and specific dose adjustments are not provided and must be determined as part of the clinical decision-making process. Therefore, the primary literature would also have to be consulted and interpreted. Another source for pharmacogenomics information is in the CPIC guidelines, when available for the particular drug/gene pair of interest. These guidelines are maintained and updated on the Pharmacogenomics Knowledge Base website (www.pharmgkb.com). This website also contains other valuable pharmacogenomics information even when guidelines are not yet available. In the future, these specific recommendations would ideally also be incorporated into clinical guidelines for the management of individual diseases.

REFERENCES

1. Evans DA, Manley KA, Mc KV. Genetic control of isoniazid metabolism in man. *Br Med J.* 1960;2:485-491.

2. Hughes HB, Biehl JP, Jones AP, Schmidt LH. Metabolism of isoniazid in man as related to the occurrence of peripheral neuritis. *Am Rev Tuberc.* 1954;70:266-273.

3. Alving AS, Carson PE, Flanagan CL, Ickes CE. Enzymatic deficiency in primaquine-sensitive erythrocytes. *Science.* 1956;124:484-485.

4. Vesell ES, Page JG. Genetic control of the phenobarbital-induced shortening of plasma antipyrine half-lives in man. *J Clin Invest.* 1969;48:2202-2209.

5. Zineh I, Pebanco GD, Aquilante CL, et al. Discordance between availability of pharmacogenetics studies and pharmacogenetics-based prescribing information for the top 200 drugs. *Ann Pharmacother.* 2006;40:639-644.

6. Zineh I, Johnson JA. Pharmacogenetics of chronic cardiovascular drugs: applications and implications. *Expert Opin Pharmacother.* 2006;7:1417-1427.

7. Guidelines and Recommendations for Laboratory Analysis and Application of Pharmacogenetics to Clinical Practice. http://www.aacc.org/members/nacb/lmpg/onlineguide/publishedguidelines/laacp/pages/default.aspx#. Accessed March 6, 2012.

8. Relling MV, Klein TE. CPIC: Clinical Pharmacogenetics Implementation Consortium of the Pharmacogenomics Research Network. *Clin Pharmacol Ther.* 2011;89:464-467.

9. Roses AD. Pharmacogenetics and the practice of medicine. *Nature.* 2000;405:857-865.

10. Haga SB, Burke W. Pharmacogenetic testing: not as simple as it seems. *Genet Med.* 2008;10:391-395.

11. Zineh I, Beitelshees AL, Gaedigk A, et al. Pharmacokinetics and CYP2D6 genotypes do not predict metoprolol adverse events or efficacy in hypertension. *Clin Pharmacol Ther.* 2004;76:536-544.

12. Crews KR, Gaedigk A, Dunnenberger HM, et al. Clinical Pharmacogenetics Implementation Consortium (CPIC) Guidelines for Codeine Therapy in the Context of Cytochrome P450 2D6 (CYP2D6) Genotype. *Clin Pharmacol Ther.* 2012;91:321-326.

13. Umemura K, Furuta T, Kondo K. The common gene variants of CYP2C19 affect pharmacokinetics and pharmacodynamics in an active metabolite of clopidogrel in healthy subjects. *J Thromb Haemost.* 2008;6:1439-1441.

14. Hulot JS, Collet JP, Cayla G, et al. CYP2C19 but not PON1 genetic variants influence clopidogrel pharmacokinetics, pharmacodynamics, and clinical efficacy in post-myocardial infarction patients. *Circ Cardiovasc Interv.* 2011;4:422-428.

15. Shuldiner AR, O'Connell JR, Bliden KP, et al. Association of cytochrome P450 2C19 genotype with the antiplatelet effect and clinical efficacy of clopidogrel therapy. *JAMA.* 2009;302:849-857.

16. Mega JL, Close SL, Wiviott SD, et al. Cytochrome p-450 polymorphisms and response to clopidogrel. *N Engl J Med.* 2009;360:354-362.

17. Mega JL, Simon T, Collet JP, et al. Reduced-function CYP2C19 genotype and risk of adverse clinical outcomes among patients treated with clopidogrel predominantly for PCI: a meta-analysis. *JAMA.* 2010;304:1821-1830.

18. Scott SA, Sangkuhl K, Gardner EE, et al. Clinical Pharmacogenetics Implementation Consortium guidelines for cytochrome P450-2C19 (CYP2C19) genotype and clopidogrel therapy. *Clin Pharmacol Ther.* 2011;90:328-332.

19. Westlind-Johnsson A, Hermann R, Huennemeyer A, et al. Identification and characterization of CYP3A4*20, a novel rare CYP3A4 allele without functional activity. *Clin Pharmacol Ther.* 2006;79:339-349.

20. Xie HG, Wood AJ, Kim RB, Stein CM, Wilkinson GR. Genetic variability in CYP3A5 and its possible consequences. *Pharmacogenomics.* 2004;5:243-272.

21. Purinethol [package insert]. Research Triangle Park, NC: GlaxoSmithKline; 2004.

22. Relling MV, Gardner EE, Sandborn WJ, et al. Clinical Pharmacogenetics Implementation Consortium guidelines for thiopurine methyltransferase genotype and thiopurine dosing. *Clin Pharmacol Ther.* 2011;89:387-391.

23. Fargher EA, Tricker K, Newman W, et al. Current use of pharmacogenetic testing: a national survey of thiopurine methyltransferase testing prior to azathioprine prescription. *J Clin Pharm Ther.* 2007;32:187-195.

24. Winter JW, Gaffney D, Shapiro D, et al. Assessment of thiopurine methyltransferase enzyme activity is superior to genotype in predicting myelosuppression following azathioprine therapy in patients with inflammatory bowel disease. *Aliment Pharmacol Ther.* 2007;25:1069-1077.

25. Diasio RB, Beavers TL, Carpenter JT. Familial deficiency of dihydropyrimidine dehydrogenase. Biochemical basis for familial pyrimidinemia and severe 5-fluorouracil-induced toxicity. *J Clin Invest.* 1988;81:47-51.

26. Tuchman M, Stoeckeler JS, Kiang DT, O'Dea RF, Ramnaraine ML, Mirkin BL. Familial pyrimidinemia and pyrimidinuria associated with severe fluorouracil toxicity. *N Engl J Med.* 1985;313:245-249.

27. Yen JL, McLeod HL. Should DPD analysis be required prior to prescribing fluoropyrimidines? *Eur J Cancer.* 2007;43:1011-1016.

28. Daly AK, Aithal GP. Genetic regulation of warfarin metabolism and response. *Semin Vasc Med.* 2003;3:231-238.

29. Daly AK, Day CP, Aithal GP. CYP2C9 polymorphism and warfarin dose requirements. *Br J Clin Pharmacol.* 2002;53:408-409.

30. Furuya H, Fernandez-Salguero P, Gregory W, et al. Genetic polymorphism of CYP2C9 and its effect on warfarin maintenance dose requirement in patients undergoing anticoagulation therapy. *Pharmacogenetics.* 1995;5:389-392.

31. Lee CR, Goldstein JA, Pieper JA. Cytochrome P450 2C9 polymorphisms: a comprehensive review of the in-vitro and human data. *Pharmacogenetics.* 2002;12:251-263.

32. Takahashi H, Echizen H. Pharmacogenetics of warfarin elimination and its clinical implications. *Clin Pharmacokinet.* 2001;40:587-603.

33. Takahashi H, Kashima T, Nomizo Y, et al. Metabolism of warfarin enantiomers in Japanese patients with heart disease having different CYP2C9 and CYP2C19 genotypes. *Clin Pharmacol Ther.* 1998;63:519-528.

34. Aithal GP, Day CP, Kesteven PJ, Daly AK. Association of polymorphisms in the cytochrome P450 CYP2C9 with warfarin dose requirement and risk of bleeding complications. *Lancet.* 1999;353:717-719.

35. Sconce EA, Khan TI, Wynne HA, et al. The impact of CYP2C9 and VKORC1 genetic polymorphism and patient characteristics upon warfarin dose requirements: proposal for a new dosing regimen. *Blood.* 2005;106:2329-2333.

36. Wadelius M, Chen LY, Downes K, et al. Common VKORC1 and GGCX polymorphisms associated with warfarin dose. *Pharmacogenomics J.* 2005;5:262-720.

37. Klein TE, Altman RB, Eriksson N, et al. Estimation of the warfarin dose with clinical and pharmacogenetic data. *N Engl J Med.* 2009;360:753-764.

38. Coumadin [package insert]. Princeton, NJ: Bristol-Myers Squibb; 2011.

39. Johnson JA, Gong L, Whirl-Carrillo M, et al. Clinical Pharmacogenetics Implementation Consortium Guidelines for CYP2C9 and VKORC1 genotypes and warfarin dosing. *Clin Pharmacol Ther.* 2011;90:625-629.

40. Anderson JL, Horne BD, Stevens SM, et al. Randomized trial of genotype-guided versus standard warfarin dosing in patients initiating oral anticoagulation. *Circulation.* 2007;116(22):2563-2570.

41. Kroese M, Zimmern RL, Pinder SE. HER2 status in breast cancer—an example of pharmacogenetic testing. *J R Soc Med.* 2007;100:326-329.

42. Wolff AC, Hammond ME, Schwartz JN, et al. American Society of Clinical Oncology/College of American Pathologists guideline recommendations for human epidermal growth factor receptor 2 testing in breast cancer. *J Clin Oncol.* 2007;25:118-145.

43. Shah SS, Ketterling RP, Goetz MP, et al. Impact of American Society of Clinical Oncology/College of American Pathologists guideline recommendations on HER2 interpretation in breast cancer. *Hum Pathol.* 2010;41:103-106.

44. Ellis IO, Bartlett J, Dowsett M, et al. Best Practice No 176: Updated recommendations for HER2 testing in the UK. *J Clin Pathol.* 2004;57:233-237.

45. Yaziji H, Goldstein LC, Barry TS, et al. HER-2 testing in breast cancer using parallel tissue-based methods. *JAMA.* 2004;291:1972-1977.

46. Herceptin [package insert]. South San Francisco, CA: Genetech; 2000.

47. Gately K, O'Flaherty J, Cappuzzo F, et al. The role of the molecular footprint of EGFR in tailoring treatment decisions in NSCLC. *J Clin Pathol.* 2012;65:1-7.

48. Lynch TJ, Bell DW, Sordella R, et al. Activating mutations in the epidermal growth factor receptor underlying responsiveness of non-small-cell lung cancer to gefitinib. *N Engl J Med.* 2004;350:2129-2139.

49. Pao W, Chmielecki J. Rational, biologically based treatment of EGFR-mutant non-small-cell lung cancer. *Nat Rev Cancer.* 2010;10:760-774.

50. Tanner NT, Pastis NJ, Sherman C, et al. The role of molecular analyses in the era of personalized therapy for advanced NSCLC. *Lung Cancer.* 2012;76(2):131-137.

51. Pao W, Ladanyi M. Epidermal growth factor receptor mutation testing in lung cancer: searching for the ideal method. *Clin Cancer Res.* 2007;13:4954-4955.

52. Pao W, Iafrate AJ, Su Z. Genetically informed lung cancer medicine. *J Pathol.* 2010.

53. Curran MP. Crizotinib: in locally advanced or metastatic non-small cell lung cancer. *Drugs.* 2012;72:99-107.

54. Ou SH. Crizotinib: a drug that crystallizes a unique molecular subset of non-small-cell lung cancer. *Expert Rev Anticancer Ther.* 2012;12:151-162.

55. Sasaki T, Rodig SJ, Chirieac LR, Janne PA. The biology and treatment of EML4-ALK non-small cell lung cancer. *Eur J Cancer.* 2010;46:1773-1780.

56. Shaw AT, Solomon B, Kenudson MM. Crizotinib and testing for ALK. *J Natl Compr Canc Netw.* 2011;9:1335-1341.

57. Pillai RN, Ramalingam SS. The biology and clinical features of non-small cell lung cancers with EML4-ALK translocation. *Curr Oncol Rep.* 2012;14(2):105-110.

58. Fecher LA, Cummings SD, Keefe MJ, Alani RM. Toward a molecular classification of melanoma. *J Clin Oncol.* 2007;25:1606-1620.

59. Chapman PB, Hauschild A, Robert C, et al. Improved survival with vemurafenib in melanoma with BRAF V600E mutation. *N Engl J Med.* 2011;364(26):2507-2516.

60. Dienstmann R, Vilar E, Tabernero J. Molecular predictors of response to chemotherapy in colorectal cancer. *Cancer J.* 2011;17:114-126.

61. Sierra JR, Cepero V, Giordano S. Molecular mechanisms of acquired resistance to tyrosine kinase targeted therapy. *Mol Cancer.* 2010;9:75.

62. Mega JL, Hochholzer W, Frelinger AL et al. Dosing clopidogrel based on CYP2C19 genotype and the effect on platelet reactivity in patients with stable cardiovascular disease. *JAMA.* 2011;306(20):2221-2228.

63. Mallal S, Nolan D, Witt C, et al. Association between presence of HLA-B*5701, HLA-DR7, and HLA-DQ3 and hypersensitivity to HIV-1 reverse-transcriptase inhibitor abacavir. *Lancet.* 2002;359:727-372.

64. Mallal S, Phillips E, Carosi G, et al. HLA-B*5701 screening for hypersensitivity to abacavir. *N Engl J Med.* 2008;358:568-579.

65. Guidelines for the use of antiretroviral agents in HIV-1 infected adults and adolescents. Department of Health and Human Services. Available at http://www.aidsinfo.nih.gov/ContentFiles/AdultandAdolescentGL.pdf. Accessed March 20, 2013.

66. McCormack M, Alfirevic A, Bourgeois S, et al. HLA-A*3101 and carbamazepine-induced hypersensitivity reactions in Europeans. *N Engl J Med.* 2011;364:1134-1143.

67. Ozeki T, Mushiroda T, Yowang A, et al. Genome-wide association study identifies HLA-A*3101 allele as a genetic risk factor for carbamazepine-induced cutaneous adverse drug reactions in Japanese population. *Hum Mol Genet.* 2011;20:1034-1041.

68. Ruschoff J, Hanna W, Bilous M, et al. HER2 testing in gastric cancer: a practical approach. *Mod Pathol.* 2012;25(5):637-650.

69. Schumacher GE, Barr JT. Total testing process applied to therapeutic drug monitoring: impact on patients' outcomes and economics. *Clin Chem.* 1998;44:370-374.

70. Miller CR, McLeod HL. Pharmacogenomics of cancer chemotherapy-induced toxicity. *J Support Oncol.* 2007;5:9-14.

CHAPTER 8

THE KIDNEYS

DOMINICK P. TROMBETTA

Objectives

After completing this chapter, the reader should be able to

- Describe the normal physiology of the kidneys

- Differentiate the renal handling of urea and creatinine

- Describe clinical situations where blood urea nitrogen (BUN) and/or serum creatinine (SCr) is/are elevated

- Describe the evolving role of cystatin C in estimating glomerular filtration rate (GFR)

- Describe the limitations in the usefulness of the SCr concentration in estimating kidney function

- Understand the clinical utility of the Cockcroft-Gault equation, the Modification of Diet in Renal Disease (MDRD) equation, and the CKD-EPI equations to assess kidney function

- Determine creatinine clearance (CrCl) given a patient's 24-hour urine creatinine (UCr) excretion and SCr

- Estimate CrCl given a patient's height, weight, sex, age, and SCr and identify limitations of the methods for estimation of kidney function

- Discuss the various components assessed by macroscopic, microscopic and chemical analysis of the urine

- Assess the utility of urine protein measurements as an indicator of kidney disease

- Describe the role of commonly obtained urinary electrolytes and the fractional excretion of sodium (FENa) in the diagnostic process

Through the excretion of water and solutes, the kidneys are responsible in large part for maintaining homeostasis within the body. They also function in the activation and synthesis of many substances that affect blood pressure (BP), mineral metabolism, and red cell production. The purpose of this chapter is to provide insight to the interpretation of laboratory tests in the assessment of kidney function, as well as provide an overview of the interpretation of a urinalysis.

KIDNEY PHYSIOLOGY

The functional unit of the kidneys is the nephron (Figure 8-1), and each of the two kidneys contains about 1 million nephrons. The major components of the nephron include the glomerulus, proximal tubule, loop of Henle, distal tubule, and collecting duct. Blood is delivered to the glomerulus, the filtering portion of the nephron, via the afferent arteriole. Acting as microfilters, the pores of glomerular capillaries allow substances with a molecular weight of up to 40,000 daltons to pass through them. Plasma proteins, such as albumin (mw 65,000 daltons) and red blood cells (RBCs) do not normally pass through the glomerulus. Ionic charge also affects filtration as the glomerulus selectively retains negatively charged proteins such as albumin. In kidney disease involving the glomerulus, the effect of ionic charge becomes less discriminate and albuminuria develops. Most drugs are small enough to be freely filtered at the glomerulus, with the exception of large proteins and drugs bound to plasma proteins.[1]

The proximal tubule reabsorbs large quantities of water and solute. Sodium passively follows the reabsorption of water back into the blood. Glucose, uric acid, chloride, bicarbonate, amino acids, urea, hydrogen, phosphate, calcium and magnesium are also primarily reabsorbed by the proximal tubule. Sodium, chloride, magnesium, and water are further reabsorbed in the loop of Henle. The distal tubule controls the amounts of sodium, potassium, bicarbonate, phosphate, and hydrogen that ultimately are excreted, and the collecting duct regulates the amount of water in the urine as a result of the effect of antidiuretic hormone (ADH), which facilitates water reabsorption.[1]

As shown in Figure 8-1, substances can enter the nephron from the peritubular blood or interstitial space via secretion. In addition, substances can be reabsorbed from primarily the distal tubule back into the systemic circulation via the peritubular vasculature. Tubular secretion occurs via two primary pathways in the proximal tubule: the organic acid transport (OAT) system and the organic cation transport (OCT) system. While each system is somewhat specific for anions and cations, respectively, some drugs, such as probenecid, are excreted by both pathways. Creatinine enters the tubule primarily by filtration through the glomerulus. However, a small amount of creatinine is also secreted by the OCT system into the proximal tubule. This becomes important when using the renal clearance of creatinine to estimate kidney function.[1]

Blood flow to the kidneys is determined, in large part, by cardiac output with about 20% or 1.2 L/min directed to the kidneys. Renal plasma flow (RPF) is directly related to renal blood flow (RBF) by taking the patient's hematocrit into consideration as follows:

$$RPF = RBF \times (1-Hct) \qquad (1)$$

where RPF = renal plasma flow; RBF = renal blood flow; and Hct = hematocrit.

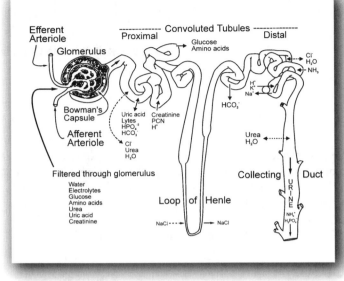

FIGURE 8-1. The nephron. Arrows pointing toward the nephron represent substances entering from the peritubular blood or interstitial space. Arrows heading away represent reabsorption. Solid arrows represent an active (energy-requiring) process, and dashed arrows represent a passive process. PCN = penicillin; lytes = electrolytes.

The normal value for RPF is about 625 mL/min. Of the plasma that reaches the glomerulus, about 20% is filtered and enters the proximal tubule, resulting in a glomerular filtration rate (GFR) of about 125 mL/min. The GFR is often used as a measure of the degree of kidney excretory function in a patient. The kidneys filter about 180 L of fluid each day; of this amount, they excrete only 1.5 L as urine. Thus, more than 99% of the GFR is reabsorbed back into the bloodstream. Many solutes, such as creatinine and many renally eliminated drugs, are concentrated in the urine.[1]

ASSESSMENT OF KIDNEY FUNCTION

Classification of kidney disease as well as dosing of medications depends on an accurate and reliable method of assessing kidney function.[2] Direct measurement of GFR using markers such as inulin and iothalamate is the most accurate assessment of kidney function but is not used routinely in clinical practice due to cost and practical concerns. Measurement of timed 24-hour urine creatinine (UCr) collections are difficult by design, flawed by collection errors, and inconvenient. The estimation of creatinine clearance (CrCl) through equations such as Cockcroft-Gault has been the "gold standard" for drug dosing. Recently, serum concentrations of cystatin C, an endogenous amino acid, have been evaluated as an alternative method to predict GFR in children as well as adults.[3-5] The estimation of GFR (eGFR) has been validated using the Modification of Diet in Renal Disease (MDRD) equation and is used to stage and monitor chronic kidney disease (CKD).[6-10] Recently, the Food and Drug Administration Guidance to Industry draft revision has proposed that both the eGFR and CrCl be incorporated into the package insert dosage recommendations for

patients with decreased renal function.[11] With more clinical laboratories reporting eGFR values and as pharmacokinetic data reference both eGFR and CrCl for new medications, the use of eGFR to adjust medication doses may become more commonplace.

Exogenous Markers

Inulin Clearance

Normal range: men = 127 mL/min/m²; women = 118 mL/min/m²

Inulin is a fructose polysaccharide, an inert carbohydrate, with a molecular weight of 5200 daltons, which is not bound to plasma proteins. Inulin is freely filtered through the glomerulus and not metabolized, secreted, or reabsorbed and can be regarded as the gold standard for measuring GFR in adults and older children.[12] Neonates and younger children may present logistical problems in obtaining accurate urine flow rates.[9] This test is fairly invasive because inulin must be administered intravenously, and it requires special analytical methods that limit its practical application in many healthcare facilities.[9]

Iothalamate and Cr-EDTA Clearance

Normal range: men = 127 mL/min/m²; women = 118 mL/min/m²

The urinary clearance of the radioactive marker *I-Iothalamate* is being more commonly used in research settings. The test involves injection of the radioactive exogenous marker, repeated blood sampling, and timed urine collection. The invasiveness and associated costs prohibit widespread application. The administration of ⁵¹*Cr-EDTA (ethylenediamine tetra-acetic)* has been used in the past as an alternative to I-Iothalamate. As with inulin, the need for intravenous (IV) administration and timed urine collections for both these markers make them impractical for routine use.

Endogenous Markers

Cystatin C

Cystatin C is a protease inhibitor produced at a steady-state by all nucleated cells that is filtered by the glomerulus and neither reabsorbed or secreted by the kidney.[13] It had been originally proposed that cystatin C may be more sensitive than SCr in tracking changes in kidney function, and that it is unaffected by diet or muscle mass. Serum cystatin C concentrations would be expected to be inversely proportional to GFR. Changes in serum cystatin C concentrations may be an indirect reflection of GFR. Combining SCr with cystatin C, age, sex, and race in estimating GFR have provided better results than equations based upon a single filtration marker.[14] The practical utility of these serum concentrations in clinical practice warrants further investigation. The standardization of this assay must be completed before cystatin C equations are adopted for use in patient care decisions.[15] Cystatin C concentrations have been used in equations for estimating GFR in pediatric patients.[3] Research has validated the use of cystatin C in these special populations over traditional SCr-based equations. Further data may support the use of cystatin C concentrations in adolescents, obstetrics, and geriatric patients.[16] Data also supports the correlation of elevated cystatin C levels and cardiovascular disease mortality.[17] Initial findings may also expand the clinical utility of measuring cystatin C concentrations to detect early kidney impairment in patients with prediabetes and diabetes and to provide more accurate estimation of renal function for patients with human immunodeficiency virus (HIV) or liver disease.[16]

CKD-EPI cystatin equation and creatinine adjusted for age, sex, and race[16]:

$$eGFR = 177.6 \times SCr^{-0.65} \times CysC^{-0.57} \times age^{-0.20} \times 0.80 \text{ (if female)}$$
$$\times 1.11 \text{ (if African American)} \qquad (2)$$

Serum Creatinine

Normal range: 0.6–1.2 mg/dL or 53–106 µmol/L for adults; 0.2–0.7 mg/dL or 18–62 µmol/L for young children

Creatinine and its precursor creatine are nonprotein, nitrogenous biochemicals of the blood. After synthesis in the liver, creatine diffuses into the bloodstream. Creatine then is taken up by muscle cells, where some of it is stored in a high-energy form, creatine phosphate. Creatine phosphate acts as a readily available source of phosphorus for regeneration of adenosine triphosphate (ATP) and is required for transforming chemical energy to muscle action.

Creatinine, which is produced in the muscle, is a spontaneous decomposition product of creatine and creatine phosphate. The daily production of creatinine is about 2% of total body creatine, which remains constant if muscle mass is not significantly changed. In normal patients at steady-state, the rate of creatinine production equals its excretion. Therefore, creatinine concentrations in the serum (SCr) vary little from day-to-day in patients with healthy kidneys. Although there is an inverse relationship between SCr and kidney function, SCr should not be the sole basis for the evaluation of renal function.[9] There are several issues to consider when evaluating a patient's SCr. Some of factors that affect SCr concentrations are muscle mass, sex, age, race, medications, method of laboratory analysis, and low-protein diets. Additionally, acute changes in a patient's GFR such as in acute kidney injury may not be initially manifested as an increase in SCr concentration since it takes time for new steady-state concentrations of SCr to be achieved. The time required to reach 95% of steady-state in patients with 50%, 25%, and 10% of normal kidney function is about 1, 2, and 4 days respectively. Steady-state concentrations of SCr become very important as they are integral in clinical practice estimations of renal function.

A SCr concentration within the reference ranges as reported by clinical laboratories does not necessarily indicate normal kidney function. For example, a SCr concentration of 1.5 mg/dL in a 45-year-old male who weighs 150 pounds and a 78-year-old female who weighs 92 pounds would correspond to different GFRs.

Clinicians can surmise that as long as no abnormalities exist in muscle mass and there has been no recent protein ingestion, an increased SCr almost always reflects a decreased GFR. The converse is not always true; a normal SCr does not necessarily imply a normal GFR. As part of the aging process, both muscle

mass and renal function diminish. Therefore, SCr may remain in the normal range because as the kidneys become less capable of filtering and excreting creatinine, they also are presented with decreasing amounts of creatinine. Thus, practitioners should not rely solely on SCr as an index of renal function.

Besides aging and alterations in muscle mass, some pathophysiological changes can affect the relationship between SCr and kidney function. For example, renal function may be overestimated on the basis of SCr alone in cirrhotic patients. In this patient population, the low SCr is due to a decreased hepatic synthesis of creatine, the precursor of creatinine. In cirrhotic patients, it is prudent to perform a measured 24-hour CrCl. If the patient also has hyperbilirubinemia, assay interference by elevated bilirubin also may contribute to a low SCr.

Laboratory measurement and reporting of SCr. Historically, the laboratory methods used to measure SCr included the alkaline picrate method, inorganic enzymatic methods, and high-pressure liquid chromatography (HPLC). The alkaline picrate assay (Jaffe) was the most commonly used method to measure SCr; however, interfering substances such as noncreatinine chromogens can often lead to underestimation of kidney function. Causes of falsely elevated SCr results included unusually large amounts of noncreatinine chromogens (e.g., uric acid, glucose, fructose, acetone, acetoacetate, pyruvic acid, and ascorbic acid) in the serum. For example, an increase in glucose of 100 mg/dL (5.6 mmol/L) could falsely elevate SCr by 0.5 mg/dL (44 µmol/L) in some assays. Likewise, serum ketones high enough to spill into the urine may falsely increase SCr and UCr. In diabetic patients in diabetic ketoacidosis (DKA), false elevation could precipitate unnecessary evaluation for renal failure when presenting with ketoacidosis. Like ketones, acetoacetate may have been elevated enough to cause falsely elevated SCr after a 48-hour fast or in patients with DKA. Another endogenous substance, bilirubin, could falsely lower SCr results with both the alkaline picrate and enzymatic assays. At low GFRs, however, creatinine secretion overtakes the balancing effects of measuring noncreatinine chromogens, causing an overestimation of GFRs by as much as 50%.[5]

Reliable and accurate measurement and subsequent reporting of SCr concentrations is very important. The MDRD equation utilizes as one of its variables the SCr concentration to stage kidney damage based on the estimation of GFR. The Cockcroft-Gault equation, which is highly dependent on the SCr concentration, has been used as the accepted methodology for drug dosing based on estimation of CrCl.[18] The greater the imprecision of the assay the less accurate the resultant GFR estimations. The primary source of measurement errors included systematic bias and interlaboratory, intralaboratory, and random variability in daily calibration of SCr values. Interlaboratory commutability is also problematic secondary to the variations in assay methodologies. Recently, a report from the Laboratory Working Group of the National Kidney Disease Program, made recommendations to improve and standardize measurement of SCr.[19,20] As of 2011, creatinine standardization is reported to be nationwide (in the United States) and calibration should be traceable to isotope dilution mass spectrometry

TABLE 8-1. Common Causes of True BUN Elevations (Azotemia)

Prerenal causes

Decreased renal perfusion: dehydration, blood loss, shock, severe heart failure

Intrarenal (intrinsic) causes

Acute kidney failure: nephrotoxic drugs, severe hypertension, glomerulonephritis, tubular necrosis

Chronic kidney dysfunction: pyelonephritis, diabetes, glomerulonephritis, renal tubular disease, amyloidosis, arteriosclerosis, collagen vascular disease, polycystic kidney disease, overuse of nonsteroidal anti-inflammatory drugs (NSAIDs)

Postrenal causes

Obstruction of ureter, bladder neck, or urethra

(IDMS). Of note, SCr concentrations are lower than had been previously reported with older methods. Calculations of renal function using Cockcroft-Gault or MDRD should use the standardized creatinine value. Calculated GFRs above 60 mL/min/1.73 m^2 using the MDRD equation should be simply reported as "greater than 60 mL/min/1.73 m^2."

Urea (Blood Urea Nitrogen)

Normal range: 8–23 mg/dL or 2.9–8.2 mmol/L

Blood urea nitrogen (BUN) is actually the concentration of nitrogen (as urea) in the *serum* and not in RBCs as the name implies. Although the renal clearance of urea can be measured, it cannot be used by itself to assess kidney function. Its serum concentration depends on urea production (which occurs in the liver) and tubular reabsorption in addition to glomerular filtration. Therefore, clinicians must consider factors other than filtration when interpreting changes in BUN.

When viewed with other laboratory and clinical data, BUN can be used to assess or monitor hydration, renal function, protein tolerance, and catabolism in numerous clinical settings (Table 8-1). Also, it is used to predict the risk of uremic syndrome in patients with severe renal failure. Concentrations above 100 mg/dL (35.7 mmol/L) are associated with this risk.

Elevated BUN

Urea production is increased by
- A high-protein diet (including amino acid infusions)
- Upper gastrointestinal (GI) bleeding
- Administration of corticosteroids, tetracyclines, or any other drug with antianabolic effects

Usually, about 50% of the filtered urea is reabsorbed, but this amount is inversely related to the rate of urine flow in the tubules. In other words, the slower the urine flows, the more time the urea has to leave the tubule and re-enter surrounding capillaries (reabsorption). Urea reabsorption tends to change in parallel with sodium, chloride, and water reabsorption. Since patients with volume depletion avidly reabsorb sodium, chloride, and water, larger amounts of urea are also absorbed.

Urine flow, in turn, is affected by fluid balance and BP. For example, patients who are dehydrated with low urine flow may develop high concentrations of urea nitrogen in the blood. Likewise, a patient with a pathologically low BP may develop diminished urine flow secondary to decreased RBF with a subsequently diminished GFR. Congestive heart failure and reduced RBF, despite increased intravascular volume, is a common cause of elevated BUN. Causes of abnormally high BUN (also called *azotemia*) are listed in Table 8-1.

Decreased BUN

In and of itself, a low BUN does not have pathophysiological consequences. BUN may be low in patients who are malnourished or have profound liver damage (due to an inability to synthesize urea). Intravascular fluid overload may initially dilute BUN (causing low concentrations), but many causes of extravascular volume overload, which are associated with third spacing of fluids into tissues (e.g., congestive heart failure, renal failure, and nephrotic syndrome) result in increased BUN because effective circulating volume is decreased.

Concomitant BUN and SCr

Simultaneous BUN and SCr determinations are commonly made and can furnish valuable information to assess kidney function. This is particularly true for acute kidney injury. In acute kidney injury due to volume depletion, both BUN and SCr are elevated. However, the BUN:SCr ratio is often >20:1 (SI: 0.08:1 or higher). This observation is due to the differences in the renal handling of urea and creatinine. Recall that urea is reabsorbed with water, and under conditions of decreased renal perfusion both urea and water reabsorption are increased. Since creatinine is not reabsorbed, it is not affected by increased water reabsorption. So the concentrations of both substances may increase in this setting, but the BUN would be increased to a greater degree, leading to a BUN:SCr >20:1.

In summary, when acute changes in kidney function are observed, and both BUN and SCr are greater than normal limits, BUN:SCr ratios greater than 20:1 suggest prerenal causes of acute renal impairment (Table 8-1), whereas ratios from 10:1 to 20:1 (SI: from 0.04:1 to 0.08:1) suggest intrinsic kidney damage. Furthermore, a ratio greater than 20:1 is not clinically important if both SCr and BUN are within normal limits (e.g., SCr = 0.8 mg/dL and BUN = 20 mg/dL).

Measurement of CrCl

A complete 24-hour urine collection to measure CrCl is difficult to obtain outside of research facilities and is prone to errors in collection. In addition, the National Kidney Foundation indicates that these measured CrCls are not better than the estimates of CrCl provided through equations such as the Cockcroft-Gault or the MDRD.[9,21] However, a 24-hour, timed urine measurement of CrCl may be useful in the following clinical situations: patients starting dialysis; in the presence of acute changes in kidney function; during evaluation of dietary intake and nutrition or malnutrition; patients with extremes in muscle mass; health enthusiasts taking creatinine supplementation; vegetarians; patients with quadriplegia or paraplegia; and patients who have undergone amputations.[2,9]

Interpreting CrCl Values with Other Renal Parameters

As noted previously, the most common clinical uses for CrCl and SCr include

- Assessing kidney function in patients with acute or CKD
- Monitoring the effects of drug therapy on slowing the progression of kidney disease
- Monitoring patients on nephrotoxic drugs
- Determining dosage adjustments for renally eliminated drugs

Because the relationship between SCr and CrCl is inverse and geometric as opposed to linear (Figure 8-2), significant declines in CrCl may occur before SCr rises above the normal range. For example, as CrCl slows, SCr rises very little until more than 50% of the nephrons have become nonfunctional. Therefore, SCr alone is not a sensitive indicator of early kidney dysfunction.

Calculating CrCl from a Timed Urine Collection

Although shorter collection periods (3–8 hours) appear to be adequate and may be more reliable, CrCl is routinely calculated using a 12- or 24-hour urine collection.[22] Creatinine excretion is normally 20–28 mg/kg/24 hr in men and 15–21 mg/kg/24 hr in women. In children, normal excretion (mg/kg/24 hr) should be approximately 15 + (0.5 × age), where age is in years.

Because its excretion remains relatively consistent within these ranges, UCr is often used as a check for the completion of the urine collection. In adults, some clinicians discount a urine sample if it contains less than 10 mg of creatinine/kg/24 hr; they assume that the collection was incomplete. However, 8.5 mg/kg/day might be a better cutoff, especially in critically ill elderly patients. Urine creatinine assays are affected by most of the same substances that affect SCr. To interfere significantly, however, the substance must appear in the urine in concentrations at least equal to those found in the blood.

Measured CrCl is calculated using the following formula:

$$\text{CrCl (mL/min)} = [\text{UCr} \times V]/[\text{SCr} \times T] \times \frac{1.73}{\text{BSA}} \quad (3)$$

where CrCl is the CrCl in mL/min/1.73 m²; UCr = urine creatinine concentration (mg/dL); V = volume of urine produced during the collection interval (mL); SCr = serum creatinine concentration (mg/dL); T = time of the collection interval (minutes), and BSA = body surface area (m²).

BSA can be estimated using the standard method of Dubois and Dubois:

$$\text{BSA (m}^2) = 0.20247 \times \text{height(m)}^{0.725} \times \text{weight(kg)}^{0.425} \quad (4)$$

BSA also can be estimated using the following equations from Mosteller[23]:

$$BSA(m)^2 = \sqrt{[height(cm) \times weight(kg)]/3600)} \quad (5)$$

$$BSA(m)^2 = \sqrt{[height(in) \times weight(lb)]/3131} \quad (6)$$

Adjustment of CrCl to a standard BSA (1.73 m²) allows direct comparison with normal CrCl ranges since such tables are in units of milliliters per minute per 1.73 m². The CrCl value adjusted for BSA is the number of milliliters cleared per minute for each 1.73 m² of the patient's BSA. Therefore, such

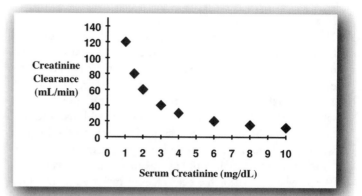

FIGURE 8-2. This plot represents the inverse relationship between SCr and CrCl. Relatively small changes in SCr at lower levels represent significant change in kidney function as assessed by CrCl.

adjustment in a large person (>1.73 m²) reduces the original nonadjusted clearance value since the assumption is that clearance would be lower if the patient were smaller. In practice, it is only important to adjust CrCl for BSA in patients who are much smaller or larger than 1.73 m².

Estimation of CrCl

In practice, dosage recommendations for medications excreted through the kidney have been traditionally based on the Cockcroft-Gault estimation of CrCl and the corresponding dosing information in the product information. With the implementation of standardized reporting of creatinine values, calculated CrCl values may be 5% to 20% higher and may not correlate with dosage guidelines based on renal dose adjustments on creatinine values obtained from older assay methodologies.

Cockcroft-Gault Equation

This formula provides an estimation of CrCl.[18] The patient's age, total body weight (TBW), and SCr concentration are necessary for the estimation. Calculations of CrCl using standardized creatinine values will result in higher and less reliable estimations of renal function. There is some controversy regarding which patient weight to use in the formula. Few patients are close to their ideal body weight (IBW). There are weight adjustment formulas that have empirically attempted to improve the estimation of CrCl by calculating an adjusted body weight. Additional attempts to improve the Cockcroft-Gault equation such as rounding SCr to 1.0, using adjusted or lean body weight have all been attempted without clinical validation. This equation should be used cautiously in patients with unstable renal function.

$$\frac{\text{CrCl}}{\text{(mL/min)}} = \frac{(140 - \text{age}) \times \text{weight (kg)}}{72 \times \text{SCr (mg/dL)}} \times 0.85 \text{ (if female)} \quad (7)$$

$$\frac{\text{CrCl}}{\text{(mL/min)}} = \frac{(140 - \text{age}) \times \text{weight (kg)}}{72 \times \text{SCr (mg/dL)}} \times \frac{0.85}{\text{(if female)}} \times \frac{1.73 \text{ m}^2}{\text{BSA}} \quad (8)$$

Cockcroft-Gault IBW, where IBW (kg) =
(2.3 × inches >5 feet) + 50 (if male),
or (2.3 × inches >5 feet) + 45.5 (if female)

Cockcroft-Gault TBW= TBW for weight in CG equation

Pediatric Patients

The National Kidney Foundation Kidney Disease Outcome Quality Initiative (KDOQI) guidelines recommend use of either the Schwartz or Counahan-Barratt equations to estimate kidney function in patients less than 12 years of age.[9] The Schwartz equation provides an estimation of CrCl whereas the Counahan-Barratt equation provides an estimation of the GFR. The older version of the Schwartz equation was derived from inulin clearance and measured creatinine concentrations, which could overestimate the true value.[24,25] The Schwartz equation has been recently modified to integrate the newer standardized SCr values.[26,27] The bedside formula may be more practical since the majority of clinical laboratories may not be able to report cystatin C values in a timely manner. The Counahan-Barratt equation was developed using 51Cr-EDTA plasma clearance.[10] Both equations are imprecise to some degree; however, they represent a more practical alternative than using SCr alone. There is a clear need for a more precise formula for estimating kidney functions in the pediatric population.[4]

Bedside IDMS-traceable Schwartz equation[26]:

$$GFR\ (mL/min/1.73m^2) = (0.413 \times Height\ (cm)/serum\ creatinine\ (mg/dL) \tag{9}$$

IDMS-traceable Schwartz equation[26]:

$$GFR\ (mL/min/1.73m^2) = 39.1\ [(height\ (m)/SCr\ (mg/dL)]^{0.516} \times [(1.8/cystatin\ C\ (mg/L)^{0.294}\ [30/BUN\ (mg/dL)]^{0.169} [1.099]^{male}\ [height\ (m)/1.4)^{0.188} \tag{10}$$

Counahan-Barratt equation[10]:

$$GFR\ (mL/min/1.73m^2) = 0.43\ [(height\ (cm)/SCr\ (mg/dL)] \tag{11}$$

In a prospective cohort study in critically ill children, urine neutrophil gelatinase-associated lipocalcin (uNGAL) has exhibited promise as an early signal of acute kidney insult when compared to SCr alone.[28] Future research may validate or better define the usefulness of this biomarker, which is currently limited to research facilities.

Estimation of GFR—MDRD Equation

The MDRD equation had been developed as a tool to identify those patients at risk for complications arising from CKD.[9,29] See Table 8-2 for the stages of chronic kidney disease. Estimated GFR values less than 60 mL/min/1.73 m² are considered to be consistent with kidney disease. The MDRD equation

TABLE 8-2. Chronic Kidney Disease Stages[2]

STAGE	GFR (mL/min/ 1.73 m²)	INTERPRETATION
1	>90	Normal or kidney damage and normal GFR
2	60–89	Slightly diminished GFR with kidney damage
3	30–59	Moderately decreased GFR with kidney damage
4	15–29	Significantly decreased GFR with kidney damage
5	<15	Kidney failure or on dialysis

GFR = glomerular filtration rate.

provides an estimated GFR, which was developed using measured GFR I-Iothalamate reference values. The original MDRD equation accounted for urea and albumin concentrations but the KDOQI guidelines recommend that clinical laboratories report the estimated GFR as calculated using the abbreviated MDRD equation.[9] Patients at age extremes may be particularly vulnerable to errors of estimated GFR.[4,8] The abbreviated MDRD equation has been re-expressed to include standardized SCr traceable to IDMS values.[6,20,30–32] Validation in clinical trials in special populations, pediatric, geriatric, and obese patients may be warranted before further applicability and clinical use. In addition, results of the MDRD equation should be interpreted cautiously in patients with low muscle mass (e.g., cachectic patients). One limitation identified with the MDRD equation that is well known is the underestimation of renal function for patients with eGFR greater than 60 mL/min/1.73 M².[33] This can lead to more patients being falsely identified with CKD.

Abbreviated MDRD using revised calibration for SCr:

$$GFR\ (mL/min/1.73\ m^2) = 175 \times standardized\ SCr^{-1.154} \times age^{-0.203} \times 1.210\ (if\ African\ American) \times 0.742\ (if\ female) \tag{12}$$

Estimation of GFR—CKD Epidemiology Collaboration Creatinine Equation

Introduced in 2009, the CKD-EPI (CKD-EPI) equation also based upon standardized SCr, age, sex, and race. This equation performs with the same degree of accuracy as the MDRD equation for patients with eGFR less than 60 mL/min/1.73M².[34,35] However, it corrects the inadequacy of the MDRD, which leads to underestimations in those patients with eGFR greater than 60 mL/min/1.73 M². Both the CKD-EPI and the MDRD equation account for the age of the patient. Like all SCr-based equations, Cockcroft-Gault, MDRD, and CKD-EPI succumb to the same inherent problems associated with this endogenous surrogate marker. At the same SCr, younger patients who have more muscle mass will have a higher GFR than older adults with low muscle mass. Clinical labs may begin reporting eGFR based upon CKD-EPI rather than MDRD.[36] The usefulness of the CKD-EPI may be particularly evident in younger patients without kidney disease, younger type 1 diabetics without microalbuminuria, or those considering kidney donation with GFR rates approximating normal values. The CKD-EPI equation may eventually replace the MDRD equation in clinical practice.

CKD-EPI equation[34,35]:

$$GFR\ (mL/min/1.73\ M^2) = 141 \times min\ (S_c/\kappa,1)^\alpha \times max (Sc/\kappa,\ 1)^{-1.209} \times 0.993^{age} \times 1.018\ (if\ female) \times 1.159\ (if\ African\ American) \tag{13}$$

S_c = standardized serum creatinine
κ = 0.7 for females and 0.9 for males
α = -0.329 for females and -0.411 for males
min indicates the minimum of Sc/κ or 1
max indicates the maximum of Sc/κ or 1

MINICASE 1

Estimating Equations for GFR

HENRY G., A 30-YEAR-OLD MAN (non-African American), has a significant history for diabetes mellitus type 1.

Laboratory tests were as follows:

Sodium, 140 mEq/L (136–145 mEq/L)

Potassium, 4.5 mEq/L (3.5–5.0 mEq/L)

Chloride, 101 mEq/L (96–106 mEq/L)

Carbon dioxide, 28 mEq/L (24–30 mEq/L)

Magnesium, 2.0 mEq/L (1.5–2.2 mEq/L)

Glucose, 98 mg/dL (70–110 mg/dL)

BUN, 12 mg/dL (8–20 mg/dL)

SCr, 1.45 mg/dL (0.7–1.5 mg/dL)

Question: Why would his eGFR vary between the MDRD and CKD-EPI estimating equations?

Discussion: Using the MDRD and CKD-EPI equations, the calculated eGFR for Henry G. are 57 mL/min/1.73 M^2 (stage III CKD) and 64 mL/min/1.73 M^2 (stage II CKD), respectively. First, it has to be recognized that the study equations were developed in different populations. The MDRD was developed in patients with CKD (average eGFR 40 mL/min/1.73 M^2) and the CKD-EPI in more diverse patients with and without kidney disease (average eGFR 68 mL/min/1.73 M^2). In a recent systematic review, inherent biases were identified in both equations. The MDRD exhibited more bias at eGFR greater than 60 mL/min/1.73 M^2 and the CKD-EPI at eGFR less than 60 mL/min/1.73 M^2. One universal equation has not been found to be optimal for all populations or ethnic populations. The CKD-EPI equation may permit more effective utilization of resources by better identification of those patients who should be under the care of a nephrologist.[37]

Clinical Controversy: Cockcroft-Gault Versus MDRD for Drug Dosing

The appropriate dosing of renally eliminated medications is necessary to prevent overdosage or underdosage of medications. Overdosage of a medication can cause significant clinical consequence and contribute to poor patient outcomes. Similarly, underdosing medications can lead to therapeutic failures. In both scenarios, inappropriate medication dosing can lead to increased length of stay, higher healthcare costs, and preventable medication-related problems. The MDRD equation provides a more accurate estimation of kidney excretory function than the Cockcroft-Gault equation.[6,30,38] At this time, the optimal single best equation that can be used universally in all populations does not exist. The usefulness of the MDRD equation in staging kidney disease is indisputable. Recently, manufacturers have provided some dosage guidance based upon eGFR for patients with deteriorating kidney function. Recent studies support the agreement of the MDRD equation with measured GFR and FDA assigned kidney function categories for medication dose adjustment.[39] The National Kidney Disease and Education Program in 2009 has suggested the use of either the CrCl as estimated by Cockcroft-Gault or the eGFR for dosing medications in CKD for most patients.[40] The eGFR needs to be individualized in patients at the extremes in body size by multiplying the eGFR/1.73 M^2 by the patients' body surface area (BSA) to convert units to mL/min:

$$\text{Individualized MDRD} = \text{eGFR}/1.73 \text{ m}^2 \times \text{estimated BSA (m}^2) = \text{eGFR for drug dosing} \quad (14)$$

Alternatively, in patients who are considered to be high risk for adverse medication events, in patients who are taking drugs that have a narrow therapeutic index, or where estimations of kidney function vary or are inaccurate, consider measuring CrCl or GFR using exogenous markers.[40] The Nephrology Practice and Research Network of the American College of Clinical Pharmacy (ACCP) has suggested an algorithm for dosing medications eliminated by the kidneys using SCr-based equations.[41] Additionally, safety and efficacy considerations affect decisions regarding dosing of renally eliminated medications that include both patient factors (clinical condition, cachexia) and drug specifics properties (therapeutic index). In summary, clinical assessment of the benefits and risks will continue to provide dosing recommendations for patients with kidney impairment.

URINALYSIS

Urinalysis is a commonly used clinical tool for the evaluation of various renal and nonrenal problems (e.g., endocrine, metabolic, and genetic). A routine urinalysis is done as a screening test during many hospital admissions and initial physician visits. It is also performed periodically in patients in nursing homes and other settings. The most common components of the urinalysis are discussed here.

An accurate interpretation of a urinalysis can be made only if the urine specimen is properly collected and handled. Techniques are fairly standardized and, keeping in mind that urine is normally sterile, aim to avoid contamination by normal flora of the external environment (mucous membranes of the vagina or uncircumcised penis or by microorganisms on the hands). Therefore, these areas are cleansed and physically kept away from the urine stream. During menses or heavy vaginal secretions, a fresh tampon should be inserted before cleansing. A first-morning, midstream collection is customarily used as the specimen.[42]

Once voided, the urine should be brought to the laboratory as soon as possible to prevent deterioration. If the sample is not refrigerated, bacteria multiply and use glucose (if present) as a food source. Subsequently, glucose concentrations decrease and ketones may evaporate with prolonged standing. Another problem is that formed elements (see Microscopic Analysis

MINICASE 2

Heart Failure

RUTH K., AN 83-YEAR-OLD FEMALE with a long history of congestive heart failure, was admitted to Community Hospital with complaints of shortness of breath (she needed to sleep in her recliner and was unable to sleep in her bed despite using two pillows), 15-pound weight gain, and fluid retention in her lower extremities. She also had anorexia, nausea, fatigue, and weakness. All had worsened over the past 2 weeks.

PMH: hypertension, osteoarthritis, atrial fibrillation

Physical examination revealed a frail (5'3"; 78 kg) woman in moderate distress; heart rate of 108 BPM; BP of 96/60 mm Hg; S3/S4 heart sounds; + three pitting edema bilateral lower extremities. Chest x-ray reveals bilateral pleural effusions.

Current medications:

Lisinopril, 20 mg PO daily
Metoprolol succinate, 100 mg PO daily
Furosemide, 40 mg PO daily
KCl, 10 mEq PO BID
Ibuprofen, 400 mg PO 4 times daily PRN for knee pain

Laboratory tests were as follows:

Sodium, 130 mEq/L (136–142 mEq/L)
Potassium, 3.2 mEq/L (3.8–5.0 mEq/L)
Chloride, 96 mEq/L (95–103 mEq/L)
Carbon dioxide, 30 mEq/L (24–30 mEq/L or mmol/L)
Magnesium, 1.3 mEq/L (1.3–2.1 mEq/L)
Glucose, 78 mg/dL (70–110 mg/dL)
Hemoglobin (Hgb), 11.5 g/dL (12.3–15.3 g/dL)
BUN, 76 mg/dL (8–23 mg/dL)
SCr, 2.5 mg/dL (0.6–1.2 mg/dL)

Urinalysis: normal

BNP: 1200 pg/mL (<100 pg/mL)

Over the next 2 days, Ruth K. received aggressive diuretic therapy (furosemide 80 mg IV twice a day), and all electrolyte abnormalities were corrected. Her physical exam was much improved. She was no longer short of breath. On the morning of day 4, her test results were

Sodium, 135 mEq/L
Potassium, 3.2 mEq/L
Chloride, 100 mEq/L
Carbon dioxide, 34 mEq/L
Magnesium, 1.4 mEq/L
Glucose, 80 mg/dL
Hgb, 11.4 g/dL
BUN, 35 mg/dL
SCr, 1.4 mg/dL
BNP, 400 pg/mL

Question: What type of renal dysfunction was Ruth K. experiencing on admission to the hospital? What were the likely causes of her elevated BUN and SCr? How often should BUN and SCr be interpreted?

Discussion: This case is rather complex because of the involvement of the kidneys in heart failure. Initially, the elevated BUN and SCr could be attributed to a prerenal state secondary to increased edema (hypervolemia) caused by worsening heart failure. This is supported by her clinical presentation (weight gain, symptoms of heart failure, CXR, elevated BNP, and an elevated BUN:SCr ratio with a ratio of greater than 20:1. The urinalysis did not reveal any cells that might indicate an intrinsic acute kidney injury (see Urinalysis section). In addition, diuretics may increase the BUN, which may complicate the picture, but the other evidence supports the diagnosis of prerenal azotemia. Assessment of kidney function on day 1 is difficult since the Cockcroft-Gault, MDRD, or CKD-EPI equations should not be used in patients with acute alterations in kidney function. In suspected acute kidney injury and when there is a need to assess GFR, measurement of CrCl through collection of urine should be considered.

Question: What was the trigger of Ruth K.'s heart failure?

Discussion: Ruth K. has several risk factors that can worsen heart failure. She has a history of hypertension and atrial fibrillation. She may have been using more ibuprofen more frequently and for an extended period for increased osteoarthritic knee pain. Additional risk factors that could also contribute to exacerbation of heart failure include noncompliance with fluid restriction (2 liters) and diet (2 g sodium/day).

Question: What other electrolyte abnormalities resulted?

Discussion: There are several electrolyte abnormalities identified during initial presentation and then subsequent lab analysis: increased BUN and SCr, increased serum bicarbonate, hypokalemia, hypomagnesemia, and hyponatremia. On admission, worsening heart failure resulted in decreased RBF. As with creatinine, there will be a reduction in BUN filtration at the glomerulus; however, urea is avidly reabsorbed in the proximal tubule (following sodium and water) resulting in an elevated ratio of BUN out of proportion to the creatinine (>20:1). Ruth K. also presented initially with hypervolemic hyponatremia. This most likely caused by the worsening heart failure, diminished blood flow to the kidney, and peripheral edema and subsequent weight gain. As Ruth K. becomes euvolemic, the hyponatremia will gradually be corrected. After aggressive diuresis with IV furosemide, hypokalemia and hypomagnesemia required replacement therapy. Loop diuretics can also cause metabolic alkalosis (increased serum bicarbonate). Overaggressive diuresis can cause elevations in BUN and SCr without evidence of overt heart failure.

---

section) begin decomposing within 2 hours. With excessive exposure to light, bilirubin and urobilinogen are oxidized. Unlike other substances, however, protein is minimally affected by prolonged standing.

After the urine sample is collected, it may undergo three types of testing: macroscopic, microscopic, and chemical (dipstick).

Macroscopic Analysis (General Appearance)

The color of normal urine varies greatly—from totally clear to dark yellow or amber—depending on the concentration of solutes. Color comes primarily from the pigments urochrome and urobilin. Fresh normal urine is not cloudy or hazy, but urine may become cloudy if urates (in an acid environment) or phosphates (in an alkaline environment) crystallize or precipitate out of solution. These salts become less soluble as the urine cools from body temperature.

Turbidity may also occur when large numbers of RBCs or white blood cels (WBCs) are present. An unusual amount of foam may be from protein or bile acids. Table 8-3 lists causes of different urine colors. Some of the changes noted may be urine pH-dependent. In general, drug-induced changes in urine color are fairly rare. Drugs that cause or exacerbate any of the medical problems listed in Table 8-3 can also be considered indirect causes of discolored urine.

Microscopic Analysis (Formed Elements)

Microscopic analysis typically involves[43]

1. Centrifuging the urine (12 mL) at 2000 revolutions per minute for 5 minutes
2. Pouring off all "loose" supernatant
3. Mixing the sediment with the residual supernatant
4. Examining the resulting suspension under 400–440x magnification (also described as high-power field)

Microscopic analysis can be done either routinely or selectively. In either case, one should look for the three "Cs"—cells, casts, and crystals.

Cells

Theoretically, no cells should be seen during microscopic examination of urine. In practice, however, an occasional cell or two is found. These cells include microorganisms, RBCs, WBCs, and tubular epithelial cells.

Microorganisms (normal range: zero to trace). If bacteria are found in the urine sediment, contamination should be the first consideration. Of course, fungi, bacteria, and other single-cell organisms can be seen in patients with a urinary tract infection or colonization. Even if ordered, some laboratories do not perform urine cultures unless there is significant bacteriuria. *Significant bacteriuria* may be defined as an initial positive dipstick screen for leukocyte esterase and/or nitrites (Chemical Analysis section). Likewise, some laboratories do not process cultures further (e.g., identification, quantification, and susceptibility) if more than one or two different bacterial species is seen on initial plating. Additionally, some labs do not perform susceptibility testing if more than one organism (some more than two) is isolated or if less than 100,000 (some use 50,000 as the cutoff) colony-forming units (cfu) per milliliter per organism are measured with a midstream, clean-catch sample. The common cutoff for urine obtained through a catheter is less than 10,000. If multiple types of bacteria are present, contamination by flora from vaginal, rectal, hand, skin, or other body sites is assumed.

Red blood cells (erythrocytes) (normal range: one to three per high-power field). Hematuria is the abnormal renal excretion of erythrocytes detected in two of three urine samples. A few RBCs are occasionally found in the urine of a healthy man or woman, particularly after exertion, trauma, or fever. If persistent, even small numbers (greater than two to three per high-powered field) may reflect urinary tract pathology. Increased numbers of RBCs are seen (among others) in glomerulonephritis, infection (pyelonephritis), renal infarction or papillary necrosis, tumors, stones, and coagulopathies. In some of these disorders, hematuria may turn the urine

TABLE 8-3. Potential Causes of Various Urine Coloring[43-45]

COLOR	CAUSE	POSSIBLE UNDERLYING ETIOLOGIES
Red to orange	Myoglobin	Crush injuries, electric shock, seizures, cocaine-induced muscle damage
	Hemoglobin/erythrocytes	Hemolysis (malaria, drugs, strenuous exercise), menstrual contamination; kidney stones
	Porphyrins	Porphyria, lead poisoning, liver disease
	Drugs/chemicals	Drugs/chemicals causing above diseases; as dyes: rifampin, phenazopyridine, daunorubicin, doxorubicin, phenolphthalein, phenothiazines, senna, chlorzoxazone
	Food	Beets, rhubarb, blackberries, cold drink dyes, carrots
Blue to green	Biliverdin	Oxidation of bilirubin (poorly preserved specimen)
	Bacteria	*Pseudomonas* or *Proteus* in urinary tract infections (rare), particularly in urine drainage bags
	Drugs/chemicals	As dyes: amitriptyline, azuresin, methylene blue, Clorets® abuse, Clinitest® ingestion, mitoxantrone, triamterene, resorcinol
Brown to black	Myoglobin	Crush injuries, electric shock, seizures, cocaine-induced muscle damage
	Bile pigments	Hemolysis, bleed into tissues, liver disease
	Melanin	Melanoma (prolonged exposure to air)
	Methemoglobin	Methemoglobinemia from drugs, dyes, etc.
	Porphyrins	Porphyria and sickle cell crisis
	Drugs/chemicals	As dyes: cascara, chloroquine, clofazimine, emodin, senna; as chemicals: ferrous salts, methocarbamol, metronidazole, nitrofurantoin, sulfonamides

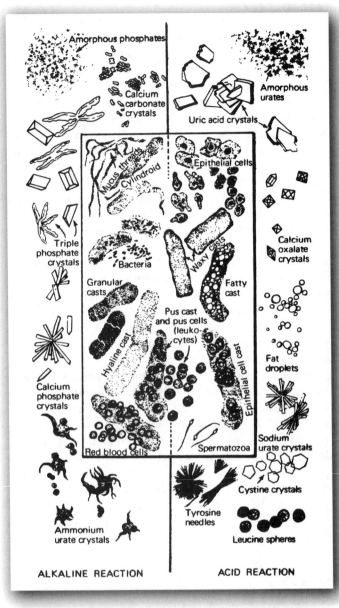

FIGURE 8-3. Possible microscopic (100–200x) findings (mostly normal) in urine sediment. Elements on the left are more likely to be seen in alkaline urine; those on the right are more likely in acid urine. (Reproduced with permission from Krupp MA, Sweet NJ, Jawetz E, et al. *Physician's Handbook.* 19th ed. Norwalk. CT: Lange Medical Publications; 1979.)

pink or red (gross hematuria). If the specimen is not collected properly, vaginal blood may contaminate the urine. Many squamous epithelial cells also appear in this case, suggesting that the erythrocytes did not originate from the urinary tract, but probably from the vaginal walls.[45-47]

White blood cells (leukocytes) (normal range: zero to two per high-power field). Potentially significant pyuria has been defined as three or more WBCs per high-power field of centrifuged urine sediment. Pyuria is usually associated with urinary tract infections (upper or lower). However, inflammatory

conditions (glomerulonephritis, interstitial nephritis) may also lead to this finding.[43,45]

Tubular epithelial cells (normal range: zero or one per high-power field). One epithelial cell per high-power field is often found in normal subjects. Cells originating from the renal tubules are small, oval, and mononuclear. Their quantity increases dramatically when the tubules are damaged (e.g., acute tubular necrosis) or when there is inflammation from interstitial nephritis or glomerulonephritis.[43]

Casts

Casts are cylindrical masses of glycoproteins (e.g., Tamm-Horsfall mucoprotein) that form in the tubules. As shown in Figure 8-3, casts have relatively smooth and regular margins (as opposed to clumps of cells) because they conform to the shape of the tubular lumen. Under certain conditions, casts are released into the urine (called *cylindruria*). Even normal urine can contain a few clear casts. These formed elements are fragile and dissolve more quickly in warm, alkaline urine. Types include hyaline, cellular, granular, waxy, and broad; their causes are listed in Table 8-4.

Hyaline casts. Being clear, hyaline casts are difficult to observe under a microscope and are, by themselves, not indicative of disease. Hyaline casts can be seen in concentrated urine or with the use of diuretics.[45,47]

Cellular casts. In contrast to hyaline casts, cellular casts are seen with intrinsic renal disease. They form when leukocytes, RBCs, or renal tubular epithelial cells become entrapped in the gelatinous matrix forming in the tubule. Their clinical significance is the same as that of the cells themselves; unlike free cells, however, cells in casts originate from within the kidneys. The identification of a particular cast-type is often used to assist in diagnosis. White blood cell casts suggest intrarenal inflammation (for example acute interstitial nephritis) or pyelonephritis. Epithelial cell casts suggest tubular destruction; they may also be noted in glomerulonephritis. Red blood cell casts are seen in glomerulonephritis.[43,47]

Granular and waxy casts. Granular and waxy casts are older, degenerated forms of the other types. Granular (also called *muddy brown*) casts can be seen in many conditions such as acute tubular necrosis, glomerulonephritis, and tubulointerstitial disease. Since waxy casts occur in many diseases, they do not offer much diagnostic information.[43,47]

Crystals

The presence of *crystals* in the urine depends on urinary pH, the degree of saturation of the urine by the substance that is forming crystals, and the presence of other substances in the urine that may promote crystallization. There are numerous types of crystals that can be detected in the urine. Crystalluria, if differentiated by type, can help to identify patients with certain local and systemic diseases. Cystine crystals occur with the condition cystinuria and struvite (magnesium ammonium phosphate) crystals are seen with struvite stones. Calcium oxalate, calcium phosphate and uric acid crystals are also suggestive of stones. Many crystals can be detected in otherwise healthy patients.[44,47]

TABLE 8-4. Causes of Various Types of Casts in Urine[43,45,46]

CAST	CAUSE
Red cell	Classically with acute glomerulonephritis; can be seen in patients who play contact sports and uncommonly with tubular interstitial disease
White cell	Classically seen with pyelonephritis; also seen with glomerulonephritis and interstitial nephritis
Tubular epithelial cell	Nonspecific; acute tubular necrosis, glomerulonephritis, tubulointerstitial disease; also seen with cytomegalovirus infection and toxicity from salicylates and heavy metals, ethylene glycol
Hyaline casts	Nonspecific and may not be pathogenic; seen with prerenal azotemia and strenuous exercise
Granular casts	Nonspecific but pathogenic; may be seen in acute tubular necrosis; volume depletion, glomerulonephritis, tubulointerstitial disease
Waxy and broad casts	Nonspecific for kidney disease

CHEMICAL ANALYSIS (SEMIQUANTITATIVE TESTS)

For this discussion, biochemical analysis of urine includes protein; pH; specific gravity; bilirubin, bile, and urobilinogen; blood and hemoglobin; leukocyte esterase; nitrite; glucose; and ketones. All of these semiquantitative tests can be performed quickly using modern dipsticks containing one or more reagent-impregnated pads. When using these strips, the clinician must carefully apply the urine to the pads as instructed and wait the designated time before comparing pad colors to the color chart. Possible results associated with various colors are displayed in Table 8-5.

Protein

Normal range: zero to trace on dipstick or <200 mg/g (urine protein to creatinine ratio)

The normal urinary proteins are albumin and low molecular weight serum globulins. The glomerulus is freely permeable to substances with a molecular weight of less than 20,000 daltons. However, albumin with a molecular weight of 65,000 daltons is typically restricted from passing through the glomerulus into the urine. The smaller serum globulins that are filtered in the nephron are generally reabsorbed in the proximal tubule. Therefore, healthy individuals excrete very small amounts of protein in the urine (about 80–100 mg of protein per day). In the presence of kidney damage, larger quantities of protein may be excreted. Increased excretion of albumin is associated with diabetic nephropathy, glomerular disease, and hypertension. If low molecular globulins are detected, it is more likely a tubulointestinal process. The term *proteinuria* is a general term that refers to the renal loss of protein (albumin and/or globulins). The term *albuminuria* specifically refers to the abnormal renal excretion of albumin. Clinical proteinuria is defined as the loss of >500 mg/day of protein urine. Patients with microalbuminuria are excreting relatively small, but still pathogenic, amounts (30–300 mg/day) of albumin. Common causes of proteinuria are listed in Table 8-6. It should be noted that proteinuria is sometimes intermittent and is not always pathologic (for example, after exercise and fever).

The KDOQI Clinical Practice Guidelines for Chronic Kidney Disease provides recommendations for screening, evaluating, and monitoring patients for kidney disease. For adult patients without risk factors for kidney disease (i.e., diabetes, hypertension), the standard dipstick for urine protein is the initial screen. If 1+ (30 mg/dL), the patient should be further evaluated with a spot total protein/creatinine ratio. If the spot total

TABLE 8-5. Examples of Tests Available and Possible Results from Multitest Urine Dipstick (Bayer Multistix 10 SG)

TEST	RESULT						
Leukocyte esterase	Negative	Trace	Small +	Moderate ++	Large +++		
Nitrite	Negative	Positive					
Urobilinogen	Normal 0.2 mg/dL	Normal 1 mg/dL	2 mg/dL	4 mg/dL	8 mg/dL		
Protein	Negative	Trace	30 mg/dL +	100 mg/dL ++	300 mg/dL +++	2000 mg/dL ++++	
pH	5	6	6.5	7	7.5	8	8.5
Blood (Hgb)	Negative	Nonhemolyzed Trace	Hemolyzed Trace	Small +	Moderate ++	Large +++	
Specific gravity	1.000	1.005	1.010	1.015	1.020	1.025	1.030
Ketones	Negative	Trace 5 mg/dL	Small 15 mg/dL	Moderate 40 mg/dL	Large 80 mg/dL	Large 160 mg/dL	
Bilirubin	Negative	Small +	Moderate ++	Large +++			
Glucose	Negative	1/10 g/dL (trace) 100 mg/dL	1/4 g/dL 250 mg/dL	1/2 g/dL 500 mg/dL	1 g/dL 1000 mg/dL	2 g/dL 2000 mg/dL	

TABLE 8-6. Causes of Proteins in Urine[41]

Mild proteinuria (<0.5 g/day)

High blood pressure

Lower urinary tract infection

Fever

Renal tubular damage

Exercise

Moderate proteinuria (0.5–3 g/day)

Congestive heart failure

Chronic glomerulonephritis

Acute glomerulonephritis (sometimes major)

Diabetic nephropathy

Pyelonephritis

Multiple myeloma

Preeclampsia of pregnancy

Significant proteinuria (>3 g/day)

Glomerulonephritis

Amyloid

Chronic glomerulonephritis (severe)

Diabetic nephropathy

Lupus nephritis

---

protein creatinine ratio is greater than 200 mg of albumin/gram of creatinine, then the patient should undergo diagnostic evaluation for kidney disease. For those patients already at increased risk, the initial screen should be performed with an albumin-specific dipstick. If positive, then further quantitative evaluation should be performed using a spot albumin/creatinine ratio. If the ratio is >30 mg/g on two or more occasions spaced over 3 months, then a diagnostic evaluation for CKD should be performed.[2]

Due to difficulties with overnight and 24-hour collections, KDOQI recommends spot (untimed) urine testing. The protein (or albumin)-to-creatinine ratio is convenient and accounts for urine volume effects on protein concentration and standardizes the protein or albumin excretion to creatinine excretion. The ratio of protein (or albumin) to creatinine in an untimed urine sample is a very accurate estimate of the total amount of protein (or albumin) excreted in the urine over 24 hours.[2]

Color indicator test strips (e.g., Albustix, Multistix) used to detect and measure protein in the urine contain a buffer mixed with a dye (usually tetrabromophenol blue). In the absence of albumin, the buffer holds the pH at 3, maintaining a yellow color. If albumin is present, it reduces the activity coefficient of hydrogen ions (the pH rises), producing a blue color. Of note, these tests are fairly insensitive to the presence of low molecular globulins including Bence-Jones proteins. Results can be affected by the urinary concentration. At both extremes of urinary concentrations, false positives and false negatives may occur. The potential for this can be easily assessed if specific gravity is measured concomitantly. Substances that

cause abnormal urine color may affect the readability of the strips. These include blood, bilirubin, phenazopyridine nitrofurantoin, and riboflavin.[48] Standard dipsticks do not detect microalbuminuria; however, newer dye-impregnated strips are available that can detect lower concentrations of albumin. Despite the availability of these products, KDOQI guidelines do not recommend their routine use.

pH

Normal range: 4.6–8.0

Sulfuric acid, resulting from the metabolism of sulfur-containing amino acids, is the primary acid generated by the daily ingestion of food. The pH is usually estimated in 0.5 unit increments by use of test strips containing methyl red and bromthymol blue indicators. These strips undergo a series of color changes from orange to blue over a pH range of 5.0–8.5. In addition, pH can be precisely measured with electronic pH meters. Normally, the kidneys can eliminate the acid load by excreting acid itself and sodium hydroxide ions. In fact, healthy persons can acidify the urine to pH 4.5, although the average pH is around 6. Any pH close to the reference range can be interpreted as normal as long as it reflects the kidneys' attempts at regulating blood pH. The urinary pH can be affected by the various acid–base disorders. Determination of the urinary pH is often used in the setting of a urinary tract infection.[46,47]

In general, acidic (versus neutral) urine deters bacterial colonization. Alkaline urine may be seen with either

- urinary tract infections caused by urea-splitting bacteria such as *Proteus mirabilis* (via ammonia production), or
- tubular defects causing decreased net tubular hydrogen ion secretion, as in renal tubular acidosis.

By their intended or unintended pharmacological actions, drugs also can cause true pH changes; they do not interfere with the reagents used to estimate urine pH. Drugs that induce diseases associated with pH changes are indirect causes. These and other causes of acidic and alkaline urine are listed in Table 8-7. Persistent pHs greater than 7.0 are associated with calcium carbonate, calcium phosphate, and magnesium–ammonium phosphate stones; pHs below 5.5 are associated with cystine and uric acid stones.

Specific Gravity

Normal range: 1.016–1.022 (normal fluid intake)

The kidneys are responsible for maintaining the blood's osmolality within a narrow range (285–300 mOsm/kg). To do so, the kidneys must vary the osmolality of the urine over a wide range. Although osmolality is the best measure of the kidneys' concentrating ability, determining osmolality is difficult. Fortunately, it correlates well with specific gravity when the urine contains normal constituents. Specific gravity is the ratio of the weight of a given fluid to the weight of an equal volume of distilled water. Sodium, urea, sulfate, and phosphate contribute most to the specific gravity of urine. Because specific gravity is related to the weight (and not the number) of particles in solution, particles with a weight different from that of sodium chloride (the solute usually in the highest concentration there) can widen the disparity. Patients with normal kidney function

TABLE 8-7. Factors Affecting Urine pH[42,45]

URINE pH AND FACTORS	CAUSES AND COMMENTS
Alkaline urine	
Postprandial	Specimens voided shortly after meals
Vegetarianism	Vegetables do not produce fixed acid residues
Alkalosis (metabolic or respiratory)	Hyperventilation, severe vomiting, GI suctioning
Urinary tract infection	Some bacteria (e.g., *Proteus*) split urea to ammonia, which is alkalinizing
Renal tubular acidosis	Impaired tubular acidification of urine and low bicarbonate and pH in blood
Drugs	Acetazolamide, bicarbonate salts, thiazides, citrate, and acetate salts
Acidic urine	
Drugs	Ammonium chloride, ascorbic acid (high dose), methenamine
Food	Cranberries, prunes, plums, fruit juices
Ketoacidosis	Diabetes mellitus, starvation, high fever
Metabolic acidosis	Increased ammonium excretion and cellular hypoxia with lactic acid production (shock)
Sleep	Mild respiratory acidosis

GI = gastrointestinal.

can dilute urine to approximately 1.001 and concentrate urine to 1.035, which correlates to an osmolality of 50–1000 mOsm/kg, respectively. A urinary specific gravity of 1.010 is considered isosthenuric; that is, the urinary osmolality is the same as plasma.[43,45,46]

Specific gravity can be measured by reagent strips (dipstick), a urinometer (hydrometer), or a refractometer. The reagent strips change color based on the pK_a change of the strips in relation to the ionic concentration of the urine. The indicator substance on the strip changes color, which can be then correlated to the specific gravity. Specific gravity measured by reagent strips is not affected by high concentrations of substances like glucose, protein, or radiographic contrast media, which may elevate readings with refractometers and urinometers. The urinometer is akin to a graduated buoy; it requires sufficient urine volume to float freely. The reading is adjusted according to the urine temperature. The refractometer uses the refractive index as a basis and needs only a few milliliters of urine and no temperature adjustment.[42,45,46]

Several conditions can affect specific gravity. In general, *urinary* specific gravity should be considered abnormal if it is the opposite (high verus low and vice versa) of that which should be produced based on the concurrent *plasma* osmolality. Patients who are volume depleted should present with a concentrated urine (specific gravity ≥1.020) as a normal compensatory mechanism. Patients with prerenal disease will likely have relatively concentrated urine while those with intrinsic damage to the renal tubules are more likely to produce urine, which is isosthenuric (the tubules are unable to dilute or concentrate the urine so the urine is the same concentration as the filtrate). The urine of patients with diabetes insipidus has low values (<1.005) despite a relatively hypertonic plasma. On the other hand, patients with the syndrome of inappropriate secretion of antidiuretic hormone (SIADH) have concentrated urine and relatively hypotonic serum.[43,45,46]

Urobilinogen

Normal range: 0.3 to 1.0 Erlich Unit

Urobilinogen (formed by bacterial conversion of conjugated bilirubin in the intestine) is normally present in urine and increases when the turnover of heme pigments is abnormally rapid, as in hemolytic anemia, congestive heart failure with liver congestion, cirrhosis, viral hepatitis, and drug-induced hepatotoxicity. Elevated urobilinogen may be premonitory of early hepatocellular injury, such as hepatitis, because it is evident in urine before serum bilirubin levels increase. Alkaline urine is also associated with increased urobilinogen concentrations due to enhanced renal elimination. Urobilinogen may decrease (if previously elevated) in patients started on antibiotics (e.g., neomycin, chloramphenicol, and tetracycline) that reduce the intestinal flora producing this substance. Urobilinogen is usually absent in total biliary obstruction, since the substance cannot be formed. Increased urobilinogen in the absence of bilirubin in the urine suggests a hemolytic process.

Bilirubin

Normal range: negative

A dark yellow or greenish-brown color generally suggests *bilirubin* in the urine (bilirubinuria). Most test strips rely on the reaction between bilirubin with a diazotized organic dye to yield a distinct color. Bilirubinuria may be seen in patients with intrahepatic cholestasis or obstruction of the bile duct (stones or tumor). Patients on phenazopyridine and some phenothiazines may have false-positive results. False-negative results may occur in patients taking ascorbic acid.

Blood and Hemoglobin

Normal range: negative

Dipsticks for blood are dependent on the oxidation of an indicator dye due to the peroxidase activity of hemoglobin. A dipstick test can detect as few as one to two RBCs per high-power field.

MINICASE 3

Renal Drug Dosing

JANE L., A 75-YEAR-OLD, 5'6", 175-LB FEMALE, was admitted to the hospital from a long-term care facility where she has been residing after hip fracture surgery 2 months ago. She usually looks forward to her physical therapy sessions and participates in many resident group activities. Recently, on the day of admission she had been lethargic, confused, and needed assistance with eating and dressing. Vital signs were BP 100/60, HR 110, and temperature 96°F. Jane L. has a PMH of long-standing CKD secondary to diabetes and hypertension. Her SCr had typically been 2.40 mg/dL and her BUN 45 mg/dL. She is allergic to ciprofloxacin, which causes hives.

A urine analysis demonstrated >100,000 cfu, WBC 40, and nitrite and leukocyte esterase were positive. Culture and sensitivity revealed *Pseudomonas aeruginosa* sensitive to imipenem and ciprofloxacin. Empiric therapy with imipenem 500 mg IV q 6 hr was initiated.

Three days later Jane L. suffered a seizure; BUN and SCr concentration were obtained and were 40 mg/dL and 2.50 mg/dL, respectively. Upon recognition of this reaction from improperly dosed imipenem, the physician discontinues the imipenem and orders IV tobramycin as per hospital pharmacist.

Question: How should Jane L.'s kidney function be estimated to dose tobramycin?

Discussion: The most conservative estimation of CrCl should be used to dose this known nephrotoxic medication. The National Kidney foundation has suggested the use of either the CG or the MDRD equation to dose drugs eliminated by the kidney. In this scenario, all of the estimations of CrCl are relatively close, between 18–24 mL/min. The most conservative estimate of 18 mL/min should be used to calculate/estimate tobramycin dosing.

Cockcroft-Gault TBW: $\frac{(140 - age) \times wt\ (kg)}{72 \times SCr} \times 0.85\ (female) = 24\ mL/min$

Cockcroft-Gault IBW, where IBW (kg) = (2.3 × inches >5 feet) + 50 (if male), or (2.3 × inches >5 feet) + 45.5 (if female) = 18.2 mL/min

MDRD (mL/min/1.73 M²) = 175 × $SCr^{-1.154}$ × $age^{-0.203}$ × 1.21 (if African American) × 0.742 (if female)

= 19 mL/min/1.73 M²

Individualized MDRD: eGFR/1.73 m² × estimated BSA (m²) = eGFR for drug dosing = 19 mL/min/1.73 M² × 1.923 M² = 21.1 mL/min

CKD-EPI: GFR= 141 × min $(S_c/k,1)^\alpha$ × max (Sc/k, 1)$^{-1.209}$ × 0.993^{age} × 1.018 (if female) × 1.159 (if African American) = 18 mL/min/1.73 M²

Question: What dose and interval of tobramycin should be recommended?

Discussion: Jane L. is not a candidate for once-daily aminoglycoside dosing since CrCl is less than 60 mL/min. More conventional dosing of tobramycin is appropriate with the frequency adjusted for her decreased renal function and a goal peak of 4–5 and a trough of 0.5. A loading dose of 1 mg/kg is based on her total body weight. The maintenance dose should be adjusted based on changes in BUN, SCr, and pharmacokinetic analysis of drug levels usually beginning with the third dose every 3–4 days. Therefore, Jane L. should receive a loading dose of 1 mg/kg (80 mg); then for a GFR 10–50 mL/min, she should receive a maintenance dose of 30% to 70% of the loading dose every 12 hours.[49]

Even small amounts of blood noted on dipstick require further investigation. It is important to note that in addition to hemoglobin, myoglobin can also catalyze this reaction so that a positive dipstick for blood may indicate hematuria (blood), hemoglobinuria (free hemoglobin in urine), or myoglobinuria. Microscopic examination of the urine is needed to distinguish hematuria. The presence of ascorbic acid in the urine may lead to a false negative with these tests; this is usually associated with a fairly large oral intake of vitamin C.[45,46,49]

Hemoglobinuria suggests the presence in intravascular hemolysis or directed damage to the small blood vessels. The presence of myoglobin in the urine is highly suggestive of rhabdomyolysis, the acute destruction of muscle cells. With rhabdomyolysis, myoglobin is cleared rapidly by the kidneys and can be detected in the urine.[45]

The clinical distinction between hematuria, hemoglobinuria, and myoglobinuria is important because the clinical conditions that cause them are very different. The color of the urine is not specific; all three may lead to red or dark brown urine. As noted, with dipsticks for blood, all three conditions will lead to a positive test. Microscopic analysis will demonstrate many more erythrocytes with hematuria, but RBCs can be seen with hemoglobinuria and myoglobinuria. Erythrocytes may be few in number in hematuria due to lysis of the RBCs if the urine has a low specific gravity (<1.005).

Leukocyte Esterase

Normal range: negative to trace

Many dipsticks can detect leukocyte esterase, give a semiquantitative estimate of pyuria (pus in the urine), and thus can be considered an indirect test for urinary tract infections. The presence of esterase activity correlates well with significant numbers of neutrophils (either present or lysed) in the urine. The leukocyte esterase test is important because the presence of actual neutrophils in the urine is not a specific indicator for urinary tract infection.[45,46]

Nitrite

Normal range: negative

The presence of nitrite in the urine is another indirect indicator of a urinary tract infection. Many organisms such as *Escherichia coli*, *Klebsiella*, *Enterobacter*, *Proteus*, *Staphylococcus*, and *Pseudomonas* are able to reduce nitrate to nitrite, and thus a positive urine test would suggest a urinary tract infection. If nitrite-positive, a culture of the urine should be obtained. A first-morning urine specimen is preferred since an incubation period is necessary for the bacteria to convert urinary nitrate to nitrite. A positive test is suggestive of a urinary tract infection, but a negative test cannot rule out a urinary tract infection (i.e., the test is specific but not highly sensitive). False-positive tests may be due to strips that are exposed to air. False negatives occur with infections caused by non-nitrite producing organisms (*Enterococcus*).[45,46]

Glucose and Ketones

Normal range: none

Although glucose is filtered in the glomerulus, it is almost completely reabsorbed in the proximal tubule so that glucose is generally absent in the urine. However, at glucose concentrations greater than approximately 180 mg/dL, the capacity to reabsorb glucose is exceeded and glycosuria will occur. Glucose in the urine is suggestive of diabetes mellitus although other, less common conditions can cause glycosuria. The use of urinary glucose to screen and monitor for diabetes is no longer a standard of care.[45-47]

Ketones in the urine typically indicate a derangement of carbohydrate metabolism resulting in utilization of fatty acids as an energy source. Ketonuria in association with glucose in the urine is suggestive of uncontrolled type 1 diabetes mellitus. Ketonuria can also occur with pregnancy, carbohydrate-free diets and starvation. Aspirin has been reported to cause a false-negative ketone test, whereas levodopa and phenazopyridine may cause false-positive ketone results.[45-47]

Urinary Electrolytes

Like most laboratory tests, urinary electrolytes are rarely definitive for any diagnosis. They can confirm suspicions of a particular medical problem from the history, physical examination, and other laboratory data. Along with the results of a urinalysis and serum electrolytes, urinary electrolyte tests allow the practitioner to rule in or out possible diseases of the differential diagnosis. These tests are relatively simple to perform and widely used in the clinical setting.

"Normal" values for urinary electrolytes are a bit of a misnomer since the kidney should be retaining or excreting electrolytes based on intake and any endogenous production. So any concentration in the urine is *normal* if it favors a normal fluid and serum electrolyte status. A related test, the urinary fractional excretion of sodium (%FE_{Na}), can assist with common diagnostic dilemmas involving the kidneys' ability to regulate electrolytes.

Urinary Sodium, Potassium, and Chloride

The electrolyte that is most commonly measured in the urine is sodium. Occasionally, it is also useful to measure potassium and chloride. For these electrolytes, there is no conversion factor to International System (SI) of units since milliequivalents per liter are equivalent to millimoles per liter.

Sodium

Normal range: varies widely

Regulation of urinary excretion of sodium maintains an effective systemic circulating volume. For this reason, the urinary sodium concentration is often used to assess volume status in a patient. Less often, a 24-hour assessment of sodium excretion (via a urine collection) can be used to assess adherence to sodium restriction in a patient with hypertension and/or heart failure.[50,51] This is because the total urinary sodium excretion should equal the amount of sodium taken in through the diet.

Sodium and water balance is an extremely complex process, and only the most common disorders that may alter sodium and water balance (and hence urine sodium) are discussed here. *Hyponatremia* is the most common electrolyte disorder seen in clinical practice. Hyponatremia is most often observed in volume depletion (GI loss and diuretics) and in SIADH, which is not uncommon; in particular it can be seen in the elderly who are maintained on drugs known to cause excess secretion of ADH, such as the selective serotonin reuptake inhibitors (SSRIs). Urine sodium concentrations of <20 mEq/L generally suggest volume depletion—the kidney is responding to the low volume by reabsorbing sodium. In the case of SIADH, which is characterized by inappropriate retention of water in the distal tubule, the urine sodium is generally greater than 20–40 mEq/L. *Hypernatremia* is less common and occurs when there is a limited access to free water since otherwise healthy adults will become thirsty in the face of hypernatremia. Diabetes insipidus, which is characterized by a decreased production or response to ADH, is another cause of hypernatremia. With diabetes insipidus, the urine sodium concentration will be low despite the presence of clinical euvolemia. This is due to dilution of the urinary sodium secondary to inappropriate loss of water in the urine.[51-53]

Urine sodium concentrations are also useful in the diagnosis of acute kidney injury. In the presence of prerenal azotemia, urine sodium concentrations are low. This is due to the kidneys' attempt to maintain volume and/or blood flow to the kidney. On the other hand, with acute tubular necrosis, the urinary sodium is generally >40 mEq/L because the damaged renal tubules are unable to reabsorb sodium and concentrate urine.[51,52]

Diuretics can interfere with the assessment of urinary sodium. Even with volume depletion, the urinary sodium can be high due to the effect of the diuretic on renal sodium handling.[51,52]

Potassium

Normal range: varies widely

As is the case with sodium, the urinary excretion of potassium varies based on dietary intake and other factors that may affect serum potassium concentrations. For patients with unexplained hypokalemia, urinary potassium may provide useful information. Concentrations greater than 10 mEq/L in a hypokalemic patient usually mean that the kidneys are responsible for the loss. This may occur with potassium-wasting diuretics, high-dose sodium penicillin therapy (e.g., ticarcillin/clavulanate and piperacillin/tazobactam), metabolic acidosis or alkalosis, and a few intrinsic renal disorders. Concomitant hypokalemia and low urinary potassium (<10 mEq/L) suggest GI loss (including chronic laxative abuse) as the cause of low serum potassium. In the setting of hyperkalemia, assessment of urinary potassium concentrations is less useful. Hyperkalemia is often due to kidney failure (with or without drugs that affect potassium homeostasis) so potassium concentrations in the urine would be low.[3,51,52]

%FE$_{Na}$ Test

Although assessment of urine sodium concentrations is very useful in determining volume status, the concentration of sodium in the urine is affected by the degree of water reabsorption in the tubules. The FE$_{Na}$ is the % of sodium (fraction) that is filtered in the glomerulus that eventually is excreted in the urine and thus corrects for the amount of water in the filtrate. An FE$_{Na}$ can be estimated off a spot (random) urine sample with a concomitant serum sample. The calculation is

$$FE_{Na} (\%) = \frac{U_{Na} \times S_{cr}}{S_{Na} \times U_{cr}} \times 100 \qquad (15)$$

where U$_{Na}$ and S$_{Na}$ are urine and serum sodium in milliequivalents per liter or millimoles per liter, and U$_{Cr}$ and S$_{Cr}$ are in milligrams per deciliter or micromoles per liter.

In the face of acute kidney injury, the FE$_{Na}$ can be useful to discriminate between a prerenal process (i.e., volume depletion) and acute tubular necrosis. In the hypovolemic, prerenal state, the kidneys will conserve sodium and the FE$_{Na}$ will be less than 1%. With tubular damage, the FE$_{Na}$ will generally be greater than 2% to 3%. As with the assessment of urine sodium, the FE$_{Na}$ can be affected by diuretic therapy and may be somewhat high despite volume depletion.[51,52]

SUMMARY

The kidneys play a major role in the regulation of fluids, electrolytes, and the acid–base balance. Kidney function is affected by the cardiovascular, pulmonary, endocrine, and central nervous systems. Therefore, abnormalities in these systems may be reflected in renal or urine tests. The urinalysis is useful as a mirror for organ systems that generate substances (e.g., blood/biliary system and urobilinogen) ultimately eliminated in the urine. A urinalysis allows indirect examination without invasive procedures.

A rise in BUN without a simultaneous rise in SCr is not specific for kidney dysfunction. However, concomitant elevations in BUN and SCr almost always reflect some disturbance in the kidneys' ability to clear substances from the body. Renal functions should be estimated based on the patient's SCr and demographic characteristics using either the MDRD or Cockcroft-Gault equations. These equations are a more reliable index of kidney function than SCr alone. A thoughtful examination of the urine (macroscopic, microscopic, and chemical) is an indispensable tool in identifying kidney and other pathological processes that may be present in a patient.

Learning Points

1. What are the concerns or issues when estimating renal function with equations?

Answer: All of the estimating equations use the endogenous filtration marker SCr. Creatinine is not an ideal marker for kidney function since it undergoes tubular secretion, is subject to change under non-steady-state conditions, and it is not ideal for patients outside of the normal 1.73 m² BSA. A significant decline in GFR must occur before SCr exceeds most reference ranges. An abrupt change in SCr such as occurs with acute kidney injury will not be immediately evident. Additional factors affecting SCr values are age, gender, ethnicity, diet, muscle mass, malnutrition, muscle wasting, or limb amputation.

2. Which is better to use for drug dosing—the Cockcroft-Gault or the MDRD equation?

Answer: Either the CrCl using CG or the eGFR may be used to calculate drug doses for most patients. The eGFR should be individualized for those patients that are at the extremes in body habitus. For patients that are considered to be high risk (youngest and very old), for patients receiving drugs that have a narrow therapeutic index, or for patients in whom estimations of kidney function vary or are likely to be inaccurate, consider measuring CrCl or measure GFR using exogenous markers.

3. What is the clinical relevance of a urinary fractional excretion of sodium (% FE$_{Na}$)?

Answer: The FE$_{Na}$ reflects the percent of filtered sodium that is ultimately excreted in the urine. Low FE$_{Na}$ values indicate that the kidney is attempting to conserve sodium and water, thus the patient is in a prerenal state. Other indicators of prerenal kidney dysfunction include a low urinary sodium value and a high urine osmolality (indicating a concentrated urine). A high FE$_{Na}$ is less specific. This may occur in a well-hydrated patient, a patient with acute tubular necrosis, or in a patient on diuretics.

REFERENCES

1. Eaton DC, Pooler J, Vander AJ. *Vander's Renal Physiology.* 6th ed. New York, NY: McGraw-Hill; 2002.

2. Levey AS, Coresh J, Balk E, et al. National Kidney Foundation practice guidelines for chronic kidney disease: evaluation, classification, and stratification. *Ann Intern Med.* 2003;139:137-147.

3. Zappitelli M, Parvex P, Joseph L, et al. Derivation and validation of cystatin C-based prediction equations for GFR in children. *Am J Kidney Dis.* 2006;48:221-230.

4. Zappitelli M, Joseph L, Gupta IR, et al. Validation of child serum creatinine-based prediction equations for glomerular filtration rate. *Pediatr Nephrol.* 2007;22:272-281.

5. Oh MS. Evaluation of renal function, water, electrolyte and acid-base. In: McPherson RA, Pincus MR, eds. *Henry's Clinical Diagnosis and Management by Laboratory Methods.* 21st ed. Philadelphia, PA: Saunders Elsevier; 2007:147-169.

6. Levey AS, Coresh J, Greene T, et al. Using standardized serum creatinine values in the modification of diet in renal disease study equation for estimating glomerular filtration rate. *Ann Intern Med.* 2006;145:247-254.

7. Brosius FC III, Hostetter TH, Kelepouris E, et al. Detection of chronic kidney disease in patients with or at increased risk of cardiovascular disease: a science advisory from the American Heart Association Kidney and Cardiovascular Disease Council; the Councils on High Blood Pressure Research, Cardiovascular Disease in the Young, and Epidemiology and Prevention; and the Quality of Care and Outcomes Research Interdisciplinary Working Group: developed in collaboration with the National Kidney Foundation. *Circulation.* 2006;114:1083-1087.

8. Lamb EJ, Webb MC, Simpson DE, et al. Estimation of glomerular filtration rate in older patients with chronic renal insufficiency: is the modification of diet in renal disease formula an improvement? *J Am Geriatr Soc.* 2003;51:1012-1017.

9. K/DOQI clinical practice guidelines for chronic kidney disease: evaluation, classification, and stratification. Kidney Disease Outcome Quality Initiative. *Am J Kidney Dis.* 2002;39:S1-S246.

10. Counahan R, Chantler C, Ghazali S, et al. Estimation of glomerular filtration rate from plasma creatinine concentration in children. *Arch Dis Child.* 1976;51:875-878.

11. US Food and Drug Administration. Guidance for industry: pharmacokinetics in patients with impaired renal function—study design, data analysis, and impact on doing and labeling, draft guidance. March 2010. Available at http://www.fda.gov/downloads/Drugs/GuidanceComplianceRegulatoryInformation/Guidances/ucm204959.pdf. Accessed January 17, 2012.

12. Briggs JP, Kriz W, Schnermann JB. Overview of kidney function and structure. In: Greenberg A, Cheung AK, Coffman TM, et al., eds. *Primer on Kidney Diseases.* 4th ed. Philadelphia, PA: Elsevier Saunders; 2005:2-25.

13. Perkins BA, Nelson RG, Ostrander BE, et al. Detection of renal function decline in patients with diabetes and normal or elevated GFR by serial measurements of serum cystatin C concentration: results of a 4-year follow-up study. *J Am Soc Nephrol.* 2005;16:1404-1412.

14. Stevens LA, Coresh J, Schmid CH, et al. Estimating GFR using serum cystatin c alone and in combination with serum creatinine: a pooled analysis of 3,418 individuals with CKD. *Am J Kidney Dis.* 2008;51:395-406.

15. National Kidney Disease Education Program. Laboratory professions. Cystatin C standardization (update as of July 2010). Available at http://www.nkdep.nih.gov/labprofessionals/update-cystatin-c.htm. Accessed January 17, 2012.

16. National Kidney Foundation. Cystatin C. What is its role in estimating GFR? Available at http://www.kidney.org/professionals/tools/pdf/CystatinC.pdf. Accessed January 17, 2012.

17. Menon V, Shlipak MG, Wang X, et al. Cystatin C as a risk factor for outcomes in chronic kidney disease. *Ann Intern Med.* 2007;147:19-27.

18. Cockcroft DW, Gault MH. Prediction of creatinine clearance from serum creatinine. *Nephron.* 1976;16:31-41.

19. Myers GL, Miller WG, Coresh J, et al. Recommendations for improving serum creatinine measurement: a report from the Laboratory Working Group of the National Kidney Disease Education Program. *Clin Chem.* 2006;52:5-18.

20. Wade WE, Spruill WJ. New serum creatinine assay standardization: implications for drug dosing. *Ann Pharmacother.* 2007;41:475-480.

21. Briggs JP, Kriz W, Schnerman JB. Clinical evaluation of kidney function and structure. In: Greenberg A, Cheung AK, Coffman TM, et al., eds. *Primer on Kidney Diseases.* 4th ed. Philadelphia, PA: Elsevier Saunders; 2005:20-25.

22. Lemann J, Bidani AK, Bain RP, et al. Use of the serum creatinine to estimate glomerular filtration rate in health and early diabetic nephropathy. Collaborative Study Group of Angiotensin Converting Enzyme Inhibition in Diabetic Nephropathy. *Am J Kidney Dis.* 1990;16:236-243.

23. Mosteller RD. Simplified calculation of body-surface area. *New Eng J Med.* 1987;317(17)1098.

24. Schwartz GJ, Feld LG, Langford DJ. A simple estimate of glomerular filtration rate in full-term infants during the first year of life. *J Pediatr.* 1984;104:849-854.

25. Schwartz GJ, Gauthier B. A simple estimate of glomerular filtration rate in adolescent boys. *J Pediatr.* 1985;106:522-526.

26. Schwartz GJ, Munoz A, Schneider MF, et al. New equations to estimate GFR in children with CKD. *J Am Soc Nephrol.* 2009;20:629-637.

27. Schwartz GJ, Work DF. Measurement and estimation of GFR in children and adolescents. *Clin J Am Soc Nephrol.* 2009;4:1832-1843.

28. Zappitelli M, Washburn KK, Arikan AA, et al. Urine neutrophil gelatinase-associated lipocalcin is an early marker of acute kidney injury in critically ill children: a prospective cohort study. *Crit Care.* 2007;11:R84.

29. Levey AS, Bosch JP, Lewis JB, et al. A more accurate method to estimate glomerular filtration rate from serum creatinine: a new prediction equation. Modification of Diet in Renal Disease Study Group. *Ann Intern Med.* 1999;130:461-470.

30. Verhave JC, Fesler P, Ribstein J, et al. Estimation of renal function in subjects with normal serum creatinine levels: influence of age and body mass index. *Am J Kidney Dis.* 2005;46:233-241.

31. Levey AS, Coresh J, Greene T, et al. Expressing the Modification of Diet in Renal Disease Study equation for estimating glomerular filtration rate with standardized serum creatinine values. *Clin Chem.* 2007;53:766-772.

32. Fadem S; Nepron.com. National Kidney Foundation GFR Calculator. October 24, 0007.

33. National Kidney Foundation. Frequently asked questions about GFR estimates. Available at http://www.kidney.org/professionals/kls/pdf/KBA_FAQs_AboutGFR.pdf. Accessed January 17, 2012.

34. Levey AS, Stevens LA, Schmid CH, et al. A new equation to estimate glomerular filtration rate. *Ann Intern Med.* 2009;150:604-612.

35. Levey AS, Stevens LA. Estimating GFR using the CKD epidemiology collaboration (CKD-EPI) equation: more accurate GFR estimates, lower CKD prevalence estimates, and better risk prediction. *Am J Kid Dis.* 2010;55 (4):622-627.

36. Becker RN, Vassalotti JA. A software upgrade: CKD testing in 2010. *Am J Kid Dis.* 2010;56(1):32-38.

37. Earley A, Miskulin D, Lamb EJ, et al. Estimating equations for glomerular filtration rate in the era of creatinine standardization. A systematic review. (published online ahead of print February 6, 2012) *Ann Intern Med.* 2012. Available at http://www.annals.org/content/early/2012/02/06/0003-4819-156-6-201203200-00391.long. Accessed June 4, 2012.

38. Froissart M, Rossert J, Jacquot C, et al. Predictive performance of the modification of diet in renal disease and Cockcroft-Gault equations for estimating renal function. *J Am Soc Nephrol.* 2005;16:763-773.

39. Stevens LA, Nolin TD, Richardson MM, et al. Comparison of drug dosing recommendations based upon measured GFR and kidney function estimating equations. *Am J Kidney Dis.* 2009;54(1):33-42.

40. National Kidney Disease Education Program. National Institute of Diabetes and Digestive and Kidney Diseases. Chronic kidney disease and drug dosing: information for providers (revised January 2010). Available at http://www.nkdep.nih.gov/professionals/drug-dosing-information.htm. Accessed January 17, 2012.

41. Nyman HA, Dowling TC, Hudson JQ, et al. Comparative evaluation of the Cockcroft-Gault Equation and the Modification of Diet in Renal Disease (MDRD) Study Equation for drug dosing: An opinion of the Nephrology Practice and Research Network of the American College of Clinical Pharmacy. *Pharmacotherapy.* 2011;31(11):1130-1144.

42. Sacher RA, McPherson RA. Laboratory assessment of body fluids. *Widmann's Clinical Interpretation of Laboratory Tests.* 11th ed. Philadelphia, PA: F.A. Davis Company; 2000:924-1014.

43. Greenberg A. Urinalysis. In: Greenberg A, Cheung AK, Coffman TM, et al., eds. *Primer on Kidney Diseases.* 4th ed. Philadelphia, PA: Elsevier Saunders; 2005:26-35.

44. Wallach J. Urine. In: *Interpretation of Diagnostic Tests.* 8th ed. Philadelphia, PA: Lippincott Williams & Wilkins; 2007:89-110.

45. McPherson RA, Ben-Ezra J, Zhao S. Basic examination of urine. In: McPherson RA, Pincus MR, eds. *Henry's Clinical Diagnosis and Management by Laboratory Methods.* 21st ed. Philadelphia, PA: Saunders Elsevier; 2007:393-425.

46. Simerville JA, Maxted WC, Pahira JJ. Urinalysis: a comprehensive review. *Am Fam Physician.* 2005;71:1153-1162.

47. Post TW, Rose BD. Urinalysis in the diagnosis of renal disease. In: Rose BD, ed. *UpToDate.* Waltham, MA: UpToDate; 2007.

48. Multistix® (various) Reagent Strips [product information]. Elkhart, IN: Bayer HealthCare LLC; 2005.

49. Tobramycin. In: DRUGDEX ® SYSTEM [internet database]. Greenwood Village, CO: Thomson Healthcare. Updated periodically. Available at http://www.thomsonhc.com/micromedex2/librarian/ND_T/ evidencexpert/ND_PR/evidencexpert/CS/11BBA9/ND_AppProduct/ evidencexpert/DUPLICATIONSHIELDSYNC/E905A5/ND_PG/ evidencexpert/ND_B/evidencexpert/ND_P/evidencexpert/PFActionId/ evidencexpert.DisplayDrugdexDocument?docId=0019&contentSetId =31&title=Tobramycin&servicesTitle=Tobramycin&topicId=dosingIn formationSection&subtopicId=adultDosageSection. Accessed May 31, 2012.

50. Glassock RJ. Hematuria and proteinuria. In: Greenberg A, Cheung AK, Coffman TM, et al., eds. *Primer on Kidney Diseases.* 4th ed. Philadelphia, PA: Elsevier Saunders; 2005:36-46.

51. Rose BD, Post TW. Meaning of urine electrolytes. In: Rose BD, ed. *UpToDate.* Waltham, MA: UpToDate; 2007.

52. Rose BD. Meaning and application of urine chemistries. *Clinical Physiology of Acid-Base and Electrolyte Disorders.* 5th ed. New York, NY: McGraw-Hill Inc; 2001:405-414.

53. Foote EF. Syndrome of inappropriate antidiuretic hormone secretion and diabetes insipidus. In: Tisdale JE, Miller DA, eds. *Drug-Induced Diseases.* Bethesda, MD: American Society of Health-System Pharmacists; 2005:611-624.

CHAPTER 9

ARTERIAL BLOOD GASES AND ACID–BASE BALANCE

ANASTASIA L. ROBERTS

Maintenance of normal pH in the body is required for normal organ function. Cellular metabolism continually produces acidic substances that must be excreted to prevent acid accumulation. The lungs, kidneys, and a complex system of buffers allow the body to maintain acid–base homeostasis. Arterial blood gases (ABGs) include pH, arterial partial pressures of oxygen (PaO_2) and carbon dioxide ($PaCO_2$), and bicarbonate (HCO_3^-) concentration. By evaluating ABGs, the clinician can assess a patient's acid–base status. The serum anion gap and lactate concentrations, combined with the patient's history and presentation, provide additional information to classify and evaluate the most likely causes of acid–base disorders.

This chapter reviews acid–base physiology and control, discusses laboratory tests used to assess acid–base status, and provides a method to evaluate potential causes of acid–base disorders. This chapter also reviews the use of ABGs to evaluate the oxygenation and ventilation functions of the lungs.

ACID–BASE PHYSIOLOGY

The pH of arterial blood is normally maintained within the narrow range of 7.38–7.44.[1,2] Values of arterial pH 7.35 and lower are termed *acidemia*, and values of arterial pH 7.45 and higher are termed *alkalemia*. A disorder that lowers pH is an *acidosis,* and a disorder that raises pH is an *alkalosis.* The distinction between these terms is often blurred. However, recognition of these concepts is critical to a thorough understanding of acid–base physiology. The arterial pH may be normal in mixed acid–base disorders (e.g., respiratory acidosis plus metabolic alkalosis) or only mildly altered even in significant acid–base disorders due to compensatory mechanisms.

Generally, the lungs and kidneys maintain acid–base homeostasis. Acid–base disorders are categorized according to the primary abnormality—the underlying pathophysiologic event that disturbs the pH. The lungs excrete carbon dioxide (CO_2), which is the primary volatile acid in the body. When the lungs fail to adequately excrete carbon dioxide and the blood level of CO_2 rises as the primary abnormality, the disorder is termed *respiratory acidosis.* Conversely, when the lungs excessively excrete CO_2 and blood CO_2 levels fall, *respiratory alkalosis* is produced. The kidneys regulate blood concentrations of bicarbonate (HCO_3^-). When the primary abnormality is a deficit of bicarbonate, the disorder is termed *metabolic acidosis*; an excess of bicarbonate is termed *metabolic alkalosis.* Laboratory assessment of acid–base status is usually performed on samples of arterial blood, which accurately reflect acid–base status in the body under most conditions.

Acid–Base Balance

Metabolism of glucose, fats, and protein as energy sources result in the daily production of 15,000 mmol of carbon dioxide, which acts as an acid in the body, and 50–100 mEq of nonvolatile acids (e.g., sulfuric acid).[3] This continual load of acidic substances must be buffered initially to prevent acute acidosis. After being buffered, these acids must be excreted to prevent exceeding the body's buffer capacity. Carbon dioxide is excreted by the lungs and the nonvolatile acids are excreted by the kidneys.

The principal buffer in the body is the carbonic acid/bicarbonate system. Other buffers, including proteins, phosphate, and hemoglobin (Hgb), also contribute to the body's buffer capacity and to maintenance of normal pH. However, the carbonic acid/bicarbonate buffer system is particularly important in understanding acid–base physiology for two reasons:

1. The key components of this system, CO_2 as the acid and HCO_3^- as the base, are easily accessible in serum and are easily measured in clinical laboratories. These parameters are used to estimate the overall acid–base status of the body. Because all buffer systems exist in equilibrium in the body, analysis of any buffer system accurately reflects the pH. Thus, even though other buffers are important, accurate assessment of acid–base status may be made using only one buffer system.

2. The lungs and kidneys closely regulate the concentrations of CO_2 and HCO_3^-, allowing rapid and precise control over acid–base equilibrium. Pathology in these organs often is associated with acid–base disorders. In addition to allowing accurate assessment of acid–base status, careful evaluation of the levels of CO_2 and HCO_3^- provides important information about the most likely underlying causes of the acid–base disorder.

Carbonic Acid/Bicarbonate Buffer System

Carbonic acid (H_2CO_3), a weak acid, and its conjugate base, *bicarbonate* (HCO_3^-), exist in equilibrium with hydrogen ions (H^+):

$$HCO_3^- + H^+ \leftrightarrow H_2CO_3$$

If hydrogen ions are added to the body or released as a result of cellular metabolism, the H^+ concentration rises and is reflected by a fall in pH. However, a large portion of the hydrogen ions combines with bicarbonate to form carbonic acid, lessening the effect on pH. The effect of the acid is buffered, and the pH remains at or near normal.

In aqueous solutions, carbonic acid reversibly dehydrates to form water and carbon dioxide. This reaction is catalyzed in the body by the enzyme carbonic anhydrase (CA), which is present in many tissues:

$$HCO_3^- + H^+ \leftrightarrow H_2CO_3 \overset{CA}{\leftrightarrow} CO_2 + H_2O$$

Nearly all carbonic acid in the body exists as carbon dioxide gas. Therefore, carbon dioxide is the acid form of the carbonic acid/bicarbonate buffer system. When hydrogen ions are released, the concentration of bicarbonate falls, and the concentration of carbon dioxide gas rises as the acid is buffered.

The Henderson-Hasselbalch equation for the carbonic acid/bicarbonate buffer system describes the mathematical relationship among pH, bicarbonate concentration in milliequivalents per liter, and partial pressure of carbon dioxide (pCO_2), a measure of the concentration of carbon dioxide gas in fluid) in millimeters of mercury:

$$pH = 6.1 + \log\left(\frac{HCO_3^-}{0.03 \times pCO_2}\right)$$

This equation demonstrates an important point: the *ratio* of the bicarbonate and carbon dioxide concentrations, not the absolute values, determines pH. The concentration of bicarbonate or carbon dioxide can change dramatically, but if the other value changes proportionately in the same direction, pH remains unchanged.

For arterial blood, the most commonly sampled medium, the normal ratio of bicarbonate (in milliequivalents per liter) to $PaCO_2$ (in millimeters of mercury) is 0.6:1. This ratio results in a pH of 7.40 when the bicarbonate concentration is normal (24 mEq/L or 24 mmol/L) and the $PaCO_2$ is normal (40 mm Hg or 5.3 kPa). It is impossible to predict the pH accurately or to assess a patient's acid–base status from either the bicarbonate concentration or $PaCO_2$ alone. If both are known, however, the pH can be calculated from this equation. In fact, when clinical laboratories evaluate ABGs, only the pH and $PaCO_2$ are measured. The bicarbonate concentration is then calculated from this equation.

Role of Kidneys and Lungs

The kidneys regulate the concentration of bicarbonate in extracellular fluid, and the lungs regulate the $PaCO_2$. An understanding of the functions of these organs is necessary to evaluate ABGs and acid–base status.

Kidneys

The principal role of the *kidneys* in maintaining acid–base homeostasis is to regulate the concentration of bicarbonate in the blood. Since bicarbonate is readily filtered at the glomerulus, the kidneys reabsorb filtered bicarbonate to prevent depletion. Approximately 90% of this reabsorption takes place in the proximal tubule and is catalyzed by carbonic anhydrase (Figure 9-1). Filtered bicarbonate combines with hydrogen ions secreted by the tubule cell to form carbonic acid. The enzyme carbonic anhydrase, located in the brush border of the tubule, catalyzes conversion of carbonic acid to carbon dioxide. The uncharged CO_2 readily crosses the cell membrane and passively diffuses into the renal tubule cell. Inside the cell, carbonic acid and bicarbonate are reformed, also catalyzed by carbonic anhydrase. The bicarbonate is reabsorbed into capillary blood. The net result of this process is reabsorption of sodium and bicarbonate. Drugs that inhibit carbonic anhydrase (e.g., acetazolamide) can cause metabolic acidosis by inhibiting this process, causing excessive quantities of bicarbonate to be lost in the urine.

The other major role of the kidneys, as discussed previously, is to excrete the 50–100 mEq/day of nonvolatile acids that are produced by the body. This process occurs primarily in the distal tubule and also requires carbonic anhydrase. The hydrogen ions that are secreted into the tubule lumen are buffered by phosphates and ammonia, so the urine pH is usually acidic but typically not less than 4.50.

Lungs

The principal role of the *lungs* in maintaining acid–base balance is to regulate the $PaCO_2$. After blood returns from the tissues to the right side of the heart, it is pumped through the pulmonary artery to the lungs. In the capillaries, carbon dioxide readily

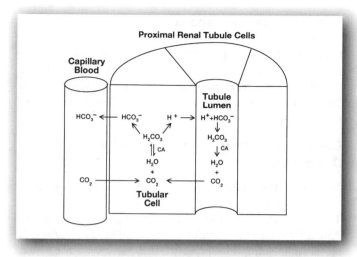

FIGURE 9-1. Reabsorption of bicarbonate from the proximal renal tubule cell.

diffuses from the blood into the alveoli of the lungs and is excreted in exhaled air.

The rate of carbon dioxide excretion is directly proportional to the rate of air passing into and out of the lungs. Under resting conditions, normal individuals take 14–18 breaths/min. The amount of air in each breath, known as the *tidal volume*, is about 500 mL. Ventilation can be increased by increasing either the rate of respiration or the tidal volume.

Chemoreceptors in the arteries and the medulla in the brain are capable of rapidly increasing or decreasing ventilation in response to changes in pH and the arterial partial pressures of oxygen (PaO_2) and carbon dioxide ($PaCO_2$). This ability allows rapid response to changes in acid–base status and is one reason that the carbonic acid/bicarbonate buffer system is physiologically important. An elevated $PaCO_2$ is usually associated with hypoventilation, and a low $PaCO_2$ is usually associated with hyperventilation.

The other major function of the lungs is to oxygenate the blood. Inspired oxygen diffuses from the alveoli into capillary blood and is bound to Hgb in red blood cells. The oxygen is carried throughout the body via the arterial system and is released to tissues for utilization. Oxygen in arterial blood is present in three forms:

1. Oxygen gas (measured as PaO_2)
2. Dissolved oxygen
3. Oxygen bound to Hgb (oxy-Hgb)

Over 90% of the total arterial oxygen content is as oxy-Hgb. As the oxygenated blood passes through the capillaries, dissolved and gaseous oxygen are taken up by tissues, and additional oxygen rapidly dissociates from Hgb and becomes available for tissue uptake.

Arterial Blood Gases

Arterial blood gas evaluations include measurements of the arterial pH, PaO_2, and $PaCO_2$. The bicarbonate concentration is calculated from the pH and $PaCO_2$ using the equations listed previously. Proper evaluation of ABG results requires specific knowledge about each test.

Arterial pH

Normal range: 7.38–7.44

The pH of arterial blood is the first value to consider when using the ABGs to assess a patient's acid–base status. As stated previously, pH values of 7.37 and lower represent acidemia, and pH values of 7.45 and higher represent alkalemia. When a patient's acid–base status is evaluated, the patient must first be classified as having normal pH, acidemia, or alkalemia. It is important to recognize that a normal pH does not exclude the possibility of an acid–base disorder. Mixed acid–base disorders may result in a normal pH.

Critical values of pH are difficult to specify. More frequently, other manifestations of the underlying disorder producing the acid–base disturbance will dictate the urgency with which treatment must be initiated. For example, in sepsis syndrome with metabolic acidosis, the negative effects of infection and organ failure are typically more deleterious than the effect of low pH. Severe acidemia causes myocardial depression, hypotension, and impairs central nervous system (CNS) activity. Severe alkalemia impairs cerebral and coronary blood flow and causes respiratory depression. In general, pH values <7.20 or >7.60 represent levels that may require therapy to reverse these specific detrimental effects of the pH value.[4]

Spurious values of pH are most commonly due to inadvertent sampling of venous, rather than arterial blood. The pH of venous blood is slightly more acidic than arterial blood.

Arterial Partial Pressure of Carbon Dioxide

Normal range: 35–40 mm Hg or 4.7–5.3 kPa

Evaluation of the $PaCO_2$ (commonly seen on lab reports as pCO_2) provides information about the adequacy of lung function in excreting carbon dioxide, the acid form of the carbonic acid/bicarbonate buffer system. Because carbon dioxide is a small, uncharged molecule, it diffuses readily from pulmonary capillary blood into the alveoli in normal lungs. Therefore, an elevated $PaCO_2$ usually implies inadequate ventilation.

It is the pH, not the absolute value of $PaCO_2$ that determines the criticality of the patient's situation. Like the pH, spurious values for $PaCO_2$ are usually due to inadvertent venous sampling, which has a higher carbon dioxide content.

Arterial Partial Pressure of Oxygen

Normal range: 95–100 mm Hg or 12.7–13.3 kPa

Evaluation of the PaO_2 (commonly seen on lab reports as pO_2) provides information about the level of oxygenation of arterial blood. If effective circulation is achieved, a normal PaO_2 generally means that oxygen delivery to tissues is adequate. PaO_2 is commonly reduced in conjunction with an elevated $PaCO_2$ in states associated with hypoventilation. In fact, the PaO_2 is more likely to be diminished because carbon dioxide is much more freely diffusible across the pulmonary capillary and alveolar membranes. Therefore, diseases that impair gas exchange in the lungs can produce hypoxemia, which stimulates increased ventilation. Hyperventilation may fail to correct the hypoxemia but may produce a normal or low $PaCO_2$.

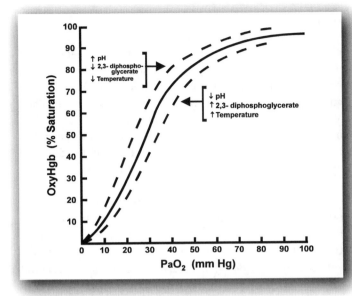

FIGURE 9-2. Oxygen–Hgb dissociation curve.

Figure 9-2 shows the sigmoid relationship between the percentage of available oxygen-binding sites on Hgb that are occupied and the PaO_2. The Hgb saturation remains above 90% as long as the PaO_2 is above 60 mm Hg (8 kPa). Since most oxygen in arterial blood is present as oxy-Hgb, oxygen delivery to tissues generally remains adequate even though the PaO_2 drops to as low as 60 mm Hg. However, PaO_2 values less than 60 mm Hg are associated with rapid falls in Hgb saturation and dramatic decreases in oxygen delivery to tissues.

This relationship is important to remember because ABGs measure PaO_2. Even though PaO_2 values between 60 mm Hg (8 kPa) and normal (95–100 mm Hg or 12.7–13.3 kPa) indicate that a disease process is present, oxygen therapy may not be urgently needed since Hgb saturation is still above 90%. However, PaO_2 values less than 60 mm Hg indicate a more significant reduction in Hgb saturation and impaired tissue oxygen delivery. This impairment may require rapid supplemental oxygen therapy. The atmosphere contains 21% oxygen, and increasing this concentration with supplemental oxygen therapy frequently reverses hypoxemia. Oxygen is administered by increasing the fraction of inspired oxygen (FiO_2) from 24% to 100%.

Spuriously low values of PaO_2 are seen with inadvertent venous blood samples or when the arterial blood sample is not stored in ice before the test is run. If kept at room temperature, cellular metabolism results in significant oxygen consumption, lowering the PaO_2 value. Conversely, air bubbles in the syringe may result in oxygen diffusion into the sample, spuriously raising the PaO_2 value.

Several conditions can alter oxygen–Hgb dissociation. Acidosis, fever, and increased concentrations of 2,3-diphosphoglycerate (2,3-DPG) shift the curve in Figure 9-2 to the right, making oxygen more readily available for delivery to tissues. Alkalosis and decreased 2,3-DPG concentrations shift the curve to the left, increasing oxygen binding to Hgb and potentially reducing oxygen delivery to tissues.

Arterial Serum Bicarbonate
Normal range: 19–24 mEq/L or 19–24 mmol/L
Once the $PaCO_2$ and pH are measured, the bicarbonate concentration is calculated and reported with the ABG results. Either the bicarbonate from the ABG determination or the total carbon dioxide content of serum (discussed below) can be used to assess acid–base disorders.

Other Tests to Assess Acid–base Balance and Oxygenation

Venous Total Carbon Dioxide (Serum Bicarbonate)
Normal range: 24–30 mEq/L or 24–30 mmol/L
The total carbon dioxide concentration is frequently determined by acidifying serum to convert all of the bicarbonate present in the sample to carbon dioxide. However, since 95% of total serum carbon dioxide consists of converted bicarbonate, this value is actually a measure of the bicarbonate concentration. The total carbon dioxide content typically can be expected to be 0–2 mEq/L higher than the bicarbonate concentration. Therefore, the term *serum bicarbonate* is used interchangeably with *total carbon dioxide*, even though clinical laboratories may report the test with the more precise term *total carbon dioxide*. Although the name total carbon dioxide implies that it is a measure of acid, it is important to recognize that this test represents bicarbonate, the base form of the carbonic acid/bicarbonate buffer system. Like the $PaCO_2$ test, the urgency of need for response to abnormal total carbon dioxide values is determined by the pH.

Anion Gap
Normal range: 3–16 mEq/L or 3–16 mmol/L
The *anion gap* is a calculated value that is helpful in categorizing and evaluating possible causes of metabolic acidosis.[5,6] For the body to remain electrically neutral, the numbers of all positively and negatively charged ions must be equal. However, clinical laboratories do not routinely measure all ions. Many positively charged ions (e.g., sodium, potassium, calcium, and magnesium) are measured. Sodium ($Na+$) typically accounts for the majority of cations in extracellular fluids. Some anions (e.g., chloride, bicarbonate, and phosphate) are routinely measured, but others (e.g., sulfate, lactate, and pyruvate) are not. Serum proteins are also sources of negative charges that are difficult to quantify.

The number of *unmeasured* anions normally exceeds the number of *unmeasured* cations. When this difference is increased above the upper limit of normal, it often reflects an increase in negatively charged, weak acids. The presence of an increased anion gap in conjunction with metabolic acidosis provides the clinician with useful information about possible causes of acidosis. By convention, the anion gap is calculated using sodium to approximate the measured cations, and chloride (Cl^-) and bicarbonate to approximate the measured anions:

$$anion\ gap = Na^+ - (Cl^- + HCO_3^-)$$

In conditions that cause metabolic acidosis either by production of hydrochloric acid (HCl) or by excessive loss of bicarbonate, which the kidneys primarily replace with chloride, the anion gap remains normal. The normal anion gap exists in these disorders because chloride anions replace bicarbonate, and both values are included in the calculation of the anion gap. These conditions are termed *hyperchloremic* or *normal anion gap* metabolic acidosis.

In other conditions, organic acids are formed that dissociate into unmeasured anions. In diabetic ketoacidosis, lipid catabolism produces the ketone bodies beta-hydroxybutyrate and acetoacetate. In methanol intoxication, methanol is metabolized to formic acid, which dissociates to produce formate and hydrogen ions. The anions beta-hydroxybutyrate, acetoacetate, and formate are not measured in routine electrolyte panels and are not included in the calculation of the anion gap. They produce acidemia, a decrease in serum bicarbonate as this buffer is consumed, and an increase in the calculated anion gap. These conditions are examples of *elevated anion gap* metabolic acidosis. The presence of an elevated anion gap in any patient is highly suggestive of a metabolic acidosis.

The normal value for the anion gap can vary based on the clinical chemistry methodologies for measuring chloride ions. The normal value at most institutions will be in the range of 3–16 mEq/L (3–16 mmol/L). However, this range may vary due to the variability in normal ranges of the values used to calculate anion gap. Clinicians should verify the normal range for anion gap at their institutions.

Various factors can alter the anion gap, making interpretation more difficult.[6,7] In particular, hypoalbuminemia, hyperlipidemia, lithium intoxication, and multiple myeloma decrease the anion gap. Albumin is one principal source of unmeasured anions, so hypoalbuminemia decreases unmeasured anions and the anion gap. Hyperlipidemia reduces the anion gap both by occupying space in the plasma volume and by interfering with the laboratory assay for chloride. Lithium is a positively charged ion not included in the anion gap calculation. In cases of intoxication, it can decrease the anion gap. Multiple myeloma produces positively charged proteins and reduces the anion gap by increasing unmeasured cations.

The anion gap can also be altered by many electrolyte abnormalities. In particular, abnormalities involving ions not included in the calculation of the anion gap (e.g., potassium and calcium) can affect the anion gap. Therefore, the anion gap must always be interpreted cautiously.

Serum Lactate
Normal ranges: 0.6–2.2 mEq/L or 0.6–2.2 mmol/L (venous) and 0.3–0.8 mEq/L or 0.3–0.8 mmol/L (arterial)
Lactate is a byproduct of the anaerobic metabolism of glucose as an energy source.[8] Metabolism of glucose yields pyruvate, which can be converted to lactate in a reaction catalyzed by lactate dehydrogenase (LDH) (Figure 9-3). Lactate is transported to the liver and converted back to pyruvate.

When tissues are normally oxygenated, pyruvate is converted to acetyl coenzyme A (acetyl CoA) and is utilized as an energy source via aerobic metabolism. In patients with inadequate tissue perfusion (e.g., septic shock) or increased tissue metabolic rates (e.g., status epilepticus), anaerobic metabolism

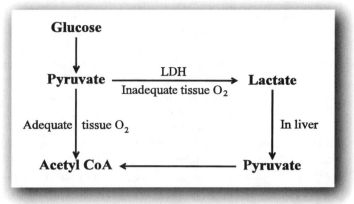

FIGURE 9-3. Lactate metabolism.

predominates. Anaerobic metabolism increases the conversion of pyruvate to lactate, increasing lactate concentrations. When inadequate tissue perfusion is present, lactate is not transported to the liver, further increasing lactate concentrations. If these processes are severe or not reversed, lactic acidosis (a type of metabolic acidosis) can occur. Drugs or other conditions that impair lactate or pyruvate metabolism can also produce elevated lactate concentrations. Lactate levels above 4 mEq/L are usually associated with critical illness and require urgent treatment.

Venous Partial Pressure of Oxygen
Normal range: 70 mm Hg or 9.3 kPa
It has been recognized for many years that in critically ill patients or during cardiopulmonary resuscitation, venous blood gases may provide a more accurate measure of the adequacy of tissue oxygenation than ABGs. In particular, the *venous partial pressure of oxygen* has been suggested as a test that better reflects tissue oxygenation. This is because the amount of oxygen remaining in venous blood after passing through the tissues reflects both oxygen delivery (DO_2) and oxygen consumption (VO_2). When venous partial pressure of oxygen is measured in pulmonary arterial blood, which reflects mixed venous blood from all tissues in the body, it is termed *mixed venous oxygen (SvO_2)*. The normal value for SvO_2 is 70 mm Hg. Values below this indicate that tissues are extracting an unusually large fraction of the delivered oxygen, and that increasing oxygen delivery or reducing tissue metabolic activity may be indicated. In particular, treatment of low SvO_2 values early in the management of patients with severe sepsis has been shown to improve mortality, and has been accepted as a standard of care for this patient population.[9]

Oxygen Saturation by Pulse Oximetry
Normal range: >94%
As an alternative to PaO_2 values obtained with ABGs, measuring the oxygen-Hgb saturation with pulse oximetry can also assess the level of oxygenation.[10] Pulse oximetry is based on the principle that oxy-Hgb molecules absorb different amounts of light than nonoxygenated Hgb. In pulse oximetry a probe is placed on the finger or earlobe. Light of specific wavelength is transmitted through the tissues, and the light intensity is measured on the opposite side of the tissue. The amount of light

absorption is proportional to the relative amounts of oxy-Hgb and Hgb present in arterial blood. The instrument calculates oxygen saturation from this ratio. This method is commonly used when frequent, noninvasive monitoring of oxygenation is needed (e.g., for patients receiving intravenous midazolam or opiates to provide moderate sedation for invasive procedures). Pulse oximetry provides a continuous estimate of oxygen saturation without the need for frequent arterial blood sampling. It is important to remember that the PaO_2 can fall dramatically, and the oxygen saturation will stay above 90%. Significant impairment of oxygenation may occur with minimal change in oxygen saturation. The results of pulse oximetry must be interpreted with this understanding.

Several factors can interfere with the accuracy of pulse oximetry. Presence of large amounts of carboxyhemoglobin (CO-Hgb), seen in heavy smokers and in carbon monoxide poisoning, falsely increases the estimated oxygen saturation. Hyperbilirubinemia also produces CO-Hgb and can falsely increase the oxygen saturation measured by pulse oximetry. Methemoglobinemia, often produced due to exposure to oxidizing substances, can produce false elevations or decreases in pulse oximetry measurements. Methylene blue produces significant decreases in the estimated oxygen saturation as measured by pulse oximetry. Physical factors such as excessive motion, skin pigmentation, and nail polish can affect the pulse oximetry measurement. Finally, hypoperfusion or use of potent vasoconstrictors can interfere with the pulse oximetry reading.

BASIC PRINCIPLES IN ACID–BASE ASSESSMENT

Table 9-1 summarizes the expected laboratory results in the four simple acid–base disorders. For each disorder, the primary laboratory abnormality is accompanied by a compensatory change. For example, the primary abnormality in metabolic acidosis is a fall in serum bicarbonate, and the compensatory change is a fall in $PaCO_2$. These compensatory changes reflect the body's attempts to return the bicarbonate/carbon dioxide ratio and pH closer to the normal range.

An important principle in interpreting these laboratory tests is to recognize that the body never overcompensates and rarely completely compensates for an acid–base disorder. The only exception is chronic respiratory alkalosis in which the kidneys can completely compensate. Therefore, the pH and direction of change from normal of the $PaCO_2$ and serum bicarbonate generally can be used to classify simple acid–base disorders.

Although respiratory compensation for metabolic acid–base disorders occurs within minutes to hours because the lungs can alter carbon dioxide excretion rapidly, renal compensation for respiratory disorders is slower. Acute respiratory acidosis and alkalosis are associated with minimal compensation (Table 9-1). Tissue buffers (e.g., protein and Hgb) are responsible for this compensation. Renal compensation, accomplished by altering the bicarbonate excretion, requires 6–12 hours to be initiated and is not complete for 3–5 days.

Pharmacists should use a standard, stepwise method to assess patients' acid–base status. Table 9-1 can be used as a guide to acid–base evaluation.

1. **Evaluate the pH from the ABGs.** As noted earlier, a pH of 7.35 or lower is acidemia and 7.45 or higher is alkalemia. In acidemia, at least one simple acidosis must be present and in alkalemia at least one alkalosis must be present. A normal pH does not mean that acid–base status is normal; complete evaluation is still required.

2. **Evaluate the total carbon dioxide (serum bicarbonate) and $PaCO_2$ values.** In patients with acidemia, a low bicarbonate suggests metabolic acidosis, and an elevated $PaCO_2$ suggests respiratory acidosis. Evaluation of Table 9-1 will demonstrate that all four simple acid–base disorders are associated with a unique pattern of alteration of total carbon dioxide and $PaCO_2$. In patients with normal pH, bicarbonate or $PaCO_2$ levels outside the normal range suggest that an acid–base disorder may be present. In particular, this situation suggests that an acidosis and alkalosis may both be present.

3. **Evaluate the degree of compensation.** Normal levels of compensation are within 10% of the estimates noted in Table 9-1. For example, in an alkalemic patient with an elevated serum bicarbonate of 32 mEq/L (consistent with metabolic alkalosis), the bicarbonate is 8 mEq/L above normal. Normal compensation is for the $PaCO_2$ to rise by 4–6 mmHg, to a value of 44–46 mmHg (0.6 x 8 plus/minus 10%, rounded to the nearest mmHg).

TABLE 9-1. Laboratory Results in Simple Acid–Base Disorders

DISORDER	pH	PRIMARY ALTERATION[a]	COMPENSATORY ALTERATION	NORMAL LEVEL OF COMPENSATION[b]
Metabolic acidosis	↓	↓↓↓ HCO_3^-	↓↓ $PaCO_2$	↓ $PaCO_2$ = 1.2 × ↓ HCO_3^-
Metabolic alkalosis	↑	↑↑↑ HCO_3^-	↑↑ $PaCO_2$	↑ $PaCO_2$ = 0.6 × ↑ HCO_3^-
Respiratory acidosis (acute)	↓↓	↑↑↑ $PaCO_2$	↑ HCO_3^-	↑ HCO_3^- = 0.1 × ↑ $PaCO_2$
Respiratory acidosis (chronic)	↓	↑↑↑ $PaCO_2$	↑↑ HCO_3^-	↑ HCO_3^- = 0.4 × ↑ $PaCO_2$
Respiratory alkalosis (acute)	↑↑	↓↓↓ $PaCO_2$	↓ HCO_3^-	↓ HCO_3^- = 0.2 × ↓ $PaCO_2$
Respiratory alkalosis (chronic)	↑	↓↓↓ $PaCO_2$	↓↓ HCO_3^-	↓ HCO_3^- = 0.4 × ↓ $PaCO_2$

[a]Arrows signify direction and relative magnitude of change from normal values of $PaCO_2$ (40 mm Hg) and venous HCO_3^- (24 mEq/L). Total carbon dioxide may be used in place of bicarbonate using a value of 24 as normal.

[b]Normal compensation can vary by approximately ±10% from calculated values.

4. **Assess causes of abnormal levels of compensation.** A level of compensation outside of the expected range suggests that a mixed acid–base disorder may be present. Compensatory changes less than expected for a simple acid–base disorder suggests a mixed acid–base disorder of the same type; either combined metabolic and respiratory acidosis or combined metabolic and respiratory alkalosis. A level of compensation *greater* than expected suggests that a form of acidosis and alkalosis may both be present.

The formulas listed in Table 9-1 for normal levels of compensation are estimates only; variability exists in the normal response. In addition, use of total carbon dioxide to estimate serum bicarbonate may slightly alter the expected value. In patients with metabolic acidosis, comparing the decrease in serum bicarbonate with the increase in the anion gap is useful. If the anion gap is elevated but not to the same degree that the bicarbonate has fallen, a combination of anion gap and hyperchloremic metabolic acidosis, caused by two underlying disorders, may be present.

In the case of renal compensation for respiratory acid–base disorders, values intermediate between acute and chronic compensation may indicate either that a mixed disorder is present or that adequate time for compensation has not elapsed. Information from the patient's history and physical examination, including temporal relationships, must be assessed to help evaluate the laboratory data. The minicases and discussions that follow build on this overview to demonstrate evaluation of patients with acid–base disorders.

Metabolic Acidosis

Patients with metabolic acidosis display an arterial pH less than 7.36 (acidemia) and a low serum bicarbonate concentration, determined either with ABGs or as the total carbon dioxide concentration on the serum chemistry panel. Under most circumstances, the body compensates by hyperventilating to increase carbon dioxide excretion, resulting in a low $PaCO_2$ value (Table 9-1).

Common causes of metabolic acidosis are listed in Table 9-2. Once metabolic acidosis is diagnosed, the next step in patient assessment is calculation of the anion gap. This step helps to determine the cause of the acidosis. As shown in Table 9-2, some causes of metabolic acidosis typically produce an increased anion gap, while others produce a normal gap. With a normal anion gap, the serum chloride is elevated, producing a hyperchloremic metabolic acidosis.

Several drugs can cause metabolic acidosis and are listed in Table 9-2. Several of the nucleoside reverse-transcriptase inhibitors used to treat human immunodeficiency virus (HIV) infection have been reported to cause lactic acidosis.[11,20] Propofol has been reported to cause metabolic acidosis as a component of what has been described as propofol infusion syndrome. This syndrome was initially reported primarily in critically ill pediatric patients, but has now been reported in critically ill adults. The syndrome typically appears with higher doses of propofol when used for ICU sedation for a prolonged period of time.[12,13,20] Prolonged, high dose infusion of intravenous lorazepam, which contains propylene glycol, has also been reported to cause lactic acidosis in critically ill patients.[14] Many other drugs have also been reported to cause metabolic acidosis, although the frequency and strength of association are lower. In addition, metabolic acidosis may appear as one complication of drug-induced acute tubular necrosis or acute renal failure. A complete review of the patient's medication list is required to rule out potential drug-induced causes.

MINICASE 1

A Patient With Diarrhea

ROBERT W., A 66-YEAR-OLD MALE, has been hospitalized for the past 2 weeks following a triple coronary artery bypass graft surgery. His hospital stay was complicated by the development of ventilator associated pneumonia 7 days ago, which required broad spectrum antibiotics. For the past 48 hours, he has been having high temperatures and a significant amount of stool output. His most recent stool sample has tested positive for *C. difficile* toxin. Current laboratory data include sodium 137 mEq/L (136–142 mEq/L), potassium 3.6 mEq/L (3.8–5.0 mEq/L), chloride 115 mEq/L (95–103 mEq/L), SCr 1.5 mg/dL (0.6–1.2 mg/dL), total carbon dioxide 14 mEq/L (24–30 mEq/L) and white blood cell count 15,000 cells/mm³ (4400–11,000 cells/mm³). Arterial blood gases were pH 7.30 (7.38–7.44), $PaCO_2$ 28 mm Hg (35–40 mm Hg), PaO_2 100 mm Hg (95–100 mm Hg), and serum bicarbonate 14 mEq/L (24–30 mEq/L).

Question: What acid–base disorder does Robert W. exhibit? What is his anion gap? What is the cause of his acid–base disorder?

Discussion: Robert W.'s pH of 7.30 is clearly in the acidemic range. Further evaluation of the ABGs reveals a low bicarbonate value, suggesting metabolic acidosis. The low $PaCO_2$ value, representing respiratory compensation, confirms this assessment. The level of respiratory compensation is consistent with the expected degree of compensation described in Table 9-1. The bicarbonate value has fallen by approximately 10 mEq/L from a normal value of 24 mEq/L, and the $PaCO_2$ has been reduced by 12 (1.2 x 10 mEq/L, as predicted in Table 9-1) to 28 mm Hg from the normal of 40 mm Hg. These values suggest that Robert W. has only metabolic acidosis and not a mixed acid–base disorder.

The importance of compensation for acid–base disorders can be appreciated by calculating the expected pH in Robert W. if respiratory compensation had not occurred. If the $PaCO_2$ had stayed at 40 mm Hg with a serum bicarbonate of 14 mEq/L, the pH would be 7.16 (Henderson-Hasselbalch equation).

Robert W.'s anion gap of 8 mEq/L (137 – [115 + 14]) is normal, allowing classification of the disorder as a metabolic acidosis with normal anion gap. The most likely cause is diarrhea (Table 9-2), as suggested by his recent development of *C. difficile*-induced diarrhea.

MINICASE 2

A Patient with Shortness of Breath

ANDREW B., A 65-YEAR-OLD MALE, presented to the emergency department complaining of shortness of breath and cough with increased sputum production that has worsened over the past 2 weeks.

Andrew B. has a history of chronic obstructive pulmonary disease (COPD) and hypertension (HTN). His current medications include lisinopril 20 mg PO daily, hydrochlorothiazide 25mg PO daily, fluticasone/salmeterol 250/50 mcg inhaled every 12 hours, and albuterol 1–2 puffs every 6 hours as needed for shortness of breath.

Vital signs included HR 100 beats/min with BP 150/90 mm Hg and respiratory rate 28 breaths/min. His laboratory data include sodium 134 mEq/L (136–142 mEq/L), potassium 4.2 (3.8–5.0 mEq/L), chloride 94 mEq/L (95–103 mEq/L), total carbon dioxide 32 mEq/L (24–30 mEq/L), SCr 1.3 (0.6–1.2 mg/dL), and glucose 135 mg/dL (70–110 mg/dL). Arterial blood gases on room air were pH 7.30 (7.38–7.44), $PaCO_2$ 60 mm Hg (35–40 mm Hg), PaO_2 70 mm Hg (95–100 mm Hg), and serum bicarbonate 32 mEq/L (24–30 mEq/L).

Question: What acid–base disorder does Andrew B. have and what is the cause? Is this disorder acute or chronic?

Discussion: Inspection of the ABGs reveals that Andrew B. is acidemic, with a slightly low pH of 7.30. If he had a metabolic acidosis, his serum bicarbonate would be expected to be low. Instead, both the serum bicarbonate and the $PaCO_2$ are elevated. These values are consistent with a compensated respiratory acidosis. The level of renal compensation is consistent with the expected degree of compensation described in Table 9-1. The $PaCO_2$ value has increased by approximately 20 mm Hg from a normal value of 40 mm Hg, and the bicarbonate has increased by 8 (0.4 x 20 mEq/L, as predicted in Table 9-1) to 32 mm Hg from the normal of 24 mEq/L. Patients with COPD commonly exhibit chronic respiratory acidosis due to impaired ventilation (Table 9-4).[18] The body compensates by avidly reabsorbing bicarbonate to return the bicarbonate/carbon dioxide ratio and pH nearer to normal. The degree of renal compensation, as well as the history of chronic, stable symptoms, is consistent with a chronic disorder (Table 9-1). The anion gap is normal at 8 mEq/L (134 – [94 + 32]), as expected in patients with respiratory acidosis.

TABLE 9-2. Common Causes of Metabolic Acidosis[1–3,5,11–20]

ELEVATED ANION GAP	NORMAL ANION GAP (HYPERCHLOREMIC)
Renal failure	**Renal tubular acidosis**
Ketoacidosis	**Diarrhea**
Diabetes mellitus	**Drugs/toxins**
Starvation	Carbonic anhydrase inhibitors (e.g., acetazolamide)
Ethanol	Amphotericin B
Lactic acidosis	Lithium carbonate
Shock—septic, cardiogenic, hypovolemic	Lead
Severe hypoxemia	Ammonium chloride
Carbon monoxide poisoning	Arginine hydrochloride
Tonic-clonic seizures	Topiramate
Liver disease	Zonisamide
Drugs	Propofol
Linezolid	Salicylates
Metformin	
Nucleoside reverse-transcriptase inhibitors	
Intravenous lorazepam (due to vehicle)	
Nitroprusside (cyanide accumulation)	
Intoxications	
Methanol	
Ethylene glycol	

TABLE 9-3. Common Causes of Metabolic Alkalosis[1–3]

Loss of gastric acid
  Vomiting
  Nasogastric suction

Mineralocorticoid excess
  Hyperaldosteronism
  Exogenous mineralocorticoids

Hypokalemia

Alkali administration
  Oral
  Parenteral nutrition with excessive acetate
  Excessive administration of bicarbonate in metabolic acidosis

Diuretic therapy
  Loop diuretics (e.g., furosemide)
  Thiazide diuretics (e.g., hydrochlorothiazide)

Metabolic Alkalosis

An elevated pH with an elevated serum bicarbonate concentration confirms the presence of *metabolic alkalosis*. Although some respiratory compensation occurs as a result of hypoventilation and carbon dioxide retention, compensation is relatively minor in metabolic alkalosis. The most common causes of metabolic alkalosis (Table 9-3) are

- Loss of gastric acid as a result of persistent vomiting or nasogastric suction
- Loss of intravascular volume and chloride ion as a result of diuretic use

Metabolic alkalosis due to loss of gastric acid may be prevented by administration of proton pump inhibitors (e.g., omeprazole) or histamine-2 antagonists (e.g., famotidine), which block gastric acid secretion.

TABLE 9-4. Common Causes of Respiratory Acidosis[1–3,22]

CNS disorders
Cerebral vascular accident
Tumor
Sleep apnea
Drugs (e.g., opioids and sedatives/hypnotics)

Lung disorders
Airway obstruction
Asthma
Chronic obstructive pulmonary disease (e.g., chronic bronchitis)
Pulmonary edema

Neuromuscular disorders
Myasthenia gravis
Guillain-Barré syndrome
Hypokalemia
Hypophosphatemia
Neuromuscular blocking drugs

TABLE 9-5. Common Causes of Respiratory Alkalosis[1–3,23]

Hypoxemia

Lung disease
Pneumonia
Pulmonary embolism

CNS–respiratory stimulation
Cerebrovascular accident
Fever
Lung disease
Anxiety-hyperventilation syndrome
Pregnancy
Progesterone derivatives
Salicylate intoxication

Metabolic alkalosis also occurs in hospitalized patients as a result of improper anion balance in parenteral nutrition solutions or overtreatment of metabolic acidosis with sodium bicarbonate. In parenteral nutrition solutions, anions are typically provided as acetate and chloride. Because acetate is metabolized to bicarbonate, excessive acetate and inadequate chloride administration can produce metabolic alkalosis. In patients with metabolic acidosis due to circulatory failure, administration of sodium bicarbonate initially returns the pH toward normal. However, after restoration of adequate circulation, excessive bicarbonate and metabolic alkalosis may be present until the kidneys excrete the excess bicarbonate and return the concentration to normal.

Respiratory Acidosis

Respiratory acidosis is usually synonymous with hypoventilation.[22] This condition can be a result of numerous causes (Table 9-4) in three general categories:

1. Impaired CNS respiratory drive
2. Impaired gas exchange in the lungs
3. Impaired neuromuscular function affecting the diaphragm and chest wall

Laboratory results consistent with respiratory acidosis are a low pH with an elevated $PaCO_2$, indicating inadequate

MINICASE 3

A Case of Syncope

ROBERT M., A 60-YEAR-OLD MALE, was brought to the emergency department from home for evaluation of chest pain and shortness of breath. He underwent total knee replacement 2 weeks ago and has not been participating in physical therapy. His vital signs included heart rate 120 beats/min, blood pressure 100/60 mm Hg, and respiratory rate 30 breaths/min. A V/Q scan reveals a high probability of pulmonary embolism.

His laboratory data included sodium 140 mEq/L (136–142 mEq/L), potassium 4.0 mEq/L (3.8–5.0 mEq/L), chloride 102 mEq/L (95–103 mEq/L), total carbon dioxide 24 mEq/L (24–30 mEq/L), SCr 1.0 (0.6–1.2 mg/dL), and glucose 160 mg/dL (70–110 mg/dL). Robert M.'s ABGs were pH 7.60 (7.38–7.44), $PaCO_2$ 25 mm Hg (35–40 mm Hg), PaO_2 70 mm Hg (95–100 mm Hg), and serum bicarbonate 23 mEq/L (24–30 mEq/L).

Question: What acid–base disorder does Robert M. exhibit?

Discussion: Robert M.'s arterial pH is in the alkalemic range. Since the serum bicarbonate concentration is not elevated, this condition is not likely to be metabolic alkalosis. However, his $PaCO_2$ is low—consistent with respiratory alkalosis. The most likely cause is pulmonary embolism (Table 9-5). Because the alkalosis developed acutely, the kidneys did not have adequate time to compensate.

excretion of carbon dioxide. Because the kidneys require 6–12 hours to initiate and 3–5 days to complete compensation, acute respiratory acidosis is associated with much greater alterations in pH than chronic respiratory acidosis. For example, a typical patient with an acute rise in $PaCO_2$ to 60 mm Hg (8 kPa) will have a pH of 7.26 with a serum bicarbonate of 26 mEq/L (26 mmol/L; Table 9-1 and Henderson-Hasselbalch equation). If the same patient's $PaCO_2$ remains at 60 mm Hg for 3–5 days when full renal compensation occurs, the serum bicarbonate will rise to 32 mEq/L (32 mmol/L). This returns the arterial pH to a nearly normal value of 7.35. While acute respiratory acidosis associated with hypoxemia may be life-threatening, chronic compensated respiratory acidosis often requires no therapeutic intervention.

Respiratory Alkalosis

Increased ventilation results in increased carbon dioxide excretion (low $PaCO_2$), elevated pH, and *respiratory alkalosis*. Typically, the symptoms of respiratory alkalosis are mild and consist of dizziness, lightheadedness, and paresthesias. Acute respiratory alkalosis, commonly produced by the anxiety-hyperventilation syndrome, is usually a benign disorder and reverses either spontaneously or as a result of rebreathing expired air. Mild chronic respiratory alkalosis is also usually a benign disorder, but in some situations it may have more serious consequences.[23]

Common causes of respiratory alkalosis are listed in Table 9-5. As noted previously, carbon dioxide more readily diffuses from the capillary blood to the alveoli than does oxygen.

MINICASE 4

A Possible Drug Ingestion

BRITTANY C., AN 18-YEAR-OLD-FEMALE, was brought to the emergency department after her roommate found her unconscious in their apartment. The roommate reports that Brittany C. has been depressed for the past 3 months after breaking up with her boyfriend and dropping out of college. During ambulance transfer, Brittany C. vomited, and the emesis contained several white tablet fragments.

The roommate reports that Brittany C. takes only oral contraceptives, and there are no other prescription medications in the apartment. She does state that there are over-the-counter bottles of acetaminophen, ibuprofen, aspirin, and cough and cold products in the apartment.

Brittany C.'s vital signs included HR 100/min with BP 120/70 mm, respiratory rate 30/min, and temperature 101°F. (38.3°C). Her physical exam was remarkable only for dry mucous membranes. Bowel sounds were present but hypoactive, and rebound tenderness was absent. She was noted to be somnolent and responded to questions only with moans.

Laboratory data included sodium 136 mEq/L (136–142 mEq/L), potassium 3.2 mEq/L (3.8–5.0 mEq/L), chloride 98 mEq/L (95–103 mEq/L), total carbon dioxide 15 mEq/L (24–30 mEq/L), SCr 1.0 mg/dL (0.6–1.2 mg/dL), and glucose 120 mg/dL (70–110 mg/dL). Her ABGs were pH 7.36 (7.38–7.44), $PaCO_2$ 28 mm Hg (35–40 mm Hg), PaO_2 100 mm Hg (95–100 mm Hg), and serum bicarbonate 15 mEq/L (24–30 mEq/L).

Question: What acid–base disorder is present? What is the most likely cause?

Discussion: Inspection of the pH reveals that the arterial pH is normal. However, both the $PaCO_2$ and serum bicarbonate are low. This combination of tests suggests that a mixed acid–base disorder may be present and emphasizes the need to fully evaluate the ABG results. The $PaCO_2$ is approximately 12 mm Hg below the normal value, which is consistent with respiratory alkalosis. The expected degree of renal compensation for this degree of decline in $PaCO_2$ is 2–5 mEq/L, depending on the time available for compensation to have occurred. This would result in a serum bicarbonate level of 19–22 mEq/L (based on equation discussed in Table 9-1). The serum bicarbonate level is lower than would be expected in renal compensation, and the anion gap is elevated, so the patient must also have metabolic acidosis. The patient is displaying a mixed acid–base disorder, respiratory alkalosis combined with elevated anion gap metabolic acidosis. This combination of acid–base disorders is often seen in patients with salicylate toxicity. Large salicylate doses stimulate respiration, as displayed in Brittany C. by her tachypnea, producing respiratory alkalosis. Salicylates also impair oxidative metabolism, producing an anion gap metabolic acidosis.

Therefore, some conditions (e.g., pulmonary embolism) may produce hypoxemia, which stimulates increased ventilation. The increased ventilation may more than offset any reduction in carbon dioxide excretion produced by the lung disease, producing respiratory alkalosis.

SUMMARY

This chapter reviews acid–base physiology and disorders and presents a method of evaluating a patient's acid–base status. The lungs regulate the concentration of carbon dioxide, the acid form of the carbonic acid/bicarbonate buffer system. The kidneys regulate the concentration of bicarbonate.

Evaluation of ABGs requires identification of whether the patient is acidemic, alkalemic, or has a normal pH. Once this determination is made, the disorder can be categorized into a metabolic or respiratory type by examining both the $PaCO_2$ and serum bicarbonate. Assessment of the degree of compensation and comparison with expected levels of compensation, along with an evaluation of other patient information, allows detection of mixed acid–base disorders. These basic skills enable the clinician to assess a patient's acid–base status quickly and effectively.

Learning Points

1. What is the key buffer system in the body and how are the components of that system used to assess acid–base status?

Answer: The carbonic acid/bicarbonate buffer system is the key buffer system in the body. It provides the majority of buffer capacity. Carbonic acid is hydrolyzed to produce carbon dioxide, the predominant acid form of this buffer system. The arterial partial pressure of carbon dioxide ($PaCO_2$), as measured on ABG reports, is used to assess the acid level in the body. The base form of the buffer system is bicarbonate (HCO_3^-), which is assessed by measuring the venous serum bicarbonate or total carbon dioxide level. Along with the pH, assessment of these laboratory tests is key to accurate assessment of a patient's acid–base status.

2. What are the appropriate steps to follow in using the ABGs to assess acid–base status?

Answer: The first step is to determine if the patient is acidemic, alkalemic, or has a normal pH (7.36–7.44). Once the correct categorization is made, the arterial partial pressure of carbon dioxide ($PaCO_2$) and serum bicarbonate (HCO_3^-) levels should be evaluated. Acidemia with an elevated $PaCO_2$ and elevation in HCO_3^- as a compensatory mechanism is consistent with respiratory acidosis. Acidemia with a low HCO_3^- level and low $PaCO_2$ as a compensatory mechanism is consistent with metabolic acidosis. Metabolic alkalosis is characterized by elevated pH and bicarbonate, while respiratory alkalosis is characterized by elevated pH and low $PaCO_2$.

3. Is it possible for a patient to have a normal pH on ABGs and yet have an acid–base disorder?

Answer: Yes, patients with normal pH may have mixed acid–base disorders. For example, patients may have disease processes that produce both metabolic acidosis and respiratory alkalosis. In this situation, the effect of each disorder on arterial pH may offset each other, producing an arterial pH in the normal range. However, evaluation of the values for $PaCO_2$ and serum bicarbonate will reveal abnormalities. These laboratory values must be assessed, including checking levels of compensation for the primary disorder. This information is combined with the patient's history, physical examination, and other laboratory test results to accurately identify the acid–base disorders present.

REFERENCES

1. Narins RG, Emmett M. Simple and mixed acid–base disorders: a practical approach. *Medicine*. 1980;59:161-187.
2. Hammond RW. Acid–base disorders. In: Koda-Kimble MA, Young LY, Kradjan WA, et al., eds. *Applied Therapeutics: The Clinical Use of Drugs*. 8th ed. Philadelphia, PA: Lippincott Williams & Wilkins; 2005:11.1-11.15.
3. Rose BD, Post TW. *Clinical Physiology of Acid–base and Electrolyte Disorders*. 5th ed. New York, NY: McGraw-Hill; 2001.
4. Adrogué HJ, Madias NE. Management of life-threatening acid–base disorders. *N Engl J Med*. 1998;338:26-34, 107-111.
5. Goodkin DA, Gollapudi GK, Narins RG. The role of the anion gap in detecting and managing mixed metabolic acid–base disorders. *Clin Endocrinol Metab*. 1984;13:333-349.
6. Kraut JA, Madias NE. Serum anion gap: its uses and limitations in clinical medicine. *Clin J Am Soc Nephrol*. 2007;2:162-174.
7. Salem MM, Mujais SK. Gaps in the anion gap. *Arch Intern Med*. 1992;152:1625-1629.
8. Mizrock BA. Lactic acidosis in critical illness. *Crit Care Med*. 1992;20:80-93.
9. Rivers E, Nguyen B, Havstad S, et al. Early goal-directed therapy in the treatment of severe sepsis and septic shock. *N Engl J Med*. 2001;345:1368-1377.
10. Sinex JE. Pulse oximetry: principles and limitations. *Am J Emerg Med*. 1999;17:59-67.
11. Carr A, Miller J, Law M, et al. A syndrome of lipoatrophy, lactic acidemia and liver dysfunction associated with HIV nucleoside analogue therapy: contribution to protease inhibitor-related lipodystrophy syndrome. *AIDS*. 2000;14:F25-F32.
12. Wysowski DK, Pollock ML. Reports of death with use of propofol (Diprivan®) for nonprocedural (long-term) sedation and literature review. *Anesthesiology*. 2006;105:1047-1051.
13. Fudickar A, Bein B, Tonner PH. Propofol infusion syndrome in anaesthesia and intensive care medicine. *Curr Opin Anaesthesiol*. 2006;19:404-410.
14. Reynolds HN, Teiken P, Regan M, et al. Hyperlactatemia, increased osmolar gap, and renal dysfunction during continuous lorazepam infusion. *Crit Care Med*. 2000;28:1631-1634.
15. Humphrey SH, Nash DA. Lactic acidosis complicating sodium nitroprusside therapy. *Ann Intern Med*. 1978;88:58-59.
16. Yaucher NE, Fish JT, Smith HW, et al. Propylene glycol-associated renal toxicity from lorazepam infusion. *Pharmacotherapy*. 2003;23:1094-1099.
17. Arenas-Pinto A, Grant AD, Edwards S, et al. Lactic acidosis in HIV infected patients: a systematic review of published cases. *Sex Transm Infect*. 2003;79:340-344.
18. Garris SS, Oles KS. Impact of topiramate on serum bicarbonate concentrations in adults. *Ann Pharmacother*. 2005;39:424-426.
19. 19. Mirza NS, Alfirevic A, Jorgensen A, et al. Metabolic acidosis with topiramate and zonisamide: as assessment of its severity and predictors. *Pharmacogenet Genomics*. 2011; 21(5): 297-302.
20. 20. Liamis G, Milionis HJ, Elisaf M. Pharmacologically-induced metabolic acidosis: a review. *Drug Saf*. 2010;33(5): 371-391.
21. Laffey JG, Kavanagh BP. Hypocapnia. *N Engl J Med*. 2002;347:43-53.
22. Weinberger SE, Schwartzstein RM, Weiss JW. Hypercapnia. *N Engl J Med*. 1989;321:1223-1231.
23. Laffey JG, Kavanagh BP. Hypocapnia. *N Engl J Med*. 2002;347:43-53.

QUICKVIEW | Venous Serum Bicarbonate (HCO$_3^-$)

PARAMETER	DESCRIPTION	COMMENTS
Common reference range		
Adults	19–24 mEq/L	Venous bicarbonate can be 1–2 mEq/L higher than arterial measure of bicarbonate
Critical value	<8 mEq/L	
Inherent activity	Yes	Primary substance responsible for buffering acids
Location		
Production	Byproduct of typical cell metabolism	
Storage	Exchanged via circulation	
Secretion/excretion	Renal excretion (reabsorption occurs at proximal tubule)	
Causes of abnormal values		
High	Metabolic alkalosis and respiratory acidosis	Change in HCO$_3^-$ is the primary method of compensation in metabolic disorders
Low	Metabolic acidosis and respiratory alkalosis	
Signs and symptoms		
High level	Related to primary process	
Low level	Related to primary process	
After event, time to....		
Initial elevation	6–12 hr to initiate compensation	Assumes acute insult
Peak values	None (will rise until pH balanced)	Assumes insult not yet removed
Normalization	3–5 days to complete compensation	Assumes insult removed and nonpermanent damage
Causes of spurious results	Inadvertent venous sampling	

QUICKVIEW | Arterial Partial Pressure of Carbon Dioxide (PaCO$_2$)

PARAMETER	DESCRIPTION	COMMENTS
Common reference range		
Adults	35–40 mg Hg (40)	
Critical value	>70 mm Hg (may require mechanical ventilation)	
Inherent activity	Yes	Primary volatile acid in the body
Location		
Production	Generated intracellularly from carbon dioxide and water	
Storage	N/A	
Secretion/excretion	Excreted by the lungs during expiration	
Causes of abnormal values		
High	Respiratory acidosis and metabolic alkalosis	Change in PaCO$_2$ is the primary method of compensation in respiratory disorders
Low	Respiratory alkalosis and metabolic acidosis	
Signs and symptoms		
High level	Respiratory failure	
Low level	Related to primary process	
After event, time to....		
Initial elevation	Minutes to hours	Assumes acute insult
Peak values	None	Assumes insult not yet removed
Normalization	Hours to days	Assumes insult removed and nonpermanent damage
Causes of spurious results	Inadvertent venous sampling	Higher carbon dioxide content

CHAPTER 10

PULMONARY FUNCTION AND RELATED TESTS

LORI A. WILKEN, MIN J. JOO

Objectives

After completing this chapter, the reader should be able to

- Identify common pulmonary function tests (PFTs) and list their purpose and limitations

  a. Spirometry

  b. Peak expiratory flow rate (PEFR)

  c. Body plethysmography

  d. Carbon monoxide diffusion capacity (DLCO)

  e. Airway reactivity tests

  f. Six-minute walk test (6MWT)

  g. Specialized tests

     i. Infant pulmonary function testing

     ii. CO breath test

     iii. Sputum inflammatory markers

- Describe how PFTs are performed and discuss factors affecting the validity of the results

- Interpret commonly used PFTs, given clinical and other laboratory data

- Discuss how PFTs provide objective measurement to aid in the diagnosis of pulmonary diseases

- Discuss how PFTs assist with monitoring efficacy and toxicity of various drug therapies

Pulmonary function tests (PFTs) provide objective and quantifiable measures of lung function and are useful in the diagnosis, evaluation, and monitoring of respiratory disease. In addition, PFTs can assess response or effectiveness of therapy and detect pulmonary side effects of medications. Spirometry, a test that measures the movement of air into and out of the lungs during various breathing maneuvers, is the most frequently used PFT. Other tests of lung function include lung volume assessment, carbon monoxide diffusion capacity (DLCO), exercise testing, and bronchoprovocation challenge tests. Arterial blood gases (ABGs) also are useful to assess lung function. Interpretation of ABGs is discussed later in this chapter.

Diagnosis and monitoring of many pulmonary diseases, including diseases of gas exchange, often require measurement of the flow or volume of air inspired and expired by the patient. Appropriate pharmacotherapeutic agents can be chosen based on PFT results. Clinicians frequently use these tests to aid in the diagnosis of respiratory diseases such as asthma and chronic obstructive pulmonary disease (COPD). Pulmonary function tests can also be used to monitor lung function after thoracic radiation, lung transplantation, or during administration of pharmacotherapy with potential toxicity to the lungs. This chapter discusses the mechanics and interpretation of PFTs.

ANATOMY AND PHYSIOLOGY OF LUNGS

The purpose of the lungs is to take oxygen from the atmosphere and exchange it for carbon dioxide in the blood. The movement of air in and out of the lungs is called *ventilation;* the movement of blood through the lungs is termed *perfusion.*

Air enters the body through the mouth and nose and travels through the pharynx to the trachea. The trachea splits into the left and right main stem bronchi, and these bronchi deliver inspired air to the respective lungs. The left and right lungs are in the pleural cavity of the thorax. These two spongy, conical structures are the primary organs of respiration. The right lung has three lobes while the left lung has only two lobes, thus leaving space for the heart. The thoracic cavity is separated from the abdominal cavity by the diaphragm. The diaphragm—a thin sheet of dome-shaped muscle—contracts and relaxes during breathing. The lungs are contained within the rib cage but rest on the diaphragm. Between the ribs are two sets of intercostal muscles. These muscles attach to each upper and lower rib.

During inhalation, the intercostal muscles and the diaphragm contract, enlarging the thoracic cavity. This action generates a negative intrathoracic pressure, allowing air to rush in through the nose and mouth down into the pharynx, trachea, and lungs. During exhalation, these muscles relax and a positive intrathoracic pressure causes air to be pushed out of the lungs. Normal expiration is a passive process that results from the natural recoil of the expanded lungs. However, in people with rapid or labored breathing or obstruction, the accessory muscles and abdominal muscles often must contract to help force air out of the lungs more quickly or completely. Within the lungs, the main bronchi continue to split successively into smaller bronchi, bronchioles, terminal bronchioles, and finally alveoli. In the alveoli, carbon dioxide is exchanged for oxygen across a thin membrane separating capillary blood from inspired air.

TABLE 10-1. Types of Pulmonary Disease

TYPE	PATHOPHYSIOLOGY	EXAMPLE
Obstructive	Reversible (e.g., bronchoconstriction) Irreversible (e.g., airway collapse, mucus)	Asthma COPD
Restrictive	Parenchymal infiltration	Idiopathic pulmonary fibrosis, interstitial pneumonias, sarcoidosis
	Loss of lung volume	Pneumothorax, pneumonectomy, pleural effusions
	Extrathoracic compression	Kyphosis, morbid obesity, ascites, chest wall deformities
Mixed obstructive and restrictive	Combinations of the above	
Decreased Diffusion capacity	Parenchymal infiltration or fibrosis	Interstitial pneumonia, emphysema
	V:Q mismatch	Pulmonary embolism, pulmonary edema

COPD = chronic obstructive pulmonary disease.

The ability of the lungs to expand and contract to inhale and exhale air is affected by the compliance of the lungs which is a measure of the ease of expansion of the lungs and thorax. Processes that result in scarring of lung tissue (e.g., pulmonary fibrosis) can decrease compliance, thus decreasing the flow and volume of air moved by the lungs. The degree of ease in which air travels through the airways is known as *resistance*. The length and radius of the airways as well as the viscosity of the gas inhaled determine resistance. A patient with a high degree of airway resistance may not be able to take a full breath in or to exhale fully (some air may become trapped in the lungs).

To have an adequate exchange of the gases, there must be a matching of ventilation (V) and perfusion (Q) at the alveolar level. An average V:Q ratio, determined by dividing total alveolar ventilation (4 L/min) by cardiac output (5 L/min), is 0.8. A mismatch of ventilation and perfusion may result from a shunt or dead space. A shunt occurs when there is flow of blood adjacent to alveoli that are collapsed. This could be physiologic (e.g., at rest some alveoli are collapsed but perfused) or pathologic when alveoli are filled with fluid (e.g., pneumonia) or collapsed (e.g., from mucous obstruction). In a shunt, blood moves from the venous circulation to the arterial circulation without being oxygenated. Dead space occurs when there is ventilation of functional alveoli without adjacent blood flow. Dead space can be physiologic (e.g., the trachea) or pathologic due to obstruction of blood flow. (e.g., pulmonary embolism).

TABLE 10-2. Selected Uses of PFTs

Diagnosis

Signs and symptoms of respiratory disease

Followup of historical or laboratory findings

Disease effects on pulmonary function

Evaluation

Medical/legal issues (e.g., disability, clearance for surgery)

Rehabilitation

Monitoring

Respiratory disease progression

Prognosis

Occupational or environmental exposure to toxins

Therapeutic drug effectiveness (e.g., inhaled corticosteroids or bronchodilators for asthma)

Adverse drug effects on pulmonary function (e.g., amiodarone)

Source: Adapted from reference 1.

For the respiration process to be complete, gas *diffusion* must occur in the alveoli. By the diffusion mechanism, gases in the alveoli equilibrate from areas of high concentration to areas of low concentration. Hemoglobin (Hgb) releases carbon dioxide and adsorbs oxygen through the alveolar walls. If these walls thicken, diffusion is hampered potentially causing carbon dioxide retention, hypoxia, or both. Membrane formation with secondary thickening of the alveolar wall may result from an acute or chronic inflammatory process such as interstitial pneumonia and pulmonary fibrosis. The pulmonary diffusing capacity is reduced in the presence of a V:Q mismatch.

The various PFTs can measure airflow in or out of the lungs, indicate how much air is in the lungs, and provide information on gas diffusion, or specific changes in airway tone or reactivity.

CLINICAL USE OF PULMONARY FUNCTION TESTING

Pulmonary function tests are useful in many clinical situations. They aid in the diagnostic differentiation of various pulmonary diseases. For example, with obstructive lung diseases (e.g., asthma or COPD), the underlying pathophysiology is a reversible or irreversible blockage to airflow in the airways. Obstructive diseases usually decrease the flow of air but not its volume. In restrictive diseases (e.g., kyphosis or sarcoidosis), the lungs are limited in the amount of air they can contain. Restrictive diseases usually decrease the volume of air and flow of air (Table 10-1).

In addition, serial PFTs allow tracking of the progression of pulmonary diseases and the need for or response to various treatments. They also help to establish a baseline of respiratory function prior to surgical, medical, or radiation therapy. Subsequent serial measurements then aid in the detection and tracking of changes in lung function caused by these therapies. Similarly, serial PFTs can be used to evaluate the risk of

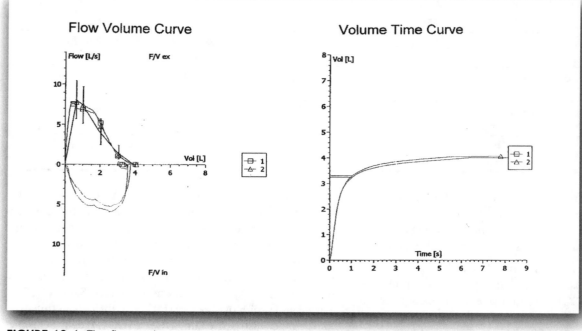

FIGURE 10-1. The flow-volume curve and volume-time curve from an effort meeting ATS acceptability criteria. The flow-volume curve has a deep inspiratory effort with a sharp complete expiratory flow. The volume-time curve demonstrates both a plateau and an exhalation time of greater than 6 seconds.

lung damage from exposure to environmental or occupational hazards.

In brief, PFTs are performed to

- Evaluate respiratory symptoms
- Assess disease severity
- Preoperatively determine the risk of thoracic or upper abdominal surgery
- Monitor the progression of lung disease
- Evaluate the response to therapy
- Assess the effect of pulmonary exposure to environmental toxins
- Monitor drug or radiation pulmonary toxicity

Table 10-2 summarizes the selected uses of PFTs.

PULMONARY FUNCTION TESTS AND MEASUREMENTS

Spirometry

Spirometry is a PFT that helps detect airway obstruction, manifested in asthma or COPD. Spirometry measures the maximum amount of air that can be exhaled by the patient after complete inhalation. The physical forces of the airflow and the total amount of air inhaled and/or exhaled are converted by transducers to electrical signals and displayed on a computer screen.

During this maneuver, a *volume-time curve,* a plot of the volume exhaled against time and a *flow-volume curve* or *flow-volume loop,* a diagram with flow (L/sec) on the vertical axis and volume expired on the horizontal axis (L), are generated as the report (Figure 10-1). After the data is generated, the patient's spirometry results are generally compared to the predicted values for people of similar age, height, gender, and

race. The predicted values are data gathered from the National Health and Nutrition Examination Survey, the Centers for Disease Control and Prevention, and the National Center for Health Statistics. The flow-volume curve is visually useful for diagnosing airway obstruction.

Spirometry is recommended in patients over the age of 40 years with any of the following characteristics: presence of risk factors including cigarette smoking or exposure to occupational dust or chemicals, symptoms of breathlessness, chronic sputum production, or chronic cough.[2] Once diagnosed with COPD, spirometry can be used on an annual basis to monitor disease state severity. Use of spirometry for asthma is recommended at the time of diagnosis, after the initiation of medications and stabilization of symptoms, during periods of uncontrolled asthma, and at least every 1–2 years to monitor asthma control.[3]

Spirometry Measurements

Spirometry routinely assesses the following:

- Forced vital capacity (FVC)
- Forced expiratory volume in 1 second (FEV_1)
- FEV_1/FVC

Forced Vital Capacity

The *forced vital capacity (FVC)* is the total volume of air, measured in liters, forcefully and rapidly exhaled in one breath (from maximum inhalation to maximum exhalation). When the full inhalation-exhalation procedure is repeated slowly—instead of forcefully and rapidly—it is called the *slow vital capacity (SVC).* This value is the maximum amount of air exhaled after a full and complete inhalation. In patients with normal airway function, FVC and SVC are usually similar and constitute the *vital capacity (VC).* In patients with diseases such

TABLE 10-3. Pulmonary Disease States and Common PFT Findings

Disease	FEV$_1$/FVC	FEV$_1$	FVC	RV	TLC
Obstructive lung disease, chronic	Decreased	Decreased	Normal or decreased	Normal or increased	Normal or increased
Obstructive lung disease, reversible and stable	Normal	Normal	Normal	Normal	Normal
Restrictive lung disease	Normal or increased	Decreased	Decreased	Decreased	Decreased
Combined restrictive and obstructive	Decreased or normal	Decreased	Decreased	Increased, normal, or decreased	Decreased

as COPD, the FVC may be lower than the SVC due to collapse of narrowed or floppy airways during forced expiration. Because of this, some guidelines recommend using the FEV$_1$/SVC ratio to determine the presence of airway obstruction.

Forced Expiratory Volume in 1 Second

The full, forced inhalation-exhalation procedure was already described as the FVC. During this maneuver, the computer can discern the amount of air exhaled at specific time intervals of the FVC. By convention, FEV$_{0.5}$, FEV$_1$, FEV$_3$, and FEV$_6$ are the amounts of air exhaled after 0.5, 1, 3, and 6 seconds, respectively. Usually, a patient's value is described in liters and as a percentage of a predicted value based on population normal values adjusted for age, height, and gender.

Of these measurements, FEV$_1$ has the most clinical relevance, primarily as an indicator of airway function. A value greater than 80% of the predicted normal value is considered normal. Normal values are often seen in patients with reversible airway obstruction when the disease is mild or well controlled. Values less than or equal to 80% are abnormal and may indicate airway obstruction.

When the postbronchodilator FEV$_1$/FVC is low, the postbronchodilator FEV$_1$ is used to determine the severity of airway obstruction in COPD. Mild airway obstruction is a FEV$_1$ greater than 80% of the predicted value, moderate airway obstruction is a FEV$_1$ of 50% to 80%, severe is 30% to 50% and very severe is less than 30% of the predicted value.[2,4] Both intermittent and mild persistent asthma have a FEV$_1$ greater than 80% the predicted value for the patient. Moderate and persistent asthma have a FEV$_1$ between 60% and 80% of the predicted value; and severe persistent asthma has a FEV$_1$ less than 60% of the predicted value.

FEV$_6$ is a useful and validated measure comparable to FVC. In patients without airway obstruction, FEV$_6$ and FVC would be the same. FEV$_6$ is especially useful for those patients with severe airway obstruction that may take more than double the normal amount of time to exhale a full breath. For patients with severe airway obstruction, using the FEV$_1$/FVC instead of the FEV$_1$/FEV$_6$ may underestimate the severity of airway obstruction. Therefore, many newer spirometers incorporate the FEV$_1$/FEV$_6$ into the report.

FEV$_1$/FVC

The ratio of FEV$_1$ to the FVC is used to estimate the presence and amount of obstruction in the airways. This ratio indicates the amount of air mobilized in 1 second as a percentage of the total amount of movable air. Normal, healthy individuals can exhale approximately 50% of their FVC in the first 0.5 second, about 80% in 1 second, and about 98% in 3 seconds. Patients with obstructive disease usually show a decreased ratio, and the actual percentage reduction varies with the severity of obstruction. In COPD, the American Thoracic Society (ATS)/European Respiratory Society (ERS) and the Global Initiative for Chronic Obstructive Lung Disease (GOLD) define chronic airway obstruction as an FEV$_1$/FVC ratio of less than 70%.

For asthma, the National Asthma Education Prevention Program (NAEPP) evaluates both FEV$_1$/FVC and FEV$_1$ in assessing asthma severity. In children 5–11 years of age, FEV$_1$/FVC greater than 85% predicted is consistent with intermittent asthma, greater than 80% is mild or well-controlled asthma, 75% to 80% is moderate or not well-controlled asthma and less than 75% is severe or very poorly controlled asthma. In children older than 12 and adults, a normal FEV$_1$/FVC can be seen in intermittent and mild persistent disease. In children older than 12 and adults, a reduction in the measured FEV$_1$/FVC of 5% from normal is consistent with moderate persistent asthma. A reduction in the measured FEV$_1$/FVC of greater than 5% from normal is consistent with severe persistent asthma using the following as normal FEV$_1$/FVC values: age 8–19 years is 85%; 20–39 years is 80%; 40–59 years is 75%; and 60–80 years is 70%. However, pulmonary function alone is not sufficient to diagnose or assess asthma severity. Frequency of asthma symptoms and "quick relief" medication use is also necessary to assess asthma severity.

Generally, the FEV$_1$/FVC is normal (or high) in patients with restrictive diseases. In mild restriction the FVC alone may be decreased resulting in a high ratio. Oftentimes in restrictive lung disease, both the FVC and FEV$_1$ are similarly reduced from normal resulting in a normal ratio. The effects of pulmonary disease on some common PFT measures are presented in Table 10-3.

There have been discussions in the pulmonary community to abandon the set cutoff of 70% in favor of using an FEV$_1$/FVC ratio compared to the lower limit of normal to define obstruction. The lower limit of normal is statistically defined as the lower 5th percentile of a reference population and is age corrected. The FEV$_1$/FVC ratio decreases with age and the set cutoff of 70% may overdiagnose COPD in the elderly population who may have age appropriate normal FEV$_1$/FVC ratios of less than 70%. In fact the ATS/ERS endorse this in the interpretation of pulmonary function testing guidelines, separate from the COPD guidelines.[8] General acceptance of the lower limit of normal to define COPD is a possibility in the near future.

Forced Expiratory Flow

Forced expiratory flow (FEF) measures airflow rate during forced expiration. While FEV measures the volume of air per specific unit of time at the beginning of expiration, FEF measures the rate of air movement during a later portion. The FEF from 25% to 75% of VC is known as FEF_{25-75}. This test is thought to measure the flow rate of air in the medium and small airways (bronchioles and terminal bronchioles). The FEF_{25-75} was used as a measure of small airways obstruction, but this relationship has fallen out of favor due to its limited utility.

The flow from 75% to 100% of VC (i.e., the end of expiration) is called *alveolar airflow*. This parameter may markedly diminish as airways collapse with increased intrathoracic pressure. Such pressure occurs in severe acute asthma when large obstructions are present in terminal bronchioles.

Flow-Volume Curves

Figure 10-2 shows several *flow-volume curves* where the expiratory flow is plotted against the exhaled volume. As explained earlier, these curves are graphic representations of inspiration and expiration. The shape of the curve indicates both the type of disease and the severity of obstruction.

Obstructive changes result in decreased airflow at lower lung volumes, revealing a characteristic concave appearance. In obstructive cases, the loop size is similar to that of a healthy individual unless there is severe, acute obstruction. Restrictive changes result in a shape similar to that of a healthy individual, but the size is considerably smaller. The flow-volume loop also reveals mixed obstructive and restrictive disease by a combination of the two patterns.

Standardization of Spirometry Measurements

Spirometry is performed by having a person breathe into a tube (mouth piece) connected to a machine (spirometer) that measures the amount and flow of inhaled and/or exhaled air. Prior to performing spirometry, the appropriate technique is explained and demonstrated to the patient. Spirometry results are highly dependent on the completeness and speed of the patient's inhalation and exhalation, so the importance of completely filling and emptying the lungs of air during the test is emphasized. During spirometry, nose clips are worn to minimize air loss through the nose. The patient is seated comfortably without leaning or slumping and any restrictive clothing (such as ties or tight belts) are loosened or removed. The patient is instructed to take a full deep breath in and then blast the air out as quickly and forcefully as possible and to keep blowing the air out until all the air is exhaled. In general, the effort should last for 6 seconds.

Like most medical tests, spirometry has seen changes over the years in equipment, computer support, and recommendations for standardization. In an effort to maximize the usefulness of spirometry results, the ATS, in conjunction with the ERS developed and updated recommendations for the standardization of spirometry.[5,6] These recommendations are intended to decrease the variability of spirometry testing by improving the performance of the test. The recommendations cover equipment, quality control, training and education of people conducting the test, and training of patients performing the test. The recommendations also provide criteria for acceptability and reproducibility of the patient's spirometry efforts and guidelines on interpreting the spirometry test results. Because the results of spirometry depend on the patient's effort, at least three acceptable efforts are obtained with a goal of having the two highest measurements of FVC and FEV_1 vary by less than 0.15 L.[6]

Other acceptability criteria include

- Satisfactory start of test (no excessive hesitation or false start)
- No coughing during the first second of the effort
- No early termination of the effort
- No interruption in airflow (e.g., glottic closure)
- No evidence of a leak (mouth not tightly sealed around mouthpiece)
- No evidence of an obstructed mouthpiece (tongue, false teeth)

Spirometry and the Pediatric Population

Children 2–6 years of age are able to perform spirometry with specific equipment and personnel trained to work with this population.[7] Although clinical application remains debatable, spirometry for this age population is becoming more prominent in clinical research. Adult criterion for testing is not applicable to this age group. For instance, at this age full exhalation is complete prior to 1 second and therefore the $FEV_{0.5}$, (forced expiratory volume in 0.5 second) may be more appropriate to measure than the FEV_1. Repeatability of two flow curves for the FVC and FEV_1 is defined as two measurements within 0.1 L or 10% of each other. Flexibility because of poor repeatability is recommended with the young child. Reference data equations for this age group have not been endorsed by ATS or ERS.

Peak Expiratory Flow Rate

The *peak expiratory flow rate (PEFR)*, or peak flow, occurs within the first milliseconds of expiratory flow and is a measure of the maximum airflow rate. The PEFR can be measured with simple hand-held devices (peak flow meters) and is easily and inexpensively measured at a patient's home, in the clinician's office, or in the emergency department. Therefore, PEFR is widely used as an indicator of large airway obstruction and to determine the severity of an asthma exacerbation. PEFR is likely to be used during an acute exacerbation of asthma in the emergency department over the use of spirometry as most patients are unable to perform spirometry during an exacerbation.

The NAEPP recommends using peak flow and/or symptom-based home monitoring plans for asthma patients.[3] Long-term, peak flow monitoring is useful to assess asthma medication changes and to identify worsening asthma control. Peak flow

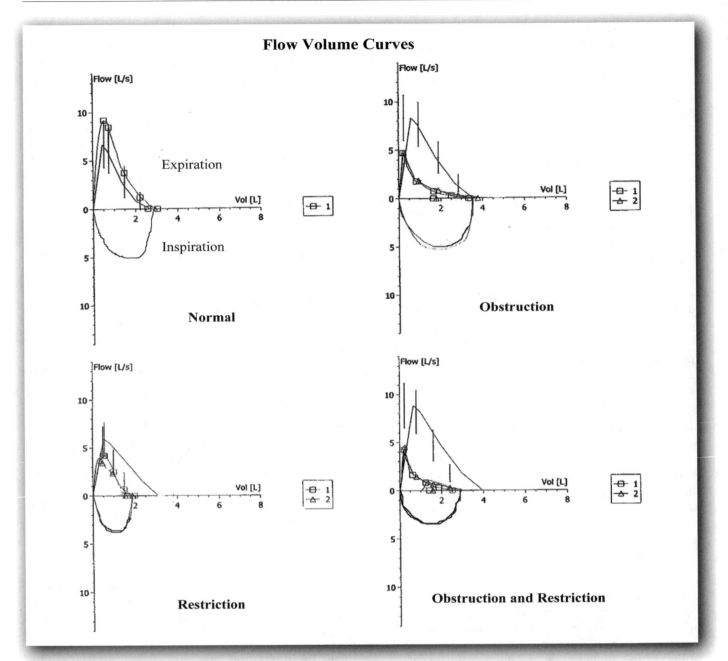

FIGURE 10-2. Flow-volume curves seen with obstructive and restrictive pulmonary diseases. This figure illustrates the flow-volume curves observed for normal adults, obstructive, restrictive, and mixed disease. Flow-volume curve number 1 represents baseline spirometry. Flow-volume curve number 2, if present, is a repeat of the spirometry after a bronchodilator is administered. (Refer to bronchodilator studies under Airway Reactivity Tests.) The curve with the vertical lines represents the predicted normal values. In these examples, there is no improvement in the flow-volume curves after bronchodilator administration. The normal flow-volume curve shows that the curve is larger than expected based on predicted values and is, therefore, normal. Concavity of the expiratory portion of the curve, consistent with limitation in flow compared to the predicted, is illustrated in the obstruction flow-volume curve. The restriction flow-volume curve shows a FVC that is smaller than expected. The predicted volume is approximately 3 L; however, the patient's FVC is 2 L. In restriction, although the forced expiratory flows are often decreased, there is no concavity such as seen in the obstruction curve. It is important to note that spirometry does not diagnose restriction. The flow-volume loop will demonstrate findings such as this consistent with restriction; however, lung volumes are needed to define restriction. Concavity in the expiratory phase and a decreased FVC volume is consistent with a combination of an obstruction and restriction flow-volume curve.

MINICASE 1

Peak Flow Monitoring in a Patient with Asthma

JOEY C. IS A 7-YEAR-OLD BOY with asthma. He is at the pharmacy with his mother to pick up a peak flow meter and a refill of his albuterol. Joey C.'s mother has a hard time telling when Joey C. needs to take his albuterol for worsening asthma symptoms. His doctor would like Joey C. and his mother to learn how to use a peak flow meter and an asthma action plan.

Question: How should Joey C. check his peak flow reading? How can Joey C.'s mother use the readings to help her monitor his asthma control?

Discussion: Peak flow meters are useful objective indicators of large airway function. Peak flow meters are used to monitor (not diagnose) airway obstruction. It is important to provide Joey C. with a pediatric or low range peak flow meter and not an adult or full range meter. By instructing Joey C. on the proper use of the peak flow meter, his mother is able to objectively determine worsening asthma.

Instructions for using a peak flow meter:

- Stand up.
- Move the indicator on the peak flow meter to the end nearest the mouthpiece.
- Hold the meter and avoid blocking the movement of the indicator and the holes on the end of the meter.
- Take a deep breath in and then seal mouth around the mouthpiece.
- Blow out into the meter as hard and as fast as possible without coughing into the meter (like blowing out candles on a cake).
- Examine the indicator on the meter to identify the number corresponding to the peak flow measurement.
- Repeat the test two more times remembering to move the indicator to the base of the meter each time.
- Record the highest value of the three measurements in a diary.

Joey C. demonstrated the proper use of the peak flow meter at the pharmacy and obtained values of 150 L/min, 145 L/min, and 145 L/min.

Establishing the patient's personal best peak flow:

- Measure the peak flow over a 2-week period of time when asthma symptoms and treatment are stable.
- Readings in the morning and afternoon are ideal.
- The highest value over the 2-week period of time is the personal best.

Joey C. recorded his peak flow for 2 weeks ranging from 120–150 L/min. So, his personal best is identified as 150 L/min.

Using an asthma action plan with peak flow readings:

All patients with asthma need an asthma action plan. An asthma action plan provides directions based on the patient's symptoms and peak flow readings so the patient knows when to use a quick-relief medication, when to call the doctor, and when to go to the emergency department. Patients are instructed to follow the directions of the plan for the worst indicator, either the peak flow reading or the asthma symptoms. See Figure 10-3 for Joey C.'s asthma action plan.

---

monitoring is patient- and clinician-specific and is less useful in preschool and elderly populations. Patients with moderate-to-severe persistent asthma, a history of severe asthma exacerbations, or those who are unable to detect symptoms of worsening asthma are encouraged to check peak flow measurements. For asthma patients not meeting the previous criteria, a symptom-based asthma action plan is sufficient.

Peak flow meters must measure PEFR within an accuracy of ±10% of a reading or ±20 L/min, whichever is greater.[3] Peak flow meters are designed for both pediatric and adult patients with PEFR between 60–400 L/min for children and between 60–850 L/min for adults. Because the calibration of peak flow meters cannot be checked, the package insert for a specific device should provide the average life span of the instrument and cleaning and maintenance instructions. Like FEV_1, the PEFR has a wide normal range and is based on the patient's age, height, gender, and race. Ethnicity may also influence PEFR, similar to FEV_1, but it is not currently factored into the predicted values for PEFR or FEV_1. The charts showing normal values that are included with the peak flow meter are based on population normal values and are not reflective of peak flow readings of a typical asthma patient. Therefore, establishing the patient's personal best peak flow reading and using this value to monitor and change asthma medications are the most appropriate uses of the peak flow readings. Minicase 1 demonstrates the use of the peak flow meter and establishing a patient's personal best peak flow value.

Body Plethysmography

Body plethysmography is a method used to obtain lung volume measures. Lung volume tests indicate the amount of gas contained in the lungs at the various stages of inflation. The lung volumes and capacities may be obtained by several methods, including body plethysmography, gas dilution, and imaging techniques.[9] Different methods can have small but significant effects on the values reported. Gas dilution methods only measure ventilated areas, whereas body plethysmography measures both ventilated and nonventilated areas. Therefore, body plethysmography values may be larger in patients with nonventilated or poorly ventilated lung areas. Computed tomography and magnetic resonance can estimate lung volumes with additional detail of the lung tissue. As body plethysmography is the most commonly used method, this technique will be discussed in more detail.

In body plethysmography, a patient sits in an airtight box and is told to inhale and exhale against a closed shutter. Inside, a mouthpiece contains a pressure transducer. This is done to measure the change in pressure within the box during respiration. It senses the intrathoracic pressure generated when the patient rapidly and forcefully puffs against the closed mouthpiece. These data are then placed into Boyle's law:

My Best Peak Flow Reading is 150 L/min

GREEN ZONE	FEELING GOOD

Symptoms
- Breathing is good
- No cough or wheeze
- Sleeps all night
- I can do all my usual activities

Daily Controller Medications
Medicine: fluticasone   How much to take: two inhalations, 110 mcg   When to take: morning and night

Peak Flow Reading: <120 L/min
(80% or more of my best peak flow reading)

YELLOW ZONE	FEELING SICK

Symptoms
- Cough, wheeze, chest tightness
- I am waking at night due to asthma
- I can do some, but not all, of my usual activities

Peak Flow Reading: 75 L/min to 120 L/min
(50% to 80% of my best peak flow reading)

1st

ADD Quick-Relief Medicine and CONTINUE your Daily Controller Medications.
Add albuterol **two puffs** to daily controller medicine. Repeat albuterol dose in 20 min, if needed.

2nd

IF YOUR SYMPTOMS AND PEAK FLOW RETURN TO THE ZONE AFTER THE ABOVE TREATMENT:

1) Return to taking daily controller medications as directed.

IF YOUR SYMPTOMS AND PEAK FLOW DO NOT RETURN GREEN TO THE GREEN ZONE AFTER THE ABOVE TREATMENT:

1) Take: **albuterol** two puffs q 4 hr for 1–2 days
2) Add: **prednisone** 20 mg daily until you return to the Green Zone for 2 days then stop the prednisone
3) Call your primary care doctor *today* for further instructions. Dr. Breathe Easy 312-222-2222

Continue to take your daily controller medications as directed.

RED ZONE	FEELING VERY ILL

Symptoms
- Lots of problems breathing
- I cannot do usual activities
- Quick-relief medicines have not helped
- Cough, wheeze, and chest tightness are getting worse

Take these medications:
Four puffs NOW and go to the hospital   **Prednisone** 20 mg NOW and go to the hospital

Peak Flow Reading: <75 L/min (50% of my personal best peak flow reading)

FIGURE 10-3. Asthma self-management action plan.

$$P_1 \times V_1 = P_2 \times V_2$$

where

P_1 = pressure inside the box where the patient is seated (atmospheric pressure)

V_1 = volume of the box

P_2 = intrathoracic pressure generated by the patient

V_2 = calculated volume of the patient's thoracic cavity

Because temperature (T_1 and T_2) is constant throughout testing, it is not included in the calculations.

By applying Boyle's law, this test will provide a measure of the functional residual capacity (FRC) or the volume of gas remaining at the end of a normal breath. Once the FRC is determined, the other lung volumes and capacities can be calculated based on this FRC and volumes obtained in static spirometry. After these data are generated, the patient's plethysmography results are usually compared to references from a presumed normal population. This comparison necessitates the generation of predicted values for that patient if he or she were completely normal and healthy. Through complex mathematical formulas, sitting and standing height, age, gender, race, barometric pressure, and altitude are factored in to give predicted values for the pulmonary functions being assessed.[6] The patient's results are compared to the percentage of predicted values based on the results of these calculations.

Body Plethysmography and Lung Volumes

Lung volumes include the following:

- Tidal volume (TV)
- Inspiratory reserve volume (IRV)
- Expiratory reserve volume (ERV)
- Residual volume (RV)

These four volumes in various combinations make up lung capacities, which include the following:

- Inspiratory capacity (IC)
- Vital capacity (VC)
- Functional residual capacity (FRC)
- Total lung capacity (TLC)

Tidal Volume, Residual Volume, and Inspiratory and Expiratory Reserve Volumes

The *tidal volume (TV)* is the amount of air inhaled and exhaled at rest in a normal breath. It is usually a very small proportion of the lung volume and is infrequently used as a measure of respiratory disease. The volume measured from the "top" of the TV (i.e., initial point of normal exhalation) to maximal inspiration is known as the *inspiratory reserve volume (IRV)*. During exhalation, the volume from the "bottom" of the TV (i.e., initial point of normal inhalation) to maximal expiration is referred to as the expiratory reserve volume (ERV). The residual volume (RV) is the volume of air left in the lungs at the end of forced expiration to the bottom of ERV. Without the RV, the lungs would collapse like deflated balloons. In diseases characterized by obstructions that trap air in the lungs (e.g., COPD), the RV increases; the patient is less able to mobilize air trapped behind these obstructions. These four volumes are depicted graphically in Figure 10-4.

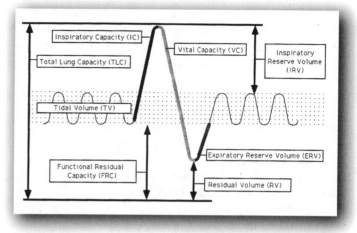

FIGURE 10-4. Lung volumes and capacities—a schematic representation of various lung compartments based on a typical spirogram. (Graphic artwork by Michele Betterton.)

Inspiratory Capacity, Functional Residual Capacity, Slow Vital Capacity, and Total Lung Capacity

The volume measured from the point of the TV where inhalation normally begins to maximal inspiration is known as the *inspiratory capacity (IC)* and is a summation of TV and IRV. The *functional residual capacity (FRC)* is the summation of the ERV and RV. It is the volume of gas remaining in the lungs at the end of the TV. It also may be defined as a balance point between chest wall forces that increase volume and lung parenchymal forces that decrease volume. An increased FRC represents hyperinflation of the lungs and usually indicates airway obstruction. The FRC may be decreased in diseases that affect many alveoli (e.g., pneumonia) or by restrictive changes, especially those due to fibrotic pulmonary tissue changes. The *slow vital capacity (SVC)* is the volume of air that is exhaled as much as possible after inhaling as much as possible. It is a summation of the IRV, TV, and ERV and was described in more detail under spirometry measurements. The *total lung capacity (TLC)* is the summation of all four lung volumes (IRV+TV+ERV+RV). It is the total amount of gas contained in the lungs at maximal inhalation.

Lung Flow Tests

Compliance, Resistance, and Conductance

Compliance and resistance of the lungs are measures that are currently not commonly used but are important in understanding pulmonary function. The elasticity of the lungs and/or thorax is measured by pulmonary compliance. *Compliance* is the change in volume divided by the change in pressure. Pulmonary compliance varies with the amount of air contained in the lungs. Therefore, compliance is often normalized relative to the FRC (the ratio of compliance to the FRC). This ratio is also helpful in comparing patients with normal lung function to those with disease. Pressure is related to the effort needed to expand the lungs. When blowing up a balloon, more effort is needed initially when the balloon is deflated and at the end when the balloon is almost fully inflated. This is also true of the lungs as compliance is the lowest at very low or very high lung volumes, more pressure is needed to produce the same change in volume compared to moderate lung volumes where the compliance is the greatest. As the pulmonary tissue nears its maximal elastic stretch, greater pressure is needed to stretch farther.

Decreased compliance is observed in patients with pulmonary fibrosis, edema, atelectasis, and some pneumonia. Decreased compliance is also seen with the loss of pulmonary surfactant (e.g., hyaline membrane disease). Pulmonary compliance increases in conditions where less pressure is needed to inflate the lungs. Because patients with emphysema have obstructed and damaged small airways, the functional RV increases resulting in the appearance of a barrel chest. This is an example of increased pulmonary compliance compared to normal lungs.

When the change in pressure is divided by the change in flow, the result is *airway resistance*. This value may be useful in differentiating obstructive from restrictive pulmonary disease or from normal pulmonary function. In obstructive diseases, resistance related to blockage of airflow increases. The magnitude of this increase is related to the amount and severity of the obstruction and, because of airway narrowing, resistance may increase during acute asthma attacks. Increases also may be seen in emphysema and bronchitis due to obstructive changes. Decreased resistance is rarely clinically meaningful.

Some clinicians prefer to speak in terms of conductance rather than resistance. *Conductance* is the inverse of resistance. To compare resistance or conductance from one time or patient to another, the value is divided by the lung volume when the measurement was made. These new normalized values are referred to as the *specific airway resistance* or *specific airway conductance*.

Diffusion Capacity Tests

Tests of gas exchange measure the ability of gases to cross (diffuse) the alveolar-capillary membrane and are useful in assessing interstitial lung disease.[10] (See Minicase 2.) Typically, these tests measure the per minute transfer of a gas, usually carbon monoxide (CO), from the alveoli to the blood. Carbon monoxide is used because it is a gas that is not normally present in the lung, has a high affinity for Hgb in red blood cells, and is easily delivered and measured. The *diffusion capacity* may be lessened following losses in the surface area of the alveoli or thickening of the alveolar-capillary membrane. Membrane thickening may be due to infiltration of inflammatory cells or fibrotic changes.

These test results can be confounded by a loss of diffusion capacity due to poor ventilation, which may be related to closed or partially closed airways (as with airway obstruction) or to a ventilation-perfusion mismatch (as with pulmonary emboli or pulmonary hypertension). The diffusion capacity of the lungs to carbon monoxide (DLCO) can be measured by either a single-breath or steady-state test.

In the single-breath test, the patient deeply inhales—to vital capacity—a mixture of 0.3%, CO, 10% helium, and air. After holding the breath for 10 seconds, the patient exhales fully;

the concentrations of CO and helium are measured during the end of expiration (i.e., alveolar flow). These concentrations are compared to the inspired concentrations to determine the amount diffusing across the alveolar membrane. The mean value for CO is about 25–30 mL/min/mm Hg.

In the steady-state test, the patient breathes a 0.1% to 0.2% concentration of CO for 5–6 minutes. In the final 2 minutes, the expired gases are collected and an ABG is obtained. The exhaled gas is measured for total volume and concentrations of CO, carbon dioxide, and oxygen. The ABG is analyzed for carbon dioxide. These values are used to calculate the amount of gas transferred across the alveolar membrane per unit of time, usually a minute. The usual mean value may be slightly less with the steady-state method than the single-breath method. Furthermore, females typically have slightly lower values than males, probably due in part to slightly smaller lung volumes.

These tests of diffusion capacity are useful for assessing gas exchange. Diffusion capacity is decreased in diseases that cause alveolar fibrotic changes. Changes may be idiopathic, such as those seen with sarcoidosis or environmental or occupational disease (asbestosis and silicosis), or be induced by drugs (e.g., nitrofurantoin, amiodarone, and bleomycin).[11,12] Anything that alters Hgb, decreases the red blood cell Hgb concentration, or changes diffusion across the red blood cell membrane may alter the DLCO. The DLCO also reflects the pulmonary capillary blood volume. An increase in this volume (pulmonary edema or asthma) may increase the DLCO.

Airway Reactivity Tests

Bronchodilator (Reversibility) Studies

One of many criteria used in the diagnostic workup of asthma is spirometry with *reversibility*. The patient is asked to perform spirometry immediately before and 15–30 minutes after the administration of an inhaled short-acting beta-2 adrenergic agonist. Definitions for a positive bronchodilator response vary. The ATS defines a positive bronchodilator response as an improvement of FEV_1 and/or FVC by at least 12% and/or 200 mL, respectively. NAEPP recommends FEV_1, FEV_6, FEV_1/FVC measurements before and after a short-acting bronchodilator is given to diagnose and determine the severity of asthma in patients 5 years old or older.[6] The NAEPP defines airway reversibility as an increase in FEV_1 of at least 12% from baseline or an increase in FEV_1 of at least 10% of the predicted FEV_1.[3] FEV_6 may be used in place of FVC in older patients with airway obstruction where a full exhalation takes longer.

Postbronchodilator FEV_1 is a useful measurement in children to monitor lung growth since children with asthma may have decreased lung growth.[13] Reversibility studies (together with the FEV_1/FVC ratio) are particularly useful to help differentiate an asthma patient from the patient with COPD.

Bronchoprovocation Challenge Testing

A bronchial provocation test (BPT) measures the reactivity of the airways to known concentrations of agents that induce airway narrowing. These tests are often referred to as *challenges,* as the airways are challenged with increasing doses of a provoking agent until a desired drop (usually 20%) in lung

MINICASE 2

Using Pulmonary Function Tests to Evaluate a Patient with Interstitial Lung Disease

JACOB K. IS A 55-YEAR-OLD MAN who presents to the medicine clinic with complaints of progressive dyspnea on exertion and minimal dry cough for the past 3 months. He has a history of rheumatoid arthritis and was started on methotrexate 4 months ago. The CT of the chest shows diffuse ground glass opacities consistent with active inflammation and some minimal fibrosis at the bases. Jacob K. had a PFT performed over a year ago that was completely normal. A repeat PFT was ordered and included spirometry, lung volumes, and diffusion capacity.

Jacob K.'s PFT reveals the following results and the flow-volume curve in Figure 10-2 labeled Restriction.

Question: How are these PFTs useful in the diagnosis, evaluation, and management of Jacob K.?

Discussion: Looking at Jacob K.'s spirometry in the table below, the FVC is 63.6% of predicted (reduced), FEV$_1$ is 61.6% of predicted (reduced), and FEV$_1$/FVC ratio is 82.2% (normal). This is consistent with a restrictive pattern. A TLC was 55% of predicted (reduced) verifying a restrictive pulmonary defect and the DLCO was only 29% of predicted (normal range is 70% of predicted). These findings are helpful in the diagnosis of interstitial lung disease in the setting of an abnormal CT scan and change from previous normal spirometry. The severity of restriction can also be determined by the amount of decrease in TLC.

Jacob K. was diagnosed with methotrexate-induced lung disease. The methotrexate was discontinued, and he was treated with prednisone. A repeat PFT was performed after 3 months of therapy. The FVC was 75% of predicted, FEV$_1$ was 72% of predicted, and the FEV$_1$/FVC ratio was 80%. The TLC increased to 65%, and the DLCO increased to 40% of predicted. The repeat PFT shows that Jacob K. is responding to pharmacotherapy. He reports improvement in his symptoms. The followup PFT is used to help evaluate the response to discontinuing the offending medication and to establish a new pulmonary function status.

| PFT | Prebronchodilator | | | Postbronchodilator | |
	Predicted	Measured	% Predicted	Measured	% Change
FVC	3.09	1.97	63.58	1.87	−4.99
FEV$_1$	2.62	1.62	61.60	1.53	−5.45
FEV$_1$/FVC		82.20		81.80	−0.49
TLC	4.57	2.54	55.58		
VC	3.09	1.83	59.09		
RV	1.50	0.71	47.74		
FRC	2.56	1.64	64.00		
DLCO	22.95	6.66	29.01		

function occurs. Agents used to provoke the lung include inhaled methacholine, histamine, adenosine, and specific allergens.[14–17] The ATS has published guidelines for methacholine and exercise challenge testing to enhance the safety, accuracy, and validity of the tests.[18]

Bronchial provocation testing begins by measuring baseline spirometry parameters to ensure it is safe to conduct the test. Bronchial provocation tests should not be performed if the FEV$_1$ is less than 60% of predicted.[18] Most BPTs then begin with nebulization of a solution of phosphate buffered saline. This both serves as a placebo to assess the airway effect of nebulization and establishes baseline airway function from which the amount of pulmonary function to be reduced is calculated. Then an extremely low concentration of the selected bronchoconstrictor agent is nebulized followed by spirometry at 30 and 90 minutes from the end of the nebulization. Additional spirometry efforts may be done to meet or exceed ATS criteria. Optimally, the FEV$_1$ values should be within 0.10 L of each other.[18] The patient inhales gradually increasing concentrations of the bronchoconstrictor at specific time intervals (usually 5

minutes) until a predesignated amount of airway restriction is attained. This is usually defined as a reduction in FEV$_1$ by at least 20% from the saline control. The challenge data is then summarized into a single number, the PC$_{20}$FEV$_1$ (mg/mL). This refers to the provocation concentration of the bronchoconstriction agent that would produce a 20% reduction in FEV$_1$.

For methacholine, a PC$_{20}$FEV$_1$ of <1.0 mg/mL indicates moderate to severe bronchial hyperresponsiveness (BHR), 1.0–4.0 mg/mL as mild BHR, 4.0–16 mg/mL as borderline BHR, and >16 mg/mL as normal bronchial responsiveness. During a BPT, patients may experience transient respiratory symptoms such as cough, shortness of breath, wheezing, and chest tightness. An inhaled, short acting beta-2 adrenergic agonist or anticholinergic agent may be administered to alleviate symptoms and quicken the return of the FEV$_1$ to the baseline value. Because BPTs can elicit severe, life-threatening bronchospasm, trained personnel and medications to treat severe bronchospasm should be on-hand in the testing area.

Bronchial provocation tests are used to aid in the diagnosis of asthma, when the more common tests (symptom history, spirometry with reversibility) cannot confirm or reject the diagnosis, to evaluate the effects of drug therapy on airway hyperreactivity, and in research to evaluate potential drug effectiveness. Using this technique in research, the magnitude and duration of different drugs' effects on the airways may be compared.[14,16,17]

Exercise Challenge Testing

Exercise- or exertion-induced bronchospasm (EIB) occurs in the majority of patients with uncontrolled asthma. The etiology of EIB is thought to be related to the cooling and drying of the airways caused by the rapid breathing during exercise. *Exercise challenge testing* is used to confirm or rule out EIB and to evaluate the effectiveness of medications used to treat or prevent EIB.

Exercise tests are usually done with a motor driven treadmill (with adjustable speed and grade) or an electromagnetically braked cycle ergometer. Heart rate should be monitored throughout the test. Nose clips should be worn and the room air should be dry and cool, to promote water loss from the airways during the exercise test. In most patients, symptoms are effectively blocked by use of an inhaled bronchodilator immediately prior to beginning exercise or other exertion causing the problem. After obtaining baseline spirometry, the exercise test is started at a low speed that is gradually increased over 2–4 minutes until the heart rate is 80% to 90% of the predicted maximum or the work rate is at 100%. The duration of the exercise is age and tolerance dependent. Children less than 12 years of age generally take 6 minutes while older children and adults take 8 minutes to complete the test. After the exercise is completed, the patient does serial spirometry at 5-minute intervals for 20–30 minutes. FEV_1 is the primary outcome variable. A 10% or more decrease in FEV_1 from baseline is generally accepted as an abnormal response, though some clinicians feel a 15% decrease is more diagnostic of EIB.[18]

Six-Minute Walk Test

The *six-minute walk test (6MWT)* is a test used to measure the distance a patient can walk on a flat, hard surface in 6 minutes.[19] The results of the test have been correlated to the patient's quality of life and abilities to complete daily activities. The results of the 6MWT also help predict morbidity and mortality for patients with congestive heart failure, COPD, and primary pulmonary hypertension.[20-22] Pulmonary hypertension studies use this test to monitor the efficacy of interventions with medications.[23] While performing the 6MWT, the patient is educated that the goal of the test is to walk as far as possible in 6 minutes, allowing the patient to select the intensity of exercise. Stopping and resting is allowed during the test. Pulse oximetry is optional during the test but is often used. Reference equations for healthy adults have been published and normal values in young healthy children have been studied.[24-26] Normal values in healthy adults range from 500–630 meters and healthy children 4–11 years of age had a mean distance walked of 470 meters (±59 meters). Clinical improvement has been correlated with an increase in distance of 54 meters; alternatively, percent change from baseline may be calculated.[27] Practice

tests, younger age, taller height, less weight, male gender, longer corridor length, and encouragement all improve test results. Unstable angina and myocardial infarction in the past month, a resting heart rate greater than 120 beats per minute, or a blood pressure reading greater than 180/100 are all contraindications for performing the 6MWT. In practice, the 6MWT is also used to assess the amount of oxygen needed with exertion. Patients with mild-to-moderate pulmonary disease may have normal oxygen saturation at rest but poor saturation with exertion. An oxygen saturation of 88% or lower indicates the need for supplemental oxygen.

Specialized Tests

Infant Pulmonary Function Testing

With advances in respiratory technology, use of *infant pulmonary function testing* is re-emerging as a possible tool for investigating the development of the lungs, the progression of lung disease, and the response to pulmonary treatment interventions. The equipment is expensive and requires specialized training. As the equipment, procedures, measurements, and interpretation of results are becoming more standardized, the role of this test in diagnosing, monitoring, and treating lung disease in infants should become clearer.[28-30]

Carbon Monoxide Breath Test

Carbon monoxide is a poisonous gas emitted from anything burning, including cigarette smoke. As mentioned under the DLCO section, CO binds more readily to Hgb than oxygen, causing increased fatigue and shortness of breath. With a simple breath test by a hand-held CO meter, the patient can see how much CO is in the body (parts per million [ppm]) and in the blood (% COHgb). In clinical studies, 10 ppm or less is often defined as a nonsmoker; however, in clinical practice 1 or 2 ppm is a nonsmoker level. This objective reading is thought to be a motivator for some to quit smoking and remain abstinent.[31] However, a Cochrane review found no significant increase in abstinence rates with CO measurements.[32] Calculating lung age using the measured FEV_1 and discussing this with the smoker was found to be a motivator for smokers to quit smoking in a clinical trial and may be applicable to clinical practice.[33] Minicase 3 uses CO testing during a smoking cessation visit.

Testing exhaled CO is a simple breath test where patients hold their breath for 15 seconds then exhale into a meter. The meter is able to indicate how much CO is in the patients' lungs and estimate how much is attached to Hgb in the patients' blood. The test is an objective value that patients can visually see the effects of inhaling smoke with higher values of CO detected. After 8–12 hours without smoking, CO levels become undetectable.

Inflammatory Markers

Airway inflammation is involved in a number of airway diseases. The ability to easily measure markers or indicators of this inflammatory process would improve our understanding of airway disease and its treatment.

MINICASE 3

Using Spirometry and Carbon Monoxide Testing in a Patient with COPD

JAMES S., IS A 56-YEAR-OLD MAN, who presents at the smoking cessation clinic today for assistance with his tobacco dependence. He is currently smoking one pack of cigarettes a day and started smoking when he was 13 years old. He has complaints today of a constant, persistent increased cough with clear phlegm and increased shortness of breath when he carries his groceries up steps. At the clinic James S. completes both a CO breath test and a spirometry test. His CO reading today is 30 ppm and his carboxyhemoglobin percentage is estimated to be 5.4%.

James S.'s spirometry revealed the following results (see table below) and the flow-volume curve in Figure 10-2 labeled Obstruction:

Question: How is spirometry and CO testing useful tests in smokers?

Answer: Looking at James S.'s spirometry flow-volume curve, a concave-pattern is visible indicating airway obstruction. His FEV_1 is decreased compared to values of another person that is the same gender, height,

race, and age as James S. (In patients susceptible to COPD and who continue to smoke, a loss of FEV_1 of 63 mL/yr may occur compared to 34 mL/yr in one who has quit tobacco, and 25 mL/yr in one who never smoked and is without COPD.[34,35]) His FVC is normal. He does not have bronchodilator reversibility. This is calculated by the following example:

- Percent FEV_1 reversibility = (the postbronchodilator FEV_1 – prebronchodilator FEV_1)/prebronchodilator FEV_1 x100
- Percent FEV_1 reversibility= (1.79–1.64 L)/1.64 L X 100
- Percent FEV_1 reversibility= 9.15%, which is less than the 12% definition
- There is 150 mL difference in the postbronchodilator and the prebronchodilator FEV_1, which is less than the defined value of 200 mL for airway reversibility.

Showing James S. the results and explaining that 5.4% of his blood has a poisonous gas instead of oxygen and that this is contributing to his shortness of breath may be a motivating factor for him to quit smoking. Education that quitting smoking is the only treatment at this time to slow the expedited loss in lung function is an empowering tool.

| PFT | Prebronchodilator | | | Postbronchodilator | | |
---	Predicted	Measured	% Predicted	Measured	% Predicted	% Change
FVC	3.54	3.34	94.28	3.78	106.69	13.17
FEV_1	2.84	1.64	57.88	1.79	63.10	9.15
FEV_1/FVC		49.20		47.40		–3.67

Bronchial alveolar lavage. Bronchial alveolar lavage (BAL) is a method of collecting cells or proteins found in pulmonary secretions for measurement. Samples are attained during bronchoscopy. This procedure is the direct visualization of the lumen of the airways, and it can be accomplished with a flexible bronchoscope. Flexible bronchoscopy may be performed while the patient is consciously sedated.

When there is a desire to understand what is in the pulmonary secretions of the patient, a small amount of fluid—usually a buffered, warmed, and sterile normal saline—is flushed into the airways and then drawn back out and sent to a laboratory for analysis. The microscopic analysis usually looks for cellular components and proteins found in the airways although it may be specific for other markers. Common cellular analysis items include numbers and types of eosinophils, neutrophils, lymphocytes, mast cells, and macrophages while protein matter includes histamine and subcellular components. The invasiveness of this method limits its use, especially for monitoring changes in lung inflammation over short period of times.

Induced sputum. In the past, sputum samples were thought to be difficult to obtain and often unreliable. Patients were asked to cough a sample of sputum into a collection cup. However, many patients could not produce enough sputum for analysis, and often the sample contained more saliva than sputum. With the introduction of newer methods of inducing sputum production and processing the resultant sample, sputum indices are

being evaluated for diagnosing and tracking the progression of disease and for comparing responses to various therapies.[36] Induced sputum generally gives a higher recovery of viable cells and produces better slides for cell differential and counting than sputum samples obtained from the patient just trying to cough up sputum. From the sputum sample, total cell counts, cytokines, chemokines, adhesion molecules, and other inflammatory mediators can be measured. To induce sputum, patients inhale nebulized hypertonic saline. Patients can be pretreated with a short-acting beta-2 adrenergic agonist to prevent airway bronchospasm from the hypertonic saline. Sputum samples should be kept in ice and processed as soon as possible. The finding of alveolar macrophages and other inflammatory cells is consistent with lower respiratory tract sampling. The presence of many epithelial cells indicates contamination with upper airway secretions and therefore an inadequate sample. Sputum cultures are also obtained to identify bacterial or fungal infections in the lungs, to test for antibiotic sensitivity to the organism, and to monitor treatment.

Fractional exhaled nitric oxide. Measurement of exhaled concentrations of nitric oxide (NO) is being evaluated as a possible noninvasive test of airway inflammation for both diagnosing and monitoring asthma. To aid the advancement of this test, ATS published recommendations for standardizing the test procedures.[37] A device to measure fractional exhaled oxide (FENO) was recently approved by the Food and Drug

Administration. A prospective study using FENO monitoring demonstrated that the cumulative dose of inhaled corticosteroids was significantly reduced in chronic asthma patients compared to assessing PFT and symptoms alone.[38]

SUMMARY

This chapter discusses the importance of pulmonary function testing as it relates to the diagnosis, treatment, and monitoring of respiratory disease states. After a review of the anatomy and physiology of the lungs, the mechanics of obtaining PFTs were emphasized. By understanding these mechanics, a clinician can better understand the interpretation of PFTs, use findings from different PFTs to help differentiate among diagnoses, and assist in making optimal therapeutic recommendations. Pulmonary function test results are not interpreted in isolation, but they need to be assessed within the context of the other findings from the medical history and from other laboratory or clinical test results.

Common tests of airflows and lung volumes are primarily used to characterize airway functions and diseases. These measurements may indicate the need for specific pharmacotherapeutic interventions. For example, clinicians recommending a peak flow meter for home monitoring of severe asthma will find the information obtained useful when considering appropriate therapeutic interventions.

Other tests, such as diffusion capacity, indicate the ability of a gas to diffuse through lung tissues and the general thickness of the membranes lining the alveoli. Specialized tests, such as bronchoprovocational and bronchodilator studies, are used to guide treatment choices. Clearly, the PFTs are an important tool to aid the clinician in decision-making.

Learning Points

1. **What is a PFT?**

   Answer: A PFT is an assessment of lung function that is composed of several different components (e.g., spirometry, volumes, diffusion capacity). The component of the PFT to be ordered is determined by the information needed. For example, spirometry is performed to reveal the presence of obstructive disease. Lung volumes determine the presence of restrictive disease, and the diffusion capacity test is completed to ascertain the adequacy of gas exchange.

2. **Why is spirometry an important test in the diagnosis and management of COPD and asthma?**

   Answer: In COPD, spirometry is used to determine the presence of obstruction and the degree of disease severity. Physical exam and history alone are often not adequate to detect airway obstruction. Therefore, an objective test with spirometry can confirm a clinical suspicion. Based on GOLD, the ATS/ERS guidelines medical management of COPD is based in part on spirometry results and will often guide therapy.

   In asthma, spirometry results can be useful to determine the severity of the disease as well as the level of control. Based on NAEPP guidelines, spirometry results along with other patient factors, such as the presence of symptoms, guide management.

3. **How is restrictive lung disease diagnosed?**

   Answer: It is important to note that spirometry can only provide evidence consistent with restrictive disease such as a decrease in FEV_1 and FVC with a normal or elevated FEV_1/FVC ratio. However, restriction is a decrease in lung volume as defined by a decrease in the TLC, which is obtained by lung volume tests, such as body plethysmography, and such test results are needed to diagnose restrictive lung disease.

REFERENCES

1. Crapo RO. Pulmonary function testing. *N Engl J Med*. 1994; 331:25-30.

2. Global Strategy for the Diagnosis, Management, and Prevention of COPD, Global Initiative for Chronic Obstructive Lung Disease (Revised 2011). http://www.goldcopd.org. Accessed July 31, 2012.

3. National Asthma Education and Prevention Program. Expert panel report 3 (EPR3): guidelines for the diagnosis and management of asthma. http://www.nhlbi.nih.gov/guidelines/asthma/asthgdln.htm. Accessed July 31, 2012.

4. Celli BR, MacNee W. Standards for the diagnosis and treatment of patients with COPD: a summary of the ATS/ERS position paper. *Eur Respir J*. 2004;23(6):932-946.

5. American Thoracic Society and the European Respiratory Society. General considerations for lung function testing. *Eur Respir J*. 2005;26:153-161.

6. American Thoracic Society and the European Respiratory Society. Standardisation of spirometry. *Eur Respir J*. 2005;26:319-338.

7. American Thoracic Society Documents. An official American Thoracic Society/European Respiratory Society Statement: Pulmonary function testing in preschool children. *Am J Respir Crit Care Med*. 2007;175:1304-1345.

8. Pellegrino R, Viegi G, Brusasco V, et al. Interpretative strategies for lung function tests. *Eur Respir J.* 2005;26:948-968.

9. Wanger J, Clausen JL, Coates CA, et al. Standardisation of the measurement of lung volumes. *Eur Respir J.* 2005;26:511-522.

10. MacIntyre N, Crapo RO, Viegi G. Standardisation of the single-breath determination of carbon monoxide uptake in the lung. *Eur Respir J.* 2005;26:720-735.

11. Cooper JA, White DA, Matthay RA. Drug-induced pulmonary disease. Part 1: cytotoxic drugs. *Am Rev Respir Dis.* 1986;133:321-340.

12. Cooper JA, White DA, Matthay RA. Drug-induced pulmonary disease. Part 2: noncytotoxic drugs. *Am Rev Respir Dis.* 1986;133:488-505.

13. Covar RA, Spahn JD, Murphy JR, et al. Childhood Asthma Management Program Research Group. Progression of asthma measured by lung function in the childhood asthma management program. *Am J Respir Crit Care Med.* 2004:170(3):234-241.

14. Ahrens RC, Hendeles L, Clarke WR, et al. Therapeutic equivalence of Spiros dry powder inhaler and Ventolin metered-dose inhaler. A bioassay using methacholine. *Am J Respir Crit Care Med.* 1999;160:1238-1243.

15. Cockcroft DW, Killian DN, Mellon JJ, et al. Bronchial reactivity to inhaled histamine: a method and clinical survey. *Clin Allergy.* 1977;7:235-243.

16. Taylor DA, Jensen MW, Kannar V, et al. A dose-dependent effect of the novel inhaled corticosteroids ciclesonide on airway responsiveness to adenosine-5'-monophosphate in asthmatic patients. *Am J Respir Crit Care Med.* 1999;160:237-243.

17. Swystun VA, Bhagat R, Kalra S, et al. Comparison of 3 different doses of budesonide and placebo on the early asthmatic response to inhaled allergen. *J Allergy Clin Immunol.* 1998;102:363-367.

18. American Thoracic Society. Guidelines for methacholine and exercise challenge testing: 1999. *Am J Respir Crit Care Med.* 2000;161:309-329.

19. American Thoracic Society. Statement guidelines for the six-minute walk test. *Am J Respir Crit Care Med.* 2002;166:111-117.

20. Cahalin LP, Mathier MA, Semigran MJ, et al. The six-minute walk test predicts peak oxygen uptake and survival in patients with advanced heart failure. *Chest.* 1996;110:325-332.

21. Kessler R, Faller M, Fourgaut G, et al. Predictive factors of hospitalization for acute exacerbations in a series of 64 patients with chronic obstructive pulmonary disease. *Am J Respir Crit Care Med.* 1999;159:158-164.

22. Kadikar A, Maurer J, Kesten S. The six-minute walk test a guide to assessment for lung transplant. *J Heart Lung Transplant.* 1997;16:313-319.

23. Badesch DB, Abman SH, Simonneau G, et al. Medical therapy for pulmonary arterial hypertension: updated ACCP evidence-based clinical practice guidelines. *Chest.* 2007;131(6):1917-1928.

24. Enright PL, Sherrill DL. Reference equations for the six-minute walk in healthy adults. *Am J Respir Crit Care Med.* 1998;158(5):1384-1387.

25. Troosters T, Gosselink R, Decramer M. Six-minute walk distance in healthy elderly subjects. *Eur Respir J.* 1999;14:270-274.

26. Lammers AE, Hislop AA, Flynn Y, et al. The 6-minute walk test: normal values for children 4–11 years of age. *Arch Dis Child.* 2008; 93:464-468.

27. Redelmeier DA, Bayoumi AM, Goldstein RS, et al. Interpreting small differences in functional status: the six minute walk test in chronic lung disease patients. *Am J Respir Crit Care Med.* 1997;155:1278-1282.

28. Series—Standard for Infant Respiratory Function Testing. ERS/ATS Task Force: tidal breath analysis for infant pulmonary function testing. *Eur Respir J.* 2002;16:1180-1192.

29. Series—Standard for Infant Respiratory Function Testing. ERS/ATS Task Force: specifications for equipment used for infant pulmonary function testing. *Eur Respir J.* 2002;16:731-740.

30. Series—Standard for Infant Respiratory Function Testing. ERS/ATS Task Force: specifications for signal processing and data handling used for infant pulmonary function testing. *Eur Respir J.* 2002;16:1016-1022.

31. Audrain J, Boyd NR, Roth J, et al. Genetic susceptibility testing in smoking-cessation treatment: one-year outcomes of a randomized trial. *Addict Behav.* 1997;22:741-751.

32. Bize R, Burnand B, Mueller Y, et al. Biomedical risk assessment as an aid for smoking cessation. *Cochrane Database Syst Rev.* 2005;4:CD004705.

33. Parkes G, Greenhalgh T, Griffen M, et al. Effect on smoking quit rate of telling patients their lung age: the Step2quit randomised controlled trial. *BMJ.* 2008;336(7644):598-604.

34. Anthonisen NR, Connett JE, Kiley JP, et al. Effects of smoking intervention and the use of an inhaled anticholinergic bronchodilator on the rate of decline of FEV_1. The Lung Health Study. *JAMA.* 1994;272:1497-1505.

35. Scanlon P, Connet J, Waller L, et al. Smoking cessation and lung function in mild-to-moderate chronic obstructive pulmonary disease: the Lung Health Study. *Am J Respir Crit Care Med.* 2000;161:381-390.

36. Green RH, Brightling CE, Mckenna S, et al. Asthma exacerbations and sputum eosinophil counts: a randomised controlled trial. *Lancet.* 2002;360(9347):1715-1721.

37. American Thoracic Society. Recommendations for standardized procedures for the online and offline measurement of exhaled lower respiratory nitric oxide and nasal nitric oxide in adults and children: 1999. *Am J Respir Crit Care Med.* 1999;160:2104-2117.

38. Smith AD, Cowan JO, Brassett KP, at el. Use of exhaled nitric oxide measurements to guide treatment in chronic asthma. *N Engl J Med.* 2005;352(21):2163-2173.

CHAPTER 11

THE HEART: LABORATORY TESTS AND DIAGNOSTIC PROCEDURES

WAFA Y. DAHDAL, SAMIR Y. DAHDAL

Objectives

After completing this chapter, the reader should be able to

- Describe the normal physiology of the heart

- Describe the electrocardiogram (ECG) changes reflected by myocardial ischemia and infarction

- Explain the roles of the different biochemical markers in the diagnosis of coronary artery disease (CAD), acute coronary syndrome (ACS), and heart failure

- Given a patient's history, clinical presentation, cardiac biochemical markers, and electrocardiographic findings, assess the presence and type of ACS

- Given a patient case, assess the presence and type of heart failure

- Describe the role of pharmacologic agents in noninvasive imaging studies

- Describe other diagnostic procedures used for the evaluation of CAD, ACS, and heart failure

The heart has two basic properties: electrical and mechanical. The two work in harmony to propel blood, delivering oxygen and nutrients to all body tissues. Heart cells responsible for these properties are (1) pacemaker cells or the "electrical power" of the heart, (2) electrical conducting cells, or the "hardwiring circuitry" of the heart, and (3) myocardial cells or the contractile units of the heart. Disturbances in the electrical system result in rhythm disorders, also known as *arrhythmias* or *dysrhythmias*. The pumping action is accomplished by means of striated cardiac muscle, which largely composes the myocardium. A number of diseases disrupt the mechanical function of the heart including coronary artery disease (CAD), acute coronary syndrome (ACS), and heart failure.

The management of ACS, heart failure, and potential complications of each contributes greatly to the overall health of and cost incurred by society. Laboratory tests are essential for the diagnosis and prognosis of patients. Accurate and expeditious assessment of a patient presenting with symptoms suggestive of ACS guides individualized treatment to optimize his or her short- and long-term outcomes. Conversely, rapid exclusion of the diagnosis permits early discharge from the coronary care unit or hospital. Laboratory and other diagnostic tests used in evaluating the patient with possible ACS and heart failure are discussed in this chapter.

CARDIAC PHYSIOLOGY

The heart consists of two pumping units that operate in parallel, one on the right side and the other on the left side. Each is composed of an upper chamber, the atrium,

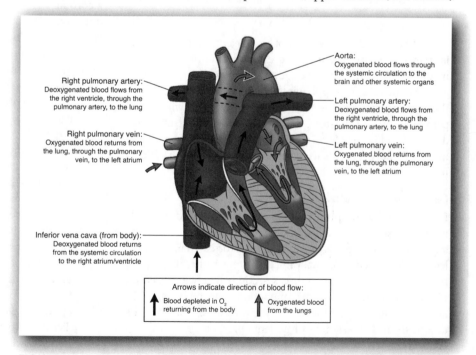

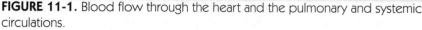

FIGURE 11-1. Blood flow through the heart and the pulmonary and systemic circulations.

and a lower chamber, the ventricle. The atrium serves as a passive portal to the ventricle and is a weak pump that helps move blood into the ventricle. The atrial contraction or kick is responsible for 20% to 30% of ventricular filling. The right and left ventricles supply the primary force that propels blood through the pulmonary and peripheral circulation, respectively (Figure 11-1).

The functional unit of the heart is comprised of a network of noncontractile cells that form the conduction system, which is responsible for originating and conducting action potentials from the atria to the ventricles. This leads to the excitation and contraction of the cardiac muscle, which is responsible for the pumping of the blood to the other organs.

The normal adult human heart contracts rhythmically at approximately 70 beats per minute (bpm). Each cardiac cycle is divided into a systolic and diastolic phase. During each cycle, blood from the systemic circulation is returned to the heart via the veins, and blood empties from the superior and inferior vena cavae into the right atrium. During the diastolic phase, blood passively fills the right ventricle through the tricuspid valve with an active filling phase by atrial contraction just prior to end-diastole. During systole, blood is then pumped from the right ventricle through the pulmonary artery to the lungs where carbon dioxide is removed and the blood is oxygenated. From the lungs, blood returns to the heart via the pulmonary veins and empties into the left atrium. Again, during diastole, blood empties from the left atrium through the mitral valve into the main pumping chamber, the left ventricle. With systole the left ventricle contracts and blood is forcefully propelled into the peripheral circulation via the aorta (Figure 11-1). At rest, the normal heart pumps approximately 4–6 L of blood per minute. Maintaining normal cardiac output (CO) is dependent on the heart rate (HR) and stroke volume (SV).

$$CO = HR \times SV$$

The SV, defined as the volume of blood ejected during systole, is determined by intrinsic and extrinsic factors including myocardial contractility, preload, and afterload. The coronary arteries, the arteries supplying the heart muscle, branch from the aorta just beyond the aortic valve and are filled with blood primarily during diastole. The major coronary arteries are depicted in Figure 11-2. In the face of increased myocardial metabolic needs, the heart is able to increase coronary blood flow by vasodilation to meet myocardial oxygen demand.

Cardiac Dysfunction

Decreased CO compromises tissue perfusion, and depending on the severity and duration, may lead to significant acute and chronic complications. A number of cardiac diseases lead to decreased CO, including hypertensive heart diseases, heart failure, valvular heart diseases, congenital heart diseases, diseases of the myocardium, conduction abnormalities, CAD, and ACS. This chapter focuses on the various tests used in the diagnosis and assessment of patients presenting with CAD, ACS, and heart failure.

Also known as *ischemic heart disease (IHD)*, CAD is caused by atherosclerosis of the coronary arteries, resulting in lumen

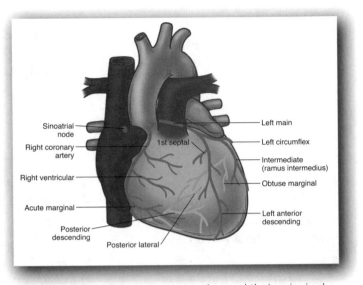

FIGURE 11-2. Major coronary arteries and their principal branches.

narrowing and blood flow reduction to the myocardium perfused by the affected artery. This leads to tissue ischemia and chest pain. Severe reduction in or total interruption of blood flow may lead to severe tissue ischemia or infarction, resulting in a clinical presentation as a type of ACS.

Patients with severe symptoms of myocardial ischemia or acute myocardial infarction (AMI) may be experiencing one of three types of ACS: unstable angina (UA), non-ST-segment elevation MI (NSTEMI), or ST-segment elevation MI (STEMI). The most common cause for ACS is atherosclerotic plaque rupture and subsequent obstruction of the coronary lumen by thrombosis composed of platelet aggregates, fibrin, and entrapped blood cells leading to myocardial ischemia. When a coronary artery is occluded, the location, extent, rate, and duration of occlusion determine the severity of myocardial ischemia resulting in UA, NSTEMI, or STEMI.

According to the universal definition of myocardial infarction (MI), MI may be classified clinically into different types[1]:

- **Type 1:** Spontaneous MI related to ischemia due to a primary coronary event such as plaque erosion and/or rupture, fissuring, or dissection
- **Type 2:** Myocardial infarction secondary to ischemia due to either increased oxygen demand or decreased supply (e.g., coronary artery spasm, coronary embolism, anemia, arrhythmias, hypertension, or hypotension)
- **Type 3:** Sudden unexpected cardiac death, including cardiac arrest, often with symptoms suggestive of myocardial ischemia accompanied by presumably new ST elevation or new left bundle branch block (LBBB), or evidence of fresh thrombus in a coronary artery by angiography and/or autopsy, but death occurring before blood samples could be obtained, or at a time before the appearance of cardiac biomarkers in the blood
- **Type 4a:** Myocardial infarction associated with percutaneous coronary intervention (PCI)
- **Type 4b:** Myocardial infarction associated with stent thrombosis as documented by angiography or at autopsy

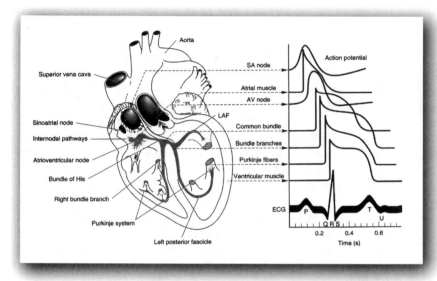

FIGURE 11-3. Conduction system of the heart. Typical transmembrane action potentials for the sinoatrial (SA) and atrioventricular (AV) nodes, other parts of the conduction system, and the atrial and ventricular muscles are shown along with the correlation to the extracellularly recorded electrical activity (i.e., the electrocardiogram [ECG]). The action potentials and ECG are plotted on the same time axis but with different zero points on the vertical scale. The PR interval is measured from the beginning of the P wave to the beginning of the QRS. (LAF, left anterior fascicle.) (Reproduced with permission from Kusumoto F. Cardiovascular disorders: heart disease. In: McPhee SJ, Lingappa VR, Ganong WF, et al. *Pathophysiology of Disease: An Introduction to Clinical Medicine.* 3rd ed. New York, NY: McGraw-Hill; 2000.)

- **Type 5:** Myocardial infarction associated with coronary artery bypass graft (CABG)

Complications of AMI include cardiogenic shock, congestive heart failure (CHF), ventricular and atrial arrhythmias, ventricular rupture or ventricular septal defect formation, cardiac tamponade, pericarditis, papillary muscle rupture, mitral regurgitation, and embolism. Initial assessment of the patient presenting with ACS may be complicated by the presence and severity of the above complications.

Heart failure is a syndrome in which the heart is unable to pump blood at a rate sufficient to meet the demands of the body or unable to accept the fluid volume with which it is presented. Heart failure may be due to reduced systolic (ventricular contraction) function defined as left ventricular ejection fraction (LVEF) less than 50%. Common etiologies for systolic heart failure include CAD, ACS, valvular diseases, or long-term hypertension. A substantial number of patients with heart failure have preserved LVEF. Those with preserved LVEF and abnormal diastolic function (abnormal relaxation, filling or stiffness) are diagnosed with diastolic heart failure.[2] Signs and symptoms consistent with heart failure may be attributed to volume overload and congestion (e.g., elevated jugular venous pressure, peripheral edema, pulmonary congestion and edema, and dyspnea) and/or hypoperfusion (e.g., tachycardia (HR >100 bpm), cold extremities, cyanosis, and fatigue).

ELECTROCARDIOGRAPHY

Electrocardiography is the recording of the electrical activity of the heart on an electrocardiogram (ECG).

Normal Conduction System and Electrocardiogram Recording

The conduction system is composed of specialized, noncontractile cells that serve to originate and conduct action potentials in the appropriate sequence and at an appropriate rate from the atria to the ventricles. At rest, the cardiac cells are more negatively charged intracellularly than extracellularly, or polarized, with a voltage difference of 60–90 mV. When excited, ionic currents across cell membranes lead to charge shifting where the interior of the cells become more positive (depolarization) and an action potential is generated. Calcium influx leads to the excitation-contraction coupling of the cells. Subsequently, the action potential is propagated and the cells return to a normal resting state (repolarization). *Depolarization* is the electrical phenomenon that leads to myocardial contraction, and *repolarization* is the electrical phenomenon that leads to myocardial relaxation. The ECG provides a pictorial presentation of the depolarization and repolarization of atrial and ventricular cells that can be assessed by reviewing a number of waves and intervals.

Normally, an electrical impulse originates in the sinoatrial (SA) node and is propagated through Bachmann bundle and internodal tracts, the atrioventricular (AV) node, His bundle, the left and right bundle branches, and the Purkinje fibers resulting in one cardiac cycle. Each cardiac cycle is presented on ECG by the P wave reflecting atrial depolarization, the QRS complex reflecting ventricular depolarization, and the T wave reflecting ventricular repolarization (Figure 11-3). By placing multiple leads on the patient, the electrical impulses of the heart are recorded from different views. The standard ECG is composed of 12 leads: six limb leads (I, II, III, AVR, AVL, and AVF) and six chest leads (V_1–V_6). Different leads provide specific information on different aspects of heart chambers and coronary arteries.

Electrocardiographic Findings in Acute Coronary Syndrome

In patients with ACS, the ECG is an essential diagnostic tool providing immediate and invaluable data vital for expeditious diagnosis, prognosis, and management. A 12-lead ECG should be obtained within 10 minutes of a patient's presentation to the emergency department if ACS is suspected. Careful reading of the ECG by an experienced clinician provides information on the presence of myocardial ischemia, injury, or infarction. The leads in which ECG changes consistent with ACS occur

TABLE 11-1. Localization of Left Ventricular Myocardial Infarction by Anatomical Relationships of Leads

ANATOMIC SITE	CORONARY ARTERY MOST LIKELY INVOLVED	ECG LEADS WITH ISCHEMIC CHANGES
Inferior wall	RCA	II, III, and aVF
Anterior wall	LAD	V_1 to V_4
Lateral wall	CX	I, aVL, V_5, and V_6
Posterior	RCA	$V_1 - V_3$

CX = circumflex branch of the left coronary artery; ECG = electrocardiogram; LAD = left anterior descending artery; RCA = right coronary artery.

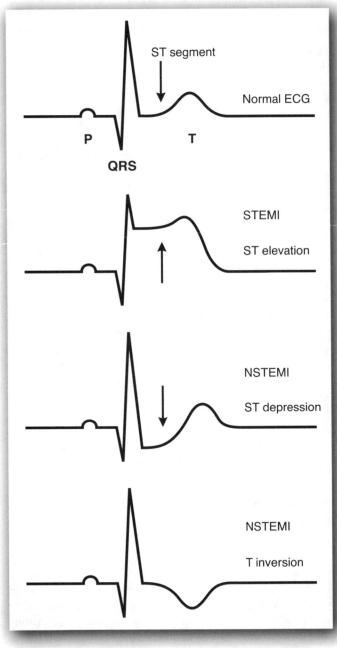

FIGURE 11-4. ECG changes consistent with STEMI and NSTEMI.

provide information on the occluded coronary artery most likely causing the ischemia or infarction (Table 11-1).

The classic ECG changes consistent with acute presentation of myocardial ischemia or infarction are (1) T-wave inversion, (2) ST-segment elevation, and (3) ST-segment depression (Figure 11-4). Q waves, defined by a width of greater than 1 mm and a depth of greater than 25% of the QRS complex height, are also indicative of MI and loss of electrically functioning cardiac tissue. Pathologic Q waves may appear within 1–2 hours of onset of symptoms, often 12 hours, and, occasionally, up to 24 hours.[3] Among patients presenting with ST-segment elevation, most ultimately develop a Q-wave MI (QwMI) whereas most patients presenting with NSTEMI ultimately develop a non-Q wave MI (NQMI).[4]

Electrocardiogram manifestations of non-ST elevation ACS are ST depression and or T-wave inversion without ST segment elevation or pathologic Q waves. Electrocardiogram criteria for the diagnosis of ST elevation MI (in the absence of LBBB and left ventricular hypertrophy [LVH]) include ≥2 mm of ST segment elevation in the two contiguous leads for men and ≥1.5 mm for women (who tend to have less ST elevation) in leads V_2-V_3 and/or ≥1 mm in other leads. Criteria for ST depression include ≥0.5 mm horizontal or down-sloping ST depression and/or T inversion of ≥1 mm in two contiguous leads with prominent R-wave or R/S ratio >1.[1]

During an acute STEMI, the EKG evolves through three stages:

1. T-wave peaking with subsequent T-wave inversion (with the onset of infarction, the T waves become hyperacute or tall and narrow, commonly known as "peaking." Shortly thereafter, usually within hours, the T waves invert. T wave changes are reflective of myocardial ischemia, but they are not indicative of myocardial infarct.

2. ST-segment elevation signifies myocardial injury, likely reflecting a degree of cellular damage beyond that of mere ischemia; however, this is potentially reversible. A more reliable sign that is diagnostic of true infarction. Persistent ST segment elevation may indicate other cardiac injury such as ventricular aneurysm.

3. Appearance of new Q-waves that are indicative of irreversible myocardial cell death (diagnostic of an MI).

Any one of these changes may be present without any of the others.

In addition to diagnosing ACS, ECG findings provide prognostic information. Patients presenting with UA/NSTEMI who experience angina at rest with transient ST-segment changes greater than 0.05 mm, new or presumed bundle-branch block, or sustained ventricular tachycardia are at high risk of short-term death or nonfatal MI.[4]

LABORATORY TESTS USED IN THE EVALUATION OF ACUTE CORONARY SYNDROME

Three criteria for the diagnosis of AMI were identified by the World Health Organization and, subsequently, modified by the

Global Task Force for the Redefinition of Myocardial Infarction, convened by the European Society of Cardiology, the American College of Cardiology (ACC), the American Heart Association (AHA), and World Heart Federation (WHF), to include clinical presentation, electrocardiography, and elevated biochemical markers of myocardial necrosis.[1,5]

Clinical presentation does not distinguish among UA, NSTEMI, and STEMI. The ECG differentiates between NSTEMI and STEMI. Unstable angina/non-ST-segment elevation MI (NSTEMI) is defined by ST-segment depression or prominent T-wave inversion and/or positive biomarkers of necrosis (e.g., troponin) in the absence of ST-segment elevation and in an appropriate clinical setting (chest discomfort or anginal equivalent).[1] The distinction between UA and NSTEMI is ultimately made on the basis of the absence or presence, respectively, of biochemical cardiac markers in the blood. The release of detectable quantities of biochemical markers in the peripheral circulation indicates myocardial injury and is more consistent with MI than UA. Markers are detected in the peripheral circulation within a few hours after the initial insult in NSTEMI and STEMI.

In the era of reperfusion therapy, diagnosing ACS accurately and without delay is crucial for risk stratification and appropriate, life-saving treatment implementation. This section describes the laboratory tests used in the diagnosis of ACS. Special emphasis is placed on cardiac biomarkers. Other noncardiac-specific tests are presented briefly.

Biochemical Cardiac Markers

Infarction of myocardial cells disrupts membrane integrity, leaking intracellular macromolecules into the peripheral circulation where they are detected. The criteria of an ideal biochemical marker for the diagnosis of ACS include the following[5]:

1. *High specificity:* present in high concentrations in the myocardial tissues and absent from nonmyocardial tissue
2. *High sensitivity:* detects minor injury to the myocardium
3. *Release and clearance kinetics provide expedient and practical diagnosis:*
   a. Rapidly released into the blood after injury to facilitate early diagnosis
   b. Persists for sufficient time to provide convenient diagnostic time window
4. Measured level of the marker is in direct proportional relationship to the extent of myocardial injury.

5. Assay technique is commercially available and is easy to perform, inexpensive, and rapid.

Several biochemical cardiac markers are used in the diagnosis and evaluation of ACS. The cardiac-specific troponins have a number of attractive features and have gained acceptance as the biochemical markers of choice in the evaluation of patients with ACS.[1,4,6,7]

Cardiac-Specific Troponin I
Diagnostic level: ≥0.30 ng/mL (assay dependent)

Cardiac-Specific Troponin T
Diagnostic level: ≥0.1 ng/mL (assay dependent)

Troponin is a protein complex consisting of three subunits: troponin C (TnC), troponin I (TnI), and troponin T (TnT). The three subunits are located along thin filaments of myofibrils, and they regulate Ca^{+2}-mediated interaction of actin and myosin necessary for the contraction of cardiac muscles. Troponin C binds Ca^{+2}, TnI inhibits actomyosin ATPase, and TnT attaches to tropomyosin on the thin filaments. The TnC expressed by myocardial cells in cardiac and skeletal muscle is identical. On the contrary, TnI and TnT expressed by cardiac cells are encoded by distinct genes different from those in skeletal muscle cells. Distinct amino acid sequences between the two isoforms allow for specific antibody development without cross-reactivity. Monoclonal antibody-based immunoassays have been developed to detect cardiac-specific TnI (cTnI) and cardiac-specific TnT (cTnT). Quantitative and qualitative assays are commercially available.

Cardiac-specific TnI and cTnT are highly specific and sensitive for MI.[8-10] Following myocardial injury, serum cTnI and cTnT begin to rise above the upper reference limit within 3–12 hours, peak in 24 hours (cTnI) or 12 hours to 2 days (cTnT), and return to normal in 5–10 days (cTnI) or 5–14 days (cTnT) (Table 11-2). The initial rise of troponin is due to the release of cytoplasmic troponin whereas the later sustained rise is due to the release of complexed troponin from disintegrating myofilaments (Figure 11-5).[11] Troponins are most beneficial in identifying AMI 6 hours or more after symptom onset. Patients with normal serum levels at presentation should be reassessed between 6–12 hours after onset of symptoms if the clinical index of suspicion is high.[7] Levels typically increase more than 20 times above the reference limit. The prolonged time course of elevation of cTnI and cTnT is useful for the late diagnosis of AMI.

TABLE 11-2. Biochemical Markers Used in the Diagnosis of ACS

MARKER	MOLECULAR WEIGHT (daltons)	RANGE OF TIME TO INITIAL ELEVATIONS (hr)	MEAN TIME TO PEAK ELEVATIONS (nonthrombolysis)	TIME TO RETURN TO NORMAL RANGE
cTnI	23,500	3–12	24 hr	5–10 days
cTnT	33,000	3–12	12 hr–2 days	5–14 days
CK-MB	86,000	3–12	24 hr	2–3 days
Myoglobin	17,800	1–4	6–7 hr	24 hr

CK-MB = creatinine kinase isoenzyme MB; cTnI = cardiac-specific troponin I; cTnT = cardiac-specific troponin T.

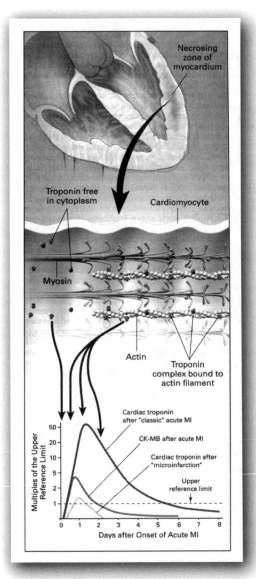

FIGURE 11-5. Release of cardiac troponins in AMI. The zone of necrosing myocardium is shown at the top of the figure, followed in the middle portion of the figure by a diagram of a cardiomyocyte that is in the process of releasing biomarkers. Most troponin exists as a tripartite complex of C, I, and T components that are bound to actin filaments, although a small amount of troponin is free in the cytoplasm. After disruption of the sarcolemmal membrane of the cardiomyocyte, the cytoplasmic pool of troponin is released first (left-most arrow in bottom portion of figure), followed by a more protracted release from the disintegrating myofilaments that may continue for several days (three-headed arrow). Cardiac troponin levels rise to about 20–50 times the upper reference limit (the 99th percentile of values in a reference control group) in patients who have a classic AMI and sustain sufficient myocardial necrosis to result in abnormally elevated levels of the MB fraction of creatine kinase (CK-MB). Clinicians can now diagnose episodes of microinfarction by sensitive assays that detect cardiac troponin elevations above the upper reference limit, even though CK-MB levels may be still in the normal reference range. (Reproduced with permission from reference 11.)

Two cutoff limits for interpreting levels of troponin have been identified: (1) upper reference limit defined as the 97.5th percentile of the values measured in normal controls without myocardial necrosis, and (2) AMI decision limit defined as a level of troponin measurement consistent with AMI, as defined by the World Health Organization and on the basis of the creatine kinase isoenzyme MB (CK-MB). Later, a standardized upper reference limit was defined as an abnormally increased level of cTnI and cTnT exceeding that of 99% of a reference control group.[12]

Several analytical factors should be considered with troponin assays. The first-generation troponin assay T ELISA was limited by lack of specificity to cardiac troponin and long turnaround time (90 minutes at 20°C and 45 minutes at 37°C). Second-generation troponin assay T ELISA was improved by changing the antibody detected to the cardiac-specific antibody M11.7, resulting in enhanced specificity.[13] The currently available third-generation assay (Elecsys, Roche Diagnostics) uses recombinant human cardiac troponin T as standard material enabling reproducibility and standardization of cTnT assays with a normal cutoff concentration of 0.1 mcg/L and a turnaround time of 9–12 minutes.[14]

In contrast to cTnT, cTnI assays lack the standardization between multiple commercially available assays developed by different manufacturers. A number of factors complicate the standardization of the assays including (1) cTnI released from disintegrating myocytes may be free cTnI, complexed with cTnC, or a combination of the two forms as well as free-cTnI degradation products; (2) the different forms undergo oxidation, phosphorylation, and proteolysis after release from cells; and (3) the differences in the matrices used and the commutability from an artificial matrix to a physiologic one.[15] Despite these differences, most commercial immunoassays measure cTnI. Contemporary cTnI assays have an analytical sensitivity almost 100-fold higher than that of the first available commercial assays. Different specificities of the antibodies used for detecting free and complexed cTnI may lead to variations in the cutoff concentration or abnormal levels of cTnI in the available immunoassays. Considerable variation (up to 20-fold) in cTnI levels may be observed when measured by different methods causing ambiguity in clinical interpretation.[16–19]

Commercially available troponin assays vary widely in lower detection limits, upper reference limits, diagnostic cut points, and assay imprecision (coefficient of variation). The upper reference limit is established by each laboratory and is set at the 99th percentile of normal population. An increased value for cardiac troponin is defined as a measurement exceeding the 99th percentile of a reference control group. Acceptable imprecision at the 99th percentile for each assay is defined as less than or equal to 10.[12] However, not all commercially available assays can achieve this precision level. Thus, when interpreting results, clinicians should employ the upper reference limit and AMI diagnostic cutoff values for the particular assay used in each institution's laboratory. Table 11-3 provides an example of one institution's interpretive data for cTnI.

TABLE 11-3. An Example of Interpretive Data for Troponin I

Reference range: 0.00–0.02 ng/mL

Comments
The 99th percentile for healthy adults is ≥0.02 ng/mL.
Probable MI is indicated at ≥0.30 ng/mL.

Hours postadmit	0–6	6–12	12–24
% sensitivity	60	79	92
% specificity	95	95	95

MI = myocardial infarction.

Cardiac troponins have been endorsed internationally as the standard biomarkers for the detection of myocardial injury, diagnosis of MI, and risk stratification in patients with suspected ACS.[4,20] Significant prognostic information may be inferred from troponin levels. In a study of patients presenting to the emergency department with chest pain, negative qualitative bedside testing of cTnI and cTnT was associated with low risk for death or MI within 30 days (event rates of 0.3 and 1.1, respectively).[21] Other large, clinical trials have documented that elevated troponin levels are strong, independent predictors of mortality and serious adverse outcome 30–42 days after ACS.[22-26] Troponin levels should always be used in conjunction with other clinical findings. In one study, in-hospital mortality was as high as 12.7% in a troponin-negative subgroup of patients with ACS.[27]

High-sensitivity troponin I (hsTnI) and troponin T (hsTnT) assays have been developed to increase the clinical sensitivity for detection of myocardial injury. However, no consensus exists on how to define a "high-sensitivity assay," in analytical or clinical terms.[28,29] Studies suggest that high-sensitivity troponins may enhance early diagnosis of AMI. In one study, hsTnT was superior to TnT but equivalent to third-generation TnI for the diagnosis of AMI. High-sensitivity TnT was the most likely assay to be elevated at baseline. The study also showed that changes in troponin levels (delta troponin) increases specificity but reduces sensitivity.[30] Another study comparing hsTnI (Architect STAT hsTnI assay, Abbott Diagnostics) and cTnI (Architect STAT cTnI assay, Abbott Diagnostics) revealed that measurement at three hours after admission may help rule out AMI. Troponin measured using either assay was superior to other biomarkers (including CK and CK-MB) in ruling in or ruling out AMI. The sensitivity and negative predictive value of the hsTnI assay were higher than the cTnI assay at admission (82.3% and 94.7% versus 79.4% and 94.0%, respectively); however, the negative predictive value of both assays was 99.4% at 3 hours. For patients with detectable troponin on admission (using the 99th percentile diagnostic cutoff value) and a 250% increase in troponin at 3 hours, the probability of AMI was 95.8%.[31] The use of hsTnI assay in early diagnosis of AMI in patients presenting soon after symptom onset is currently in clinical use in Europe.[20] The clinical use of delta troponin in addition to troponin levels may further enhance diagnostic accuracy. Studies have evaluated delta troponin using high-sensitivity troponin assays in patients presenting with AMI, with promising findings.[30,32,33] High-sensitivity troponin assays

TABLE 11-4. Causes of Detectable Serum Levels of Troponins in the Absence of Acute Coronary Syndrome

Aortic dissection

Bradycardia or tachycardia

Burns affecting >30% of body surface area

Cardiac contusion or trauma (cardiac surgery, ablation, pacing, implantable cardioverter-defibrillator shocks, cardioversion, endomyocardial biopsy)

Cardiomyopathy

Cardiotoxicity (doxorubicin, fluorouracil, trastuzumab)

Cardiopulmonary resuscitation

Coronary angioplasty or vasospasm

Critical illness (respiratory failure, sepsis)

Heart failure (chronic and acute decompensation)

Heart transplant rejection

Infiltrative disorders with cardiac involvement (amyloidosis, sarcoidosis)

Left ventricular hypertrophy

Myocarditis or pericarditis

Neurological diseases, acute (cerebrovascular accident, subarachnoid hemorrhage)

Pulmonary embolism or severe pulmonary hypertension

Rhabdomyolysis with cardiac injury

Renal failure and hemodialysis

Source: Adapted from references 34–36.

are not commercially available in the United States, and their role over contemporary assays is being debated. Further investigation is needed before they are incorporated into clinical practice.

A number of cardiac and noncardiac conditions have been reported to cause detectable serum levels of troponins in the absence of ACS (Table 11-4).[34-36] The use of cardiac troponin levels in patients with renal dysfunction has been controversial.[37-40] Most data indicate that cTnI is highly specific, but it should be considered as a useful but an imperfect marker in patients with renal insufficiency and end-stage renal disease.[37] In patients with end-stage renal disease and no evidence of acute myocardial necrosis, less than 10% will have elevated cTnI and a significantly higher number will have elevated cTnT. This is thought to be due to silent subendocardial ischemia, decreased clearance, or other metabolic abnormalities. Regardless of cause, it is well-established that these patients with elevated cardiac troponin levels have a higher risk of mortality even in the absence of symptoms.[39]

In high-risk patients with UA/NSTEMI undergoing PCI, cTnI re-elevation, defined as a postprocedural elevation >1 times admission levels, was associated with a significant increase in in-hospital and 6-month mortality.[41] Another study showed elevated cTnI after successful PCI to be an independent predictor of mortality at 12 months in patients with chronic renal insufficiency (as defined by a serum creatinine of at least 1.8 mg/dL but not on dialysis). Patients with cTnI >3 times normal values were particularly at higher risk.[42] A recent meta-analysis showed that troponin elevation after

TABLE 11-5. Causes of Elevated CK Levels

SKELETAL MUSCLE CAUSES	CARDIAC CAUSES
Dermatomyositis	Myocarditis
Polymyositis	Pericarditis
Muscular dystrophy	AMI
Myxedema	
Malignant hyperpyrexia	
Vigorous exercise	
Malignant hyperthermia syndrome	
Rhabdomyolysis	
Delirium tremens	
Seizures	
Trauma	

MEDICATIONS	OTHER CAUSES
HMG-CoA reductase inhibitors	Hypothyroidism
Amphotericin B	Renal failure
Clofibrate	Cerebrovascular accident
Ethanol (binge drinking)	Pulmonary embolism
Lithium	Severe hypokalemia
Halothane	
Succinylcholine	
Barbiturate poisoning	
Large doses of aminocaproic acid	
IM injections	

AMI = acute myocardial infarction; CK = creatine kinase; HMG-CoA = 3-hydroxy-3-methylglutaryl-coenzyme A; IM = intramuscular.

PCI was associated with increased mortality and that mortality or nonfatal MI was more likely to occur in patients with post-PCI troponin elevation.[43]

Creatine Kinase

Normal range: males, 55–170 International Units/L or 919–2839 nmol sec/L; females, 30–135 International Units/L or 501–2254 nmol sec/L

Creatine kinase (CK) is an enzyme that stimulates the transfer of high-energy phosphate groups, and it is found in skeletal muscle, myocardium, and the brain. Circulating serum CK is directly related to the individual's muscle mass.

Serum CK concentrations rise sharply 4–8 hours after the onset of chest pain associated with AMI, peak in 24 hours, and return to normal in 3–4 days. Maximum concentrations of CK may reach 5–7 times the normal values. Serial CK measurements following AMI provide excellent sensitivity (98%) but poor specificity (67%). Other causes for increased serum CK concentrations include any musculoskeletal injury or diseases, intramuscular (IM) injections, and a number of medications (Table 11-5).

Creatine Kinase Isoenzymes

Normal range: CK-MB ≤6.0 ng/mL

The enzyme CK is a dimer of two B monomers (CK-BB), two M monomers (CK-MM), or a hybrid of the two (CK-MB). The three isoenzymes are found in different sources: CK-BB, found in the brain, lungs, and intestinal tract; CK-MM, found primarily in skeletal and cardiac muscle; and CK-MB, found predominantly in the myocardium but also in skeletal muscle. Fractionation of total CK into three isoenzymes increases the diagnostic specificity of the test for AMI.

The CK-MB isoenzyme is most specific for myocardial tissue and has been used for the diagnosis of AMI. Serum CK-MB concentrations begin to rise 3–12 hours after the onset of symptoms, peak in 24 hours, and return to baseline in 2–3 days. Other causes for elevated CK-MB levels include trauma, skeletal muscle injury, or surgical procedures involving the small intestine, tongue, diaphragm, uterus, or prostate.[44]

Electrophoretic separation followed by fluorometric analysis of isoenzyme bands is used to determine the actual CK-MB concentration in International Units per liter (International Units/L). The cutoff for the upper limit of normal when the actual CK-MB concentration is determined ranges between is 5–25 International Units/L. Alternatively, CK-MB as a percentage of the total CK concentration is determined by dividing the CK-MB concentration by the total CK concentration. The cutoff for the upper limit of normal for this value is usually 3% to 6%. The diagnosis of AMI is strongly suggested when CK-MB as a percentage of total CK is greater than 5% or when the actual CK-MB concentration is greater than 10 International Units/L.

Laboratory artifacts may cause false-positive elevations of CK-MB. When using column chromatography assays, false-positive results may be caused by carryover of elevated CK-MM isoenzyme into fractions that normally contain CK-MB. In addition, variant isoenzymes that migrate as a band between CK-MM and CK-MB on electrophoresis may be interpreted as CK-MB on quantitative assays. These variants are usually due to immunoglobulin G complexed to CK-BB or to a mitochondrial source of CK, which differs slightly from cytoplasmic CK. An uncommon problem of qualitative electrophoretic assays is nonspecific fluorescence from other proteins (especially albumin), which may exhibit migration similar to that of other fractions.

Most laboratories currently use the newer CK-MB immunoassay using direct chemiluminometric technology. The assay measures the immunological activity of CK-MB using two monoclonal antibodies and reports the concentration in mass units (ng/mL) or SI units (nmol/L). The conversion formula is 1.0 ng/mL = 0.0125 nmol/L. These new monoclonal antibody immunoassay methodologies are highly sensitive and specific. Furthermore, they do not show the interferences common to earlier immunoassay or traditional electrophoretic and chromatographic methods.

When interpreting serum CK-MB levels, the timing of blood specimen collections in relation to the onset of symptoms must be assessed. Lack of absolute cardiac specificity (skeletal muscle, healthy persons) limits CK-MB interpretation. Other causes for elevated CK-MB levels are listed in Table 11-6 and are usually not associated with the typical rise and fall in serum levels as seen in AMI.[45,46] To differentiate between cardiac and noncardiac sources of CK-MB elevation, the relative index (RI),

TABLE 11-6. Causes of Elevated CK-MB Levels in the Absence of Acute Coronary Syndrome

Athletic activity (e.g., marathons)
Cardiac surgery
Hyperthermia/Hypothermia with cardiac involvement
Hypothyroidism
Malignancy
Muscular dystrophy
Myocardial puncture/trauma
Myocarditis
Myositis
Pericarditis
Pulmonary embolism
Renal failure
Rhabdomyolysis
Storke and subarachnoid hemorrhage
Surgery (gastrointestinal, prostate)

or the ratio of CK-MB to total CK concentrations, can be used and is calculated using the following equation:

$$RI = \frac{CK\text{-}MB}{Total\ CK} \times 100$$

This index is usually calculated only when both total CK and CK-MB are elevated above the normal value. It is useful in differentiating MB released from cardiac versus skeletal muscle. An index greater than 5 indicates significant myocardial injury.

CK-MB Isoforms

Once *CK-MB*, also known as the *CK-MB$_2$* isoform while in the myocardial tissue, is released into the circulation following an AMI, it undergoes metabolism by lysine carboxypeptidase producing the more negatively charged isoform CK-MB$_1$. In healthy individuals, the two isoforms are in equilibrium and the normal levels are 0.5–1 International Units/L for each isoform. One study showed that elevated CK-MB$_2$ levels of >1.0 International Units/L and an increased ratio of CK-MB$_2$ to CK-MB$_1$ of 1.5 has a sensitivity of AMI diagnosis in the emergency department of 59% when measured at 2–4 hours and 92% at 4–6 hours post-onset of symptoms.[47] Another study showed that CK-MB isoforms were most sensitive and specific (91% and 89%) when measured 6 hours after onset of chest pain in patients with MI presenting to the emergency department.[48] Similar to CK-MB, the isoforms lack absolute cardiac specificity. In addition, assays are not widely available for clinical use. The role of CK-MB isoforms among other biochemical markers remains to be defined.[49]

Myoglobin

Myoglobin is a low-molecular-weight heme protein found in cardiac and skeletal muscle. This protein is one of two preferred markers for the early detection of AMI, and automated immunoassays are commercially available. Serum levels are detected within 1–4 hours and peak 6–7 hours after the onset of symptoms. The early rise of myoglobin levels after onset of symptoms makes it most appropriate and convenient test for early detection of AMI. Myoglobin is cleared rapidly by renal glomerular filtration, and levels return to the reference value 24

MINICASE 1

Acute Coronary Syndrome

JOHN S., A 68-YEAR-OLD MAN, presented to the emergency department complaining of chest pain that started 3 hours ago. The pain is characterized as substernal pressure across his chest with radiation to his left arm and jaw. The pain was associated with slight shortness of breath. His past medical history includes hypertensive heart disease and dyslipidemia.

On physical examination, John S. had a blood pressure of 148/90 mm Hg and a pulse of 98 bpm. Heart and lung examinations were normal. Initial 12-lead ECG revealed sinus rhythm at 92 bpm and a 1-mm ST-segment depression in leads II, III, and aVF. Biochemical markers tested are as follows:

	TROPONIN I (0.00–0.02 ng/mL)
At presentation	0.01
6 hr later	1.4

Question: What is the most likely assessment of John S.'s presentation?

Discussion: On presentation, the ECG findings are consistent with ST-segment depression representing ischemia in the inferior leads. Cardiac troponin level, however, is within the reference range, using the 99th percentile of normal controls. According to the ECG findings and baseline troponin level, John S. may be diagnosed as having UA.

However, the assumption that John S. has UA based on normal markers may be erroneous since his symptoms started 3 hours prior to presentation and the release kinetics of troponin I are such that the levels begin to rise between 3–12 hours after onset of AMI. Because the clinical presentation is highly suspicious, a second level should be drawn between 6–12 hours later. The second troponin level was positive for myocardial infarct (MI diagnostic cutoff at ≥0.30 ng/mL). Thus, the clinical picture is consistent with a non-ST-segment elevation myocardial infarction (NSTEMI) rather than UA.

hours following AMI. The fast rise and fall of myoglobin levels make it an appropriate marker to detect a reinfarction if occurring 24 hours after the initial insult. In addition, in patients presenting with AMI receiving thrombolytic therapy, elevated baseline or 12–hour myoglobin levels predict 30-day mortality and may be useful in triaging patients following reperfusion.[50,51]

Because of its release kinetics and high sensitivity to myocardial ischemia, myoglobin used to be most useful in ruling out AMI. However, lack of specificity to cardiac muscle limits the interpretation of myoglobin levels. Several conditions lead to false-positive results including skeletal muscle injury of any cause, trauma, and renal failure. In addition, studies using myoglobin used the WHO definition of Acute MI. New guidelines put forth by ACC and ESC recommend troponin as the standard biomarker for AMI because of its substantially higher sensitivity and specificity rendering myoglobin measurement essentially obsolete in current era.[4,20]

Lactate Dehydrogenase

Normal range: 100–190 International Units/L or
1667–3167 nmol sec/L

Lactate dehydrogenase (LDH) is an enzyme that catalyzes the reversible formation of lactate from pyruvate. Following AMI, serum LDH rises in 24–48 hours, peaks at 2–3 days, and returns to normal in 8–14 days after the onset of chest pain. The major limitation to LDH is the lack of specificity as it is found in numerous organs and tissues including the heart, liver, lungs, kidneys, skeletal muscle, red blood cells, and lymphocytes. Electrophoretic fractionation of LDH to its five major isoenzymes (LDH_1–LDH_5) better distinguishes the site of origin, but these tests are not specific for AMI. The heart contains mainly LDH_1 and to a lesser extent LDH_2. In the past, elevation of LDH_1 or a ratio of LDH_1:LDH_2 greater than one was used in the differential diagnosis of AMI. Since the development of more cardiac-specific markers, LDH and LDH isoenzymes are no longer recommended for the evaluation of the patient with ACS.[7]

Aspartate Aminotransferase

Normal range: 8–33 International Units/L or
134–551 nmol sec/L

Aspartate aminotransferase (AST) is an enzyme involved in amino acid synthesis. It is widely distributed in the liver, heart, skeletal muscle, red blood cells, kidneys, and pancreas. Serum levels of AST rise within 12 hours of AMI, peak in 24–48 hours, and return to baseline in 3–4 days. Poor specificity of AST for myocardial cell damage led to its replacement by more cardiac-specific markers.

Recommendations for Measurement of Biochemical Markers

Given the release and clearance kinetics of the different biochemical markers, the time of the patient's presentation in relation to the onset of AMI should always be considered when interpreting laboratory results. Until recently, early-rising biochemical markers (myoglobin or CK-MB isoforms) were considered most appropriate for patients presenting within 6 hours of onset of symptoms whereas troponins were considered most appropriate for patients presenting 6 hours or later after AMI. A combination of an early marker with troponins was acceptable practice and was adopted by most laboratories.[7] The advent of contemporary and high-sensitivity troponin assays have rendered myoglobulin and CK-MB measurements unnecessary. Currently, cTnI and cTnT have emerged as the preferred cardiac biochemical markers for the evaluation of patients with ACS.[4,7,20] In settings where cardiac troponin assays are not available, CK-MB is the preferred alternative biomarker.

Cardiac troponins should be measured at presentation. Patients with normal serum levels at presentation should be reassessed after 6–12 hours or 6–9 hours.[20] High-sensitivity troponins have been suggested to enhance early diagnostic performance in patients with suspected ACS. The European Society of Cardiology has recommended a protocol using high-sensitivity troponins, measured at presentation and then 3 hours afterward. Baseline troponin levels greater than the upper limit of normal using the 99th percentile of healthy controls, as well as the relevant change in troponin level at 3 hours from baseline, are used for detecting early AMI. The relevant change in levels is assay dependent and is greatly debated.[20] High-sensitivity troponin assays are not available in the United States.

Other Biochemical Markers

Two other biochemical markers have been shown useful in patients with ACS: B-type natriuretic peptide (BNP) and c-reactive protein (CRP).

B-type natriuretic peptide is a neurohormone released by ventricular myocardium in response to volume overload. Its primary utilization is for the evaluation of patients with heart failure. However, it has been shown to be a strong predictor of short- and long-term mortality in patients with ACS. A detailed discussion of BNP is presented later in the chapter.

C-reactive protein is a nonspecific acute-phase reactant that is released in the presence of inflammatory processes caused be various etiologies (e.g., infections, malignancy, trauma, rheumatoid arthritis, and other inflammatory processes). It is synthesized in the liver and is normally present in trace amounts in the peripheral circulation. In the presence of inflammation, CRP production is stimulated by systemic cytokines. Since inflammation plays a role in the pathophysiologic processes leading to atherosclerosis and plaque rupture, serum and plasma levels of CRP are elevated in patients with CAD and ACS. In fact, several studies have reported CRP to be a strong predictor of mortality in patients presenting with ACS.[52-56] In addition, the risk of recurrent MI and death in patients with ACS receiving aggressive statin therapy were decreased significantly more in patients with low CRP levels than those with higher CRP levels regardless of the low-density lipoprotein cholesterol level.[57]

Several CRP qualitative and quantitative assays are commercially available. The diagnostic level cutoff is assay dependent. CRP assays lack the sensitivity necessary to measure low levels of the protein that might be found in healthy individuals for prognostic purposes; they are intended for use in the acute setting for the evaluation of the presence of infection, tissue injury, and inflammatory disorders. In addition, as a nonspecific marker of inflammation, the test is used to indicate the presence of inflammation, but it is not useful in the delineation among the many causes of inflammation. Measuring CRP for the diagnosis of CAD or ACS or cardiovascular risk stratification is not recommended for routine use in clinical practice.

High-sensitivity C-reactive protein (hsCRP) is a more sensitive CRP test with an ability to detect low levels (0.2–0.4 mg/L) with sufficient precision needed for accurate atherosclerotic cardiovascular risk assessment in otherwise healthy individuals. High-sensitivity C-reactive protein levels have been shown to be a strong independent predictor of cardiovascular and peripheral vascular disease risk and of recurrent cardiac events in patients with history of CAD or ACS. In patients presenting with ACS, a cutoff level of 10 mg/L or greater has been identified as a marker of high risk for death and MI, a cutoff level between 3 mg/L and 10 mg/L has been identified as intermediate risk, and a cutoff level of less than 3 mg/L has been identified as low risk.[58] In patients with stable CAD, a cutoff level of greater than 1 mg/L has been identified as a strong predictor of adverse cardiovascular events regardless of baseline characteristics and treatments.[59] The evaluation of hsCRP should be performed in conjunction with the standard cholesterol evaluation for cardiovascular disease risk stratification. The average of two measurements of hsCRP performed 2 weeks apart should be used. Patients with active infections or systemic inflammatory processes have increased hsCRP levels. To enhance the accuracy of cardiovascular risk assessment in these patients, hsCRP measurement should be postponed until the acute phase of the active infection or systemic inflammatory process has subsided and the patients are metabolically stable.[60]

The role of CRP in hypertension has also been investigated, and it has been suggested to upregulate angiotensin type 1 receptors in vascular smooth muscle.[61] Elevated levels of hsCRP have been shown to be a useful marker of arterial stiffness in hypertensive patients.[62] Moreover, treatment with valsartan, an angiotensin receptor blocker has been shown to reduce hsCRP levels.[63] Further evaluation of the clinical benefit of routine CRP use in the evaluation and management of hypertensive patients is needed.

In 2005, the Food and Drug Administration (FDA) delineated another type of designation to a high-sensitivity CRP assay, the cardiac CRP (cCRP).[64] The guidance provided manufacturers with recommendations for development of CRP assays, specifically that cCRP is exclusively indicated for the assessment and stratification of individuals at risk for cardiovascular disease, whereas hsCRP is indicated for the evaluation of other conditions thought to be associated with inflammation, in otherwise healthy individuals. In essence, the FDA defines cCRP as "high-sensitivity CRP with evidence of efficacy for identification and assessment/stratification of individuals at risk for future cardiovascular disease." The diagnostic cutoff for cCRP is the same as that of hsCRP. The need to differentiate between the two types of CRP assays has been debated.[65-66] Even though it has no role in the diagnosis of ACS, when used in conjunction with standard clinical laboratory evaluation of ACS, cCRP may be useful as an independent marker of prognosis for recurrent events, in patients with stable coronary disease, or ACS.[67-70]

Other biochemical markers include serum amyloid A and interleukin-6, which are acute phase inflammation markers and have been shown to predict an increased risk of adverse outcomes of ACS patients.[72,72] Fibrinopeptide and fibrinogen, two markers of coagulation cascade activity, also appear to be associated with an increased risk and a poor clinical outcome in patients with UA.[73,74] Myeloperoxidase, a hemoprotein with microbicidal activity has been shown to have pro-atherogenic properties, leading to CAD and ACS. Several studies have revealed that elevated serum and plasma levels of myeloperoxidase are independent predictors of outcomes in patients presenting with ACS.[75-77] In addition, microalbuminuria has been shown in a limited number of studies to be an independent predictor of CAD and a strong prognostic marker in patients with AMI.[78-81]

Miscellaneous Laboratory Tests

A number of noncardiac specific laboratory abnormalities may be manifested in patients with AMI. These include nonspecific elevation of serum glucose, white blood cells, and erythrocyte sedimentation rate (ESR), and alterations in lipid profile findings. Recognition of these abnormalities as secondary to AMI precludes misinterpretation or misdiagnosis of other disorders.

Serum Glucose
Normal range: 70–110 mg/dL or 3.9–6.1 mmol/L, preprandial
Following AMI, patients may present with elevations of serum glucose, apparently related to stress, and may persist for several weeks. Hyperglycemia may be found in diabetic as well as nondiabetic patients. Measurement of glycosylated hemoglobin may help to differentiate hyperglycemia associated with AMI versus uncontrolled diabetes mellitus.[82,83] Hyperglycemia on admission and fasting glycemia during early hospitalization in patients with AMI has been shown to be a strong predictor of mortality even in nondiabetic patients.[84,85]

White Blood Cells
Normal range: $4.4–11.0 × 10^3$ cells/mm^3 or
$4.4–11.0 × 10^9$ cells/L for adults
White blood cell count may be increased in patients presenting with AMI in response to myocardial tissue necrosis or secondary to increased adrenal glucocorticoid secretion due to stress. Polymorphonuclear leukocytosis of 10,000–20,000 cells/mm^3 ($10–20 × 10^9$ cells/L) may be seen 12–24 hours after onset of symptoms and may last for 1–2 weeks depending on extent of tissue necrosis. Fever may accompany leukocytosis.

Erythrocyte Sedimentation Rate
Normal range: males, 1–15 mm/hr females; 1–20 mm/hr
The *erythrocyte sedimentation rate (ESR)* is related to levels of acute phase reactants that increase in patients with AMI. The ESR usually peaks on day 4 or 5 and may remain elevated for 3–4 weeks post-AMI.

Lipid Panel
Total cholesterol and low-density lipoprotein may be decreased when measured 48–72 hours post-MI and may persist for 6–8 weeks afterward.

LABORATORY TESTS USED IN THE EVALUATION OF HEART FAILURE

Natriuretic Peptides

Natriuretic peptides are naturally-secreted hormones that are released by various cells in response to increased volume or pressure. A number of natriuretic peptides have been identified, including atrial natriuretic peptide (ANP), BNP, C-type natriuretic peptide (CNP), Dendroaspis natriuretic peptide (DNP), and urodilatin. The latter were recently isolated from the venom of Dendroaspis angusticeps (green mamba snake) and human urine, respectively. However, their clinical utilization in patients with cardiovascular diseases is not well-defined as of this writing. A structurally related peptide to ANP and BNP, CNP is secreted by the heart and vascular endothelium and exerts vasodilating effects.[86] Limited evidence suggests that plasma CNP levels are increased in patients with heart failure, but further investigation of the clinical utilization of CNP levels and their interpretation in the diagnosis and assessment of heart failure is warranted.[87]

Atrial natriuretic peptide and BNP are known cardiac-specific peptides. The two are structurally similar and exert potent diuretic, natriuretic, and vascular smooth muscle-relaxing effects. A 28-amino acid (aa) peptide, ANP is primarily secreted by the atrial myocytes in response to increased atrial wall tension. A 32-aa peptide, BNP was first identified in porcine brain extracts (hence the name brain natriuretic peptide).[88] Subsequently, it was found in much higher concentrations in cardiac ventricles and is primarily secreted by the left ventricular myocytes in response to volume overload and increased ventricular wall tension.

The precursor for BNP is PreproBNP, a 134-aa peptide that is enzymatically cleaved into proBNP, a 108-aa peptide. The latter is then further cleaved into the biologically active C-terminal 32-aa BNP and the biologically inactive amino-terminal portion of the prohormone, N-terminal-proBNP (NT-proBNP). Plasma levels of both BNP and NT-proBNP are elevated in response to increased volume and ventricular myocyte stretch in patients with heart failure. Once released into the peripheral circulation, BNP is cleared by enzymatic degradation via endopeptidase and natriuretic peptide receptor-mediated endocytosis, whereas NT-proBNP is cleared renally. The elimination half-life of BNP is significantly shorter than that of NT-proBNP (20 minutes versus 120 minutes, respectively).

The quantitative measurements of BNP and NT-proBNP levels are indicated for the evaluation of patients suspected of having heart failure, assessment of the severity of heart failure, and risk stratification of patients with heart failure and ACS.[89] In conjunction with standard clinical assessment, BNP and NT-proBNP levels at the approved cutoff points are highly sensitive and specific for the diagnosis of acute heart failure and correlate well with the severity of heart failure symptoms as evaluated by the New York Heart Association (NYHA) Classification.[90,91] In addition, BNP and NT-proBNP are strong independent markers of clinical outcomes in patients with heart failure, IHD, and ACS even in the absence of previous history of CHF or objective evidence of left ventricular dysfunction during hospitalization.[92-98]

There is growing interest in the value of serial BNP and NT-proBNP measurements to guide optimal heart failure therapy.[99] Several randomized trials of chronic heart failure patients have compared standard heart failure therapy plus BNP or NT-proBNP- guided therapy to standard heart failure treatment alone.[100-104] A meta-analysis of these trials confirmed the findings that BNP-guided heart failure therapy reduces all-cause mortality in patients with chronic heart failure, compared

with usual clinical care in patients younger than 75 years, but not in those older than 75 years of age. Mortality reduction might be attributable to the higher percentage of patients achieving target doses of angiotensin-converting enzyme inhibitors (ACE-I) and beta blockers, classes of agents shown to delay or halt progression of cardiac dysfunction and improve mortality in patients with heart failure.[105] A greater than 30% reduction in BNP levels in response to heart failure treatment indicates a good prognosis.[106] B-type natriuretic peptide levels cannot be used in the assessment of patient receiving therapy with the synthetic BNP, Natrecor® (nesiritide, Scios). Assays measuring NT-pro-BNP are not affected by the presence of synthetic BNP and thus may be used in the assessment of patients.

Several factors impact the BNP and NT-proBNP levels, including gender, age, renal function, and obesity. Plasma BNP and NT-proBNP levels in normal volunteers are higher in women and increase with age. In addition, renal insufficiency at an estimated glomerular filtration rate (GFR) below 60 mL/min may impact the interpretation of the measured natriuretic peptides. Significant correlation between NT-proBNP level, and GFRs have been shown, more so than that between BNP level and GFRs. This is because renal clearance is the primary route of elimination of NT-proBNP, and the measured levels of the biomarker are elevated in patients with mild renal insufficiency. Yet, evaluation of patients with GFRs as low as 14.8 mL/min revealed that the test continues to be valuable for the evaluation of the dyspneic patient irrespective of renal function.[107] Higher diagnostic cutoffs for different GFR ranges may be necessary for optimal interpretation in patients with renal insufficiency.

Plasma levels of BNP and NT-proBNP are reduced in obese patients, limiting the clinical interpretation of the tests in these patients. An inverse relation between the levels of these markers and body mass index (BMI) is observed.[108,109] The exact mechanism for this is not known, but a BMI-related defect in natriuretic peptide secretion has been suggested.[110] In one study, NT-proBNP levels were found to be lower in obese patients presenting with dyspnea (with or without acute heart failure), but the test seemed to retain its diagnostic and prognostic capacity across all BMI categories.[111] Similarly, in patients with advanced systolic heart failure, although BNP levels were relatively lower in overweight and obese patients, the test predicted worse symptoms, impaired hemodynamics, and higher mortality at all levels of BMI. Optimal BNP cutoff levels for prediction of death or urgent transplant in lean, overweight, and obese patients were reported to be 590 pg/mL, 471 pg/mL, and 342 pg/mL, respectively.[112] In order to increase the specificity of BNP levels for heart failure in obese and lean patients, a diagnostic cutoff level of greater than or equal to 54 pg/mL for severely obese patients and a cutoff level of greater than or equal to 170 pg/mL in lean patients have been suggested.[113]

Despite the fact that BNP and NT-proBNP have no role in the diagnosis of ACS, they are powerful prognostic markers and predictors of mortality in these patients.[20,106,114-117] The use

TABLE 11-7. Interpretation of BNP and NT-proBNP Levels in Patients with Acute Dyspnea

	HEART FAILURE UNLIKELY	GREY ZONE	HEART FAILURE LIKELY	
BNP[a]	<100 pg/mL	100–500 pg/mL	>500 pg/mL	
NT-pro-BNP[b]	<300 pg/mL		<50 yr	>450 pg/mL
			50–75 yr	>900 pg/mL
			>75 yr	>1800 pg/mL

[a]In patients with estimated glomerular filtration rate <60 mL/min/1.73 m² and body mass index <35 kg/m², different decision limits must be used.
[b]In patients with estimated glomerular filtration rate <60 mL/min/1.73 m², different decision limits must be used.
Source: Adapted from reference 106.

of BNP levels in the assessment of cardiotoxicity associated with anthracycline chemotherapy is under investigation.[118-121]

B-Type Natriuretic Peptide

Diagnostic cutoff: 100 pg/mL (or ng/L)
The clinical diagnostic cutoff level for heart failure is a B-type natriuretic peptide (BNP) level of greater than 100 pg/mL. In addition to standard clinical evaluation, a BNP level of greater than 100 pg/mL is associated with sensitivity and specificity of 90% for heart failure in a patient presenting with shortness of breath.[122] The test has a high negative predictive value in ruling out heart failure as a primary cause for the presentation. A BNP level of 100–500 pg/mL is suggestive of heart failure and a level greater than 500 pg/mL is indicative of heart failure as the likely etiology of acute dyspnea (Table 11-7).[106]

Several assays using various technologies are currently available in the United States for the quantitative measurement of BNP including the AxSYM (Abbott Laboratories), which utilizes microparticle enzyme immunoassay; the ADVIA Centaur (Bayer Diagnostics), which utilizes direct chemiluminescent sandwich immunoassay; the Triage BNP (Biosite, Inc.), which utilizes single use fluorescence immunoassay; and the Beckman Coulter (Biosite, Inc.), which utilizes two-site chemiluminescent immuno-enzymatic assay. The Biosite Triage BNP Test is a point-of-care test with a turnaround time of 15 minutes, making it readily available for use in emergency rooms and physicians' offices.

N-Terminal-ProBNP

Diagnostic cutoff: 300 pg/mL (or ng/L)
N-terminal-proBNP (NT-proBNP) is a more stable form of BNP that correlates well with BNP in patients with heart failure, and its levels are typically higher than BNP levels. In addition, NT-proBNP levels are elevated in the elderly and, accordingly, the clinical diagnostic cutoff level for heart failure is higher in older patients. An NT-proBNP level less than 300 pg/mL was optimal for ruling out acute CHF, with a negative predictive value of 99%. For cut points of greater than 450 pg/mL for patients younger than 50 years of age and greater than 900 pg/mL for patients 50 years of age or older, NT-proBNP levels were highly sensitive and specific for the diagnosis of acute heart failure (Table 11-7).[106,123]

Several NT-proBNP assays utilizing various technologies are currently available in the United States including the Elecsys (Roche Diagnostics, Inc.), which utilizes electrochemiluminescent immunoassay and the Dimension (Dade Behring), which utilizes microparticle enzyme immunoassay. In addition, a point-of-care NT-proBNP assay is commercially available.

Other Biochemical Markers

Elevated cardiac troponin levels in patients with heart failure have been shown to be related to the severity of heart failure and worse outcomes.[124-126] In patients presenting with acute decompensated heart failure, routine measurement of troponin levels is recommended.[127] In addition to baseline troponin levels, serial troponin measurements may be useful in predicting outcomes.[128] In a recent study of patients hospitalized for acute heart failure, 60% of patients had detectable cTnT levels (>0.01 ng/mL) levels and 34% had positive values (>0.03 ng/mL) at baseline. Of the patients with negative troponin at baseline, 21% had elevated cTnT levels by day 7. Positive troponin levels at baseline and conversion to detectable levels were associated were associated with poor prognosis.[129]

IMAGING STUDIES

A number of imaging modalities contribute to the diagnosis and assessment of ACS, including chest roentgenography, echocardiography, cardiac catheterization, perfusion imaging, computed tomography (CT), magnetic resonance imaging (MRI), and positron-emission tomography (PET). For patients presenting with ACS, these tests may be used when clinical presentation, biochemical markers, and ECG are nondiagnostic with high clinical suspicion.

Chest Roentgenogram

Chest radiography taken at the initial presentation of patients with ACS provides an early estimation of the size of the left heart chambers. In addition, presence and degree of pulmonary congestion indicates elevated left-ventricular end-diastolic pressure, which may result from a sizeable infarction of the left ventricle. In addition, chest radiography is a standard study in evaluating patients presenting with symptoms suggestive of heart failure. *Chest roentgenogram* findings of heart failure include cardiac enlargement, vascular redistribution, interstitial and alveolar edema, peribronchial cuffing, and pleural effusions. Cardiac enlargement on chest roentgenogram in patients with heart failure is associated with a higher morbidity rate.

Echocardiography

Echocardiography is based on sound transmitted to and through the heart. Different tissues present different acoustical impedance (resistance to transmitting sound). Transthoracic echocardiography (TTE) involves sound waves from a transducer positioned on the anterior chest directed across cardiac tissues. The sound is reflected back in different frequencies, and images of cardiac anatomy are displayed on an oscilloscope or an electronic monitor.

Two-dimensional (2D) echocardiography records multiple views providing cross-sectional images of the heart. Clinical uses include anatomic assessment of the heart and functional assessment of cardiac chambers and valves. Contrast agents may be injected for better visualization of endocardial borders. M-mode, or motion-mode, records the motion of individual structures. Doppler echocardiography uses sound or frequency ultrasound to record the velocity and direction of blood and wall motion; it is based on the principle of bouncing ultrasound waves off of a moving object (e.g., red blood cells). This method permits the assessment of valvular and wall motion abnormalities.

As a noninvasive test that measures cardiac hemodynamics and filling pressures, TTE plays an important role in assessing patients with ACS presenting with apparent large infarct and hemodynamic instability. Information provided includes wall motion abnormalities to assess the extent of the infarct or the level of function of the remaining myocardium, recognition of complications such as postinfarction ventricular septal defect, and the presence of left ventricular thrombi.[130] In addition, TTE can be combined with exercise and pharmacologic stress testing to assess stress-induced structural or functional abnormalities (e.g., wall motion abnormality associated with ischemia) in patients with IHD.

Left ventricular ejection fraction is a valuable diagnostic and prognostic index in patients with failure, and it is defined as the fraction of end-diastolic volume ejected from the left ventricle during each systolic contraction. The normal range for LVEF is 55% to 75%. Patients may have heart failure due to diastolic ventricular dysfunction with a normal LVEF. In clinical practice, TTE is currently the modality most utilized and accepted for the evaluation of systolic and diastolic cardiac function.

Newer and sophisticated techniques such as speckle tracking and strain rate are now utilized in 2D echocardiography to aid in evaluation of the dynamic nature of the myocardial function and provide more precise quantitative myocardial function assessment. Three-dimensional (3D) echocardiography provides improved accuracy over 2D echocardiography and is recommended for left ventricular function assessment (volume and ejection fraction).[131] Further investigation is needed before 3D echocardiography is recommended for routine in clinical practice.

Transesophageal echocardiography (TEE) involves mounting the transducer at the end of a flexible endoscope and passing it through the esophagus to position it closer to the heart. Transesophageal echocardiography provides higher resolution of the posterior cardiac structures making it ideal for viewing the atria, cardiac valves, and aorta. Clinical indications include detection of atrial appendage thrombi, native and prosthetic

valvular function and morphology, cardiac masses, or thoracic aortic dissection, and TEE has no role in the diagnosis or assessment of patients with ACS. Appropriateness criteria for use of TTE and TEE in the evaluation of cardiac structure and function has been published.[132]

Noninvasive Stress Testing

Exercise Stress Testing

In patients with chronic stable CAD who are capable of physical exercise, myocardial perfusion imaging is used in conjunction with exercise testing. Physical exercise is performed using a graded exercise protocol on a treadmill or upright bicycle. The most widely used protocol is the Bruce protocol. Nonimaging endpoints include reproduction of anginal symptoms, exhaustion, hypertension or 20 mm Hg decrease in systolic blood pressure, ventricular arrhythmias, or severe ST-segment depression on ECG. Exercise allows for several useful measurements including the duration of exercise, total workload, maximum HR, exercise-induced symptoms, ECG changes, and blood pressure response. Limitations include patients with orthopedic, neurological, or peripheral vascular problems. Patients receiving agents that may blunt HR response to exercise (beta blockers or nondihydropyridine calcium channel blockers) may not be able to achieve the target *heart rate* necessary for diagnostic and prognostic purposes.

Pharmacologic Stress Testing

Patients who are unable to exercise may be stressed pharmacologically using either (1) vasodilating agents such as adenosine or dipyridamole or (2) positive inotropic agents such as dobutamine. Both modalities produce a hyperemic (vasodilatory response or increased blood flow) response leading to heterogeneity of myocardial blood flow between vascular areas supplied by normal and significantly stenosed coronary arteries. Heterogeneity is visualized with radionuclide myocardial perfusion agents.

Adenosine is an endogenous vasodilator. Coronary vasodilation is mediated through the activation of A_{2a} receptors. Dipyridamole blocks the cellular reabsorption of endogenous adenosine. Vasodilation, by both adenosine and dipyridamole, increases coronary blood flow in normal arteries 3–5 times baseline with little or no increase in blood flow to stenotic arteries. Dobutamine increases myocardial oxygen demand by increasing myocardial contractility, HR, and blood pressure. Following dobutamine administration, coronary blood flow in normal arteries is increased 2–3 times baseline, which is similar to that achieved with exercise. Myocardial uptake of thallium-201, a radiopharmaceutical agent, is directly proportional to coronary blood flow (see Myocardial Perfusion Imaging). Administration of the above pharmacologic agents causes relatively less thallium-201 uptake in myocardial areas supplied by stenotic arteries. Therefore, a greater difference is seen between tissue supplied by normal arteries and tissue supplied by stenotic arteries.

Cardiac Catheterization

Cardiac catheterization involves the introduction of a catheter through the femoral or brachial artery, which is advanced to the heart chambers or great vessels guided by fluoroscopy. Measurements collected include intracardiac pressures, hemodynamic data, and blood flow in the heart chambers and coronary arteries.

Coronary Angiography

Coronary angiography, also referred to as *angiocardiography* or *coronary arteriography*, is a diagnostic test in which contrast media is injected into the coronary arteries. X-ray exposures of the coronary arteries are then examined to assess the location and severity of coronary atherosclerotic lesions. Therapeutic interventions or PCI may be performed during the catheterization including percutaneous transluminal coronary angioplasty (PTCA) and bare-metal or drug-eluting stent placement.

Left Ventriculography

Left ventriculography is the injection of contrast media into the left ventricle to assess its structure and function. The test is often performed as part of a diagnostic cardiac catheterization to evaluate ventricular wall motion and measure LVEF.

Nuclear Imaging

Nuclear imaging involves the injection of trace amounts of radioactive elements that concentrate in certain areas of the heart. A gamma camera is then rotated around the patient, and multiple planar images are taken to detect the radioactive emissions and form an image of the deployment of the tracer in the different regions of the heart. Single-photon emission CT (SPECT) is the most common imaging technique.

Nuclear imaging is used to assess blood flow through the heart and myocardial perfusion, locate and assess severity of myocardial ischemia and infarction, and evaluate myocardial metabolism.

Myocardial Perfusion Imaging

Thallium-201 (^{201}Tl) became available in 1974 and was the conventional radiopharmaceutical agent used until the early 1990s, at which time technetium-99m (^{99m}Tc)-labeled compounds such as ^{99m}Tc-sestamibi and ^{99m}Tc-tetrofosmin were introduced for visualization of myocardial perfusion. The imaging agents measure the relative distribution of myocardial blood flow between normal and stenotic coronary arteries.

^{201}Tl, a potassium analog is taken up by healthy functioning tissue in a manner similar to potassium. ^{201}Tl is taken up at reduced rates by ischemic myocardial tissue and is not distributed to or taken up by regions of MI. Imaging with ^{201}Tl for detection of infarction is accomplished with the patient at rest and is optimal within 6 hours of symptom onset. ^{201}Tl is injected intravenously and imaging is initiated 10–20 minutes after injection; imaging is repeated 2–4 hours later to determine whether redistribution occurred. The diagnosis of AMI must be inferred by a lack of regional myocardial uptake of the radiotracer. ^{201}Tl imaging for a perfusion defect has a sensitivity of about 90% if applied within the first 24 hours after symptom onset and falls sharply thereafter.

^{99m}Tc is an infarct-avid agent. It concentrates in necrotic myocardial tissue, presumably because it enters myocardial cells and selectively binds to calcium and calcium complexes. Abnormal intracellular uptake of calcium is a feature of irreversible cell death and begins as early as 12 hours after AMI and may persist for 2 weeks. ^{99m}Tc scans may be positive as early as 4 hours after the onset of AMI symptoms. The peak sensitivity for the scan is between 48–72 hours, but it generally remains positive for up to 1 week post AMI. When obtained within 24–72 hours after onset of infarction, the scan has a diagnostic sensitivity of 90% to 95% in patients with Q-wave AMI or 38% to 92% in patients with non-Q-wave AMI. ^{99m}Tc imaging has moderate specificity, with an overall range of 60% to 80%.

^{201}Tl perfusion imaging is widely utilized in patients with atypical chest pain following a nondiagnostic (symptoms or findings consistent with CAD are not evident during the test due to inability to achieve target HR or a technically-limited study) or false-positive stress test to determine if coronary artery atherosclerosis is the cause of symptoms. In addition, since redistribution is a marker of jeopardized but viable myocardial tissue, ^{201}Tl can be used to indicate the probable success of revascularization or angioplasty and for preoperative prognostic stratification of patients. Transient defects (redistribution) indicate hemodynamically significant coronary lesions with the risk of cardiac death.

Nuclear imaging in conjunction with stress testing provides further information on myocardial perfusion and function. ^{99m}Tc-sestamibi may be used in combination with ^{201}Tl to assess rest and stress myocardial perfusion sequentially in 1 day. The patient's rest study is done first with ^{201}Tl; imaging is started immediately after tracer injection and is completed within about 45 minutes. Stress testing (pharmacologically or with exercise) is begun after the rest study, and ^{99m}Tc-sestamibi is injected at peak cardiac stress.

Since ^{99m}Tc-sestamibi emits higher energy photons than ^{201}Tl, its images are not subject to cross-interference from the previously administered ^{201}Tl. Both ^{201}Tl and ^{99m}Tc-sestamibi undergo first-pass extraction from blood by myocardial cells; both provide a *stop-frame* image of regional myocardial blood flow at the time of tracer injection. ^{99m}Tc-sestamibi does not leak appreciably from myocardial cells, thus imaging may be delayed to allow blood and lung concentrations to diminish. Consequently, ^{99m}Tc-sestamibi imaging can be completed between 1–4 hours after tracer injection without significantly reducing diagnostic reliability.

The clinically most important application of myocardial perfusion imaging is detection of an AMI. Images are interpreted qualitatively and quantitatively and assessment of myocardial perfusion to the different areas is reported as normal, defect, reversible defect, fixed defect, or reverse redistribution. Myocardial perfusion imaging may also be used for the assessment of thrombolytic therapy effectiveness and early risk stratification of patients presenting with AMI or ACS who were treated conservatively at initial presentation. Electrocardiogram-gated myocardial perfusion SPECT studies enhance the interpretive confidence and accuracy and provide

MINICASE 2

Heart Failure

MARTIN G., A 64-YEAR-OLD MAN with a history of chronic obstructive pulmonary disease, presents to the emergency department with complaints of worsening shortness of breath. He reports that his symptoms have worsened over the past four weeks. He now has shortness of breath at rest and has noticed increased swelling in his feet. He is an active smoker and has consumed one pack of cigarettes per day for over 40 years.

On examination, Martin G. was unable to complete full sentences. His BP was 150/90 mm Hg and pulse was 100 bpm. His jugular venous pressure was increased at 11 cm H_2O. Lungs revealed poor air exchange with diffuse rhonchi and crackles. Lower extremities showed 2 + edema. His ECG revealed sinus tachycardia at 110 bpm. Troponin I level was less than 0.02 ng/mL and BNP level was 900 pg/mL. Chest x-ray was limited and revealed changes consistent with COPD along with mild cardiomegaly and possible mild vascular redistribution.

Question: How should Martin G.'s findings and laboratory values be interpreted?

Discussion: Given Martin G.'s history of pulmonary disease, his presentation could be easily attributed to COPD exacerbation. However, his presentation is consistent with signs and symptoms of new onset heart failure (tachycardia, elevated JVP, crackles, lower extremity edema and shortness of breath). The troponin I level is within the normal reference range and is consistent with the lack of any evidence of myocardial ischemia or infarction on ECG. His BNP level is elevated well above the diagnostic level of 100 pg/mL, and the 500 pg/mL level is indicative of heart failure. Based on the symptoms and the BNP level, Martin G.'s presentation is consistent with heart failure. An echocardiography is needed to further evaluate his LVEF and possible etiologies of heart failure.

information critical for the diagnosis, prognosis, and management decisions, including global left ventricular function and regional wall motion and thickening.

Computed Tomography

Computed tomography (CT) involves an intense, focused electron beam that is swept along target rings by electromagnets. When the electron beam strikes the target ring, a fan of x-rays is produced and moves around the patient. Computed tomography of the heart is limited by cardiac motion, which may be overcome by gating of the CT scan with a simultaneous ECG recording. Alternatively, Ultrafast CT (cine-CT) allows scanning in real time without gating. The main advantage of CT is enhanced resolution and special definition of structures.

In recent years, there has been rapid advancement in state-of-the-art, noninvasive cardiac imaging technology and increased demand for its use. Cardiac CT (CCT) is useful in the assessment of cardiac structure including cardiac masses, pericardial conditions, and evaluation of aortic (e.g., dissection or aneurysm) and pulmonary disease. It is also appropriate in the evaluation of chest pain syndrome in patients with low to intermediate pretest probability of CAD.[133]

Magnetic Resonance Imaging

Magnetic resonance imaging (MRI) is a noninvasive imaging technique capable of detailed tissue characterization and blood flow measurements. The procedure involves placing patients in a device generating a powerful magnetic field and aligning the protons of the body's hydrogen atoms relative to the magnetic field. Radio waves pulsed through the field and force the protons to shift their orientation. When the radio waves stop, the protons return to their previous orientation, releasing energy in the form of radio waves. The waves are detected by a scanner and converted into images. The images are physiologically gated to an ECG.

During the procedure, the patients are required to remain motionless. Claustrophobic patients may not be able to undergo the procedure. Sedation may be necessary. In addition, patients with metal prostheses (e.g., pacemakers and ferromagnetic intracerebral clips) should not undergo MRI.

Clinical uses of cardiac MRI (CMR) include assessment of congenital, aortic, and pericardial diseases, tumors, and intravascular thrombus. Magnetic resonance imaging has become more available, but restricted to some medical centers because of the cost, scan time, and need for specialized equipment and personnel. Current recommendations for CMR use include the evaluation of chest pain syndrome with use of vasodilator perfusion CMR or dobutamine stress function CMR in patients with intermediate pretest probability of IHD in the setting of uninterpretable ECG or an inability to exercise. Cardiac MRI is also recommended for the evaluation of suspected coronary anomalies. There is no clear acceptable use for CMR in the setting of acute chest pain.[134]

Positron Emission Tomography

Positron emission tomography (PET) is a nuclear imaging technique capable of measuring myocardial blood flow and cellular metabolism of substrates such as fatty acids, glucose, and oxygen in vivo. The technique uses the properties of short-lived, positron-emitting, isotope-labeled compounds (nitrogen-13, oxygen-15, carbon-11, or fluorine-18) coupled with mathematical models of physiological function. Its most relevant clinical use for cardiovascular evaluation is detection of ischemic, but viable (or *hibernating*), myocardium that appears irreversibly necrotic by other diagnostic tests.

Blood Pool Imaging

Blood pool scintigraphy is used to evaluate ventricular wall motion and function as well as left ventricular volume. Human serum albumin or the patient's red blood cells are tagged with Tc-99m and injected intravenously into the patient. A scintillation camera records the radioisotope as it passes through the ventricle. Imaging can be gated or linked with a simultaneous ECG recording. Multiple images are taken and are combined to produce a cine film permitting the evaluation of ventricular chamber size, wall motion, filling defects, and ventricular ejection fraction.

SUMMARY

The heart is a muscular pump that circulates blood to the lungs for oxygenation and throughout the vascular system to supply oxygen and nutrients to every cell in the body. Many diseases affect the heart's function including ACS and heart failure.

The classic laboratory workup for ACS includes the measurement of serum cTnI or cTnT, and/or CK-MB, a more specific isoenzyme of CK. Classic ECG changes such as T-wave inversion, ST-segment depression or elevation, and Q-wave appearance may also be present and are useful in evaluating patients presenting with ACS. In addition to confirming an equivocal diagnosis, imaging techniques may localize and estimate the size of MIs. After an AMI, LVEF may be determined for prognostic information. Measurement of BNP and CRP provides additional prognostic information. For the diagnosis and assessment of heart failure, BNP or NT-proBNP measurement is considered the gold standard test. Determination of LVEF is essential for differentiating systolic, preserved LVEF and diastolic heart failure and targeting therapy accordingly.

The clinician must be well-informed of the various tests used to diagnose and assess patients with CAD, ACS and its potential complications, and heart failure. Knowledge of these tests and their clinical significance greatly impacts decisions regarding implementation of appropriate management strategies and preventative measures.

Learning Points

1. **Summarize the criteria used in the assessment of patients presenting with ACS.**

   Answer: Three criteria are used to evaluate patients presenting with possible ACS. These are clinical presentation or symptoms, ECG changes, and cardiac biochemical markers such as cardiac troponins and CK-MB. The latter two are used to distinguish between a diagnosis of UA/NSTEMI and STEMI. Classic ECG changes include ST-segment elevation, consistent with STEMI, or ST-segment depression or T-wave inversion, consistent with NSTEMI. Elevated levels of plasma cardiac biomarkers are consistent with infarction and distinguish UA from NSTEMI.

2. **Discuss the release kinetics of cardiac specific troponins and recommendations for measurement of this lab test in patients presenting with chest pain.**

   Answer: cTnI and cTnT levels are detectable above the upper reference limit by 3 hours from the onset of symptoms. Mean to peak elevation levels without reperfusion therapy is 24 hours for cTnI and 12 hours to 2 days for cTnT. Due to continuous release from injured myocytes, cTnI levels may remain elevated for 7–10 days after an MI versus 10–14 days for cTnT. Levels are obtained at initial presentation of patients with chest discomfort and repeated at approximately every 6–12 hours in order to confirm the diagnosis of MI within 12 hours.

3. **Define the utility of BNP levels in the clinical assessment of patients presenting with heart failure.**

   Answer: The BNP levels are a good marker of left ventricular dysfunction and a strong marker to predict morbidity and mortality in patients with heart failure. In conjunction with the standard clinical assessment, BNP is used to establish or exclude the diagnosis of heart failure in patients presenting to emergency departments for evaluation of acute dyspnea. Serum BNP levels correlate with the clinical severity of heart failure as assessed by NYHA classification.

REFERENCES

1. Thygesen K, Alpert JS, White HD; Joint ESC/ACCF/AHA/WHF Task Force for the Redefinition of Myocardial Infarction. Universal definition of myocardial infarction. *Eur Heart J.* 2007;28:2525-2538.

2. Swedberg K, Cleland J, Dargie H, et al. Guidelines for the diagnosis and treatment of chronic heart failure: executive summary (update 2005): The Task Force for the Diagnosis and Treatment of Chronic Heart Failure of the European Society of Cardiology. *Eur Heart J.* 2005;26:1115-1140.

3. Morris F, Brady WJ. ABC of clinical electrocardiography: acute myocardial infarction-Part I. *BMJ.* 2002;324:831-834.

4. Anderson JL, Adams CD, Antman EM, et al. ACC/AHA 2007 guidelines for the management of patients with unstable angina/non–ST-elevation myocardial infarction: a report of the American College of Cardiology/American Heart Association Task Force on Practice Guidelines (Writing committee to revise the 2002 guidelines for the management of patients with unstable angina/non-ST-elevation myocardial infarction). *J Am Coll Cardiol.* 2007;50:e1-e157.

5. World Health Organization. Nomenclature and criteria for diagnosis of ischemic heart disease. Report of the Joint International Society and Federation of Cardiology/World Health Organization task force on standardization of clinical nomenclature. *Circulation.* 1979;59(3):607-609.

6. Adams JE III, Abendschein DR, Jaffe AS. Biochemical markers of myocardial injury: is MB creatine kinase the choice for the 1990s? *Circulation.* 1993;88(2):750-763.

7. Wu AH, Apple FS, Gibler WB, et al. National Academy of Clinical Biochemistry Standards of Laboratory Practice: recommendations for the use of cardiac markers in coronary artery diseases. *Clin Chem.* 1999;45:1104-1121.

8. Adams JE III, Bodor GS, Davila-Roman VG, et al. Cardiac troponin I: a marker with high specificity for cardiac injury. *Circulation.* 1993;88:101-106.

9. Apple FS. Tissue specificity of cardiac troponin I, cardiac troponin T and creatine kinase-MB. *Clin Chim Acta.* 1999;284:151-159.

10. Mair J, Morandell D, Genser N, et al. Equivalent early sensitivities of myoglobin, creatine kinase MB mass, creatine kinase isoform ratios, and cardiac troponins I and T for acute myocardial infarction. *Clin Chem.* 1995;41:1266-1272.

11. Antman EM. Decision-making with cardiac troponin tests. *N Engl J Med.* 2002;346(26):2079–2082.

12. The Joint European Society of Cardiology/American College of Cardiology Committee: myocardial infarction redefined: a consensus document of the Joint European Society of Cardiology/American College of Cardiology Committee for the redefinition of myocardial infarction. *J Am Coll Cardiol.* 2000;36(3):959-969.

13. Muller-Bardorff M, Hallermayer K, Schroder A, et al. Improved troponin T ELISA specific for cardiac troponin T isoform: assay development and analytical and clinical validation. *Clin Chem.* 1997;43(3):458-466.

14. Hallermayer K, Klenner D, Vogel R. Use of recombinant human cardiac troponin T for standardization of third generation troponin T methods. *Scand J Clin Lab Invest Suppl.* 1999;230:128-131.

15. Christenson RH, Duh SH, Apple FS, et al. Standardization of cardiac troponin I assays: round Robin of ten candidate reference materials. *Clin Chem.* 2001;47(3):431-437.

16. Wu AH, Feng YJ, Moore R, et al. American Association for Clinical Chemistry Subcommittee on cTnI Standardization. Characterization of cardiac troponin subunit release into serum after acute myocardial infarction and comparison of assays for troponin T and I. *Clin Chem.* 1998;44(6):1198-1208.

17. Apple FS, Maturen AJ, Mullins RE, et al. Multicenter clinical and analytical evaluation of the AxSYM troponin-I immunoassay to assist in the diagnosis of myocardial infarction. *Clin Chem.* 1999;45:206–212.

18. Laurino JP. Troponin I: an update on clinical utility and method standardization. *Ann Clin Lab Sci.* 2000;30(4):412-421.

19. Venge P, Lagerqvist B, Diderholm E, et al. Clinical performance of three cardiac troponin assays in patients with unstable coronary artery disease (a FRISC II substudy). *Am J Cardiol.* 2002;89(9):1035-1041.

20. Hamm CW, Bassand JP, Agewall S, et al. ESC Guidelines for the management of acute coronary syndromes in patients presenting without persistent ST-segment elevation: The Task Force for the management of acute coronary syndromes (ACS) in patients presenting without persistent ST-segment elevation of the European Society of Cardiology (ESC). *Eur Heart J.* 2011;32(23):2999-3054.

21. Hamm CW, Goldmann BU, Heeschen C, et al. Emergency room triage of patients with acute chest pain by means of rapid testing of cardiac troponin T or troponin I. *N Engl J Med.* 1997;337:1648-1653.

22. Antman EM, Tanasijevic MJ, Thompson B, et al. Cardiac-specific troponin I levels to predict the risk of mortality in patients with acute coronary syndromes. *N Engl J Med.* 1996;335:1342-1349.

23. Ohman EM, Armstrong PW, Christenson RH, et al. Cardiac troponin T levels for risk stratification in acute myocardial ischemia. GUSTO IIA Investigators. *N Engl J Med.* 1996;335:1333-1341.

24. Hamm CW, Braunwald E. A classification of unstable angina revisited. *Circulation.* 2000;102:118-122.

25. Kontos MC, de Lemos JA, Ou FS, et al. Troponin-positive, MB-negative patients with non-ST-elevation myocardial infarction: an undertreated but high-risk patient group: results from the National Cardiovascular Data Registry Acute Coronary Treatment and Intervention Outcomes Network—Get With The Guidelines (NCDR ACTION-GWTG) Registry. *Am Heart J.* 2010;160:819-825.

26. James SK, Lindahl B, Siegbahn A, et al. N-terminal pro-brain natriuretic peptide and other risk markers for the separate prediction of mortality and subsequent myocardial infarction in patients with unstable coronary artery disease: a Global Utilization of Strategies to Open Occluded Arteries (GUSTO)-IV Substudy. *Circulation.* 2003;108:275-281.

27. Steg PG, FitzGerald G, Fox KA. Risk stratification in non-ST-segment elevation acute coronary syndromes: troponin alone is not enough. *Am J Med.* 2009;122:107-108.

28. Apple FS, Collinson PO; for the IFCC Task Force on Clinical Applications of Cardiac Biomarkers: analytical characteristics of high-sensitivity cardiac troponin assays. *Clin Chem.* 2012 Jan;58(1):54-61.

29. Wu A, Collinson P, Jaffe A, et al. High-sensitivity cardiac troponin assays: what analytical and clinical issues need to be addressed before Introduction into clinical practice? Interview by Fred S. Apple. *Clin Chem.* 2010;56(6):886-891.

30. Aldous SJ, Florkowski CM, Crozier IG, et al. Comparison of high sensitivity and contemporary troponin assays for the early detection of acute myocardial infarction in the emergency department. *Ann Clin Biochem.* 2011;48(3):241-248.

31. Keller T, Zeller T, Ojeda F, et al. Serial changes in highly sensitive troponin I assay and early diagnosis of myocardial infarction. *JAMA.* 201;306:2684-2693.

32. Mueller M, Biener M, Vafaie M, et al. Absolute and relative kinetic changes of high-sensitivity cardiac troponin T in acute coronary syndrome and in patients with increased troponin in the absence of acute coronary syndrome. *Clin Chem.* 2012;58(1):209-218.

33. Apple FS, Morrow DA. Delta cardiac troponin values in practice: are we ready to move absolutely forward to clinical routine? *Clin Chem.* 2012;58(1):8-10.

34. Goldmann BU, Christenson RH, Hamm CW, et al. Implications of troponin testing in clinical medicine. *Curr Control Trials Cardiovasc Med.* 2001;2(2):75-84.

35. Jaffe AS, Babuin L, Apple FS. Biomarkers in acute cardiac disease. *J Am Coll Cardiol.* 2006;48:1-11.

36. French JK, White HD. Clinical implications of the new definition of myocardial infarction. *Heart.* 2004;90:99-106.

37. Watnick S, Perazella MA. Cardiac troponins: utility in renal insufficiency and end-stage renal disease. *Semin Dial.* 2002;15(1):66-70.

38. Aviles RJ, Askari AT, Lindahl, et al. Troponin T levels in patients with acute coronary syndromes, with or without renal dysfunction. *N Engl J Med.* 2002;346:2047-2052.

39. Freda BJ. Tang WH, Van Lente F, et al. Cardiac troponins in renal insufficiency: review and clinical implications. *J Am Coll Cardiol.* 2002;40:2065-2071.

40. deFilippi C, Wasserman S, Rosanio S, et al. Cardiac troponin T and c-reactive protein for predicting prognosis, coronary atherosclerosis, and cardiomyopathy in patients undergoing long-term hemodialysis. *JAMA.* 2003;290:353-359.

41. Fuchs S, Gruberg L, Singh S, et al. Prognostic value of cardiac troponin I re-elevation following percutaneous coronary intervention in high-risk patients with acute coronary syndromes. *Am J Cardiol.* 2001;88(2):129-133.

42. Gruberg L, Fuchs S, Waksman R, et al. Prognostic value of cardiac troponin I elevation after percutaneous coronary intervention in patients with chronic renal insufficiency: a 12-month outcome analysis. *Catheter Cardiovasc Interv.* 2002;55(2):174-179.

43. Nienhuis MB, Ottervanger JP, Bilo HJ, et al. Prognostic value of troponin after elective percutaneous coronary intervention: A meta-analysis. *Catheter Cardiovasc Interv.* 2008 Feb 15;71(3):318-324.

44. Tsung SH. Several conditions causing elevation of serum CK-MB and CK-BB. *AM J Clin Pathol.* 1981;75:711-715.

45. Lee TH, Goldman L. Serum enzyme assays in the diagnosis of acute myocardial infarction. *Ann Intern Med.* 1986;105(2):221-233.

46. Stein PD, Janjua M, Matta F, et al. Prognosis based on creatine kinase isoenzyme MB, cardiac troponin I, and right ventricular size in stable patients with acute pulmonary embolism. *Am J Cardiol.* 2011;107(5):774-777.

47. Puleo PR, Meyer D, Wathen C, et al. Use of a rapid assay of subforms of creatine kinase-MB to diagnose or rule out acute myocardial infarction. *N Engl J Med.* 1994;331(9):561-566.

48. Zimmerman J, Fromm R, Meyer D, et al. Diagnostic marker cooperative study for the diagnosis of myocardial infarction. *Circulation.* 1999;99(13):1671-1677.

49. Weissler AM. Diagnostic marker cooperative study for the diagnosis of myocardial infarction (letter). *Circulation.* 2000;102(6):E40.

50. De Lemos JA, Antman EM, Giugliano RP, et al. Very early risk stratification after thrombolytic therapy with a bedside myoglobin assay and the 12-lead electrocardiogram. *Am Heart J.* 2000;140(3):373-378.

51. Srinivas VS, Cannon CP, Gibson CM, et al. Myoglobin levels at 12 hr identify patients at low risk for 30-day mortality after thrombolysis in acute myocardial infarction: a thrombolysis in myocardial infarction 10B substudy. *Am Heart J.* 2001;142(1):29-36.

52. Morrow DA, Rifai N, Antman EM, et al. C-reactive protein is a potent predictor of mortality independently of and in combination with troponin T in acute coronary syndromes: a TIMI 11A substudy. Thrombolysis in Myocardial Infarction. *J Am Coll Cardiol.* 1998;31(7):1460-1465.

53. Oltrona L, Ardissino D, Merlini PA, et al. C-reactive protein elevation and early outcome in patients with unstable angina pectoris. *Am J Cardiol.* 1997;80(8):1002-1006.

54. Haverkate F, Thompson SG, Pyke SD, et al. Production of C-reactive protein and risk of coronary events in stable and unstable angina. European Concerted Action on Thrombosis and Disabilities Angina Pectoris Study Group. *Lancet.* 1997;349(9050):462-466.

55. de Winter RJ, Bholasingh R, Lijmer JG, et al. independent prognostic value of C-reactive protein and troponin I in patients with unstable angina or non-Q-wave myocardial infarction. *Cardiovasc Res.* 1999;42:240-245.

56. Ridker PM, Glynn RJ, Hennekens CH. C-reactive protein adds to the predictive value of total and HDL cholesterol in determining risk of first myocardial infarction. *Circulation.* 1998;97:2007-2011.

57. Ridker PM, Cannon CP, Morrow D, et al. C-reactive protein levels and outcomes after statin therapy. *N Engl J Med.* 2005;352:20-28.

58. Myers GL, Rifai N, Tracy RP, et al. CDC/AHA Workshop on markers of inflammation and cardiovascular disease: application to clinical and public health practice. Report from the laboratory science group. *Circulation.* 2004;110:e545-e549.

59. Sabatine MS, Morrow DA, Jablonski KA, et al. Prognostic significance of the Centers for Disease Control/American Heart Association high-sensitivity c-reactive protein cut points for cardiovascular and other outcomes in patients with stable coronary artery disease. *Circulation.* 2007;115:1528-1536.

60. Pearson TA, Mensah GA, Alexander W, et al. Markers of inflammation and cardiovascular disease: application to clinical and public health practice: a statement for healthcare professionals from the centers for disease control and prevention and the American Heart Association. *Circulation.* 2003;107:499-511.

61. Wang CH, Li SH, Weisel RD, et al. C-reactive protein upregulates angiotensin type 1 receptors in vascular smooth muscle. *Circulation.* 2003;107:1783-1790.

62. Kim JS, Kang TS, Kim JB, et al. Significant association of C-reactive protein with arterial stiffness in treated non-diabetic hypertensive patients. *Atherosclerosis.* 2007;192:401-406.

63. Ridker PM, Danielson E, Rifai N, et al. Valsartan, blood pressure reduction, and C-reactive protein: primary report of the Val-MARC trial. *Hypertension.* 2006;48:73-79.

64. US Food and Drug Administration. Guidance for Industry and FDA Staff: Criteria for assessment of C-reactive protein (CRP), high sensitivity C-reactive protein (hsCRP) and cardiac C-reactive protein (cCRP) assays. http://www.fda.gov/MedicalDevices/DeviceRegulationandGuidance/GuidanceDocuments/ucm077167.htm. Accessed January 30, 2012.

65. Rifai N, Ballantyne CM, Cushman M, et al. High-sensitivity c-reactive protein and cardiac c-reactive protein assays: Is there a need to differentiate? *Clin Chem.* 2006;52:1254-1256.

66. Callaghan J, Gutman SI. Food and Drug Administration guidance for c-reactive protein assays: matching claims with performance data. *Clin Chem.* 2006;52:1256-1257.

67. Heeschen C, Hamm CW, Bruemmer J, et al. Predictive value of C-reactive protein and troponin T in patients with unstable angina: a comparative analysis. CAPTURE Investigators. Chimeric c7E3 antiplatelet therapy in unstable angina REfractory to standard treatment trial. *J Am Coll Cardiol.* 2000;35:1535-1542.

68. Morrow DA, Rifai N, Antman EM, et al. C-reactive protein is a potent predictor of mortality independently of and in combination with troponin T in acute coronary syndromes: a TIMI 11A substudy—thrombolysis in myocardial infarction. *J Am Coll Cardiol.* 1998;31:1460-1465.

69. Lindahl B, Toss H, Siegbahn A, et al. Markers of myocardial damage and inflammation in relation to long-term mortality in unstable coronary artery disease. FRISC Study Group. Fragmin during Instability in Coronary Artery Disease. *N Engl J Med.* 2000;343:1139-1147.

70. Currie CJ, Poole CD, Conway P. Evaluation of the association between the first observation and the longitudinal change in C-reactive protein, and all-cause mortality. *Heart.* 2008;94:457-462.

71. Morrow DA, Rifai N, Antman EM, et al. Serum amyloid A predicts early mortality in acute coronary syndromes: A TIMI 11A substudy. *J Am Coll Cardiol.* 2000;35(2):358-362.

72. Biasucci LM, Vitelli A, Liuzzo G, et al. Elevated levels of interleukin-6 in unstable angina. *Circulation.* 1996;94(5):874-877.

73. Ardissino D, Merlini PA, Gamba G, et al. Thrombin activity and early outcome in unstable angina pectoris. *Circulation.* 1996;93(9):1634-1639.

74. Becker RC, Cannon CP, Bovill EG, et al. Prognostic value of plasma fibrinogen concentration in patients with unstable angina and non-Q-wave myocardial infarction (TIMI IIIB Trial). *Am J Cardiol.* 1996;78(2):142-147.

75. Baldus S, Heeschen C, Meinertz T, et al. Myeloperoxidase serum levels predict risk in patients with acute coronary syndromes. *Circulation.* 2003;108:1440-1445.

76. Cavusoglu E, Ruwende C, Eng C, et al. Usefulness of baseline plasma myeloperoxidase levels as an independent predictor of myocardial infarction at two years in patients presenting with acute coronary syndrome. *Am J Cardiol.* 2007;99:1364-1368.

77. Mocatta TJ, Pilbrow AP, Cameron VA, et al. Plasma concentrations of myeloperoxidase predict mortality after myocardial infarction. *J Am Coll Cardiol.* 2007;49:1993-2000.

78. Borch-Johnsen K, Feldt-Rasmussen B, Strandgaard S, et al. Urinary albumin excretion: An independent predictor of ischemic heart disease. *Thromb Vasc Biol.* 1999;19:1992-1997.

79. Berton G, Cordiano R, Palmieri R, et al. Microalbuminuria during acute myocardial infarction: A strong predictor for 1-year mortality. *Eur Heart J.* 2001;22:1466-1475.

80. Sonmez K, Eskisar AO, Demir D, et al. Increased urinary albumin excretion rates can be a marker of coexisting coronary artery disease in patients with peripheral arterial disease. *Angiology.* 2006;57:15-20.

81. Klausen KP, Scharling H, Jensen JS. Very low level of microalbuminuria is associated with increased risk of death in subjects with cardiovascular or cerebrovascular diseases. *J Intern Med.* 2006;260:231-237.

82. Soler NG, Frank S. Value of glycosylated hemoglobin measurements after acute myocardial infarction. *JAMA.* 1981;246(15):1690-1693.

83. Husband DJ, Alberti KG, Julian DG. "Stress" hyperglycaemia during acute myocardial infarction: an indicator of pre-existing diabetes? *Lancet.* 1983;2(8343):179-181.

84. Aronson D, Hammerman H, Suleiman M, et al. Usefulness of changes in fasting glucose during hospitalization to predict long-term mortality in patients with acute myocardial infarction. *Am J Cardiol.* 2009;104:1013-1017.

85. Suleiman M, Hammerman H, Boulos M, et al. Fasting glucose is an important independent risk factor for 30-day mortality in patients with acute myocardial infarction: a prospective study. *Circulation.* 2005;111:754-760.

86. Tokudome T, Horio T, Soeki T, et al. Inhibitory effect of C-type natriuretic peptide (CNP) on cultured cardiac myocyte hypertrophy: interference between CNP and endothelin-1 signaling pathways. *Endocrinology.* 2004;145:2131-2140.

87. Del Ry S, Passino C, Maltinti M, et al. C-type natriuretic peptide plasma levels increase in patients with chronic heart failure as a function of clinical severity. *Eur J Heart Fail.* 2005;7:1145-1148.

88. Sudoh T, Kangawa K, Minamino N, et al. A new natriuretic peptide in porcine brain. *Nature.* 1988;32:78-81.

89. Tang WH, Francis GS, Morrow DA, et al. National academy of clinical biochemistry laboratory medicine practice guidelines: clinical utilization of cardiac biomarker testing in heart failure. *Circulation.* 2007;116:e99-e109.

90. Maisel A, Krishnaswamy P, Nowak RM, et al. Rapid measurement of B-type natriuretic peptide in the emergency diagnosis of heart failure. *N Engl J Med.* 2002;347:161-167.

91. Janzurri JL, Camargo CA, Anwaruddin S, et al. The N-terminal pro-BNP investigation of dyspnea in the emergency department (PRIDE) study. *Am J Cardiol.* 2005;95:948-954.

92. Berger R, Huelsman M, Strecker K, et al. B-type natriuretic peptide predicts sudden death in patients with chronic heart failure. *Circulation.* 2002;105:2392-2397.

93. Masson S, Latini R, Anand IS, et al. Direct comparison of B-type natriuretic peptide (BNP) and amino-terminal proBNP in a large population of patients with chronic and symptomatic heart failure: the Valsartan Heart Failure (Val-HeFT) data. *Clin Chem.* 2006;52:1528-1538.

94. Richards M, Nicholls MG, Espiner EA, et al. Comparison of B-type natriuretic peptides for assessment of cardiac function and prognosis in stable ischemic heart disease. *J Am Coll Cardiol.* 2006;47:52-60.

95. Jernberg T, Stridsberg M, Venge P, Lindahl B. N-terminal pro brain natriuretic peptide on admission for early risk stratification of patients with chest pain and no ST-segment elevation. *J Am Coll Cardiol.* 2002;40:437-445.

96. James SK, Lindahl B, Siegbahn A, et al. N-terminal pro-brain natriuretic peptide and other risk markers for the separate prediction of mortality and subsequent myocardial infarction in patients with unstable coronary artery disease: a Global Utilization of Strategies to Open Occluded Arteries (GUSTO)-IV Substudy. *Circulation.* 2003;108:275-281.

97. Morrow DA, de Lemos JA, Sabatine MS, et al. Evaluation of B-type natriuretic peptide for risk assessment in unstable angina/non-STelevation myocardial infarction: B-type natriuretic peptide and prognosis in TACTICS-TIMI 18. *J Am Coll Cardiol.* 2003;41:1264-1272.

98. Galvani M, Ottani F, Oltrona L, et al. N-terminal pro-brain natriuretic peptide on admission has prognostic value across the whole spectrum of acute coronary syndromes. *Circulation.* 2004;110:128-134.

99. Balion CM, McKelvie RS, Reichert S, et al. Monitoring the response to pharmacologic therapy in patients with stable chronic heart failure: is BNP or NT-proBNP a useful assessment tool? *Clin Biochem.* 2008;41:266-276.

100. Troughton R, Frampton CM, Yandle EA, et al. Treatment of heart failure guided by plasma aminoterminal brain natriuretic peptide (N-BNP) concentrations. *Lancet.* 2000;355:1126-1130.

101. Jourdain P, Jondeau G, Funck F, et al. Plasma brain natriuretic peptide-guided therapy to improve outcome in heart failure; the STARS-BNP multicenter study. *J Am Coll Cardiol.* 2007;49:1733-1739.

102. Berger R, Moertl D, Peter S, et al. N-terminal pro-B-type natriuretic peptide-guided, intensive patient management in addition to multidisciplinary care in chronic heart failure a 3-arm, prospective, randomized pilot study. *J Am Coll Cardiol.* 2010;55(7):645-653.

103. Lainchbury JG, Troughton RW, Strangman KM, et al. N-terminal pro-B-type natriuretic peptide-guided treatment for chronic heart failure: results from the BATTLESCARRED (NT-proBNP-assisted treatment to lessen serial cardiac readmissions and death) trial. *J Am Coll Cardiol.* 2009;55(1):53-60.

104. Pfisterer M, Buser P, Rickli H, et al. TIME-CHF Investigators. BNP-guided vs symptom-guided heart failure therapy: the trial of intensified vs. standard medical therapy in elderly patients with congestive heart failure (TIME-CHF) randomized trial. *JAMA.* 2009;301(4):383-392.

105. Porapakkham P, Porapakkham P, Zimmet H, et al. B-type natriuretic peptide-guided heart failure therapy: a meta-analysis. *Arch Intern Med.* 2010;170(6):507-514.

106. Thygesen K, Mair J, Mueller C, et al. Recommendations for the use of natriuretic peptides in acute cardiac care: a position statement from the Study Group on Biomarkers in Cardiology of the ESC Working Group on Acute Cardiac Care. *Eur Heart J.* 2011;10:1093/eurheartj/ehq509.

107. Anwaruddin S, Lloyd-Jones DM, Baggish A, et al. Renal function, congestive heart failure, and amino-terminal pro-brain natriuretic peptide measurement: results from the ProBNP investigation of dyspnea in the emergency department (PRIDE) study. *J Am Coll Cardiol.* 2006;47:91-97.

108. Mehra MR, Uber PA, Park MH, et al. Obesity and suppressed B-type natriuretic peptide levels in heart failure. *J Am Coll Cardiol.* 2004;43:1590-1595.

109. McCord J, Mundy BJ, Hudson MP, et al. Relationship between obesity and B-type natriuretic peptide levels. *Arch Intern Med.* 2004;164:2247-2252.

110. Krauser DG, Lloyd-Jones DM, Chae CU, et al. Effect of body mass index on natriuretic peptide levels in patients with acute congestive heart failure: a ProBNP investigation of dyspnea in the emergency department (PRIDE) study. *Am Heart J.* 2005;149:744-750.

111. Bayes-Genis A, Lloyd-Jones DM, van Kimmenade RR, et al. Effect of body mass index on diagnostic and prognostic usefulness of amino-terminal pro-brain natriuretic peptide in patients with acute dyspnea. *Arch Intern Med.* 2007;167:400-407.

112. Horwich TB, Hamilton MA, Fonarow GC. B-type natriuretic peptide levels in obese patients with advanced heart failure. *J Am Coll Cardiol.* 2006;47:85-90.

113. Daniels LB, Clopton P, Bhalla V, et al. How obesity affects the cut-points for B-type natriuretic peptide in the diagnosis of acute heart failure. Results from the breathing not properly multinational study. *Am Heart J.* 2006;151:999-1005.

114. de Lemos JA, Morrow DA, Bentley JH, et al. The prognostic value of B-type natriuretic peptide in patients with acute coronary syndromes. *N Engl J Med.* 2001; 345:1014-1021.

115. Morrow DA, de Lemos JA, Blazing MA, et al. Prognostic value of serial B-type natriuretic peptide testing during follow-up of patients with unstable coronary artery disease. *JAMA.* 2005;294:2866-2871.

116. Richards AM, Nicholls MG, Yandle TG, et al. Plasma N-terminal pro-brain natriuretic peptide and adrenomedullin: new neurohormonal predictors of left ventricular function and prognosis after myocardial infarction. *Circulation.* 1998;97:1921-1929.

117. James SK, Lindahl B, Siegbahn A, et al. N-terminal pro-brain natriuretic peptide and other risk markers for the separate prediction of mortality and subsequent myocardial infarction in patients with unstable coronary artery disease: a Global Utilization of Strategies to Open Occluded Arteries (GUSTO)-IV Substudy. *Circulation.* 2003;108:275-281.

118. Poutanen T, Tikanoja T, Riikonen P, et al. Long-term prospective follow-up study of cardiac function after cardiotoxic therapy for malignancy in children. *J Clin Oncol.* 2003;21:2349-2356.

119. Vogelsang TW, Jensen RJ, Hesse B, et al. BNP cannot replace gated equilibrium radionuclide ventriculography in monitoring of anthracycline-induced cardiotoxicity. *Int J Cardiol.* 2008;124(2):193-197.

120. Feola M, Garrone O, Occelli M, et al. Cardiotoxicity after anthracycline chemotherapy in breast carcinoma: effects on left ventricular ejection fraction, troponin I and brain natriuretic peptide. *Int J Cardiol.* 2011;148(2):194-198.

121. Goel S, Simes RJ, Beith JM. Exploratory analysis of cardiac biomarkers in women with normal cardiac function receiving trastuzumab for breast cancer. *Asia Pac J Clin Oncol.* 2011;7(3):276-280.

122. Morrison LK, Harrison A, Krishnaswamy P, et al. Utility of a rapid B-natriuretic peptide assay in differentiating congestive heart failure from lung disease in patients presenting with dyspnea. *J Am Coll Cardiol.* 2002;39(2):202-209.

123. Januzzi JL Jr, Camargo CA, Anwaruddin S, et al. The N-terminal Pro-BNP investigation of dyspnea in the emergency department (PRIDE) study. *Am J Cardiol.* 2005;95(8):948-954.

124. Perna ER, Macín SM, Cimbaro Canella JP, et al. Minor myocardial damage detected by troponin T is a powerful predictor of long-term prognosis in patients with acute decompensated heart failure. *Int J Cardiol.* 2005;99:253-261.

125. Demir M, Kanadasi M, Akpinar O, et al. Cardiac troponin T as a prognostic marker in patients with heart failure: a 3-year outcome study. *Angiology.* 2007;58:603-609.

126. 126. Latini R, Masson S, Anand IS, eta l. Prognostic value of very low plasma concentrations of troponin T in patients with stable chronic heart failure. *Circulation.* 2007;116:1242-1249.

127. Lindenfeld J, Albert NM, Boehmer JP, et al. Executive summary: HFSA 2010 comprehensive heart failure practice guideline. *J Card Fail.* 2010;16:475-539.

128. WL, Hartman KA, Burritt MF, et al. Profiles of serial changes in cardiac troponin T concentrations and outcome in ambulatory patients with chronic heart failure. *J Am Coll Cardiol.* 2009;54:1715-1721.

129. O'Connor C.M., Fiuzat M., Lombardi C., et al. Impact of serial troponin release on outcomes in patients with acute heart failure: analysis From the PROTECT pilot study. *Circ Heart Fail.* 2011;4:724-732.

130. Popp RL. Echocardiography (second of two parts). *N Engl J Med.* 1990;323(3):165-172.

131. Lang RM, Badano LP, Tsang W, et al. EAE/ASE Recommendations for Image Acquisition and Display Using Three-Dimensional Echocardiography. *J Am Soc Echocardiogr.* 2012;25(1):3-46.

132. ACCF/ASE/AHA/ASNC/HFSA/HRS/SCAI/SCCM/SCCT/SCMR 2011 Appropriate use criteria for echocardiography. A report of the American College of Cardiology Foundation Appropriate Use Criteria Task Force, American Society of Echocardiography, American Heart Association, American Society of Nuclear Cardiology, Heart Failure Society of America, Heart Rhythm Society, Society for Cardiovascular Angiography and Interventions, Society of Critical Care Medicine, Society of Cardiovascular Computed Tomography, and Society for Cardiovascular Magnetic Resonance Endorsed by the American College of Chest Physicians. *J Am Coll Cardiol.* 2011;57(9):1126-1166.

133. Taylor AJ, Cerqueira M, Hodgson JM, et al. ACCF/SCCT/ACR/AHA/ASE/ASNC/NASCI/SCAI/SCMR 2010 appropriate use criteria for cardiac computed tomography. A report of the American College of Cardiology Foundation Appropriate Use Criteria Task Force, the Society of Cardiovascular Computed Tomography, the American College of Radiology, the American Heart Association, the American Society of Echocardiography, the American Society of Nuclear Cardiology, the North American Society for Cardiovascular Imaging, the Society for Cardiovascular Angiography and Interventions, and the Society for Cardiovascular Magnetic Resonance. *J Am Coll Cardiol.* 2010;56(22):1864-1894.

134. Hendel RC, Berman DS, Di Carli MF, et al. ACCF/ASNC/ACR/AHA/ASE/SCCT/SCMR/SNM 2009 appropriate use criteria for cardiac radionuclide imaging: A report of the American College of Cardiology Foundation Appropriate Use Criteria Task Force, the American Society of Nuclear Cardiology, the American College of Radiology, the American Heart Association, the American Society of Echocardiography, the Society of Cardiovascular Computed Tomography, the Society for Cardiovascular Magnetic Resonance, and the Society of Nuclear Medicine. *J Am Coll Cardiol.* 2009;53(23):2201-2229.

QUICKVIEW | Troponins I and T

PARAMETER	DESCRIPTION	COMMENTS
Common reference ranges	Troponin I: ≤0.02 ng/mL	Assay dependent; see Table 11-3
	Troponin T: <0.1 ng/mL	Assay dependent
Critical value	Troponin I: ≥0.30 ng/mL	Assay dependent; see Table 11-3
	Troponin T: ≥0.1 ng/mL	Assay dependent
Inherent activity	Yes	Regulates calcium-medicated interaction of actin and myosin
Location	Cardiac and skeletal muscle	Cardiac troponins I and T and skeletal muscle troponins I and T have different amino acid sequences
Cause of abnormal values		
High	MI; myocardial ischemia produces mild elevations of troponin levels, which indicate increased risk for cardiac events	
Low	Normal finding	No lower limit for normal
Signs and symptoms		
High	Chest pain, nausea, vomiting, diaphoresis	Decreased or increased HR and BP, anxiety, and confusion, depending on AMI size, location, and duration
Low	None	Does not cause signs and symptoms
After AMI, time to…		
Initial elevation	4 hr	Time course studies of release needed
Peak values	12 hr–2 days	
Normalization	5–14 days	
Causes of spurious results	Table 11-4	

AMI = acute myocardial infarction; BP = blood pressure; HR = heart rate; MI = myocardial infarction.

QUICKVIEW | CK-MB

PARAMETER	DESCRIPTION	COMMENTS
Common reference ranges		
Adults	6.0 ng/mL <3% to 6% of total CK	Assay dependent
Critical value	>6.0 ng/mL >5% of total CK	Assay dependent
Inherent activity	Yes	Catalyzes transfer of high-energy phosphate groups
Location		
Production	Primarily cardiac muscle	Release from traumatized skeletal muscle can be incorrectly interpreted as cardiac in origin
Storage	Small amounts in skeletal muscle	
Secretion/excretion	Excreted via glomerular filtration	Eliminated at slightly faster rate than total CK
Causes of abnormal values		
High	MI	
Low	Not significant	No lower limit for normal
Signs and symptoms		
High level	AMI: chest pain, nausea, vomiting, diaphoresis	Decreased or increased HR and BP, anxiety, and confusion, depending on AMI size, location, and duration
Low level	None	Does not cause signs and symptoms
After AMI, time to...		
Initial elevation	3–12 hr	
Peak values	12–20 hr	
Normalization	2–3 days	
Causes of spurious results	Table 11-6	

AMI = acute myocardial infarction; BP = blood pressure; CK = creatine kinase; HR = heart rate; MI = myocardial infarction.

QUICKVIEW | BNP/NT-proBNP

PARAMETER	DESCRIPTION	COMMENTS
Common reference ranges		
Adults	BNP: <100 pg/mL	
	NT-proBNP: <300 pg/mL	
Critical value	BNP: >500 pg/mL	Affected by age, gender, renal function, and obesity
	NT-proBNP: >450 pg/mL in patients <50 years of age; >900 pg/mL in patients 50–75 years of age; >1800 pg/mL in patients >75 years of age	
Inherent activity	Yes	Diuretic, natriuretic, and vascular smooth muscle-relaxing effects
Location		
Production/storage	Ventricular myocyte	Released in response to increased ventricular wall tension
Secretion/excretion	BNP: enzymatic degradation via endopeptidase and natriuretic peptide receptor-mediated endocytosis	
	NT-proBNP: renal elimination	
Causes of abnormal values		
High	Heart failure	
Low	Not significant	
Signs and symptoms		
High level	Shortness of breath, pulmonary and peripheral edema	
Low level	None	
Causes of spurious results	Pulmonary embolism, pulmonary hypertension, pericarditis, sepsis	

BNP = B-type natriuretic peptide; NT-proBNP = N-terminal-proBNP.

CHAPTER 12

LIVER AND GASTROENTEROLOGY TESTS

PAUL FARKAS, JOANNA SAMPSON, BARRY SLITZKY, BRIAN ALTMAN

Objectives

After completing this chapter, the reader should be able to

- Discuss how the anatomy and physiology of the liver and pancreas affect interpretation of pertinent laboratory test results

- Classify liver test abnormalities into cholestatic and hepatocellular patterns and understand the approach to evaluating patients with these abnormalities

- Explain how hepatic and other diseases, as well as drugs and analytical interferences, cause abnormal laboratory test results for bilirubin

- Understand hepatic encephalopathy and the role of serum ammonia in its diagnosis

- Design and interpret a panel of laboratory studies to determine if a patient has active, latent, or previous viral hepatitis infection

- Understand the significance and utility of amylase and lipase in evaluating abdominal pain and pancreatic disorders

- Discuss the role of *Helicobacter pylori* in peptic ulcer disease and the tests used to diagnose it

- Discuss the tests and procedures used to diagnose *Clostridium difficile* colitis

Hepatic and other gastrointestinal (GI) abnormalities can cause a variety of clinically significant diseases, in part because of their central role in the body's biochemistry. This chapter provides an introduction to common laboratory studies used to investigate these diseases. Studies of the liver are roughly divided into those associated with (1) synthetic liver function, (2) excretory liver function and cholestasis (3) hepatocellular injury, and (4) detoxifying liver function and serum ammonia. Specific tests may also be used to investigate specific disease processes including viral hepatitis and primary biliary cirrhosis (PBC). This chapter also covers several tests for specific nonhepatic disease processes (including pancreatitis, *Helicobacter pylori* infection, and *Clostridium difficile* colitis).

ANATOMY AND PHYSIOLOGY OF THE LIVER AND PANCREAS

Liver

The *liver*, located in the right upper quadrant of the abdomen, is the largest solid organ in the human body.[1] It has two sources of blood:

1. The hepatic artery, originating from the aorta, supplies arterial blood rich in oxygen.
2. Portal veins shunt the venous blood from the intestines to the liver. This transports absorbed toxins, drugs, and nutrients directly to the liver for metabolism.

The liver is divided into thousands of lobules (Figure 12-1). Each lobule is comprised of plates of hepatocytes (liver cells) that radiate from the central vein much like spokes in a wheel. Between adjacent liver cells formed by matching grooves in the cell membranes are small bile canaliculi. The hepatocytes continually form and secrete bile into these canaliculi, which empty into terminal bile ducts. Subsequently, like tiny streams forming a river, these bile ducts empty into larger and larger ducts until they ultimately merge into the common duct. Bile then drains into either the gallbladder for temporary storage or directly into the duodenum.

The liver is a complex organ with a prominent role in all aspects of the body's biochemistry. It takes up amino acids absorbed by the intestines, processes them, and synthesizes them into circulating proteins including albumin and clotting factors. The liver is also involved in the breakdown of excess amino acids and processing of byproducts including ammonia and urea. The liver plays a similar role in absorbing carbohydrates from the gut, storing them in the form of glycogen, and releasing them as needed to prevent hypoglycemia. Most lipid and lipoprotein metabolism, including cholesterol synthesis, occurs in the liver. The liver is the primary location for detoxification and excretion of a wide variety of endogenous substances produced by the body (including sex hormones) as well as exogenous substances absorbed by the intestines (including a panoply of drugs and toxins). Thus, in patients with liver failure, standard dosing of some medications can lead to dangerously high serum concentrations and toxicity. The role of the liver in bilirubin metabolism is explored further below.

With its double blood supply, large size, and critical role in regulating body metabolic pathways, the liver is affected by many systemic diseases. Although numerous illnesses affect the liver, it has tremendous reserve capacity and can often maintain its function in spite of significant disease. Furthermore, the liver is one of the few human organs capable of regeneration.

Pancreas

The *pancreas* is an elongated gland located in the retroperitoneum. Its head lies in close proximity to the duodenum, and the pancreatic ducts empty into the duodenum. The pancreas has both exocrine glands (which secrete digestive enzymes into the duodenum) and endocrine glands (which secrete hormones directly into the circulation).

The pancreatic exocrine glands produce enzymes that aid in digestion of proteins, fats, and carbohydrates (including trypsin, chymotrypsin, lipase, and amylase). Insufficient enzyme production (i.e., pancreatic exocrine insufficiency) is associated with malabsorption of nutrients, leading to progressive weight loss and severe diarrhea.

The pancreatic endocrine glands produce many hormones including insulin and glucagon. Insufficient insulin production leads to diabetes mellitus. Thus, the pancreas plays an important role in digestion and absorption of food as well as metabolism of sugar. Like the liver, the pancreas has a tremendous reserve capacity; over 90% glandular destruction is required before diabetes or pancreatic insufficiency develops.

AN INTRODUCTION TO LIVER TESTS AND THE LFT PANEL

Investigation of liver disease often begins with obtaining a panel of liver tests generally referred to as the *LFT panel* or *LFTs (liver function tests)*. This panel may vary slightly between hospitals and labs but generally includes the *aminotransferases*, also referred to as *transaminases, AST* and *ALT* (which stand for aspartate aminotransferase and alanine aminotransferase, respectively), bilirubin, alkaline phosphatase (ALP), and albumin. The term *liver function test* is a misnomer because not all of these tests actually measure liver function (specifically, transaminases reflect liver *injury*). Additionally, the liver has several functions, and different tests reflect these different functions. Table 12-1 divides liver tests into rough categories. Although there is considerable overlap between these categories, these divisions may provide an initial framework for understanding the LFT panel.

This grouping of tests mirrors a division of liver diseases into two broad categories: cholestatic and hepatocellular. In cholestatic disease, there is an abnormality in the *excretory* function of the liver (i.e., namely secretion of bile by hepatocytes and passage of bile through the liver and bile ducts into the duodenum). In hepatocellular disease, there is primary inflammation and damage to the hepatocytes themselves (e.g.,

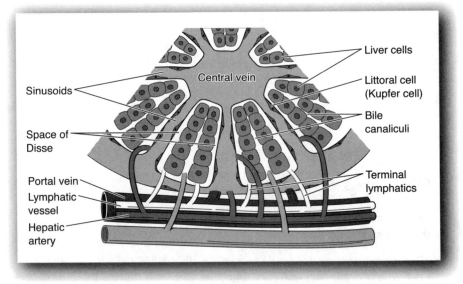

FIGURE 12-1. Basic structure of a liver lobule including the lymph flow system comprised of the spaces of Disse and interlobular lymphatics. (Reproduced with permission from Guyton AC. *Medical Physiology.* 5th ed. Philadelphia, PA: WB Saunders; 1976.)

due to viral infection of the hepatocytes). These two categories may overlap because disease of the hepatocytes (hepatocellular processes), if severe enough, will also lead to derangement of bile secretion. However, the distinction between primarily cholestatic versus primarily hepatocellular diseases and in turn LFT patterns remains useful and fundamental.[2] Perhaps further confusing this is that liver tests may be abnormal in patients with diseases that do not affect the liver.

The range of normal laboratory values used here is taken from *Harrison's Principles of Internal Medicine*, 18th edition, and *Nelson's Textbook of Pediatrics*, 19th edition. Reference ranges may vary slightly between different laboratories, and most laboratories will list their reference ranges along with lab results. Listed normal ranges are for adult patients, and

TABLE 12-1. Categories of Liver Tests

PROCESS	MOST CLOSELY RELATED TESTS
Protein synthesis	Albumin
	Prealbumin
	PT/INR (clotting proteins)
Excretion into the bile ducts and drainage into the duodenum (impairment of this process is defined as cholestasis)	Bilirubin
	ALP
	5'-nucleotidase
	GGT
Hepatocellular injury	Transaminases
	AST
	ALT
Detoxification	Ammonia (NH_3+)

ALP = alkaline phosphatase; ALT = alanine aminotransferase; AST = aspartate aminotransferase; GGT = gamma-glutamyl transpeptidase; INR = international normalized ratio; PT = prothrombin time.

pediatric patients will often have different ranges of normal values.

TESTS OF SYNTHETIC LIVER FUNCTION

As discussed above, one of the functions of the liver is to synthesize proteins that circulate in the blood, including albumin and clotting proteins. Measurement of the levels of these proteins in the blood provides a direct reflection of the ability of the liver to synthesize them. The liver has an enormous reserve function, so that it may synthesize normal amounts of proteins despite significant liver damage. Therefore, tests of synthetic function are not sensitive to low levels of liver damage or dysfunction. Inadequate protein synthetic function is mainly limited to hepatic cirrhosis, scarring of the liver that can result from years of alcohol abuse, inflammation, or massive liver damage (e.g., due to alcoholic liver disease, severe acute viral hepatitis, unrecognized and untreated chronic hepatitis, or potentially lethal toxin ingestion). In these situations, measuring synthetic function may be useful in determining prognosis by reflecting the degree of hepatic failure. The most commonly used tests of protein synthetic function are albumin and prothrombin time (PT).

Albumin

Normal range[3]: 4.0–5.0 g/dL

Albumin is a major plasma protein that is involved in maintaining plasma oncotic pressure and the binding and transport of numerous hormones, anions, drugs, and fatty acids.[4] The normal serum half-life of albumin is about 20 days, with about 4% degraded daily.[5] Because of albumin's long half-life, serum albumin measurements are slow to fall after the onset of hepatic dysfunction (e.g., complete cessation of albumin production results in only a 25% decrease in serum concentrations after 8 days).[1] For this reason, levels are often *normal* in acute viral hepatitis or drug-related hepatotoxicity.[2] Alternatively, albumin is commonly reduced in patients with chronic synthetic dysfunction due to cirrhosis.

Albumin levels may be low due to a variety of other abnormalities in protein synthesis, distribution, and excretion in addition to liver dysfunction. These include malnutrition/malabsorption, protein loss from the gut, kidney, or skin (as in nephrotic syndrome, protein-losing enteropathy, or severe burns, respectively), or increased blood volume (e.g., following administration of large volumes of intravenous [IV] fluids).[6–9] Albumin is a *negative acute phase reactant* meaning that in the setting of systemic inflammation (e.g., as due to infection or malignancy), the liver will produce less albumin. Severely ill hospitalized patients commonly have low albumin levels due to a combination of poor nutrition, systemic inflammation, and IV fluid administration. Extremely low albumin concentrations carry a poor prognosis for this reason irrespective of any particular liver disease. Given the numerous causes of a low albumin level, it is important to interpret it within the context of each patient. For example, in a patient with metastatic cancer and no known liver disease, a low albumin level suggests decreased nutritional intake and advanced malignancy

with systemic inflammation. Alternatively, in a patient with known cirrhosis a low albumin level suggests severe chronic liver failure. In a patient with no known medical disease, a low albumin level suggests the presence of significant disease and requires further investigation.

Hypoalbuminemia itself is usually not associated with specific symptoms or findings until concentrations become quite low. At very low concentrations (<2–2.5 g/dL), patients can develop peripheral edema, ascites, or pulmonary edema. Albumin normally generates oncotic pressure, which holds fluid in the vasculature. Under conditions of low albumin, fluid leaks from the vasculature into the interstitial spaces of subcutaneous tissues or into the body cavities. Finally, low albumin concentrations affect the interpretation of total serum calcium and concentrations of drugs that are highly protein bound (e.g., phenytoin and salicylates).

Hyperalbuminemia is seen in patients with marked dehydration (which concentrates their plasma), where it is associated with concurrent elevations in blood urea nitrogen (BUN) and hematocrit. Patients taking anabolic steroids may demonstrate truly increased albumin concentrations, but those on heparin or ampicillin may have falsely elevated results with some assays. Hyperalbuminemia is asymptomatic.

Prealbumin (Transthyretin)

Normal range[3]: 17–34 mg/dL

Prealbumin is similar to albumin in several respects: it is synthesized primarily by the liver; it is involved in the binding and transport of various solutes (thyroxin and retinol); and it is affected by similar factors that affect albumin levels. The primary difference between the two proteins is that prealbumin has a short half-life (2 days, compared to 20 days for albumin) and a smaller body pool than albumin, making the former more rapidly responsive than albumin.[10] Additionally, due to its high percentage of tryptophan and essential amino acids, prealbumin is more sensitive to protein nutrition than albumin and is less affected by liver disease or hydration state than albumin.[11] In practice, prealbumin is generally used to assess protein calorie nutrition. Prealbumin is generally regarded as the best laboratory test of protein nutrition, and it is routinely used to monitor patients receiving IV or tube feeding.[12–14]

International Normalized Ratio and Prothrombin Time

Normal range: INR 0.9–1.1, PT 12.7–15.4 sec

For an introduction to *international normalized ratio (INR)* and *prothrombin time (PT)*, please see Chapter 16: Hematology: Blood Coagulation Tests. These two tests measure the speed of a set of reactions in the extrinsic pathway of the coagulation cascade. A coagulation deficit correlates with prolonged reaction times, and increased values of INR and PT. Both PT and INR are two different measures of the same set of reactions, with the INR being a derived index that takes into account variations between test reagents used in different laboratories. As such, INR is more precise and easily interpretable, and it is replacing the use of the PT.

The liver is required for the synthesis of clotting factors (with the exception of factor VIII), many of which require a

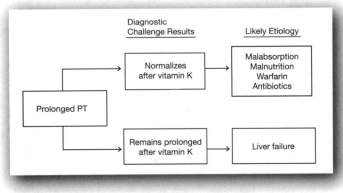

FIGURE 12-2. Evaluation of a prolonged PT.

vitamin K cofactor for their activation. Therefore, either hepatic impairment or vitamin K deficiency may lead to a deficiency in activated coagulation factors with subsequent prolongation of PT/INR. Both synthetic failure and vitamin K deficiency may also cause prolongation of activated partial thromboplastin time (aPTT which measures a different set of coagulation reactions in the intrinsic coagulation cascade) but to a much lesser degree than PT/INR.

The prolongation of PT/INR alone is not specific for liver disease. It can be seen in many situations, most of which interfere with the utilization of vitamin K, a cofactor required for the proper posttranslational activation of clotting factors II, VII, IX, and X. Because vitamin K is a fat soluble vitamin, inadequate vitamin K in the diet or fat malabsorption as caused by cholestasis may cause hypovitaminosis.[15] Many broad-spectrum antibiotics, including tetracyclines, may eliminate vitamin K-producing flora in the gut. The anticoagulant agent warfarin interferes directly with vitamin K dependent activation of clotting factors.

If the etiology of elevated PT/INR remains unclear despite obtaining additional coagulation tests, then the clinical approach is to provide parenteral vitamin K (generally subcutaneously).[16] If the PT/INR is prolonged due to malabsorption, warfarin, perturbed gut flora, or the absence of vitamin K in the diet, the PT/INR usually corrects by at least 30% within 24 hours.[9] Alternatively failure of PT/INR to normalize despite parenteral vitamin K suggests impaired synthetic liver function (see Figure 12-2).[4] Other factors that may cause a prolonged PT/INR that does not respond to parenteral vitamin K include inherited clotting factor deficiencies.

Because clotting factors are produced in excess of need and because the liver has tremendous synthetic reserves, only substantial hepatic impairment (>80% loss of synthetic capability) leads to decreased synthesis of these factors and subsequent clotting abnormalities.[6] Thus, PT/INR, albumin, and prealbumin levels lack sensitivity and may remain normal in the face of substantial liver damage.[4] However, they have considerable prognostic value if liver damage is sufficient to affect them. Unlike albumin (which responds slowly to hepatic insult), PT responds within 24 hours to changes in hepatic status due to the short half-life of certain clotting proteins (i.e., factor VII has a half-life of less than 6 hours).[17] Thus, the PT may become elevated days before other manifestations of liver failure and,

likewise, may normalize prior to other evidence of clinical improvement.[18] The primary utility of PT in liver disease is to provide prognostic data, generally in situations where the cause of the elevated PT/INR is known, for example, acute acetaminophen overdose leading to hepatic failure.

In addition to serving as a liver function test, PT/INR has direct clinical relevance in accessing the patient's tendency to bleed spontaneously, or due to surgical or diagnostic procedures. Bleeding is a dramatic complication of hepatic failure. When the PT/INR is significantly elevated, bleeding may be controlled or at least diminished by fresh frozen plasma, which contains the needed activated clotting factors and often corrects the PT/INR temporarily.

Des-gamma-carboxy prothrombin (DCP) is an abnormal prothrombin form that is released in the absence of vitamin K, in the presence of vitamin K antagonists (warfarin), and by certain tumors (hepatocellular carcinoma). White it has been used to evaluate the risk of hepatocellular carcinoma, DCP has a lower sensitivity than alpha fetoprotein for tumors under 3 cm. in size.[19]

CHOLESTATIC LIVER DISEASE

Cholestasis is a deficiency of the excretory function of the liver. As described above, bile is normally secreted by hepatocytes into bile canaliculi, where it flows into larger bile ducts, and eventually empties into the duodenum. Excretion of bile from the liver serves multiple purposes. Certain large lipophilic toxins, drugs, and endogenous substances are eliminated by secretion into the bile with eventual elimination in the feces. Bile salts also play an important role in dissolving and absorbing dietary fat-soluble vitamins and nutrients within the small intestine.

Failure of the excretory functions of the liver leads to a predictable set of consequences. Substances normally secreted in the bile accumulate, resulting in jaundice (from bilirubin), pruritus (from bile salts), or xanthomas (from lipid deposits in skin). Absence of bile salts to dissolve fat-soluble nutrients leads to deficiencies of fat-soluble vitamins A, D, E, and K. This may result in osteoporosis, due to lack of vitamin D, and PT/INR elevation, due to lack of vitamin K.

Cholestatic syndromes may be subclassified as either anatomic obstructions to macroscopic bile ducts (*extrahepatic cholestasis*) or disorders of hepatocytes and microscopic bile ducts (*intrahepatic cholestasis*).[20] The approach to a patient with cholestasis generally begins with a radiographic study, often a right upper-quadrant ultrasound, to look for dilation of large bile ducts within or outside the liver. Dilation of such large bile ducts indicates extrahepatic cholestasis; otherwise extrahepatic cholestasis is largely excluded, and the next step is to investigate for various causes of intrahepatic cholestasis.

Intrahepatic Cholestasis

Intrahepatic cholestasis includes a variety of processes that interfere with hepatocyte secretion of bile, as well as diseases of the micro- and macroscopic bile ducts within the liver. Etiologies involving impaired hepatocyte secretion of bile overlap to some extent with hepatocellular diseases as noted above; such processes include viral hepatitis (especially type A), alcoholic hepatitis, and even cirrhosis. Processes that cause a more pure cholestatic pattern include a variety of drugs (see Table 12-2), pregnancy, severe infection (cholestasis of sepsis), and certain nonhepatic neoplasms, especially renal cell carcinoma. Infiltrative process of the liver will produce a primarily cholestatic pattern, and these include granulomatous diseases and amyloidosis. Primary biliary cirrhosis causes inflammatory scarring of the microscopic bile ducts, whereas sclerosing cholangitis is a similar process that may affect micro- or macroscopic bile ducts within the liver. Masses within the liver, including tumors or abscesses, may block the flow of bile as well.

Extrahepatic Cholestasis

Extrahepatic cholestasis involves obstruction of the large bile ducts outside of the liver. The most common cause is stones in the common bile duct; other causes include obstruction by strictures (after surgery), or tumors (of pancreas, ampulla of Vater, duodenum, or bile ducts), chronic pancreatitis with scarring of the ducts as they pass through the pancreas, and parasitic infections of the ducts. Another cause is sclerosing cholangitis, a disease causing diffuse inflammation of the bile ducts, often both intrahepatic and extrahepatic. Of note is that sclerosing cholangitis is associated with inflammatory bowel disease, especially involving the colon. Some patients with HIV can develop a picture similar to sclerosing cholangitis, referred to as *AIDS cholangiopathy*. Although previously referred to as surgical cholestasis, *extrahepatic cholestasis* can now often be treated or at least palliated using endoscopic means (e.g., dilation of strictures with or without stent placement).

Tests Associated with Excretory Liver Function and Cholestasis

Laboratory tests do not distinguish between intra- and extrahepatic cholestasis. This distinction is usually made radiographically. In most instances of extrahepatic cholestasis, a damming effect causes dilation of bile ducts above the obstruction, which can be visualized via a computed tomography (CT) scan, a magnetic resonance imaging (MRI) scan, or ultrasound. Laboratory abnormalities primarily associated with cholestasis include elevation of ALP, 5'-nucleotidase, gamma-glutamyl transpeptidase (GGT), and bilirubin.

Alkaline Phosphatase

Normal range[3]: 33–96 units/L
Alkaline phosphatase (ALP) refers to a group of isoenzymes whose exact function remains unknown. These enzymes are found in many body tissues including the liver, bone, small intestine, kidneys, placenta, and leukocytes. In the liver they are found primarily in the bile canicular membranes of the liver cells. In adults, most serum ALP comes from the liver and bone (~80%), with the remainder mostly contributed by the small intestine.

Normal ALP concentrations vary primarily with age. In children and adolescents, elevated ALP concentrations result from bone growth, which may be associated with elevations as

TABLE 12-2. Classification of Liver Disease[a]

HEPATOCELLULAR	CHOLESTATIC
Viral hepatitis	Intrahepatic
Autoimmune hepatitis	Cholestasis of sepsis
Impaired blood flow	Extra-hepatic neoplasms
Hypotension (shock liver)	(i.e., renal cell)
Congestive heart failure	Cholestasis of pregnancy
Metabolic diseases	Infiltrative liver diseases
Hemochromatosis	Granulomatous (sarcoid, TB)
Wilson disease	Lymphoma
Alcoholic hepatitis	Metastatic carcinoma
NAFLD	Inflammatory diseases of bile ducts
Drugs	PBC
Acetaminophen	PSC
ACE Inhibitors	Drugs
Allopurinol	Allopurinol
Amiodarone	Antibiotics
Antiepileptic agents	Erythromycin
Carbamazepine	Beta-lactams
Phenytoin	Rifampin
Valproic acid	Cardiovascular
Antimicrobial agents	Amiodarone
Amoxicillin–clavulanic acid	Captopril
Azole antifungals	Diltiazem
Dapsone	Quinidine
INH	Carbamazepine
Nitrofurantoin	Hormonal agents
Protease inhibitors	Estrogens
Azathioprine	Methyltestosterone
Cisplatin	Anabolic steroids
Glyburide	Niacin
Heparin	NSAIDs
Labetalol	Penicillamine
Methotrexate	Phenothiazines
Niacin	Sulfa drugs
NSAIDs	TPN (hyperalimentation)
Phenothiazines	**Extrahepatic**
Trazodone	Biliary stricture
Statin medications	Gallstone-obstructing bile duct
Sulfonamides	Tumors
Herbal medications	Pancreatic cancer
Nutritional supplements	Cholangiocarcinoma of bile duct
Illicit drugs	PSC
Toxins	AIDS cholangiopathy

ACE = angiotensin-converting enzyme; AIDS = acquired immune deficiency syndrome; INH = isoniazid; NAFLD = nonalcoholic fatty liver disease; NSAIDs = nonsteroidal anti-inflammatory drugs; PBC = primary biliary cirrhosis; PSC = primary sclerosing cholangitis; TB = tuberculosis; TPN = total parenteral nutrition.

[a]Please note that listings of drugs contain more commonly used agents and are not exhaustive. For any particular patient, potentially causative drugs should be specifically researched in appropriate databases to determine any hepatotoxic effects.

TABLE 12-3. Initial Evaluation of Elevated ALP Concentrations in Context of Other Test Results

ALP	GGT, 5' NUCLEOTIDASE	AMINOTRANSFERASES (ALT AND AST)	DIFFERENTIAL DIAGNOSIS
Mildly elevated	Within normal limits	Within normal limits	Pregnancy; nonhepatic causes (Table 12-4)
Moderately elevated[a]	Markedly elevated	Within normal limits or minimally elevated	Cholestatic syndromes
Mildly elevated[b]	Mildly elevated	Markedly elevated	Hepatocellular disease

[a]Usually greater than 4 times normal limits.
[b]Usually less than 4 times normal limits.

high as 3 times the adult normal range. Similarly, the increase during late pregnancy is due to placental ALP.[21,22] In the third trimester, concentrations often double and may remain elevated for 3 weeks postpartum.[23]

The mechanism of hepatic ALP release into the circulation in patients with cholestatic disease remains unclear. Bile accumulation appears to increase hepatocyte synthesis of ALP, which eventually leaks into the bloodstream.[8,24] The ALP concentrations persist until the obstruction is removed and then normalize within 2–4 weeks.

Clinically, ALP elevation is associated with cholestatic disorders and, as mentioned previously, does not help to distinguish between intra- and extrahepatic disorders. ALP concentrations more than 4 times normal suggest a cholestatic disorder, and 75% of patients with primarily cholestatic disorders have ALP concentrations in this range (Table 12-3). Concentrations of 3 times normal or less are nonspecific and can occur in all types of liver disease. Mild elevations, usually less than 1½ times normal, can be seen in normal patients and are less significant.

When faced with an elevated ALP concentration, a clinician must determine whether it is derived from the liver. One approach is to fractionate the ALP isoenzymes using electrophoresis, but this method is expensive and often unavailable. Thus, the approach usually taken is to measure other indicators of cholestatic disease, 5'-nucleotidase or GGT. If ALP is elevated, an elevated 5'-nucleotidase or GGT indicates that at least part of the elevated ALP is of hepatic origin. Alternatively,

a normal 5'-nucleotidase or GGT suggests a nonhepatic cause (Table 12-3).

Nonhepatic causes of elevated ALP include bone disorders (e.g., healing fractures, osteomalacia, Paget disease, rickets, tumors, hypervitaminosis D, or vitamin D deficiency as caused by celiac sprue), hyperthyroidism, hyperparathyroidism, sepsis, diabetes mellitus, renal failure, and neoplasms (which may synthesize ALP ectopically, outside tissues that normally contain ALP) (Table 12-4). Some families have inherited elevated concentrations (2–4 times normal), usually as an autosomal dominant trait.[25] Markedly elevated concentrations (greater than 4 times normal) are generally seen only in cholestasis, Paget disease, or infiltrative diseases of the liver. Due to an increase in intestinal ALP, serum ALP concentrations can be falsely elevated in patients of blood type O or B whose blood is drawn 2–4 hours after a fatty meal.[26]

Alkaline phosphatase concentrations can be lowered by a number of conditions including hypothyroidism, hypophosphatemia, pernicious anemia, and zinc or magnesium deficiency.[8] Also, ALP may be confounded by a variety of drugs.

5'-Nucleotidase
Normal range: 0–11 units/L
Although *5'-nucleotidase* is found in many tissues (including liver, brain, heart, and blood vessels), serum 5'-nucleotidase is elevated most often in patients with hepatic diseases.[19] It has a response profile parallel to ALP and similar utility in differentiating between hepatocellular and cholestatic liver disease. Since it is only elevated in the face of liver disease, the presence of an elevated ALP in the face of a normal 5'-nucleotidase suggests that the ALP is elevated secondary to nonhepatic causes.

Gamma-Glutamyl Transpeptidase
Normal range: 9–58 units/L
Gamma-glutamyl transpeptidase (GGT, also GGTP), a biliary excretory enzyme, can also help determine whether an elevated ALP is of hepatic etiology. Similar to 5'-nucleotidase, it is not elevated in bone disorders, adolescence, or pregnancy. It is rarely elevated in conditions other than liver disease.

Generally, GGT parallels ALP and 5'-nucleotidase levels in liver disease. Additionally, GGT concentrations are usually elevated in patients who abuse alcohol or have alcoholic liver disease. Therefore, this test is potentially useful in differential diagnosis with a GGT/ALP ratio greater than 2.5 being highly indicative of alcohol abuse.[16,27] With abstinence, GGT concentrations often decrease by 50% within 2 weeks.

TABLE 12-4. Some Nonhepatic Illnesses Associated With Elevated ALP

BONE DISORDERS	OTHER DISORDERS AND DRUGS
Healing fractures	Acromegaly
Osteomalacia	Anticonvulsant drugs (e.g., phenytoin and phenobarbital)
Paget disease	
Rickets	Hyperthyroidism
Tumors	Lithium (bone isoenzymes)
	Neoplasia
	Oral contraceptives
	Renal failure
	Small bowel obstruction
	Pregnancy
	Sepsis

Although GGT is often regarded as the most sensitive test for cholestatic disorders, unlike 5'-nucleotidase it lacks specificity. In one study of nonselected patients, only 32% of GGT elevations were of hepatic origin.[18] Gamma-glutamyl transpeptidase is found in the liver, kidneys, pancreas, spleen, heart, brain, and seminal vesicles. Elevations may occur in pancreatic diseases, myocardial infarction, severe chronic obstructive pulmonary diseases, some renal diseases, systemic lupus erythematosus, hyperthyroidism, certain cancers, rheumatoid arthritis, and diabetes mellitus. Gamma-glutamyl transpeptidase may be confounded in patients on a variety of medications, some of which overlap with the medications that confound ALP test results. Thus, elevated GGT (even with concomitant elevated ALP) does not necessarily imply liver injury when 5'-nucleotidase is normal, but rather both elevations in GGT and ALP may be due to a common confounding medication (e.g., phenytoin, barbiturates) or medical conditions (e.g., myocardial infarction).

Bilirubin

Total bilirubin: 0.3–1.3 mg/dL

Indirect (unconjugated, insoluble) bilirubin: 0.2–0.9 mg/dL (bound to albumin in the blood)

Direct (conjugated, water soluble) bilirubin[3]: 0.1–0.4 mg/dL (excreted by the kidney)

Understanding the various laboratory studies of *bilirubin* requires knowledge of the biochemical pathways for bilirubin production and excretion (see Figure 12-3). Bilirubin is a breakdown product of heme pigments, which are large, insoluble organic compounds. Most of the body's heme pigments are located in erythrocytes, where they are a component of hemoglobin. Breakdown of erythrocytes releases hemoglobin into the circulation, which is converted to bilirubin (predominantly in the spleen), where it is initially a large lipophilic molecule bound to albumin.

The liver plays a central role in excretion of bilirubin, similar to its role in the metabolism and excretion of a wide variety of lipophilic substances. Prior to excretion, bilirubin must be converted into a form that is water-soluble. The liver achieves this covalently linking it to a water-soluble sugar molecule (glucuronic acid) using an enzyme glucuronyl transferase. The conjugate of bilirubin linked to glucuronic acid is water soluble, so it may then be excreted into the bile and eventually eliminated in the feces. Incidentally, bilirubin and some of its breakdown products are responsible for coloring feces brown (such that with complete obstruction of the bile ducts or cessation of bile synthesis by the liver, stool will take on a pale color).

Indirect Versus Direct Bilirubin

The total amount of bilirubin in the serum can be divided into *direct* and *indirect* fractions. Bilirubin conjugated to glucuronic acid (water-soluble bilirubin) reacts quickly in the van der Bergh reaction and is thus called *direct-reacting* or *direct bilirubin*. Alternatively, unconjugated bilirubin, because it is water insoluble, requires the presence of dissolving agents to be detected by this assay and is thus called *indirect-reacting* or *indirect bilirubin*. Although this nomenclature system is

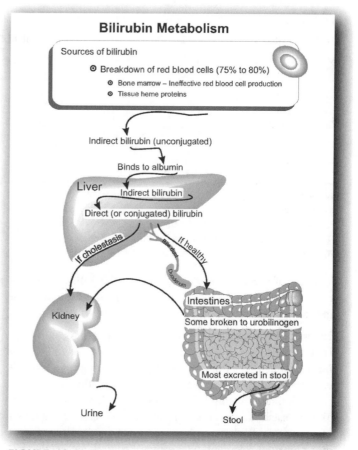

FIGURE 12-3. Overview of bilirubin production and metabolism. Most bilirubin is produced by the breakdown of heme pigments in erythrocytes (red blood cells) and to a lesser extent other tissues. The indirect bilirubin is carried in the circulation to the liver where it is conjugated and becomes direct or conjugated bilirubin. In health this is largely excreted via the biliary system into the gut. In disease it will "back up" into the circulation, causing elevated levels of direct/conjugated bilirubin and ultimately jaundice. (With thanks to Esta Farkas.)

slightly awkward, it is the standard terminology used in clinical practice today. Only the water-soluble direct bilirubin can be excreted in the urine, and therefore urine dipsticks will only measure this fraction. In fact, urine dipsticks may be more sensitive than most serum tests for detecting a slight elevation of direct bilirubin.

Elevated bilirubin causes abnormal yellow coloration of the skin (jaundice) and sclera of the eyes (icterus). Excess carotenes (as due to large amounts of carrot consumption) may cause a similar effect on the skin but spare the eyes. Icterus usually becomes visible when total bilirubin concentrations exceed 2–4 mg/dL. In infants, extremely elevated concentrations of bilirubin (for example, >20 mg/dL) may have neurotoxic effects on the developing brain, but in adults a direct toxic effect of bilirubin is quite rare.[28]

The first step in evaluating an elevated serum bilirubin is to determine if only the indirect fraction is elevated, or if there is involvement of the direct fraction. Given the sequential

TABLE 12-5. Evaluation of Elevated Bilirubin Concentrations in Context of Other Test Results

TOTAL BILIRUBIN	DIRECT BILIRUBIN	INDIRECT BILIRUBIN	ALT, AST, GGT	DIFFERENTIAL DIAGNOSIS
Moderately elevated	Within normal limits or low	Moderately elevated	Within normal limits	Hemolysis,[a] Gilbert syndrome,[a] Crigler-Najjar syndrome,[b] neonatal jaundice
Moderately elevated	Moderately elevated	Within normal limits	Within normal limits	Congenital syndromes[c]: Dubin-Johnson,[d] Rotor
Mildly elevated	Mildly elevated	Moderately elevated	Moderately elevated	Hepatobiliary disease

ALT = alanine aminotransferase; AST = aspartate aminotransferase; GGT = gamma-glutamyl transpeptidase.
[a]Usually indirect bilirubin is less than 4 mg/dL but may increase to 18 mg/dL.
[b]Usually indirect bilirubin is greater than 12 mg/dL and may go as high as 45 mg/dL.
[c]These syndromes are distinguished in the laboratory by liver biopsy.
[d]Usually direct bilirubin is 3–10 mg/dL.

location of these two molecules within the pathway of bilirubin metabolism, elevated levels of the molecules may have markedly different significance (Table 12-5).

Indirect Hyperbilirubinemia (unconjugated, insoluble)

Indirect bilirubin is mostly produced by the breakdown of erythrocytes and is removed from the circulation by conversion to direct bilirubin by glucuronyl transferase in the liver. Therefore, elevated levels may result from increased breakdown of red blood cells (hemolysis) or reduced hepatic conversion to direct bilirubin.[18] Patients with primarily *unconjugated hyperbilirubinemia* (>70% indirect) generally do *not* have serious liver disease. The most common causes of elevated indirect bilirubin are hemolysis, Gilbert syndrome, Crigler-Najjar syndrome, or various drugs, including probenecid and rifampin.[29] In infants this can be physiologic (neonatal jaundice), although very high levels may require medical intervention.

Hemolysis refers to increased destruction of erythrocytes, which increases the production of indirect bilirubin and may overwhelm the liver's ability for conjugation and excretion. However, the liver's processing mechanisms are intact so that serum bilirubin generally doesn't climb too high (rarely >5 mg/dL). Hemolysis may result from a wide variety of hematologic processes including sickle cell anemia, spherocytosis, hematomas, mismatched blood transfusions, or intravascular fragmentation of blood cells. Evaluation will include various hematologic tests as described in further detail in another chapter.

Gilbert syndrome is an inherited, benign trait present in 3% to 5% of the population. It is due to reduced production of hepatic glucuronyl transferase enzymes, resulting in intermittent elevation of indirect bilirubin and mild jaundice (increased with fasting, stress, or illness). The primary significance is that it may cause elevation of bilirubin when there is in fact no significant hepatic or hematologic disease. Bilirubin elevation is generally mild, with values less than 5 mg/dL.[2]

Direct Hyperbilirubinemia (conjugated, soluble)

Conjugated hyperbilirubinemia is defined as bilirubinemia with >50% in the direct fraction (although absolute levels of unconjugated bilirubin may also be elevated).[17] In the normal course of bilirubin metabolism, direct bilirubin is synthesized in hepatocytes and secreted into bile. Therefore, elevated direct bilirubin implies hepatic or biliary tract disease that interferes with secretion of bilirubin from the hepatocytes or clearance of bile from the liver.

Direct hyperbilirubinemia is generally classified as a positive cholestatic liver test, although as discussed earlier, it may be elevated to some extent in hepatocellular processes as well. In cholestatic disease bilirubin is primarily conjugated, whereas in hepatocellular processes significant increases in both conjugated and unconjugated bilirubin may result. The most reliable method of determining the cause of hyperbilirubinemia considers the magnitude and pattern of abnormalities in the entire liver function panel. It should be noted that direct bilirubin is generally readily cleared by the kidney, such that its levels never rise very high even in severe cholestatic disease if the patient has normal renal function. Very rarely, congenital disorders (e.g., Dubin-Johnson and Rotor syndromes) may cause elevations of primarily conjugated bilirubin.

It should be noted that a gray area exists between indirect and direct hyperbilirubinemia. Most authors agree that greater than 50% direct bilirubin indicates direct hyperbilirubinemia whereas less than 30% direct fraction indicates indirect hyperbilirubinemia.[2] For cases where the fraction falls between 30% to 50%, other liver tests and hematologic tests may be required to determine the etiology. Patients with elevated direct bilirubin levels may have some binding of the bilirubin to the albumin, referred to as *delta bilirubin*. This explains delayed resolution of jaundice during recovery from acute hepatobiliary diseases, for while the "free" bilirubin is rapidly metabolized, the bilirubin linked to albumin is metabolized at a much slower rate. Delta bilirubin has a half-life similar to albumin, of 14–21 days.[30,]

HEPATOCELLULAR INJURY

As discussed earlier, the liver is a large organ with diverse biochemical roles, which require its cells to be in close communication with the bloodstream. These properties place the hepatocytes at risk of injury due to a variety of processes. Toxin and drug metabolism produce cascades of metabolic byproducts, some of which may damage hepatocytes. Likewise, the liver plays a central role in the body's biochemical homeostasis, so metabolic disorders tend to involve the liver. Finally, the close relationship of the hepatocytes to the blood supply places them at risk for a variety of infectious agents.

Hepatitis is a term that technically refers to a histologic pattern of inflammation of hepatocytes. It may also be used to refer to a clinical syndrome due to diffuse liver inflammation. The laboratory reflection of hepatitis is a hepatocellular injury pattern, which is marked primarily by elevated aminotransferases.

There are multiple causes of hepatitis. One common type is viral hepatitis, which is classified A, B, C, D (delta hepatitis), E, or G based on the causative virus. These viruses, and the tests for them, are discussed in detail in the Viral Hepatitis section. Less commonly viral hepatitis may be caused by the Epstein-Barr virus, herpes virus, or cytomegalovirus.

Hepatitis may also be caused by various medications, and such drug-induced hepatitis can be either acute or chronic.[28] Some drugs commonly implicated in cellular hepatotoxicity are listed in Table 12-2. In addition, elevation of aminotransferases has been reported in patients receiving heparin.[31] ALT is elevated in up to 60% of these patients, with a mean maximal value of 3.6 times the baseline. A vast number of drugs can cause hepatic injury, especially drugs that are extensively metabolized by the liver. Although numerous drugs may result in aminotransferase elevations, such elevations are usually minor, transient, not associated with any symptoms, and of no clinical consequence.[32]

Perhaps the most common cause of abnormal aminotransferases in ambulatory patients is that of fatty liver. Estimates are that 30% to 40% of adults in the United States have fatty liver, which can vary from hepatic steatosis (fat in the liver) to nonalcoholic steatohepatitis (NASH), where the extra fat in the liver is associated with inflammation. It is potentially serious as up to one-quarter of these patients can progress to cirrhosis. Fatty liver and NASH are mostly related to increased body mass index (BMI), but they can also be associated with rapid weight loss or drugs such as tamoxifen, amiodarone, diltiazem, nifedipine, corticosteroids, and petrochemicals. Fatty liver/NASH can also be seen in hepatitis C and patients on total parenteral nutrition (TPN), and it is associated with hypothyroidism and short bowel syndrome. It is important to note that although mild hepatic inflammation is often of minimal significance, it may signal the presence of a chronic and serious disease process. Some other causes of hepatic inflammation and injury are listed in Table 12-2.

It is often difficult to determine the exact etiology of hepatic inflammation or hepatitis. A careful history—especially for exposure to drugs, alcohol, or toxins—and detailed physical examination are crucial. Additional laboratory studies are usually necessary to distinguish one form of hepatitis from another (Figure 12-4). Radiological testing or liver biopsy may be indicated, not only to determine the etiology of the liver

disease, but also to help determine the indications for (and results of) therapy and prognosis.

Aminotransferases: AST and ALT

AST: 12–38 units/L; ALT: 7–41 units/L (normal values vary from lab to lab but tend to be in the range of <30 units/L for men and <20 units/L for women)

The *aminotransferases* (also known as *transaminases*) are used to assess hepatocellular injury. These enzymes are primarily located inside hepatocytes, where they assist with various metabolic pathways. They are released into the serum in greater quantities when there is hepatocyte damage, and they are very sensitive and may be elevated even with minor levels of hepatocyte damage.[33] However, this renders them relatively nonspecific, and slightly elevated levels may not be clinically significant (particularly in an ill, hospitalized patient who is on many medications and has a variety of active medical problems).

Aminotransferases will often be slightly increased in cholestatic liver diseases, but in this situation they will generally be overshadowed by a greater elevation of cholestatic liver tests (i.e., ALP and total bilirubin to produce a predominantly cholestatic pattern of liver tests). If both transaminases and cholestatic tests are elevated in a similar pattern, it suggests a severe hepatocellular process, which interferes with bile secretion at the level of the hepatocytes. Finally, it should be noted that aminotransferases may rise into the thousands within 24–48 hours following common bile duct obstruction, after which they decline rapidly. This is one instance in which a cholestatic process may transiently cause a hepatocellular injury LFT profile.

Both AST and ALT have half-lives of 17 and 47 hours, respectively, so they reflect *active* hepatocyte damage, and not, for example, damage to hepatocytes that occurred weeks, months, or years previously. This may lead to some counterintuitive relationships between aminotransferase levels and the overall state of the liver. For example, a drop in aminotransferase levels in the setting of acute massive (*fulminant*) hepatitis may reflect a depletion of viable hepatocytes with poor prognosis.[18] Extremely high concentrations (>1000 International Units/L) are usually associated with acute viral hepatitis, severe drug or toxic reactions, or ischemic hepatitis (inadequate blood flow to the liver). Lesser elevations are caused by a vast number of hepatic insults and are less specific.[34]

The ratio of AST to ALT may be of value in diagnosing alcoholic hepatitis, where the AST is generally at least twice the ALT and the AST is rarely above 300 International Units/L. In alcoholic liver disease, a mitochondrial isoform of AST with a relatively long half-life (87 hours) is released from hepatocytes, increasing the AST/ALT ratio. Alcoholic liver disease is also suggested by an elevation in GGT as previously reviewed.

Aspartate aminotransferase is not solely located in hepatocytes but rather is also found in cardiac muscle, skeletal muscle, kidneys, brain, lungs intestines, and erythrocytes. Consequently, AST may be elevated due to a variety of situations including musculoskeletal diseases (e.g., muscular dystrophy,

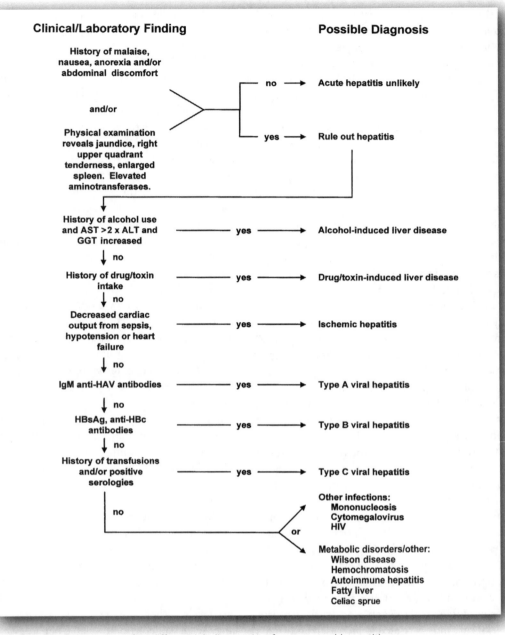

FIGURE 12-4. Algorithm for differential diagnosis of suspected hepatitis.

dermatomyositis, heavy exercise, trichinosis, gangrene, and muscle damage secondary to hypothyroidism), myocardial infarction, renal infarction or failure, brain trauma or cerebral infarction, hemolysis, pulmonary embolism, necrotic tumors, burns, and celiac sprue.[6,7,18] Alanine aminotransferase is more localized to the liver than AST, so it is more specific to liver injury. Elevation of AST without elevation of the ALT or other liver test abnormality suggests cardiac or muscle disease.[17] A muscular origin of aminotransferases may also be indicated by increases in aminotransferases above 300 International Units/L with concomitant increases in serum creatine kinase (CK) activity.[25,35]

Measurement of AST may be affected by a bewildering variety of medications. Almost any prescription drug (as well as various herbal compounds and illegal drugs) can cause an elevation of aminotransferases, and the significance of these elevations is often unclear.[26] Furthermore, the in vitro assay may be confounded by a variety of factors including uremia, hyperlipidemia, and hemolysis.[36] False elevations in the in vitro test may be also seen in patients on acetaminophen, levodopa, methyldopa, tolbutamide, para-aminosalicylic acid, or erythromycin.[8,37,38]

Other factors may interfere with the test's accuracy. Levels may be elevated to 2–3 times normal by vigorous exercise in males and decreased to about half following dialysis.[7] Complexing of AST with immunoglobulin (known as *macro-AST*) may occasionally produce a clinically irrelevant elevation of AST. Testing for macro-AST is not a clinical lab test used in practice. Given the array of factors that can cause an abnormal result, unexplained false positives often occur. In healthy individuals, an isolated elevated ALT returns to normal in repeat studies one-half to one-third of the time.[39] For this reason, prior to an evaluation of mildly elevated aminotransferases in low-risk healthy patients, a practitioner should see either elevation of more than one test (i.e., both AST and ALT) or repeated elevations of a single test.

TESTS ASSOCIATED WITH DETOXIFICATION

Hepatic Encephalopathy

Hepatic encephalopathy refers to a diffuse metabolic dysfunction of the brain that may occur in acute or chronic liver failure. Clinically it ranges from subtle changes in personality to coma and death.

The etiology of hepatic encephalopathy remains controversial and has undergone significant revision recently. Many theories ascribe a major role to ammonia. The majority of serum ammonia enters the blood from the intestines, where it is formed by bacterial catabolism of protein within the gut lumen as well as conversion of serum glutamine into ammonia by enterocytes of the small intestine.[40] Normally, the liver removes >90% of this ammonia via first-pass metabolism.[41] In liver failure, ammonia, along with possibly other toxic substances may avoid this first-pass metabolism and gain immediate access to the brain where it has a variety of toxic effects.[42] While serum ammonia is currently the "standard" lab test for assessing hepatic encephalopathy, other tests are being developed. Elevated serum levels of 3-nitro-tyrosine may be a marker for minimal hepatic encephalopathy (cirrhotic patients with mild cognitive impairment). In a pilot study using a cutoff of 14 nm, 3-nitro-tyrosine levels had a 93% sensitivity and an 89% specificity in identifying these patients.[43]

Ammonia

Normal range[3]: 19–60 mcg/dL

Ammonia levels do not correlate well with hepatic encephalopathy in the setting of chronic liver failure (i.e., patients with cirrhosis). This is likely because hepatic encephalopathy also involves an increase in the permeability of the blood–brain barrier to ammonia.[6,44] There is a large overlap between ammonia levels in patients with and without hepatic encephalopathy among patients with chronic liver disease making this a poor test in this situation.[45] A very high ammonia level (i.e., greater than 250 mcg/dL) is suggestive of hepatic encephalopathy, but most cirrhotic patients suspected of having encephalopathy will have normal or slightly elevated ammonia levels, which adds little diagnostic information. In this situation, hepatic encephalopathy is a clinical diagnosis based on history, physical exam, and exclusion of other possibilities.

Some recent studies have suggested that ammonia may have more significance in the setting of acute liver failure (e.g., due to overwhelming infection of the liver by viral hepatitis). In these patients, the degree of ammonia elevation correlates with severity of hepatic encephalopathy and the likelihood of death, and may be a useful marker for predicting which patients require emergent liver transplant.[46,47]

TABLE 12-6. Groups at Higher Risk of Infection by Various Hepatitis Viruses

Hepatitis A virus

Contacts with infected persons

Daycare workers and attendees

Institutionalized persons

Travelers to countries with high rate of hepatitis A infections

Military personnel

Men who have sex with men

IV drug users

Hepatitis B virus

Contacts of infected persons

Unvaccinated healthcare professionals and morticians

Hemodialysis patients

Male homosexuals

IV drug users

Multipartner heterosexuals

Tattooed/body-pierced persons

Newborns of HBsAg-carrier mothers

Hepatitis C virus

Dialysis patients

Healthcare professionals

IV drug users (primary cause) (even once)

Snorting cocaine

Recipients of clotting factors before 1987

Recipients of transfusion or organ transplant before July 1992

Tattooed/body-pierced persons

Children born to HCV-positive mothers

Hepatitis D virus

Only individuals with chronic HBV infection

Hepatitis E virus

Travelers to Latin America, Egypt, India, and Pakistan

Contacts with infected persons

HBV = hepatitis B virus; HCV = hepatitis c virus; IV = intravenous.

Ammonia concentration may also be elevated in patients with Reye syndrome, inborn disorders of the urea cycle, various medications (most notably valproic acid), impaired renal function, uterosigmoidostomy, or urinary tract infections with bacteria that convert urea to ammonia. In cirrhotic patients or patients with mild liver disease, elevated ammonia and hepatic encephalopathy may be precipitated by such factors as increased dietary protein, GI bleeding, constipation, and *Helicobacter pylori* infection.[7]

VIRAL HEPATITIS

The onset of acute *viral hepatitis* may be quite dramatic and present as an overwhelming infection, or it may pass unnoticed by the patient. In the usual prodromal period, the patient often has a nonspecific flu-like illness that may include nausea,

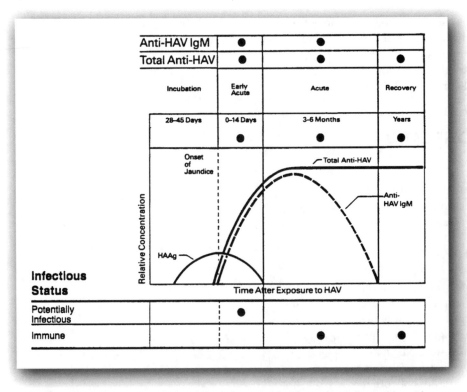

FIGURE 12-5. Temporal relationships of serologies for type A hepatitis with onset of jaundice and infectious status. Anti-HAV IgM is the IgM antibody against the hepatitis A virus. HAAg is the hepatitis A antigen (virus). Total anti-HAV is primarily IgG antibodies (and some IgM in acute phase) against hepatitis A virus. (Adapted with permission from educational material of Abbott Laboratories, North Chicago, IL.)

vomiting, fatigue, or malaise. This period may be followed by clinical hepatitis with jaundice. During this time, the most abnormal laboratory studies are usually the aminotransferases, which can be in the thousands (normal values vary, in range of <30 units/L for men and <20 units/L for women). Bilirubin may be quite elevated, while ALP only mildly so.

The major types of viral hepatitis are reviewed here, but they are often clinically indistinguishable. Thus, serologic studies of antibodies, molecular assays to detect viral genetic material, and knowledge of the epidemiology and risk factors for different viruses (Table 12-6) are central to diagnosis.

Type A Hepatitis

Hepatitis A virus (HAV) is spread primarily by the fecal-oral route by contaminated food or water or by person-to-person contact. It has an incubation period of 3–5 weeks with a several-day prodrome (preicteric phase) before the onset of jaundice and malaise, or the icteric phase. The icteric phase generally lasts 1–3 weeks, although prolonged courses do occur. Hepatitis A is responsible for about 50% of acute hepatitis in the United States (more than all other hepatotropic viruses combined), generally due to person-to-person contact within community-wide outbreaks.[48,49] Interestingly the incidence of new cases has diminished with the wide spread use of the HAV vaccine (see below).

Unlike types B, C, and D hepatitis virus, HAV does not cause chronic disease, and recovery usually occurs within one month. Many patients who get type A hepatitis never become clinically ill. Perhaps 10% of all patients become symptomatic, and only 10% of those patients become jaundiced.[4] The majority of patients have a full recovery, but there is a substantial mortality risk in elderly patients, very young patients, as well as in patients with chronic hepatitis B or C and patients with chronic liver disease of other etiologies.[50-52]

A vaccine for HAV is now available. It is recommended for those traveling to endemic regions (i.e., Central and South America), men who have sex with men, users of street drugs, those with occupational exposure, susceptible patients requiring clotting factors, those from endemic regions, and patients with chronic liver diseases. This vaccine is increasingly being recommended as a universal vaccine for pediatric patients. While this vaccine is generally preferred for postexposure prophylaxis, use of immunoglobulin should be considered in the very young (under 12 months) or patients who cannot use the vaccine.

Presently, the only two tests available measure antibodies to HAV, either immunoglobulin M (IgM) or total (all isotypes of) antibody. Detection of IgM is the more clinically relevant test as it reveals acute or recent infection. These antibodies are present at the onset of jaundice and decline within 12 (usually 6) months.[52] Total antibody, which is comprised of antibody of all isotypes against HAV, indicates present or previous infection or immunization (Figure 12-5).

Type B Hepatitis

Hepatitis B virus (HBV) is a DNA virus spread by bodily fluids, most commonly as a sexually transmitted disease, but also via contaminated needles (as with drug abuse or needle stick accidents), shared razor blades or toothbrushes, nonsterile tattooing or body piercing, blood products, or vertical transmission (transmission from mother to child, generally at birth). This disease is 50–100 times more contagious than HIV. The incubation period of HBV varies from 2–4 months, much longer than that of HAV. Geographically, there is a markedly increased prevalence of hepatitis B in Southeast Asia, China, and sub-Saharan Africa with 10% to 20% of the populations being hepatitis B carriers. In contrast, the incidence of hepatitis B carriers in the United States is approximately 0.5%.

The clinical illness is generally mild and self-limited but can be quite severe. Unfortunately, up to 5% of infected adults and

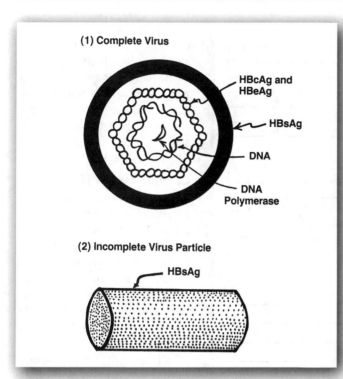

FIGURE 12-6. Hepatitis B virus and its antigenic components. The complete and infectious virus (1), originally known as the *Dane particle,* is composed of the outer layer (HBsAg) and inner nucleocapsid core. The inner core is comprised of HBcAg intermeshed with HBeAg and encapsulates the viral DNA. HBeAg may be an internal component or degradation product of the nucleocapsid core. An incomplete and noninfectious form (2) is composed exclusively of HBsAg and is cylindrical in shape.

90% of infected neonates develop a chronic illness. Chronic HBV infection is often mild but may progress to cirrhosis, liver failure, or hepatocellular carcinoma, thereby contributing to premature death in 15% to 25% of cases.[53]

Viral Antigens and Their Antibodies

Three HBV antigens and antibody systems are relevant to diagnosis and management (HBsAg, HBcAg, and HBeAg). The HBV surface antigen (HBsAg) is present on the outer surface of the virus, and neutralizing antibodies directed against this protein (anti-HBs) are central to natural and vaccine-induced immunity (Figure 12-6).

Neither the core protein (HBcAg) nor the e antigen (HBeAg) are on the surface of the virion, and thus antibodies against these antigens are not protective. Nevertheless, antibodies are directed against these proteins and may serve as markers of infection. Of these antigens, only HBsAg and HBeAg can be detected in the serum by conventional techniques.[53] HBsAg is detected for a greater window of time during infection and reveals active infection. Detection of HBeAg indicates large amounts of circulating hepatitis B virus; these patients are 5–10 times more likely to transmit the virus than are HBeAg

TABLE 12-7. Interpretation of Common Hepatitis B Serological Test Results

HBsAg	ANTI-HBs	ANTI-HBc	INTERPRETATION
Positive	Negative	Positive	Acute infection or chronic hepatitis B
Negative	Positive	Positive	Resolving hepatitis B or previous infection
Negative	Positive	Negative	Resolving or recovered hepatitis B or patient after vaccination

negative persons. HBsAg levels are often used to determine a given patient's suitability for hepatitis B therapy, and subsequently to monitor for effectiveness of hepatitis B therapy.

In response to infection with HBV, the body may produce antibodies to the antigens: antisurface antibody (anti-HBs), anticore antibody (anti-HBc), and anti-e antibody (anti-HBe). All of these antibodies can be detected in clinical laboratories, and in the case of anti-HBcAg separate tests are available to detect IgM or total antibody (all isotypes). Anti-HBs is associated with resolved type B hepatitis, or patients who have responded to vaccination for HBV. Anti-HBc is a bit more challenging to interpret, as it can be seen in acute type B hepatitis, after recovery from type B hepatitis (often in concert with Anti-HBs), in chronic infection (often with HBsAg, and HBeAg), and there can be false-positive results as well. As shown in Table 12-7 and Figure 12-7, levels of antigens and antibodies show complex patterns in the course of HBV infection and thus can yield considerable information about the infection's course and chronology (Table 12-7).

In addition to serological tests, sensitive molecular assays may be used to detect HBV DNA, revealing active viral replication in either acute or chronic infection.[55] These assays may be useful for early detection, as in screening blood donors, since DNA is detectible an average of 25 days before seroconversion.[49] Additionally, some assays allow the quantification of serum viral load, which may be used in the decision to treat and, subsequently, monitor therapy. Presently eight genotypes of HBV have been identified and identification of these genotypes can be of real value in terms of determining appropriate therapy for chronic infection. For example genotype A, most prevalent in the United States, seems to respond better to interferon than the others, and patients with this genotype might benefit from starting with interferon as opposed to the oral agents available. Genotype C is more prevalent in Asia. For the details of these assays (PCR, RNA:DNA hybrid capture assay, nucleic acid cross-linking assay, and branched DNA assay), the reader is referred to a recent review by Pawlotsky et al.[56]

Acute Type B Hepatitis

HBsAg titers usually develop within 4–12 weeks of infection and may be seen even before elevation of aminotransferases or clinical symptoms (see Figure 12-7). Subsequently, HBsAg levels decline as anti-HBs titers develop, which indicates resolution of the acute symptomatic infection and development

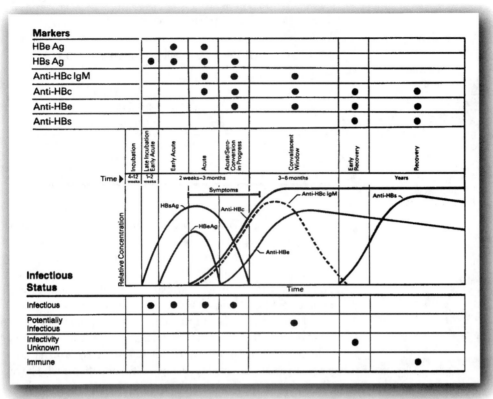

FIGURE 12-7. Serological profile, including temporal relationships integrated with infectious status and symptoms, in 75% to 85% of patients with acute type B hepatitis. (Adapted with permission from educational material of Abbott Laboratories, North Chicago, IL.)

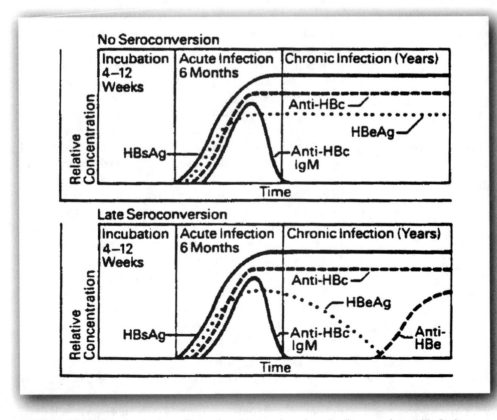

FIGURE 12-8. Serological profiles of patients who chronically carry hepatitis B virus. (Reproduced with permission from Abbott Laboratories, North Chicago, IL.)

of immunity. In between the decline of HBsAg and the rise of anti-HBs, there is often a window when neither is present during which time anti-HBcAg may be used to diagnose infection. IgM anti-HBcAg may be used to reveal acute infection as opposed to a flare of chronic HBV.[55]

Chronic Type B Hepatitis

Chronic hepatitis is defined as persistently elevated LFTs for 6 months. The development of chronic hepatitis B is suggested by the persistence of elevated LFTs (aminotransferases) and is supported by persistence of HBsAg for more than 6 months after acute infection. Persistence of HBeAg also suggests chronic infection, but some chronically infected patients produce anti-HBeAg and, subsequently, clear HBeAg well after the acute phase is over (late seroconversion; see Figure 12-8). Clearance of the HBeAg is associated with a decrease in viral DNA, and some degree of remission in chronic hepatitis B. This, however, can be confusing as HBeAg is a precore protein, and in patients infected with certain mutations developed during the course of the disease (precore and core promoter) HBeAg may not be produced. Yet even in the face of anti-HBe, there may be active disease with ongoing fibrosis and development of cirrhosis. Although chronically infected individuals usually lack anti-HBsAg, in some cases low levels of non-neutralizing antibodies may be present. Additionally, low levels of IgM anti-HBcAg may persist.[48]

Hepatitis B Vaccine

The *HBV vaccine* consists of recombinant HBsAg, which is not infectious, and it stimulates the production of protective anti-HBs. Generally, this is a safe vaccine, with efficacy of over 90%. It is indicated for people at high risk of acquiring type B hepatitis or its complications including neonates of mothers with hepatitis B, men who have sex with men, injection drug abusers, dialysis patients, healthcare workers, HIV patients, family and household contacts of patients with type B hepatitis, sexually active people with multiple partners, and patients with chronic liver disease. More recent efforts, especially in endemic countries, are leading to this being accepted as a universal vaccine. This vaccine, for example, is often required for students in the United States before entering public school. A vaccine product directed against both HAV and HBV is available. In analyzing serologic data, successful vaccination may be distinguished from previous infection by the presence of anti-HBs and absence of antibodies against other antigens (e.g., HBcAg, HBeAg). Testing for antibodies after vaccination is not generally recommended, with exceptions including healthcare workers, dialysis patients, spouses or sexual partners of infected patients. If these individuals test negative for the antibody to HBV, they should receive a second series of vaccine doses. While some patients will fail to develop antibodies for a number of reasons, including anergy, if antibody tests are negative after the second vaccine series the patient should be evaluated for the possibility of occult HBV infection. The vaccine has a prolonged duration of action. Routine booster injections are not recommended except, perhaps, for dialysis patients when their titers of anti-HBs are less than 10 International Units/L.

Type C Hepatitis

Hepatitis C virus (HCV) is an RNA virus mainly spread parenterally, although it may also be transmitted vertically and sexually.[54] While 70% to 80% of acute infections are asymptomatic, 70% to 80% of patients develop chronic disease.[49] Given the mildness of the acute attack and the tendency to develop into chronic hepatitis, it is understandable why many patients with this disease first present decades later with cirrhosis or more commonly chronic elevations of aminotransferases. Because chronic HCV infection is often asymptomatic and LFTs may be normal or intermittently elevated, it is recommended that patients at high risk for HCV be screened appropriately. Patients for whom screening would be appropriate include those with a history of illegal drug use, including snorting cocaine, as well as parenteral drug abuse. Additionally patients who received clotting factors before 1987 or blood products or organ transplants before July 1992, and patients with a history of hemodialysis should be screened.

Acute hepatitis C is often asymptomatic, and when symptoms are present they are mild. Diagnosis of acute hepatitis C, however, is important as evidence suggests that prompt treatment with antiviral medications can prevent progression to chronic hepatitis C in a majority of cases.

In chronic hepatitis C infection, the LFTs are usually minimally elevated with ALT and AST values commonly in the 60–100 International Units/L range. These values can fluctuate and occasionally return to normal for a year or more, only to rebound when next checked.[57] The primary clinical concern in chronic HCV is that if untreated, within 20 years 20% to 30%

of patients develop cirrhosis and 1% to 5% develop hepatocellular carcinoma.[49]

The first screening test used is often an ELISA (also referred to as *anti-HCV*), which detects antibodies against a cocktail of HCV antigens. Positive tests can be seen in patients who have passively acquired these antibodies (but not the infection), as in after transfusions, or children of mothers with hepatitis C. Due to possible cross-reactivity with one of the antigens in the assay, this test has a considerable false-positive rate, and thus positive results need to be confirmed with a more specific assay. One such assay is the recombinant immunoblot assay (RIBA), which is similar to ELISA in principle, but tests antibody reactivity to a panel of antigens individually. Binding to two or more antigens is considered a positive test.[51] Binding to one antigen is considered indeterminate. Presently the approach to a positive ELISA is to skip the RIBA and go directly to the reverse transcriptase polymerase chain reaction (RT-PCR) assay.

Qualitative RT-PCR, often referred to as just *PCR*, detects viral RNA in the blood. It is a very sensitive assay that may be used in diagnosis and subsequent management of hepatitis C. RT-PCR has several advantages compared to serologic tests. It can detect HCV within 1–2 weeks of exposure and weeks before seroconversion, symptoms, or the elevation of LFTs. This may be useful because seroconversion has only occurred in 70% to 80% of patients at the onset of symptoms, and it may never occur in immunosuppressed patients.[57] Additionally there is now evidence suggesting that treating acute hepatitis C may be of value. Some immunocompromised patients with hepatitis C (as above) may have false-negative ELISA studies, and thus the PCR is recommended for consideration in patients with hepatitis or chronic liver disease who are immunosuppressed. Furthermore, unlike serologic assays, RT-PCR is not confounded by passively acquired antibodies that may be present in uninfected infants or recipients of blood products, and RT-PCR can distinguish between resolved and chronic infection.

Once a diagnosis of HCV infection is established, various quantitative molecular assays that monitor viral load may be useful in following viral titers during treatment or assessing likelihood of response to therapy. A major consideration with these tests is that the methodology is not yet standardized, and there is lab-to-lab variability. These tests are not preferred for initial diagnosis since they are less sensitive than qualitative RT-PCR. They include a quantitative PCR assay and a branched-chain DNA assay (for more information, see Pawlotsky et al.).[56] Presently most labs report HCV PCR measurements in International Units/mL, with pretreatment levels often in the millions.

There are at least six major genotypes of the type C virus and multiple subtypes. Viral genotype determination is useful since genotype is known to affect the likelihood of response to certain treatments. Additionally, while the treatment for the most common genotypes found in the United States (type 1) is 1 year in duration, current recommendations suggest that some other genotypes (notably type 2 or 3) can be successfully treated with only 6 months of therapy. As newer therapies become available, length of treatment may vary depending not only on genotype but on the rapidity of a patient's response to therapy.[58] Presently two protease inhibitors are approved for treatment of hepatitis C, when used in conjunction with ribavirin-interferon therapy, telaprevir and boceprevir. Genotype determination may be done via direct sequencing or hybridization of PCR amplification products.[57]

Type D Hepatitis

Hepatitis D virus (HDV) is caused by a defective virus that requires the presence of hepatitis B surface antigen (HBsAg) to cause infection. Therefore, people can only contract type D hepatitis concomitantly with HBV infection (coinfection) or if chronically infected with HBV (superinfection). Coinfection presents as an acute infection that may be more severe than HBV infection alone.[49] Alternatively, the picture of superinfection is that of a patient, with known or unknown chronic HBV, who develops an acute flare with worsening liver function and increases in HBsAg.[51] Acute coinfection is usually self-limited with rare development of chronic hepatitis, while superinfection becomes chronic in more than 75% of cases and increases the risk of negative sequelae such as cirrhosis. Transmission of HDV is generally by parenteral routes, although no obvious cause can be determined in some cases.

Testing for HDV is usually only indicated in known cases of HBV infection. The single, widely available assay detects anti-HDV antibodies of all isotypes (Figure 12-9). This test is unable to distinguish between acute, chronic, or resolved infection and lacks sensitivity since only about 38% of infected patients have detectible anti-HDV within the first 2 weeks of illness.[55] Because seroconversion may occur as late as 3 months after infection, testing may be repeated if the clinical picture suggests HDV.[48] Tests are also available for HDV RNA, and stains are available to assess the D antigen in hepatocytes.

Type E Hepatitis

Hepatitis E virus (HEV) is generally quite similar to hepatitis A. It is a hardy, protein-coated RNA virus that is spread via a fecal-oral route often by contaminated food or water. Like HAV, HEV causes an acute illness that is generally self-limited, and HEV is endemic in parts of Asia. It is becoming increasingly recognized in the United States. Unlike HAV, HEV is notable

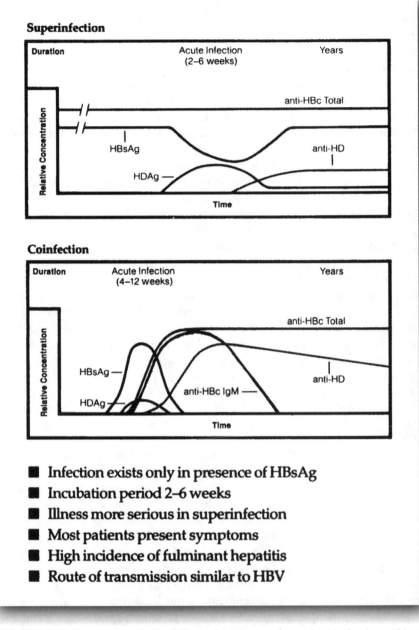

- ■ **Infection exists only in presence of HBsAg**
- ■ **Incubation period 2–6 weeks**
- ■ **Illness more serious in superinfection**
- ■ **Most patients present symptoms**
- ■ **High incidence of fulminant hepatitis**
- ■ **Route of transmission similar to HBV**

FIGURE 12-9. Two serological profiles of patients infected with the hepatitis D virus. HDAg = hepatitis D antigen (the virus); anti-HD = antibodies against hepatitis D virus. (Reproduced with permission from Abbott Laboratories, North Chicago, IL.)

for a predilection for causing life-threatening illness in women who are in their third trimester of pregnancy. Recently, testing for antibodies to hepatitis E has become available, including HEVAg, or hepatitis E antigen. Work is underway to develop a vaccine for hepatitis E.

Primary Biliary Cirrhosis

Primary biliary cirrhosis (PBC) is a chronic disease involving progressive destruction of small intrahepatic bile ducts leading to cholestasis and progressive fibrosis over a period of decades. It can progress to cirrhosis and liver failure, necessitating transplantation. Ninety percent of affected individuals are female,

TABLE 12-8. Selected Drugs That May Cause Pancreatitis

5-ASA drugs[a]	Nitrofurantoin
Asparaginase	Pentamidine
Atypical antipsychotics	Ranitidine
Azathioprine	Sitagliptin
Cimetidine	Statins
Didanosine	Steroids
Estrogens	Sulfonamides
Exenatide	Sulindac
Furosemide	Tetracycline
Isoniazid	Thiazides
Mercaptopurine	Valproic acid
Methyldopa	
Metronidazole	

[a]5-ASA drugs refers to 5-aminosalicylic acid agents (e.g., olsalazine, mesalamine, and sulfasalazine).

with onset occurring between the early twenties and late eighties.[59,60] The etiology of the disease is unknown, although it seems to involve an autoimmune component, and has associations with a variety of autoimmune disorders including Sjögren syndrome, rheumatoid arthritis, and scleroderma. The initial symptoms of the disease are often those of progressive cholestasis with fatigue, pruritus, jaundice, and deficiencies in fat-soluble vitamins.[60]

The most useful laboratory test in diagnosing PBC is the detection of antimitochondrial antibody (AMA), with a sensitivity of 95%.[61] This assay is also highly specific, although patients with autoimmune and drug-induced hepatitis occasionally have low antibody titers. PBC usually presents with a predominantly cholestatic laboratory picture, initially with an elevated ALP and GGT, and later, with an elevated bilirubin. Aminotransferases tend to be minimally elevated or normal.

TESTS TO ASSESS PANCREATIC INFLAMMATION/PANCREATITIS

Pancreatitis describes inflammation of the pancreas (either acute or chronic) and is the most common disease associated with this gland. Although there are multiple causes of pancreatitis, the clinical presentation is often the same. Acute pancreatitis generally presents with severe midepigastric abdominal pain developing over an hour, often radiating to the back. The pain tends to be continuous and can last for several days.

This condition is often associated with nausea and vomiting; in severe cases, fever, ileus, and hypotension can occur. Ultimately, there can be progressive anemia, hypocalcemia, hypoglycemia, hypoxia, renal failure, and death. The clinician faces the challenge of rapidly establishing this diagnosis, because many conditions (e.g., ulcers, biliary disease, myocardial infarction, and intestinal ischemia or perforation) can present in a similar manner. Most individuals with acute pancreatitis can make full recoveries; however, the long-term inflammation associated with chronic pancreatitis can lead to fibrosis and calcification of the pancreas causing irreversible damage, occasionally leading to the development of diabetes mellitus or

malabsorption due to deficiencies in the production of pancreatic enzymes.

Gallstones and alcohol abuse are causative factors in 60% to 80% of acute pancreatitis cases.[62] Medications can also cause acute pancreatitis (Table 12-8). Other possible causes include autoimmune diseases, trauma (a typical example being an injury due to a bicycle handlebar), penetrating ulcers, hypercalcemia, hypertriglyceridemia, pancreatic neoplasm, and hereditary or autoimmune pancreatitis. Often, however, it is impossible to determine the definite cause of a patient's attack.

The tests discussed in this section, amylase and lipase, are primarily used to diagnose pancreatitis, although they may be clinically useful in the diagnosis of other pathologies.

Amylase

Normal range: 20–96 units/L (method dependent)
Amylase helps break starch into its individual glucose molecules. The enzyme's most frequent clinical use is in the diagnosis of acute and chronic pancreatitis. While amylase levels are often used for this diagnosis, increasingly lipase (see below) is preferred in part due to the longer half-life of the latter.

As with any serum protein, concentrations result from the balance between entry into circulation and rate of clearance. Most circulating amylase originates from the pancreas and salivary glands. These sources are responsible for approximately 40% and 60% of serum amylase, respectively. However, the enzyme is also found in the lungs, liver, fallopian tubes, ovary, testis, small intestine, skeletal muscle, adipose tissue, thyroid, tonsils, and certain cancers, and various pathologies may increase secretion from these sources. The kidneys are responsible for about 25% of the metabolic clearance, with the remaining extrarenal mechanisms being poorly understood. The serum half-life is between 1–2 hours.[63,64] Patients with azotemia can have decreased amylase clearance, and elevated amylase levels. More than half of the patients who have a creatinine clearance between 13–39 mL/min have elevated amylase levels.[65] Although there is no amylase activity in neonates and only small amounts at 2–3 months of age, concentrations increase to the normal adult range by 1 year.

Amylase concentrations rise within 2–6 hours after the onset of acute pancreatitis and peak after 12–30 hours if the underlying inflammation has not recurred. In uncomplicated disease, these concentrations frequently return to normal within 3–5 days. More prolonged, mild elevations occur in up to 10% of patients with pancreatitis and may indicate ongoing pancreatic inflammation or associated complications (e.g., pancreatic pseudocyst).

Although serum amylase concentrations do not correlate with disease severity or prognosis, a higher amylase may indicate a greater likelihood that the patient has pancreatitis.[66] For example, serum amylase concentrations may increase up to 25 times the upper limit of normal in acute pancreatitis while elevations from opiate-induced spasms of the sphincter of Oddi generally are less than 2–10 times the upper limit of normal. Unfortunately, the magnitude of enzyme elevation can overlap in these situations, and ranges are not very specific.

MINICASE 1

A Case of a Prolonged PT and Low Serum Albumin

JANE M., A 50-YEAR-OLD WOMAN, presented to her physician complaining of increasing fatigue and a 20-lb weight loss over the past 4 months. Initial evaluation showed an albumin of 2 g/dL (4.0–5.0 g/dL) and a PT of 18 seconds (12.7–15.4 seconds). Jane M. was referred for evaluation of possible cirrhosis. On further questioning, she denied any history of hepatitis, exposure to hepatotoxins, alcohol use, family history of liver disease, or liver disease.

Jane M.'s physical examination did not suggest liver disease; there was no evidence of ascites, palmar erythema, asterixis, hepatomegaly, splenomegaly, or spider angiomata. It was noted that she had pedal edema. Liver function studies were otherwise normal: ALT, 12 International Units/L (7–41 International Units/L); AST, 20 International Units/L (12–38 International Units/L); total bilirubin, 1 mg/dL (0.3–1.3 mg/dL); and ALP, 56 International Units/L (33–96 International Units/L).

An IM dose of vitamin K 10 mg corrected the PT (12 seconds) within 48 hours. Workup showed that Jane M. had malabsorption due to sprue, a disease of the small bowel. With proper dietary management, her symptoms resolved and she gained weight. At a followup visit 3 weeks later, her albumin concentration was 3.7 g/dL and her edema had resolved.

Question: Why did Jane M. develop a low albumin and a prolonged PT? What caused her pedal edema?

Discussion: This case demonstrates that while low albumin and a prolonged PT suggest advanced liver disease, other causes need to be considered. Administration of vitamin K promptly corrected Jane M.'s PT, suggesting malabsorption of vitamin K. If she had had cirrhosis, her PT would not have corrected with the vitamin K. Similarly, her hypoalbuminemia was not due to her liver's inability to synthesize albumin but to the malabsorptive disorder that was interfering with protein absorption. Therefore, Jane M. had a low albumin and elevated PT in the absence of liver disease. Her pedal edema was due to hypoalbuminemia secondary to malabsorption.

MINICASE 2

Jaundice Due to Oral Contraceptives

AMBER S., A 16-YEAR-OLD, was found by her pediatrician to be slightly jaundiced during a routine school physical. She denied any history of liver disease, abdominal pain, illicit drug abuse, alcohol use, or abdominal trauma. Lab evaluation showed a moderately elevated bilirubin of 2.3 mg/dL (0.3–1.3 mg/dL) along with ALP and GGT concentrations of about 4 times normal. Her AST was 23 International Units/L (12–38 International Units/L).

Amber S. denied being on any medications (except for vitamins), or being exposed to toxins. Nothing suggested the possibility of a neoplastic or infectious process (temperature of 98.9°F [37.2°C] and WBC count of 7.5 x 10³ cells/mm³ [3.54–9.06 x 10³ cells/mm³]). Ultrasound of the liver and biliary system was normal, with no evidence of biliary dilation.

Her parents then took her to a pediatric hepatologist. After much discussion (and threat of a liver biopsy), Amber S. tearfully revealed that she had gone to a local family planning clinic and was using birth control pills.

Question: How might oral contraceptives cause a cholestatic picture? What was the importance of the ultrasound? What is the usual outcome of patients who develop jaundice while taking oral contraceptives?

Discussion: This case demonstrates that oral contraceptives, primarily because of their estrogen content, can cause alterations in cholestatic test results (manifested by an elevated bilirubin, GGT, and ALP) with relatively normal aminotransferases. The ultrasound helped to distinguish between intra- and extrahepatic cholestasis. The absence of biliary dilation suggested intrahepatic cholestasis. The normal AST suggested that jaundice was not due to hepatitis.

Amylase has a relatively low sensitivity, with about 20% of patients with acute pancreatitis having normal levels. This is especially common in patients with alcoholic pancreatitis or pancreatitis due to hypertriglyceridemia. Additionally, amylase has relatively low specificity and may be elevated in a wide range of conditions. These include a variety of diseases of the pancreas, salivary glands, GI tract (including hepatobiliary injury, perforated peptic ulcer, and intestinal obstruction or infarction), and gynecologic system (e.g., ovarian or fallopian cysts), as well as pregnancy, trauma, renal failure, various neoplasms, and diabetic ketoacidosis. Additionally, alcohol and a variety of medications (including but not limited to: aspirin, cholinergics, thiazide diuretics, and oral contraceptives, may also cause increased values.[67] In diagnosing acute pancreatitis, other useful laboratory tests include lipase (since it is confounded by fewer factors) and fractionation of serum amylase into pancreatic and salivary isoenzymes (although its utility has been questioned).[68,69]

Another condition that may cause elevated amylase concentrations is macroamylasemia, a benign condition present in 2% to 5% of patients with hyperamylasemia.[70] In this condition, amylase molecules are bound by immunoglobulins or complex polysaccharides, forming aggregates that are too large to enter the glomerular filtrate and be cleared by the kidneys. This results in serum concentrations up to 10 times the normal limit.[71] Macroamylasemia can be detected by fractionating serum amylase or by measuring urine amylase.

Urine amylase concentrations (normal range: <32 International Units for 2-hour collection or <384 International Units for 24-hour collection) usually peak later than serum concentrations, and elevations may persist for 7–10 days. This is useful if a patient is hospitalized after acute symptoms have subsided at which point serum amylase may already have returned to normal, leaving only urinary amylase to indicate pancreatitis. As discussed below, lipase may also persist after serum amylase levels decline. Urine amylase levels may also be useful in revealing macroamylasemia, in which case serum amylase is elevated while urinary amylase is normal or decreased.[69] However, this pattern of elevated serum amylase without elevated urinary amylase is also consistent with renal failure.

One cause of amylase's relatively low sensitivity is that marked hypertriglyceridemia may cause amylase measurements to be artificially low, masking an elevation in serum amylase. This finding is clinically relevant since hypertriglyceridemia (>800 mg/dL) is a potential cause of acute pancreatitis. Fortunately, however, urinary amylase and serum lipase would typically be abnormal in this situation. Additionally in this situation, one can serially dilute the serum ultimately finding elevated amylase values.

Lipase

Normal range: 3–43 units/L

Lipase is an enzyme secreted by the pancreas that is transported from the pancreatic duct into the duodenum where it aids in fat digestion. Lipase catalyzes the hydrolysis of triglycerides into fatty acids and glycerol, simpler lipids which are more readily absorbed and transported throughout the body. Although mostly secreted by the pancreas, lipase can also be found in the tongue, esophagus, stomach, small intestine, leukocytes, adipose tissue, lung, breast milk, and liver. In healthy individuals, serum lipase tends to be mostly of pancreatic origin.[72]

Lipase initially parallels amylase levels in acute pancreatitis, increasing rapidly and peaking at 12–30 hours. However, lipase has a half-life of 7–14 hours so that it declines much more slowly, typically returning to normal after 8–14 days. Thus, one utility of lipase (similar to urinary amylase) is the detection of acute pancreatitis roughly 3 or more days after onset at which point amylase levels may no longer be elevated. As with amylase, peak lipase concentrations typically range from 3–5 times the upper limit of the reference range.

A comparison of the sensitivity and specificity of amylase versus lipase, and the utility of these tests alone or in combination remains under debate. This issue is complicated by the fact that the sensitivity and specificity of any laboratory test vary depending on where the cutoff is chosen (e.g., choosing a higher cutoff increases specificity at the cost of lower sensitivity). In general, serum lipase appears to be superior, particularly with respect to specificity.[68-70,73-75] However, simultaneous determination of both lipase and amylase may increase overall specificity because different factors confound the different assays.[76] For example, an elevated amylase with a normal lipase suggests amylase of salivary origin, or may represent macroamylasemia. Similarly, an elevated lipase with normal amylase has been shown to often not be due to pancreatitis, although in the case of pancreatitis it could be caused by delayed laboratory evaluation or artificial lowering of amylase levels by hypertriglyceridemia.[77]

Lipase concentrations may be elevated in patients with nonpancreatic abdominal pain such as a ruptured abdominal aortic aneurysm, and a variety of disorders of the alimentary tract and liver such as intestinal infarction. This is because lipase is located in these organs. Renal failure, nephrolithiasis,

---

MINICASE 3

A 36-Year-Old Executive with Abnormal LFTs

DANA D., A 36-YEAR-OLD EXECUTIVE, was referred to a prominent medical center for a second opinion. Her physician had found an elevated AST of 180 International Units/L (12–38 International Units/L) on a routine screening exam. Dana D. had no symptoms; her physical examination had been normal, without any signs of liver disease or hepatomegaly.

Additional studies showed an ALT of 60 International Units/L (7–41 International Units/L), a markedly elevated GGT of 380 International Units/L (9–58 International Units/L), and a minimally elevated ALP of 91 International Units/L (33–96 International Units/L). Her WBC count was elevated at 20×10^3 cells/mm^3 (3.54–9.06×10^3 cells/mm^3). After much discussion, she revealed that she was drinking 1 pint of vodka a day.

Dana D. then enrolled in Alcoholics Anonymous and stopped drinking. Three months later, all of her tests were normal: ALT, 28 International Units/L; GGT, 54 International Units/L; and ALP, 54 International Units/L.

Question: What findings suggested alcoholic liver disease? Why did all of Dana D.'s lab test results return to normal? What else might have happened in this situation?

Discussion: This case demonstrates several aspects of alcoholic liver disease. The diagnosis was suggested by an elevated AST out of proportion to the ALT, as well as by a markedly elevated GGT with a normal (or virtually so) ALP. An elevated MCV, if present, also would have supported this diagnosis. Patients with alcoholic liver disease may have markedly elevated WBC counts.

Alcoholic liver disease tends to have several different stages. The earliest manifestation may be just a "fatty liver," which is generally reversible with cessation of alcohol intake. Alcoholic hepatitis and cirrhosis can follow with excessive alcohol intake. Unfortunately, alcoholic cirrhosis can develop without any warning signs. If Dana D. had alcoholic cirrhosis, stopping alcohol consumption probably would not have significantly altered her abnormal test results.

Clinicians should remember that a patient does not need to be a "skid row" alcoholic to develop alcoholic cirrhosis. Women are more susceptible to the hepatotoxic effects of alcohol than are men, and as few as two or three drinks a day can cause significant liver disease in susceptible persons, this being due to metabolizing differences.

---

diabetic ketoacidosis, and alcoholism are conditions where lipase elevations tend to be present; however usually in concentrations less than 3 times the upper limit of the reference range. Drug-induced elevations in lipase can be attributed to certain opioids (codeine, morphine), NSAIDs (indomethacin), and cholinergics (methacholine and bethanechol).[67] In the condition of macrolipasemia, similar to macroamylasemia but far less frequent, macromolecular complexes of lipase to

MINICASE 4

A Jaundiced College Student

JACOB N., A 19-YEAR-OLD COLLEGE STUDENT, anxiously reported to the infirmary when his girlfriend noticed that he was becoming yellow. He felt well and had a normal physical examination. On discussion, he indicated that he had recently embarked on a rigorous crash diet in anticipation of winter break in Florida.

Evaluation showed an elevated total bilirubin of 4.8 mg/dL (0.3–1.3 mg/dL), of which 90% was unconjugated (4.3 mg/dL). The absence of hemolysis was established by microscopic examination of a blood smear, normal reticulocyte count, and LDH, which was 112 International Units/L (115–221 International Units/L). Jacob N.'s other LFTs were normal: ALT, 21 International Units/L (7–41 International Units/L); and ALP, 76 International Units/L (33–96 International Units/L).

Question: What was the most likely cause of Jacob N.'s signs and symptoms? How should his condition be managed? What is his prognosis?

Discussion: Elevated bilirubin concentrations do not necessarily indicate severe liver disease. The normal ALT and ALP ruled out hepatocellular and cholestatic liver diseases. If done, AST would have been normal. The normal LDH, RBC microscopic exam, and reticulocyte count ruled out hemolysis as a cause of the elevated bilirubin. The normal LDH was also consistent with a lack of intrinsic liver disease.

Jacob N. should be reassured that he has Gilbert syndrome and might become somewhat jaundiced with fasting or acute or chronic illness. Gilbert syndrome is not associated with any symptoms, is totally benign, and requires no treatment. When a patient has an elevated bilirubin, a practitioner should always obtain LFTs before either providing a diagnosis or performing unnecessary tests.

immunoglobulin prevent excretion and elevate serum lipase concentrations.[78]

Cholestasis from oral contraceptives is generally benign and reverses promptly when the medication is withdrawn. Patients often omit mentioning their use of birth control pills.

Other Test Results in Pancreatitis

In severe cases of acute pancreatitis, occasionally several days after the insult, fat necrosis may result in the formation of *organic soaps* that bind calcium. Serum calcium concentrations then decrease (low albumin may also contribute), sometimes enough to cause tetany. When pancreatitis is of biliary tract origin, typical elevations in ALP, bilirubin, AST, and ALT are seen. Some researchers believe that in acute pancreatitis an increase of ALT to 3 times baseline or higher is relatively specific for gallstone-induced pancreatitis.[79]

Pancreatitis also may be associated with hemoconcentration and subsequent elevations of the BUN or hematocrit. Depending on the severity of the attack, lactic acidosis, azotemia, anemia, hyperglycemia, hypoalbuminemia, and hypoxemia also may occur.

Despite the performance of amylase and lipase assays for acute pancreatitis, the sensitivity and specificity of these tests are often regarded as unsatisfactory, and in some patients pancreatitis is only diagnosed on autopsy. For this reason, several new tests have been investigated (e.g., serum trypsin and trypsinogen), although they are not yet widely available.[75,80] Ultimately it is recognized that the lack of sensitivity for both amylase and lipase implies that these tests can be used to support a diagnosis of acute pancreatitis, but may not definitively provide a secure diagnosis, particularly if the levels are not dramatically elevated.[64] A CT scan or an MRI may be of value in demonstrating pancreatitis (or excluding other processes) when serum markers are not helpful.

ULCER DISEASE

Up to 10% of the U.S. population will develop *ulcers* at some point in life. For many decades ulcers were believed to be primarily due to acid. Traditional therapy with antacids, histamine$_2$-antagonists, and proton pump inhibitors has been effective in treating ulcers, but are not as effective in preventing recurrences.

Helicobacter Pylori

Helicobacter pylori has been identified as a cause of ulcer disease, and studies into its detection and treatment are still in a state of rapid development. *H. pylori* is a gram-negative bacillus, usually acquired during childhood, that establishes lifelong colonization of the gastric epithelium in affected individuals. Transmission seems to be via a fecal-oral or oral-oral route. Prevalence increases with age and correlates with poor sanitation.[81] In developed countries up to 40% to 50% of people harbor these bacteria by the age of 50, whereas in developing countries the prevalence is over 90% by this age.[82]

H. pylori infection may be found in more than 90% of patients with duodenal ulcers and more than 80% of patients with gastric ulcers.[86] Furthermore, the bacterium has been associated with the development of antral gastritis, gastric cancer, and certain types of gastric lymphoma.[83-85] It has not been associated with nonulcer dyspepsia. The most common lymphoma associated with *H. pylori* is referred to as *MALT* (*mucosa-associated lymphoid tissue*) and is often curable just by treating the underlying *H. pylori* infection. However, most infected individuals (>70%) are asymptomatic, and eradication therapy is not a standard recommendation for asymptomatic colonization.[82] From the other perspective, *H. pylori*-infected individuals have a 10% to 20% chance of developing peptic ulcers and a 1% to 2% chance of developing gastric cancer during their lifetime.[87] Routine screening for *H. pylori* is recommended in those with active ulcer disease, history of ulcer disease, and certain gastric lymphomas. It should be considered prior to long-term therapy with NSAIDs. One problem in managing patients with *H. pylori* infection is that treatment is not always successful in eradicating this bacterium, in part due to increasing resistance to antibiotics. In the United States rates of resistance to metronidazole (20% to 40%) and clarithromycin (10% to 15%) have been documented.[88]

MINICASE 5

Hepatic Encephalopathy

STEPHEN F., A 47-YEAR-OLD ALCOLHOLIC, was admitted after being found on a park bench surrounded by empty beer bottles. Known to have cirrhosis, Stephen F. was thought to be showing signs of hepatic encephalopathy as he slowly lapsed into a deep coma over the first 4 days of hospitalization. His physical examination was significant in that he had hepatomegaly and splenomegaly.

Lab evaluation showed a negative urine drug screen for central nervous system (CNS) depressants with serum glucose mildy elevated at 120 mg/dL. All serum electrolytes also were normal: sodium, 140 mEq/L; potassium, 4 mEq/L; chloride, 98 mEq/L; carbon dioxide, 25 mEq/L; and magnesium, 1.5 mEq/L. Stephen F.'s blood alcohol concentration on admission was 150 (normal: 0). His serum GGT was 321 International Units/L (9–58 International Units/L), and his AST was 87 International Units/L (12–38 International Units/L).

Unfortunately, efforts at treating hepatic encephalopathy did not reverse his coma. When it was noted that his ammonia concentration was normal at 48 mcg/dL (19–60 mcg/dL), further examination and testing were undertaken. A large bruise was then noticed on the side of Stephen F.'s head, and a CT scan revealed a large subdural hematoma. With surgical treatment of the hematoma, he promptly awoke and began asking for more beer.

Question: How does one establish the diagnosis of hepatic encephalopathy for this patient? What is the role of the serum ammonia concentration in the diagnosis?

Discussion: This case demonstrates that the diagnosis of hepatic encephalopathy is not always straightforward. Hepatic encephalopathy is only one cause of altered mental function in patients with advanced liver disease. Other causes may include accumulation of drugs with CNS depressant properties, head trauma, hypoglycemia, delirium tremens, and electrolyte imbalance. The diagnosis of hepatic encephalopathy is suggested by

- Elevated ammonia concentrations
- Presence (in early stages) of asterixis or a flapping tremor of the hands
- Absence of other causative factors
- Characteristic electroencephalographic findings (rarely used)

The response to therapy (usually correction of electrolyte imbalances, rehydration, and lactulose or neomycin) further supports this diagnosis. Serum ammonia concentrations, therefore, are just one piece of this puzzle. An elevated concentration suggests—but does not establish—this diagnosis. Furthermore, although normal ammonia concentrations may cause one to question the diagnosis of hepatic encephalopathy, they can occur in this condition.

Diagnosis

The diagnostic tests for *H. pylori* are classified as *noninvasive* (serology, urea breath test, and fecal antigen test) or *invasive* (histology, culture, and rapid urea test), the latter depending on upper endoscopy and biopsy.

The serological test for *H. pylori* detects circulating immunoglobulin G (IgG) antibody against bacterial proteins. It has a relatively low sensitivity and specificity (80% to 95%) but has advantages of being widely available and inexpensive.[82,89] Although useful to establish an initial diagnosis of *H. pylori*, it should not be used to monitor the success of eradication therapy as antibody titers decrease slowly in the absence of bacteria.

The urea breath test is based on the ability of the bacteria to produce urease, an enzyme that breaks down urea, releasing ammonia and carbon dioxide. In the breath test, ^{13}C- or ^{14}C-labeled urea is given by mouth. If the bacteria are present, the radiolabeled urea is metabolized to radiolabeled CO_2, which may be measured in exhaled air. The tests have high sensitivity and specificity (both 90% to 95% for ^{13}C and 86% to 95% for ^{14}C).[82,86] However, the ^{14}C isotope has the drawback of being radioactive, and the ^{13}C isotope requires the use of sophisticated detection methods such as isotope ratio mass spectrometry (although samples are stable and may be mailed away for analysis).[90] The fecal antigen test detects *H. pylori* proteins in stool via ELISA. It has high sensitivity and specificity (both 90% to 95%) and, like the urea breath test, is a very accurate noninvasive measure that is used primarily to monitor the success of eradication therapy, although it may be used

as a test for infection when endoscopy is not indicated.[91] The fecal antigen test is not appropriate for patients with active GI bleeding because of a cross-reactivity with blood constituents in the immunoassay, presenting a high incidence of false-positive results.[92] Patients need to be off proton pump inhibitors (PPIs) for 2 and preferably 4 weeks before these tests as PPIs may decrease numbers of *H. pylori* in the stomach and hence the accuracy of the tests.

Upper endoscopy with biopsy of gastric tissue and subsequent histological examination has high sensitivity and specificity (88% to 95% and 90% to 95%, respectively) with the added advantage of allowing detection of gastritis, intestinal metaplasia, or other histological features. Although not commonly done, biopsy specimens may also be used to culture *H. pylori*. By performing various tests on the cultured bacteria, this test may be rendered highly specific (95% to 98%), but the bacterium is difficult to culture making this the least sensitive test (80% to 90%).[81,82] The main advantage of culture is that it allows for antibiotic sensitivity testing, which can help optimize therapy and possibly prevent treatment failure. Rapid urease tests involve incubating a biopsy specimen in the presence of urea and a pH indicator. As mentioned above, *H. pylori* metabolizes urea, releasing ammonia, which in this case may be detected by its effect of increasing the pH. This test allows for rapid results (e.g., 1-hour incubation time following endoscopy), high sensitivity and specificity (both 90% to 95% respectively), and low cost.[82,94] One proposed strategy is to take several biopsies at the time of endoscopy and first check the rapid urease test, sending specimens for detailed pathologic

MINICASE 6

Laboratory Diagnosis of Acute Hepatitis

MICHAEL C., A 45-YEAR-OLD EXECUTIVE, presented to his physician after noticing that he was turning yellow. Other than increased fatigue, he felt well. His physical examination was normal except for his jaundice and tenderness over a slightly swollen liver. Initial laboratory studies showed elevations of the aminotransferases with an ALT of 1235 International Units/L (7–41 International Units/L) and an AST of 2345 International Units/L (12–38 International Units/L). His total bilirubin was 18.6 mg/dL (0.3–1.3 mg/dL).

The tentative diagnosis was acute hepatitis. However, Michael C. had not had any transfusions, used parenteral drugs, or had recent dental work. No exposure to medications or occupational exposure accounted for the disease, and there was no family history of liver disease. Careful review of his history offered no explanation for his development of hepatitis.

Ultimately, serologies showed a positive HBsAg and anti-HBc antibody. A diagnosis of acute type B hepatitis was established. After much questioning, Michael C. revealed that he had a "brief encounter" with a prostitute on a recent business trip. His wife was treated with the vaccine and hepatitis B immunoglobulin, a gamma-globulin with high concentrations of antibodies to HBsAg. Although Michael C.'s wife did not develop hepatitis, she did divorce him after learning that his secretary developed type B hepatitis about 3 months later.

Question: How was this diagnosis established? How should Michael C. be followed and what is the likely outcome?

Discussion: This case demonstrates why a determination of the etiology of hepatitis is often difficult. The practitioner must obtain a detailed history of exposures to medicines, drugs, alcohol, infected people, family members with similar illness, and ongoing medical illness. In this case, the exposure to the prostitute put Michael C. at risk for hepatitis B, C, and D and for human immunodeficiency virus (HIV). The diagnosis was established by the serologies. Had just the anti-HBc antibody been present, he could have

- Been in the "window" phase of the acute disease where this antibody is positive and HBsAg is negative
- Previously recovered from hepatitis B
- Been a chronic carrier

Although the additional presence of HBsAg helped to secure the diagnosis, the clinical picture still had to be considered. Both HBsAg and anti-HBc also can be positive in patients with chronic hepatitis B. Determination of the type of hepatitis has prognostic value and, in this case, made it possible to administer prophylactic medications to people who might have been exposed.

HBsAg	ANTI-HBs	ANTI-HBc	INTERPRETATION
Positive	Negative	Positive	Acute infection or chronic hepatitis B
Negative	Positive	Positive	Resolving hepatitis B or previous infection
Negative	Positive	Negative	Resolving or recovered hepatitis B or patient after vaccination

There is no generally accepted drug therapy for acute viral hepatitis. Michael C. should have repeated examinations and LFTs (specifically albumin, PT, AST, ALT, and bilirubin). There is a less than 1% chance that he will develop fulminant hepatitis and die. Most likely, he will recover completely, with his LFTs normalizing over 1–2 months. However, there is a 10% to 20% chance that he will develop chronic hepatitis, which could lead to cirrhosis.

The prostitute probably had chronic active hepatitis, but her HIV status was unknown. Unfortunately, even after this case was reported to the public health department, nothing could be done to prevent the prostitute from spreading these diseases to other contacts.

---

analysis only if the urease test is negative (or tissue diagnosis is needed to sort out other diagnoses). One other invasive test requires a nasogastric catheter; PCR detection of *H. pylori* DNA may be performed on gastric juice extracted via the catheter.[81]

These tests, with the exception of serology, tend to be confounded by a common set of factors that lower bacterial burden. In patients with achlorhydria (no acid production by the stomach) or patients being treated with antisecretory drugs (e.g., PPIs), increased stomach pH decreases bacterial levels and may lead to false-negative results.[90,93,95,96] Similarly, use of bismuth or antibiotics (including recent, unsuccessful eradication therapy) may decrease test sensitivity. Recommendations advise waiting 2–3 months after therapy before performing these tests to determine whether or not *H. pylori* has been successfully eradicated, and additionally holding PPIs for 2–4 weeks and antibiotics for 4 weeks prior to testing.

While GI bleeding may confound the rapid urea test as well as the fecal antigen test, urea breath tests remain a viable diagnostic option in patients with active bleeding, detecting 86% of *H. pylori*-positive patients.[91-95]

Generally routine testing is not recommended for confirmation of bacterial clearance after therapy. Exceptions to this include those patients with *H. pylori*-induced ulcer, patients not responding clinically, and those with *H. pylori*-associated MALT lymphoma or gastric cancer.

COLITIS

Colitis—acute or chronic inflammation of the colon—often presents quite dramatically with profound and bloody diarrhea, urgency, and abdominal cramping. It is generally distinguished from noninflammatory causes of diarrhea on the basis of physical signs (fever, abdominal tenderness) as well as laboratory abnormalities (elevated white blood cell [WBC] count in the blood).

There are many causes of colitis. Infectious colitis may be caused by invasive organisms including *Campylobacter jejuni*,

MINICASE 7

Laboratory Diagnosis of Hepatitis Type C

KATHERINE M., A 48-YEAR-OLD WOMAN, received a notice 2 weeks after donating blood that it could not be used because her aminotransferases were elevated and a test for hepatitis C was positive. She was referred to a specialist who found that her ALT was 87 International Units/L (7–41 International Units/L) and her AST was 103 International Units/L (12–38 International Units/L). Her bilirubin was 0.8 mg/dL (0.3–1.3 mg/dL).

A liver biopsy demonstrated chronic active hepatitis. After considerable discussion, Katherine M. was placed on a new regimen of triple drug therapy. After 3 months of therapy, however, her aminotransferases were not responding and she was referred for a second opinion.

Type C hepatitis was excluded when her RIBA and RT-PCR studies were negative. Additional history then was obtained. Katherine M. had been reluctant to tell her local family physician that, about 6 months previously, she had a positive skin test for tuberculosis (TB) after discovering that her partner was HIV positive. Being embarrassed, she had sought treatment in a nearby city and been placed on isoniazid. Although she had finished the prescriptions, she had never returned to the clinic.

Question: What are the roles of the second- and third-generation tests in the diagnosis of hepatitis C? What other nonviral forms of hepatitis can present as chronic hepatitis?

Discussion: This case demonstrates several points. Many patients with chronic active hepatitis remain totally asymptomatic, their disease first being detected during routine blood work or when symptoms of cirrhosis or liver failure develop. Now that all blood donors are checked for hepatitis C and abnormal aminotransferases, many patients with chronic liver disease are detected before symptoms are present. Unfortunately, however, the blood banks tend to use the less expensive and less accurate ELISA test for hepatitis C, which (as in this case) gives many false-positive results. Before starting interferon therapy or establishing a diagnosis of type C hepatitis, a practitioner should confirm the diagnosis with either a RIBA or RNA polymerase.

There are many nonviral causes of chronic hepatitis including medications such as isoniazid, methyldopa, nitrofurantoin, and dantrolene. A similar picture also may be seen in autoimmune hepatitis, Wilson disease, alpha-1 antitrypsin deficiency, and hemochromatosis. Isoniazid, a common medication for TB, can cause serious liver damage that may be clinically and histologically indistinguishable from viral chronic active hepatitis. Therefore, aminotransferases need to be carefully monitored in patients on this drug. This problem tends to occur in patients over the age of 50, particularly women.

The aminotransferases may be only minimally elevated, as in this patient. Generally, hepatitis develops after about 2–3 months of drug therapy. With withdrawal of the medication, the numbers usually return to normal over an additional 1–2 months. When the diagnosis of chronic active hepatitis is considered, a patient's medications must be very carefully reviewed.

Shigella, Salmonella, and invasive *Escherichia coli.* Amoeba can present in this manner as can certain infections associated with HIV/AIDS, for example, cytomegalovirus and herpes virus. Noninfectious colitis includes ischemic colitis (insufficient blood flow to the colon), drug-induced colitis (as with gold salts or NSAIDs), inflammatory bowel disease (Crohn disease or ulcerative colitis), and radiation injury. *Clostridium difficile* (*C. diff*), which will be discussed in the next section, is a relatively new disease that has emerged as a major cause of hospital-acquired infection over the past 40 years largely due to the widespread use of broad spectrum antibiotics.[97]

CLOSTRIDIUM DIFFICILE

Clostridium difficile (*C. diff* colitis) is a toxin-induced bacterial disease, which is becoming increasingly common and increasingly difficult to treat. It is surpassing methicillin-resistant *Staphylococcus aureus* (MRSA) as the leading cause of hospital-acquired infections. Most infections follow antibiotic use, which reduces the normal bacterial content of the colon producing a niche for supra-infection by *C. difficile*. As such, *C. difficile* infection only became common following widespread use of broad-spectrum antibiotics in the 1960s.[97] *C. difficile* infection is most commonly associated with, but not limited to, exposure to fluoroquinolones, clindamycin, cephalosporins, and beta-lactamase inhibitors.[98] Clinical symptoms of infection form a spectrum of disease ranging from an asymptomatic carrier state, to chronic diarrhea, to acute colitis, to life-threatening colitis with sepsis. Severe *C. difficile* colitis is marked by a characteristic appearance of *pseudomembranes*, which consist of inflammatory exudates or yellowish plaques on the colonic mucosa, and is thus referred to as *pseudomembranous colitis*. Milder cases present with inflammation limited to the superficial colonic epithelium; however, in severe cases there can be necrosis of the full thickness of the colonic wall.[99]

Clostridia species have the ability to form spores that can survive extreme environmental conditions and remain viable for years. Spores tend to persist within the hospital environment where they may infect patients receiving antibiotics, causing *C. difficile* to be the most common cause of infectious diarrhea in hospitalized patients.[97]

Clostridium difficile produces clinical disease by secreting various toxins within the colon. Toxins A and B are the most common toxins produced, with >90% of pathogenic strains producing toxin A. These toxins affect the permeability of enterocytes, trigger apoptosis, and stimulate inflammation. Some emerging strains also produce a binary toxin of unclear significance, but which is associated with a more severe illness. The bacterium itself is not pathogenic, and some strains of *C. difficile* do not produce toxins and are therefore harmless.[100]

About 3% of healthy adults and 20% of hospitalized patients are asymptomatically colonized with *C. difficile* bacteria.[101] Unlike other similar hospital-infections (e.g., *Staphylococcus*

MINICASE 8

A Case of Acute Liver Failure

MATTHEW Z. WAS IN HIS LAST YEAR OF HIGH SCHOOL when he noticed he was becoming increasingly tired and somewhat weak. He initially was taken to a local clinic where he was reassured that most likely he was getting the "flu" and was sent home. Over the next day he became progressively weaker and finally his family noticed that he was becoming yellow. He was taken to his physician.

He denied being on any medications or supplements. There was no family history of liver disease. Matthew Z. denied alcohol use. There had been no recent history of unusual travel.

Initial physical examination was unremarkable except for his being markedly icteric (jaundiced), and that his liver seemed somewhat enlarged.

Laboratory evaluation included an ALT of 1354 International Units/L (7–41 International Units/L), an AST of 1457 International Units/L (12–38 International Units/L), and a total bilirubin of 12.5 mg/dL (0.3–1.3 mg/dL). Serum ALP was 245 International Units/L (33–96 International Units/L).

The initial tentative diagnosis was acute viral hepatitis. However, as the labs came back, this diagnosis was increasingly under question. Labs showed negative serologies for hepatitis A, B, C, and E. Evaluation for autoimmune hepatitis was negative as well with a negative ANA (antinuclear antibody) and ASMA (anti-smooth muscle antibody). Serologies for mononucleosis and cytomegalovirus (CMV) were negative as well.

Matthew Z. was admitted to the hospital and over the next 2 days his total bilirubin progressively climbed to 23.4 mg/dL. His INR increased to 4 (0.9–1.1). He became increasingly confused and lethargic, and a serum ammonia level was found to be elevated at 348 mcg/dL (19–60 mcg/dL).

A diagnosis of acute liver failure was made, and he was transferred to a liver transplant center. It was only there that he admitted that in the days before the onset of his illness he had visited his girlfriend in college and they both took some ecstasy (MDMA, 3,4-methylenedioxy-N-methylamphetamine).

Question: What is acute liver failure and what generally causes it?

Discussion: Acute liver failure refers to the rapid development (typically within 8 weeks) of severe liver injury with associated failure of the liver to perform its usual synthetic/detoxifying functions. In this case that is evident by the elevated bilirubin, prolonged INR, and the development of hepatic encephalopathy. There are many potential causes. Most common are drug or toxin related, with acetaminophen being among the most common culprits. Viral hepatitis can cause this picture as can ischemia of the liver, sepsis, autoimmune hepatitis, malignancy, and certain conditions associated with pregnancy.

MDMA hepatotoxicity is increasingly common in young people, as this drug is increasingly used. It can cause subclinical liver damage including fibrosis and is rarely associated with a picture of fulminant liver failure as in Matthew Z. Treatment is largely supportive and may involve liver transplantation.

---

aureus), asymptomatic carriage of *C. difficile* bacteria actually *reduces* the likelihood of developing clinical disease, even following antibiotic exposure. This is probably because people who are asymptomatically colonized have developed antibody that neutralizes the *C. difficile* toxins, or have harmless strains of *C. difficile,* which produce no toxin (yet occupy a niche in the colon preventing infection by toxigenic strains).[102]

Recently, a number of outbreaks have resulted from a new strain of *C. difficile* bacteria, which is resistant to new classes of fluoroquinolones (e.g., gatifloxacin and moxifloxacin).[103-105] This strain expresses a binary toxin (until now generally not seen in clinical isolates), as well as up-regulates its expression of toxins A and B by about 20-fold. Clinically, this correlates with ominous increases in morbidity and mortality. The continued emergence of *C. difficile* strains with resistance to commonly utilized antibiotics and increased expression of virulence factors suggests that this bacterium will continue to be a serious complication of antibiotic use until a toxin vaccine can be developed. Current treatment consists of metronidazole (oral or IV), vancomycin (oral or rectal), and various probiotics, depending on severity; however 20% to 30% of patients who receive therapy will face recurrent *C. difficile* infection.[106] Fidaxomicin, a recently FDA-approved narrow spectrum macrolide for *C. difficile* infection may serve as a beneficial alternative therapy.[107]

Prevention of *C. difficile* infection is largely based on avoidance of antibiotic therapy, unless absolutely necessary, and careful hand washing in hospitals and other institutional settings (including in-home patient care). *C. difficile* spores are somewhat resistant to alcohol-based hand disinfectants, so washing with soap and water is preferred.

Diagnosis

The diagnosis of *C. difficile* is challenging. For example, culturing this bacteria is difficult, hence the name. Similar to *H. pylori*, there are a variety of modalities available that vary in sensitivity, specificity, cost, availability, and timeliness. One important difference compared to *H. pylori* is that patients with pseudomembranous colitis may deteriorate rapidly, so making a prompt and accurate diagnosis is important. In some situations that clearly point to a diagnosis of *C. difficile* in an acutely ill patient, it may be reasonable to initiate treatment on an empiric basis before the test results are even available. Diagnosis may also be made during lower endoscopy on encountering the characteristic white or yellow pseudomembranes on the colonic wall.

Until recently, the most commonly used tests for *C. difficile* infection have been ELISA assays for toxin or *C. difficile* antigen within the stool. These tests are available in various commercial kits and have the advantage of being rapid (available within

Antibiotic-Induced Pseudomembranous Colitis

JULIA T. PRESENTED TO HER PHYSICIAN after several days of crampy abdominal pain, diarrhea, persistent fever up to 102.5°F (39.2°C), and chills. On physical examination, she was noted to be well hydrated. Her abdomen was soft and nontender. Stools were sent for pathogenic bacterial cultures including *Shigella, Salmonella, Campylobacter,* entero-invasive *E. coli,* and *Yersinia;* meanwhile, Julia T. was given a prescription for diphenoxylate.

Twenty-four hours later, Julia T. presented to the emergency room doubled over with severe abdominal pain. Her abdomen was distended and tender with diffuse rigidity and guarding. Clinically, she was dehydrated. Her WBC count was elevated at 23,000 cells/mm³ (3.54–9.06 x 10³ cells/mm³), and her BUN was 34 mg/dL (7–20 mg/dL). Abdominal x-rays showed a dilated colon (toxic megacolon) and an ileus. The emergency room physician then learned that, about 6 weeks earlier, Julia T. had taken two or three of her sister's amoxicillin pills because she had thought she was developing a urinary tract infection. Although pseudomembranous colitis was tentatively diagnosed, Julia T. could not take oral medication because of her ileus. Therefore, IV metronidazole and rectal vancomycin were started. She continued to get sicker; early the next day, most of her colon was removed (the rectum was left intact), and an ileostomy was created.

Question: What is the time course of pseudomembranous colitis? Did the use of diphenoxylate influence the outcome?

Discussion: Pseudomembranous colitis can occur even after only one or two doses of a systemic antibiotic or after topical antibiotic use. Moreover, it can occur up to 6 weeks later. A complete history of antibiotic use is critical when dealing with patients with diarrhea.

Diphenoxylate or loperamide use in the face of colitis is associated with a risk, although small, of toxic megacolon. In this medical emergency, the colon has no peristalsis; together with the inflammation in the colon wall (colitis), this condition leads to progressive distention. If untreated, perforation and death ensue. The development of a megacolon or ileus in this patient is especially worrisome because the best treatment—oral antibiotics—would be of little benefit. However, IV metronidazole is excreted into the bile in adequate bactericidal levels to eradicate the bacteria.

A Case of NASH

ALLEN K. WAS A 48-YEAR-OLD executive for a major software company when he presented for his required company physical examination. He had no medical complaints, a negative past medical history, and was on no medications.

On examination he was noted to weigh 240 lb and was 5'10" tall. His blood pressure was elevated at 154/98. The rest of his physical examination was normal.

Laboratory data included a normal CBC and kidney function. It was noted that a fasting glucose was 129 and that his cholesterol was elevated as well. Of concern to the examining physician was that his LFTs were elevated with an ALT of 134 International Units/L (<30 International Units/L), an AST of 105 International Units/L (<30 International Units/L). His serum bilirubin, albumin, ALP, and INR were all normal.

He was referred for evaluation of his abnormal liver panel, and further testing showed no evidence of viral hepatitis, hemochromatosis, or autoimmune liver disease. The possibility of fatty liver was raised, and a liver biopsy was performed which showed NASH with early cirrhosis.

QUESTION: What is NASH (nonalcoholic steatohepatitis) and how is it treated?

DISCUSSION: Our society is experiencing a marked increase in the incidence of obesity. Many of these patients develop what is defined as metabolic syndrome, which must have three of the following: abdominal obesity, elevated blood pressure, impaired glucose tolerance, or hyperlipidemia). Obese patients, particularly those with the "metabolic syndrome" are at a higher risk of developing what has been termed *NAFLD* (nonalcoholic fatty liver disease) or fatty liver. Some patients with fatty liver can progress to NASH and ultimately to cirrhosis and liver failure. While many drugs have been tried in these cases, ultimately the only accepted treatment is weight loss through diet, and occasionally with assistance of surgery, including laparoscopic gastric bypass or banding. Fatty liver can also be caused by rapid weight loss, hyperalimentation, medications (such as steroids, estrogens, amiodarone) and short bowel syndrome.

hours) and relatively inexpensive. Tests for toxin detect toxin A or both toxins A and B; have high specificity (typically >95%) but variable sensitivity (60% to 95%). For this reason, a negative test may be followed by one to two repeat tests to increase the composite sensitivity to the 90% range and exclude infection with more certainty.[101,108] Testing for both toxins has a diagnostic advantage over testing for toxin A, because a minority of strains are toxin A-negative and toxin B-positive.[109]

ELISA assays for *C. difficile* common antigen (glutamate dehydrogenase) have improved sensitivity but are less specific because they will detect nontoxigenic species as well as some species of closely related anaerobes. Therefore, a positive assay for *C. difficile* antigen does not prove pseudomembranous colitis and must be followed up with a toxin assay to prove the presence of a pathogenic *C. difficile* strain.[110] The advantage of this assay for *C. difficile* antigen is that the sensitivity is better, such that a single negative assay may be used to exclude the presence of pseudomembranous colitis. The availability, performance, and appropriate use of these assays may vary between hospital laboratories, and inquiries should be made with the laboratory regarding which tests are available and the appropriate strategy for their use.

The "gold standard" test for pseudomembranous colitis has been the detection of toxin A or B in stool samples by demonstrating its cytopathic effect in cell cultures and inhibition of cytopathic effect by specific antiserum.[111,112] Referred to as *cell cytotoxicity assay*, this test has excellent sensitivity (94% to 100%) and specificity (99%). However, these performance characteristics may be laboratory-dependent.[108,113] Moreover, this test is limited by high cost, a requirement for meticulously maintained tissue culture facilities, and a time delay of 1–3 days.[112]

C. difficile can be cultured from stools with selective medium and identified with more traditional microbiologic techniques including colony morphology, fluorescence, odor, gram stain, and/or signature gas liquid chromatography. Interestingly, this is not the most sensitive test for the organism (the bacterium is named *difficile* because of *difficulty* in culturing it). Another drawback is that isolated bacteria must then be tested for toxin production to avoid confusing it with nontoxic *C. difficile* strains.[114] Altogether, these factors make bacterial culture and toxin profiling a costly, time-consuming process, and thus they are rarely used. The primary advantage of this approach is that it isolates the organism, allowing genetic tests, which may aid in tracking mutant strains and determining the source of epidemics.[115]

The FDA recently approved three RT-PCR assays for the gene toxin B, which not only provide fast and accurate diagnosis of *C. difficile*, but also provide the ability to identify if the pathogen is in the epidemic 027/NAP1/BI strain.[116] This test is rapidly becoming the standard test for initial evaluation for *C. difficile* infections.

SUMMARY

Analysis of liver tests is complex and may be frustrating. Most tests in the LFT panel check for the presence of two broad categories of liver diseases: cholestasis versus hepatocellular injury, and therefore an abnormal value may raise more questions than it answers. None of the tests are 100% sensitive, and most may be confounded by a variety of factors. How, then, can these tests be used to answer clinical questions with any certainty?

Probably the most important point to bear in mind when interpreting LFTs is that they are but one piece of the puzzle. Correct interpretation relies on interpreting the test within the greater context of the patient, other laboratory data, historical information, and the physical exam.[2,19] For example, mildly elevated bilirubin and ALP in the setting of a critically ill, septic patient is likely cholestasis of sepsis and does not necessarily require extensive evaluation. The same set of laboratory tests (mildly elevated bilirubin and ALP) in an ambulatory patient could be a sign of serious chronic illness such as PBC. However, if this same ambulatory patient had a history of normal LFTs and had recently started taking a medication known to cause cholestasis, then the abnormality would most likely be a side effect of the medication. Thus, the same set of liver tests in three different settings may have widely differing significance.

It is also important to interpret an abnormal value within the context of other laboratory tests, and this is why LFTs are often obtained as a group (the *LFT panel*). For example, a mildly elevated AST in the setting of an otherwise normal LFT panel might be of nonhepatic origin (e.g., muscle disease). Alternatively, a mildly elevated AST combined with mildly elevated ALT might raise a concern about a mild hepatocellular process, perhaps chronic viral hepatitis or NASH. Finally, mildly elevated ALT and AST in combination with dramatically elevated ALP and bilirubin would point instead to a cholestatic process.

Therefore, liver tests should always be interpreted with a clear understanding of the clinical context and other laboratory abnormalities. Although the LFT panel will rarely yield an exact diagnosis, it may indicate the type of process (e.g., cholestatic versus hepatocellular) and the severity of the process (e.g., fulminant liver failure versus mild hepatic inflammation). This will lead the practitioner to a group of possibilities that may be further evaluated based on the information at hand, along with other labs or studies (e.g., radiographs, endoscopic procedures, or tissue biopsies) as needed. The diagnostic yield of these tests also depends on their appropriateness and the thoughtfulness of their selection. Liver studies obtained to answer a specific clinical question (e.g., "does this patient have liver inflammation due to initiation of statin medications?") are more likely to yield interpretable information than a less guided question ("is this patient sick?").

Some other aspects of gastroenterology and related laboratory tests are also reviewed in this chapter: amylase and lipase may reflect pancreatic inflammation; *H. pylori* may be related to ulcer disease; and *C. difficile* is a major cause of hospital-acquired colitis. Although these tests are less convoluted than the LFT panel, it is still paramount to obtain them in a thoughtful manner and interpret the results in the appropriate clinical setting. For example, colonization with *H. pylori* may be of no significance in an asymptomatic patient, whereas it may mandate a course of multiple antibiotics in a patient with recurrent significant gastric ulcer bleeding.

Learning Points

1. Why is the term *liver function test* a misnomer?

Answer: Often, the term *liver function test (LFT)* is used to describe a panel of tests including AST, ALT, bilirubin, ALP, and albumin. However, the term is a misnomer because not all of these tests measure liver function. The liver has several functions and different tests reflect these different functions. The table below divides liver tests into rough categories by function and type.

FUNCTION/TYPE	LAB TESTS
Synthetic liver function	Albumin, prealbumin, PT, INR
Excretory function	ALP, 5' nucleotidase, GGT, bilirubin
Hepatocellular injury	AST, ALT
Detoxification	Ammonia

2. Identify common disorders that cause increased indirect bilirubinemia versus direct bilirubinemia. Explain the pathophysiologic cause of the lab abnormality in each case.

Answer: Indirect bilirubin is produced by the breakdown of erythrocytes. Indirect bilirubin is delivered to the liver, where it is converted to direct bilirubin by glucuronyl transferase. Thus, an elevated level of indirect bilirubin may result from increased breakdown of red blood cells (hemolysis) or reduced hepatic conversion of indirect bilirubin to direct bilirubin. Common causes include hemolysis, Gilbert syndrome, or drugs including probenecid or rifampin.

Increased direct bilirubin implies hepatic disease, which interferes with secretion of bilirubin from the hepatocytes or clearance of bile from the liver. Direct bilirubinemia, therefore, is generally classified as a positive cholestatic liver test, although it may also be due to a hepatocellular process. In cholestatic disease, the bilirubin is primarily conjugated, whereas in hepatocellular processes, significant increases in both conjugated and unconjugated bilirubin may result. Cholestasis may be intrahepatic or extrahepatic. Intrahepatic cholestasis may be due to viral hepatitis, alcoholic hepatitis or cirrhosis, pregnancy, severe infection, or PBC. Extrahepatic cholestasis involves obstruction of the large bile ducts outside of the liver, which can be due to strictures, stones, or tumors.

3. Should serum ammonia levels be used to diagnose hepatic encephalopathy?

Answer: Ammonia levels do not correlate well with hepatic encephalopathy in the setting of chronic liver failure. This is likely because hepatic encephalopathy also involves an increase in the permeability of the blood–brain barrier to ammonia. A large overlap between ammonia levels in patients with and without hepatic encephalopathy among patients with chronic liver disease makes this a poor test in this situation.

REFERENCES

1. Sherlock S, Dooley J. *Diseases of the Liver and Biliary System.* 9th ed. London, England: Blackwell Scientific; 1993.
2. Smellie WSA, Ryder SD. Biochemical liver function tests. *Br Med J.* 2006;333:481-483.
3. Fauci AS, Braunwald E, Kasper DL. et al. *Harrison's Principles of Internal Medicine.* 17th ed. New York, NY: McGraw Hill; 2008:A2-A15.
4. Johnson PJ, McFarlane IG. *The Laboratory Investigation of Liver Disease.* London, England: Bailliere Tindall; 1989.
5. Chopra S, Griffin PH. Laboratory tests and diagnostic procedures in evaluation of liver disease. *Am J Med.* 1985;79:221-230.
6. Johnston DE. Special considerations in interpreting liver function tests. *Am Fam Phys.* 1999;59:2223-2230.
7. Dufour DR, Lott JA, Nolte FS, et al. Diagnosis and monitoring of hepatic injury I: performance characteristics of laboratory tests. *Clin Chem.* 2000;46:2027-2049.
8. Aranda-Michael J, Sherman KE. Tests of the liver: use and misuse. *Gastroenterologist.* 1998;6:34-43.
9. Gopal DV, Rosen HR. Abnormal findings on liver function tests. *Postgrad Med.* 2000;107:100-114.
10. Neyra NR, Hakim RM, Shyr Y, et al. Serum transferrin and serum prealbumin are early predictors of serum albumin in chronic hemodialysis patients. *J Renal Nutr.* 2000;10:184-90.
11. Spiekerman AM. Nutritional assessment (protein nutriture). *Anal Chem.* 1995;67:429R-36R.
12. Spiekerman AM. Proteins used in nutritional assessment. *Clin Lab Med.* 1993;13:353-369.
13. Mittman N, Avram MM, Oo KK, et al. Serum prealbumin predicts survival in hemodialysis and peritoneal dialysis: 10 years of prospective observation. *Am J Kidney Dis.* 2001;38:1358-1364.
14. Beck FK, Rosenthal TC. Prealbumin: a marker for nutritional evaluation. *Am Fam Phys.* 2002;65:1575-78.
15. Beckingham IJ, Ryder SD. Investigation of liver and biliary disease. *Br Med J.* 2001;322:33-36
16. Giannini EG, Testa R, Savarino V. Liver enzyme alteration: a guide for clinicians. *CMAJ.* 2005;172:367-379.
17. Kamath PS. Clinical approach to the patient with abnormal liver test results. *Mayo Clin Proc.* 1996;71:1089-1095.
18. Pratt DS, Kaplan MM. Evaluation of the liver: laboratory tests. In: Schiff ER, ed. *Schiff's Diseases of the Liver.* 8th ed. Philadelphia, PA: Lippincott; 1999.
19. McPherson RA, Pincus MR. *Henry's Clinical Diagnosis and Management by Laboratory Methods.* 22nd ed. Philadelphia, PA: Elsevier, Saunders; 2011:302.
20. Green RM, Flamm S. AGA Technical Review on the Evaluation of Liver Chemistry Tests. *Gastroenterology.* 2002;123:1367-1384.
21. Reichling JJ, Kaplan MM. Clinical use of serum enzymes in liver disease. *Dig Dis Sci.* 1988;33:1601-1614.
22. Birkett DJ, Done J, Neale FC, et al. Serum alkaline phosphatase in pregnancy: an immunologic study. *Br Med J.* 1966;1:1210-1212.
23. Moss DW, Henderson AR. Clinical enzymology. In: Burtis CA, Ashwood ER, eds. *Tietz Textbook of Clinical Chemistry.* 3rd ed. Philadelphia, PA: WB Saunders Company; 1999.
24. Bakerman S, Bakerman P, Strausbauch P. *ABC's of Interpretive Laboratory Data.* 3rd ed. Myrtle Beach, SC: Interpretive Laboratory Data; 1994.
25. Wilson JW. Inherited elevation of alkaline phosphatase activity in the absence of disease. *N Engl J Med.* 1979;301:983-984.
26. Pratt DS, Kaplan MM. Evaluation of abnormal liver-enzyme results in asymptomatic patients. *N Engl J Med.* 2000;342:1266-1271.

27. Kaplan MM, Matloff DS, Selinger MJ, et al. Biochemical basis for serum enzyme abnormalities in alcoholic liver disease. In: Chang NC, Chan NM, eds. *Early Identification of Alcohol Abuse. NIAAAA Research Monograph 17.* Rockville, MD: US Department of Health and Human Services; 1985:186-198.

28. Berg CL, Crawford JM, Gollan JL. Bilirubin metabolism and the pathophysiology of jaundice. In: Schiff ER, ed. *Schiff's Diseases of the Liver.* 8th ed. Philadelphia, PA: Lippincott; 1999.

29. Ockner RK. Drug induced liver disease. In: Zakim D, Boyer TD, eds. *Hepatology: A Textbook.* Philadelphia, PA: WB Saunders Company; 1982:691-723.

30. Friedman LS, Keefee EB. *Handbook of Liver Disease.* 3rd ed. Philadelphia, PA: Elsevier Saunders; 2012:2.

31. Dukes GE, Sanders SW, Russo J, et al. Transaminase elevations in patients receiving bovine or porcine heparin. *Ann Intern Med.* 1984;100:646-650.

32. Jick H. Drug-associated asymptomatic elevations of transaminase in drug safety assessments. *Pharmacotherapy.* 1995;15(1):23-25.

33. Fregia A, Jensen D. Evaluation of abnormal liver tests. *Compr Ther.* 1994;20(1):50-54.

34. Whitehead MW, Hawkes ND, Hainsworth I, et al. A prospective study of the causes of notably raised aspartate aminotransferase of liver origin. *Gut.* 1999;45:129-133.

35. Ayling RM. Pitfalls in the interpretation of common biochemical tests. *Postgrad Med J.* 2000;76:129-132.

36. Cohen GA, Goffinet JA, Donabedian RK, et al. Observations on decreased serum glutamic oxaloacetic transaminase (SGOT) activity in azotemic patients. *Ann Intern Med.* 1976;84:275-280.

37. Glynn KP, Cefaro AF, Fowler CW, et al. False elevations of serum glutamic oxaloacetic transaminase due to para-aminosalicylic acid. *Ann Intern Med.* 1970;72:525-527.

38. Young DS. *Effects of Drugs on Clinical Laboratory Tests.* 3rd ed. Washington, DC: American Association for Clinical Chemistry Press; 1990.

39. Friedman LS, Martin P, Munoz SJ. Liver function tests and the objective evaluation of the patient with liver disease. In: Zakim D, Boyer TD, eds. *Hepatology: A Textbook of Liver Disease.* Philadelphia, PA: WB Saunders Company; 1996.

40. Shawcross D, Jalan R. Dispelling myths in the treatment of hepatic encephalopathy. *Lancet.* 2005;365:431-433.

41. Mas A. Hepatic encephalopathy: from pathophysiology to treatment. *Digestion.* 2006;73:86-93.

42. Gammal SH, Jones EA. Hepatic encephalopathy. *Med Clin North Am.* 1989;73:793-813.

43. Montoliu C, Cauli O, Urios A, et al. 3-nitro-tyrosine as a peripheral biomarker of minimal hepatic encephalopathy in patients with liver cirrhosis. *Am J Gastroenterol.* 2011;106(9):1629.

44. Zieve L. The mechanism of hepatic coma. *Hepatology.* 1981;1:360-365.

45. Ong JP, Aggarwal A, Krieger D, et al. Correlation between ammonia levels and the severity of hepatic encephalopathy. *Am J Med.* 2003;114:188-193.

46. Kundra A, Jain A, Banga A, et al. Evaluation of the plasma ammonia levels in patients with acute liver failure and chronic liver disease and its correlation with the severity of hepatic encephalopathy and clinical features of raised intracranial tension. *Clin Biochem.* 2005;38:696-699.

47. Bhatia V, Singh R, Acharya SK. Predictive value of arterial ammonia for complications and outcome of acute liver failure. *Gut.* 2006;55:98-104.

48. Saab S, Martin P. Tests for acute and chronic viral hepatitis. *Postgrad Med.* 2000;107:123-130.

49. Wolk DM, Jones MF, Roesnblatt JE. Laboratory diagnosis of viral hepatitis. *Infect Dis Clin N Am.* 2001;15:1109-1126.

50. Lemon SM. Type A viral hepatitis: new developments in an old disease. *N Engl J Med.* 1985;313:1059-1067.

51. Waite J. The laboratory diagnosis of the hepatitis viruses. *Int J STD AIDS.* 1996;7:400-408.

52. Lemon SM. Type A viral hepatitis: epidemiology, diagnosis, and prevention. *Clin Chem.* 1997;43:1494-1499.

53. Mahoney FJ. Update on diagnosis, management, and prevention of Hepatitis B virus infection. *Clin Microbiol Reviews.* 1999;12:351-366.

54. Alter HJ. Transmission of hepatitis C virus—route, dose, and titer. *N Engl J Med.* 1994;330:784-786.

55. Sjögren MH. Serologic diagnosis of viral hepatitis. *Med Clin N Am.* 1996;80:929-956.

56. Pawlotsky JM. Molecular diagnosis of viral hepatitis. *Gastroenterology.* 2001;122: 554-568.

57. Moyer LA, Mast EE, Alter MJ. Hepatitis C: routine serologic testing and diagnosis. *Am Fam Phys.* 1999;59:79-88.

58. Ghany MG, Nelson DB, et al. An update on treatment of genotype 1 chronic hepatitis C virus infection: 2011 practice guideline by the American Association for the Study of Liver Diseases. *Hepatology.* 2011;54:1433.

59. Nishio A, Keeffe EB, Gershwin ME. Primary biliary cirrhosis: lessons learned from an organ-specific disease. *Clin Exp Med.* 2001;1:165-178.

60. Heathcote J. Update on primary biliary cirrhosis. *Can J Gastroenterol.* 2000;14:43-48.

61. Worman JH. Molecular biological methods in diagnosis and treatment of liver diseases. *Clin Chem.* 1997;43:1476-1486.

62. Gregory PB. Diseases of pancreas. *Sci Am Med.* 1994;4(V):1-15.

63. Soergel K. Acute pancreatitis. In: Sleisenger MH, Fordtran JS, eds. *Gastrointestinal Disease.* 5th ed. Philadelphia, PA: WB Saunders Company; 1993:1638-1639.

64. Pieper-Bigelow C, Strocchi A, Levitt MD. Where does serum amylase come from and where does it go? *Gastroenterol Clin North Am.* 1990;19:793-810.

65. Anon. AGA Institute technical review on acute pancreatitis. *Gastroenterology.* 2007;2022-2044.

66. Lankisch PG. Underestimation of acute pancreatitis: patients with only a small increase in amylase/lipase levels can also have or develop severe acute pancreatitis. *Gut.* 1999;44:542-544.

67. Frossardl JL, Steer ML, Pastor CM. Acute Pancreatitis. *The Lancet.* 2008;371(9607):143-152.

68. Treacy J, Williams A, Bais R, et al. Evaluation of amylase and lipase in the diagnosis of acute pancreatitis. *ANZ J Surg.* 2001;71:577-582.

69. Ransom JH. Diagnostic standards for acute pancreatitis. *World J Surg.* 1997;21:136-142.

70. Vissers RJ, Abu-Laban RB, McHugh DF. Amylase and lipase in the emergency department evaluation of acute pancreatitis. *J Emerg Med.* 1999;17:1027-1037.

71. Gumaste VV. Diagnostic tests for acute pancreatitis. *Gastroenterologist.* 1994;2:119-130.

72. Gumaste VV, Dave P, Sereny G. Serum lipase: a better test to diagnose acute alcoholic pancreatitis. *Am J Med.* 1992;92:239-242.

73. Rogers AI. Elevated lipase levels always means pancreatitis? *Postgrad Med.* 2002;111:104.

74. Gumaste VV, Roditis N, Mehta D, et al. Serum lipase levels in nonpancreatic abdominal pain versus acute pancreatitis. *Am J Gastroenterol.* 1993;88:2051-2055.

75. Munoz A, Katerndahl DA. Diagnosis and management of acute pancreatitis. *Am Fam Phys.* 2000;62:164-174.

76. Keim V, Teich N, Fiedler F, et. al. A comparison of lipase and amylase in the diagnosis of acute pancreatitis in patients with abnormal pain. *Pancreas.* 1998;16:45-49.

77. Frank B, Gottlieb K. Amylase normal, lipase elevated: Is it pancreatitis? *Am J Gastro.* 1999;94:463-469.

78. Bode C, Riederer J, Brauner B, et al. Macrolipasemia: a rare cause of persistently elevated serum lipase. *Am J Gastroenterol.* 1990;85:412-416.

79. Ros E, Navarro S, Bru C, et al. Occult microlithiasis in "idiopathic" acute pancreatitis: prevention of relapses by cholecystectomy or ursodeoxycholic acid therapy. *Gastroenterology.* 1991;101:1701-1709.

80. Kemppainen EA, Hedstrom JI, Puolakkainen PA, et al. Advances in the laboratory diagnostics of acute pancreatitis. *Ann Med.* 1998;30:169-175.

81. Nakamura RM. Laboratory tests for the evaluation of *Helicobacter pylori* infections. *J Clin Lab Anal.* 2001;15:301-307.

82. Logan RP, Walker MM. Epidemiology and diagnosis of *Helicobacter pylori* infection. *Brit J Med.* 2001;323:920-922.

83. Vaira D, Gatta L, Ricci C, et al. Review article: diagnosis of *Helicobacter pylori* infection. *Ailment Pharmacol Ther.* 2002;16:16-23.

84. Nomura A, Stemmermann GN, Chyou PH, et al. *Helicobacter pylori* infection and gastric carcinoma among Japanese Americans in Hawaii. *N Engl J Med.* 1991;325:1132-1136.

85. Parsonnet J, Friedman GD, Vandersteen DP, et al. *Helicobacter pylori* infection and the risk of gastric carcinoma. *N Engl J Med.* 1991;325:1127-1131.

86. Vaira D, Vakli N. Blood, urine, stool, breath, money, and *Helicobacter pylori. Gut.* 2001;28:287-289.

87. Klusters JG, Vliet HA, Kuipers EJ. Pathogenesis of *Helicobacter pylori* infection. *Clin Microbiol Rev.* 2006;19(3):449-490.

88. F Megraud. *H pylori* antibiotic resistance; prevalence, importance, and advances in testing. *Gut.* 2004;53:1374-1384.

89. Vakil N. Review article: the cost of diagnosing *Helicobacter pylori* infection. *Aliment Pharmacol Ther.* 2001;15:10-15.

90. Savarino V, Vigneri S, Celle G. The ¹³C urea breath test in the diagnosis of *Helicobacter pylori* infection. *Gut.* 1999;45(Suppl 1):18-22.

91. Gisbert JP, Pajares JM. Diagnosis of *Helicobacter pylori* infection by stool antigen determination: a systematic review. *Am J Gastro.* 2001;96:2829-2838.

92. Lin HJ, Lo WC, Perng CL, et al. *Helicobacter pylori* stool antigen test in patients with bleeding peptic ulcers. *Helicobacter.* 2004; 9(6):663.

93. Vaira D, Vakil N, Menegatti M, et al. The stool antigen test for detection of *Helicobacter pylori* after eradication therapy. *Ann Int Med.* 2002;136:280-287.

94. Marshall BJ, Warren JR, Francis GJ, et al. Rapid urease test in the management of *Campylobacter pyloridis* associated gastritis. *Am J Gastroenterol.* 1987;82:200.

95. Gisbert JP, Esteban C, et al. 13C-urea breath testing during hospitalization for the diagnosis of *Helicobacter pylori* infection in peptic ulcer bleeding. *Helicobacter.* 2007;12(3):231.

96. Hebrick P, van Doorn LJ. Serological methods for diagnosis of *Helicobacter pylori* infection and monitoring of eradication therapy. *Eur J Clin Microbiol Infect Dis.* 2000;19:164-173.

97. Kelly CP, LaMont JT. *Clostridium difficile* infection. *Ann Rev Med.* 1998;49:375-390.

98. Clabots C, Johnson S, et al. Acquisition of *Clostridium difficile* by hospitalized patients; Evidence for colonized new admissions as a source of infection. *J Infect Dis.* 1992; 166(3):561-567.

99. Price AB, Davies DR. Pseudomembranous colitis. *J Clin Pathol.* 1977;30(1):1-12.

100. Lee VR. *Clostridium difficile* infection in older adults: A review and update on its management. *Am J Geriatr Pharmacother.* 2012;Feb; 10(1):14-24.

101. Fekety R, Shah AB. Diagnosis and treatment of *Clostridium difficile* colitis. *JAMA.* 1993;269:71-75.

102. Yassin SY, Young-Fadok TM, Zein NN, et al. *Clostridium difficile*-associated diarrhea and colitis. *Mayo Clin Proc.* 2001;76:725-730.

103. Hookman P, Barkin JS. Review: *Clostridium difficile*-associated diarrhea and *Clostridium difficile* colitis: The emergence of a more virulent era. *Dig Dis Sci.* 2007;52:1071-1075.

104. Cookson B. Hypervirulent strains of *Clostridium difficile. Postgrad Med J.* 2007;83:291-295.

105. Blossom DB, McDonald LC. The challenges posed by reemerging *Clostridium difficile* infection. *Clin Infect Dis.* 2007;45:222-227.

106. Kelly CP, LaMont JT. *Clostridium difficile*—more difficult than ever. *N Engl J Med.* 2008;359:1932-1940.

107. Louie TJ, Miller MA et al. Fidaxomicin vs vancomycin for *Clostridium difficile* infection. *N Engl J Med* 2011;364:422-432.

108. Kelly CP, Pothoulakis C, LaMont JT. Current concepts: *Clostridium difficile* colitis. *N Engl J Med.* 1994;330:257-262.

109. Brazier JS. The diagnosis of *Clostridium difficile*-associated disease. *J Antimicro Chemother.* 1998;41:29-40.

110. Wilkins TD, Lyerly DM. *Clostridium difficile* testing: after 20 years, still challenging. *J Clin Micro.* 2003;41:531-534.

111. Aslam S, Musher DM. An update on diagnosis, treatment, and prevention of *Clostridium difficile*-associated disease. *Gastroenterol Clin North Am.* 2006;35:315-335.

112. Barbut F, Kajzer C, Planas N, et al. Comparison of three enzyme immunoassays, a cytotoxicity assay, and toxigenic culture for diagnosis of *Clostridium difficile* associated diarrhea. *J Clin Microbiol.* 1993;31:963-967.

113. Delmee M. Laboratory diagnosis of *Clostridium difficile* disease. *Clin Micro Infect.* 2001;7:411-415.

114. Mylonakis E, Ryan ET, Calderwood SB. *Clostridium difficile*-associated diarrhea. *Arch Intern Med.* 2001;161:525-533.

115. Sunenshine RH, McDonald LC. *Clostridium difficile*-associated disease: new challenges from an established pathogen. *Cleveland Clin J Med.* 2006;73:187-197.

116. Bababy NE, Stiles J et al. Evaluation of the Cephoid Xpert *Clostridium difficile* Epi assay for diagnosis of *Clostridium difficile* infection and typing of the NAP1 strain at a cancer hospital. *J Clin Microbiol.* 2010;48(12)4519-4524. Epub 2010 Oct 13.

QUICKVIEW | Albumin

PARAMETER	DESCRIPTION	COMMENTS
Common reference ranges		
Adults	4.0–5.0 g/dL	
Pediatrics	1.9–4.9 g/dL	<1 yr old
	3.4–4.2 g/dL	1–3 yr old
Critical value	<2.5 g/dL	In adults
Natural substance?	Yes	Blood protein
Inherent activity?	Increases oncotic pressure of plasma; carrier protein	
Location		
Production	Liver	
Storage	Serum	
Secretion/excretion	Catabolized in liver	Half-life, approximately 20 days
Major causes of...		
High or positive results	Dehydration	
	Anabolic steroids	
Associated signs and symptoms	Limited to underlying disorder	No toxicological activity
Low results	Decreased hepatic synthesis	Seen in liver disease
	Malnutrition or malabsorption	Substrate deficiency
	Protein losses Pregnancy or chronic illness	Via kidney in nephrotic syndrome or via gut in protein-losing enteropathy
Associated signs and symptoms	Edema, pulmonary edema, ascites	At levels <2–2.5 g/dL
After insult, time to...		
Initial depression or positive result	Days	
Lowest values	Weeks	Half-life, approximately 20 days
Normalization	Days	Assumes insult removed and no permanent damage
Drugs often monitored with test	Parenteral nutrition	Goal is increased levels
Causes of spurious results		
Falsely elevated	Ampicillin and heparin	
Falsely lowered	Supine patients, icterus, penicillin	

QUICKVIEW | PT/INR

PARAMETER	DESCRIPTION	COMMENTS
Common reference ranges		
Adults and pediatrics	INR: 0.9–1.1	
	PT: 12.7–15.4 sec	
Critical value	INR: >5	Unless on warfarin
Natural substance?	Yes	
Inherent activity?	Indirect measurement of coagulation factors	
Location		
Production	Coagulation factors produced in liver	
Storage	Carried in bloodstream	
Secretion/excretion	None	
Major causes of…		
Prolonged elevation	Liver failure	Liver unable to produce coagulation factors; prolonged PT or increased INR does not correct with vitamin K
	Malabsorption or malnutrition	Vitamin K aids in activation of coagulation factors and is not absorbed; defect corrects with parenteral vitamin K supplementation
	Warfarin	Corrects with vitamin K supplementation
	Antibiotics	Interfere with vitamin K production by bacteria in the GI tract, or metabolism, or activation of clotting factors
Associated signs and symptoms	Increased risk of bleeding and ecchymoses	Easy bruising
Low results	None	
After insult, time to…		
Initial elevation or positive result	6–12 hr	
Peak values	Days to weeks	Depends on etiology
Normalization	4 hr if vitamin K responsive (due to malabsorption, maldigestion, warfarin, etc.) but 2–4 days if due to liver disease and liver disease reverses	
Drugs often monitored with test	Warfarin	
Causes of spurious results	Improper specimen collection	

GI = gastrointestinal; INR = international normalized ratio; PT = prothrombin time.

QUICKVIEW | ALP

PARAMETER	DESCRIPTION	COMMENTS
Common reference ranges		
Adults	Varies with assay	Elevated in pregnancy
Pediatrics	Varies; can be 2- to 3-fold higher than in adults	Elevated with developing bone
Natural substance?	Yes	Metabolic enzyme (intracellular)
Inherent activity?	Elevation alone causes no symptoms	Intracellular activity only
Location		
Production	Intracellular enzyme	
Storage	Liver, placenta, bone, small intestine, leukocytes	These tissues are rich in ALP
Secretion/excretion	None	
Major causes of...		
High or positive results	Cholestasis	Hepatic; associated with elevation of GGT
	Bone disease	Paget disease, bone tumors, rickets, osteomalacia, healing fracture
	Pregnancy	Placental ALP
	Childhood	Related to bone formation
Associated signs and symptoms	Limited to underlying disorder	Reflects tissue or organ damage
Low results	Vitamin D intoxication	
	Scurvy	
	Hypothyroidism	
Associated signs and symptoms	Limited to underlying disorder	
After insult, time to...		
Initial elevation or positive result	Hours	
Peak values	Days	
Normalization	Days	Assumes insult removed and no ongoing damage
Drugs often monitored with test	None	
Causes of spurious results	Blood drawn after fatty meal and prolonged serum storage	

ALP = alkaline phosphatase; GGT = gamma-glutamyl transpeptidase.

QUICKVIEW | AST

PARAMETER	DESCRIPTION	COMMENTS
Common reference ranges		
Adults	12–38 International Units/L	Varies with assay
Newborns/infants	30–100 International Units/L	Varies with assay
Critical value	>80 International Units/L	2 times upper limit of normal
Natural substance?	Yes	Metabolic enzyme
Inherent activity?	None in serum	Intracellular activity only
Location		
Production	Intracellular enzyme	
Storage	Liver, cardiac muscle, kidneys, brain, pancreas, lungs	These tissues are rich in AST
Secretion/excretion	None	
Major causes of...		
High or positive results	Hepatitis	Elevated in any disease with hepatocyte inflammation (liver cells)
	Hemolysis	Elevated in any disease with damage to tissues rich in enzyme
	Muscular diseases	
	Myocardial infarction	
	Renal infarction	
	Pulmonary infarction	
	Necrotic tumors	
Associated signs and symptoms	Varies with underlying disease	Reflects tissue or organ damage
Low results	None	
After insult, time to...		
Initial elevation or positive result	2–6 hr	
Peak values	24–48 hr (without further cell damage)	With extensive liver or cellular damage, levels can go up to thousands
Normalization	24–48 hr	Assumes insult removed and no ongoing damage
Drugs often monitored with test	Isoniazid, HMG-COA inhibitors, allopurinol, methotrexate, ketoconazole, and valproic acid	Monitoring frequency varies with drug
Causes of spurious results		
Falsely elevated	Heparin, levodopa, methyldopa, tolbutamide, para-aminosalicylic acid, erythromycin, diabetic ketoacidosis	
Falsely lowered	Metronidazole, trifluoperazine, vitamin B_6 deficiency	

AST = aspartate aminotransferase.

QUICKVIEW | ALT

PARAMETER	DESCRIPTION	COMMENTS
Common reference ranges		
Adults	3–30 International Units/L	Varies with assay
Newborns/infants	6–40 International Units/L	Decreases to adult values within a few months
Critical value	>60 International Units/L	Greater than 2 times normal limit
Natural substance?	Yes	Metabolic enzyme
Inherent activity?	None in serum	Intracellular activity only
Location		
Production	Intracellular enzyme	
Storage	Liver, muscle, heart, kidneys	These tissues are rich in ALT
Secretion/excretion		Normally contained intracellularly, but with cell damage, serum concentrations increase
Major causes of...		
High or positive results	Hepatitis	Elevated in any disease with hepatocyte inflammation (liver cells)
	Hemolysis	Elevated in any disease with damage to tissues rich in enzymes
	Muscular diseases	
	Myocardial infarction	
	Renal infarction	
Associated signs and symptoms	Varies with underlying disease	Reflects tissue or organ damage
Low results	Patients deficient in vitamin B_6	
Associated signs and symptoms	None	
After insult, time to...		
Initial elevation or positive result	2–6 hr	
Peak values	24–48 hr (without further cell damage)	With extensive liver or cellular damage, levels can go up to thousands
Normalization	24–48 hr	Assumes insult removed and no ongoing damage
Drugs often monitored with test	Isoniazid and cholesterol-lowering agents (e.g., HMG COA inhibitors, allopurinol, ketoconazole, valproic acid, and methotrexate)	Monitoring frequency varies with drug
Causes of spurious results	Heparin (false elevation)	

ALT = alanine aminotransferase.

QUICKVIEW | Bilirubin

PARAMETER	DESCRIPTION	COMMENTS
Common reference ranges		
Adults	0.3–1.3 mg/dL	Varies slightly with assay
Pediatrics	2–4 mg/dL	24-hr infant
	5–6 mg/dL	48-hr infant
	0.3–1.3 mg/dL	>1 month old
Critical value	>4 mg/dL	In adults
Natural substance?	Yes	Byproduct of Hgb metabolism
Inherent activity?	Yes	CNS irritant or toxin in high levels in newborn (not adult)
Location		
Production	Liver	
Storage	Gallbladder	Excreted into bile
Secretion/excretion	Stool and urine	Bilirubin and urobilinogen
Major causes of...		
High or positive results	Liver disease, both hepatocellular and cholestatic	
	Hemolysis	
	Metabolic abnormalities (e.g., Gilbert syndrome)	
Associated signs and symptoms	Jaundice	
Low results	No important causes	
After insult, time to...		
Initial elevation or positive result	Hours	
Peak values	3–5 days	Assumes insult not removed
Normalization	Days	Assumes insult removed and no evolving damage
Drugs often monitored with test	None	
Causes of spurious results	Fasting, levodopa, phenelzine, methyldopa, ascorbic acid (false elevation)	

CNS = central nervous system; Hgb = hemoglobin.

QUICKVIEW | Ammonia

PARAMETER	DESCRIPTION	COMMENTS
Common reference ranges		
Adults and pediatrics	30–70 mcg/dL	Varies with assay
Newborns	<100 mcg/dL	Varies with assay
Critical value	Varies, generally 1.5 upper limit of normal	
Natural substance?	Yes	Product of bacterial metabolism of protein (in the gut)
Inherent activity?	Probably	Progressive deterioration in neurologic function
Location		
Production	In gut (by bacteria)	
Storage	None	
Secretion/excretion	Liver metabolizes to urea	Urea cycle; diminished in cirrhosis
Major causes of...		
High or positive results	Liver failure	
	Reye syndrome	
	Metabolic abnormalities (urea cycle)	
Associated signs and symptoms	Hepatic encephalopathy	
Low results	No important causes	
After insult, time to...		
Initial elevation or positive result	Hours	
Peak values	No peak value; rises progressively	
Normalization	Days	After appropriate therapy or resolution of underlying liver disease
Drugs often monitored with test	Valproic acid	
Causes of spurious results	Sensitive test (discussed in text)	

CHAPTER 13

ENDOCRINE DISORDERS

EVA M. VIVIAN, BRADY BLACKORBAY

Objectives

After completing this chapter, the reader should be able to

- Identify patients who should be screened for diabetes mellitus (DM) and determine the diagnostic tests that should be employed

- Recognize and differentiate between the subjective and objective data consistent with a diagnosis of type 1 and type 2 DM and relate this data to the pathogenesis of type 1 and type 2 DM

- Explain the major differences between laboratory values found in diabetic ketoacidosis (DKA) and in a hyperosmolar hyperglycemic state

- Identify common medications or chemicals that may induce hyperglycemia or hypoglycemia

- Describe the use of glycosylated hemoglobin (A1c), fasting plasma glucose (FPG), and oral glucose tolerance tests as diagnostic tools

- Describe the actions of thyroxine (T_4), triiodothyronine (T_3), and thyroid-stimulating hormone (TSH) and the feedback mechanisms regulating them

- Recognize the signs and symptoms associated with abnormally high and low concentrations of thyroid hormones

- Given a case description including thyroid function test results, identify the type of thyroid disorder, and describe how tests are used to monitor and adjust related therapy

(continued on 284)

The endocrine system consists of hormones that serve as regulators, which stimulate or inhibit a biological response to maintain homeostasis within the body. Endocrine disorders often result from a deficiency or an excess of a hormone, leading to an imbalance in the physiological functions of the body. Usually, negative feedback mechanisms regulate hormone concentrations (Figure 13-1). Therefore, laboratory assessment of an endocrine disorder is based on the concentrations of a plasma hormone and on the integrity of the feedback mechanism regulating that hormone. In this chapter, the relationship between a hormone (insulin) and a target substrate (glucose) serves as an example of these concepts. The evaluation of the function of the thyroid and adrenal glands is also described. The relationships between vasopressin (antidiuretic hormone [ADH]) and serum and urine osmolality are used to demonstrate the basis for the water deprivation test in diagnosing diabetes insipidus (DI).

GLUCOSE HOMEOSTASIS

Glucose serves as the fuel for most cellular functions and is necessary to sustain life. Carbohydrates ingested from a meal are metabolized in the body into glucose. Glucose is absorbed from the gastrointestinal (GI) tract into the bloodstream where it is utilized in skeletal muscle for energy.

Glucose is also stored in the liver in the form of glycogen (glycogenesis) and is converted in adipose tissue to fats and triglycerides (lipogenesis). Insulin, which is produced, stored, and released from beta cells of the pancreas, facilitates these anabolic processes. The liver, skeletal muscle, brain, and adipose tissue are the main tissues affected by insulin. To induce glucose uptake, insulin must bind to specific cell-surface receptors. Most secreted insulin is taken up by the liver, while the remainder is metabolized by the kidneys. About 80% of glucose uptake is independent of insulin. These insulin-independent cells include nerve tissue, red blood cells (RBCs), mucosal cells of the GI tract, and exercising skeletal muscle.[1,2]

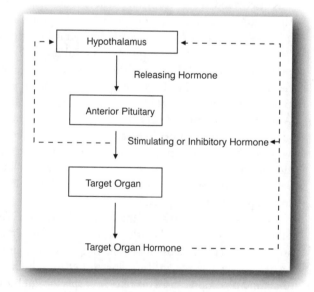

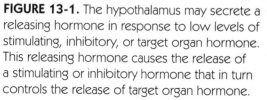

FIGURE 13-1. The hypothalamus may secrete a releasing hormone in response to low levels of stimulating, inhibitory, or target organ hormone. This releasing hormone causes the release of a stimulating or inhibitory hormone that in turn controls the release of target organ hormone.

Objectives

- Describe the relationship between urine osmolality, serum osmolality, and antidiuretic hormone (ADH) as it relates to diabetes insipidus (DI)
- Describe the lab tests used to diagnose Addison disease and Cushing syndrome

In the fasting state, insulin levels decrease, resulting in an increase in glycogen breakdown by the liver (glycogenolysis) and an increase in the conversion of free fatty acids to ketone bodies (lipolysis).[1,2]

When glucose concentrations fall below 70 mg/dL, an event known as *hypoglycemia* occurs resulting in the release of glucagon by the alpha cells of the pancreas. Glucagon stimulates the formation of glucose in the liver (gluconeogenesis) and glycogenolysis. Glucagon also facilitates the breakdown of stored triglycerides in adipose tissue into fatty acids (lipolysis), which can be used for energy in the liver and skeletal muscle. In addition to glucagon secretion, hypoglycemia leads to secretion of counter regulatory hormones such as epinephrine, cortisol, and growth hormone. Glucagon and, to a lesser degree, epinephrine promote an immediate breakdown of glycogen and the synthesis of glucose by the liver. Cortisol increases glucose levels by stimulating gluconeogenesis. Growth hormone inhibits the uptake of glucose by tissues when glucose levels fall below 70 mg/dL.[3,4]

Other hormones, amylin and incretin, affect glucose concentrations. Amylin, a beta-cell hormone co-secreted with insulin at a molar ratio of 1:20–50 in response to a glucose challenge, was discovered in 1987. Amylin is a neuroendocrine hormone that complements the actions of insulin by restraining the vagus nerve-mediated rate of gastric emptying, thereby slowing intestinal carbohydrate absorption and resulting in lower postprandial glucose (PPG) levels. This delay in gastric emptying has been found to be the same in patients with type 1 and type 2 DM mellitus (DM) that were without complications. Amylin also suppresses hepatic glucose output by inhibiting glucagon after ingestion of a meal.[5-8] In animal studies, amylin was found to induce postprandial satiety in direct proportion to food intake.[6] The administration of amylin has been reported to decrease food intake, thereby resulting in weight loss in patients with type 2 DM.[9,10]

Recent studies have shown that beta-cell response is greater after food ingestion or when glucose is given orally versus after intravenous (IV) glucose infusion. This difference in insulin secretion has been termed the *incretin effect*, which implies that food ingestion causes the release of specific gut hormones known as *incretins* that enhance insulin secretion beyond the release caused by the rise in glucose secondary to absorption of digested nutrients.[11,12] Studies in humans and animals have shown that the incretin hormones glucagon-like peptide-1 (GLP-1) and glucose-dependent insulinotropic peptide (GIP) stimulate insulin release when glucose levels are elevated.[12-14]

After food is ingested, GIP is released from K cells in the proximal gut (duodenum), and GLP-1 is released from L cells in the distal gut (ileum and colon). Under normal circumstances, dipeptidyl-peptidase 4 (DPP-4) rapidly degrades these incretins to their inactive forms after their release into the circulation. As a result, the plasma half-life of GIP and GLP is less than 5 minutes.[12]

GLP-1 and GIP stimulate insulin response in pancreatic beta cells, and GLP-1 (but not GIP) also suppresses glucagon production in pancreatic alpha cells when the glucose level is elevated. The subsequent increase in glucose uptake in muscles and reduced glucose output from the liver help maintain *glucose homeostasis*. Thus, the incretins GLP-1 and GIP are important glucoregulatory hormones that positively affect glucose homeostasis by physiologically helping to regulate insulin in a glucose-dependent manner.[12,15] The kidney contributes to glucose homeostasis primarily by the reabsorption and return of glucose to the circulation. Glucose is freely filtered by the glomerulus, and in healthy individuals, approximately 180 g of glucose are filtered daily and almost all of this is reabsorbed by the proximal tubule. Glucose reabsorption by the kidney is mediated by a class of specific glucose transport proteins, the sodium glucose cotransporters (SGLTs). One member of this family, SGLT2, is responsible for the majority of renal glucose reabsorption and is located on the luminal side of cells in the initial part of the nephron, the early proximal convoluted tubule. Another member of this family, SGLT1, is expressed mainly in the intestine, but it is also present in skeletal muscle, heart, and, based on animal studies, in the late proximal tubule where it accounts for additional glucose reabsorption from the glomerular filtrate. Glucose is taken up into the cell by SGLTs and exits across the basolateral membrane into the interstitium by facilitative diffusion via the facilitative glucose transporters GLUT2 and GLUT1.[16]

In individuals without diabetes, once plasma glucose concentrations exceed approximately 180 mg/dL (the renal threshold), renal glucose reabsorption is saturated and glucose starts to appear in the urine. In hyperglycemic individuals, the renal threshold may be exceeded, and large amounts of glucose may be excreted in the urine. However, the kidneys continue to reabsorb glucose, and in patients with type 2 DM, the renal capacity to reabsorb glucose may be increased, which further contributes to hyperglycemia.[17]

In summary, glucose concentrations are affected by any factor that can influence glucose production or utilization, glucose absorption from the GI tract, glycogen catabolism, insulin production, or secretion. Fasting suppresses the rate of insulin secretion, and feasting generally increases insulin secretion. Increased insulin secretion lowers serum glucose concentrations, while decreased secretion raises glucose concentrations.[1-4]

DIABETES MELLITUS

The three most commonly encountered types of DM:
- Type 1 DM (formally known as *insulin-dependent diabetes mellitus [IDDM]*)

TABLE 13-1. General Characteristics of Type 1 and Type 2 Diabetes Mellitus

CHARACTERISTICS	TYPE 1	TYPE 2
Age of onset	Childhood or adolescence	>40 yr old
Rapidity of onset	Abrupt	Gradual
Family studies	Increased prevalence of type 1	Increased prevalence of type 2
Body weight	Usually thin and undernourished	Obesity is common
Islet cell antibodies and pancreatic cell-mediated immunity	Yes	No
Ketosis	Common	Uncommon; if present associated with severe stress or infection
Insulin	Markedly diminished early in disease or totally absent	Levels may be low, normal, or high (indicating insulin resistance)
Symptoms	Polyuria, polydipsia, polyphagia, weight loss	May be asymptomatic; polyuria, polydipsia, polyphagia may be present

- Type 2 DM (formerly known as *adult onset* or *noninsulin dependent diabetes mellitus [NIDDM]*)[18]
- Gestational DM

Type 1 DM is characterized by a lack of endogenous insulin, predisposition to ketoacidosis, and an abrupt onset. Some patients present with ketoacidosis after experiencing polyuria, polyphagia, and polydipsia for several days. Typically, this type of DM is diagnosed in children and adolescents but may also occur at a later age. In contrast, patients with type 2 DM are not normally dependent on exogenous insulin to sustain life and are not ketosis prone, but they are usually obese and are more than 40 years old. There is an alarming increase in the number of children and adolescents diagnosed with type 2 DM. Although there is a genetic predisposition to the development of type 2 DM, environmental factors such as high-fat diets and sedentary lifestyles contribute to the disorder. Type 2 DM patients are both insulin deficient and insulin resistant (Table 13-1).[1,2]

Many type 2 DM patients are asymptomatic so diagnosis often depends on laboratory studies. Concentrations of ketone bodies in the blood and urine are typically low or absent, even in the presence of hyperglycemia. This finding is common because the lack of insulin is not severe enough to lead to abnormalities in lipolysis and significant ketosis or acidosis.

Because of the chronicity of asymptomatic type 2 DM, many patients with type 2 DM present with evidence of microvascular complications (neuropathy, nephropathy, and retinopathy) and macrovascular complications (coronary artery, cerebral vascular, and peripheral arterial disease) at the time of diagnosis. Type 2 DM is often discovered incidentally during glucose screening sponsored by hospitals and other healthcare institutions.[1,2]

Gestational diabetes mellitus, a third type of glucose intolerance, develops during the third trimester of pregnancy. Patients with gestational DM have a 30% to 50% chance of developing type 2 DM.[19] A woman with diabetes who becomes pregnant, or a woman diagnosed with diabetes early in her pregnancy, are not included in this category.

Pathophysiology

Type 1 DM usually develops in childhood or early adulthood and accounts for up to 10% of all patients with diabetes. Patients are usually thin, have an absolute lack of insulin, and require exogenous insulin to prevent diabetic ketoacidosis (DKA) and sustain life. Genetics as well as environmental and immune factors are the major factors thought to cause type 1 DM.[20]

Over 90% of all type 1 DM patients have a combination of human leukocyte antigen (HLA)-DQ coded genes, which increase the risk of developing type 1 DM. Type 1 DM may result from a trigger, which could be environmental or viral. Viral infections may stimulate monocytes and macrophages that activate T cells, which attack beta cells, thereby decreasing insulin production. Bovine serum albumin has also been identified as an environmental trigger. Therefore, it is believed that exposure to cow's milk may increase the risk of developing type 1 DM in patients with a genetic predisposition. An immunologic attack against insulin may also occur. The combination of an autoimmune attack on beta cells and on circulating insulin results in insulin insufficiency.[20-22]

Type 2 DM involves multiple organ dysfunction that results in insulin resistance and insulin deficiency. During the early stages of type 2 DM, the ability of insulin to facilitate the diffusion of glucose into the cell is impaired. Defects in insulin receptor function, insulin receptor-signal transduction pathway, glucose transport and phosphorylation, and glycogen synthesis and oxidation contribute to muscle insulin resistance. The pancreas compensates for this deficiency by secreting larger amounts of insulin. Patients remain euglycemic until the pancreatic beta cells are no longer able to compensate for the insulin resistance. Hence, insulin is unable to suppress hepatic glucose production and hyperglycemia results (Figure 13-2).[1,22-24]

Recently, other causes for the excessive postprandial increase in plasma glucose levels have been identified. Because amylin is co-secreted with insulin, there is an absolute deficiency of this hormone in patients with type 1 DM. In patients with type 2 DM, amylin levels decrease progressively. Whether due to

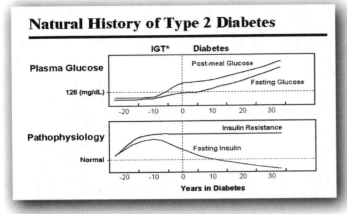

FIGURE 13-2. In the early stages of type 2 DM, the pancreatic beta cells compensate for insulin resistance by secreting more insulin. Over time, these cells burn out resulting in insulin deficiency and hyperglycemia. IGT = impaired glucose tolerance. (Source: Adapted from International Diabetes Center [IDC], Minneapolis, MN.)

the destruction of pancreatic beta cells in patients with type 1 DM or the progressive exhaustion of beta-cell function in patients with type 2 DM, amylin deficiency is now recognized as a contributor to the development of DM.[12-15]

The incretin effect is abnormal in those with type 2 DM mellitus. The diminished incretin effect observed in patients with type 2 DM may be due to reduced responsiveness of pancreatic beta cells to GLP-1 and GIP or to impaired secretion of the relevant incretin hormone.[13]

Secondary Causes

Diabetes mellitus may be the result of other pancreatic and hormonal diseases, medications, and abnormalities of the insulin receptor.[13] Pancreatic cell destruction may be related to diseases, such as cystic fibrosis, or autoimmune conditions. It can be related to drugs (e.g., L-asparaginase, streptozocin, and pentamidine). Similarly, hyperglycemia may result from hormonal disease in which concentrations of circulating catecholamines and glucocorticoids are increased (e.g., catecholamine-secreting pheochromocytoma and Cushing syndrome, respectively).[13]

Various medications or chemicals may induce hyperglycemia and glucose intolerance. Beta-adrenergic blocking agents may decrease or impair insulin secretion in patients with diabetes. Beta-adrenergic blocking agents may decrease glycogenolysis and gluconeogenesis. Diazoxide and phenytoin may decrease insulin secretion resulting in increased glucose levels. High doses of thiazides and loop diuretics may cause hyperglycemia by an unknown mechanism.[24] It should be noted that potassium-sparing diuretics have little or no effect on glucose levels.

Estrogen products influence glucose tolerance to varying degrees, depending on the formulation. In one study, women taking combination oral contraceptives for at least 3 months had plasma glucose concentrations 43% to 61% higher than controls.[25] Monophasic and triphasic combination products diminished glucose tolerance, whereas progestin-only products

did not. Insulin resistance was the proposed mechanism, and fasting plasma glucose (FPG) concentrations were not adversely affected. Table 13-2 lists medications with the potential to cause hyperglycemia.

Diagnostic Laboratory Tests

C-Peptide

Fasting range: 0.78–1.89 ng/mL (0.26–0.62 nmol/L SI unit)
Range 1 hr after a glucose load: 5.00–12.00 ng/mL (during a glucose tolerance test)

C-peptide levels are used to evaluate residual beta-cell function. A C-peptide test is done to

- Distinguish between type 1 and type 2 DM
- Identify the cause of hypoglycemia
- Check to see whether a tumor of the pancreas (insulinoma) was completely removed

Insulin is synthesized in the beta cells of the islets of Langerhans as the precursor, proinsulin. Proinsulin is cleaved to form C-peptide and insulin, and both are secreted in equimolar amounts into the portal circulation. By measuring the levels of C-peptide, the level of insulin can also be calculated. High levels of C-peptide generally indicate high levels of endogenous insulin production. This may be a response to high levels of blood glucose caused by glucose intake and/or insulin resistance. High levels of C-peptide also are seen with insulinomas (insulin-producing tumors) and may be seen with hypokalemia, pregnancy, Cushing syndrome, and renal failure.

Low levels of C-peptide are associated with low levels of insulin production. This can occur when insufficient insulin is being produced by the beta cells, when production is suppressed by exogenous insulin, or with suppression tests that involve substances such as somatostatin.[26]

A C-peptide test can be done when DM has just been found and it is not clear whether type 1 or type 2 DM is present. A patient with type 1 DM has a low level of insulin and C-peptide. A patient with type 2 DM has a normal or high level of C-peptide. When a patient has newly diagnosed type 1 or type 2 DM, C-peptide can be used to help determine how much insulin the patient's pancreas is still producing. With type 2 DM, the test may be ordered to monitor the status of beta-cell function and insulin production over time and to determine if/when insulin injections may be required.

A C-peptide test can also help identify the cause of hypoglycemia, such as excessive use of medicine to treat diabetes or a noncancerous growth (tumor) in the pancreas (insulinoma). Because synthetic insulin does not have C-peptide, a patient with hypoglycemia from taking too much insulin will have a low C-peptide level. An insulinoma causes the pancreas to release too much insulin, which causes hypoglycemia. Such a patient will have a high level of C-peptide in the blood.[26]

Even though they are produced at the same rate, C-peptide and insulin leave the body by different routes. Insulin is processed and eliminated mostly by the liver, while C-peptide is removed by the kidneys. The half-life of C-peptide is about 30 minutes as compared to the half-life of insulin, which is 5

TABLE 13-2. Medications and Chemicals That May Cause Hyperglycemia[11,25,26]

Diuretics

Chlorthalidone	Metolazone
Loop diuretics[a]	Thiazides

Steroids/hormones

Estrogens	Oral contraceptives[c]
Glucocorticoids	Thyroid hormones

Antihypertensives

Calcium antagonists[b]	Diazoxide
Clonidine[b]	Beta blockers

Miscellaneous drugs

Amiodarone[b]	Epinephrine[d]
L-asparaginase	Lithium[b]

Phenothiazines[b]

Nicotinic acid	

Protease Inhibitors

Ritonavir	Tipranavir
Indinavir	Atazanavir
Saquinavir	Fosamprenavir
Nelfinavir	Amprenavir
Darunavir	Pentamidine[e]

Nucleoside Reverse transcriptase Inhibitors

Didanosine	Zidovudine
Emtricitabine	Phenytoin
Lamivudine	Cyclosporine
Stavudine	Tacrolimus
Tenofovir	Streptozocin

Atypical Antipsychotics

Aripiprazole	Olanzapine
Clozapine	Risperidone

[a]Loop diuretics are furosemide, bumetanide, torsemide, and ethacrynic acid. Torsemide has less effect on glucose concentrations.[24]

[b]Clinical significance is less clear.

[c]Progestin-only products do not affect glucose tolerance.

[d]Oral sympathomimetics, such as those found in decongestants, are unlikely to be more of a cause of increased glucose than the "stress" from the illness for which they are used.

[e]After initial hypoglycemia, which occurs in about 4–14 (average 11) days.

minutes. Thus, there will be usually about 5 times as much C-peptide in the bloodstream as insulin.[26]

Diabetes-Related Autoantibody Testing

Diabetes-related (islet) autoantibody testing is used to distinguish between type 1 DM and type 2 DM. Determining which type of diabetes is present allows for early treatment with the most appropriate therapy to avoid complications from the disease. The four most common autoantibody tests used to distinguish between type 1 DM and type 2 DM are islet cell cytoplasmic autoantibodies (ICA), glutamic acid decarboxylase

autoantibodies (GADA), insulinoma-associated-2 autoantibodies (IA-2A), and insulin autoantibodies (IAA).

The autoantibodies seen in children are often different than those seen in adults. Insulin autoantibodies is usually the first marker to appear in young children. As the disease evolves, this may disappear and ICA, GADA, and IA-2A become more important. Insulinoma-associated-2 autoantibodies is less commonly positive at the onset of type 1 DM than either GADA, or ICA. Whereas about 50% of children with new-onset type 1 DM will be IAA positive, IAA positivity is not common in adults.

A combination of these autoantibodies may be ordered when a person is newly diagnosed with diabetes and the healthcare provider wants to distinguish between type 1 and type 2 DM. In addition, these tests may be used when the diagnosis is unclear in persons with diabetes who have been diagnosed as type 2 DM but who have great difficulty in controlling their glucose levels with oral medications. If ICA, GADA, and/or IA-2A are present in a person with symptoms of DM, the diagnosis of type 1 DM is confirmed. Likewise, if IAA is present in a child with DM who is not insulin-treated, type 1 DM is the cause. If no diabetes-related autoantibodies are present, then it is unlikely that the diabetes is type 1 DM. Some people who have type 1 DM will never develop detectable amounts of islet autoantibodies, but this is rare. The majority of people, 95% or more, with new-onset type 1 DM will have at least one islet autoantibody.[26]

Laboratory Tests to Assess Glucose Control

The two most common methods used for evaluating glucose homeostasis are the FPG and glycosylated hemoglobin (A1c). The oral glucose tolerance test (OGTT) is mainly used to assess equivocal results from these two tests. Glycosylated hemoglobin and fructosamine tests are used to monitor long- and medium-term glucose control, respectively. Urine glucose monitoring in patients with DM has been replaced by fingerstick blood glucose tests. Therefore, discussion of this test is relatively brief.

With all of these tests, proper collection and storage of the sample and performance of the procedure are important. Improper collection and storage of samples for glucose determinations can lead to false results and interpretations. After collection, RBCs and white blood cells (WBCs) continue to metabolize glucose in the sample tube. This process occurs unless (1) the RBCs can be separated from the serum using serum separator tubes, or (2) metabolism is inhibited using sodium fluoride–containing (gray-top) tubes or refrigeration. Without such precautions, the glucose concentration drops by 5–10 mg/dL (0.3–0.6 mmol/L) per hour, and the measured glucose level will not reflect the patient's FPG at collection time. In vitro, metabolic loss of glucose is hastened in samples of patients with leukocytosis or leukemia.[27]

Fasting Plasma Glucose and 2-Hour Postprandial Glucose

The categories of *fasting plasma glucose (FPG)* values are as follows:

- FPG <100 mg/dL (5.5 mmol/L) represents normal fasting glucose
- FPG ≥100 (5.5 mmol/L) and <126 mg/dL (7.0 mmol/L) represents *prediabetes* (previously termed *impaired fasting glucose [IFG])*
- FPG ≥126 mg/dL (7.0 mmol/L) represents provisional diagnosis of diabetes (the diagnosis must be confirmed as described below)[18]

An FPG concentration is the best indicator of glucose homeostasis. This test measures the ability of endogenous or exogenous insulin to prevent fasting hyperglycemia by regulating glucose anabolism and catabolism. Fasting plasma glucose may be used to monitor therapy in patients being treated for glucose abnormalities. For this test, the patient maintains his or her usual diet, and the assay is performed on awakening (before breakfast). This timing usually allows for an 8-hour fast. An FPG greater than 126 mg/dL (>7.0 mmol/L), found on at least two occasions, is diagnostic for DM (Table 13-3).

The diagnosis of DM usually can be made if the *2-hour post-prandial glucose (PPG)* is equal to or greater than 200 mg/dL (>11.2 mmol/L), especially if previous tests reveal fasting hyperglycemia (Table 13-3).[28] Testing in asymptomatic people should be considered in adults of any age who are overweight or obese (BMI ≥25 kg/m²) with one or more risk factors[18]:

- Physical inactivity
- A1c ≥5.7%, impaired glucose tolerance or impaired fasting glucose on a previous testing
- First-degree relative with diabetes
- Polycystic ovary syndrome
- Vascular disease, hypertension, or dyslipidemia
- High-risk ethnic groups (e.g., Native Americans, Latino/Hispanics, African Americans, Pacific Islanders)
- Women with a prior history of gestational DM)
- Individuals without these risk factors should be screened no later than 45 years of age. The American College of Endocrinology recommends that individuals from high-risk groups, aged greater than 30 years, be screened for DM every 3 years.[29]

Oral Glucose Tolerance Test

The categories for the *oral glucose tolerance test (OGTT)* are as follows:

- 2-hour postload glucose (PG), <140 mg/dL represents normal glucose tolerance
- 2-hour PG 140–199 mg/dL represents prediabetes (previously termed *impaired glucose tolerance [IGT])*
- 2-hour PG ≥200 mg/dL represents provisional diagnosis of diabetes (the diagnosis must be confirmed as described above)

The OGTT is used to assess patients who have signs and symptoms of DM but whose FPG is normal or suggests prediabetes (<126 mg/dL or <7.0 mmol/L). The OGTT measures both the ability of the pancreas to secrete insulin following a glucose load and the body's response to insulin. Interpretation of the test is based on the plasma glucose concentrations drawn before and during the exam. This exam may also be used in diagnosing DM with onset during pregnancy if the disease threatens the health of the mother and fetus. The OGTT is not required for patients who have FPG levels greater than 126 mg/dL on at least two separate occasions as such values confirm the diagnosis of DM.[28]

The OGTT is performed by giving a standard 75-g dose of an oral glucose solution over 5 minutes following an overnight fast. The pediatric dose is 1.75 g/kg up to a maximum of 75 g. Blood samples commonly are drawn before the test, between 0 and 2 hours, and at 2 hours. The samples should be collected into tubes containing sodium fluoride, unless the assay will be performed immediately.[28]

If the patient vomits the test dose, the exam is invalid and must be repeated. The OGTT is diagnostic for DM if the 2-hour plasma glucose is at least 200 mg/dL (11.2 mmol/L). The patient is considered to have prediabetes if the 2-hour concentration is 140–199 mg/dL (7.8–11.2 mmol/L).

Pregnant women with risk factors (overweight or obese with a BMI greater than 25, family history of type 2 DM, hypertension, hyperlipidemia, high-risk ethnic group [Hispanic, African American, Native American, South or East Asian, or of Pacific Island descent]) should be screened at the first prenatal visit using standard diagnostic criteria. Pregnant women not previously known to have DM or risk factors, can be screened for gestational DM at 24–28 weeks gestation. A screening test is performed that measures plasma glucose fasting and plasma glucose at 1 and 2 hours after a 75-g oral glucose load. The diagnosis of gestational DM can be made when any of the following plasma glucose values are exceeded:

- FPG ≥92 mg/dL

TABLE 13-3. Diagnosis of Diabetes Mellitus Based on Fasting Plasma Glucose Concentration, Oral Glucose Tolerance Test, and Glycosylated Hemoglobin[18]

Level of Glucose Tolerance	FPG	VENUS PLASMA GLUCOSE[a] (mg/dL)		A1c
		OGTT Value at 30, 60, or 90 min	OGTT Value at 2 hr	
"Normal"	<100	<200	<140	<5.7%
Prediabetes	100–125	>200	140–199	5.7% to 6.4%
DM	≥126	>200	>200	≥6.5%
Gestational DM	<92	>180 (1 hr)	>153	

DM = diabetes mellitus; FPG = fasting plasma glucose; A1c = glycosylated hemoglobin; OGTT = oral glucose tolerance test.
[a]Multiply number by 0.056 to convert glucose to International System (SI) units (mmol/L).

- 1 hour ≥180 mg/dL
- 2 hour ≥153 mg/dL[18]

The OGTT should not be performed on individuals who are chronically malnourished, consume inadequate carbohydrates (<150 g/day), or are bedridden. Alcohol consumption and medications that cause hyperglycemia (Table 13-2) should be stopped if possible 3 days prior to the examination. Coffee and smoking are not permitted during the test.[28]

Glycosylated Hemoglobin

Normal range: 4% to 5.6%

A1c, also known as *glycosylated* or *glycated A1c*, is a component of the hemoglobin molecule. During the 120-day lifespan of an RBC, glucose is irreversibly bound to the hemoglobin moieties in proportion to the average serum glucose. The process is called *glycosylation*. Measurement of A1c is, therefore, indicative of glucose control during the preceding 2–3 months. The entire hemoglobin A1 molecule—composed of A1a, A1b, and A1c—is not used because subfractions A1a and A1b are more susceptible to nonglucose adducts in the blood of patients with opiate addiction, lead poisoning, uremia, and alcoholism.[30,31] Because the test is for hemoglobin, the specimen analyzed is RBC and not serum or plasma.

Results are not affected by daily fluctuations in the blood glucose concentration, and a fasting sample is not required. Results can reflect overall patient compliance to various treatment regimens. With most assays, 95% of a normal individual's hemoglobin is 4% to 6% glycated. An A1c ≥7% suggests poor glucose control. Patients with persistent hyperglycemia may have an A1c up to 20% (Table 13-4).[30]

For years, the A1c has been used to monitor glucose control in people already diagnosed with DM. Initially it was not recommended for diagnosis since the test variability from laboratory to laboratory was too great for a diagnostic test. The A1c cut point of ≥6.5% identifies one-third fewer cases of undiagnosed DM than a fasting glucose cut point of ≥126 mg/dL. However, the lower sensitivity of the test at the cut point is offset by the test's greater practicality, and wider use of this more convenient test may result in an increase in the number of diagnoses made.[18]

A few situations confound interpretation of test results. False elevations in A1c may be noted with uremia, chronic alcohol intake, and hypertriglyceridemia.[31] Patients who have diseases with chronic or episodic hemolysis (e.g., sickle cell disease and thalassemia) generally have spuriously low A1c concentrations caused by the predominance of young RBCs (which carry less A1c) in the circulation. In splenectomized patients and those with polycythemia, A1c is increased. If these disorders are stable, the test still can be used, but values must be compared with the patient's previous results rather than published normal values. Both falsely elevated and falsely lowered measurements of A1c may also occur during pregnancy. Therefore, A1c should not be used to screen for gestational DM.[32-34]

Affinity chromatography and colorimetric assay methods measure total A1c including subfractions A1a and A1b. Ion-exchange chromatography and high-performance liquid chromatography only measure the subfraction. The Cholestech GDX® and the Metrika A1cNow® are portable analyzers, which provide A1c results within 5–8 minutes.[34] The American Diabetes Association (ADA) recommends A1c testing 1–2 times a year for patients with good glycemic control and quarterly in patients with poor control or whose therapy has changed.[18]

Fructosamine

Normal range: <285 μmol/L

Fructosamine is a general term that is applied to any glycosylated protein. Unlike the A1c test, only glycosylated proteins in the serum or plasma (e.g., albumin)—not erythrocytes—are measured. In nondiabetics, the unstable complex dissociates into glucose and protein. Therefore, only small quantities of fructosamine circulate. In patients with DM, higher glucose concentrations favor the generation of more stable glycation, and higher concentrations of fructosamine are found.

Fructosamine has no known inherent toxicological activity but can be used as a marker of medium-term glucose control. Fructosamine correlates with glucose control over 2–3 weeks based on the half-lives of albumin (14–20 days) and other serum proteins (2.5–23 days). As a result, high fructosamine concentrations may alert caregivers to deteriorating glycemic control earlier than increases in A1c.

Falsely elevated results may occur when

- Serum (not whole blood) hemoglobin concentrations are greater than 100 mg/dL (normally <15 mg/dL)
- Serum bilirubin is greater than 4 mg/dL
- Serum ascorbic acid is greater than 5 mg/dL[36]

Methyldopa and calcium dobesilate (the latter is used outside the United States to minimize myocardial damage after an acute infarction) may also cause falsely elevated results. Serum fructosamine concentrations are lower in obese patients with DM as compared to lean patients with DM.[36] Some clinicians advocate the use of fructosamine concentrations as a monitoring tool for short-term changes in glycemic control (e.g., gestational DM). However, more clinical studies are required to determine if this test provides useful clinical information.[37,38]

TABLE 13-4. Correlation Between A1c Level and Estimated Average Glucose (eAG) Levels

Level A1c (%)	ESTIMATED AVERAGE GLUCOSE LEVEL (mg/dL)[a]	mmoL/L
5	97 (76–120)	5.4 (4.2–6.7)
6	126 (100–152)	7.0 (5.5–8.5)
7	154 (123–185)	8.6 (6.8–10.3)
8	183 (147–217)	10.2 (8.1–12.1)
9	212 (170–249)	11.8 (9.4–13.9)
10	240 (193–282)	13.4 (10.7–15.7)
11	269 (217–314)	14.9 (12.0–17.5)
12	298 (246–347)	16.5 (13.3–19.3)

[a]Data in parentheses are 95% CIs. Linear regression eAG (mg/dL) = 28.7 × A1c − 46.7.

Source: Adapted from reference 35.

Urine Glucose

Normal range: negative

Glucose "spills" into the urine when the serum glucose concentration exceeds the renal threshold for glucose reabsorption (normally 180 mg/dL). However, a poor correlation exists between *urine glucose* and concurrent serum glucose concentrations. This poor correlation occurs because urine is "produced" hours before it is tested, unless the inconvenient double-void method (urine is collected 30 minutes after emptying of the bladder) is used. Furthermore, the renal threshold varies among patients and tends to increase in diabetes over time, especially if renal function is declining.

Urine testing gradually has been replaced by convenient fingerstick blood sugar testing, Urine glucose testing should be recommended only if the patient is unable or unwilling to perform blood glucose monitoring.[39]

The presence and amount of glucose in the urine can be determined by two different techniques. Commercial products that use copper-reducing methods (e.g., Clinitest®) provide the most quantitative estimate of the degree of glycosuria. Therefore, this method is preferred for patients who spill large quantities of glucose into the urine. The two-drop method can detect higher concentrations of glucose up to 5% as compared to the five-drop method, which can quantitate up to only 2%. Generally, copper-reducing products have poor specificity for glucose.

Contrary to popular belief, isoniazid, methyldopa, and ascorbic acid do not interfere with Clinitest®. The literature is unclear on whether chloral hydrate, nitrofurantoin, probenecid, and nalidixic acid interfere with this method. Patients should be aware that a "pass-through" phenomenon occurs with this test when more than 2% glucose is in the urine. During the test, a fleeting orange color may appear at the climax of the reaction and fade to a greenish-brown when the reaction is complete. The latter color (0.75% to 1%) may be incorrectly used to assess glucose levels, and the glucose concentration actually may be underestimated.

The second method of urine glucose testing is specific for glucose and provides a more qualitative assessment of it in the urine. Commercial products of this type (e.g., Tes-Tape®, Clinistix®, Diastix®, and Chemstrip®) consist of plastic dipsticks with paper pads that have been impregnated with glucose oxidase. These tests are sensitive to 0.1% glucose (100 mg/dL). Substances that may cause false-negative results with this type of test include ascorbic acid (high dose), salicylates (high dose), and levodopa. Interference also has been reported with phenazopyridine and radiographic contrast media, but the likelihood is less clear.[40,41]

Self-Monitoring Tests of Blood Glucose

Blood glucose meters and *reagent test strips* are commercially available so that patients may perform blood glucose monitoring at home. These systems are also used frequently in hospitals, where nurses rely on quick results for determining insulin requirements. The meters currently marketed are lightweight, relatively inexpensive, accurate, and user-friendly.

The first generation of self-monitoring blood glucose (SMBG) meters relied on a photometric analysis that was based on a dye-related reaction. This method, also termed *reflectance photometry, light reflectance,* or *enzyme photometric,* involves a chemical reaction between capillary blood and a chemical on the strip that produces a change in color. The amount of color reflected from the strip is measured photometrically. The reflected color is directly related to the amount of glucose in the blood. The darker color the test strip, the higher the glucose concentration. The disadvantages of this method are that the test strip has to be developed after a precise interval (the blood has to be washed away), a large sample size of blood (>12 microliter) is required, and the meter requires frequent calibration.[42]

Most SMBG meters today utilize an electrochemical or enzyme electrode process, which determine glucose levels by measuring an electric charge produced by the glucose-reagent reaction. These second-generation glucometers can further be subdivided according to the electrochemical principle used: amperometry or colorimetry. Amperometry biosensor technology requires a large sample size (4–10 µL). Furthermore, alterations in temperature or hematocrit levels may result in inaccurate results with this method. Such SMBG meters that employ the amperometry method include Sidekick Testing System® and Prestige IQ®.[42]

The *colorimetry* method involves converting the glucose sample into an electrochemical charge, which is then captured for measurement. An advantage of this system is that a small amount of blood (e.g., 0.3 mL) is enough to determine the blood glucose level. The colorimetry method is not influenced by changes in temperature and hematocrit levels. These monitors can use blood samples extracted from the arm and thigh too. At these alternative sites, there are fewer capillaries and nerve endings, allowing for a less painful needle stick. Some examples of second-generation glucometers that use the colorimetry method include Reli-On Ultima®, OneTouch Ultra®, and Freestyle® (Table 13-5).

While new SMBG meters report as plasma values, older meters may report whole blood values, which are approximately 10% to 15% lower than plasma values. The ADA recommends whole blood fasting readings of 80–120 mg/dL and bedtime readings between 100–140 mg/dL. Plasma fasting readings should be between 90–130 mg/dL and bedtime readings between 110–140 mg/dL.[43]

Special features of glucose meters. Blood glucose testing can be challenging for adults with poor vision or limited dexterity as well as children with small hands. Patients should try out several meters by checking their ease of use with the lancing device and lancets, test strips, and packaging, and meter features before committing to one. Meters with a backlight or test strip port light should be recommended for individuals with visual impairment. Many meters also offer an audio function that is available in several different languages. Persons with limited dexterity, such as patients with arthritis, neuropathy, Parkinson disease, etc., may consider either the Breeze 2, which has a disk that holds 10 strips, or the Accu

TABLE 13-5. Blood Glucose Monitors[a]

COMPANY AND CONTACT INFORMATION	METER NAME	KEY FEATURES	BLOOD SAMPLE SIZE (MICROLITER)	USER CODING NEEDED?
Abbott Diabetes Care (www.abbotdiabetescare.com)	FreeStyle Freedom Lite	C	0.3	No
	FreeStyle Lite	B, C	0.3	No
	Precision Xtra	B, C, K	0.6	Yes
AgaMatrix (www.wavesense.info)	WaveSense Jazz	B, C	0.5	No
	WaveSense KeyNote	B, C	0.5	Yes
	WaveSense KeyNote Pro	B, C	0.5	Yes
	WaveSense Presto	B, C	0.5	No
Arkray (customerservice@arkrayusa.com)	Glucocard 01	C	0.3	No
	Glucocard 01-mini		0.3	No
	Glucocard Vital	C	0.5	No
Bayer (www.simplewins.com)	Breeze2	C	1.0	No
	Contour	C	0.6	No
	Contour TS[b]	C	0.6	No
	Contour USB	C	0.6	No
Bionime (www.bionimeusa.com)	Rightest GM100		1.4	No
	Rightest GM300[b]	C	1.4	Yes
	Rightest GM550	B, C	1.0	No
Biosense Medical Devices (www.solometers.com)	Solo V2	A, C	0.7	No
Diabetic Supply of Suncoast (www.dsosi.com)	Advocate Redi-Code Dash		0.7	No
	Advocate Redi-Code Duo	A, BP, C	0.7	No
Diagnostic Devices (www.prodigymeter.com)	Prodigy Autocode	A, C	0.7	No
	Prodigy Pocket	C	0.7	No
	Prodigy Voice	A, C	0.7	No
Entra Health Systems (www.myglucohealth.net)	MyGlucoHealth Wireless	A, C	0.3	No
Fifty50 Medical (www.fifty50.com)	Fifty50 Blood Glucose Monitoring System 2.0	C	0.5	No
Fora Care (www.foracare.com/usa)	Fora D10	A, BP, C	0.7	Yes
	Fora D15	BP, C	0.7	Yes
	Fora D20	A, BP, C	0.7	Yes
	Fora G20	C	0.5	No
	Fora G71[a]		0.5	No
	Fora G90	B, C, K	0.7	No
	Fora Premium V10	A, C	0.5	No
	Fora V20	A, C	0.7	No
Gluco Com (www.glucocom.com)	Codefree	C	0.7	No
Infopia www.infopiausa.com	Eclipse	C	1.0	Yes
	Element	C	0.3	No
	Element Plus	A C	0.3	No
	Envision	C	1.5	No
	Evolution	C	0.3	No
	GlucoLab	C	1.0	Yes
	Xpres		0.3	No

TABLE 13-5. Blood Glucose Monitors[a], continued

COMPANY AND CONTACT INFORMATION	METER NAME	KEY FEATURES	BLOOD SAMPLE SIZE (MICROLITER)	USER CODING NEEDED?
LifeScan (www.onetouch.com)	OneTouch Ping[a]	B, C, P	1.0	Yes
	OneTouch Select[b]	C	1.4	Yes
	OneTouch Ultra2	B, C	1.0	Yes
	OneTouch UltraMini	C	1.0	Yes
	OneTouch UltraSmart	B, C	1.0	Yes
Nipro Diagnostics (www.niprodiagnostics.com)	Sidekick		1.0	No
	True2Go		0.5	No
	Trubalance[b]	C	1.0	No
	Trueresult	C	0.5	No
	Truetrack	C	1.0	Yes
Nova Biomedical (www.novacares.com)	Nova Max Link	C, P	0.3	No
	Nova Max Plus	C, K	0.3 for blood glucose; 0.8 for ketones	No
Oak Tree International Holdings (www.oaktreeint.com)	EasyMax Light	B, C	0.6	No
	EasyMax No Code	C	0.6	No
	EasyMax Voice	C	0.6	No
	EasyMax Voice 2nd Generation	C	0.6	No
	EasyPlus T2	C	0.6	No
Omnis Health (www.omnishealth.com)	Embrace	A	0.6	No
Roche www.accu-chek.com/us	Accu-Chek Aviva	C	0.6	Yes
	Accu-Chek Compact Plus	C	1.5	No
U.S. Diagnostics (www.usdiagnostics.net)	Acura		0.5	No
	Control	C	1.0	Yes
	EasyGluco		1.5	Yes
	EasyGluco Plus	B	0.5	No
	Infinity	C	0.5	No
	Maxima		0.5	Yes
Walmart (www.relion.com)	ReliOn Confirm	C	0.3	No
	ReliOn Micro		0.3	No
	ReliOn Ultima	B, C	0.6	Yes

A = audio capability; B = backlight on display; BP = dual meter that measures both blood glucose and blood pressure; C = computer download capability; K = also tests blood ketones; P = communicates with insulin pump.
[a]Available by mail order only.
[b]Adapted from the American Diabetes Association Resource Guide 2002. Blood glucose monitors and data management. *Diabetes Forecast.* 2012;36-51.

Check Compact Plus meter, which holds a drum of test strips. The test strip for these meters is easily dispensed with a push of a button. Individuals with visual impairment may benefit from larger display screen, screen back light, or test strip port light. Examples of meters that offer a screen back light include the Freestyle Lite, OneTouch Ultra 2, ReliOn Ultima, and WaveSense KeyNote. The Contour USB and Freestyle Lite meters also have a test strip port light.

Some children are more comfortable monitoring their blood glucose than others. Some children may like glucometers that come in bright or "cool" colors. The Arkray's Glucocard 01-mini and Diabetic Supply of Suncoast's Advocate Redi-Code Dash come in fun colors and patterns that may be appealing to younger patients. Many "auto-code" or "no-code" meters, which do not require manually programming the meter to recognize a specific group of test strips, are ideal choices for children who are learning how to monitor their blood glucose levels. Parents should select a meter that requires a very small blood sample size. Children or adolescents who enjoy video games might enjoy the Didget meter, which plugs into a handheld Nintendo DS system.

TABLE 13-6. Continuous Glucose Monitoring Systems[45-49]

PRODUCT NAME (MANUFACTURER/ DISTRIBUTOR)	COMPONENTS	DESCRIPTION
DexCom Seven Plus Continuous Blood Glucose Monitor (DexCom)	Sensor, wireless transmitter, receiver	The DexCom Seven Plus consists of a small, wire-like sensor that continuously measures glucose levels, which are transmitted to the Seven Plus receiver; the sensor is inserted under the skin 2 inches from the naval and can be worn for up to 7 days before it needs to be replaced; the receiver displays glucose measurements averaged every 5 min; the device must be calibrated every 12 hr with blood glucose readings ranged from 40–400 mg/dL; it alerts the user when blood glucose level drop below 55 mg/dL; DexCom Seven Plus is compatible with Data Manager 3 (DM3) software
Minimed Paradigm Real-Time (RT) Revel (Medtronic Diabetes)	Sensor, transmitter, remote control, blood glucose meter (optional)	The Minimed Paradigm RT Revel is a combination of a continuous blood glucose monitor and an insulin pump; the sensor is inserted in the subcutaneous layer of the skin at a site where there is adequate fatty tissue (abdominal area) and should be replaced every 3 days; the device measures blood glucose levels and can deliver insulin doses ranging from 0.0–25.0 units; the device must be calibrated every 12 hr after initial calibration; it alerts the user 30 min prior to reaching programmed upper or lower glucose limits; MiniMed Paradigm RT Revel is compatible with Carelink Personal software
Guardian Real-Time (RT) Glucose Monitoring System (Medtronic Diabetes)	Sensor, wireless transmitter, monitor	The Guardian RT consists of three components: sensor, wireless transmitter, and monitor; the sensor is inserted in the subcutaneous layer of the skin at a site where there is adequate fatty tissue (abdominal area) and should be replaced every 3 days; glucose readings are taken in time increments based on 3-, 6-, 12-, and 24-hr device selections; data is graphed on the monitor and can be saved and transferred to Carelink Personal software; the device must be calibrated every 12 hr after initial calibration; it alerts the user 30 min prior to reaching programmed upper or lower glucose limits

Most meters hold from 100 to 450 test results, though a few save well over 1000. This makes it easier to track blood glucose control over time. Many meters on the market have computer download capability through a USB connection. These meters come with their own software that can be downloaded directly to a desktop on both Mac and PC computers. Meter results can also be exported to an Excel file.[44]

An additional method to assess glucose control is called *continuous glucose monitoring (CGM)*, which provides readings every few minutes throughout the day. This method allows patients and providers an opportunity to observe trends in glucose levels throughout the day and make the appropriate adjustments to medication, meal, or exercise regimens. A small sterile disposable glucose-sensing device called a *sensor* is inserted into the subcutaneous tissue. This sensor measures the change in glucose levels in interstitial fluid and sends the information to a monitor that can store 3–7 days worth of data. The monitor must be calibrated daily by entering at least three blood glucose readings obtained at different times using a standard blood glucose meter. The monitors have an alert system to warn patients if their blood glucose level is dangerously low or high (Table 13-6).[45]

Generally, blood glucose concentrations determined by these methods are clinically useful estimates of corresponding plasma glucose concentrations measured by the laboratory. Therefore, home blood glucose monitoring is preferred to urine testing. Home blood testing clarifies the relationship between symptomatology and blood glucose concentrations. The best meter for a patient is an individual decision. Patients should be encouraged to try different brands of meters to find the device with which they are most comfortable.[42,43]

Quality control, which consists of control solution testing, calibration, and system maintenance, is a necessary component of accurate glucose testing. Most manufacturers supply control solutions with SMBG meters that can be used to assess the accuracy of the test strip. This method of verifying accuracy operates the same way that the patient analyzes a drop of blood. A few meters require manual calibration prior to use, but most have an automatic calibration mode for ease of use. In photometric meters, the blood sample intended for the strip may come in contact with the meter and soil the optic window resulting in inaccurate results. Pharmacists should guide patients through the instructions for cleaning the meter that are usually provided by the manufacturer.

Factors affecting glucose readings. Environmental factors such as temperature, humidity, altitude, and light may influence the accuracy of glucose readings. Exposing glucometers to extremes of temperature can alter battery life and performance. Therefore, glucometers should be stored at room temperature to ensure accuracy (most will function at temperatures between 50°F and 104°F). The ReliOn Precision Xtra will function at higher temperatures (122°F maximum) while the Sidekick glucose meter is ideal for lower temperatures (34°F minimum).[40,51] Temperature changes and humidity may decrease the shelf life of test strips resulting in inaccurate test results. Test strips should not be stored in areas of high humidity, such as a bathroom, or in areas with notable temperature changes, such as the car. Individuals should check the expiration date of the test strips. Because test strips are costly, patients are often tempted to use expired strips that result in inaccurate readings.[51] Most test strips expire within 90–180 days after being opened.

At higher altitudes, changes in oxygen content and temperature alter glucose testing results. Results of studies evaluating the accuracy of glucometers at altitudes greater than 10,000 feet have revealed major alterations in blood glucose levels. These changes were attributed to variations in metabolic rate, hydration, diet, physical exercise, hematocrit, and temperature associated with higher altitudes. Patients should be educated on how to use glucometers at high altitudes. Changes in light exposure can also alter results with photometric glucometers.[43] Additional variables such as hypotension, hypoxia, high triglyceride concentrations, and various drugs can alter readings; each patient should be evaluated for the presence of such variables and medication-related effects.

User error is the most common reason for inaccurate results. Some of the most common errors include not putting enough blood on the reagent. Patients should be asked periodically to demonstrate how they operate the meter.[43]

Frequency of glucose monitoring. Glucose monitoring requirements may vary based on the pharmacologic therapy administered. Patients who are well-controlled on oral medications should monitor blood glucose levels at least daily and more frequently if there are any changes in drugs or drug doses. Patients who are poorly controlled on oral medications should monitor blood glucose levels 2–4 times daily. Patients taking insulin injections twice a day should check blood glucose levels at least twice a day. Patients on intensive insulin therapy should monitor blood glucose levels 3–4 times a day. Patients on insulin pumps need monitoring 4–6 times a day to determine the effectiveness of the basal and bolus doses. In general, premeal glucose measurements are needed to monitor the effectiveness of the basal insulin dose (e.g., glargine or detemir) dose. Two-hour PPG readings are needed to monitor rapid-acting insulins (e.g., lispro, glulisine, and aspart). Oral blood glucose lowering agents, such as metformin, thiazolidinediones, sitagliptin, and glipizide, are evaluated using the 2-hour postprandial readings. Pregnancy requires frequent monitoring of blood glucose levels 4–6 times a day to ensure tight control, and premeal testing is required during acute illness to determine the need for supplemental insulin.[53-60]

Diagnosis of Hyperglycemia

The diagnosis of patients with hyperglycemia commonly falls into one of three categories: (1) DM or prediabetes, (2) DKA, and (3) hyperosmolar hyperglycemia state (HHS).

Diabetes Mellitus or Prediabetes

Goals of therapy. Once DM is diagnosed, the clinician needs to establish a therapeutic goal with respect to glucose control. The ideal goal would be to maintain concentrations at normal physiological levels. For type 1 patients, this effort requires tight control. Tight control could include preprandial plasma glucose concentrations of 90–130 mg/dL (5.0–7.2 mmol/L) and postprandial concentrations of less than 180 mg/dL (less than 10 mmol/L). Tight control requires intensive therapy and monitoring (i.e., three or more insulin injections per day and self-monitoring of glucose concentrations).[5]

Data from the Diabetes Control and Complications Trial (DCCT) suggest that this approach leads to significant health benefits.[61] Overall, the study showed that in patients with type 1 DM, intensive therapy delays the onset and slows progression of microvascular complications (e.g., diabetic retinopathy, nephropathy, and neuropathy), and macrovascular diseases (e.g., large vessel, peripheral vascular diseases, stroke, and ischemic heart disease).

The United Kingdom Prospective Diabetes Study (UKPDS 33) compared the effects of intensive drug therapy with a sulfonylurea (e.g., chlorpropamide and glipizide) insulin and conventional therapy (diet) in 3867 patients with newly diagnosed type 2 DM from 1977 until 1991.[62] The results of the UKPDS show that intensive drug therapy decreased the risk of microvascular complications when compared with conventional therapy. The investigators reported that patients in the intensive group with a 1% median reduction in A1c had a 25% reduction in risk of microvascular complications (p=0.0099).

Basal secretion of insulin from the pancreas occurs at a rate of 0.5–1 unit/hr. Bolus secretion of insulin occurs when blood sugar levels are above 100 mg/dL after ingestion of food. Therefore, the normal physiologic release pattern of insulin is one of valleys or basal secretion and peaks or bolus secretions (Figure 13-3a). The normal pancreas secretes 25–50 units of insulin daily.[63-64]

Because the most common and effective means to manage insulin deficiency is with insulin, the importance of the relationship between insulin injection and interpretation of glucose concentrations is briefly discussed. In general, 1 unit of any type of insulin produces the same metabolic response. Every 1–2 unit increase in the insulin dose usually leads to a 30–50 mg/dL decrease in the glucose concentration. Although the amount of *total* activity is equal for any given number of units of any insulin, the activity is not elicited evenly over time. A clinician must know the activity-over-time profiles of various insulin types at various injection sites to anticipate correctly a dose's effect on glucose concentrations at a particular time (Table 13-7).[63]

The starting dose of insulin is based on clinical assessment of insulin deficiency and insulin resistance, as well as the patient's lifestyle (i.e., eating patterns, exercise, and waking/sleep patterns). In general, insulin requirements for patients with type 1 DM with a BMI less than 25 kg/m² are 0.5–1.0 unit/kg/day. Insulin requirements may vary during illness or stress. Insulin requirements may decrease during the "honeymoon phase," a remission period that occurs early in the course of the disease.[28] Insulin requirements for patients with type 2 DM vary based on the degree of insulin resistance and insulin deficiency. In general, a single or bedtime dose of insulin can be given to patients with type 2 DM who do not achieve glycemic control with noninsulin agents. The noninsulin agents should be continued at the same dose in most cases. Patients with a BMI less than 25 kg/m² can be started on 5–10 units of intermediate or long-acting insulin at bedtime. Patients with a BMI greater than 25 kg/m² should be started on 10–15 units of

TABLE 13-7. Comparisons of Human Insulins and Insulin Analogues

INSULIN	ONSET (min)	PEAK ACTION (hr)	DURATION (hr)
Rapid-acting			
Lispro/aspart/glulisine	5–15	0.5–1.5	4–6
Short-acting			
Human regular	30–60	2–4	6–10
Intermediate-acting			
Human NPH	60–120	4–8	10–18
Combinations			
70/30; 50/50; 75/25	30–60	2–8	14–18
Long-acting			
Detemir	60–180	6–8	6–23
Glargine	60–180	Peakless	24

intermediate (NPH) or long-acting (glargine, detemir) insulin at bedtime or combination insulin (70/30) before dinner.[64]

Figures 13-3b and 13-3c illustrate the use of short-acting (regular) or rapid-acting (lispro, glulisine, or aspart) insulin before breakfast, lunch, and dinner and a long-acting basal insulin (detemir or glargine) given at bedtime. This regimen, often referred to as "the poor man's pump," is ideal for patients with unusual schedules. Figures 13-3d and 13-3e illustrate insulin therapy administered by an insulin pump. The pump is programmed to administer insulin (rapid- or short-acting) throughout the day, and the patient activates the pump to give a bolus of insulin prior to meals. Intensive regimens require more frequent monitoring and are accompanied by an increased risk of hypoglycemia.

In a single daily injection regimen (Figure 13-3f), one injection of intermediate or long-acting insulin is administered at bedtime. This regimen is ideal for a patient with type 2 DM who has failed to obtain glycemic control on oral agents. The oral agents can be continued and long-acting insulin can be administered at bedtime.

In a twice-a-day injection regimen (Figure 13-3g), an injection of intermediate-acting insulin is administered before breakfast and at bedtime. The administration of intermediate-acting insulin before bedtime decreases the risk of hypoglycemia in the early morning.

An average regimen (Figure 13-3h) combines a mixed injection of intermediate-acting and regular insulin given before breakfast, an injection of regular insulin at dinner, and another injection of intermediate-acting insulin given before bedtime, which provides safer, more effective overnight glucose control. Without regular insulin administered before dinner, however, glucose concentrations may become unacceptably high after dinner.

Regular insulin should be given 30–45 minutes before meals unless the preprandial glucose concentration is below 70 mg/dL (<3.9 mmol/L). If the concentration is less than 70 mg/dL, the patient should consume 15 g of carbohydrates (e.g., 4 ounces

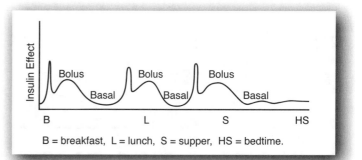

B = breakfast, L = lunch, S = supper, HS = bedtime.

FIGURE 13-3A. Normal physiologic release pattern of insulin in adult. Adapted with permission from reference 64.

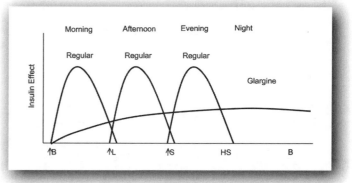

FIGURE 13-3B. Effect of short-acting insulin before meals and long-acting insulin at bedtime. Adapted with permission from reference 64.

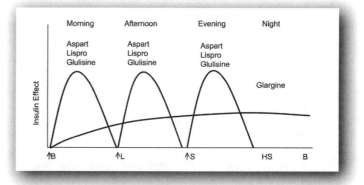

FIGURE 13-3C. Effect of rapid-acting insulin before meals and a long-acting insulin at bedtime. Adapted with permission from reference 64.

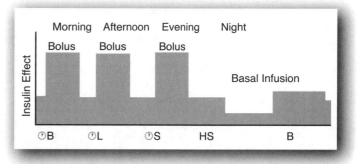

FIGURE 13-3D. Effect of short-acting insulin boluses at meals and basal insulin pump. Adapted with permission from reference 64.

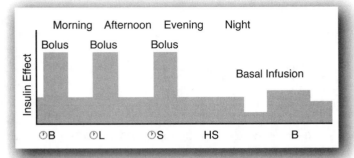

FIGURE 13-3E. Effect of rapid-acting insulin boluses at meals and basal insulin pump. Adapted with permission from reference 64.

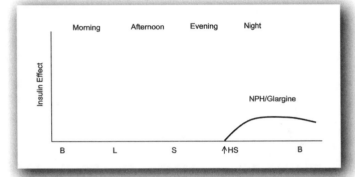

FIGURE 13-3F. Effect of a single bedtime dose of long-acting insulin. Adapted with permission from reference 64.

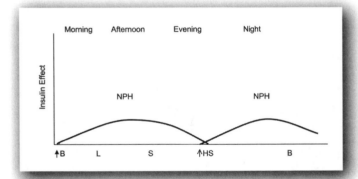

FIGURE 13-3G. Effect of intermediate-acting insulin before breakfast and at bedtime. Adapted with permission from reference 64.

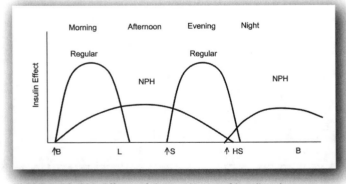

FIGURE 13-3H. Effect of three doses of insulin: short-acting, intermediate-acting, and mixed. Adapted with permission from reference 64.

of orange juice, regular soda, or skim milk) immediately, and check glucose levels 15 minutes later. In all regimens, regular insulin doses are adjusted on the basis of self-monitored preprandial glucose concentrations. Lispro, glulisine, and aspart insulin should be given 5–15 minutes before a meal. Insulin should be used along with diet, exercise, and stress management for best effects.[62-64]

Oral agents in the management of type 2 DM. Currently, there are several classes of oral agents available for the management of diabetes. All lower blood glucose concentrations in responsive patients (Table 13-8).

The sodium glucose cotransporter inhibitors (SGLT-2 inhibitors), which inhibit the SGLT in the renal tubules represent a novel class of drugs currently under development. Inhibition of SGLT-2 promotes renal glucose excretion resulting in improved glycemic control. Dapagliflozin is the first of the new class of agents that recently underwent review by the FDA. In addition to its glucose lowering effect, dapagliflozin appears to have favorable impacts on weight and blood pressure (BP), and has a low risk of causing hypoglycemia. However, as with all new treatments, long-term safety is unknown. Clinical trials have shown that dapagliflozin may cause urinary tract infection, headache, diarrhea, nasopharyngitis, and back pain.[16] The FDA recently requested more data on dapagliflozin's safety due to concerns regarding a possible increased incidence of breast and bladder cancer in patients on dapagliflozin. Nine cases of bladder cancer occurred in male patients who took dapagliflozin in clinical trials, compared with one case among patients treated with a placebo. Breast cancer occurred in nine patients who took the new drug, and in one patient in the control group. Further clinical investigation will confirm or refute whether these concerns are valid.[16,17]

Diabetic Ketoacidosis

Insulin deficiency after ingestion of a meal can result in impaired glucose utilization by peripheral tissues and the liver. Prolonged insulin deficiency results in protein breakdown and increased hepatic glucose production (gluconeogenesis) by the liver and increased release of counter regulatory hormones such as glucagon, catecholamines (e.g., epinephrine and norepinephrine), cortisol, and growth hormones. In the face of lipolysis, free fatty acids are converted by the liver to ketone bodies (beta-hydroxybutyric acid and acetoacetic acid), which results in metabolic acidosis. Diabetic ketoacidosis, which occurs most commonly in patients with type 1 DM, is initiated by insulin deficiency. (See Minicase 1.) The most common causes of DKA are[70]

- Infections, illness, and emotional stress
- Nonadherence or inadequate insulin dosage
- Undiagnosed type 1 DM
- Unknown or no precipitating event

Clinically, patients with DKA typically present with dehydration, lethargy, acetone-smelling breath, abdominal pain, tachycardia, orthostatic hypotension, tachypnea, and, occasionally, mild hypothermia, and lethargy or coma. Because of the patient's tendency toward low body temperatures, fever strongly suggests infection as a precipitant of DKA.

TABLE 13-8. Antidiabetic Agents[65-69]

CLASS	AGENT	MECHANISM	SIDE EFFECTS	DOSAGE RANGE AND ROUTE OF ADMINISTRATION	LAB TESTS FOR MONITORING
Sulfonylureas		Increases insulin secretion by binding to sulfonylurea receptor on pancreatic beta cell and blocking ATP-K channels	Hypoglycemia, weight gain, water retention, hematologic reactions, skin reactions (particularly rashes), purpura, nausea, vomiting and cholestasis, constipation, headache, photosensitivity		Directly affects FPG and PPG; A1c should be monitored to assess overall glycemic control
1st generation	Chlorpropamide Diabinese®		Disulfiram-like reaction when combined with alcohol; excessive hypoglycemia in patients with renal insufficiency so avoid	100–500 mg PO daily; max: 750 mg/day	
	Tolazamide Tolinase®			100–1000 mg PO in 1 or 2 divided doses daily	
	Tolbutamide Orinase®			500–2500 mg PO in 1–3 divided doses daily	
2nd generation	Glipizide Glucotrol®		Increased risk of rash when compared to other sulfonylureas	5–10 mg PO daily; titrate to maximum dose of 40 mg daily; usually not above 20 mg/day; give 30 min before meals	
	Glyburide Diabeta®, Glynase®, Micronase®		Dizziness, blurred vision; avoid in patients with renal insufficiency (do not use if CrCl <50 mL/min)	5 mg PO daily; titrate to maximum dose of 20 mg daily; usually not above 10 mg/day	
	Glimepiride Amaryl®		Mild incidence of hypoglycemia, fullness, heartburn, blood dyscrasias	1–2 mg PO daily; titrate to maintenance; usually not above 8 mg/day	
D-phenylalanine derivative	Nateglinide Starlix®	Increases insulin secretion by blocking ATP-K channels on the pancreatic beta cells	Mild hypoglycemia (primarily postprandial), nausea, diarrhea, weight gain	60–360 mg PO daily; give before meals	Directly affects PPG; FPG and A1c should be monitored to assess overall glycemic control
Meglitinide	Repaglinide Prandin®	Increases insulin secretion by blocking ATP-K channels on the pancreatic beta cells	Mild hypoglycemia (primarily postprandial), nausea, diarrhea, upper respiratory infection, headache, rhinitis, bronchitis, back pain, tooth disorder, chest pain, hyperglycemia, heartburn, epigastric fullness, weight gain	0.5–2 mg (maximum of 4 mg) should be taken 15 min prior to meals, but may vary from immediately preceding a meal to as long 30 min prior; dosed up to 4 times daily in response to meal pattern; max: 16 mg/day	Directly affects PPG; FPG and A1c should be monitored to assess overall glycemic control

TABLE 13-8. Antidiabetic Agents[65-69], continued

CLASS	AGENT	MECHANISM	SIDE EFFECTS	DOSAGE RANGE AND ROUTE OF ADMINISTRATION	LAB TESTS FOR MONITORING
Biguanide	Metformin Glucophage®	Inhibits gluconeo-genesis, increases insulin sensitivity by increasing tyrosine kinase activity, increases glycogen synthesis	GI side effects including abdominal discomfort and diarrhea are most common; interference with vitamin B$_{12}$ absorption; rarely lactic acidosis (especially when hypoperfusion is present (e.g., renal impairment and heart failure); do not use if SCr 1.5 (males), ≥1.4 (females) or eGFR 50 mL/min	500 mg PO once a day to start (decreases incidence of diarrhea), increase by 500 mg increments per week as tolerated; given in divided dose q 8–12 hr; maximum dose: 2550 mg/day	FPG, A1c, SCr
Alpha-glucosidase inhibitors		Inhibits alpha-glucosidase enzyme, which metabolizes complex carbohydrates and sucrose (cane sugar)	Bloating, abdominal discomfort/pain, diarrhea and flatulence in up to 30% of patients; abnormal liver function tests	25 mg PO daily with first bite of food; titrate slowly to 3 times a day; maximum dose 50 mg 3 times a day for patients <60 kg and 100 mg TID for patients >60 kg; do not take without a meal	Directly affects PPG; FPG and A1c should be monitored to assess overall glycemic control, liver function tests
	Acarbose Precose®				AST and ALT every 3 months for 1 yr
	Miglitol Glyset®		Skin rash, no reports of hepatic toxicity to date		
Thiazolidinediones		Facilitates muscle cell response to insulin by acting on the PPAR, thereby allowing glucose to diffuse into the cell more effectively	Hepatotoxicity, edema; contraindicated in patients with congestive heart failure NYHA class III or IV, rash, weight gain, decrease in hemoglobin and hematocrit; possible increase in LDL chol-esterol; potential increase in heart attacks and heart-related chest pain; do not use if ALT >2.5x ULN		Directly affects PPG and FPG; A1c should be monitored to assess overall glycemic control liver function tests, hemoglobin, and hematocrit
	Rosiglitazone Avandia®		Do not use in combination with insulin or nitrates (may increase risk of myocardial infarction)	4 mg PO daily; maximum dose of 8 mg daily; 4 mg BID more effective than 8 mg daily	
	Pioglitazone Actos®		May increase risk of bladder cancer with long-term use (>2 yr use)	15–30 mg PO daily; maximum dose 45 mg (30 mg max if on insulin)	

TABLE 13-8. Antidiabetic Agents[65-69], continued

CLASS	AGENT	MECHANISM	SIDE EFFECTS	DOSAGE RANGE AND ROUTE OF ADMINISTRATION	LAB TESTS FOR MONITORING
GLP-1 agonists		GLP-1, a naturally occurring peptide, which enhances insulin secretion in response to elevated plasma glucose levels	Hypoglycemia when combined with sulfonylureas; nausea is common; vomiting, diarrhea, dizziness, headache, jitteriness, weight loss		
	Exenatide Byetta®	Mimetic of GLP-1		Subcutaneous injection of 5–10 mcg twice a day 60 min before morning and evening meals (do not use if CrCl <30 mL/min)	FPG, PPG, A1c
	Bydureon®	Mimetic of GLP-1		Subcutaneous injection of once a week	
	Liraglutide Victoza®	Analog of GLP-1	Black-box warning: can increase risk of thyroid C-cell tumors, MTC, and multiple endocrine neoplasia syndrome type 2	Subcutaneous injection of 0.6 mg once a day; max daily dose of 1.8 mg daily	FPG, PPG, A1c
DPP-4 inhibitor		Inhibits DPP-4; increases levels of GLP-1, suppresses glucagon secretion	Hypoglycemia when used in combination with sulfonylurea, nausea, diarrhea, headache, upper respiratory tract infection		Directly affects PPG; FPG and A1c should be monitored to assess overall glycemic control
	Sitagliptin Januvia®			100 mg PO once daily (50 mg PO once daily if CrCl 30–50 mL/min, 25 mg PO once daily if CrCl <30 mL/min)	
	Saxagliptin Onglyza®			5 mg PO once daily (2.5 mg PO once daily if CrCl <50 mL/min)	
	Linagliptin Tradjenta®			5 mg PO once daily	

TABLE 13-8. Antidiabetic Agents[65-69], continued

CLASS	AGENT	MECHANISM	SIDE EFFECTS	DOSAGE RANGE AND ROUTE OF ADMINISTRATION	LAB TESTS FOR MONITORING
Amylin analog	Pramlintide Symlin®	Improves glycemic control by slowing the rate of gastric emptying, preventing postprandial rise in glucagon levels, and increasing sensations of satiety, thereby reducing caloric intake and potentiating weight loss	Nausea, headache, vomiting, anorexia, weight loss	Subcutaneous injection; preprandial, rapid-acting, short-acting, and fixed-mix insulin doses should by decreased by 50% when pramlintide is initiated; for type 1 patients, initial recommended dosing is 15 mcg, which should be titrated at 15-mcg increments to a maintenance dose of 30 mcg or 60 mcg as tolerated; for type 2 patients, initial dose should be 60 mcg, with a single increment increase to 120 mcg as tolerated	Directly affects PPG; FPG and A1c should be monitored to assess overall glycemic control
Bile acid Sequestrants	Colesevelam Welchol®	Binds bile acids, cholesterol	Constipation, ↑ triglycerides; may interfere with the absorption of other medications	1875 mg (three 625 mg tablets PO twice a day or 3750 (six 625 mg tablets) PO once a day	FPG, A1c, triglycerides, LDL, HDL
Dopamine agonists	Bromocriptine Cycloset®	Increases dopamine levels; inhibits excessive sympathetic tone within the CNS; this enhances suppression of hepatic glucose production and reduces postmeal plasma glucose levels	Somnolence, hypotension, syncope, nausea, vomiting, fatigue	0.8 mg PO once a day in the morning; may increase dose each week with a maximum dose of 4.8 mg/day	Directly affects PPG; monitor FPG and A1c to assess glycemic control

A1c = glycosylated hemoglobin; ALT = alanine aminotransferase; AST = aspartate aminotransferase; ATP-K = adenosine triphosphate–potassium; BID = twice a day; CNS = central nervous system; CrCl = creatinine clearance; DPP-4 = dipeptidyl peptidase-4; eGFR = estimated glomerular filtration rate; FPG= fasting plasma glucose; GI = gastrointestinal; GLP-1 = glucagon-like peptide-1; HDL = high density lipoprotein; LDL = low density lipoprotein; MTC = medullary thyroid carcinoma; NYHA = New York Heart Association; PO = oral; PPAR = peroxisome proliferator-activated receptor; PPG = postprandial glucose; SCr = serum creatinine; TID = three times a day; ULN = upper limit of normal.

Chemically, DKA is characterized by a high glucose concentration. This concentration is typically greater than 300 mg/dL or 16.8 mmol/L. The plasma glucose concentration is not related to the severity of DKA. Some patients who continue to administer insulin, are pregnant, have not eaten adequately, or have vomited excessively, may present with lower glucose concentrations. As insulin is given, the glucose concentrations decline at a rate of about 75–100 mg/dL/hr.[71]

Diabetic ketoacidosis is also characterized by low venous bicarbonate 0–15 mEq/L) and a decreased arterial pH (<7.20).

Hyperglycemia can lead to osmotic diuresis resulting in hypotonic fluid losses, dehydration, and electrolyte loss. Sodium and potassium concentrations may be low, normal, or high. Sodium concentrations are reflective of the amount of total body water and sodium lost and replaced. In the presence of hyperglycemia, sodium concentrations may be decreased because of the movement of water from the intracellular space to the extracellular space. The potassium level reflects a balance between the amount of potassium lost in the urine and insulin deficiency, which causes higher concentrations of serum potassium as potassium shifts from intracellular spaces to extracellular fluid. Hypertonicity and acidosis can cause potassium to move from the intracellular space to the extracellular space resulting in elevated potassium levels. However, total potassium depletion always occurs regardless of the initial potassium level. Patients with low or normal potassium levels should be monitored closely because treatment can result in a severe total body potassium deficit that may place the patient at risk for cardiac dysrhythmia.

The phosphate level is usually normal or slightly elevated.[71,72] Creatinine and blood urea nitrogen (BUN) are usually elevated due to dehydration. These levels usually return to normal after rehydration unless there was pre-existing renal insufficiency. Hemoglobin, hematocrit, and total protein levels are mildly elevated due to decreased plasma volume and dehydration. Amylase levels may be increased due to increased secretion by the salivary glands. Liver function tests are usually elevated, but return to normal in 3–4 weeks.

Initially, potassium concentrations may be elevated due to metabolic acidosis. Correction of acidosis elicits the opposite effect. Potassium shifts intracellularly with insulin therapy, leading to a decrease in serum potassium concentrations. Serum osmolality is typically elevated at 300–320 mOsm/kg (normally, 280–295 mOsm/kg). Serum osmolarity (milliosmoles per liter), which is practically equivalent to osmolality (milliosmoles per kilogram), can be estimated using the following formula:

$$\text{serum osmolarity (mOsm/L)} = (2 \times \text{sodium}) + \text{glucose}/18 + \text{BUN}/2.8$$

where glucose and BUN units are milligrams per deciliter.

Blood and urine ketones. Ketones are present in the blood and urine of patients in DKA, as the name of this disorder implies. Formation of ketone bodies, acetoacetate, acetone, and beta-hydroxybutyrate, is the main cause of acidosis in DKA.[72,73] Diabetic ketoacidosis can be prevented if patients are educated about detection of hyperglycemia and ketonuria. It is recommended that all patients with DM test their urine for ketones during acute illness or stress, when blood glucose levels are consistently >250 mg/dL (14 mmol/L), during pregnancy, or when any symptoms of ketoacidosis—such as nausea, vomiting, or abdominal pain—are present.[73,74]

All of the commercially available urine testing methods are based on the reaction of acetoacetic acid with sodium nitroprusside (nitroferricyanide) in a strongly basic medium. The colors range from beige or buff-pink for a "negative" reading to pink and pink-purple for a "positive" reading (Acetest®, Ketostix®, Labstix®, and Multistix®). These nitroprusside-based (nitroferricyanide) assays do not detect beta-hydroxybutyrate and are 15–20 times more sensitive to acetoacetate than to acetone. In a few situations (e.g., severe hypovolemia, hypotension, low partial pressure of oxygen [PO$_2$], and alcoholism) where beta-hydroxybutyrate predominates, assessment of ketones may be falsely low. As DKA resolves, beta-hydroxybutyric acid is converted to acetoacetate, the assay-reactive ketone

body. Therefore, a stronger reaction may be encountered in laboratory results. However, this reaction does not necessarily mean a worsening of the ketoacidotic state.[34]

Clinicians must keep in mind that ketonuria may also result from starvation, high-fat diets, fever, and anesthesia, but these conditions are not associated with hyperglycemia. Levodopa, mesna, acetylcysteine (irrigation), methyldopa, phenazopyridine, pyrazinamide, valproic acid, captopril, and high-dose aspirin may cause false-positive results with urine ketone tests.[75–78,81] The influence of these drugs on serum ketone tests has not been studied extensively. If the ketone concentration is increased, a typical series of dipstick results is

1. Negative
2. Trace or 5 mg/dL
3. Small or 15 mg/dL
4. Moderate or 40 mg/dL
5. Large or 80 mg/dL
6. Very large or 160 mg/dL

False-negative readings have been reported when test strips have been exposed to air for an extended period of time or when urine specimens have been highly acidic, such as after large intakes of ascorbic acid.[34]

Urine ketone tests should not be used for diagnosing or monitoring treatment of DKA. Acetoacetic and beta-hydroxybutyric acids concentrations in urine greatly exceed blood concentrations. Therefore, the presence of ketone bodies in urine cannot be used to diagnose DKA. Conversely, during recovery from ketoacidosis, ketone bodies may be detected in urine long after blood concentrations have fallen.[34,81] In addition, urine testing only provides an estimate of blood ketone levels 2–4 hours before testing and is dependent on the person being able to pass urine. The ADA recommends testing blood beta-ketone because ketones are detectable in the blood far earlier than in urine, so blood beta-ketone testing can provide a patient with an early warning of impending DKA.[74] A beta-hydroxybutyric level less than 0.6 mmol/L is considered normal. Patients with levels between 0.6 and 1.0 mmol/L should take additional insulin and increase their fluid intake to flush out the ketones. Patients should contact their physician if levels are between 1.0–3.0 mmol/L. Patients should be advised to report to the emergency room immediately if their levels are greater than 3.0 mmol/L.[78,79]

Hyperosmolar Hyperglycemia State

Hyperosmolar hyperglycemia state (HHS) is a condition that occurs most frequently in elderly patients with type 2 DM, and it is usually precipitated by stress or illness when such patients do not drink enough to keep up with osmotic diuresis. Patients usually present with severe hyperglycemia (glucose concentrations greater than 600 mg/dL or greater than 33.3 mmol/L); decreased mentation (e.g., lethargy, confusion, dehydration); neurologic manifestations (e.g., seizures and hemisensory deficits); and an absence of ketosis. Insulin deficiency is not as severe in HHS as in DKA. Therefore, lipolysis—which is necessary for the formation of ketone bodies—does not occur. (See Minicase 2.) The absence of ketosis results in significantly milder GI symptoms than patients with DKA. Therefore,

MINICASE 1

Diabetic Ketoacidosis

VERA K. IS A 29-YEAR-OLD FEMALE with a 20-year history of type 1 DM. She presents to the ED with a pH of 7.15, HCO3 of 9, and blood glucose greater than 600 mg/dL. Vera K.'s husband brought her into the ED after finding her "out of it" when attempting to wake her. Two days ago, she developed fever, chills, and polyuria. She has not been monitoring her blood glucose levels regularly.

Vera K. recently switched to a new insulin pump but did not receive any formal training on how to use the pump. The ED physician noticed that the pump was disconnected. Physical examination revealed a lethargic female with a BP of 116/68 (which dropped to 95/50 when standing), HR 105, respiratory rate 30 (deep and regular), and oral temperature 101.4°F (38.6°C). Her skin turgor was poor, and her mucous membranes were dry. Vera K. had a fruity aromatic odor to her breath and was disoriented and confused. Her lab results were as follows:

- Sodium, 143 mEq/L (136–142 mEq/L)
- Potassium, 5.4 mEq/L (3.8–5.0 mEq/L)
- Chloride, 99 mEq/L (95–103 mEq/L)
- BUN, 38 mg/dL (8–23 mg/dL)
- SCr, 2.8 mg/dL (0.6–1.2 mg/dL)
- Phosphorus, 2.7 mg/dL (2.3–4.7 mg/dL)
- Amylase, 350 International Units/L (30–220 International Units/L)
- pH, 7.15 (7.38–7.44)
- Bicarbonate, 9.0 mEq/L (21–280 mEq/L)
- Hct, 52% (36% to 45%)
- WBCs, 16 x 10^3 cells/mm³ (4.8–10.8 × 10^3 cells/mm³)
- Calcium, 9 mg/dL (9.2–11.0 mg/dL)
- Glucose, 650 mg/dL (70–110 mg/dL)
- Ketones, 3+ @1:8 serum dilution (normal = 0)
- Osmolality, 335 mOsm/kg (280–295 mOsm/kg)
- Triglycerides, 174 mg/dL (10–190 mg/dL)
- Lipase, 1.4 units/mL (<1.5 units/mL)
- Magnesium, 2 mEq/L (1.3–2.1 mEq/L)

A urine screen with Multistix indicated a "large" (160 mg/dL) amount of ketones (the highest designation on the strip).

Question: Based on clinical and lab findings, what is the most likely diagnosis for Vera K.? What precipitated this metabolic disorder? Can interpretation of any results be influenced by her acidosis or hyperglycemia? Are there potential drug interferences with any lab tests?

Discussion: Vera K., a type 1 DM patient, developed DKA from an infection and interruption in insulin delivery. Insulin pump therapy uses only rapid- or short-acting insulin. Therefore, any interruption in insulin delivery (due to infusion set clogs, leaks, loss of insulin potency, or pump malfunction) may result in hyperglycemia (high blood glucose) within 2–4 hours and, subsequently, the rapid onset of DKA within 4–10 hours. The onset of stress or illness (caused by infection or an emotional event) can also result in a rise of blood glucose levels and the development of DKA, which rarely occurs in patients with type 2 DM. Clinically, Vera K.'s presentation is classic. Her decreased skin turgor, dry mucous membranes, tachycardia (HR of 105), and orthostatic hypotension are consistent with dehydration, a common condition in patients with DKA. Her breathing is rapid and deep. Although she is not comatose, she is lethargic, confused, and disoriented.

Chemically, Vera K. probably has a total body deficit of sodium and

potassium despite serum concentration results within normal limits. Orthostatic hypotension is consistent with decreased intravascular volume, causing hemoconcentration of these electrolytes. Therefore, these values do not reflect total body stores, and the clinician can expect them to decline rapidly if unsupplemented fluids are infused. Although Vera K.'s phosphorus concentration is in the normal range (lower end), it likely will decrease after rehydration and insulin. Serial testing should be done every 3–4 hours during the first 24 hours.

Serial glucose, ketones, and acid–base measurements, typical of DKA, should show gradual improvement with proper therapy. With use of the sodium correction factor (addition of 2 mEq/L to the sodium result for every 100 mg/dL of glucose above 200 mg/dL), Vera K.'s sodium would have been 152 mEq/L had her glucose been normal, a value more consistent with the BUN and Hct concentrations. Potassium balance is altered in patients with DKA because of combined urinary and GI losses. While total potassium is depleted, the serum potassium concentration may be high, normal, or low, depending on the degree of acidosis. Vera K.'s metabolic acidosis has resulted in an extracellular shifting of potassium, causing an elevated serum potassium concentration. Potassium supplementation may be withheld for the first hour or until serum levels begin to drop. Low serum potassium in the face of pronounced acidosis suggests severe potassium depletion requiring early, aggressive therapy to prevent life-threatening hypokalemia during treatment.

Decreased intravascular volume has led to a hemoconcentrated hematocrit and BUN, which is also elevated by decreased renal perfusion (prerenal azotemia), although intrinsic renal causes should be considered if SCr is also elevated. Fortunately, as is probably the case with Vera K., high SCr may be an artifact caused by the influence of ketone bodies on the assay. If so, SCr concentrations should decline with ketone concentrations.

Vera K. also exhibits the typical leukocytosis that often accompanies DKA in the absence of infection. Her estimated plasma osmolarity based on the osmolarity estimation formula would be $(2 \times 143) + (650/18) + (38/2.8) = 335.7$ mOsm/L, is approximately equal to the actual measured laboratory result. This value is slightly higher than usual for DKA (300–320 mOsm/kg).

The serum ketone results still would have to be interpreted as real and significant, given all of the other signs and symptoms. A urine screen also indicated the presence of ketones.

A serum amylase and lipase were measured to rule out pancreatitis, usually suspected with abdominal pain. However, elevated amylase probably originated from the salivary glands because Vera K.'s lipase was normal. An elevated amylase is observed in 20% of patients with DKA. Assessment of Vera K.'s willingness to check her blood glucose levels 4–6 times a day should be assessed before she is discharged. The frequency and timing of SMBG vary based on several factors, including an individual's glycemic goals, the current level of glucose control, and the treatment regimen. The ADA recommends SMBG (4–6 times per day) for patients receiving insulin pump therapy. Pump therapy is not recommended for patients who are unwilling or unable to perform a minimum of four blood glucose tests per day and to maintain contact with their healthcare professional. If Vera K. agrees to the terms of the self-management to receive insulin pump therapy, she should be advised to always carry an "emergency kit" of supplies (including insulin, syringes or pens, blood glucose test strips, and meter and urine ketone test strips), in case she develops a problem with her pump and her insulin delivery is stopped, putting her at risk for hyperglycemia.

patients often fail to seek medical attention. Patients with HHS are usually more dehydrated on presentation than patients with DKA due to impairment in the thirst mechanism, which results in prolonged diuresis and dehydration.[72]

In some cases, patients are taking drugs that cause glucose intolerance (e.g., diuretics, steroids, and phenytoin). Stroke and infection are nondrug predisposing factors. Initially, electrolytes are within normal ranges, but BUN routinely is elevated. Serum osmolalities characteristically are higher than those in diabetic ketoacidosis—in the range of 320–400 mOsm/kg. Serum electrolytes (e.g., magnesium, phosphorus, and calcium) are typically abnormal and should be monitored until they return to normal range.[71-73]

Hypoglycemia

Hypoglycemia is defined as a blood glucose level of 70 mg/dL (3.9 mmol/L) or lower. The classification of hypoglycemia is based on the individual's ability to self-treat. Mild hypoglycemia is characterized by symptoms such as sweating, trembling,

---

MINICASE 2

Hyperosmolar Hyperglycemia State Secondary to Uncontrolled Type 2 DM

EARL V. IS A 63-YEAR-OLD AFRICAN-AMERICAN MALE with a 19-year history of T2DM, hypertension, and dyslipidemia. He lives alone. His medication lists includes glipizide 10 mg twice a day, simvastatin 20 mg daily at bedtime, lisinopril 20 mg daily, hydrochlorothiazide 25 mg daily, and ASA 325 mg daily. He monitors his blood glucose once a day, and his results have ranged from 215–400 mg/dL. His fasting blood glucose has averaged 200 mg/dL over the last week. He reports frequent urination throughout the day and night, which has increased over the last 6 days. He denies any nausea or vomiting but states he hasn't had much of an appetite lately. "I'm just not feeling like myself lately." His daughter accompanied him to the doctor's office because she felt he has been acting weird lately.

Physical examination revealed a very disoriented and confused man with a BP of 120/60 (which dropped to 95/50 when standing), HR 100, respiratory rate 20 (deep and regular), and oral temperature 101.4°F (38.6°C). His skin turgor was poor, and his mucous membranes were dry. His lab results were as follows:

- Sodium, 139 mEq/L (136–142 mEq/L)
- Potassium, 4.6 mEq/L (3.8–5.0 mEq/L)
- Chloride, 102 mEq/L (95–103 mEq/L)
- BUN, 50 mg/dL (8–23 mg/dL)
- SCr, 3.0 mg/dL (0.6–1.2 mg/dL)
- Phosphorus, 2.7 mg/dL (2.3–4.7 mg/dL)
- pH, 7.38 (7.36–7.44)
- Bicarbonate, 26 mEq/L (21–28 mEq/L)
- Hct, 39% (36% to 45%)
- WBCs, 9.4x 10^3 cells/mm³ (4.8–10.8 × 10^3 cells/mm³)
- Calcium, 9 mg/dL (9.2–11.0 mg/dL)
- Glucose, 715 mg/dL (70–110 mg/dL)
- Ketones, 0 @1:8 serum dilution (normal = 0)
- Osmolality, 335 mOsm/kg (280–295 mOsm/kg)
- Triglycerides, 174 mg/dL (10–190 mg/dL)
- Lipase, 1.4 units/mL (<1.5 units/mL)
- Magnesium, 2 mEq/L (1.3–2.1 mEq/L)
- Hemoglobin A1c, 9.5 (4% to 5.6%)

Question: Based on the subjective and objective data provided, what is the most likely diagnosis for Earl V.? What signs and symptoms support the diagnosis? What could have precipitated this disorder?

Discussion: Earl V. is over 60 years of age. Hyperosmolar hyperglycemia state occurs most frequently in the elderly population. He complains of symptoms for more than 5 days. He has decreased skin turgor, dry mucous membranes, tachycardia (HR 100), and orthostatic hypotension (a fall of systolic BP of 20 mm Hg after 1 minute of standing), which are consistent with dehydration. He is lethargic, confused, and disoriented (HHS patients are generally more dehydrated; therefore, mentation changes are more commonly seen in HHS than in DKA). The elderly often have an impaired thirst mechanism that increases the risk of HHS. Earl V. has lost fluids over a longer period of time.

Earl V.'s plasma glucose level is greater than 600 mg/dL; bicarbonate concentration is normal; and pH is normal. Negative ketone bodies <2+ in 1:1 dilution confirms the diagnosis of HHS (and not DKA where ketones are present in the blood and urine of patients). Insulin deficiency is less profound in HHS; therefore, lipolysis resulting in the production of ketone bodies does not occur. Earl V.'s plasma osmolarity can be estimated using a formula:

$$pOsm = (2 \times serum\ sodium) + glucose/18 + BUN/2.8$$

The estimated osmolality is (2 × 139) + (715/18) + 50/2.8 = 335 mOsm/kg, which is close to the actual lab value. Massive fluid loss due to prolonged osmotic diuresis secondary to hyperglycemia may have precipitated the onset of HHS.

Earl V. should be rehydrated with oral fluids since he has no complaints of GI discomfort. Insulin should be administered. Although Earl V.'s sodium and potassium are within normal limits, the presence of orthostatic hypotension is consistent with decreased intravascular volume, causing hemoconcentration of sodium and potassium. Potassium shifts out of cells when the pH of the blood is acidic due to an increased influx of hydrogen ions. The total potassium concentration appears normal because potassium has shifted from the intracellular compartment to the circulation. These levels may decline when the patient is rehydrated with fluids. Potassium replacement will probably be required. Phosphorus is also within normal limits but may decrease after rehydration and insulin. Decreased intravascular volume has led to hemoconcentration of hematocrit and Bun, which is also elevated by decreased renal perfusion (prerenal azotemia), although intrinsic renal causes should be considered if SCr is also elevated.

Although metformin is considered the first-line therapy for patients with type 2 DM, not all patients with type 2 DM are candidates for metformin. Patients must have good renal, hepatic, respiratory, and cardiac function to be considered a candidate for metformin therapy. One injection of long-acting insulin administered at breakfast or bedtime is a ideal regimen for a patient with type 2 DM who has failed to obtain glycemic control on oral agent(s). The oral agents can be continued and long-acting insulin can be administered at bedtime.

shaking, rapid heartbeat, heavy breathing, and difficulty concentrating. The symptoms associated with mild hypoglycemia vary in severity and does not imply that the symptoms experienced by the individual are minor or easily tolerated. While patients may experience profuse sweating, dizziness, and lack of coordination, they still may be able to self-treat. These symptoms resolve after consuming carbohydrates (e.g., fruit juice, milk, or hard candy).[82,83]

Severe hypoglycemia is characterized by an inability to self-treat due to mental confusion or unconsciousness. Emergency medical treatment is required to raise the blood glucose level out of a dangerously low range.[82,83]

Increased release of counter regulatory hormones is responsible for most hypoglycemic symptoms. Most of the early signs of hypoglycemia (e.g., trembling, shaking, rapid heartbeat, fast pulse, heavy breathing, and changes in body temperature) are mediated by the adrenergic system. Sweating, another cardinal sign of hypoglycemia, is mediated by the cholinergic system.[84]

Glucagon and epinephrine are the primary counter regulatory hormones responsible for increasing blood glucose concentrations in the presence of hypoglycemia. Glucagon enhances glycogenolysis and epinephrine increases gluconeogenesis and inhibits glucose utilization by tissues. Defects in hormonal counter regulation can diminish autonomic symptoms resulting in hypoglycemia unawareness. Glucagon secretion may become impaired after the first few years of type 1 DM, resulting in epinephrine as the primary mechanism for raising low blood glucose levels. Frequent episodes of hypoglycemia can cause temporary deficits in epinephrine response, resulting in an absence of autonomic symptoms for several days. Epinephrine response returns to normal when patients avoid low blood glucose levels over a period of 3–6 weeks. Patients with diabetes must be taught the importance of maintaining a balanced diet and monitoring their blood glucose levels regularly to decrease the risk of developing hypoglycemia.[82,84]

Neuroglycopenia occurs during hypoglycemic episodes due to decreased glucose supply to the central nervous system (CNS). The earliest signs of neuroglycopenia include slow thinking and difficulty concentrating and reading. Patients report that it takes more effort to perform routine tasks (e.g., brushing teeth, combing hair, or taking a bath). As the blood glucose levels decrease further, mental confusion, disorientation, slurred or rambling speech, irrational behavior, and extreme fatigue and lethargy may occur. Neuroglycopenia is usually the cause of physical injuries and accidents that occur during hypoglycemic episodes. Most patients with deficits in epinephrine will only experience signs of neuroglycopenia. Patients and their family/caregivers should be taught the early warning signs of neuroglycopenic symptoms (e.g., slow thinking, blurred vision, slurred speech, numbness, trouble concentrating, dizziness, fatigue, and sleepiness).[83] Patients should be encouraged to keep a symptom diary and record their symptoms whenever they measure their blood glucose.

Hypoglycemic episodes are usually caused by excess in blood glucose lowering medications (e.g., insulin and insulin secretagogues), physical activity, or inadequate carbohydrate intake. It is important to carefully examine the individual's insulin regimen. Hypoglycemia frequently occurs when insulin action is peaking. Individuals should also check their blood glucose levels after exercising. Alcohol consumption in the absence of food intake may also result in hypoglycemia.[84]

Sulfonylureas used concomitantly with sulfa-type antibiotics (e.g., trimethoprim-sulfamethoxazole) can cause severe and refractory hypoglycemia. Patients with DM who are taking a sulfonylurea must be educated to inform their healthcare provider if a sulfa-type antibiotic is also prescribed.

Individuals with DM should be taught how to avoid a hypoglycemic episode. Consumption of a high-fat meal may slow gastric emptying and the absorption of carbohydrates. Therefore, eating a high-fat, low-carbohydrate meal after an insulin injection may result in hypoglycemia.

15/15 Rule

Individuals should be taught that all blood glucose levels below 70 mg/dL (3.9 mmol/L) should be treated, even in the absence of symptoms. Patients should eat or drink 10–15 g of glucose- or carbohydrate-containing food or beverage, which should increase blood glucose levels by 30–45 mg/dL. Foods and beverages, which contain 15 g of carbohydrate, include 4 ounces of fruit juice, 4 ounces of nondiet soda, eight to 10 Life Savers, or three to four glucose tablets. Avoid drinks and foods that are high in fat (e.g., chocolate or whole milk) that may slow absorption of carbohydrates and take longer to raise blood glucose levels. Ingesting protein such as meat will not treat hypoglycemia and will not raise blood glucose levels. Test blood glucose levels 15–20 minutes later. If blood glucose levels are still low, repeat the treatment. Patients should be informed not to miss meals and to have a bedtime snack if blood glucose levels are less than 120 mg/dL.[82-84]

Other Laboratory Tests Used in the Management of Diabetes

The leading cause of death in patients with DM is cardiovascular disease. Control of hypertension and dyslipidemia is necessary to decrease the risk of macrovascular complications.

Patients with DM tend to have a unique type of dyslipidemia, which consists of elevated low-density lipoprotein (LDL) levels, reduced high-density lipoprotein (HDL) levels, elevated triglycerides, and increased platelet adhesiveness, all of which can contribute to the development of atherosclerotic vascular disease. Aggressive treatment of dyslipidemia will reduce the risk of cardiovascular disease in patients with DM. Primary therapy should focus on obtaining LDL goals of less than 100 mg/dL, triglycerides less than 150 mg/dL, and HDL greater than 40 mg/dL for men and greater than 50 mg/dL for women.[85]

Both systolic and diastolic hypertension increases the risk of microvascular and macrovascular complications in patients with DM. Aggressive treatment of hypertension can attenuate the progression of complications. The ADA currently recommends a goal BP of <140/80 mm Hg, but a lower systolic target of <130 mm Hg may be appropriate in younger patients if it can be obtained without exposing the patient to adverse effects associated with treatment.[86]

Urinalysis for detection of proteinuria should be obtained in patients with DM on a yearly basis. This should begin at diagnosis in patients with type 2 DM and 5 years after diagnosis in patients with type 1 DM.[87] A quantitative test for urine protein should follow a positive result on urinalysis. If urinalysis is negative for proteinuria, testing for microalbuminuria should be obtained. Microalbuminuria indicates glomerular damage and is predictive of clinical nephropathy.

There are three methods available to screen for microalbuminuria. One method is measurement of the urine albumin to creatinine ratio in a spot urine sample. This method is convenient in the clinical setting, as it only requires one urine sample. A morning sample is preferred to take into account the diurnal variation of albumin excretion. A second method is a 24-hour urine collection for determination of albumin excretion. This method may be tedious and accuracy relies on proper collection techniques. An advantage of this method is that renal function can simultaneously be quantified. A third alternative method to the 24-hour collection is a timed urine collection for albumin. *Microalbuminuria* is defined as a urinary albumin excretion of 30–299 mcg/mL on a spot urine sample, 30–299 mg/24 hr on a 24-hour urine collection, or 20–199 mcg/min on a timed urine collection. Transient rises in albumin excretion can be associated with exercise, hyperglycemia, hypertension, urinary tract infection, heart failure, and fever. Therefore, if any of these conditions are present, they may result in false positives on screening tests. Variability exists in the excretion of albumin; thus, microalbuminuria must be confirmed in two repeated tests in a 3- to 6-month period. Two of three positive screening tests for microalbuminuria confirm the diagnosis.[87-89]

Based on results of landmark studies, the ADA recommends angiotension-converting enzyme inhibitors (ACEIs) or angiotension receptor blockers (ARBs) for the treatment of both micro and microalbuminuria. If one class is not tolerated, the other should be substituted. Patients with DM and hypertension should be treated with pharmacologic therapy regimen that includes either an ACEI or an ARB. While ARBs have been shown to delay the progression of nephropathy in patients with type 2 DM, hypertension, microalbuminuria, and renal insufficiency, ACEIs are the initial agents of choice in patients with type 1 DM with hypertension and any degree of albuminuria. Thiazide diuretics, beta blockers, or calcium channel blockers should be used as an add-on agent to further decrease BP.[89,90]

THYROID

Anatomy and Physiology

The *thyroid* gland is a butterfly-shaped organ composed of two connecting lobes that span the trachea. The thyroid produces the hormones thyroxine (T_4) and triiodothyronine (T_3). Approximately 80 and 30 mcg of T_4 and T_3, respectively, are produced daily in normal adults. Although T_4 is produced solely by the thyroid gland, only about 20% to 25% of T_3 is

directly secreted by this gland. Approximately 80% of T_3 is formed by hepatic and renal deiodination of T_4.

Thyroxine has a longer half-life than T_3, approximately 7 days versus 1 day, respectively. At the cellular level, however, T_3 is 3–4 times more active physiologically than T_4.[91] When the conversion of T_4 to T_3 is impaired, a stereoisomer of T_3, known as *reverse* T_3, is produced; reverse T_3 has no known biological effect.

Thyroid hormones have many biological effects, both at the molecular level and on specific organ systems. These hormones stimulate the basal metabolic rate and can affect protein, carbohydrate, and lipid metabolism. They are also essential for normal growth and development. Thyroid hormones act to

- Stimulate neural and skeletal development during fetal life
- Stimulate oxygen consumption at rest
- Stimulate bone turnover by increasing bone formation and resorption
- Promote the conversion of carotene to vitamin A
- Promote chronotropic and inotropic effects on the heart
- Increase the number of catecholamine receptors in heart muscle cells
- Increase basal body temperature
- Increase the production of RBCs
- Increase the metabolism and clearance of steroid hormones
- Alter the metabolism of carbohydrates, fats, and protein
- Control the normal hypoxic and hypercapnic respiratory drives

The synthesis of thyroid hormones depends on iodine and the amino acid tyrosine. The thyroid gland, using an energy-requiring process, transports dietary iodide (I^-) from the circulation into the thyroid follicular cell. Iodide is oxidized to iodine (I_2), and then combined with tyrosyl residues within the thyroglobulin molecule to form thyroid hormones (iodothyronine). Thus, the thyroid hormones are formed and stored within the thyroglobulin protein for release into the circulation.[91-94]

Both T_4 and T_3 circulate in human serum bound to three proteins: the majority to thyroxine-binding globulin (TBG), thyroid-binding prealbumin (TBPA), and albumin. Only 0.02% of T_4 and 0.2% of T_3 circulate unbound, free to diffuse into tissues.[95] The "free" fraction is the physiologically active component. Total and free hormones exist in an equilibrium state in which the protein-bound fraction serves as a reservoir for making the free fraction available to tissues.[96]

Thyroid hormone secretion is regulated by a feedback mechanism involving the hypothalamus, anterior pituitary, and thyroid gland itself (Figure 13-4). The release of T_4 and T_3 from the thyroid gland is regulated by *thyrotropin*, also called *thyroid-stimulating hormone (TSH)*, which is secreted by the anterior pituitary. The intrathyroidal iodine concentration also influences thyroid gland activity, and TSH secretion primarily is regulated by a dual negative feedback mechanism:

1. Thyrotropin-releasing hormone (TRH) or protirelin is released by the hypothalamus, which stimulates the synthesis and release of TSH from the pituitary gland.

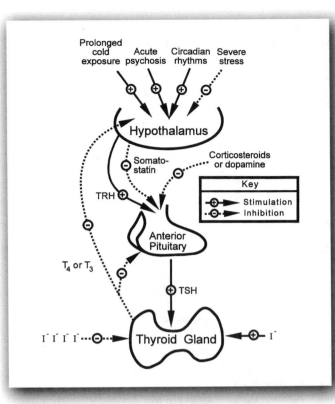

FIGURE 13-4. The hypothalamic-pituitary-thyroid axis. (Adapted with permission from Katzung BG, ed. *Basic and Clinical Pharmacology*. 4th ed. Norwalk, CT: Appleton & Lange; 1989.)

Basal TSH concentrations in persons with normal thyroid function are about 0.3–5.0 milliunits/L. The inverse relationship between TSH and free T_4 is logarithmic. A 50% decrease in free T_4 concentrations leads to a 50-fold increase in TSH concentrations and vice versa.[97]

2. Unbound T_4 and T_3 (mainly the concentration of intracellular T_3 in the pituitary) directly inhibit pituitary TSH secretion. Consequently, increased concentrations of free thyroid hormones cause decreased TSH secretion, and decreased concentrations of T_4 and T_3 cause increased TSH secretion.[98]

Prolonged exposure to cold and acute psychosis may activate the hypothalamic-pituitary-thyroid axis, whereas severe stress may inhibit it. While TRH stimulates pituitary TSH release, somatostatin corticosteroids and dopamine inhibit it. Small amounts of iodide are needed for T_4 and T_3 production, but large amounts inhibit their production and release. Most recent evidence based on the most sensitive assays suggests that no physiologically relevant change in serum TSH concentrations occurs in relation to age.[96]

Thyroid Disorders

Patients with a normally functioning thyroid gland are said to be in a *euthyroid* state. When this state is disrupted, thyroid disease may result. It occurs 4 times more often in women than in men and may occur at any age, but it peaks between the third

and sixth decades of life. A family history of this disease often is present, especially for the autoimmune thyroid diseases.

Diseases of the thyroid usually involve an alteration in the quantity or quality of thyroid hormone secretion and may manifest as *hypothyroidism* or *hyperthyroidism*. In addition to the signs and symptoms discussed below, thyroid disease may produce an enlargement of the thyroid gland known as *goiter*.

Hypothyroidism

Hypothyroidism results from a deficiency of thyroid hormone production, causing body metabolism to slow down. This condition affects about 2% of women and 0.2% of men and the incidence increases with age. Symptoms include lethargy; constipation; dry, coarse skin and hair; paresthesias and slowed deep tendon reflexes; facial puffiness; cold intolerance; decreased sweating; impaired memory, confusion, and dementia; slow speech and motor activity; and anemia and growth retardation in children. Interestingly, these typical signs and symptoms have been observed in as few as 25% of elderly hypothyroid patients.[99]

Hypothyroidism is usually caused by one of three mechanisms. Primary hypothyroidism is failure of the thyroid to produce thyroid hormone, secondary hypothyroidism is failure of the anterior pituitary to secrete TSH, and tertiary hypothyroidism is failure of the hypothalamus to produce TRH. Most patients with symptomatic primary hypothyroidism have TSH concentrations greater than 20 milliunits/L. Patients with mild signs or symptoms (usually not the reason for the visit to the doctor) have TSH values of 10–20 milliunits/L. Patients with secondary and tertiary hypothyroidism may have a low or normal TSH, but other hormones (e.g., prolactin, cortisol, and gonadotropin) can be measured to confirm pituitary insufficiency. Table 13-9 outlines the numerous etiologies of hypothyroidism.

Thyrotoxicosis

Thyrotoxicosis results when excessive amounts of thyroid hormones are circulating and is usually due to hyperactivity of the thyroid gland (hyperthyroidism). Signs and symptoms include nervousness; fatigue; weight loss; heat intolerance; increased sweating; tachycardia or atrial fibrillation; muscle atrophy; warm, moist skin; and, in some patients, exophthalmos. These signs and symptoms occur much less frequently in the elderly, except for atrial fibrillation, which occurs 3 times more often.[99] Table 13-10 summarizes the specific causes of hyperthyroidism.

Nonthyroid Laboratory Tests in Patients with Thyroid Disease

Both hypo- and hyperthyroidism may cause pathophysiology outside the thyroid gland. Table 13-11 lists nonthyroid laboratory tests that may indicate a thyroid disorder. The influence on these tests reflects the widespread effects of thyroid hormones on peripheral tissues. Findings from these tests cannot be used alone to diagnose a thyroid disorder. However, they may support a diagnosis of thyroid dysfunction when used with specific thyroid function tests and the patient's presenting signs and symptoms.

TABLE 13-9. Classification of Hypothyroidism by Etiology[91,101,102]

Primary

Iodide deficiency

Excessive iodide intake (e.g., kelp and contrast dyes)

Thyroid ablation: surgery, post 131I (radioactive Iodine I-131) treatment of thyrotoxicosis, radiation of neoplasm

Hashimoto thyroiditis

Subacute thyroiditis

Genetic abnormalities of thyroid hormone synthesis

Drugs: propylthiouracil, methimazole, thiocyanate, lithium, amiodarone

Food: excessive intake of goitrogenic foods (e.g., cabbage and turnips)

Secondary

Hypopituitarism: adenoma, ablative therapy, pituitary destruction, sarcoidosis hypothalamic dysfunction

Other

Abnormalities of T_4 receptor

Thyroid Function Tests

Tests more specific for thyroid status or function can be categorized as those that (1) measure the concentration of products secreted by the thyroid gland, (2) evaluate the integrity of the hypothalamic-pituitary-thyroid axis, (3) assess intrinsic thyroid gland function, and (4) detect antibodies to thyroid tissue.[104] Tests that directly or indirectly measure the concentrations of T_4 and T_3 include

- Free T_4
- Total serum T_4
- Serum T_3 resin uptake
- Free T_4 index
- Total serum T_3

The integrity of the hypothalamic-pituitary-thyroid axis is assessed by measuring

- TSH
- TRH

A test that assesses intrinsic thyroid gland function includes

- Radioactive iodine uptake

A test that detects antibodies to thyroid tissue includes

- Antithyroid antibodies

Free Thyroxine (T_4)

Normal range: 0.9–2.3 ng/dL

This test measures the unbound T_4 in the serum and is the most accurate reflection of thyrometabolic status. The low concentration of *free T_4* in the serum (<1% of total T_4) makes accurate measurement a difficult and laborious process. Therefore, free T_4 is assayed primarily when TBG alterations or nonthyroidal illnesses confound interpretation of conventional tests (Tables 13-11 and 13-12).

Several methods can determine free T_4. Some methods perform well only in otherwise healthy hypo- and hyperthyroid

TABLE 13-10. Classification of Hyperthyroidism by Etiology[91,99,101,102]

Overproduction of thyroid hormone

Graves disease[a]

TSH-secreting pituitary adenomas

Hydatidiform moles/choriocarcinomas[b]

Multinodular goiter

"Leaking" thyroid hormone due to thyroid destruction

Lymphocytic thyroiditis

Granulomatous thyroiditis

Subacute thyroiditis

Radiation

Drugs

Thyroid-replacement drugs (excessive), amiodarone, iodinated radiocontrast agents, kelp[c]

Ovarian teratomas with thyroid elements

Metastatic thyroid carcinoma

[a]Most frequent cause. The mechanism is production of thyroid-stimulating antibodies; usually associated with diffuse goiter and ophthalmopathy.
[b]Tumor production of chorionic gonadotropin, which stimulates the thyroid.
[c]Patients at risk of hyperthyroidism from these agents usually have some degree of thyroid autonomy.

TABLE 13-11. Nonthyroid Laboratory Tests Consistent with Thyroid Disorders[91,94,101,102]

HYPOTHYROIDISM	HYPERTHYROIDISM
Decreased	**Decreased**
Hemoglobin (Hgb)/hematocrit (Hct)[a]	Granulocytes
Serum glucose	Serum cholesterol
Serum sodium	Serum triglycerides
Urinary excretion of 17-hydroxysteroids	
Urinary excretion of 17-ketosteroids	
Increased	**Increased**
Aspartate aminotransferase (AST/SGOT)	Alkaline phosphatase
Capillary fragility	Lymphocytes
Cerebrospinal fluid protein	Serum ferritin
Lactate dehydrogenase (LDH)	Urinary calcium excretion
Partial pressure of carbon dioxide (pCO_2)	
Serum carotene	
Serum cholesterol	
Serum creatine phosphokinase (CPK)	
Serum prolactin	
Serum triglycerides	

[a]Associated with normocytic and/or macrocytic anemias.

TABLE 13-12. Free T$_4$ and TSH in Thyroidal and Nonthyroidal Disorders[a]

DIAGNOSIS	FREE T$_4$ INDEX OR DIRECT EQUILIBRIUM DIALYSIS FREE T$_4$[a]	TSH (milliunits)[a]
Hypothyroidism		
Primary		
Normal ↓ ↑		
On dopamine or glucocorticoids	↓	↓
Secondary or tertiary—functional hypopituitarism	↓	↓
Recent thyroid supplement withdrawal	↓	<0.10
Recently treated hyperthyroidism	↓	<0.10
Hyperthyroidism	↑	<0.10[b]
With severe nonthyroidal illness	↓/WNL/↑[c]	<0.10[b]
Euthyroid states	WNL	WNL
Low total T$_4$ of nonthyroidal illness	↓/WNL/↑[d]	WNL/↑
After T$_3$ therapy	↓	WNL/↓
After T$_4$ therapy	WNL	WNL
High total T$_4$ of nonthyroidal illness	↑	WNL/↑
High total T$_4$ from amiodarone or iodinated contrast media	↑	↑
Decreased T$_4$-binding proteins	↑/WNL[e]	WNL

[a] ↑ = increased; ↓ = decreased; WNL = within normal limits.
[b] Usually absent TSH response to TRH; also may be normal with hyperthyroidism from TSH-secreting tumors.
[c] Normal or low using free T$_4$ index estimation; increased using the direct equilibrium dialysis free T$_4$ assay.
[d] Decreased using free T$_4$ index estimation; normal to high using the direct equilibrium dialysis free T$_4$ assay.
[e] Decreased using free T$_4$ index estimation; normal using the direct equilibrium dialysis free T$_4$ assay.
Source: Adapted from reference 93.

patients and in euthyroid patients with mild abnormalities of TBG. However, in patients with severe alterations of T$_4$ binding to carrier proteins (e.g., severe nonthyroidal illness), only the direct equilibrium dialysis method maintains accuracy (Table 13-13).[105]

A decreased direct equilibrium dialysis free T$_4$ with an elevated TSH is diagnostic of primary hypothyroidism, even in patients with severely depressed TBG. Conversely, an increased direct equilibrium dialysis free T$_4$ with a TSH of less than 0.10 milliunit/L is consistent with nonpituitary hyperthyroidism.[53] Decreased direct equilibrium dialysis free T$_4$ with normal or decreased TSH concentrations may be seen in patients on T$_3$ therapy. Although free T$_4$ assays are becoming widely available (Table 13-13), most clinicians initially rely on the traditional total serum T$_4$ measurement by radioimmunoassay (RIA).

Total Serum Thyroxine (T$_4$)

Normal range: 5.5–12.5 mcg/dL or 71–161 nmol/L

Although ultrasensitive TSH and free T$_4$ assays are gradually supplanting this RIA methodology, total serum T$_4$ still is the standard initial screening test to assess thyroid function because of its wide availability and quick turnaround time. In most patients, the total serum T$_4$ level is a sensitive test for the functional status of the thyroid gland. It is high in 90% of hyperthyroid patients and low in 85% of hypothyroid patients. This test measures both bound and free T$_4$ and is, therefore, influenced by any alteration in the concentration or binding affinity of thyroid-binding protein.

Conditions that increase or decrease thyroid-binding protein result in an increased or decreased total serum T$_4$, respectively, but do not affect the amount of metabolically active free T$_4$ in the circulation. Therefore, thyrometabolic status may not always be truly represented by the results. To circumvent this problem, most clinicians concomitantly obtain the T$_3$ resin uptake test (discussed later) so they can factor out this interference. Table 13-14 lists factors that alter thyroid-binding protein.

Increased total serum thyroxine. An increased total serum T$_4$ may indicate hyperthyroidism, elevated concentrations of thyroid-binding proteins, or nonthyroid illness. Total serum T$_4$ elevations have been noted in patients, particularly the elderly, with relatively minor illnesses. These transient elevations may be due to TSH secretion stimulated by a low T$_3$ concentration. Similarly, up to 20% of all patients admitted to psychiatric hospitals have had transient total serum T$_4$ elevations on admission.[71,83] Thus, the differential diagnosis for a patient with this elevation must include nonthyroid illness versus hyperthyroidism if other signs and symptoms of thyroid disease are absent or inconsistent.

Decreased total serum thyroxine. A decreased total serum T$_4$ may indicate hypothyroidism, decreased concentrations of thyroid-binding proteins, or *nonthyroid illness* (also called *euthyroid sick syndrome*). Nonthyroid illness may lower the total serum T$_4$ concentration with no change in thyrometabolic status. Typically in this syndrome, total serum T$_4$ is decreased (or normal), total serum T$_3$ is decreased, reverse T$_3$ is increased, and TSH is normal. Neoplastic disease, DM, burns, trauma, liver disease, renal failure, prolonged infections, and cardiovascular disease are nonthyroid illnesses that can lower total serum T$_4$ concentrations.

Several mechanisms probably contribute to this low T$_4$ state. The concentration of serum-binding proteins may diminish hormone-binding capacity. Moreover, the conversion of T$_4$ to T$_3$ may be inhibited, causing an increase in the production of reverse T$_3$. Another theory suggests that a circulating thyroid hormone inhibitor may bind to the thyroid-binding protein.

In general, a correlation exists between the degree of total serum T$_4$ depression and the prognosis of the illness (i.e., the lower the total serum T$_4$, the poorer the disease outcome). Since severely ill patients may appear to be hypothyroid, it is important to differentiate between patients with serious nonthyroid illnesses and those who are truly hypothyroid.[82,85]

TABLE 13-13. Performance and Availability of Free T_4 Methods

ASSAY	% OF EUTHYROID PATIENTS WITH SEVERE TBG DEPRESSION OR SEVERE NONTHYROIDAL ILLNESS IN WHICH ASSAY UNDERESTIMATES FREE T_4	COMMENTS
Free T_4 index[a] or single-step 50% to 80%[106]	Available in most clinical labs	Immunoassays
Immunoextraction or radioimmunoassay[b]	10% to 30%[93]	Available in some clinical labs
Direct equilibrium dialysisc	0% to 5%[107,d]	Available in reference labs and large medical center labs; gold standard
Ultrafiltrationc	0% to 5%[107]	Available only in research labs

[a]Corrects total T_4 values using an assessment of T_4-binding proteins.
[b]Uses a T_4 analog or two-step-back titration with solid-phase T_4 antibody but does not use membranes to separate free from bound hormone.
[c]Uses minimally diluted serum that separates free T_4 from bound T_4 using a semipermeable membrane.
[d]May be underestimated in about 25% of patients on dopamine.[107]

TABLE 13-14. Factors Altering Thyroid-Binding Protein[91,94,96,98,101]

FACTORS THAT INCREASE THYROID-BINDING PROTEIN	FACTORS THAT DECREASE THYROID-BINDING PROTEIN
Acute infectious hepatitis	Acromegaly
Acute intermittent porphyria	Androgen therapy
Chronic active hepatitis	L-asparaginase
Clofibrate	Cirrhosis
Estrogen-containing oral contraceptives	Danazol
	Salsalate
Estrogen-producing tumors	Genetic deficiency of total binding protein
Estrogen therapy	
5-Fluorouracil	Glucocorticoid therapy (high dose)
Genetic excess of total binding protein	High-dose furosemide
Heroin	Hypoproteinemia
Methadone maintenance	Malnutrition
Perphenazine	Nephrotic syndrome
Pregnancy	Salicylates
Tamoxifen	Testosterone-producing tumors

TABLE 13-15. Medications That Cause a True Alteration in Total Serum T_4 and Free T_4 Measurements[a]

MECHANISM	INCREASE TOTAL SERUM T_4 AND FREE T_4	DECREASE TOTAL SERUM T_4 AND FREE T_4
Interference in central regulation of TSH secretion at hypothalamic-pituitary level	Amphetamines	Glucocorticoids (acutely)
Interference with thyroid hormone synthesis and/or iodides,[b] lithium carbonate, release from thyroid	Amiodarone,[b] iodides[b]	Aminoglutethimide, amiodarone,[b] 6-mercaptopurine, sulfonamides
Altered thyroid hormone metabolism	Amiodarone,[a] iopanoic acid, ipodate, propranolol (high dose)	Phenobarbital
Inhibition of GI absorption of exogenous thyroid hormone	Nadolol	Antacids, cholestyramine, colestipol, iron, sodium polystyrene sulfonate, soybean flour (infant formulas), sucralfate

TSH = thyroid-stimulating hormone.
[a]In true alterations, the concentration change is not due to assay interference or alteration in thyroid-binding proteins.
[b]May increase or decrease total serum T_4 and free T_4.
Source: Compiled, in part, from references 91, 94, 96, 98, and 101.

Drugs causing true alterations in total serum thyroxine. Medications can cause a true alteration in total serum T_4 and a corresponding change in free T_4 concentrations (Table 13-15). In such cases, the total serum T_4 (and free T_4) result remains a true reflection of thyrometabolic status. High-dose salicylates and phenytoin also may lower total serum T_4 significantly via decreased binding in vivo. Phenytoin may lower free T_4, and salicylates may increase it.[109]

As noted in Table 13-16, iodides can significantly alter thyroid status. They have the potential to inhibit thyroid hormone release and to impair the organification of iodine. In healthy individuals, this effect lasts only 1–2 weeks. However, individuals with subclinical hypothyroid disease may develop clinical hypothyroidism after treatment with iodides. Iodide-induced hypothyroidism has also been noted in patients with cystic fibrosis and emphysema.[96]

Iodides may also *increase* thyroid function. A previously euthyroid patient may develop thyrotoxicosis from exposure to increased quantities of iodine. Supplemental iodine causes autonomously functioning thyroid tissue to produce and secrete thyroid hormones, leading to a significant increase in T_4 and T_3 concentrations. This phenomenon commonly occurs

TABLE 13-16. Iodine-Containing Compounds That May Influence Thyroid Status

Oral radiopaque agents

Diatrizoate

Iocetamic acid

Iopanoic acid

Ipodate

Tyropanoate

Expectorants

Iodinated glycerol[a]

Potassium iodide solution

SSKI (supersaturated potassium iodide)

Parenteral radiopaque agents

Diatrizoate meglumine

Iodamide meglumine

Iopamidol

Iothalamate meglumine

Metrizamide

Miscellaneous compounds

Amiodarone

Kelp-containing nutritional supplements

[a]No longer available; most products reformulated with guaifenesin.
Source: Compiled, in part, from references 96 and 101.

during therapeutic iodine replacement in patients who live in areas of endemic iodine deficiency.

Similarly, patients with underlying goiter who live in iodine-sufficient areas may develop hyperthyroidism when given pharmacological doses of iodide. The heavily iodinated anti-arrhythmic medication amiodarone may induce hyperthyroidism (1% to 5% of patients) as well as hypothyroidism (6% to 10% of patients).[109,110] Table 13-16 lists iodine-containing compounds.

Although antithyroid drugs such as propylthiouracil and methimazole are not listed in Table 13-16, they are used in hyperthyroid patients to decrease hormone concentrations. Both T_4 and T_3 concentrations decrease more rapidly with methimazole than propylthiouracil.[111]

Serum Triiodothyronine (T_3) Resin Uptake

Normal range: 25% to 38%

The T_3 *resin uptake* test indirectly estimates the number of binding sites on thyroid-binding protein occupied by T_3. This result is also referred to as the *thyroid hormone-binding ratio*. The T_3 resin uptake is usually low when the concentration of thyroid-binding protein is high.[101,102]

In this test, radiolabeled T_3 is added to endogenous hormone. An aliquot of this mixture is then added to a resin that competes with endogenous thyroid-binding proteins for the free hormone. Radiolabeled T_3 binds to any free endogenous thyroid-binding protein; at the saturation point, the remainder binds to the resin. The amount of thyroid-binding protein can be estimated from the amount of radiolabeled T_3 taken up by the resin. The T_3 resin uptake result is expressed as a percentage of the total radiolabeled T_3 that binds to the resin. The T_3 resin uptake can verify the clinical significance of measured total serum T_4 and T_3 concentrations because it is an indicator of thyroid-binding protein-induced alterations of these measurements.[101,102]

Elevated T_3 resin uptake concentrations are consistent with hyperthyroidism, while decreased concentrations are consistent with hypothyroidism. However, this test is never used alone for diagnosis. The T_3 resin uptake is low in hypothyroidism because of the increased availability of binding sites on the TBG. However, in nonthyroidal illnesses with a low T_4, the T_3 resin uptake is elevated. Therefore, the test may be used to differentiate between true hypothyroidism and a low T_4 state caused by nonthyroid illness.[101,102]

All of the disease states and medications listed in Table 13-14 can influence thyroid-binding protein and, consequently, alter T_3 resin uptake results. Radioactive substances taken by the patient also will interfere with this test. In practice, the T_3 resin uptake test is used only to calculate the free T_4 index.

Free Thyroxine (T_4) Index

Normal range: 1.0–4.0 units

The *free T_4 index* is the product of total serum T_4 multiplied by the percentage of T_3 resin uptake:

$$\text{free } T_4 \text{ index} = \text{total serum } T_4 \text{ (mcg/dL)} \times T_3 \text{ resin uptake (\%)}$$

The free T_4 index adjusts for the effects of alterations in thyroid-binding protein on the total serum T_4 assay. The index is high in hyperthyroidism and low in hypothyroidism. Patients taking phenytoin or salicylates have low total serum T_4 and high T_3 resin uptake with a normal free T_4 index. Pregnant patients have high total serum T_4 and low T_3 resin uptake with a normal free T_4 index. Patients taking therapeutic doses of levothyroxine may have a high free T_4 index because total serum T_4 and T_3 resin uptake are high. In addition to affecting total serum T_4 and free T_4 (Table 13-15), propranolol and nadolol block the conversion of T_4 to T_3, which may cause mild elevations in the free T_4 index.[101,109]

Total Serum Triiodothyronine (T_3)

Normal range: 80–200 ng/dL or 1.2–3.0 nmol/L

This RIA measures the highly active thyroid hormone T_3. Like T_4, almost all of T_3 is protein bound. Therefore, any alteration in thyroid-binding protein influences this measurement. As with the total serum T_4 test, changes in thyroid-binding protein increase or decrease total serum T_3 but do not affect the metabolically active free T_3 in the circulation. Therefore, the patient's thyrometabolic status remains unchanged.

The total serum T_3 is primarily used as an indicator of hyperthyroidism. This measurement is usually made to detect T_3 toxicosis when T_3, but not T_4, is elevated. Generally, the serum T_3 assay is not a reliable indicator of hypothyroidism because of the lack of reliability in the low to normal range.

Drugs that affect T_4 concentrations (Table 13-15) have a corresponding effect on T_3 concentrations. Additionally, propranolol, propylthiouracil, and glucocorticoids inhibit the peripheral conversion of T_4 to T_3 and cause a decreased T_3 concentration (T_4 usually stays normal).[112]

Total serum T_3 concentrations can be low in euthyroid patients with conditions (e.g., malnutrition, cirrhosis, and uremia) in which the conversion of T_4 to T_3 is suppressed. T_3 is low in only half of hypothyroid patients because these patients tend to produce relatively more T_3 than T_4. A patient with a normal total serum T_4, a low T_3, and a high reverse T_3 has euthyroid sick syndrome.

Thyroid-Stimulating Hormone (TSH)

Normal range: 0.5–5.0 milliunits/L

Thyroid-stimulating hormone is a glycoprotein with two subunits, alpha and beta. The alpha subunit is similar to those of other hormones secreted from the anterior pituitary: follicle-stimulating hormone (FSH), human chorionic gonadotropin (HCG), and luteinizing hormone (FSH). The beta subunit of TSH is unique and renders its specific physiological properties.[101,102]

Although the older, "first-generation" TSH assays have been useful in diagnosing primary hypothyroidism, they have not been useful in diagnosing hyperthyroidism. Almost all patients with symptomatic primary hypothyroidism have TSH concentrations greater than 20 milliunits/L; those with mild signs or symptoms have TSH values of 10–20 milliunits/L. Often, TSH concentrations become elevated before T_4 concentrations decline. All assays can accurately measure *high* concentrations of TSH.[101,102]

The first-generation TSH assays, however, cannot distinguish low–normal from abnormally low values because their lower limit of detection is 0.5 milliunit/L, while the lower limit of basal TSH is 0.2–0.3 milliunit/L in most euthyroid persons. This distinction can usually be ascertained with the second-generation assays, which can accurately measure TSH concentrations as low as 0.05 milliunit/L. Occasionally, some euthyroid patients have concentrations of 0.05–0.5 milliunit/L. Therefore, supersensitive, third-generation assays have been developed; they can detect TSH concentrations as low as 0.005 milliunit/L. Concentrations below 0.05 milliunit/L are almost always diagnostic of primary hyperthyroidism in patients younger than 70 years.[101,102]

Some clinicians feel that neither a low basal TSH concentration nor a blunted TSH response to TRH discussed later is a reliable predictor of hyperthyroidism in elderly patients.[112] Although third-generation assays are usually not required to make or confirm this diagnosis, they provide a wider margin of tolerance so that discrimination at 0.1 milliunit/L can be ensured even when the assay is not performing optimally.[108]

Use in therapy. In patients with primary hypothyroidism, TSH concentrations are also used to adjust the dosage of levothyroxine replacement therapy. In addition to achieving a clinical euthyroid state, the goal should be to lower TSH into the midnormal range (Minicase 3). While TSH concentrations reflect long-term thyroid status, serum T_4 concentrations

reflect acute changes. Patients with long-standing hypothyroidism often notice an improvement in well-being 2–3 weeks after starting therapy. Significant improvements in heart rate (HR), weight, and puffiness are seen early in therapy, but hoarseness, anemia, and skin/hair changes may take many months to resolve.[114]

Unless undesirable changes in signs or symptoms occur, it is rational to wait at least 6–8 weeks after starting or changing therapy to repeat TSH and/or T_4 concentrations to refine dosing.[93,115] The hypothalamic-pituitary axis requires this time to respond fully to changes in circulating thyroid hormone concentrations.

This slow readjustment can be exploited elsewhere. One study found that greater than 50% of TSH elevations in patients being treated with levothyroxine were attributed to noncompliance; with counseling alone, TSH normalized on subsequent visits.[116] Noncompliant hypothyroid patients who take their levothyroxine pills only before being tested may have elevated TSH concentrations despite a normal T_4 concentration.[108]

Because of slow axis readjustment, patients given antithyroid drugs (e.g., methimazole) may maintain low TSH concentrations for 2–3 months after T_4 and T_3 concentrations have returned to normal. Single, daily doses of 10–20 mg of methimazole usually lead to euthyroidism within several weeks.[117] Treatment should not be adjusted too early using (low) TSH concentrations alone. However, the dose should be reduced within the first 8 weeks if TSH concentrations become elevated.

Patients with thyroid cancer are often treated with TSH suppressive therapy, usually levothyroxine. The therapeutic endpoint is a basal TSH concentration of about 0.1 milliunit/L.[118] Some clinicians suggest more complete suppression with TSH concentrations less than 0.005 milliunit/L, while others think that it leads to toxic effects of over-replacement (e.g., accelerated bone loss) (Minicase 3).[108,116]

Potential misinterpretation and drug interference. Some TSH assays may yield falsely high results whenever HCG concentrations are high (i.e., pregnancy) due to the similarity in structure of these two proteins.

Most patients who have secondary or tertiary hypothyroidism have low or normal TSH concentrations. In patients with nonthyroid illness, TSH may be suppressed by factors other than thyroid hyperfunction. As mentioned previously, the TSH concentration typically is normal in patients with euthyroid sick syndrome.

Thyroid function tests are known to be altered in depressed patients. With the advent of the third-generation TSH assays, investigators hoped that TSH concentrations could help to determine various types of depression and response to therapies. Unfortunately, neither TSH nor its response to TRH has proven useful in this way.[120]

Because endogenous dopamine inhibits the stimulatory effects of TRH, any drug with dopaminergic activity can inhibit TSH secretion. Therefore, levodopa, glucocorticoids, bromocriptine, and dopamine are likely to lower TSH results. The converse is also true—the dopamine antagonists (metoclopramide) may increase TSH concentrations.

MINICASE 3

A Case of Possible Hypothyroidism

AMY T., A 28-YEAR-OLD FEMALE, visited her physician with complaints of weakness, fatigue, weight gain, hoarseness, cold intolerance, and unusually heavy periods worsening over the past 2–3 months. Her pulse was 50, and her BP was 110/70. Her physical exam was normal, except for a mildly enlarged thyroid gland, pallor, and diminished tendon reflexes. She denied taking any medications or changing her diet.

Amy T.'s chemistry results were sodium 130 mEq/L (136–142 mEq/L), potassium 3.8 mEq/L (3.8–5.0 mEq/L), carbon dioxide 28 mEq/L (21–28 mEq/L), calcium 9.5 mg/dL (9.2–11.0 mg/dL), magnesium 2 mEq/L (1.3–2.1 mEq/L), glucose 80 mg/dL (70–110 mg/dL), BUN 20 mg/dL (8–23 mg/dL), SCr 1.1 mg/dL (0.6–1.2 mg/dL), and cholesterol 235 mg/dL (<200 mg/dL). The cholesterol concentration was elevated since a screening 6 months ago. A test for mononucleosis was negative. Hematocrit was low at 36% (36% to 45%)—close to her usual. Her total serum T_4 was 8 mcg/dL (5.5–12.5 mcg/dL), her T_3 resin uptake was 15% (25% to 38%), and her free T_4 index was 1.2 (1.0–4.0).

Question: How should these results be interpreted? Are confirmatory tests needed?

Discussion: Clinically, all of the history and physical findings point to hypothyroidism. The pallor and weakness are also consistent with anemia, but an Hct of 35% is unlikely to cause such significant symptoms. Amy T.'s cholesterol recently became elevated, consistent with primary hypothyroidism.[36] Classically, both the total serum T_4 and T_3 resin uptake should be low in hypothyroid patients. In Amy T. only the T_3 resin uptake is low, and the free T_4 index is borderline normal, making laboratory diagnosis unclear. Confirmatory tests should prove useful.

A few days later, Amy T. revisited her physician for additional tests. When questioned, she admitted that she has been taking oral contraceptives and would like to continue. The following day, her TSH was 25 milliunits/L (0.3–5.0 milliunits/L).

Question: Does this information help to elucidate the diagnosis?

Discussion: An elevated TSH confirms primary hypothyroidism. The reason for equivocal total serum T_4 and T_3 resin uptake is now apparent—the estrogens in the birth control pills. Estrogens elevate total serum T_4 and thyroid-binding protein and lower T_3 resin uptake. If Amy T. had not been taking estrogens, her total serum T_4 probably would have been below normal, and her T_3 resin uptake probably would have been higher (but still below normal). The diagnosis would have been clear earlier. If oral contraceptive use had been identified at the first visit, a TSH concentration should have been performed then.

Amy T. was started on levothyroxine 0.2 mg/day, and her TSH was 6 milliunits/L 3 weeks later. Clinically, she improved but was not fully back to normal. Six weeks after starting therapy, she complained of jitteriness, palpitations, and increased sweating. Her TSH was less than 0.3 milliunit/L. Her physician lowered the dose of levothyroxine to 0.1 mg/day, and Amy T. became asymptomatic after about 2 weeks. Eight weeks later, her TSH was 1.5 milliunits/L and she remained asymptomatic. Her cholesterol was 100 mg/dL, sodium was 138 mEq/L, and Hct was 40%.

Question: Which test(s) should be used to determine proper dosing of levothyroxine? How long after a dosage change should clinicians wait before repeating the test(s)?

Discussion: Although total serum T_4, T_3 resin uptake, and free T_4 index can be used to monitor and adjust doses of thyroid supplements in patients with a hypothyroid disorder, the highly sensitive TSH is most reliable. Chemically, the goal is to achieve a TSH in the normal range, as was ultimately achieved in Amy T. (TSH of 1.5 milliunits/L). Because of her continued use of birth control pills, TSH is the best test for her. The newer TSH assays make it possible to determine whether TSH secretion is being excessively suppressed by thyroid replacement (<0.3 milliunit/L).

With the increased availability of this sensitive test, TSH is becoming the standard for adjusting thyroid replacement therapy in most patients. The 0.2-mg levothyroxine dose was excessive, given the "hyperthyroid" symptoms and the fully suppressed TSH. Eight weeks later, after T_4 steady-state was reached on the 0.1-mg/day dose and after the hypothalamic-pituitary-thyroid axis reached homeostasis, TSH was within the desired range. Amy T.'s cholesterol, sodium, and Hct also normalized as she became euthyroid.

Thyrotropin-Releasing Hormone (TRH) Stimulation Test

Thyrotropin-releasing hormone, a hormone secreted by the hypothalamus, regulates TSH secretion from the pituitary. The TRH test measures the ability of injected TRH to stimulate the pituitary to release TSH (and prolactin). This test has been the most reliable indicator of hyperthyroidism in patients whose other thyroid function tests are equivocal, primarily with the older, less sensitive TSH assays. With second- and third-generation TSH assays becoming more widely available, this TRH test is infrequently required. Nevertheless, it is useful to distinguish primary from secondary hypothyroidism (Table 13-17).[101]

This test is performed by drawing a baseline serum TSH concentration and then administering approximately 200–400 mcg of TRH (synthetic protirelin) intravenously over 30–60

TABLE 13-17. Differentiation of Hypothyroid Disorders Based on TSH and TRH Challenge Test Results[a]

DYSFUNCTIONING TISSUE OR GLAND	TSH BEFORE TRH CHALLENGE	TSH AFTER TRH CHALLENGE
Thyroid	High	Exaggerated
Pituitary	Low/absent	No response
Hypothalamus	Low	Sluggish response

TRH = thyrotropin-releasing hormone; TSH = thyroid-stimulating hormone.
[a]Patients with hyperthyroidism have a suppressed pretest TSH and no response or a blunted response to TRH infusion.

seconds. TSH concentrations are drawn at 30–60 minutes. A normal response, indicative of the euthyroid state, is defined as a TSH rise of 5 microunits/mL over baseline. A significant increase virtually rules out hyperthyroidism. A blunted or absent TSH response suggests hyperthyroidism. However, a rise of less than 5 microunits/mL can be seen in euthyroid men over age 40, in depressed patients, and in patients with glucocorticoid excess. A blunted response may occur in euthyroid patients receiving adequate thyroid suppression therapy, dopamine, glucocorticoid, somatostatin, or L-dopa therapy.[101]

Endogenous TRH secretion is enhanced by norepinephrine and serotonin. As mentioned previously, the need for this test should decrease with the advent of the sensitive TSH immunometric assays. Patients with basal TSH concentrations less than 0.1 microunit/mL typically do not have a TSH increase after a TRH challenge.[101]

Radioactive Iodine Uptake Test

This test is used to detect the ability of the thyroid gland to trap and concentrate iodine and, thereby, produce thyroid hormone. In other words, this test assesses the intrinsic function of the thyroid gland. This test is not specific, and its reference range must be adjusted to the local population. Therefore, its use is declining. In patients with a normal thyroid gland, 12% to 20% of the radioactive iodine is absorbed by the gland after 6 hours and 5% to 25% is absorbed after 24 hours. The radioactive iodine uptake test is an indirect measure of thyroid gland activity and should not be used as a basic screening test of thyroid function. This test is most useful in distinguishing hyperthyroidism caused by subacute thyroiditis with absent or reduced uptake of iodine.[102,121,122]

A high radioactive iodine uptake is noted with[87,109,110]

- Thyrotoxicosis
- Iodine deficiency
- Post-thyroiditis
- Withdrawal rebound after thyroid hormone or antithyroid drug therapy

A low test result occurs in[102,121,122]

- Acute thyroiditis
- Euthyroid patients who ingest iodine-containing products
- Patients on exogenous thyroid hormone therapy
- Patients who are taking antithyroid drugs such as propylthiouracil
- Hypothyroidism

The radioactive iodine uptake test is affected by the body's store of iodine. Therefore, the patient should be carefully questioned about the use of iodine-containing products prior to the test. This test is contraindicated during pregnancy.

Antithyroid Antibodies

Normal range: varies with antibody

Antibodies that "attack" various thyroid tissue components can be detected in the serum of patients with autoimmune disorders such as Hashimoto thyroiditis and Graves disease. Thyroid microsomal antibody is found in 95% of patients with Hashimoto thyroiditis, 55% of patients with Graves disease, and 10% of adults without thyroid disease. In patients who have nodular and hard goiters, high antibody titers strongly suggest Hashimoto thyroiditis as opposed to cancer. In Graves disease, hyperthyroidism is caused by antibodies, which activate TSH receptors. In chronic autoimmune thyroiditis, hypothyroidism

may be caused by antibodies competitively binding to TSH receptors, thereby blocking TSH from eliciting a response.[123]

Results are reported as titers. Titers in excess of 1:100 are significant and usually can be detected even during remission.

Antibodies (>1:10) to thyroglobulin are present in 60% to 70% of adults with active Hashimoto thyroiditis, but typically are not detected during remission. Titers above 1:1000 are found only in Hashimoto thyroiditis or Graves disease (25% or 10%, respectively). Lower titers may be seen in 4% of the normal population, although the frequency increases with age in females. The thyroid microsomal antibody and thyroglobulin antibody serological tests may be elevated or positive in patients with nonthyroidal autoimmune disease.

Anti-TSH receptor antibodies are present in virtually all patients with Graves disease, but the test is usually not necessary for diagnosis. These antibodies mostly stimulate TSH receptors but also may compete with TSH and, thus, inhibit TSH stimulation. High titers allow a confirmation of Graves disease in asymptomatic patients, such as those whose only manifestation is exophthalmos.

Laboratory Diagnosis of Hypothalamic-Pituitary-Thyroid Axis Dysfunction

The laboratory diagnosis of primary hypothyroidism can be made with a low free T_4 index and an elevated TSH concentration. The presence of a low free T_4 index and a normal or low serum TSH concentration indicates secondary or tertiary hypothyroidism or nonthyroid illness. In such patients, the T_3 resin uptake may differentiate between hypothyroidism and a low T_4 state due to nonthyroid illness. An elevated reverse T_3 concentration also suggests nonthyroid illness. The TRH test may be used to pinpoint the thyroid axis defect (Table 13-17). T_3 is of limited usefulness in diagnosing hypothyroidism because it may be normal in up to one-third of hypothyroid patients.[102,104,121,122] With the availability of ultrasensitive TSH assays, many clinicians begin their evaluations with this test. One such approach is illustrated in Figure 13-5 and Minicase 3.

The newer TSH assay can also be used to diagnose hyperthyroidism (<0.1 milliunit/L). The total serum T_4 and free T_4 or free T_4 index still are commonly used and are increased in almost all hyperthyroid patients. Usually, both T_3 and T_4 are elevated. However, a few (<5%) hyperthyroid patients exhibit normal T_4 with elevated T_3 (T_3 toxicosis). Second-line tests such as antithyroid antibody serologies are necessary to diagnose autoimmune thyroid disorders. Table 13-18 summarizes test results seen with common thyroid disorders.

Adrenal Disorders

The adrenal glands are located extraperitoneally at the upper poles of each kidney. The adrenal medulla, which makes up 10% of the adrenal gland, secretes catecholamines (e.g., epinephrine and norepinephrine). The adrenal cortex, which comprises 90% of the adrenal gland, is divided into three areas:

1. The outer layer of the adrenal gland, known as the *zona glomerulosa*, makes up 15% of the adrenal gland and is responsible for production of aldosterone, a mineralocor-

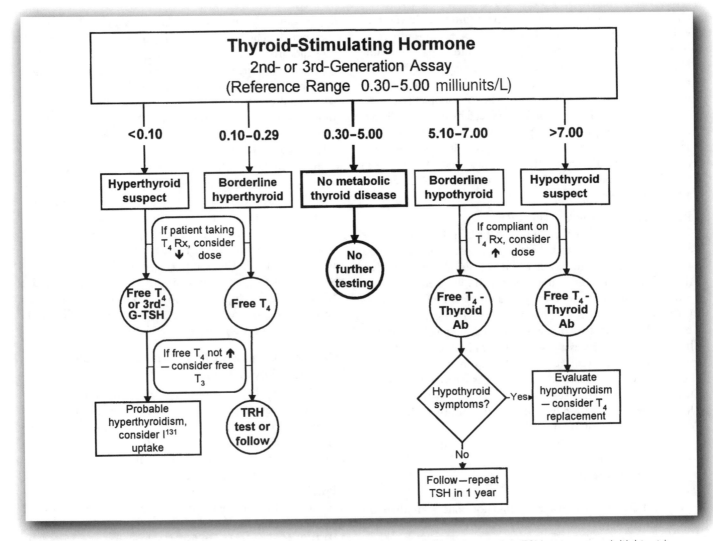

FIGURE 13-5. Algorithm for investigation of thyroid disease using second-third-generation TSH assay as an initial test in patients without pituitary or neuropsychiatric disease. (Adapted, with permission, from reference 83.)

ticoid that regulates electrolyte and volume homeostasis.

2. The *zona fasciculata*, located in the center of the adrenal gland, occupies 60% of the gland and is responsible for glucocorticoid production. Cortisol, a principal end product of glucocorticoid production, regulates fat, carbohydrate, and protein metabolism. Glucocorticoids maintain the body's homeostasis by regulating bodily functions involved in stress as well as normal activities.

3. The *zona reticularis* makes up 25% of the adrenal gland and is responsible for adrenal androgens such as testosterone and estrogens such as estradiol. These hormones influence the development of the reproductive system.[100]

Cushing Syndrome

Cushing syndrome, first described 70 years ago, is the result of excessive concentrations of cortisol. In most cases, hypercortisolism is the result of overproduction of cortisol by the adrenal glands due to an adrenocorticotropic hormone (ACTH) secreting pituitary tumor. Adrenal tumors and long-term use of glucocorticoids can also result in hypercortisolism.

Patients with hypercortisolism generally present with facial plethora (moon face) as a result of atrophy of the skin and underlying tissue. A common sign of hypercortisolism is fat accumulation in the dorsocervical area often referred to as "buffalo hump." Other cardinal signs and symptoms include hypertension, osteopenia, glucose intolerance, myopathy, bruising, and depression. Hyperpigmentation is present in patients with ACTH-secreting pituitary tumors. Hair loss, acne, and oligomenorrhea are also the result of superfluous cortical secretion.[126]

Diagnostic Tests

The following tests are employed to identify patients with Cushing syndrome: 24-hour urine-free cortisol (UFC), midnight plasma cortisol, and/or the low-dose dexamethasone suppression test (DST) using 1 mg for the overnight test or 0.5 milligrams every 6 hours for the 2-day study. The most frequently used test to identify patients with hypercortisolism is the 24-hour UFC test, which measures free cortisol levels and creatinine in a urine sample that is collected over a 24-hour period.

MINICASE 4

A Patient with Hypothyroidism

MARIE M., A 70-KG, 40-YEAR-OLD music teacher, presents to her primary care provider complaining of feeling tired all the time. She has gained 20 pounds, feels mentally sluggish, tires easily, and finds she can no longer hit high notes during choir rehearsals.

Her physical exam was normal, except for an enlarged thyroid gland, puffy facies, yellowish skin, and diminished tendon reflexes.

- Sodium, 145mEq/L (136–142 mEq/L)
- Potassium, 4.0 mEq/L (3.8–5.0 mEq/L)
- Chloride, 101 mEq/L (95–103 mEq/L)
- Carbon dioxide, 26 mEq/L (21–28 mEq/L)
- BUN, 10 mg/dL (8–23 mg/dL)
- SCr, 0.8 mg/dL (0.6–1.2 mg/dL)
- Hgb, 12 g/dL (12–16 g/dL)
- Hct, 36% (36% to 45%)
- RBCs, 3.5 M/mm³ (4.0–5.2 M/mm³)
- Antithyroid antibodies 1:200
- Mean corpuscular volume (MCV), 104 mm³ (80–100)
- WBCs, 16 x 10³ cells/mm³ (4.8–10.8 × 10³ cells/mm³)
- Calcium, 9 mg/dL (9.2–11.0 mg/dL)
- Glucose, 96 mg/dL (70–110 mg/dL)
- Free T₄, 0.6 ng/dL (0.9–2.3 ng/dL)
- TSH, 7.0 microunits/mL (0.5–5.0 microunits/mL)

Question: How should these results be interpreted? Are confirmatory tests needed?

Discussion: Marie M. presents with many of the clinical features of hypothyroidism. These include weight gain, mental sluggishness, easy fatigability, lowering of the voice pitch, a puffy facies, a yellowish tint of the skin, diminished tendon reflexes, and an enlarged thyroid. The diagnosis of hypothyroidism can be confirmed by her laboratory results of a low T₄, and an elevated TSH value.

The firm goiter, antithyroid antibodies, and clinical symptoms of hypothyroidism strongly suggest Hashimoto thyroiditis. She has no prior history of antithyroid drug use, surgery, or radioactive iodine treatment, which are common causes of hypothyroidism. She is not taking any drugs known to cause hypothyroidism. Marie M. also has macrocytic anemia. Anemia can occur in hypothyroidism because thyroid hormones stimulate erythropoiesis. Three types of anemia can occur with hypothyroidism: (a) normochromic, normocytic anemia is found in 25% of hypothyroid patients; (b) hypochromic, microcytic anemia is usually exacerbated by menorrhagia and occurs in 4% to 15% of hypothyroid patients, and (c) macrocytic anemia.

TABLE 13-18. Test Results Seen in Common Thyroid Disorders and Drug Effects on Test Results[93,104,108,124,125]

DISEASE	TOTAL SERUM T₄	TOTAL SERUM T₃	T₃ RESIN UPTAKE	FREE T₄ INDEX	RAIU	TSH	COMMENT
Hypothyroidism	↓	↓	↓	↓	↓	↑/↓ ᵃ	
Hyperthyroidism	↑	↑	↑	↑	↑	↓	
T₃ thyrotoxicosis	No change	↑	No change	No change	No change	↓	T₃ resin uptake may be slightly increased
Euthyroid sick	No change/↓	↓	↑	Variable	No change	No change syndrome	
Corticosteroids	↓	No change/↓	↑	No change	↓	No change/↓	
Phenytoin/ aspirin	↓	↓	↑	No change	↓	No change	Large salicylate dose
Radiopaque media	No change/↑	No change/↓	No change	No change/↑	↓	No change	

RAIU = radioactive iodine uptake test; T₃ = triiodothyronine; T₄ = thyroxine; TSH = thyroid-stimulating hormone; ↑ = increased; ↓ = decreased.
ᵃIncreased TSH diagnostic of primary hypothyroidism. TSH is decreased in secondary and tertiary types.

Clinically, the easiest way to make the diagnosis is to perform a dehydration test, where the patient is deprived of water for 8–12 hours. Urine osmolality, urine volume, and body weight are taken before and after the subcutaneous administration of desmopressin acetate. As compared to patients with nephrogenic DI whose urine osmolality will not rise above 300 mOsm/kg, patients with central DI have an immediate rise in urine osmolality with a decrease in urine volume when challenged with a subcutaneous injection of desmopressin.

Patients can be challenged with a test dose of ADH. Urine osmolality greater than 750 mOsm/kg in response to an ADH test dose confirms the diagnosis of central DI. A hypertonic saline solution can also be administered intravenously in an attempt to raise plasma osmolality to 300 mOsm/kg. A direct measurement of ADH can be done to determine the response to hypertonic plasma. Patients with nephrogenic DI will have normal ADH levels compared to patients with central DI, who will have a negligible response to the hypertonic solution due to a decrease or lack of endogenous ADH.[136] Cortisol levels greater than 200 mcg/mL suggest hypercortisolism. Physiological levels of cortisol usually decline between 8:00 a.m. and 11:00 p.m. Midnight serum cortisol levels greater than 7.5 mcg/mL indicate Cushing syndrome.

Of the suppression tests, the overnight DST is the least laborious test to perform. The patient is given 1 mg of dexamethasone at 11:00 p.m. followed by a plasma cortisol assay at 8 a.m. the next morning. Patients with Cushing syndrome will have high cortisol concentrations (>5 mcg/mL) due to an inability to suppress the negative-feedback mechanism of the hypothalamic-pituitary-adrenal (HPA) axis.[126-128]

Once hypercortisolism is confirmed, one of the following tests should be performed to identify the source of hypersecretion: high-dose DST, plasma ACTH via immunoradiometric assay (IRMA) or RIA; adrenal vein catheterization; metyrapone stimulation test; adrenal, chest, or abdominal computed tomography (CT); corticotropin-releasing hormone (CRH) stimulation test; inferior petrosal sinus sampling; and pituitary magnetic resonance imaging (MRI). Other possible tests and procedures include insulin-induced hypoglycemia, somatostatin receptor scintigraphy; the desmopressin stimulation test; naloxone CRH stimulation test; loperamide test; the hexarelin stimulation test; and radionuclide imaging. Additional tests should be performed to confirm the diagnosis since other factors (starvation, topical steroid application, and acute stress) influence the results of the above mentioned tests.[126]

Plasma ACTH concentrations can be measured by RIA procedures. Interpretation of the results is as follows:

- ACTH levels less than 5 mcg/mL indicate an ACTH-independent adrenal source such as an adrenal tumor or long-term use of steroids.
- ACTH levels between 5–10 mcg/mL should be followed by a CRH test.
- ACTH levels greater than 10 mcg/mL indicate an ACTH-dependent syndrome.

The CRH test can be employed to determine if the source of hypercortisolism is pituitary or ectopic (extra-pituitary). Baseline ACTH and CRH levels are obtained. Then, ACTH and cortisol levels are measured 30–45 minutes after the administration of a 1 mcg/mL dose of CRH. A 50% increase from baseline in ACTH levels indicates an ACTH- dependent syndrome.[126]

The overnight high-dose DST is also used to identify the source of hypercortisolism. A baseline plasma cortisol level is obtained the morning prior to the test. Patients are given dexamethasone 8 mg at 11:00 p.m. Plasma cortisol levels are obtained at 8:00 a.m. the following morning. Plasma cortisol levels less than 50% of baseline indicate an ACTH-dependent syndrome.[126,127]

Pharmacologic Treatment

Treatment of Cushing syndrome involves inhibition of steroid synthesis. Mitotane is the most frequently prescribed agent for the treatment of this disorder. Mitotane inhibits steroid biosynthesis as well as inhibits peripheral steroid metabolism and cortisol release. Alternative agents, metyrapone,

---

MINICASE 5

A Patient with Abnormal TSH Test Results

RITA T., A 27-YEAR-OLD FEMALE being assessed for infertility, was found to have a TSH concentration of 8.2 milliunits/L (0.5–5.0 milliunits/L) as measured by a second-generation assay. Her physical exam revealed no abnormalities, and she was clinically euthyroid. Her total serum T_4 was 10 mcg/dL (5.5–12.5 mcg/dL). She was treated with 0.125 mg/day of levothyroxine for 1 month, and a repeat TSH was 6.8 milliunits/L. Her dose was increased to 0.2 mg/day.

After 2 months, Rita T.'s TSH was 8.8 milliunits/L, while her total serum T_4 was 15 mcg/dL, her total serum T_3 was 200 ng/dL (80–200 ng/dL), her TBG was 32 nmol/L (10–26 nmol/L), and her free T_3 was 4.7 pmol/L (3.2–5.1 pmol/L). She was slightly hyperthyroid. Levothyroxine therapy was stopped and, on that day, a TRH challenge (200 mcg IV) evoked only minimal increases in TSH concentrations. An MRI of the hypothalamic-pituitary area was normal.

Question: What could have caused Rita T.'s initial elevated TSH?

Discussion: Although TSH is classically elevated in patients with primary hypothyroidism, Helen T. did not have any clinical signs or symptoms of this disorder. Inappropriate elevation of TSH can be caused by a TSH-secreting pituitary tumor, thyroid hormone resistance, or assay interference. Tumor was ruled out by the normal MRI. Hormone resistance is not consistent with her picture. If Rita T. had pituitary-confined resistance, persistent secretion of TSH and thyroid hormones would have led to clinical hyperthyroidism. If resistance had been general, she would have been euthyroid (as she was), but T_4 and T_3 concentrations would have been elevated along with TSH.[38]

Finally, transiently elevated TSH may be found in patients recovering from major physiological stress (e.g., intensive care illnesses and trauma), which was not the case here. Thyroid status should be evaluated after major medical problems have stabilized. The TRH challenge showed essentially no response, a finding that reflects the iatrogenic hyperthyroidism at the time. Therefore, by exclusion, Rita T.'s elevated TSH concentration most likely is an artifact, probably due to interfering antibodies. This condition is rare but has been described.

---

aminoglutethimide, and ketoconazole are adrenal enzyme inhibitors that inhibit enzymes necessary for the conversion of cholesterol into steroid hormones, which is a necessary step for the production of cortisol. Cyproheptadine is a neuromodulatory agent that has been used to decrease ACTH secretion. Due to a low response rate of less than 30%, cyproheptadine is reserved for patients who fail conventional therapy.[127,128]

Adrenal Insufficiency or Addison Disease

Adrenal insufficiency (Addison disease or *primary adrenal insufficiency)* is the result of an autoimmune destruction of all regions of the adrenal cortex. Tuberculosis, fungal infections, acquired immunodeficiency syndrome, metastatic cancer, and lymphomas can also precipitate adrenal insufficiency. Adrenal insufficiency results in deficiencies in cortisol, aldosterone, and androgens. Patients usually present with weakness, weight loss, increased pigmentation, hypotension, GI symptoms, postural dizziness, and vertigo.

Secondary adrenal insufficiency can result from the use of high doses of exogenous steroids, which suppress the hypothalamic-pituitary axis resulting in a decrease in the release of ACTH. Patients with secondary adrenal insufficiency maintain normal aldosterone levels and do not exhibit signs of hyperpigmentation.[129,130]

Diagnostic Tests

The cosyntropin stimulation test is used to diagnose patients with low cortisol levels. Patients are administered 250 mcg of synthetic ACTH or cosyntropin intravenously or intramuscularly. Serum cortisol levels are drawn at the time of injection and 30 minutes and 1 hour after the injection. Cortisol levels greater than 18 mcg/dL indicate an adequate response from the adrenal gland, thus ruling out adrenal insufficiency. The cosyntropin stimulation test may be normal in patients with secondary adrenal insufficiency or mild primary adrenal insufficiency due to the high dose of corticotropin given. In light of this, many endocrinologists recommend that higher cutoff values (≥22 to 25 mcg/dL) be used.

Similar results have been obtained using a lower dose of 1 mcg of cosyntropin. Cortisol levels should increase to 18 mcg/dL or more 30 minutes after the injection. Other tests used to assess patients suspected of hypercortisolism include the insulin hypoglycemia test, the metyrapone test, and the CRH stimulation test.[129-131]

Pharmacologic Treatment

Corticosteroids are used to treat adrenal insufficiency. The agents of choice include prednisone 5 mg/day, hydrocortisone 20 mg/day, or cortisone 25 mg/day given in the morning and evening. Additional mineralocorticoid (e.g., fludrocortisone acetate 0.05–2.0 mg daily) should be given to patients with primary adrenal insufficiency since there is a concomitant decrease in aldosterone production. The endpoint of therapy is the reversal of signs and symptoms of adrenal insufficiency, particularly excess pigmentation.[131]

DIABETES INSIPIDUS

Diabetes insipidus is a syndrome in which the body's inability to conserve water manifests as excretion of very large volumes of dilute urine. This section explores related pathophysiology, types of DI, and interpretation of test results to evaluate this disorder.

Physiology

Normally, serum osmolality is maintained around 285 mOsm/kg and is determined by the amounts of sodium, chloride, bicarbonate, glucose, and urea in the serum. The excretion of these solutes along with water is a primary factor in determining urine volume and concentration. In turn, the amount of water excreted by the kidneys is determined by renal function and ADH (vasopressin).

Antidiuretic hormone is synthesized in the hypothalamus and stored in the posterior pituitary gland. This hormone is released into the circulation following physiological stimulation, such as a change in serum osmolality or blood volume detected by the osmoregulatory centers in the hypothalamus.[132,133] Congestive heart failure lowers the osmotic threshold for ADH release, while nausea—but not vomiting—strongly stimulates ADH. In general, alpha-adrenergic agonists stimulate ADH release while beta-adrenergic agonists inhibit release, and acts on the distal renal tubule and the collecting duct to cause water reabsorption. Chlorpropamide potentiates the effect of ADH on renal concentrating ability. When ADH is lacking or the renal tubules do not respond to the hormone, polyuria ensues. If the polyuria is severe enough, a diagnosis of DI is considered.[133,134]

Clinical Diagnosis

Diabetes insipidus should be differentiated from other causes of polyuria such as osmotic diuresis (e.g., hyperglycemia, mannitol, and contrast media), renal tubular acidosis, diuretic therapy, and psychogenic polydipsia. Patients usually excrete 16–24 L of dilute urine in 24 hours. The urine specific gravity is less than 1.005 and urine osmolality <300 mOsm/kg.[134,135] As long as the thirst mechanism is intact and the patient can drink, no electrolyte problems result. However, if the patient is unable to replace fluids lost through excessive urine output, the patient can develop dehydration.

While DI is usually caused by a defect in the secretion (neurogenic, also called *central*) or renal activity (nephrogenic) of ADH, it can also be caused by a defect in thirst (dipsogenic) or psychological function (psychogenic), with resultant excessive intake of water. Although DI typically does not lead to significant morbidity, the underlying cause should be sought to ensure proper diagnosis and therapy. The specific type of DI often can be identified by the clinical setting. If the diagnosis is equivocal, a therapeutic trial with an antidiuretic drug or measurement of plasma ADH is necessary.[135]

Central Diabetes Insipidus

Central DI (ADH deficiency) may be the result of any disruption in the pituitary-hypothalamic regulation of ADH. Patients often present with a sudden onset of polyuria (in the absence of hyperglycemia) and preference for iced drinks. Tumors or metastases in or around the pituitary or hypothalamus, head trauma, neurosurgery, genetic abnormalities, Guillain-Barré syndrome, meningitis, encephalitis, toxoplasmosis, cytomegalovirus, tuberculosis, and aneurysms are some of the known causes. In addition, phenytoin and alcohol inhibit ADH release from the pituitary. In response to deficient secretion of ADH and subsequent hyperosmolality of the plasma, thirst is stimulated. Thirst induces water intake, which leads to polyuria in the absence of effective ADH.[133]

Nephrogenic Diabetes Insipidus

In nephrogenic DI (ADH resistance), the secretion of ADH is normal, but the renal tubule does not respond to ADH. Causes of nephrogenic DI include chronic renal failure, pyelonephritis, hypokalemia, hypercalciuria, malnutrition, genetic defects, and sickle cell disease. Additionally, lithium toxicity, colchicine, glyburide, demeclocycline, cidofovir, and methoxyflurane occasionally cause this disorder.

Lithium leads to polyuria in about 20% of patients. Typically, polyuria occurs after 2–3 months of therapy. This antimanic drug appears to exert its nephrotoxicity by entering collecting duct cells through sodium channels. Lithium impairs ADH's ability to produce cyclic adenosine monophosphate (AMP), resulting in resistance to the renal effects of ADH on the collecting duct and water loss. Sodium reabsorption in the cortical diluting and distal tubules results in increased urine output. Amiloride, a potassium-sparing diuretic, is useful at doses of 5 mg/day in lithium-induced DI because it closes the sodium channels in the collecting duct cells and decreases lithium accumulation. Chlorpropamide potentiates ADH's effect on the collecting tubules. Chlorpropamide is usually given in doses of 125–500 mg daily; patients should be monitored for hypoglycemia. Thiazides can be used to block sodium reabsorption in the cortical diluting tubule and the distal tubule, thereby, decreasing urine output. Hydrochlorothiazide 50–100 mg daily or an equivalent dose of another thiazide diuretic can be used. Patients who are treated with thiazide diuretics must be monitored because these agents can cause hypokalemia and hypomagnesemia.[133]

Diabetes Insipidus of Pregnancy

A transient DI, originally thought to be a form of nephrogenic DI, may develop during late pregnancy from excessive vasopressinase (ADHase) activity. This kind of DI is associated with preeclampsia with liver involvement. Fortunately, vasopressinase does not metabolize DDAVP (desmopressin acetate), which is, therefore, the treatment of choice.[134]

Laboratory Diagnosis

Some clinicians avoid dehydration testing and rely on measuring plasma ADH concentrations to distinguish neurogenic from nephrogenic forms. In otherwise healthy adults, the average basal plasma ADH concentration is 1.3–4.0 pg/mL or ng/L (Figure 13-6).

Based on medical history, symptoms, and signs, an elevated basal plasma ADH level almost always indicates nephrogenic DI. If the basal plasma ADH concentration is low (<1 pg/mL) or immeasurable, the result is inconclusive and a dehydration test should be done. If the diagnosis is ambiguous based on the clinical setting and basal plasma ADH concentrations, the plan

in Figure 13-6 should elucidate the diagnosis, even in a patient with a less common form of DI.

The theory behind the water deprivation test is that, in normal individuals, dehydration stimulates ADH release and the urine becomes concentrated. An injection of vasopressin at this point does not further concentrate the urine. In contrast, the urine of patients with central DI will not be maximally concentrated after fluid deprivation but will be after vasopressin injection.

To perform the test, patients are deprived of fluid intake (up to 18 hours) until the urine osmolality of three consecutive samples varies by no more than 30 mOsm/kg. Urine osmolality and/or specific gravity are measured hourly. At this time, 5 units of aqueous vasopressin are administered subcutaneously, and urine osmolality is measured 1 hour later. Plasma osmolality is measured before the test, when urine osmolality has stabilized, and after vasopressin has been administered.

In healthy individuals, fluid deprivation for 8- to 12-hour results in normal serum osmolality and a urine osmolality of about 800 mOsm/kg. The urine osmolality plateaus after 16–18 hours. Patients with central DI have an immediate rise in urine osmolality to approximately 600 mOsm/kg, with a corresponding decrease in urine output with vasopressin injection. Patients with nephrogenic DI are unable to increase urine osmolality above 300 mOsm/kg as vasopressin injection has little effect.

In addition to being inconvenient and expensive, dehydration procedures are reliable only if the DI is severe enough that—even with induced dehydration—the urine still cannot be concentrated. Table 13-19 presents a summary of typical results of a water deprivation test.

Accurate interpretation requires consideration of potential confounding factors. If the laboratory cannot ensure accurate and precise plasma (not serum) osmolality measurements, plasma sodium should be used. Patients should be observed for nonosmotic stimuli, such as vasovagal reactions, that may affect ADH release. Lastly, if the patient has previously received ADH therapy, ADH antibodies may cause false-positive results suggestive of nephrogenic DI.[136]

SUMMARY

Endocrine disorders often result from a deficiency or excess of a hormone. Laboratory tests that measure the actual hormone, precursors, or metabolites can help to elucidate whether and why a hormonal or metabolic imbalance exists. Tests used

TABLE 13-19. Differential Diagnosis of Diabetes Insipidus Based on Water Deprivation Test[132,133]

DIAGNOSIS	URINE SPECIFIC GRAVITY	AVERAGE URINE OSMOLALITY (mOsm/kg)	PLATEAU URINE OSMOLALITY (mOsm/kg)	AVERAGE SERUM OSMOLALITY (mOsm/kg)	CHANGE IN URINE OSMOLALITY AFTER VASOPRESSIN
Normal individuals	>1.015	300–800	<1600	280–295	Little change
Central diabetes insipidus	<1.010	<300	<300	Normal or increased	Increases
Nephrogenic diabetes insipidus	<1.010	<300	<300	Normal or increased	Little change

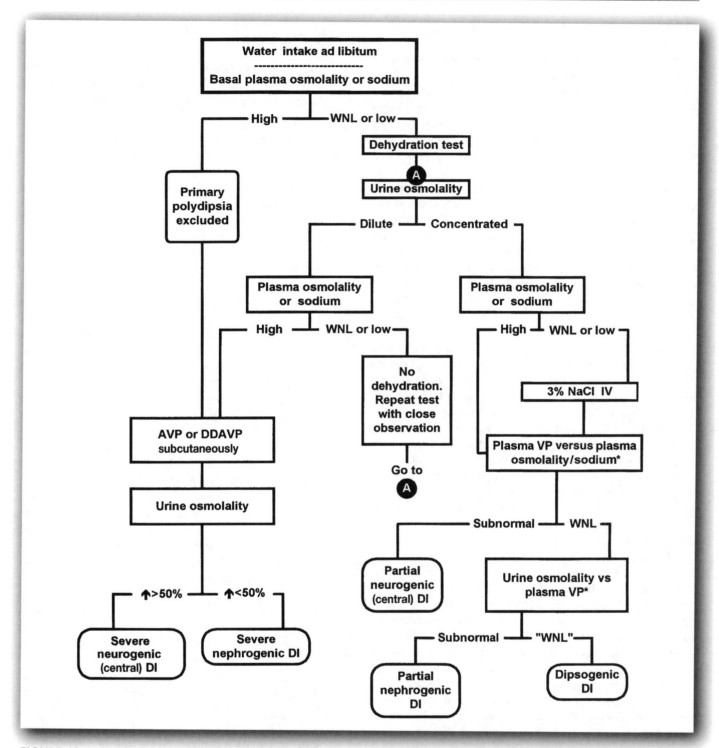

FIGURE 13-6. Evaluation of diabetes insipidus if diagnosis is ambiguous based on the clinical setting and basal plasma vasopressin concentrations. Plasma osmolality and sodium are considered high if they exceed the upper limit of normal for the laboratory (usually 295 mOsm/kg and 142 mEq/L, respectively). Urine is considered diluted if its osmolality is less than 300 mOsm/kg; it is concentrated if its osmolality is greater than 300 mOsm/kg. If indicated, hypertonic saline is infused at 0.1 mL/kg/min for 2 hours. The vasopressin (aqueous Pitressin, AVP) dose is 5 units, while the DDAVP (desmopressin) dose is 1 mcg subcutaneously. Interpretation of plasma VP versus plasma osmolality/sodium and urine osmolality versus plasma VP requires use of a nomogram. ADH = antidiuretic hormone; DI = diabetes insipidus; IV = intravenous; VP = vasopressin; WNL = within normal limits. (Adapted with permission from reference 133.)

to assess thyroid, adrenal, glucose, and water homeostasis or receptors have been discussed.

The FPG and the 2-hour PPG concentrations are the most commonly performed tests for evaluation of glucose homeostasis. If elevated (>126 mg/dL) blood glucose persists, DM is likely. However, other causes of hyperglycemia (e.g., drugs) should be considered. Glycosylated hemoglobin assesses average glucose control over the previous 2–3 months, while fructosamine assesses average control over the previous 2–3 weeks.

Diabetic ketoacidosis and hyperosmolar nonketotic hyperglycemia are the most severe disorders along the continuum of glucose intolerance. Extreme hyperglycemia (600–2000 mg/dL) with insignificant ketonemia/acidosis is consistent with hyperosmolar nonketotic hyperglycemia, while less severe (350–650 mg/dL) hyperglycemia with ketonemia and acidosis is characteristic of DKA. Conversely, hypoglycemia (glucose <50 mg/dL) most often is seen in patients with type 1 DM who have injected excessive insulin relative to their caloric intake.

Thyroid tests can be divided into those that (1) measure the concentration of products secreted by the thyroid gland (T_3 and T_4); (2) evaluate the integrity of the hypothalamic-pituitary-thyroid axis (TSH and TRH); (3) assess intrinsic thyroid gland function (radioactive iodine uptake test); and (4) detect antibodies to thyroid tissue (thyroid microsomal antibody). While TSH concentrations are usually undetectable or less than 0.3 milliunit/L (newer assays), T_4 concentrations are usually high in patients with overt hyperthyroidism. The TSH concentrations are low or undetectable in patients with hypothyroidism from hypothalamic or pituitary insufficiency and in patients with nonthyroidal illness. In contrast, TSH concentrations are high and T_4 concentrations are low in patients with primary hypothyroidism.

Glucocorticoids maintain the body's homeostasis by regulating bodily functions involved in stress and normal activities. Cortisol, androgens, aldosterone, and estrogens are all produced in the adrenal glands. Cushing syndrome is the result of excessive cortisol in the body. Addison disease occurs when there is a deficiency in cortisol production.

Diabetes insipidus is a syndrome in which the body's inability to conserve water manifests as excretion of very large volumes of dilute urine. It most often is caused by a defect in the secretion (neurogenic, also called *central*) or renal activity (nephrogenic) of ADH. Urine and plasma osmolality are key tests. With the advent of high-performance assays, the use of plasma vasopressin concentrations to distinguish neurogenic from nephrogenic types may obviate the need for provocative iatrogenic dehydration testing procedures.

Learning Points

1. **Which patients with diabetes benefit from SMBG and how can different test results (premeal, postmeal, and fasting) be used in diabetes management?**

   Answer: The ADA recommends SMBG for all people with diabetes who use insulin.[18] Self-monitoring provides information patients can use to adjust insulin doses, physical activity, and carbohydrate intake in response to high or low glucose levels. The goal of SMBG is to prevent hypoglycemia while maintaining blood glucose levels as close to normal as possible. Most people with type 1 DM must use SMBG to achieve this goal. While people with type 2 DM receiving insulin therapy benefit from SMBG, the benefit of SMBG for individuals with type 2 DM who do not use insulin is not firmly established.[136,137] The ADA states that SMBG may be desirable in patients treated with sulfonylureas or other drugs that increase insulin secretion.[136] The frequency and timing of SMBG vary based on several factors, including an individual's glycemic goals, the current level of glucose control, and the treatment regimen. The ADA recommends SMBG 3 or more times per day for most individuals who have type 1 DM and pregnant women who use insulin. More frequent testing (4–6 times per day) may be needed to monitor pump therapy.[18] In patients with type 1 DM, SMBG is most commonly recommended 4 times a day, before meals and at bedtime. A periodic 2 a.m. test is recommended to monitor for nighttime hypoglycemia. These measurements are used to adjust insulin doses and attain the fasting glucose goal. However, there is evidence that blood glucose measurements taken after lunch, after dinner, and at bedtime have the highest correlation to A1c values.[138] When premeal or fasting goals are reached but A1c values are not optimal, SMBG 2 hours after meals can provide guidance for further adjustment of insulin regimens. Postmeal measurements are also used to evaluate the effects of rapid-acting insulins (e.g., lispro, aspart), which are injected just before meals. Type 2 patients who use multiple daily injections of insulin should generally test as often as type 1 patients (at least 3 times per day). Patients on once-daily insulin and/or oral medications may also benefit from testing before meals and at bedtime when therapy is initiated or if control is poor.[139,140]

2. **What factors should a pharmacist consider when helping a patient select a SMBG meter?**

   Answer: Meters offer a variety of features that should be considered in the selection process. The key features are meter size; the amount of blood required for each test; ease of use; speed of testing; cleaning and calibration requirements; alternate site testing capability; meter and test strip cost; language choice; and the capability to store readings, average readings over time, and/or download data. Patient factors to consider include lifestyle (where they will be testing; importance of portability and speed), preferences (importance of small sample size or alternate site capability), dexterity (can they operate the meter), visual acuity, and insurance coverage.[141]

3. What factors may affect the accuracy of a A1c result?

Answer: False elevations in A1c may be noted with uremia, chronic alcohol intake, and hypertriglyceridemia. Patients who have diseases with chronic or episodic hemolysis (e.g., sickle cell disease and thalassemia) generally have spuriously low A1c concentrations caused by the predominance of young RBCs (which carry less A1c) in the circulation. In splenectomized patients and those with polycythemia, A1c is increased. If these disorders are stable, the test still can be used, but values must be compared with the patient's previous results rather than published normal values. Both falsely elevated and falsely lowered measurements of A1c may also occur during pregnancy. Therefore, it should not be used to screen for gestational DM.[32,141]

4. Which laboratory tests are recommended in the initial evaluation of thyroid disorders?

Answer: The principal laboratory tests recommended in the initial evaluation of a suspected thyroid disorder are the sensitive TSH and the free T_4 levels. Free T_4 is the most accurate reflection of thyrometabolic status. The free T_4 is the most reliable diagnostic test for the evaluation of hypothyroidism and hyperthyroidism when thyroid hormone binding abnormalities exist. If a direct measure of the free T_4 level is not available, the estimated free T_4 index can provide comparable information. Total serum T_4 is still the standard initial screening test to assess thyroid function because of its wide availability and quick turnaround time. In most patients, the total serum T_4 level is a sensitive test to evaluate the function of the thyroid gland. This test measures both bound and free T_4 and is, therefore, less reliable than the free T_4 or free T_4 index when alterations in TBG or nonthyroidal illnesses exist. The serum TSH is the most sensitive test to evaluate thyroid function. Thyroid-stimulating hormone secreted by the pituitary is elevated in early or subclinical hypothyroidism (when thyroid hormone levels appear normal) or when thyroid hormone replacement therapy is inadequate.[142]

REFERENCES

1. Buse JB. Progressive use of medical therapies in type 2 diabetes. *Diabetes Spectr.* 2000;13(4):211-220.

2. Krentz AJ, Bailey CJ. Oral antidiabetic agents: current role in type 2 diabetes mellitus. *Drugs.* 2005;65(3):385-411.

3. Gerich JE. Matching treatment to pathophysiology in type 2 diabetes. *Clin Ther.* 2000;23:646-659.

4. Dinneen S, Gerich J, Rizza R. Carbohydrate metabolism in noninsulin-dependent diabetes mellitus. *N Engl J Med.* 1992;327:707-713.

5. Symlin (pramlintide acetate) injection [package insert]. San Diego, CA: Amylin; 2005.

6. Kruger DF, Gloster MA. Pramlintide for the treatment of insulin-requiring diabetes mellitus: rationale and review of clinical data. *Drugs.* 2004;64:1419-1432.

7. Kleppinger EL, Vivian EM. Pramlintide for the treatment of diabetes mellitus. *Ann Pharmacother.* 2003;37:1082-1089.

8. Ryan GJ, Jobe LJ, Martin R. Pramlintide in the treatment of type 1 and type 2 diabetes mellitus. *Clin Ther.* 2005;27:1500-1512.

9. White JR Jr, Davis SN, Coopan R, et al. Clarifying the role of insulin in type 2 diabetes management. *Clin Diabetes.* 2003;21:14-21.

10. Thompson RG, Pearson L, Schoenfeld SL, et al. for the Pramlintide in Type 2 Diabetes Group. Pramlintide, a synthetic analog of human amylin, improves the metabolic profile of patients with type 2 diabetes using insulin. *Diabetes Care.* 1998;21:987-993.

11. Hollander PA, Levy P, Fineman MS, et al. Pramlintide as an adjunct to insulin therapy improves long-term glycemic and weight control in patients with type 2 diabetes: a 1-year randomized controlled trial. *Diabetes Care.* 2003;26:784-790.

12. Druck DJ. The biology of incretin hormones. *Cell Metab.* 2006;3:153-165.

13. Vilsboll T, Krarup T, Sonne J, et al. Incretin secretion in relation to meal size and body weight in healthy subjects and people with type 1 and type 2 diabetes mellitus. *J Clin Endocrinol Metab.* 2003;88:2706-2713.

14. Kahn SE. The relative contributions of insulin resistance and beta-cell dysfunction to the pathophysiology of type 2 diabetes. *Diabetologia.* 2003;46:3-19.

15. Gomis R, Novials A, Coves MJ, et al. Suppression by insulin treatment of glucose induced inhibition of insulin release in noninsulin dependent diabetics. *Diabetes Res Clin Pract.*1989;6:191-198.

16. Tahrani AA, Barnett AH. Dapagliflozin: a sodium glucose cotransporter 2 inhibitor in development for type 2 diabetes. *Diabetes Ther.* 2010;1(2):45-56.

17. Basile JA. New approach to glucose control in type 2 diabetes: the role of kidney sodium-glucose co-transporter 2 inhibition. *Postgrad Med.* 2011 Jul;123(4):38-45.

18. American Diabetes Association. Standards of Medical Care in Diabetes—2013. *Diabetes Care.* 2013;(suppl 1):11S-66S.

19. Metzger BE, Gabbe SG, Persson B, et al. International Association of Diabetes and Pregnancy Study Groups consensus Panel. International association of diabetes and pregnancy study groups recommendations on the diagnosis and classification of hyperglycemia in pregnancy. *Diabetes Care.* 2010;33:676-682.

20. Redondo MJ, Fain PR, Eisenbarth GS. Genetics of type 1A diabetes. *Recent Pro Horm Res.* 2001;56:69-89.

21. Ong KK, Dunger DB. Thrifty genotypes and phenotypes in the pathogenesis of type 2 diabetes. *J Pediatr Endocrinol Metab.* 2000;13(suppl 6):1419-1424.

22. Tripathy D, Carlsson AL, Lehto M, et al. Insulin secretion and insulin sensitivity in diabetic subgroups: studies in the prediabetic and diabetic state. *Diabetologia.* 2000;43:1476-1483.

23. Froguel P, Velho G. Genetic determinants of type 2 diabetes. *Recent Prog Horm Res.* 2001;56:91-105.

24. Bennett PH. Definition, diagnosis, and classification of diabetes mellitus and impaired glucose tolerance. In: Kahn CR, Weir GC, eds. *Joslin's Diabetes Mellitus.* 13th ed. Philadelphia, PA: Lea & Febiger; 1994:193-200.

25. Godsland IF, Crook D, Simpson R, et al. The effects of different formulations of oral contraceptive agents on lip and carbohydrate metabolism. *N Engl J Med.* 1990;323:1375-1381.

26. Sacks DB, Arnold M, Bakris GL, et al. Guidelines and recommendations for laboratory analysis in the diagnosis and management of diabetes mellitus. *Clin Chem.* 2011;57(6)e1-e47

27. Howanitz PJ, Howanitz JH. Carbohydrates. In: Henry JB, ed. *Clinical Diagnosis and Management by Laboratory Methods.* 17th ed. Philadelphia, PA: WB Saunders; 1984:165-203.

28. American Diabetes Association. Diagnosis and classification of diabetes mellitus. *Diabetes Care.* 2013;(Suppl 1)36:67S-74S.

29. AACE Diabetes Mellitus Clinical Practice Guidelines Task Force. American Association of Clinical Endocrinologists medical guidelines for clinical practice for the management of diabetes mellitus. *Endocr Pract.* 2009;15:540-559.

30. Goldstein DE, Little RR, Wiedmeyer HM, et al. Glycated hemoglobin: methodologies and clinical applications. *Clin Chem.* 1986;32(suppl 10):B64-B70.

31. Yarrison G, Allen L, King N, et al. Lipemic interference in Beckman Diatrac hemoglobin A1c procedure removed. *Clin Chem.* 1993;39:2351-2352.

32. Goldstein DE, Parker M, England JD, et al. Clinical application of glycosylated hemoglobin measurements. *Diabetes.* 1982;31(suppl 3):70-78.

33. American Diabetes Association. *Resource Guide 2003: Glycohemoglobin Tests Diabetes Forecast.* Alexandria, VA: American Diabetes Association; 2003:(suppl 1)67.

34. American Diabetes Association. Tests of glycemia in diabetes. *Diabetes Care.* 2003;26(suppl 1):S106-S108.

35. Nathan DM, Kuenen J, Borg R, et al. Translating the A1c assay into estimated average glucose values. *Diabetes Care.* 2008;31:1-6.

36. Ardawi MS, Nasrat HA, Bahnassy AA. Fructosamine in obese normal subjects and type 2 diabetes. *Diabet Med.* 1994;11:50-56.

37. Cefalu WT, Ettinger WH, Bell-Farrow AD, et al. Serum fructosamine as a screening test for diabetes in the elderly: a pilot study. *J Am Geriatr Soc.* 1993;41:1090-1094.

38. Tahara Y, Shima K. Kinetics of HbA1c, glycated albumin, and fructosamine and analysis of their weight functions against preceding plasma glucose level. *Diabetes Care.* 1995;18(4)440-447.

39. Laffel L. Ketone bodies: a review of physiology, pathophysiology and application of monitoring to diabetes. *Diabetes Metab Res Rev.* 1999;15:412-426.

40. Smolowitz JL, Zaldivar A. Evaluation of diabetic patients' home urine glucose testing technique and ability to interpret results. *Diabetes Educ.* 1992;18:207-210.

41. Rotblatt MD, Koda-Kimble MA. Review of drug interference with urine glucose tests. *Diabetes Care.* 1987;10:103-110.

42. American Diabetes Association. Urine glucose and ketone determinations (Position Statement). *Diabetes Care.* 1992;15(suppl. 2):38.

43. Mehta M, Vincze G, Lopez D. Emerging technologies in diabetes care. US Pharmacist [serial online]. 2002;27:11. http://www.uspharmacist. com/index.asp?show=article&page=8_995.htm. Accessed January 12, 2003.

44. Ginsberg BH. Factors affecting blood glucose monitoring: sources of errors in measurement. *J Diabetes Sci Technol.* 2009;3(4):903-913.

45. Wahowiak L. Blood glucose meters. Diabetes forecast resource guide. 2012;January 3:32-43.

46. 2012 consumer guide: continuous glucose monitors (2012). *Diabetes Forecast.* http://forecast.diabetes.org/files/images/v65n01_CGMs_0. pdf. Accessed December 30, 2011.

47. Seven Plus continuous glucose monitoring system user guide (2010). *Dexcom.* http://www.dexcom.com/sites/all/themes/dexcom/node-files/ SEVEN_Plus_Users_Guide.pdf. Accessed January 3, 2012.

48. Paradigm REAL-Time Revel user guide (2009). *Medtronic.* http:// www.medtronic.com/wcm/groups/mdtcom_sg/@mdt/@diabetes/ documents/documents/x23_user_guide.pdf January 3. Acessed January 3, 2012

49. Guardian REAL-Time continuous glucose monitoring user guide (2009). *Medtronic.* http://www.medtronic.com/wcm/groups/mdtcom_ sg/@mdt/@diabetes/documents/documents/guardian_real_time_ started.pdf. Accessed January 3, 2012.

50. Sylvester AC, Price CP, Burrin JM. Investigation of the potential for interference with whole blood glucose strips. *Ann Clin Biochem.* 1994;31:94-96.

51. Diabetes Forecast (2011). American Diabetes Association. http:// forecast.diabetes.org/magazine/features/2011-blood-glucose-meter-special-features. Accessed January 3, 2012.

52. Tonyushkina K, Nichols JH. *Glucose meters: a review* of technical challenges to obtaining accurate results. *J Diabetes Sci Technol.* 2009;3(No.4):971-980.

53. Sacks DB, Arnold M, Bakris GL, et al. Guidelines and recommendations for laboratory analysis in the diagnosis and management of diabetes mellitus. *Diabetes Care.* 2011;34:e61-e69.

54. Avignon A, Radauceanu A, Monnier L. Nonfasting plasma glucose is a better marker of diabetic control than fasting plasma glucose. *Diabetes Care.* 1997;20:1822-1826.

55. Bell DS, Ovalle F, Shadmany S. Postprandial rather than preprandial glucose levels should be used for adjustment of rapid-acting insulins. *Endocr Pract.* 2000;6:477-478.

56. McGeoch G, Derry S, Moore RA. Self monitoring of blood glucose in type 2 diabetes mellits: what is the evidence? *Diabetes Metab Res Rev.* 2007;23:423-440.

57. Benjamin EM. Self-Monitoring of blood glucose: the basics. *Clin Diabetes.* 2002;20:45-47.

58. Banerji MA. The foundation of diabetes self-management: glucose monitoring. *Diabetes Educ.* 2007;(suppl)87S-90S.

59. Daudek CD, Derr RL, Kalyani RR. Assessing glycemia in diabetes using self-monitoring blood glucose and hemoglobin A1c. *JAMA.* 2006;295:1688-1697.

60. Austin MM, Haas L, Johnson T, et al. Self-monitoring of blood glucose: benefits and utilization. *The Diabetes Educator.* 2006;32(6)835-847.

61. The Diabetes Control and Complications Trial Research Group. The effect of intensive treatment of diabetes on the development and progression of long-term complications in insulin-dependent diabetes mellitus. *N Engl J Med.* 1993;329:977-986.

62. UK Prospective Diabetes Study Group. Intensive blood glucose control with sulphonylureas or insulin compared with conventional treatment and risk of complications in patients with type 2 diabetes (UKPDS 33). *Lancet.* 1998;352:837-853.

63. Nathan DM, Buse JB, Davidson MB, et al. Medical management of type 2 diabetes. Medical management of hyperglycemia in type 2 diabetes: a consensus algorithm for the initiation and adjustment of therapy. *Diabetes Care.* 2009;32(1):193-203.

64. Skyler JS. Insulin treatment. In: Lebovitz HE, ed. *Therapy for Diabetes Mellitus and Related Disorders.* 3rd ed. Alexandria, VA: American Diabetes Association; 1998:186-203.

65. Rodbard HW, Jellinger PS, Davidson JA, et al. Statement by an American Association of Clinical Endocrinologists/American College of Endocrinology consensus panel on type 2 diabetes mellitus: an algorithm for glycemic control. *Endocr Pract.* 2009;15(No.6):540-559.

66. Nathan DM, Buse JB, Davison MB, et al. Medical management of hyperglycemia in type 2 diabetes: A consensus algorithm for the initiation and adjustment of therapy. *Diabetes Care.* 2009;32(No.1):193-203.

67. Vilsboll T, Zdravkovic M, Le-Thi T, et al. Liraglutide significantly improves glycemic control, and lowers body weight without risk of either major or minor hypoglycemic episodes in subject with type 2 diabetes [abstract]. *Diabetes.* 2006;55(suppl 1):A462. Abstract A27–A28, Abstract 115-OR.

68. Rosenstock J, Baron MA, Dejager S, et al. Comparison of vildagliptin and rosiglitazone monotherapy in patients with type 2 diabetes: a 24-week, double-blind, randomized trial. *Diabetes Care.* 2007;30:217-223.

69. Cycloset [product information]. Tiverton, RI: Veroscience; September 2010.

70. Kitabchi AE, Nyenwe EA. Hyperglycemic crises in diabetes mellitus: diabetic ketoacidosis and hyperglycemic hyperosmolar state. *Endocrinol Metab Clin North Am.* 2006;35(4):725-751.

71. DeFronzo RA, Matsuda M, Barrett E. Diabetic ketoacidosis: a combined metabolic-nephrologic approach to therapy. *Diabetes Rev.* 1994;2:209-238.

72. Matz R. Hyperosmolar nonacidotic diabetes (HNAD). In: Porte D Jr, Sherwin RS, eds. *Diabetes Mellitus: Theory and Practice.* 5th ed. Amsterdam, Netherlands: Elsevier; 1997:845-860.

73. Burge MD, Hardy KJ, Schade DS. Short-term fasting is a mechanism for the development of euglycemic ketoacidosis during periods of insulin deficiency. *J Clin Endocrinol Metab.* 1993;76:1192-1198.

74. American Diabetes Association. Hyperglycemic crises in patients with diabetes mellitus. *Diabetes Care.* 2004;27(suppl 1):S94-S102.

75. Goren MP, Pratt CB. False-positive ketone tests: a bedside measure of urinary mesna. *Cancer Chemother Pharmacol.* 1990;25:371-372.

76. Holcombe BJ, Hopkins AM, Heizer WD. False-positive tests for urinary ketones (letter). *N Engl J Med.* 1994;330:578.

77. Graham P, Naidoo D. False-positive Ketostix in a diabetic on antihypertensive therapy. *Clin Chem.* 1987;33:1490.

78. Warren SE. False-positive urine ketone test with captopril. *N Engl J Med.* 1980;303:1003-1004.

79. Foster DW, McGarry JD. The metabolic derangements and treatment of diabetic ketoacidosis. *N Engl J Med.* 1983;309:159-169.

80. Schade DS, Eaton RP. Diabetic ketoacidosis—pathogenesis, prevention and therapy. *Clin Endocrinol Metab.* 1983;12:321-338.

81. Young DS. *Effects of Drugs on Clinical Laboratory Tests.* 3rd ed. Washington, DC: American Association for Clinical Chemistry Press; 1990.

82. Cryer PE. Hypoglycemia: the limiting factor in the management of IDDM. *Diabetes.* 1994;43:1378-1389.

83. Cox DJ, Gonder-Frederick L, Antoun B, et al. Perceived symptoms in the recognition of hypoglycemia. *Diabetes Care.* 1993;6:519-527.

84. Cryer, PE. *Hypoglycemia: Pathophysiology, Diagnosis and Treatment.* New York, NY: Oxford University Press; 1997.

85. American Diabetes Association. Management of dyslipidemia in adults with diabetes. *Diabetes Care.* 2004;(suppl 1);68S-71S.

86. Executive Summary: Standards of Medical Care in Diabetes—2013. *Diabetes Care.* 2013;(suppl 1):4S-10S.

87. Moorhead JF. Lipids and progressive kidney disease. *Kidney International.* 1991;39 (suppl 31):35-40.

88. Ritz E, Orth SR. Nephropathy in patients with type 2 diabetes mellitus. *N Engl J Med.* 1999;341:1127-1133.

89. Remuzzi G, Schieppati A, Ruggenenti P. Clinical practice. Nephropathy in patients with type 2 diabetes. *N Engl J Med.* 2002;346:1145-1151.

90. Cooper-DeHoff RM, Gong Y, Handberg EM, et al. Tight blood pressure control and cardiovascular outcomes among hypertensive patients with diabetes and coronary artery disease. *JAMA.* 2010;304:61-68.

91. Petrone LR. Thyroid disorders. In: Arcangelo VP, Peterson AM, eds. *Pharmacotherapeutics for Advanced Practice, A Practical Approach.* 1st ed. Philadelphia, PA: Lippincott Williams & Wilkins; 2001:666-681.

92. Surks, MI, Sievert, R. Drugs and thyroid function. *N Engl J Med.* 1995;333:1688-1694.

93. Kaptein EM. Clinical application of free thyroxine determinations. *Clin Lab Med.* 1993;13:653-672.

94. Thomas JA, Keenan EJ. Thyroid and antithyroidal drugs. In: Thomas JA, Keenan EJ, eds. *Principles of Endocrine Pharmacology.* New York, NY: Plenum; 1986:69-91.

95. Nelson JC, Wilcox RB, Pandin MR. Dependence of free thyroxine estimates obtained with equilibrium tracer dialysis on the concentration of thyroxine-binding globulin. *Clin Chem.* 1992;38:1294-1300.

96. Singer PA. Thyroid function tests and effects of drugs on thyroid function. In: Lavin N, ed. *Manual of Endocrinology and Metabolism.* Boston, MA: Little Brown; 1986:341-354.

97. Klee GG, Hay ID. Assessment of sensitive thyrotropin assays for an expanded role in thyroid function testing: proposed criteria for analytic performance and clinical utility. *J Clin Endocrinol Metab.* 1987;64:461-471.

98. Ingbar SH, Woeber KA. The thyroid gland. In: Williams RH, ed. *Textbook of Endocrinology.* 6th ed. Philadelphia, PA: WB Saunders; 1981:117-248.

99. Mokshagundam S, Barzel US. Thyroid disease in the elderly. *J Am Geriatr Soc.* 1993;41:1361-1369.

100. Reasner CA, Talbert RL. Thyroid disorders. In: DiPiro JT, Talbert RL, Yee GC, eds. *Pharmacotherapy: A Pathophysiologic Approach.* 5th ed. New York, NY: McGraw-Hill; 2002:1359-1378.

101. Safrit H. Thyroid disorders. In: Fitzgerald PA, ed. *Handbook of Clinical Endocrinology.* Greenbrae, CA: Jones Medical Publications; 1986:122-169.

102. Hershman JM. Hypothyroidism and hyperthyroidism. In: Lavin N, ed. *Manual of Endocrinology and Metabolism.* Boston, MA: Little Brown; 1986:365-378.

103. Tunbridge WM, Evered DC, Hall R, et al. The spectrum of thyroid disease in a community: the Whickham survey. *Clin Endocrinol* (Oxf). 1977;7:481-493.

104. Becker DV, Bigos ST, Gaitan E, et al. Optimal use of blood tests for assessment of thyroid function. *JAMA.* 1993;269:2736-2737.

105. Spencer CA. Thyroid profiling for the 1990s: free T_4 estimate or sensitive TSH measurement. *J Clin Immunoassay.* 1989;12:82-85.

106. Surks MI, Hupart KH, Pan C, et al. Normal free thyroxine in critical nonthyroidal illnesses measured by ultrafiltration of undiluted serum and equilibrium dialysis. *J Clin Endocrinol Metab.* 1988;67:1031-1039.

107. Wong TK, Pekary AE, Hoo GS, et al. Comparison of methods for measuring free thyroxine in nonthyroidal illness. *Clin Chem.* 1992;38:720-724.

108. Klee GG, Hay ID. Role of thyrotropin measurements in the diagnosis and management of thyroid disease (review). *Clin Lab Med.* 1993;13(3):673-682.

109. Young DS. *Effects of Drugs on Clinical Laboratory Tests.* 3rd ed. Washington, DC: American Association for Clinical Chemistry Press; 1990.

110. Khanderia U, Jaffe CA, Theisen V. Amiodarone-induced thyroid dysfunction. *Clin Pharm.* 1993;12:774-779.

111. Okamura K, Ikenoue H, Shiroozu A, et al. Reevaluation of the effects of methylmercaptomidazole and propylthiouracil in patients with Graves' hyperthyroidism. *J Clin Endocrinol Metab.* 1987;65:719-723.

112. Franklyn JA. The management of hyperthyroidism. *N Engl J Med.* 1994;330:1731-1738.

113. Finucane P, Rudra T, Hsu R, et al. Thyrotropin response to thyrotropin-releasing hormone in elderly patients with and without acute illness. *Age Ageing.* 1991;20:85-89.

114. Toft AD. Thyroxine therapy. *N Engl J Med.* 1994;331:174-180.

115. Nicoloff JT, Spencer CA. The use and misuse of the sensitive thyrotropin assays. *J Clin Endocrinol Metab.* 1990;71:553-558.

116. McClelland P, Stott A, Howel-Evans W. Hyperthyrotropinaemia during thyroxine replacement therapy. *Postgrad Med J.* 1989;65:205-207.

117. Reinwein D, Benker G, Lazarus JH, et al. A prospective randomized trial of antithyroid drug dose in Graves' disease therapy. *J Clin Endocrinol Metab.* 1993;76:1516-1521.

118. Liewendahl K, Helenius T, Lamberg BA, et al. Free thyroxine, free triiodothyronine, and thyrotropin concentrations in hypothyroid and thyroid carcinoma patients receiving thyroxine therapy. *Acta Endocrinol.* 1987;116:418-424.

119. Stall GM, Harris S, Sokoll LJ, et al. Accelerated bone loss in hypothyroid patients overtreated with L-thyroxine. *Ann Intern Med.* 1990;113:265-269.

120. Vanelle JM, Poirier MF, Benkelfat C, et al. Diagnostic and therapeutic value of testing stimulation of thyroid-stimulating hormone by thyrotropin-releasing hormone in 100 depressed patients. *Acta Psychiatr Scand.* 1990;81:156-161.

121. Ingbar SH. Diseases of the thyroid. In: Braunwald E, Isselbacher KJ, Petersdorf RG, et al., eds. *Harrison's Principles of Internal Medicine.* 11th ed. New York, NY: McGraw-Hill; 1987:1732-1752.

122. Hershman JM, Chopra IJ, Van Herle AJ, et al. Thyroid disease. In: Hershman JM, ed. *Endocrine Pathophysiology: A Patient-Oriented Approach.* 2nd ed. Philadelphia, PA: Lea & Febiger; 1982:34–68.

123. Utiger RD. Thyrotropin-receptor mutations and thyroid dysfunction. *N Engl J Med.* 1995;332:183-185.

124. Sacher RA, McPherson RA. *Widman's Clinical Interpretation of Laboratory Tests.* 10th ed. Philadelphia, PA: FA Davis; 1991.

125. Wallach J. *Interpretation of Diagnostic Tests: A Synopsis of Laboratory Medicine.* 5th ed. Boston, MA: Little Brown; 1992.

126. Findling JW, Raff H. Newer diagnostic techniques and problems in Cushing's disease. *Endocrinol Metab Clin North Am.* 1999;28:191-210.

127. White PC. Mechanisms of disease: disorders of aldosterone biosynthesis and action. *N Engl J Med.* 1994;331:250-258.

128. Fitzgerald PA. Pituitary disorders. In: Fitzgerald PA, ed. *Handbook of Clinical Endocrinology.* Greenbrae, CA: Jones Medical Publications; 1986:22-29.

129. Dorin RI, Qualls Cr, Crapo LM. Diagnosis of adrenal insufficiency. *Ann Intern Med.* 2003;139:194-204.

130. Arlt W, Allolio B. Adrenal insufficiency. *Lancet.* 2003;361:1881-1893.

131. Ramsay DJ. Posterior pituitary gland. In: Greenspan FS, Forsham PH, eds. *Basic and Clinical Endocrinology.* 2nd ed. Los Altos, CA: Lange Medical Publications; 1986:132-142.

132. Robertson GL. Differential diagnosis of polyuria. *Ann Rev Med.* 1988;39:425-442.

133. Lightman SL. Molecular insights into diabetes insipidus. *N Engl J Med.* 1993;328:1562-1563.

134. Krege J, Katz VL, Bowes WA Jr. Transient diabetes insipidus of pregnancy. *Obstet Gynecol Surv.* 1989;44:789-795.

135. Sowers JR, Zieve FJ. Clinical disorders of vasopressin. In: Lavin N, ed. *Manual of Endocrinology and Metabolism.* Boston, MA: Little Brown; 1986:65-74.

136. Benjamin EM. Self Monitoring of blood glucose: the basics. *Clinical Diabetes.* 2002;20:45-47.

137. Banerji MA. The foundation of diabetes self-management: glucose monitoring. *The Diabetes Educator;* 2007:87S-90S.

138. Bell D, Ovalle F, Shadmany S. Postprandial rather than preprandial glucose levels should be used for adjustment of rapid-acting insulins. *Endocrine Practice.* 2000;6:477-478.

139. Daudek CD, Derr RL, Kalyani RR. Assessing glycemia in diabetes using self-monitoring blood glucose and hemoglobin A1c. *JAMA.* 2006;295:1688-1697.

140. Austin MM, Haas L, Johnson T, et al. Self-monitoring of blood glucose: benefits and utilization. *The Diabetes Educator.* 2006;32(6)835-847.

141. Daudek CD, Derr RL, Kalyani RR. Assessing glycemia in diabetes using self-monitoring blood glucose and hemoglobin A1c. *JAMA.* 2006;295:1688-1697.

142. AACE Thyroid Task Force. American Association of Clinical Endocrinologists medical guidelines for clinical practice for the evaluation and treatment of hyperthyroidism and hypothyroidism. *Endocr Pract.* 2002;8(6):457-469.

Quickview | Total Serum T$_3$

PARAMETER	DESCRIPTION	COMMENTS
Common reference ranges		
Adults and children	80–200 ng/dL	Affected by TGB changes
	(1.23–3.0 nmol/L)	SI conversion factor = 0.0154 (nmol/L)
Critical value	Not established	Extremely high or low values should be reported quickly
Natural substance?	Yes	Only 0.2% of T$_3$ is unbound
Inherent activity?	Only free portion	Total assumed to correlate with free T$_3$ activity
Location		
Production and storage	20% to 25% secreted by thyroid gland, remainder produced by conversion of T$_4$ to T$_3$	Bound mostly to thyroglobulin
Secretion/excretion	From thyroid, liver, and kidneys to blood	
Major causes of ...		
High results	Hyperthyroidism	Not truly a cause but a reflection of high result
	T$_4$/T$_3$ supplements	
	Other causes (Table 13-10)	
Associated signs and symptoms	Signs and symptoms of hyperthyroidism	Nervousness, weight loss, heat intolerance, tachycardia, diaphoresis
Low results	Hypothyroidism	Not truly a cause but a reflection of low result
	Other causes (Table 13-9)	
	Propranolol	
	Propylthiouracil	
	Glucocorticoids	
Associated signs and symptoms	Signs and symptoms of hypothyroidism	Lethargy, constipation, dry skin, cold intolerance, slow speech, confusion
After insult, time to...		
Initial elevation or depression	Weeks to months	Increases within hours in acute T$_4$ or T$_3$ overdose
Peak values	Weeks to months	Increases within hours in acute T$_4$ or T$_3$ overdose
Normalization	Usually same time as onset	Assumes insult removed or effectively treated
Drugs often monitored with test	Thyroxine (T$_4$) and triiodothyronine (T$_3$)	Other drugs (Tables 13-16 and 13-18)
Causes of spurious results	Increased or decreased TBG leads to falsely increased or decreased total serum T$_3$, respectively; nonthyroidal illness leads to falsely increased or decreased total serum T$_3$	Factors affecting TBG (Tables 13-14 and 13-15)

T$_3$ = triiodothyronine; T$_4$ = thyroxine; TBG = thyroxine-binding globulin; SI = International System of Units.

QUICKVIEW | Total Serum T_4

PARAMETER	DESCRIPTION	COMMENTS
Common reference ranges		
Adults and children	5.5–12.5 mcg/dL (71–161 nmol/L)	Affected by TBG changes with nonthyroidal illness
		SI conversion factor = 12.87 (nmol/L)
Newborn/3–5 days	11–23/9–18 mcg/dL	Affected by TBG changes with nonthyroidal illness
Critical value	Not established	Extremely high or low values should be reported quickly, especially in newborns
Natural substance?	Yes	Only 0.02% of T_4 is unbound
Inherent activity?	Only free portion	Total assumed to correlate with free T_4 activity
Location		
Production and storage	Thyroid gland	Bound mostly to thyroglobulin
Secretion/excretion	From thyroid to blood	About 33% converted to T_3 outside thyroid
Major causes of...		
High results	Hyperthyroidism	Not truly a cause but a reflection of high result
	T_4 supplements	
	Other causes (Table 13-10)	
Associated signs and symptoms	Signs and symptoms of hyperthyroidism	Nervousness, weight loss, heat intolerance, tachycardia, diaphoresis
Low results	Hypothyroidism	Not truly a cause but a reflection of low result
	Other causes (Table 13-9)	
	Signs and symptoms of hyperthyroidism	Lethargy, constipation, dry skin, cold intolerance, slow speech, confusion
After insult, time to...		
Initial elevation or depression	Weeks to months	Increases within hours in acute T_4 overdose
Peak values	Weeks to months	Increases within hours in acute T_4 overdose
Normalization	Usually same time as onset	Assumes insult removed or effectively treated
Drugs often monitored with test	Thyroxine (T_4)	Other drugs (Tables 13-16 and 13-18)
Causes of spurious results	Increased or decreased TBG leads to falsely increased or decreased total serum T_4, respectively; nonthyroidal illness leads to falsely increased or decreased total serum T_4	Factors affecting TBG (Table 13-14 and 13-15)

T_3 = triiodothyronine; T_4 = thyroxine; TBG = thyroxine-binding globulin; SI = International System of Units.

QUICKVIEW | Free T$_4$

PARAMETER	DESCRIPTION	COMMENTS
Common reference ranges		
Adults and children	1–4 units	Higher in infants <1 month; direct equilibrium dialysis assay not affected by TBG changes or severe nonthyroidal illness
	0.9–2.3 ng/dL	
	(12–30 pmol/L)	SI conversion factor = 12.87 (pmol/L)
Critical value	Not established	Extremely high or low values should be reported quickly
Natural substance?	Yes	Only 0.02% of T$_4$ is unbound
Inherent activity?	Probably	Some influence on basal metabolic rate; T$_3$ most active
Location		
Production and storage	Thyroid gland	Bound mostly to thyroglobulin
Secretion/excretion	From thyroid to blood	33% converted to T$_3$ outside thyroid
Major causes of...		
High results	Hyperthyroidism	Not truly a cause but a reflection of high result
	T$_4$ supplements	
	Other causes (Table 13-10)	
Associated signs and symptoms	Signs and symptoms of hyperthyroidism	Nervousness, weight loss, heat intolerance, tachycardia, diaphoresis
Low results	Hypothyroidism	Not truly a cause but a reflection of low result
	Other causes (Table 13-9)	
Associated signs and symptoms	Signs and symptoms of hypothyroidism	Lethargy, constipation, dry skin, cold intolerance, slow speech, confusion
After insult, time to...		
Initial elevation or depression	Weeks to months	Increases within hours in acute T$_4$ overdose
Peak values	Weeks to months	Increases within hours in acute T$_4$ overdose
Normalization	Usually same time as onset	Assumes insult removed or effectively treated
Drugs often monitored with test	Thyroxine (T$_4$)	Other drugs (Tables 13-16 and 13-18)
Causes of spurious results	Rare with direct equilibrium dialysis assay (Table 13-12)	Decreased direct equilibrium dialysis assay for free T$_4$ with decreased or normal TSH may occur in patients

T$_3$ = triiodothyronine; T$_4$ = thyroxine; TSH = thyroid-stimulating hormone.

QUICKVIEW | TSH

PARAMETER	DESCRIPTION	COMMENTS
Common reference ranges		
Adults and children	0.5–5.0 milliunits/L	Sometimes reported in milliunits/L
Critical value	Not established	Extremely high or low values should be reported quickly
Natural substance?	Yes	
Inherent activity?	Yes	Stimulates thyroid to secrete hormone
Location		
Production and storage	Anterior pituitary	
Secretion/excretion	Unknown	
Major causes of...		
High results	Primary hypothyroidism	Causes of primary hypothyroidism
	Antithyroid drugs	
Associated signs and symptoms	Signs and symptoms of hypothyroidism	Lethargy, constipation, dry skin, cold intolerance, slow speech, confusion
Low results	Primary hyperthyroidism	Must be ≤0.05 milliunit/L for definitive diagnosis of (primary hyperthyroidism); may be decreased or normal in secondary or tertiary hypothyroidism
	Other causes (Table 13-12)	
Associated signs and symptoms	Signs and symptoms of hyperthyroidism	Nervousness, weight loss, heat intolerance, HR increase, diaphoresis
After insult, time to...		
Initial elevation or depression	Weeks to months	Decreases within hours in acute T_4 overdose
Peak values	Weeks to months	Decreases within hours in acute T_4 overdose
Normalization	Usually same time as onset	Assumes insult removed or effectively treated
Drugs often monitored with test	Thyroxine (T_4) and triiodothyronine (T_3)	Also antithyroid drugs (methimazole and propylthiouracil)
Causes of spurious results	Increased TSH: dopamine antagonists	Metoclopramide and domperidone
	Decreased TSH: dopamine agonists	Dopamine, bromocriptine, levodopa, glucocorticoids
	Above TSH measurements are accurate here	These drugs decrease TSH, but the change is not reflective of primary hypo- or hyperthyroidism; therefore, the results are not truly spurious

HR = heart rate; T_3 = triiodothyronine; T_4 = thyroxine; TSH = thyroid-stimulating hormone.

QUICKVIEW | Plasma Glucose

PARAMETER	DESCRIPTION	COMMENTS
Common reference ranges		
Adults	Adult fasting: 70–110 mg/dL (3.9–6.1 mmol/L)	Multiply by 0.056 for SI units (mmol/L)
	Adult 2-hr postprandial: <140 mg/dL (8.4 mmol/L)	
	Full-term infant normal: 20–90 mg/dL	
Critical value	No previous history: >200 mg/dL	In known diabetic, increased glucose is not an immediate concern unless patient is symptomatic; an increased glucose is not critical if serial levels are decreasing over time
	Anytime: <50 mg/dL	
Natural substance?	Yes	Always present in blood
Inherent activity?	Yes	Major source of energy for cellular metabolism
Location		
Production	Liver and muscle	Dietary intake
Storage	Liver and muscle	As glycogen
Secretion/excretion	Mostly metabolized for energy	Levels >180 mg/dL spill into urine
Major causes of...		
High results	Type 1 and 2 DM	
	Drugs	Corticosteroids, thiazides, epinephrine, Also, diazoxide, L-asparaginase, total parenteral nutrition
	Excess intake	
Associated signs and symptoms	Polyuria, polydipsia, polyphagia, weakness	Long-term: damage to kidneys, retina, neurons, and vessels
Low results	Insulin secretion/dose excessive relative to diet	Most common in diabetics
	Sulfonylureas or other hypoglycemic agents	
	Insulinomas	
Associated signs and symptoms	Hunger, sweating, weakness, trembling, headache, confusion, seizures, coma	From neuroglycopenia and adrenergic discharge
After insult, time to...		
Initial elevation	Type 1 DM: months to elevation	
	Type 2 DM: years to elevation	
	After insulin: minutes to decrease	
	After meal: 15–30 min to elevation	
	After epinephrine or glucagon: minutes	
	After steroids and growth hormone: hours	
Normalization	After insulin: minutes	Depends on insulin type
	After exercise: minutes to hours	Depends on intensity and duration
Drugs often monitored with test	Insulin, sulfonylureas, biguanides (e.g., metformin), thiazolidinediones, or other hypoglycemic agents	Also, diazoxide, L-asparaginase, total parenteral nutrition
Causes of spurious results	High-dose vitamin C	With some glucometers
	Metronidazole	With some automated assays

DM = diabetes mellitus; SI = International System of Units.

QUICKVIEW | A1c

PARAMETER	DESCRIPTION	COMMENTS
Common reference ranges		
Adults and children	4% to 5.6%	Fasting not required; represents average glucose levels past 8 weeks
Critical value	Not applicable	Reflects long-term glycemic control; >13% suggests poor control
Natural substance?	Yes	Subunit of Hgb
Inherent activity?	Yes	Oxygen carrier; also carries glucose
Location		
Production	Bone marrow	In newborns in liver and spleen
Storage	Not stored	Circulates in blood
Secretion/excretion	Older cell removed by spleen	Converted to bilirubin
Major causes of...		
High results	DM	Any cause of prolonged hyperglycemia
	Chronic hyperglycemia	
Associated signs and symptoms	Signs and symptoms of diabetes	
Low results		
Associated signs and symptoms	Not clinically useful	
After insult, time to...		
Initial elevation	2–4 months	Initial insult is chronic hyperglycemia
Normalization	2–4 months	Assumes sudden and persistent euglycemia
Drugs often monitored with test	Insulin, sulfonylureas, biguanides	Also diet and exercise
Causes of spurious results	High results: alcoholism, uremia, increased triglycerides, hypertriglyceridemia, hemolysis, polycythemia	Also seen in pregnant and splenectomized patients
	Low results: sickle cell anemia, thalassemia	

DM = diabetes mellitus; Hgb = hemoglobin.

CHAPTER 14

LIPID DISORDERS

JILL S. BORCHERT, KATHY E. KOMPERDA

Objectives

After completing this chapter, the reader should be able to

- List primary and secondary causes of dyslipidemia

- Outline the pathophysiology of lipid metabolism and correlate lipid levels to the risk of atherosclerotic cardiovascular disease

- Calculate low-density lipoprotein (LDL) when provided with total cholesterol (TC), high-density lipoprotein (HDL), and triglyceride (TG) values

- Given a case study, interpret laboratory results from a lipid profile and discuss how they should guide treatment choices

Dyslipidemia, or an abnormal serum lipid profile, is a major risk factor in the development of coronary heart disease (CHD). With over 16 million people in the United States affected by CHD—accounting for nearly 1 of every 6 deaths in the United States—preventative efforts are essential to decrease associated morbidity and mortality.[1] Practitioners are being asked to assess the lipid panel in an effort to decrease overall cardiovascular risk.

Approximately one-quarter of American adults have low-density lipoprotein (LDL) cholesterol levels above the desirable range.[1] As a 10% decrease in total cholesterol (TC) levels may result in an estimated 30% reduction in the incidence of CHD, lipid monitoring is warranted, and effective treatments are indicated in selected patients. While there are millions of people with dyslipidemia and effective treatment options exist, many go untreated due to lack of physician recognition or lack of patient adherence to therapy.[2,3] As a result, less than half of patients who require lipid-lowering therapy receive such treatment, and only one-quarter of patients achieve LDL goals.[1] Some experts note that a more aggressive approach to LDL reduction is required to reduce the risk of new cardiovascular events.[4]

This chapter primarily covers the physiology of cholesterol and triglyceride (TG) metabolism, their actions as part of lipoproteins, disorders of lipids and lipoproteins, and consequences of elevated lipid levels. The effects of diet, exercise, and drugs on these lipid values are also discussed. A detailed interpretation of test results and drug therapy with regard to cardiovascular risk is beyond the scope of this chapter, but references provide additional information.[3,5-8]

PHYSIOLOGY OF LIPID METABOLISM

The major plasma lipids are cholesterol, TGs, and phospholipids. The regulation of serum lipids is determined by the synthesis and metabolism of lipoproteins. An understanding of this regulation is necessary for proper diagnosis and treatment of dyslipidemia in efforts to reduce overall cardiovascular risk.

Cholesterol serves as a structural component of cell wall membranes and is a precursor for the synthesis of steroid hormones and bile acids. It may be dietary in origin or synthesized in the liver and intestine. Cholesterol is continuously undergoing synthesis, degradation, and recycling. Approximately 40% of cholesterol consumed in the diet is absorbed.[7] Dietary cholesterol directly contributes relatively little to serum cholesterol levels. Approximately 90% of serum cholesterol is derived from cholesterol synthesis. Most cholesterol synthesis occurs during the night.[9] The rate-limiting step in cholesterol synthesis is the conversion of hepatic hydroxymethylglutaryl-coenzyme A (HMG-CoA) to mevalonic acid. This conversion is catalyzed by the enzyme HMG-CoA reductase and is inhibited by drugs designed to reduce cellular synthesis of cholesterol.[8]

Intestinal cholesterol absorption, hepatic cholesterol synthesis, and excretion of cholesterol and bile acids regulate serum cholesterol concentrations (Figure 14-1).[7,8] An inhibitory feedback mechanism modulates cholesterol synthesis. The presence of cholesterol in hepatic cells leads to decreased biosynthesis of cholesterol. Conversely,

The contribution of material written by Diana Laubenstein and Scott L. Traub in previous editions of this book is acknowledged.

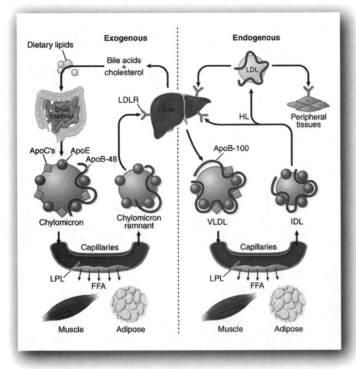

FIGURE 14-1. Lipid metabolism. (Reprinted with permission from Longo DL, Fauci AS, Kasper DL, et al., eds. *Harrison's Principles of Internal Medicine.* 18th ed. Columbus, OH: The McGraw-Hill Companies, Inc.; 2011.)

when hepatic cholesterol concentrations decrease, there is a resulting increase in hepatic cholesterol biosynthesis. However, the feedback inhibition mechanism is inadequate in preventing a rise in serum cholesterol levels in the presence of a diet high in calories and saturated fat.

Triglycerides, the esterified form of glycerol and fatty acids, constitute the main form of lipid storage in humans, and they serve as a reservoir of fatty acids to be used as fuel for gluconeogenesis or for direct combustion as an energy source. Like cholesterol, TGs can either be synthesized by the liver or absorbed. Endogenous TGs are mainly synthesized in the liver from accumulated fatty acids. Dietary fat is incorporated into chylomicrons in the small intestine and is known as *exogenous TG*.

Phospholipids are lipid molecules that contain a phosphate group. Like cholesterol, phospholipids become constituents of cell wall membranes. In contrast to cholesterol and TGs, dietary phospholipids are not absorbed. Most phospholipids originate in the liver and intestinal mucosa, but they may be synthesized by most body tissues. Phospholipids act as donors of phosphate groups for intracellular metabolism and blood coagulation.

Triglycerides, cholesterol, and phospholipid molecules complex with specialized proteins (apoproteins) to form lipoproteins, the transport form in which lipids are measured in the blood. As lipids are insoluble in aqueous plasma, they are formed into complexes with an outer hydrophilic coat of phospholipids and proteins and an inner core of fatty cholesterol and TGs. The apolipoproteins not only serve to support the formation of lipoproteins, but they also mediate binding to receptors and activate enzymes in lipoprotein metabolism. All lipoproteins contain phospholipids, TGs, and esterified and unesterified cholesterol in varying degrees. There are many ways to classify these lipoproteins, but, most frequently, lipoproteins are classified by their density, size, and major apolipoprotein composition. Table 14-1 summarizes the characteristics of TGs and cholesterol in terms of lipoprotein density.[7,8,10] In the fasting state, there are three major lipoproteins found in the serum: LDL, high-density lipoprotein (HDL), and very low-density lipoprotein (VLDL).[3] Intermediate density lipoprotein (IDL) are typically included in the LDL calculation. Typically, LDL cholesterol comprises 60% to 70% of TC, whereas HDL cholesterol comprises about one-quarter of TC. Very low-density lipoprotein cholesterol and chylomicrons are TG-rich lipoproteins, which comprise 10% to 15% of total serum cholesterol.

There is a strong correlation between dyslipidemia and the development of atherosclerotic vascular disease. Atherosclerotic vascular disease may be manifested by CHD, stroke, and peripheral vascular disease. There is a strong positive relationship between serum cholesterol levels and the risk for CHD.[3] Proper diagnosis and treatment of dyslipidemia can be an important preventative strategy. Numerous trials of effective treatment of dyslipidemia have demonstrated reductions in cardiovascular events, stroke, and total mortality in patients with a prior history of atherosclerotic vascular disease

TABLE 14-1. Characteristics of Lipoproteins[7,8,10]

LIPOPROTEIN	SIZE	DENSITY	MAJOR APOLIPOPROTEIN	ORIGIN	COMMENTS
Chylomicrons and chylomicron remnants	Largest	Least	ApoB-48	Intestines	Primarily TGs
VLDL			ApoB-100	Liver and intestines	Primarily TGs
IDL or remnants			ApoB-100	Chylomicrons and VLDL	Transitional forms
LDL			ApoB-100	End-product of VLDL	Major carrier of cholesterol
HDL	Smallest	Most	ApoA-I	Intestines and liver	Removes cholesterol from atherosclerotic plaques in arteries

HDL = high-density lipoprotein; IDL = intermediate-density lipoprotein; LDL = low-density lipoprotein; TGs = triglycerides; VLDL = very low-density lipoprotein.

TABLE 14-2. Classification of Selected Primary Dyslipidemias[7,8,18]

PRIMARY LIPID ABNORMALITY	PRIMARY DYSLIPIDEMIA	SELECTED FEATURES[a]	CLINICAL MANIFESTATIONS
Increased TC and LDL	Familial hypercholesterolemia	LDL receptor defect, may be homozygous or heterozygous, TC may be >500–1000 in homozygous	Tendinous xanthomas, premature CHD
	Familial defective ApoB-100	ApoB-100 mutation impairs LDL binding	Tendinous xanthomas, premature CHD
	Polygenic hypercholesterolemia	TG often normal, moderately elevated LDL, no clear genetic factors, influenced by environmental and metabolic factors	Premature CHD
Increased TG	Familial hypertriglyceridemia	Type IV increases TG-rich VLDL particles, TG 200–500	Often asymptomatic, associated with metabolic syndrome
	Lipoprotein lipase deficiency	TG 2000–25,000	Eruptive xanthomas, hepatosplenomegaly, pancreatitis
Increased TG and cholesterol	Familial combined hyperlipidemia	Overproduction of ApoB, increased production of VLDL, occurs in 1% to 2% of population, elevations in LDL, TG, TC, but degree varies widely	Premature CHD
	Familial dysbetalipoproteinemia	ApoE mutation, TG 300–400	Palmar and plantar xanthomas, premature CHD, peripheral vascular disease
Decreased HDL	Familial hypoalphalipoproteinemia	HDL <30 in men; HDL <35 in women	Premature CHD

CHD = coronary heart disease; HDL = high-density lipoprotein; LDL = low-density lipoprotein; TC = total cholesterol; TG = triglyceride; VLDL = very low-density lipoprotein.

[a]TG, LDL, HDL, and TC in mg/dL. Conversion factor for LDL, HDL and TC in International System (SI) units (millimoles per liter) is 0.02586. Conversion factor for TG in SI units (millimoles per liter) is 0.01129.

(secondary prevention) and in patients with asymptomatic dyslipidemia (primary prevention).[11–17]

Primary Lipid Disorders

Dyslipidemias, or abnormal concentrations of any lipoprotein type, are classified by etiology into primary or secondary disorders. Primary disorders are caused by genetic defects in the synthesis or metabolism of the lipoproteins. Table 14-2 shows the characteristics of the major primary dyslipidemias.[7,8,18] Historically, familial dyslipidemias were categorized by the Fredrickson electrophoresis profile of lipoproteins. More recently, clinicians have shifted to classification by the primary lipid parameter affected.[18] Primary lipid disorders rarely occur alone, and it is unlikely for a genetic predisposition to be the sole cause of a lipid disorder. Clinically, other causes, such as diet or medications, should be considered and minimized in all patients.

Secondary Lipid Disorders

Secondary dyslipidemias are disorders precipitated by other disease states, medications, or lifestyle (Table 14-3).[3,8,19-23] When a secondary cause is likely responsible for the lipid abnormality, treatment of the underlying cause should be strongly considered.

Common disease-related causes of dyslipidemia are diabetes and thyroid disorders. Patients with well-controlled type 1 diabetes typically do not have abnormal lipid levels;

however, patients with type 2 diabetes may present with elevated TG levels, decreased HDL cholesterol levels, and relatively normal LDL cholesterol levels.[8,24] These abnormalities may persist despite adequate glycemic control, but optimization of glycemic control is still considered an important step in the management of elevated TGs.[8] Low-density lipoprotein cholesterol concentrations and, in some cases, TG levels increase in hypothyroidism. In addition to these endocrine disorders, renal and liver disease should be excluded.[8,25] Alterations in lipid concentrations are dependent on the type of renal disorder present. For example, patients with chronic kidney disease will present similarly to diabetic dyslipidemia, while lipid profiles in patients with nephrotic syndrome will be characterized by markedly elevated LDL cholesterol and TC.[25] Different liver disorders also have varying effects on lipid profiles.[8] It is recommended that secondary causes are excluded by patient history, physical examination, and laboratory data. Laboratory tests such as fasting blood glucose, thyroid-stimulating hormone (TSH), serum creatinine, urinalysis for proteinuria, and alkaline phosphatase are useful to exclude common secondary causes of dyslipidemia.

In drug-induced dyslipidemia, withdrawal of the precipitating medication usually leads to reversal of secondary dyslipidemia. Antihypertensive agents are frequently administered to patients with cardiovascular risk. Beta-blocking agents, except agents with intrinsic sympathomimetic activity may increase

TG concentrations and reduce HDL cholesterol concentrations.[26,27] Thiazide diuretics increase TC, LDL cholesterol, and TG concentrations.[27] Thiazide effects on the lipid panel are most pronounced with higher dosages (50 mg or more daily), which are generally not recommended for use.[27] The effects of beta blockers and diuretics may be short-term, with a return to baseline levels at 1 year.[28] In contrast, other commonly used antihypertensive agents have no clinically significant effects on the lipid profile. While it is important to realize the effect of antihypertensive agents on the lipid profile, agents that adversely affect the lipid profile are not contraindicated in patients with dyslipidemia. Careful consideration of patient-specific factors is warranted.

Other drug classes have been implicated as sources of lipid abnormalities; however, effects on the lipid panel should not be considered a class effect for these medications. Atypical antipsychotics are known to cause lipid abnormalities with olanzapine possessing the greatest potential to increase LDL cholesterol, TC, and TG levels.[20] Other atypical antipsychotics have a more variable effect including beneficial effects on the lipid panel, such as ziprasidone. Similar variability has been seen among oral contraceptives, immunosuppressive drugs, and protease inhibitors. Various oral contraceptives affect lipoproteins differently. Combination oral contraceptives increase TG concentrations. Effects on LDL and HDL are variable, depending on oral contraceptive components.[22,23,29] Oral contraceptives with second-generation progestins (e.g., levonorgestrel) may increase LDL cholesterol levels and decrease HDL cholesterol levels.[22,23] However, combined oral contraceptives with third-generation progestins (e.g., desogestrel) may favorably decrease LDL levels and increase HDL.[22] Immunosuppressive drugs such as cyclosporine, sirolimus, and corticosteroids adversely affect the lipid profile, but tacrolimus does not impact the lipid profile with the same magnitude and mycophenolate mofetil has no effect.[22]

Protease inhibitors are known to primarily cause an increase in TG levels.[30] Ritonavir-boosted regimens of tipranavir, lopinavir, and fosamprenavir seem to have the greatest impact, while newer agents such as atazanavir have little to no effect. Lipid abnormalities have also been identified with other antiretroviral therapy, including nucleoside reverse transcriptase inhibitors and non-nucleoside reverse transcriptase inhibitors. However, the changes with these antiretroviral therapies tend to be modest, and agents within these classes are available that should not impact lipid levels. Though drug-associated adverse effects on the lipid profile have not been directly correlated with increased risk for CHD, it is important to assess these effects in considering laboratory data and the appropriate treatment plan for the patient.

Lifestyle also may affect lipoprotein concentrations. Besides being independent risk factors for CHD, obesity, physical inactivity, and cigarette smoking cause an increase in serum TGs and a decrease in HDL cholesterol.[3,31] Therapeutic lifestyle changes (TLC) focusing on these risk factors can aid in reversing the lipid abnormalities and reducing CHD risk.[3] A diet that is high in saturated fats, trans fatty acids, and cholesterol increases total serum cholesterol concentrations and LDL. Diets low in saturated fats and low in trans fatty acids are recommended to reduce risk of CHD.[3] Popular low-carbohydrate diets favorably change TGs and HDL cholesterol, but they may increase LDL cholesterol levels.[32] Light-to-moderate alcohol intake (one to two glasses of beer or wine or 1–2 ounces of liquor per day) increases HDL and is associated with lower mortality from CHD as compared with abstention from alcohol.[33] However, light-to-moderate alcohol consumption is associated with increases in TGs.[34] Since evidence to-date is epidemiologic in nature, alcohol is not recommended until data from controlled clinical trials is available.[35]

LABORATORY TESTS FOR LIPIDS AND LIPOPROTEINS

Dyslipidemia is a major contributor to CHD and peripheral vascular disease. Fortunately, several laboratory tests can be used to assess the concentrations of various lipids in the blood, making early detection and monitoring possible. Identification of patients at risk for CHD and peripheral vascular disease is a two-part process. First, a laboratory assessment of the lipid profile must occur. Second, an assessment of the risk determinants of CHD must occur.

The third report of the Expert Panel on Detection, Evaluation and Treatment of High Blood Cholesterol in Adults (Adult Treatment Panel III, or ATP III) by the National Cholesterol Education Program (NCEP) outlines adult screening recommendations for the detection of dyslipidemia.[3,36] A fasting lipoprotein profile is recommended once every 5 years in all adults older than 20 years of age. If the screening was nonfasting, then only the TC and HDL cholesterol data will be useable as eating causes clinically insignificant differences in these two levels.[3,36,37] In this case, if the TC >200 mg/dL or HDL <40 mg/dL, the patient should return for a fasting lipoprotein profile to determine the appropriate plan for treatment.

The Expert Panel on Integrated Guidelines for Cardiovascular Health and Risk Reduction in Children and Adolescents recently released dyslipidemia screening recommendations for pediatric patients.[38] Fasting lipoprotein profiles are recommended for children between the ages of 2 and 8 if the child has a positive family history for premature cardiovascular disease, a parent with known dyslipidemia, or the child has cardiovascular risk factors, such as hypertension, diabetes, or elevated body mass index. In addition, universal screening is recommended in all pediatric patients between the ages of 9 and 11. Either a fasting lipoprotein profile or a nonfasting sample, focusing on non-HDL cholesterol and HDL levels, can be used for universal screening in this age group. No routine screening is recommended at this time during puberty since levels may fluctuate. Reference ranges and treatment strategies for pediatric patients differ from the adult population. A review of such pediatric recommendations is beyond the scope of this chapter.

The fasting lipoprotein profile includes TC, TG, HDL, and calculated LDL. A typical sample is collected following a 9- to 12-hour fast. Patients must avoid food, as well as beverages with caloric content such as juices, sodas, or coffee with cream or sugar during the fasting period. Depending on the fat and carbohydrate content of the meal, recent food intake can cause increases in TGs of up to 50% and decreases in LDL cholesterol of 10% to 15%.[39] Ideally, the patient should remain seated 5 minutes prior to phlebotomy to avoid hemoconcentration, which may cause falsely elevated lipid levels. Serum samples are collected in collection tubes without anticoagulant; plasma samples are collected in tubes with ethylenediaminetetraacetic acid (EDTA).[39,40]

A number of factors may cause variation in obtained lipid values including sample type and tourniquet application.[39,40] Plasma concentration lipid values are approximately 3% lower than those values associated with serum measurements. Prolonged tourniquet application (longer than 1 minute) may cause venous stasis and increase total serum cholesterol concentrations by 5% to 10%. Methods used to assay total serum cholesterol vary. It is important to become familiar with the method of lipid profile measurement used by the laboratory that the clinician uses regularly.

In addition to factors specific for laboratory methods, patient-specific factors may interfere with the lipid panel results.[39] The preferred lipid panel is obtained in the absence of any acute illness. This provides levels that are not affected by deviation from a baseline stable condition. Vigorous physical activity (within the last 24 hours), pregnancy, recent weight loss, and acute illness result in levels that are not representative of the patient's usual value. Measurement of plasma lipids in the setting of acute coronary syndrome usually provides LDL values that are lower than baseline by 24 hours after an event.[41] The LDL values may continue to be decreased for weeks following the event. While these values are not representative of baseline values, the recommendations are to use these values to guide initiation of LDL-lowering therapy to reduce cardiovascular risk and continue to follow lipids postdischarge.[42,43]

Total Serum Cholesterol

For nonfasting adults >20 years[36]:
desirable, <200 mg/dL or <5.17 mmol/L;
borderline high, 200–239 mg/dL or 5.17–6.18 mmol/L;
or high, ≥240 mg/dL or ≥6.20 mmol/L

In all patient populations, including the elderly, lowering elevated serum cholesterol concentrations decreases death from CHD and results in regression of atherosclerotic lesions.[36,44,45] In young healthy adults, *total serum cholesterol* is a strong predictor of clinically evident cardiovascular events occurring 25 or more years later.[46]

Despite popular belief, a fasting sample is not necessary because total serum cholesterol is not significantly affected by a single meal. Factors that may interfere with accurate assessment include pregnancy, recent weight loss, vigorous exercise, and acute myocardial infarction (MI). Although low total serum cholesterol is usually considered a sign of good health, it can be a sign of hyperthyroidism, malnutrition, chronic anemia, cancer, or severe liver disease.

Methods used to assay total serum cholesterol vary greatly among laboratories. Therefore, clinicians should become familiar with the method used by their laboratory as well as with potential causes of misleading or erroneous results. Serum or heparinized plasma is the typical specimen collected.

Triglycerides

For adults >20 years[36]:
normal, <150 mg/dL or <1.69 mmol/L;
borderline high, 150–199 mg/dL or 1.69–2.25 mmol/L;
high, 200–499 mg/dL or 2.26–5.63 mmol/L;
or very high, ≥500 mg/dL or ≥5.64 mmol/L

Disorders leading to hypertriglyceridemia involve dysregulation of chylomicrons and/or VLDL. Chylomicrons and intermediate-density lipoproteins are present only in postprandial or pathological states, while VLDL, LDL, and HDL are present in the fasting state. *Triglycerides* in the form of chylomicrons appear in the plasma as soon as 2 hours after a meal, reach a maximum at 4–6 hours, and persist for up to 14 hours.[7,8,10] To avoid falsely elevated concentrations, measurement of TGs and lipoproteins is recommended after an overnight fast. Triglyceride concentrations occasionally become transiently or persistently elevated in patients receiving intermittent or constant infusions of intravenous lipids, respectively. However, lipid emulsion regimens are not usually stopped unless there is risk of pancreatitis. Heparin, a common additive to parenteral nutrition solutions, may facilitate faster metabolism of chylomicrons and reduce TG concentrations by a stimulatory effect on lipoprotein lipase.

As a secondary disorder, hypertriglyceridemia is associated with obesity, uncontrolled diabetes mellitus, liver disease, alcohol ingestion, and uremia. Combination oral contraceptives, corticosteroids, some antihypertensive agents, protease inhibitors and isotretinoin may also elevate TG concentrations (Table 14-3).

Extremely high concentrations of TGs—concentrations in excess of 2000 mg/dL (22.6 mmol/L)—may also lead to eruptive cutaneous xanthomas on the elbows, knees, and buttocks. Once TG concentrations are reduced, the xanthomas gradually disappear over the course of 1↑–3 months. Hypertriglyceridemia may also manifest as lipemia retinalis (a salmon-pink cast in the vascular bed of the retina). This sign is due to TG particles scattering light in the blood and is seen in the retinal vessels during an eye exam. In patients with lipemia retinalis, TG concentrations may be 4000 mg/dL (45 mmol/L) or greater.[7,47] A concentration this high requires immediate action because it causes hyperviscosity of the blood with the risk of thrombus formation.

Hypertriglyceridemia, without other lipid abnormalities, is established as an independent risk factor for CHD.[36] In addition to increased risk of cardiovascular disease, hypertriglyceridemia (concentrations >500 mg/dL or >5.64 mmol/L) may precipitate pancreatitis. In fact, many patients with hypertriglyceridemia have intermittent episodes of epigastric pain due to recurrent pancreatic inflammation. In patients with very high TGs (concentrations >500 mg/dL or 5.64 mmol/L),

TABLE 14-3. Secondary Causes of Dyslipidemia and Major Associated Changes in Lipoprotein Component[3,8,19–23]

DISORDER OR CONDITION[a]	DRUG OR DIET[a]
Acute hepatitis (↑TG)	Alcohol (↑TG)
Cholestasis (↑LDL)	Amiodarone (↑TG)
Chronic renal failure (↓HDL, ↑TG)	Atypical antipsychotics (↑TG, ↑LDL)
Cigarette use (↓HDL, ↑TG)	Beta blockers (↑TG, ↓HDL)
Diabetes mellitus (↓HDL, ↑TG)	Contraceptives (estrogen and progestin)[b] (↑TG)
Glycogen storage disease (↑TG)	Corticosteroids (↑LDL, ↑TG)
Hypothyroidism (↑LDL, ↑TG)	Cyclosporine (↑LDL, ↑TG)
Liver failure (↓LDL, ↓TG)	Diet high in saturated fats and cholesterol (↑LDL, ↑TG)
Nephrotic syndrome (↑LDL, ↑TG)	Diet high in carbohydrates (↓HDL,↑TG)
Obesity (↓HDL, ↑TG)	Estrogens (↑HDL, ↓LDL, ↑TG)
Obstructive liver disease (↑LDL)	Estrogen-receptor modulators (↓LDL, ↑TG)
Pregnancy (↑TG)	Interferons (↑TG)
Sedentary lifestyle (↓HDL, ↑TG)	Isotretinoin (↑LDL, ↓HDL, ↑TG)
	Parenteral lipid emulsions (↑TG)
	Progestins (↑LDL, ↓HDL, ↓TG)
	Protease inhibitors (↑TG)
	Sirolimus (↑LDL, ↑TG)
	Thiazide diuretics (↑LDL, ↑TG)

LDL = low-density lipoprotein; HDL = high-density lipoprotein; TG = triglyceride.
[a]↑=increase; ↓=decrease.
[b]Effect on HDL and LDL depends on specific components.

the initial goal of therapy is to prevent pancreatitis through a very low-fat diet (≤15% of calories from fat), weight reduction, increased physical activity, and drug therapy. In patients with a TG concentration of 250–750 mg/dL (2.8–8.5 mmol/L), a 10- to 20-lb weight loss usually leads to a marked reduction in TG concentrations and an increase in HDL (if low). For patients with diabetes, glycemic control may help to lower TG concentrations.[36,48] The drugs of choice for lowering TGs are fibrates, nicotinic acid, or omega-3 fatty acids. An alternative approach to drug therapy in patients with borderline high or high TGs is to intensify therapy with an LDL-lowering drug, such as a statin, which will provide some reduction in TGs. Bile acid sequestrants should be avoided since these agents are known to increase TG concentrations.

Many patients with a high TG concentration are inactive and obese. Patients encountered in clinical practice with elevated TGs often have similar lipid and nonlipid risk factors of metabolic origin termed *metabolic syndrome*.[36,47] The metabolic syndrome is characterized by abdominal obesity, insulin resistance, hypertension, low HDL, and elevations in TGs. Metabolic syndrome is managed by correcting underlying causes, such as obesity, with TLC and by treating associated lipid risk factors.

Since hypertriglyceridemia is an independent risk factor for CHD, this suggests that TG-rich lipoproteins may be atherogenic.[36] Very low-density lipoprotein is a TG-rich lipoprotein. There is recent evidence that VLDL, like LDL particles, is

atherogenic. In patients with high TGs, the sum of atherogenic particles (both VLDL and LDL) may be estimated by calculating non-HDL cholesterol. The lowering of non-HDL cholesterol (total cholesterol [LDL + VLDL] – HDL) is a secondary target of therapy in all persons with high TGs (≥200 mg/dL). VLDL is estimated to be the plasma TG level divided by five. The non-HDL cholesterol target of therapy is set at 30 mg/dL greater than the LDL goal. For example, if a patient has an LDL goal of less than 130 mg/dL, the non-HDL goal will be set at <160 mg/dL. If TGs are less than 200 mg/dL, then lifestyle modifications are appropriate. If TGs are 200–499 mg/dL, then the non-HDL goal should be the target of therapy once the LDL goal is reached. This underscores the need to assess non-HDL as a marker of atherosclerotic risk in all patients with serum TGs greater than 200 mg/dL. Very low-density lipoprotein levels are not routinely measured in practice or targeted in therapy. The TG-rich lipoprotein is assessed by use of TG or non-HDL levels instead.

Several TG assay interferences exist. The TG assay itself is susceptible to interference by glycerol, which may be a component of medications or used as a lubricant in laboratory equipment.[49] Clinically significant increases in glycerol concentrations can also occur following prolonged emotional stress or in diabetes.[39] An excess of TGs in the blood can lead to errors in other laboratory measurements. Lipemic samples can cause falsely low serum amylase results, underestimation of electrolytes, and erratic interferences with many other tests.[50]

The potential interference with amylase is especially clinically relevant since high TG concentrations can cause pancreatitis, and accurate amylase concentrations are crucial to diagnosis.

Fortunately, most technologists can identify lipemic samples as the serum specimen will appear milky. The appearance of a patient's serum sample before and after 12–16 hours of refrigeration can indicate TG-rich serum. If the sample shows a uniform turbidity or opalescence, VLDL has increased without a concurrent increase in chylomicrons. A "cream" supernatant layer atop a clear solution indicates chylomicronemia, with an excess of both chylomicrons and VLDL.

Low-Density Lipoprotein Cholesterol

For fasting adults >20 years[36]:
optimal, <100 mg/dL or <2.58 mmol/L;
near or above optimal, 100–129 mg/dL or 2.58–3.33 mmol/L;
borderline high, 130–159 mg/dL or 3.36–4.11 mmol/L;
high, 160–189 mg/dL or 4.13–4.89 mmol/L;
or very high, ≥190 mg/dL or ≥4.91 mmol/L

Since TC concentrations include both the "good" (HDL) and "bad" (LDL) cholesterol, the primary goals of therapy are stated in terms of only the "bad" cholesterol, or *low-density lipoprotein (LDL)*. The LDL must be measured while the patient is in a fasting state. Low-risk patients whose LDL cholesterol is less than the individualized goal (without drug therapy) should have their fasting lipoprotein profile measured every 5 years.[3] More frequent measurement may be desired in patients with multiple risk factors, or patients with low-risk (0–1 risk factor) but with previous LDL values only slightly below individualized goal. The total fasting lipid profile includes TC, HDL, LDL, and TGs. Direct measurement of LDL is not commonly performed due to labor-intensive centrifugation. Instead, LDL cholesterol

concentrations can be estimated indirectly by a method determined by Friedewald.[51] The formula subtracts the HDL and VLDL cholesterol from the total plasma cholesterol. The VLDL is estimated to be the plasma TG level divided by five. Using the following formula (all in milligrams per deciliter), LDL may be estimated in patients with a TG concentration less than 400 mg/dL (<4.52 mmol/L) and without familial dysbetalipoproteinemia (see Table 14-2):

LDL = total serum cholesterol − HDL − (triglycerides/5)

If a patient's serum TG concentration exceeds 400 mg/dL (4.52 mmol/L), LDL cholesterol cannot be calculated with this formula. A direct LDL measurement by laboratory would provide an LDL value. However, since treatment of hypertriglyceridemia would take priority in such a patient, most clinicians would treat hypertriglyceridemia through lifestyle modifications and medications first. Once TG values have decreased to <400 mg/dL (<4.52 mmol/L), a fasting lipid panel would provide LDL cholesterol data.

Table 14-4 lists the treatment recommendations from the 2001 report of the expert panel of the NCEP and provides intensified optional goal recommendations based on new clinical trial data.[3,6,36] LDL-cholesterol lowering is the primary goal of therapy in patients with dyslipidemia. This is because for each 1% decrease in LDL cholesterol levels, there is a corresponding 1% decrease in the relative risk for a CHD major event.[6] LDL cholesterol levels are generally considered *optimal* when maintained below 100 mg/dL. However, in a patient at very high risk for a cardiovascular event, *optimal* LDL cholesterol levels may rest at a lower threshold of below 70 mg/dL. The actual goal LDL for an individual patient is defined by a risk evaluation.

TABLE 14-4. LDL-Based Treatment Recommendations of the Expert Panel of the National Cholesterol Education Program[3,6,36]

CHD OR CHD RISK EQUIVALENTS[a]	RISK FACTORS[b]	LDL (mg/dL)[c] AT WHICH TO INITIATE LIFESTYLE CHANGES	LDL (mg/dL) AT WHICH TO CONSIDER DRUG THERAPY[d]		LDL CHOLESTEROL GOAL (mg/dL)	
			Recommended	Optional[e]	Recommended	Optional[e]
No	None or one	≥160	≥190	160–189	<160	
	Two or more: 10-yr risk <10%	≥130	≥160		<130	
	Two or more: 10-yr risk 10% to 20%		≥130	100–129	<130	<100
Yes		≥100	≥130	>100	<100	<70

[a]Coronary heart disease (CHD) includes angina, myocardial infarction (MI), and coronary angioplasty. Coronary heart disease risk equivalents include diabetes, peripheral arterial disease, abdominal aortic aneurysm, transient ischemic attack or stroke, and a 10-yr risk >20%.
[b]Risk factors in List 14-1. An increased (≥60 mg/dL) HDL concentration is a negative risk factor and negates one of the positive risk factors. Assess 10-year CHD risk with Framingham risk assessment when necessary.
[c]Conversion factor for cholesterol in the International System of Units (SI) is 0.02586 (millimoles per liter).
[d]When LDL-lowering drug therapy is initiated, intensity of therapy should provide at least 30% to 40% reduction in LDL.
[e]Optional goals indicated from the Adult Treatment Panel (ATP) considerations of recent clinical trial data.[6]

The first step is determining if a patient has CHD or a CHD risk equivalent. Examples of patients with CHD include a patient with a history of MI, unstable angina, stable angina, or coronary angioplasty. Diabetes, peripheral arterial disease, history of transient ischemic attack, and stroke are examples of CHD risk equivalents. If CHD or a CHD risk equivalent is identified, the defined goal LDL is less than 100 mg/dL. Further, current recommendations suggest that a practitioner should consider an optional intensified LDL goal of less than 70 mg/dL in patients considered very high risk. Patients with both established CHD and multiple or poorly controlled risk factors are examples of very high-risk patients. Risk factors may include acute coronary syndromes, diabetes, cigarette smoking, and presence of metabolic syndrome. Therefore, the American Diabetes Association recommends a goal LDL of less than 100 mg/dL for patients with diabetes and an intensified optional goal of less than 70 mg/dL for patients with diabetes and established CHD.[52] The American Association of Clinical Endocrinologists similarly recommends a goal LDL of less than 100 mg/dL for patients with diabetes, but recommends the intensified goal of less than 70 mg/dL for patients with diabetes and two or more major risk factors or established CHD.[24]

In patients without CHD or a CHD risk equivalent, an assessment of the patient's number of risk factors must be made (List 14-1). For patients with two or more risk factors, a Framingham risk score is calculated to determine the patient's CHD risk (Figure 14-2).[6,36] The Framingham score takes into account data from the Framingham study used to weigh individual risk factors. If a patient is determined to have a 10-year CHD risk of greater than 20%, this patient is determined to have a CHD risk equivalent and is treated to a goal LDL of less than 100 mg/dL. In patients with two or more risk factors and a 10-year CHD risk of 20% or less, an LDL goal of less than 130 mg/dL is desired. However, drug therapy may be initiated earlier in those patients with a risk of greater than 10% and an optional goal of less than 100 mg/dL may be considered. In those patients with lower risk (0–1 risk factors), the goal LDL is set at less than 160 mg/dL.

Lifestyle modifications are appropriate for all patients with dyslipidemia. Detailed education should be provided to patients regarding the adoption of a low saturated fat and low cholesterol diet, maintenance of a healthy weight, and regular physical activity. Reducing saturated fat in the diet to <7% of calories gives an approximate LDL cholesterol reduction of 8% to 10%, while an intake of <200 mg/day of dietary cholesterol would provide an additional 3% to 5% reduction in LDL.[3] A weight reduction of 10 pounds due to moderate physical activity and dietary changes may provide an approximate LDL reduction of 5% to 8%. Dietary supplementation with soluble fiber and the use of plant stanols and sterols are therapeutic dietary options to lower LDL cholesterol providing 3% to 5% and 6% to 15% reductions in LDL cholesterol, respectively. If all of these dietary modifications are employed simultaneously, a cumulative 20% to 30% reduction in LDL cholesterol may be achieved. When drug therapy is initiated, doses adequate to provide reductions to meet established LDL goals should be used. Additionally, based on trial evidence demonstrating reductions in CHD risk, it is recommended that when drug therapy is used doses that achieve at least a 30% to 40% reduction in LDL should be targeted.[6] This means that for a patient with LDL cholesterol only 15% above goal, a sufficient dose to achieve a 30% to 40% reduction should be used regardless of the fact that only a small reduction is needed to achieve goal.

High-Density Lipoprotein Cholesterol

For fasting adults >20 years[36]:
low, <40 mg/dL or <1.03 mmol/L;
high, ≥60 mg/dL or ≥1.55 mmol/L

Based on epidemiological evidence, *high-density lipoprotein (HDL)* acts as an antiatherogenic factor and is often termed "good cholesterol."[53,54] While a high HDL concentration is associated with cardioprotection, low levels are associated with increased risk of CHD. Every 1% increase in HDL cholesterol is associated with a decrease in CHD by 2% in men and 3% in women.[55] The Framingham Study demonstrated that HDL levels were predictive of cardiovascular risk independent of elevations in LDL. Examples of this atherogenic potential are best illustrated with the coronary arteries. Concentrations less than 40 mg/dL (<1.03 mmol/L) are associated with an increased risk of MI. Similarly, low HDL is also associated with an increased risk of coronary angioplasty restenosis.[54,56] In the setting of increased TG, HDL cholesterol less than 40 mg/dL (1.03 mmol/L) in men or 50 mg/dL (1.3 mmol/L) in women is considered a risk factor of metabolic syndrome.[36] The blood specimen does not need to be drawn after a 12-hour fast. However, a fast is usually required because HDL is often ordered in combination with LDL.

Most patients with low HDL levels have concomitant elevated TG levels. In these patients, lifestyle therapy or drug therapy to decrease TGs usually results in a desirable increase in HDL. However, there are also patients with isolated low HDL cholesterol. Since LDL is the primary target of therapy in the NCEP guidelines, there is no specific goal for raising HDL, which is negatively correlated with TGs, smoking, and obesity. In contrast, HDL is positively correlated with physical activity and smoking cessation. Due to beneficial effects of estrogen, women, especially premenopausal women, typically have higher HDL levels than men.

LIST 14-1. Risk Factors for Atherosclerotic Vascular Disease from High Cholesterol (Primarily LDL)[36]

Age: ≥45 years for men or ≥55 years for women
Family history of premature CHD (first-degree relative: male <55 years, female <65 years)
Cigarette smoking: any within the past month
Hypertension or on antihypertensive medication
HDL cholesterol <40 mg/dL[a]

CHD = coronary heart disease; HDL = high-density lipoprotein; LDL = low-density lipoprotein.

[a]When risk assessed, an HDL ≥60 mg/dL is considered a negative risk factor that, if present, subtracts one risk factor from the total count.

Estimate of 10-Year Risk for **Men**

Age, yr	Points
20–34	−9
35–39	−4
40–44	0
45–49	3
50–54	6
55–59	8
60–64	10
65–69	11
70–74	12
75–79	13

Total Cholesterol, mg/dL	Points				
	Age 20–39 yr	Age 40–49 yr	Age 50–59 yr	Age 60–69 yr	Age 70–79 yr
<160	0	0	0	0	0
160–199	4	3	2	1	0
200–239	7	5	3	1	0
240–279	9	6	4	2	1
≥280	11	8	5	3	1

	Points				
	Age 20–39 yr	Age 40–49 yr	Age 50–59 yr	Age 60–69 yr	Age 70–79 yr
Nonsmoker	0	0	0	0	0
Smoker	8	5	3	1	1

HDL, mg/dL	Points
≥60	−1
50–59	0
40–49	1
<40	2

Systolic BP, mm Hg	If Untreated	If Treated
<120	0	0
120–129	0	1
130–139	1	2
140–159	1	2
≥160	2	3

Point Total	10-Yr Risk, %
<0	<1
0	1
1	1
2	1
3	1
4	1
5	2
6	2
7	3
8	4
9	5
10	6
11	8
12	10
13	12
14	16
15	20
16	25
≥17	≥30

Estimate of 10-Year Risk for **Women**

Age, yr	Points
20–34	−7
35–39	−3
40–44	0
45–49	3
50–54	6
55–59	8
60–64	10
65–69	12
70–74	14
75–79	16

Total Cholesterol, mg/dL	Points				
	Age 20–39 yr	Age 40–49 yr	Age 50–59 yr	Age 60–69 yr	Age 70–79 yr
<160	0	0	0	0	0
160–199	4	3	2	1	1
200–239	8	6	4	2	1
240–279	11	8	5	3	2
≥280	13	10	7	4	2

	Points				
	Age 20–39 yr	Age 40–49 yr	Age 50–59 yr	Age 60–69 yr	Age 70–79 yr
Nonsmoker	0	0	0	0	0
Smoker	9	7	4	2	1

HDL, mg/dL	Points
≥60	−1
50–59	0
40–49	1
<40	2

Systolic BP, mm Hg	If Untreated	If Treated
<120	0	0
120–129	1	3
130–139	2	4
140–159	3	5
≥160	4	6

Point Total	10-Yr Risk, %
<9	<1
9	1
10	1
11	1
12	1
13	2
14	2
15	3
16	4
17	5
18	6
19	8
20	11
21	14
22	17
23	22
24	27
≥25	≥30

FIGURE 14-2. Framingham point scores.[36]

MINICASE 1

Primary Prevention

HENRY F., A 47-YEAR-OLD MALE, presents to the clinic to discuss his lipid profile during his annual exam. His friend recently suffered a heart attack, and he is very concerned about his own personal heart disease risk. His past medical history includes hypertension diagnosed 5 years ago, which is currently controlled with lisinopril 10 mg daily. He takes no other medications. He follows a reasonable, low-fat diet and jogs 4 times per week for exercise. He denies tobacco use; however, he reports drinking one glass of wine with dinner most nights of the week. He does not have a family history of diabetes, dyslipidemia, or CHD. At his office visit, he has a normal physical exam with a blood pressure reading of 118/78. He had his labs drawn yesterday after a 12-hour fast. The following laboratory results were obtained: TC 240 mg/dL, HDL cholesterol 61 mg/dL, TGs 145 mg/dL, LDL cholesterol 150 mg/dL, and glucose 89 mg/dL. Electrolyte, hematology, liver, renal, and thyroid tests are all normal. He is 5'10" and weighs 198 lb.

Question: How should the lipid results be interpreted?

Discussion: Henry F. is asymptomatic and follows a healthy lifestyle including a low-fat diet, daily physical activity, and avoiding tobacco products. He has no evident secondary causes of dyslipidemia. He does not have type 2 diabetes, thyroid, renal, or liver disease, and his antihypertensive medication has no effects on the lipid panel. His moderate alcohol intake may contribute to his elevated HDL; however, alcohol use should not be recommended as a preventative measure since no clinical trials support such a recommendation.

Henry F.'s TC and HDL cholesterol are in the high category, and his TGs are within the normal range. An elevated HDL cholesterol level is considered cardioprotective and needs to be considered when assessing

a patient's cardiovascular risk. An HDL cholesterol level >60 mg/dL is considered a negative risk factor, and the clinician can subtract one existing positive risk factor (List 14-1). Henry F.'s age and history of hypertension are considered risk factors that would modify his LDL goal; however, given his high HDL, Henry F. should be treated as if he had only one risk factor. His desired LDL goal is less than 160 mg/dL (Table 14-4). As direct LDL measurements are not often obtained from the laboratory, the LDL was calculated using the Friedewald formula: LDL = total serum cholesterol − HDL − (triglycerides/5).

$$LDL = 240 \text{ mg/dL} - 61 \text{ mg/dL} - (145 \text{ mg/dL}/5) = 150 \text{ mg/dL}$$

Question: Should any other laboratory tests be ordered to assess his cardiovascular risk? What should be done next?

Discussion: A number of emerging risk factors are under investigation including ApoB and hs-CRP. Higher levels of ApoB have been correlated with elevated cardiovascular risk; however, ApoB levels strongly correlate with non-HDL cholesterol levels, which is already available from the lipid panel. Thus, routine measurement of ApoB is not recommended. Increased hs-CRP levels have been associated with elevated cardiovascular risk. The ACCF/AHA guidelines recommend that it may be reasonable to measure hs-CRP in men >50 or women >60 years old with LDL <130 mg/dL or those younger but at intermediate risk. Given that Henry F.'s age is below this threshold and his low CHD risk, no emerging laboratory tests are needed to evaluate his cardiovascular risk.

Henry F. should continue with his low-fat, low-cholesterol diet and physical activity. Since his LDL is below the desired goal of 160 mg/dL, no drug therapy is required. A repeat fasting lipid profile is desired in 5 years. However, some clinicians may choose to follow up sooner since his LDL of 150 mg/dL was only slightly below the goal of less than 160 mg/dL.

Emerging Lipid Risk Factors

A number of *emerging lipid risk factors* for CHD are being investigated to varying degrees: lipoprotein remnants and lipoprotein (a), LDL particle number, HDL subspecies, and apolipoproteins, such as apolipoprotein B (ApoB), apolipoprotein AI, and apolipoprotein E.[3,57,58] Apolipoprotein B is the major component of atherogenic lipoproteins and higher levels of apo B have been correlated with an increase in CHD.[3,59] However, ApoB levels are strongly correlated with non-HDL levels. Therefore, ApoB is typically not measured in clinical practice as non-HDL is already a secondary target of therapy in the current guidelines. Further, the role of LDL particle number has been investigated.[58,59] Even with the same LDL cholesterol level, individuals with a greater number of LDL particles have a higher CHD risk. However, again, the non-HDL level was similarly able to predict CHD risk. Therefore, the current American College of Cardiology Foundation (ACCF) and American Heart Association (AHA) Guidelines for Assessment of Cardiovascular Risk in Asymptomatic Adults does not recommend routine advanced lipid testing.[59] While further investigation into these markers may help to explain some of the variation in CHD risk among individuals with similar lipoprotein profiles, currently measurements of these emerging risk

factors are not readily available in clinical practice. At this time, measurement of these risk factors is primarily employed by specialists until more evidence linking them to cardiovascular risk and risk reduction is available.

Nonlipid emerging risk factors are also under investigation.[3,60] Plasma homocysteine levels, thrombogenic factors, and inflammatory markers, all have been linked to CHD. Like the emerging lipid risk factors, NCEP provides no recommendations at this time to routinely monitor these laboratory data in patients.[36] However, the ACCF/AHA more recently recommended measurement of select nonlipid risk factors in certain patient populations.[59] Since inflammation plays a role in the pathophysiology of atherosclerosis, one of the most studied inflammatory markers is high-sensitivity C-reactive protein (hs-CRP). In a meta-analysis, elevated hs-CRP levels were linked to the risk of cardiovascular events, cerebrovascular events, and cardiovascular mortality.[61] In the JUPITER trial, men ≥50 or women ≥60 years old with an LDL cholesterol of <130 mg/dL but with elevated hs-CRP levels of >2 mg/dL treated with a statin instead of placebo were shown to have a lower rate of major cardiovascular events.[62] Therefore, the ACCF/AHA 2010 Guidelines recommends that it is reasonable to test hs-CRP in men ≥50 or women ≥60 years old with LDL

MINICASE 2

Secondary Prevention

GINA P., A 68-YEAR-OLD, 5' 4", 200-LB FEMALE, presents to the clinic following discharge from the hospital last week. Prior to her hospitalization, her past medical history was significant for obesity, hypertension treated with hydrochlorothiazide, and tobacco dependence. She does not have a history of diabetes or thyroid disorder. She presented to the emergency department with indigestion and dizziness. While she denied chest pain, she was diagnosed with an MI. Discharge prescriptions include metoprolol succinate, lisinopril, hydrochlorothiazide, atorvastatin, and low-dose aspirin daily. She has never previously taken cholesterol-lowering medication. She has not filled her discharge prescriptions as she was unsure if she needed all of the medications and wanted to check with the providers in the clinic who know her well. Since her MI last week, she has quit smoking. Gina P. states she tries to cook low-fat for her immediate family, but she often entertains for extended family and does not follow any dietary restrictions for these gatherings. She did very little exercise prior to her MI, but she plans on starting to walk regularly once she regains her energy. Her father died of a heart attack at age 54.

Her blood pressure today at the clinic was 144/86, and her heart rate was 64. Fasting lipid profile was as follows: TC 220 mg/dL; TGs 150 mg/dL; LDL 148 mg/dL; and HDL 42 mg/dL. Fasting glucose is 76 mg/dL; electrolyte, hematology, liver, renal, and thyroid tests are all normal.

Question: Was it appropriate to order a lipid profile? How should the lipid profile be interpreted? Should Gina P. have her prescription for a lipid-lowering medication filled?

Discussion: All patients with CHD, including MI, should have a lipid profile performed. It is unknown whether Gina P.'s lipid panel had been previously measured and if the results were within desired range.

Even before her MI at age 68, Gina P. was at risk for atherosclerotic disease. At that time she was an obese, female smoker—older than 55 years—with hypertension who lived a sedentary lifestyle. Her father died prematurely of atherosclerotic vessel disease; his age at death (54) meets the criteria for a risk factor (<55 years old). Of her risk factors, all except her age and family history are modifiable risk factors, meaning she has the ability to change her risk by making lifestyle changes.

Gina P. is obese, which may contribute to increase in TGs and decreases in HDL cholesterol; she has no other evidence of disease-related secondary causes of dyslipidemia (diabetes, hypothyroidism, obstructive liver disease, renal dysfunction). However, there are potential substance- or medication-related secondary causes of dyslipidemia in Gina P.'s case. While short-term use of hydrochlorothiazide may increase LDL cholesterol and TGs, long-term use is typically not associated with lipid changes.[31] She was also very recently a smoker. Smoking is associated with increases in TGs and decreases in HDL cholesterol. Gina P.'s newly prescribed beta blocker may impact the lipid profile by causing decreases in HDL and increases in TGs. However, Gina P. should still start therapy with the beta blocker as the benefits of beta blockers in reducing mortality post-MI outweigh the impact on the lipid profile. Further, Gina P.'s LDL cholesterol is elevated and will be the primary target of therapy.

Currently, Gina P. has three risk factors for cardiovascular disease that determine her LDL goal: hypertension, female age ≥55, and a premature family history. It is not necessary to calculate her Framingham risk score, as with a history of MI she has CHD. All patients with CHD have an initial LDL goal of less than 100 mg/dL. Further, based on recent clinical trials consideration of an LDL goal of less than 70 mg/dL is a therapeutic option since Gina P.'s MI places her in the very high-risk category. Therapeutic lifestyle changes (TLC) are appropriate for Gina P., including weight loss, increasing physical activity and a greater emphasis on reducing saturated fat and cholesterol intake in the diet. She should be commended for quitting smoking and encouraged to keep her new healthy habit. While TLC should definitely be initiated, even if she adheres strictly to a TLC diet, only a 10% to 15% decrease in LDL cholesterol is expected. Gina P. needs to obtain a 32% reduction in her LDL cholesterol to bring her current LDL cholesterol of 148 mg/dL to a goal of less than 100 mg/dL, or a 53% reduction to bring her to the optional goal of less than 70 mg/dL. Therefore, drug therapy should also be initiated. Statins, bile acid sequestrants, ezetimibe, and nicotinic acid are all considered LDL-lowering drug therapy. Typically, statins are considered the drug of choice for elevations in LDL cholesterol as they not only provide substantial reductions in LDL, but they also have documented evidence in reducing morbidity and mortality. Therefore, it is reasonable for Gina P. to fill her prescription for atorvastatin. Since she already had a fasting lipid panel and LFTs performed during her hospitalization, the only baseline laboratory value that could be ordered is a CK. The fasting lipid profile should be repeated in 6 weeks to determine if goals have been met or changes in drug therapy are warranted.

<130 mg/dL who are not on lipid-lowering therapy or those at a younger age but with intermediate risk.[59] The marker is also one factor in the Reynolds Risk Score. This tool, similar to the Framingham Risk Score, incorporates hs-CRP in stratification of a patient's cardiovascular risk but is not yet recommended by NCEP guidelines for clinical use.[63,64] Another nonlipid marker is lipoprotein-associated phospholipase A2 (Lp-PLA2), an enzyme produced by macrophages and lymphocytes that is found on atherogenic lipoproteins.[59] Since levels of Lp-PLA2 are correlated with increased risk of CHD, the ACCF/AHA states that it may be reasonable to measure for risk assessment in intermediate risk asymptomatic adults. However, the groups also note that there is currently no information about whether measurement of Lp-PLA2 concentrations will improve clinical outcomes. Currently, these emerging risk factors are not commonly used in the clinical setting. (See Minicases 1 and 2.)

Point-of-Care Testing Options

In addition to laboratory monitoring, there are home testing kits available to the patient for determination of lipids.[65] Some home testing kits provide results directly to the patient within 30 minutes or less; these kits typically only provide TC results. The clinical applicability of this testing method, which utilizes a fingerstick for obtaining a sample, is limited since TC alone is no longer recommended as a screening tool by NCEP.[36] Other home testing kits provide results of the full lipid panel. These tests require the patient to apply blood to a card and mail the sample into a laboratory for processing. In addition to home testing methods, there are relatively inexpensive compact devices for point-of-care testing outside the laboratory that are waived from the Clinical Laboratory Improvement Amendments (CLIA). These devices enable testing for TC, HDL cholesterol, and TGs. The LDL is calculated either by the user or the device using the Friedewald formula. Some devices use one cartridge, which can test multiple components of the panel, whereas other devices require a separate cartridge for each individual lab test necessitating multiple fingersticks.

One important consideration when evaluating studies of point-of-care testing devices is to be aware that some variability may be explained by the fact that different sample types are often compared. For example, a fingerstick provides a sample with capillary blood and a venous draw provides venous whole blood. Nevertheless, the point-of-care testing devices are accepted methods for screening for dyslipidemia and are frequently used at health fairs and other screening opportunities. However, considering that NCEP recommends the complete lipid panel for screening purposes, methods that provide only TC or portions of the lipid panel may have limited utility.[36] In any point-of-care testing setting, quality control, quality assessment, and proper training of personnel can work to improve the accuracy of testing.[66] One of the benefits of point-of-care testing is that it involves the patient in the laboratory process, which has been identified by NCEP as an intervention to improve patient adherence.[36] The laboratory visits become opportunities for the clinician to provide the patient with feedback on progress and reinforce the steps needed to achieve goals.

EFFECTS OF HYPOLIPEMIC MEDICATIONS

Clinicians must be aware of how antihyperlipidemic drugs can influence laboratory test results. The two principal approaches to management of dyslipidemia are lifestyle modifications and drug therapy. In high-risk patients drug therapy is immediately initiated along with lifestyle modifications, which are always concurrently used with drug therapy. In most patients, when lifestyle modifications do not result in appropriate reductions, drug therapy is considered. The ultimate goal of therapy is to reduce cardiovascular risk, or, in the case of elevated TGs alone, reduce the risk of pancreatitis. In general, statins, ezetimibe, niacin, and bile acid sequestrants are considered LDL-lowering drug therapy. Fibrates, niacin, and omega-3 fatty acids are considered drugs for lowering TGs or raising HDL. Specific actions of the drugs are reviewed below.

Statins

By inhibiting the enzyme that catalyzes the rate-limiting step in cholesterol synthesis, statins, or HMG-CoA reductase inhibitors lower TC and LDL (18% to 55%, depending on the drug and dose) and may raise HDL as much as 17%.[5,36,67,68] Statins may also decrease TG concentrations (by 7% to 43%). The degree of TG lowering with the statins depends on the degree of initial elevation in TGs.[48,69] With all statins, maximum effects usually are seen after 4–6 weeks. A lipid profile can be ordered 6 weeks after therapy is initiated to assess efficacy.

Rare adverse effects include serious liver injury and increases in creatine kinase (CK) with muscle pain. Previous recommendations to detect potential hepatotoxicity included routine monitoring of liver function tests (LFTs).[70] However, the FDA recently approved revised package labeling to only recommend monitoring of LFTs prior to statin initiation and when clinically indicated thereafter.[71] This change was made since serious liver injury due to statins is extremely rare and routine monitoring has not proven to be effective in preventing this adverse effect. Patients need to be educated to report any symptoms associated with liver injury (e.g., unusual fatigue, yellowing of the skin or dark-colored urine) to their healthcare provider. Myalgia, muscle pain, tenderness and/or weakness, occurs in 2% to 7% of patients on statins.[72] Myopathy occurs in 0.1% to 0.2% of patients on statins. Increased risk of myopathy is associated with the use of high-dose statins, renal insufficiency, concurrent use of fibrates, and concurrent use of cytochrome P450 inhibitors.[72] Recommendations differ with respect to baseline CK levels. ATP-III recommends that all patients have a baseline CK drawn prior to initiation of statin therapy.[3] However, newer recommendations state baseline CK monitoring is only needed in high-risk patients and can be avoided in the majority of patients.[70] In treated patients with complaints of muscle pain, tenderness or weakness, serum CK should be drawn. Elevations in CK and myalgia together are termed *myopathy*. In some cases, rhabdomyolysis has been reported. Most clinicians will discontinue the drug when CK levels are greater than 10 times the upper limit of normal. Routine monitoring of CK during therapy is not warranted.

Numerous trials document the clinical benefits of statins for primary and secondary prevention of CHD. The agents are associated with reductions in major coronary events, CHD deaths, need for coronary procedures, stroke, and total mortality.[36]

Ezetimibe

By selectively inhibiting the intestinal absorption of cholesterol, ezetimibe monotherapy reduces LDL cholesterol by approximately 18%.[73] Adding ezetimibe to therapy with a statin provides LDL reductions greater than the statin alone. In patients with primary hypercholesterolemia, ezetimibe reduces TGs by approximately 8%. Ezetimibe is generally well-tolerated. When ezetimibe is coadministered with a statin, LFTs should be performed as with statin therapy alone. The incidence of increased transaminases from coadministration of ezetimibe and a statin (1.3%) is higher than the incidence for patients treated with statins alone (0.4%). No cardiovascular outcome data have been documented.

Bile Acid Sequestrants

Agents that bind bile acids (e.g., cholestyramine, colesevelam, and colestipol) lower LDL concentrations by 15% to 30% but may raise TGs, especially if hypertriglyceridemia exists.[5] (See Minicase 3.) Because these products stay within the enterohepatic circulation, they do not directly cause other systemic effects that may be reflected in laboratory data. They do, however, interfere with the absorption of fat-soluble vitamins and some drugs (e.g., digoxin, thyroid supplements, and warfarin) and may affect serum concentrations of these drugs or prothrombin times. Bile acid sequestrants may increase TG levels and are not recommended in individuals with TGs greater than 200 mg/dL and are contraindicated in patients with TGs greater than 400 mg/dL. In clinical trials, bile acid sequestrants are associated with reduced major coronary events and CHD deaths.[36]

Niacin

Although niacin, or nicotinic acid, is associated with more bothersome side effects (e.g., flushing, pruritus, and gastrointestinal distress) than other agents, it has desirable effects on the lipid profile.[5] In therapeutic doses, this B vitamin lowers total serum cholesterol, LDL (by 5% to 25%), and TGs (by 20% to 50%) and tends to raise HDL (by 15% to 35%). Niacin may increase serum glucose, uric acid, and LFTs, and decrease serum thyroxine and thyroxine-binding globulin without causing clinical hypothyroidism.[74,75] Baseline and routine monitoring of glucose, uric acid, and LFTs is recommended.[3] Flushing can be minimized by taking aspirin prior to dosing or by taking niacin with a meal. Sustained-release formulations may also minimize flushing. However, hepatotoxicity, detected by an increase in LFTs greater than 3 times the upper limit of normal, is more often associated with sustained-release preparations of niacin.[74] Niacin is associated with reductions in major coronary events and possibly reductions in total mortality.[36]

Fibric Acid Derivatives

Fibrates—gemfibrozil, fenofibrate, and fenofibric acid—reduce TGs by 20% to 50% and increase HDL by 10% to 20%.[3,76,77] However, the effect of treatment with a fibrate on LDL is less predictable. In patients with normal-to-moderately elevated TGs, LDL may be decreased 5% to 20% by fibrates. Conversely, in patients with very high TGs, fibrates may increase LDL concentrations. Like the statins, the agents are associated with transaminase and CK elevations. Routine LFTs should be done in patients receiving these drugs. Creatine kinase should be monitored in patients with complaints of muscle aches. A higher risk of myopathy is observed in patients on combination therapy with fibrates and statins.[78] In addition, mild hematologic changes and elevations in serum creatinine have been observed with fibrates.[76,79] Complete blood count (CBC) should be done periodically during the first year of therapy. Monitoring of renal function in patients at risk for renal impairment is advised.

Omega-3 Fatty Acids

Prescription fish oil products predominantly contain the omega-3 fatty acids eicosapentaenoic acid (EPA) and docosahexaenoic acid (DHA).[80,81] Omega-3 fatty acids target TGs, with reductions of up to 45% in patients with very high TG levels. While increases in HDL cholesterol of up to 13% may be seen, the fatty acids increase conversion of VLDL to LDL resulting in LDL cholesterol increases of up to 45%.[80,81] Recently, an EPA-only product was FDA-approved that does not result in an increase in LDL.[82] In some patients, increases in transaminase levels may be seen. Aspartate aminotransferase (AST) and alanine aminotransferase (ALT) levels should be monitored

periodically.[80] Omega-3 fatty acids have an antithrombotic potential. However, in one study, there were no increases in international normalized ratio or major bleeding episodes.[83] As such, no additional laboratory coagulation testing beyond standard testing in usual practice is recommended for patients taking warfarin or antiplatelet agents.[81]

MINICASE 3

Hypertriglyceridemia

LARRY M. IS A 56-YEAR-OLD, 5'11", 280-LB MALE who had a lipid panel drawn yesterday for routine screening. The results of a lab are now available and you call him to follow up on the results. His past medical history is significant for hypertension and depression. He has no family history of cardiovascular disease or pancreatitis. Daily medications include losartan 50 mg, paroxetine 20 mg, and a multivitamin. His diet consists of hamburgers, pizza, and pasta, with two to three cans of beer each night. In addition to beer, he reports "a few shots of tequila" on the weekends. Physical activity is minimal beyond general daily activities. Larry M. denies abdominal pain, nausea, vomiting, epigastric tenderness, and fever. Lab results are as follows: TC 190 mg/dL, TGs 786 mg/dL, and HDL 44 mg/dL. The lab was drawn at 6:12 a.m.

Question: How should the lipid results be interpreted? What should be done next?

Discussion: The first action the clinician should take is to confirm with the patient that the lab result is indeed a fasting lipid profile. Often high TG values create unnecessary panic because the patient misunderstood directions and failed to fast. It is important for patients to realize that a fasting lipid panel requires abstaining from food and also beverages such as juice or coffee with sugar or cream. Larry M. confirms the lipids were drawn in the fasting state. An LDL value is unavailable since LDL can only be calculated with the Friedewald formula when TGs are less than 400 mg/dL and it is rarely directly measured.

Larry M. has very high TGs with a TG level greater than 500 mg/dL; therefore, TG lowering is the primary target of therapy. He has no physical signs or symptoms of pancreatitis. Though the risk of acute pancreatitis is greater when the TG level is greater than 1000 mg/dL, Larry M. should take immediate steps to reduce his risk. To prevent acute pancreatitis, TGs should be lowered through a very low-fat diet with ≤15% of caloric intake from fat, weight reduction, and increased physical activity. Larry M.'s current diet is high in saturated fat and carbohydrates. Abstention from all alcohol intake is important to minimize the risk of pancreatitis. Since diabetes is a common secondary cause of hypertriglyceridemia, a fasting glucose level should be obtained to determine if this is a factor in Larry M.'s case. Further, a TG-lowering drug, such as a fibrate, nicotinic acid, or omega-3 fatty acids, may also be considered. Bile acid sequestrants should be avoided as they may increase TGs. If Larry M. experiences epigastric pain or vomiting, it may be prudent to check amylase and lipase levels and proceed with further evaluation. Once TG levels have been lowered to less than 500 mg/dL, then attention can be turned to assessing LDL. Keep in mind that unless an institution has direct LDL measurements available, an indirect value cannot be calculated if TGs remain above 400 mg/dL.

SUMMARY

All adults, age 20 years or older, should have a fasting lipoprotein profile checked once every 5 years. The fasting lipid profile consists of TC, calculated LDL cholesterol, HDL cholesterol, and TGs. If total serum cholesterol, LDL cholesterol, and TGs are lowered and HDL is raised, death from CHD decreases. Additionally, hypertriglyceridemia increases the risk of pancreatitis. Dyslipidemia may be primary (genetic or familial) or secondary to other diseases or drugs. Measurement of the specific lipoproteins (LDL and HDL), which carry cholesterol and TGs, assists with diagnostic, prognostic, and therapeutic decisions. While lowering LDL is the primary goal of therapy, decreasing non-HDL is a secondary target of therapy, particularly in patients with elevated TGs. When diet and exercise fail to correct the lipid disorder, hypolipemic agents are used to impact the lipid profile.

BIBLIOGRAPHY

2010 ACCF/AHA guideline for assessment of cardiovascular risk in asymptomatic adults: a report of the American College of Cardiology Foundation/American Heart Association Task Force on Practice Guidelines. J Am Coll Cardiol. 2010;56:e50-103.

Duell PB, Illingworth DR, Connor WE, et al. Disorders of lipid metabolism. In: Felig P, Frohman LA, eds. Endocrinology & Metabolism. 4th ed. New York, NY: McGraw-Hill Health Professions Division; 2001:993-1075.

Executive Summary of The Third Report of The National Cholesterol Education Program (NCEP) Expert Panel on Detection, Evaluation, and Treatment of High Blood Cholesterol in Adults (Adult Treatment Panel III). JAMA. 2001;285:2486-2497.

Grundy SM, Cleeman JI, Mertz CNB, et al. Implications of recent clinical trials for the National Cholesterol Education Program Adult Treatment Panel III Guidelines. Circulation. 2004;110:227-239.

Rader DJ, Hobbs HH. Disorders of lipoprotein metabolism. In: Longo D, Fauci A, Kasper D, et al., eds. Harrison's Principles of Internal Medicine. 18th ed. New York, NY: McGraw-Hill; 2011:93-101.

Scolaro KL, Stamm PL, Lloyd KB. Devices for ambulatory and home monitoring of blood pressure, lipids, coagulation, and weight management, part 1. Am J Health Syst Pharm. 2005;62:1802-1812.

The Third Report of The National Cholesterol Education Program (NCEP) Expert Panel on Detection, Evaluation, and Treatment of High Blood Cholesterol In Adults (Adult Treatment Panel III). Circulation. 2002;106:3143-3421.

Learning Points

1. Who should receive cholesterol testing?

Answer: Starting at age 20, all adults should have a fasting lipoprotein profile at a minimum of every 5 years.[3] The lipoprotein profile includes TC, calculated LDL cholesterol, HDL cholesterol, and TGs. While it is reasonable to measure it once every 5 years in low-risk persons, more frequent checks are required for persons with multiple risk factors.[3] For persons with CHD or CHD risk-equivalents, the cholesterol testing should be repeated every year. Repeat testing is recommended at least every 2 years for those with two or more risk factors, or for those with one or fewer risk factors in whom the current LDL is only slightly below goal. For example, in a low-risk patient, more frequent testing is recommended if the LDL is less than 30 mg/dL below goal. Otherwise, followup every 5 years is suggested for the low-risk population.

2. If a lipid panel is drawn in the nonfasting state, which components of the lipid panel are clinically usable?

Answer: While it is recommended that patients avoid food and beverages with caloric content including juices, coffee with cream or sugar, and alcohol drinks for 12 hours prior to a lipid panel (TC, TGs, HDL, and calculated LDL), some components of the lipid profile are not significantly affected by food and drink.[3,37] The total serum cholesterol and HDL cholesterol levels are useable from a nonfasting lipid profile. The LDL cholesterol and TG levels are significantly affected by food and drink, with the level of variation depending on the fat and carbohydrate content of the meal. In patients at low-risk for cardiovascular disease with one risk factor or fewer, further testing is not required if TC is below 200 mg/dL and HDL cholesterol is above 40 mg/dL. However, a fasting lipid profile is required if persons at low-risk have values above these cut-points or for persons with multiple (two or more) cardiovascular risk factors.

3. Why was no LDL cholesterol measurement reported for a patient in whom a fasting lipid panel was ordered?

Answer: Typically, no LDL cholesterol value is reported when TGs exceed 400 mg/dL (4.52 mmol/L). Direct measurement of LDL is not commonly performed due to labor-intensive centrifugation. Instead, LDL cholesterol concentrations can be estimated indirectly by a method determined by Friedewald[51]: LDL = total serum cholesterol − HDL − (triglycerides/5). If a patient's serum TG concentration exceeds 400 mg/dL (4.5 mmol/L), LDL cholesterol cannot be calculated with this formula. A direct LDL measurement by laboratory would provide an LDL value. However, hypertriglyceridemia may cause variations in direct LDL cholesterol assays as well.[84] Further, since LDL cholesterol is not the primary target of therapy in patients with TGs in excess of 500 mg/dL, the LDL cholesterol value would provide little clinical utility.

REFERENCES

1. Roger VL, Go AS, Lloyd-Jones DM, et al. Heart disease and stroke statistics—2011 update: a report from the American Heart Association. *Circulation.* 2011;123:e18-e209.

2. McBride P, Schrott HG, Plane MB, et al. Primary care practice adherence to National Cholesterol Education Program guidelines for patients with coronary heart disease. *Arch Intern Med.* 1998;158:1238-1244.

3. The third report of the National Cholesterol Education Program (NCEP) expert panel on detection, evaluation, and treatment of high blood cholesterol in adults (Adult Treatment Panel III). *Circulation.* 2002;106:3143-3421.

4. Waters DD, Brotons C, Chiang CW, et al. Lipid treatment assessment project 2: a multinational survey to evaluate the proportion of patients achieving low-density lipoprotein cholesterol goals. *Circulation.* 2009;120:28-34.

5. Gotto AM. Management of dyslipidemia. *Am J Med.* 2002;112 Suppl 8A:10S-18S.

6. Grundy SM, Cleeman JI, Merz CN, et al. Implications of recent clinical trials for the National Cholesterol Education Program Adult Treatment Panel III guidelines. *Circulation.* 2004;110:227-239.

7. Duell PB, Illingworth DR, Connor WE. Disorders of lipid metabolism. In: Felig P, Frohman LA, eds. *Endocrinology and Metabolism.* 4th ed. New York, NY: The McGraw-Hill Companies Inc; 2001:993-1075.

8. Rader DJ, Hobbs HH. Disorders of lipoprotein metabolism. In: Longo DL, Fauci AS, Kasper DL, et al., eds. *Harrison's Principles of Internal Medicine.* 18th ed. New York, NY: The McGraw-Hill Companies Inc; 2012:3145-3161.

9. Jones PJ, Schoeller DA. Evidence for diurnal periodicity in human cholesterol synthesis. *J Lipid Res.* 1990;31:667-673.

10. Ginsberg HN. Lipoprotein physiology. *Endocrinol Metab Clin North Am.* 1998;27:503-519.

11. Scandinavian Simvastatin Survival Study Group. Randomised trial of cholesterol lowering in 4444 patients with coronary heart disease: the Scandinavian Simvastatin Survival Study (4S). *Lancet.* 1994;344:1383-1389.

12. The Long-Term Intervention with Pravastatin in Ischaemic Disease (LIPID) Study Group. Prevention of cardiovascular events and death with pravastatin in patients with coronary heart disease and a broad range of initial cholesterol levels. *N Engl J Med.* 1998;339:1349-1357.

13. Sacks FM, Pfeffer MA, Moye LA, et al. The effect of pravastatin on coronary events after myocardial infarction in patients with average cholesterol levels. *N Engl J Med.* 1996;335:1001-1009.

14. Cannon CP, Braunwald E, McCabe CH, et al. Intensive versus moderate lipid lowering with statins after acute coronary syndromes. *N Engl J Med.* 2004;350:1495-1504.

15. Miettinen TA, Pyörälä K, Olsson AG, et al. Cholesterol-lowering therapy in women and elderly patients with myocardial infarction or angina pectoris: findings from the Scandinavian Simvastatin Survival Study (4S). *Circulation.* 1997;96:4211-4218.

16. Shepherd J, Cobbe SM, Ford I, et al. Prevention of coronary heart disease with pravastatin in men with hypercholesterolemia. *N Engl J Med.* 1995;333:1301-1307.

17. Downs JR, Clearfield M, Weis S, et al. Primary prevention of acute coronary events with lovastatin in men and women with average cholesterol levels: results of AFCAPS/TexCAPS Air Force/Texas Coronary Atherosclerosis Prevention Study. *JAMA.* 1998;279:1615-1622.

18. Hachem SB, Mooradian AD. Familial dyslipidaemias: an overview of genetics, pathophysiology and management. *Drugs.* 2006;66:1949-1969.

19. Donahoo WT, Kosmiski LA, Eckel RH. Drugs causing dyslipoproteinemia. *Endocrinol Metab Clin North Am.* 1998;27:677-697.

20. Chaggar PS, Shaw SM, Williams SG. Effect of antipsychotic medications on glucose and lipid levels. *J Clin Pharmacol.* 2011;51:631-638.

21. Ross LA, Ross BS, East H. Dyslipidemia. In: Linn WD, Wofford MR, O'Keefe ME, et al., eds. *Pharmacotherapy in Primary Care.* New York, NY: The McGraw-Hill Companies Inc; 2009:91-102.

22. Mantel-Teeuwisse AK, Kloosterman JM, Maitland-van der Zee AH, et al. Drug-Induced lipid changes: a review of the unintended effects of some commonly used drugs on serum lipid levels. *Drug Saf.* 2001;24:443-456.

23. Henkin Y, Como JA, Oberman A. Secondary dyslipidemia. Inadvertent effects of drugs in clinical practice. *JAMA.* 1992;267:961-968.

24. Handelsman Y, Mechanick JI, Blonde L, et al. American Association of Clinical Endocrinologists Medical Guidelines for Clinical Practice for Developing a Diabetes Mellitus Comprehensive Care Plan. *Endocr Pract.* 2011;17(suppl 2):1-53.

25. Vaziri ND. Dyslipidemia of chronic renal failure: the nature, mechanisms, and potential consequences. *Am J Physiol Renal Physiol.* 2006;290:F262-F272.

26. Krone W, Nägele H. Effects of antihypertensives on plasma lipids and lipoprotein metabolism. *Am Heart J.* 1988;116:1729-1734.

27. Kasiske BL, Ma JZ, Kalil RS, et al. Effects of antihypertensive therapy on serum lipids. *Ann Intern Med.* 1995;122:133-141.

28. Lakshman MR, Reda DJ, Materson BJ, et al. Diuretics and beta-blockers do not have adverse effects at 1 year on plasma lipid and lipoprotein profiles in men with hypertension. Department of Veterans Affairs Cooperative Study Group on Antihypertensive Agents. *Arch Intern Med.* 1999;159:551-558.

29. Teichmann A. Metabolic profile of six oral contraceptives containing norgestimate, gestodene, and desogestrel. *Int J Fertil Menopausal Stud.* 1995;40(suppl 2):98-104.

30. Dubé MP, Cadden JJ. Lipid metabolism in treated HIV infection. *Best Pract Res Clin Endocrinol Metab.* 2011;25:429-442.

31. Stone NJ. Secondary causes of hyperlipidemia. *Med Clin North Am.* 1994;78:117-141.

32. Nordmann AJ, Nordmann A, Briel M, et al. Effects of low-carbohydrate vs low-fat diets on weight loss and cardiovascular risk factors: a meta-analysis of randomized controlled trials. *Arch Intern Med.* 2006;166:285-293.

33. Gaziano JM, Buring JE, Breslow JL, et al. Moderate alcohol intake, increased levels of high-density lipoprotein and its subfractions, and decreased risk of myocardial infarction. *N Engl J Med.* 1993;329:1829-1834.

34. Brinton EA. Effects of ethanol intake on lipoproteins and atherosclerosis. *Curr Opin Lipidol.* 2010;21:346-351.

35. Goldberg IJ, Mosca L, Piano MR, et al. Wine and your heart: a science advisory for healthcare professionals from the Nutrition Committee, Council on Epidemiology and Prevention, and Council on Cardiovascular Nursing of the American Heart Association. *Circulation.* 2001;103:472-475.

36. Executive Summary of the Third Report of The National Cholesterol Education Program (NCEP) Expert Panel on Detection, Evaluation, and Treatment of High Blood Cholesterol In Adults (Adult Treatment Panel III). *JAMA.* 2001;285:2486-2497.

37. Craig SR, Amin RV, Russell DW, et al. Blood cholesterol screening: influence of fasting state on cholesterol results and management decisions. *J Gen Intern Med.* 2000;15:395-399.

38. Expert Panel on Integrated Guidelines for Cardiovascular Health and Risk Reduction in Children and Adolescents. Expert panel on integrated guidelines for cardiovascular health and risk reduction in children and adolescents: summary report. *Pediatrics.* 2011;128 (suppl 5):S213-256.

39. Rifai N, Warnick GR, Remaley AT. Lipids, lipoproteins, apolipoproteins, and other cardiovascular risk factors. In: Burtis CA, Ashwood ER, Bruns DE, et al., eds. *Tietz Fundamentals of Clinical Chemistry.* 6th ed. St. Louis, MO: Saunders; 2008:402-430.

40. Myers GL, Cooper GR, Sampson EJ. Traditional lipoprotein profile: clinical utility, performance requirement, and standardization. *Atherosclerosis.*1994;108(suppl):S157-S169.

41. Faulkner MA, Hilleman DE, Destache CJ, et al. Potential influence of timing of low-density lipoprotein cholesterol evaluation in patients with acute coronary syndrome. *Pharmacotherapy.* 2001;21:1055-1060.

42. Spin JM, Vagelos RH. Early use of statins in acute coronary syndromes. *Curr Cardiol Rep.* 2002;4:289-297.

43. Henkin Y, Crystal E, Goldberg Y, et al. Usefulness of lipoprotein changes during acute coronary syndromes for predicting postdischarge lipoprotein levels. *Am J Cardiol.* 2002;89:7-11.

44. Grundy SM, Cleeman JI, Rifkind BM, et al. Cholesterol lowering in the elderly population. Coordinating Committee of the National Cholesterol Education Program. *Arch Intern Med.* 1999;159:1670-1678.

45. Jukema JW, Bruschke AV, van Boven AJ, et al. Effects of lipid lowering by pravastatin on progression and regression of coronary artery disease in symptomatic men with normal to moderately elevated serum cholesterol levels. The Regression Growth Evaluation Statin Study (REGRESS). *Circulation.* 1995;91:2528-2540.

46. Klag MJ, Ford DE, Mead LA, et al. Serum cholesterol in young men and subsequent cardiovascular disease. *N Engl J Med.* 1993;328:313-318.

47. Jacobson TA, Miller M, Schaefer EJ. Hypertriglyceridemia and cardiovascular risk reduction. *Clin Ther.* 2007;29:763-777.

48. Gotto AM. High-density lipoprotein cholesterol and triglycerides as therapeutic targets for preventing and treating coronary artery disease. *Am Heart J.* 2002;144(6 suppl):S33-S42.

49. Klotzsch SG, McNamara JR. Triglyceride measurements: a review of methods and interferences. *Clin Chem.* 1990;36:1605-1613.

50. Hulley SB, Newman TB. Cholesterol in the elderly. Is it important? *JAMA.* 1994;272:1372-1374.

51. Friedewald WT, Levy RI, Fredrickson DS. Estimation of the concentration of low-density lipoprotein cholesterol in plasma, without use of the preparative ultracentrifuge. *Clin Chem.* 1972;18:499-502.

52. American Diabetes Association. Standards of medical care in diabetes—2011. *Diabetes Care.* 2011;34(suppl 1):S11-S61.

53. Kwiterovich PO. The antiatherogenic role of high-density lipoprotein cholesterol. *Am J Cardiol.* 1998;82:13Q-21Q.

54. Rader DJ. Pathophysiology and management of low high-density lipoprotein cholesterol. *Am J Cardiol.* 1999;83:22F-24F.

55. Gordon DJ, Probstfield JL, Garrison RJ, et al. High-density lipoprotein cholesterol and cardiovascular disease. Four prospective American studies. *Circulation.* 1989;79:8-15.

56. Johansen O, Abdelnoor M, Brekke M, et al. Predictors of restenosis after coronary angioplasty. A study on demographic and metabolic variables. *Scand Cardiovasc J.* 2001;35:86-91.

57. Bennet AM, Di Angelantonio E, Ye Z, et al. Association of apolipoprotein E genotypes with lipid levels and coronary risk. *JAMA.* 2007;298:1300-1311.

58. El Harchaoui K, van der Steeg WA, Stroes ES, et al. Value of low-density lipoprotein particle number and size as predictors of coronary artery disease in apparently healthy men and women: the EPIC-Norfolk Prospective Population Study. *J Am Coll Cardiol.* 2007;49:547-553.

59. Greenland P, Alpert JS, Beller GA, et al. 2010 ACCF/AHA guideline for assessment of cardiovascular risk in asymptomatic adults: a report of the American College of Cardiology Foundation/American Heart Association Task Force on Practice Guidelines. *J Am Coll Cardiol.* 2010;56:e50-e103.

60. Ridker PM, Cannon CP, Morrow D, et al. C-reactive protein levels and outcomes after statin therapy. *N Engl J Med.* 2005;352:20-28.

61. Kaptoge S, Di Angelantonio E, Lowe G, et al. C-reactive protein concentration and risk of coronary heart disease, stroke, and mortality: an individual participant meta-analysis. *Lancet* 2010;375:132-140.

62. Ridker PM, Danielson E, Fonseca FA, et al. Rosuvastatin to prevent vascular events in men and women with elevated C-reactive protein. *N Engl J Med* 2008;359:2195-2207.

63. Ridker PM, Paynter NP, Rifai N, et al. C-reactive protein and parental history improve global cardiovascular risk prediction: the Reynolds Risk Score for men. *Circulation.* 2008;118:2243-2251.

64. Ridker PM, Buring JE, Rifai N, et al. Development and validation of improved algorithms for the assessment of global cardiovascular risk in women: the Reynolds Risk Score. *JAMA.* 2007;297:611-619.

65. Scolaro KL, Stamm PL, Lloyd KB. Devices for ambulatory and home monitoring of blood pressure, lipids, coagulation, and weight management, part 1. *Am J Health Syst Pharm.* 2005;62:1802-1812.

66. du Plessis M, Ubbink JB, Vermaak WJ. Analytical quality of near-patient blood cholesterol and glucose determinations. *Clin Chem.* 2000;46:1085-1090.

67. Livalo® (pitavastatin) [package insert]. Montgomery, AL: Kowa Pharmaceuticals America Inc; 2012.

68. Crestor® (rosuvastatin) [package insert]. Wilmington, DE: AstraZeneca Pharmaceuticals; 2012.

69. Garg A, Simha V. Update on dyslipidemia. *J Clin Endocrinol Metab.* 2007;92:1581-1589.

70. McKenney JM, Davidson MH, Jacobson TA, et al. Final conclusions and recommendations of the National Lipid Association Statin Safety Assessment Task Force. *Am J Cardiol.* 2006;97(suppl):89C-94C.

71. US Food and Drug Administration. FDA drug safety communication: important safety label changes to cholesterol-lowering statin drugs. Available at http://www.fda.gov/Drugs/DrugSafety/ucm293101.htm. Accessed July 17, 2012.

72. Hamilton-Craig I. Statin-associated myopathy. *Med J Aust.* 2001;175:486-489.

73. Zetia® (ezetimibe) [package insert]. Whitehouse Station, NJ: Merck & Co Inc; 2012.

74. Knopp RH. Drug treatment of lipid disorders. *N Engl J Med.* 1999;341:498-511.

75. Shakir KM, Kroll S, Aprill BS, et al. Nicotinic acid decreases serum thyroid hormone levels while maintaining a euthyroid state. *Mayo Clin Proc.* 1995;70:556-558.

76. Trilipix® (fenofibric acid) [package insert]. North Chicago, IL: Abbott Laboratories; 2011.

77. Backes JM, Gibson CA, Ruisinger JF, et al. Fibrates: what have we learned in the past 40 years? *Pharmacotherapy.* 2007;27:412-424.

78. Chatzizisis YS, Koskinas KC, Misirli G, et al. Risk factors and drug interactions predisposing to statin-induced myopathy: implications for risk assessment, prevention and treatment. *Drug Saf.* 2010;33:171-187.

79. Tricor® (fenofibrate) [package insert]. North Chicago, IL: Abbott Laboratories; 2011.

80. Lovaza® (omega-3 acid ethyl esters) [package insert]. Research Triangle Park, NC: GlaxoSmithKline; 2010.

81. McKenney JM, Sica D. Role of prescription omega-3 fatty acids in the treatment of hypertriglyceridemia. *Pharmacotherapy.* 2007;27:715-728.

82. Vascepa (icosapent ethyl) [package insert]. Bedminster, NJ: Amarin Pharma; 2012.

83. Bender NK, Kraynak MA, Chiquette E, et al. Effects of marine fish oils on the anticoagulation status of patients receiving chronic warfarin therapy. *J Thromb Thrombolysis.* 1998;5:257-261.

84. Faas FH, Earleywine A, Smith G, et al. How should low-density lipoprotein cholesterol concentration be determined? *J Fam Pract.* 2002;51:972-975.

QUICKVIEW | Serum Triglycerides

PARAMETER	DESCRIPTION	COMMENTS
Common reference ranges		
Adults	Desirable: <150 mg/dL	SI conversion factor: 0.01129 (mmol/L)
	Borderline high: 150–199 mg/dL	
	High: 200–499 mg/dL	
	Very high: >500 mg/dL	

Pediatrics	Acceptable:
	  0–9 yr: <75 mg/dL
	  10–19 yr: <90 mg/dL
	Borderline high:
	  0–9 yr: 75–99 mg/dL
	  10–19 yr: 90–129 mg/dL
	High:
	  0–9 yr: ≥100 mg/dL
	  10–19 yr: ≥130 mg/dL	

Critical value	500	High risk of pancreatitis
Inherent activity?	Intermediary for other active substances and stored energy in adipose tissue	Needed for formation of other lipids and fatty acids
Location		
Production	Liver and intestines	From ingested food
Storage	Adipose tissue	
Secretion/excretion	None	
Causes of abnormal values		
High	Excess fat intake	Tables 14-2 and 14-3
	Excess carbohydrate intake	Associated with obesity, diabetes, and metabolic syndrome
	Genetic defects	
	Drugs	
	Alcohol	
Low	Hypolipidemics	Statins, niacin, fibric acids, omega-3 fatty acids
	Lifestyle modifications	
Signs and symptoms		
High level	Pancreatitis	Increased risk of atherosclerotic vascular disease
	Eruptive xanthomas	
	Lipemia retinalis	
Low level	None	
After event, time to...		
Initial elevation	Days to weeks	Single meal has major effect on TG concentration within 2 hr
Peak values	Days to weeks	Increases with aging
Normalization	Days to weeks	After diet changes or drug treatment is started
Causes of spurious results	Glycerol, recent meal, alcohol, lipid emulsion	
Additional info	TGs are not the primary target of therapy unless TGs >500 mg/dL	

SI = International System of Units; TG = triglyceride.

QUICKVIEW | Total Cholesterol

PARAMETER	DESCRIPTION	COMMENTS
Common reference ranges		
Adults	Desirable: <200 mg/dL	SI conversion factor: 0.02586 (mmol/L)
	Borderline high: 200–239 mg/dL	
	High: ≥240 mg/dL	
Pediatrics	Acceptable: <170 mg/dL	
	Borderline high: 170–199 mg/dL	
	High: ≥200 mg/dL	
Critical value	Not acutely critical	Depends on risk factors, LDL, TG, and HDL
Inherent activity?	Intermediary for other active substances	Needed for cell wall, steroid, and bile acid production
Location		
Production	Liver and intestines	Ingested in diet
Storage	Lipoproteins	
Secretion/excretion	Excreted in bile	Also recycled to liver
Causes of abnormal values		
High	Diet high in saturated fats and cholesterol	Tables 14-2 and 14-3
	Genetic defects	
	Drugs	
Low	Hyperthyroidism	
	Liver disease	Statins, ezetimibe, niacin, fibric acids, bile acid sequestrants
	Hypolipidemics	
	Lifestyle modifications	
Signs and Symptoms		
High level	Atherosclerotic vascular disease	Angina, MI, stroke, peripheral vascular disease
	Tendon xanthomas	
Low level	None	Usually considered sign of good health
After insult, time to...		
Initial elevation	Days to weeks	Single meal has little effect on TC concentration
Peak values	Days to weeks	Can increase with aging; does not change acutely
Normalization	Weeks to months	After diet changes or drugs
Causes of spurious results	Prolonged tourniquet application	Causes venous stasis (increase 5% to 10%)
Additional Info	Not applicable	

LDL = low-density lipoprotein; HDL = high-density lipoprotein; MI = myocardial infarction; SI = International System of Units; TC = total cholesterol; TG = triglyceride.

QUICKVIEW | LDL Cholesterol

PARAMETER	DESCRIPTION	COMMENTS
Common reference ranges		
Adults	Optimal: <100 mg/dL	SI conversion factor: 0.02586 (mmol/L)
	Near or above optimal: 100–129 mg/dL	
	Borderline high: 130–159 mg/dL	
	High: 160–189 mg/dL	
	Very high: ≥190mg/dL	
Pediatrics	Acceptable: <110 mg/dL	
	Borderline high: 110–129 mg/dL	
	High: ≥130 mg/dL	
Critical Value	Not acutely critical	Depends on risk factors and CHD history
Inherent activity?	Intermediary for other active substances	Needed for cell wall, steroid, and bile acid production
Location		
Production	Liver and intestines	Ingested in diet
Storage	Lipoproteins	
Secretion/excretion	Excreted to bile	Also recycled to liver
Causes of abnormal values		
High	Diet high in saturated fats and cholesterol, genetic defects, hypothyroidism, nephrotic syndrome	Tables 14-2 and 14-3
Low	Drugs, hyperthyroidism, liver disease, hypolipidemics, lifestyle modifications	Table 14-3 Statins, ezetimibe, niacin, bile acid sequestrants
Signs and symptoms		
High level	Atherosclerotic vascular disease, tendon xanthomas	Angina, MI, stroke, peripheral vascular disease
Low level	None	Usually considered sign of good health
After event, time to...		
Initial elevation	Days to weeks	Single meal has little effect on cholesterol concentration; however, must be measured under fasting state
Peak values	Days to weeks	Can increase with aging; does not change acutely
Normalization	Weeks to months	After diet changes or medications
Causes of spurious results	Acute coronary syndrome	LDL levels decline within few hours of event and may remain low for several weeks
Additional info	LDL is the primary target of therapy	
	Indirect methods are typically used to calculate LDL cholesterol with the most common being the Friedewald equation:	
	LDL = total serum cholesterol – HDL – (triglycerides/5)	
	This equation cannot be used if the specimen is nonfasting, TG >400 mg/dL, or in patients with familial dysbetalipoproteinemia	

CHD = coronary heart disease; HDL = high-density lipoprotein; LDL = low-density lipoprotein; MI = myocardial infarction; SI = International System of Units; TG = triglyceride.

CHAPTER 15

HEMATOLOGY: RED AND WHITE BLOOD CELL TESTS

PAUL R. HUTSON, ASHLEY M. JOHNSON

Objectives

After completing this chapter, the reader should be able to

- Describe the physiology of blood cell development and bone marrow function

- Discuss the interpretation and alterations of hemoglobin (Hgb), hematocrit (Hct), and various red blood cell (RBC) indices in the evaluation of macrocytic; microcytic; and normochromic, normocytic anemias

- Describe the significance of abnormal erythrocyte morphology, including sickling, anisocytosis, and nucleated erythrocytes

- Name the different types of leukocytes and describe their primary functions

- Calculate the absolute number of various types of leukocytes from the white blood cell (WBC) count and differential

- Interpret alterations in the WBC count, differential, and CD4 lymphocyte count in acute bacterial infections, parasitic infections, and human immunodeficiency virus (HIV) infection

- Identify potential causes of neutrophilia

- Identify how leukocyte CD phenotypes are used for antitumor drug selection

This chapter reviews the basic functions and expected laboratory values of erythrocytes and leukocytes. It also discusses, in an introductory manner, selected disorders of these two cellular components of blood. It must be remembered that the ability of laboratory medicine to discriminate between leukocytes is increasing, and many methods considered investigational in this edition may become a routine component of blood examination in the future.

PHYSIOLOGY OF BLOOD CELLS AND BONE MARROW

The cellular components of blood are derived from pluripotential stem cells located in the bone marrow that can differentiate into red and white blood cells (RBCs, WBCs), as well as megakaryocytes, which produce platelets (Figure 15-1). *Bone marrow* is a highly structured and metabolically active organ of both the hematopoietic and reticuloendothelial systems. It normally produces 2.5 billion RBCs, 1 billion granulocytes, and 2.5 billion platelets/kg of body weight daily.[1] Production can vary greatly, from nearly zero to 5 to 10 times normal. Usually, however, levels of circulating cells remain in a relatively narrow range.[2]

In the fetus and children, blood cell formation or hematopoiesis occurs in the marrow of virtually all bones. With maturation, the task of hematopoiesis shifts to flat bones of the axial skeleton such as the cranium, ribs, pelvis, and vertebrae. The long bones, such as the femur and humerus, do not produce a large amount of blood cells in adulthood as the marrow is gradually replaced by fatty tissue. Radiation directed to large portions of hematopoietic bones can lead to deficient hematopoiesis in patients treated for cancerous lesions. Similarly, preparation for a bone marrow transplant will often include total body irradiation (TBI) to destroy the hematopoietic cells of the recipient in the bone, spleen, and other sites so that the grafted cells will not be destroyed by residual host defenses.

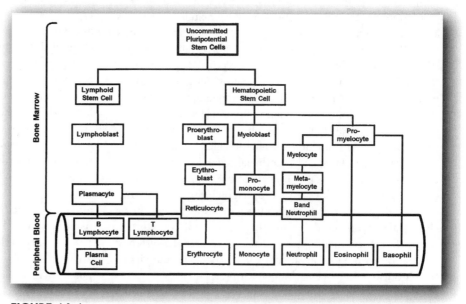

FIGURE 14-1. Schematic diagram of hematopoiesis.

Although the majority of hematopoiesis occurs in the marrow, modern methods of identifying cellular characteristics have demonstrated that pluripotential cells—identified by a cellular expression of the surface marker CD34—also normally circulate in the blood.[3,4]

Although the majority of this chapter discusses laboratory analysis of blood obtained from the vein (peripheral venipuncture), an analysis of the bone marrow itself may be needed to diagnose or monitor various disease states, most commonly the leukemias discussed later in the chapter. Bone marrow specimens are usually obtained from the posterior iliac crest of the pelvis or, less commonly because of increased risk, from the sternum. Bone marrow sampling can involve an aspirate, a core biopsy, or both. After penetrating the bone cortex with the bone marrow needle and entering the medullary cavity inside the bone containing the marrow, a heparinized syringe is attached to the needle and 1–2 mL of bone marrow is aspirated. The contents of the syringe are smeared on a series of slides that are stained and examined microscopically. If special studies such as flow cytometry or cytogenetics are requested, additional heparinized syringes are aspirated and submitted to the laboratory. The bone marrow biopsy is obtained with the same needle by advancing it further past the site of aspiration through the bone marrow to cut a sample of the bone marrow matrix for removal and examination. The biopsy provides the advantage of examining the structure of the marrow stroma, as well as the spatial relationship of the various hematopoietic cells.[5]

Blood stem cells become increasingly differentiated in the bone marrow until they are committed to develop further into erythrocytes, platelets, or various leukocytes (Figure 15-1). Many regulatory proteins are involved in the differentiation and proliferation phases of hematopoiesis, but their functions and interrelationships are not yet fully understood. In addition to the colony-stimulating factors mentioned above, proteins that stimulate hematopoiesis include erythropoietin, thrombopoietin, and various interleukins. Inhibitors of hematopoiesis are not as well-defined but include interferons and lymphotoxins. In considering the response of neutrophils or erythrocytes to exogenously administered hematopoietic stimulants (e.g., filgrastim or erythropoietin), it is important to recall that normal physiologic hematopoietic regulation is more complex than the effect of one therapeutic protein would suggest. White blood cell formation involves local production of a combination of signaling proteins by cells of the hematopoietic microenvironment (e.g., macrophages, T lymphocytes, osteoblasts, fibroblasts, and endothelial cells). Leucocyte-stimulating proteins such as granulocyte colony-stimulating factor (G-CSF) and granulocyte-macrophage colony-stimulating factor (GM-CSF) are normally directed toward adjacent or closely approximated differentiating hematopoietic cells.[4] In contrast, erythropoietin is formed and released to the systemic circulation by the kidney, affecting erythrocyte precursors in the blood-forming areas of bone marrow.

Committed blood precursor cells undergo further differentiation in the bone marrow until they develop into mature cells. These developmental stages can be identified by differing morphological or immunochemical staining characteristics. These same imaging techniques are used to identify the developmental phenotype of the cancerous white cells of leukemia and lymphoma. Generally, only mature cellular forms are found in the circulating blood, and it is from this blood that clinical specimens are usually taken. As discussed below, the presence of immature forms of white or red cells in the blood typically indicates the presence of a pathologic process.

COMPLETE BLOOD COUNT

The *complete blood count (CBC)* is a frequently ordered laboratory test. It supplies useful information regarding the concentration of the different cellular and noncellular elements of blood and applies to multiple disorders. Complete blood count is a misnomer because concentrations of cells/μL, not counts, are measured and reported. Functionally, the CBC can be thought of as a complete blood analysis because a series of tests are performed. Moreover, information besides concentrations is reported.

Most clinical laboratories utilize automated hematology analyzers to determine the CBC. Results are usually accurate, reproducible, and rapidly obtained. Numerous measured and calculated values are included in a CBC (Table 15-1). These results traditionally include

- Leukocyte (WBC) count
- Erythrocyte (RBC) count
- Hgb
- Hct
- RBC indices (mean corpuscular volume [MCV], mean corpuscular hemoglobin concentration [MCHC]), and RBC distribution width (RDW)—the RBC indices are also commonly referred to as *Wintrobe indices*
- Platelet count and mean platelet volume (MPV)
- Reticulocyte count

When a "CBC with differential" is ordered, the various types of WBCs are also analyzed (White Blood Cell Count and Differential section). The reliability of the results can be doubtful if (1) the integrity of the specimen is questionable (inappropriate handling or storage), or (2) the specimen contains substances that interfere with the automated analysis. Grossly erroneous results are usually flagged for verification by another method. Manual microscopic review of the blood smear is used to resolve unusual automated results.[1]

Mature erythrocytes have a median lifespan of 120 days under normal conditions. They are removed from the circulation by macrophages in the spleen and other reticuloendothelial organs. The erythrocytes are tested for flexibility, size, and integrity in these organs as the cells pass through areas of osmotic, pH, or hypoxic stress.[6]

Variability in the size of red cells is termed *anisocytosis*, and any variation in the normal biconcave disc shape is termed *poikilocytosis*. Such abnormalities are seen with iron deficiency or periods of increased erythrocyte production and/or red cell damage.[7]

TABLE 15-1. Reference Ranges and Interpretative Comments for Common Hematological Tests (Typical CBC)[a]

TEST NAME	RANGE[a] REFERENCE	SI UNITS	COMMENTS
RBC	Males: 4.5–5.9 × 10⁶ cells/μl Females: 4.1–5.1 × 10⁶ cells/μl	4.5–5.9×10^{12} cells/L 4.1–5.1×10^{12} cells/L	
Hgb	Males: 14–17.5 g/dL Females: 12.3–15.3 g/dL	140–175 g/L 123–153 g/L	Amount of Hgb in given volume of whole blood; indication of oxygen-transport capacity of blood; falsely elevated in hyperlipidemia
Hct	Males: 42% to 50% Females: 36% to 45%	0.42–0.50 0.36–0.45	Percentage volume of blood comprised of erythrocytes; usually approximately 3 times Hgb
MCV	80–96 fL/cell	80–96 fL/cell	Hct/RBC: increased in vitamin B_{12} and folate deficiency, reticulocytosis, myelodysplastic anemia, falsely elevated in hyperglycemia; decreased in iron deficiency, and mild thalassemias
MCHC	33.4–35.5 g/dL	334–355 g/L	Hgb/Hct: amount of Hgb in terms of percentage volume of cell; increased in hereditary spherocytosis, falsely increased in hyperlipidemia and cold agglutinins; decreased in iron deficiency
Reticulocyte count	0.5% to 2.5% of RBCs	0.005–0.025	Immature RBCs; increased in acute blood loss and hemolysis; decreased in untreated iron, vitamin B_{12}, and folate deficiency
RDW	11.5% to 14.5%	0.115–0.145	Measure of variation in red cell volumes (anisocytosis): the larger the width percent, the greater the variation in size of red cells; increased in early iron deficiency anemia and mixed anemias
WBC count	4.4–11.3 × 10³ cells/μL	4.4–11.3×10^9 cells/L	Elevated by neutrophil demargination with exercise, glucocorticoids, epinephrine; decreased with cold agglutinins
Platelet count	150,000–450,000 cells/μL	150–450×10^9 cells/L	Falsely elevated in presence of red cell fragments and microcytic erythrocytes; decreased in presence of large numbers of giant platelets and platelet clumps
MPV	6.8–10.0 fL	6.8–10.0 fL	

Hct = hematocrit; Hgb = hemoglobin; MCHC = mean corpuscular hemoglobin concentration; MCV = mean corpuscular volume; MPV = mean platelet volume; RBC = red blood cell; RDW = RBC distribution width; WBC = white blood cell.
[a]Modified from references 8 and 9.

Red Blood Cell Count

Normal adult range:
males: 4.5–5.9 × 10⁶ cells/μL or 4.5–5.9 × 10¹² cells/L;
females: 4.1–5.1 × 10⁶ cells/μL or 4.1–5.1 × 10¹² cells/L
The *red blood cell (RBC) count* is the number of red corpuscles in a given volume of blood. The International Unit for reporting blood cells is for a 1-liter volume, but it is still common to see values reported in cells/microliter (μL) or less commonly in cells/cubic millimeter (mm³). After puberty, females have slightly lower counts (and Hgb) than men, partly because of their menstrual blood loss and because of higher concentrations of androgen (an erythropoietic stimulant) in men. The RBC count in all anemias is by definition below the normal range. This decrease causes a proportionate decrease in Hct and Hgb.

The *reticulocyte* is the cell form that precedes the mature RBC or erythrocyte. During the entire maturation process, Hgb is produced, gradually filling the cytoplasm. The reticulocyte does not contain a nucleus but possesses nucleic acids that can be considered remnants of the nucleus or endoplasmic reticulum. The mature erythrocyte contains neither an organized nucleus nor nucleic acids. Reticulocytes persist in the circulation for 1–2 days before maturing into erythrocytes.[2]

White Blood Cell Count

Normal range: 4.4–11.0 × 10³ cells/mm³ or
4.4–11.0 × 10⁹ cells/L
The *WBC count* is an actual count of the number of leukocytes in a given volume of blood. Unlike RBCs, leukocytes have a nucleus and normally represent five different mature cell types. The various percentages of the five mature and WBC types comprise the WBC differential, which is discussed later in this chapter.

Hemoglobin

Normal range: males: 14–17.5 g/dL or 140–175 g/L;
females: 12.3–15.3 g/dL or 123–153 g/L
The *hemoglobin (Hgb)* value is the amount of this metalloporphyrin-protein contained in a given volume (100 mL or 1 L) of whole blood. The Hgb concentration provides a direct

indication of the oxygen-transport capacity of the blood. As the major content of the RBCs, Hgb is proportionately low in patients with anemia.

Hematocrit

Normal range: males: 42% to 50% or 0.42–0.50;
females: 36% to 45% or 0.36–0.45

Hematocrit (Hct) is the percentage volume of blood that is composed of erythrocytes. It is also known as the *packed cell volume*. To manually perform the Hct test, a blood-filled capillary tube is centrifuged to settle the erythrocytes. Then, the percentage volume of the tube that is composed of erythrocytes is calculated.[5] The Hct is usually about 3 times the value of the Hgb, but disproportion can occur when cells are substantially abnormal in size or shape. Like Hgb, Hct is low in patients with anemia.

Red Blood Cell Indices

Because the following laboratory tests specifically assess RBC characteristics, they are called *RBC indices*. These indices are useful in the evaluation of anemias, polycythemia, and nutritional disorders. Essentially, they assess the size and Hgb content of the RBC. The MCV is measured directly while the MCHC and mean corpuscular hemoglobin (MCH) are calculated from the Hgb, MCV, and RBC count using predetermined formulas. Due to its dependence on cell size, MCH is not used clinically, but rather the MCHC is used to assess RBCs for their Hgb concentration and color.

Mean Corpuscular Volume

Normal range: 80–96 fL/cell

The *mean corpuscular volume (MCV)* is an estimate of the average volume of RBCs and is the most clinically useful of the RBC indices. It can be calculated by dividing the Hct by the RBC count, but it is ordinarily determined by averaging the directly measured size of thousands of RBCs.

Abnormally large cells have an increased MCV and are called *macrocytic*. Vitamin B_{12} and/or folate deficiency cause the formation of macrocytic erythrocytes, which corresponds to a true increase in MCV. In contrast, a false increase in MCV may be observed when a patient has reticulocytosis, an increase in the number of reticulocytes in the peripheral blood, since reticulocytes are larger than mature erythrocytes.[5] The MCV may also be falsely increased in hyperglycemia due to osmotic expansion of the erythrocyte. When erythrocytes are mixed with diluting fluid to perform the test, the cells swell because the diluent is relatively hypotonic compared to the patient's hyperglycemic blood. Abnormally small cells (with a decreased MCV) are called *microcytic*. A decrease in the MCV implies some abnormality in Hgb synthesis. The most common cause of microcytic erythrocytes (microcytosis) is iron deficiency.[8]

Mean Corpuscular Hemoglobin Concentration

Normal range: 33.4–35.5 g/dL or 334–355 g/L

The *mean corpuscular hemoglobin concentration (MCHC)* is the Hgb divided by the Hct. As mentioned previously, this calculation is usually around 33 g/dL (330 g/L) because the Hct is usually 3 times the Hgb. Iron deficiency is the only anemia

in which the MCHC is *routinely* low, although it can also be decreased in other disorders of Hgb synthesis.[8,9] In this case, RBCs are described as hypochromic (pale). It can be falsely elevated in hyperlipidemia. It must be considered that the Wintrobe indices are averages for the patient's blood and that normal values may be reported by automated methods even in the presence of a mixed (normal + abnormal) erythrocyte population.

Red Blood Cell Distribution Width

Normal range: 11.5% to 14.5% or 0.115–0.145

The *RBC distribution width (RDW)* is an indication of the variation in red cell size, termed *anisocytosis*.[8] The RDW is reported as the coefficient of variation of the MCV (standard deviation/mean value). This value is used primarily with other tests to differentiate iron deficiency anemia from thalassemias. The RDW increases in macrocytic anemias and in early iron deficiency, often before other tests show signs of this kind of anemia. However, it is not specific for iron deficiency anemia. Mild forms of thalassemia often are microcytic but have a normal or only slightly elevated RDW.

Reticulocyte Count

Normal range: 0.5% to 2.5% of RBCs or 0.005–0.025

In anemia, the *reticulocyte count* or *reticulocyte index (RI)* reflects not only the level of bone marrow production but also a decline in the total number of mature erythrocytes that normally dilute the reticulocytes. Therefore, the reticulocyte count would double in a person whose bone marrow production is unchanged, but whose Hct has fallen from 46% to 23%. The RI was used with hand-counting methods to correct for a low Hct, but it is not necessary with modern, automated cell counters.[11]

In persons with anemia secondary to *acute* blood loss or hemolysis, even the corrected reticulocyte count is increased.[6] This increase reflects an attempt by the bone marrow to compensate for the lack of circulating erythrocytes. Because RBC production is increased to far above basal activity, more reticulocytes escape into the circulation earlier than normal. In contrast, persons with *untreated* anemia secondary to iron, folate, or vitamin B_{12} deficiency are unable to increase their reticulocyte count appropriate to the degree of their anemia. Similarly, appropriate treatment of an anemia should be accompanied by an increase in the reticulocyte count.

The reticulocyte count can be useful in identifying drug-induced bone marrow suppression in which the percentage of circulating reticulocytes should be close to zero. It can also be used to monitor an anemic patient's response to vitamin or iron therapy. In such patients, supplementation of the lacking factor causes rapid (5–7 days) elevation of the reticulocyte count.

ERYTHROCYTE SEDIMENTATION RATE

Normal range: males: 1–15 mm/hr; females: 1–20 mm/hr (increases with age)

Numerous physiological and disease states are associated with the rate at which erythrocytes settle from blood, termed the

TABLE 15-2. Conditions That May Alter ESR

INCREASED ESR	DECREASED ESR
Advanced age	Carcinoma
Female sex	Congestive heart failure
Infection	Corticosteroids
Macrocytic anemia	Liver disease
Multiple myeloma	Microcytic anemia
Normocytic anemia	Sickle cell anemia
Pregnancy	
Rheumatoid arthritis	

ESR = erythrocyte sedimentation rate.

erythrocyte sedimentation rate (ESR). Erythrocytes normally settle slowly in plasma but settle rapidly when they aggregate because of electrostatic forces. Each cell normally has a net negative charge and repels other erythrocytes because like charges repel each other. Many plasma proteins are positively charged and are attracted to the surface charge of one or more erythrocytes, thereby promoting erythrocyte aggregation.[12] Nonmicrocytic anemia, pregnancy, multiple myeloma, and various inflammatory diseases (including infections) can elevate the ESR (Table 15-2). Sickle cell disease, high doses of corticosteroids, liver disease, microcytosis, carcinomas, and congestive heart failure can decrease the ESR.[8]

Although the ESR may be used to confirm a diagnosis supported by other tests, it is rarely used alone for a specific diagnosis. Rather, the ESR is useful for monitoring the activity of inflammatory conditions (e.g., temporal arteritis, polymyalgia rheumatica, rheumatoid arthritis, and osteomyelitis).[12] The ESR is often higher when the disease is active due to increased amounts of circulating proteins, termed *acute phase reactants* (e.g., fibrinogen), and falls when the intensity of the disease decreases.

The ESR is usually measured using either the Wintrobe or the Westergren method. Anticoagulated blood is diluted and placed in a perfectly vertical glass tube of standard size. After 1 hour, the distance from the plasma meniscus down to the top of the erythrocyte column is recorded as the ESR in millimeters per hour.[12] A corrected sedimentation rate, called the *zeta-sedimentation rate* or *ratio*, has been developed to eliminate the effect of anemia on the ESR.[13] This value is called the *zetacrit*, and its normal range is 40% to 52%.[8] Elevations above the normal range are interpreted in the same manner as an elevated ESR by traditional methods.

PLATELET COUNT AND MEAN PLATELET VOLUME

Normal ranges: 150,000–450,000 cells/μL
The *platelet count,* often included routinely in the CBC with differential, is discussed with other coagulation tests in Chapter 16: Hematology: Blood Coagulation Tests.

LABORATORY ASSESSMENT OF ANEMIA

The functions of the erythrocyte are to transport and protect Hgb, the molecule used for oxygen and carbon dioxide transport. *Anemia* can be caused as a decrease in either the HCT or the Hgb concentration below the normal range for age and gender. Anemia is not a disease in itself but one manifestation of an underlying disease process. Appropriate treatment of the anemic patient depends on the exact cause of the condition. Signs and symptoms of anemia depend on its severity and the

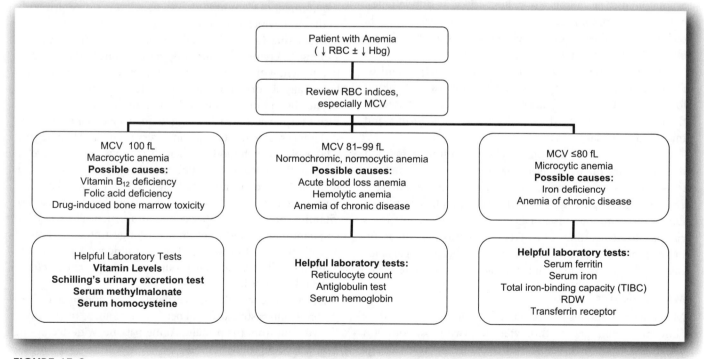

FIGURE 15-2. Use of erythrocyte morphology in differential diagnosis of anemia.

TABLE 15-3. Qualitative Laboratory Findings for Various Types of Anemia[a]

	VITAMIN B$_{12}$ DEFICIENCY	FOLATE DEFICIENCY	IRON DEFICIENCY	ACUTE BLOOD LOSS	HEMOLYTIC ANEMIA	ANEMIA OF CHRONIC DISEASE
RBC	↓	↓	↓	↓	↓	↓
Hgb	↓	↓	↓	↓	↓	↓
Hct	↓	↓	↓	↓	↓	↓
MCV	↑	↑	↓	↔	↔	↔↓
MCHC	↔	↔	↔	↔		↔↓
RDW	↑	↑	↑	↔	↔	↔
Reticulocyte count	↓	↓	↑	↑	↑	↔↓
Serum vitamin B$_{12}$	↓	↔				
Serum folate	↔	↓				
Serum methylmalonate	↑	↔				
Serum homocysteine	↑	↑				
Ferritin			↓			↔
Serum iron			↓			↓
TIBC			↑			↓
Serum haptoglobin					↓	
Plasma hemoglobin					↑	
Autoantibodies[b]					+	

Hct = hematocrit; Hgb = hemoglobin; MCHC = mean corpuscular hemoglobin concentration; MCV = mean corpuscular volume; RBC = red blood cell; RDW = RBC distribution width; TIBC = total iron-binding capacity.
[a]Some tests with no change (↔) are left empty for clarity.
[b]Autoantibodies positive for antibody-mediated immune hemolysis.

rapidity with which it has developed. Severe, acute blood loss results in more dramatic symptoms than an anemia that took months to develop because with chronic loss some compensatory adaptation may occur. Patients with mild anemia are often asymptomatic (i.e., absence of pallor, weakness, and fatigue), but severely symptomatic patients manifest shortness of breath, tachycardia, and palpitations even at rest. This contrast should be kept in mind when interpreting test results.

Anemia can be caused by decreased production and/or increased destruction of erythrocytes as well as acute blood loss. The first two situations can often be differentiated by the reticulocyte count, which is decreased in the former and increased in the latter.

Use of erythrocyte morphology is one common method to characterize the possible etiology of anemia. This method is useful because different causes of anemia lead to different erythrocyte morphology. Figure 15-2 outlines this approach. Only a few common causes of anemia are included, but others can fit into this outline. Other laboratory tests that are useful in differentiating the anemias are described below. Usual laboratory findings are also included in each section (Table 15-3).

Macrocytic Anemia

Macrocytic anemia is a lowered Hgb value characterized by abnormally enlarged erythrocytes. The two most common causes are vitamin B$_{12}$ and/or folic acid deficiencies. Drugs that cause macrocytic anemia mainly interfere with proper

utilization, absorption, and metabolism of these vitamins (Table 15-4).

Vitamin B$_{12}$ Deficiency

Vitamin B$_{12}$ is also known as *cobalamin*. The normal daily requirement of vitamin B$_{12}$ is 2–5 mcg.[14] It is stored primarily in the liver, which contains approximately 1 mcg of vitamin/g of liver tissue. Overall, the body has B$_{12}$ stores of approximately 2–5 mg. Therefore, if vitamin B$_{12}$ absorption suddenly ceased in a patient with normal liver stores, several years would pass before any abnormalities occurred due to vitamin deficiency.

The absorption of vitamin B$_{12}$ is complex, and the mechanisms responsible are still being defined. Cobalamin (vitamin B$_{12}$) is ingested in meats, eggs, and dairy products. Strict vegans, who avoid all such foods in their diet, may over time develop vitamin B$_{12}$ deficiency if supplements are not ingested. Some forms of B$_{12}$, such as those made by the blue–green algae *Spirulina*, are active vitamins in bacterial assays but are not active vitamins for humans. Other cobamides structurally related to cobalamin are found in plasma after ingesting other animal and plant-based foods. Only the cobamide with an attached 5,6-dimethylbenzimidazole group is correctly termed *cobalamin* and is active in humans.[14]

Dietary B$_{12}$ or cobalamin is usually bound nonspecifically to proteins, and gastric acid and pepsin are required to hydrolyze the vitamin from the protein. Aging patients with decreasing stomach acid production may be less able to free vitamin B$_{12}$ from meat protein. Freed B$_{12}$ is bound with very high affinity to protein R, which is a large protein secreted in saliva. The cobalamin-protein R complex moves to the duodenum where pancreatic proteases denature protein R and allow the freed vitamin to bind to intrinsic factor, which is secreted in the stomach and is resistant to the intestinal proteases. Patients may develop autoantibodies to intrinsic factor, and, thereby, develop vitamin B$_{12}$ deficiency. The cobalamin-intrinsic factor complex is transported into the ileal epithelium and dissociates, and the cobalamin enters the circulation on the basolateral side of the cell bound to transcobalamin, which is largely homologous with intrinsic factor. Clearly, there are several steps in the absorption of vitamin B$_{12}$ that may be responsible for a deficiency.

A deficiency of cobalamin (vitamin B$_{12}$) may arise from inadequate intake of the vitamin, or a deficiency of the intrinsic factor required for the effective ileal absorption of the vitamin. Inadequate dietary intake is a rare cause of vitamin B$_{12}$ deficiency, usually occurring only in vegans who abstain from all animal food including milk and eggs.[14] On the other hand, defective production of intrinsic factor is a common cause of the deficiency.[16] The gastric mucosa can fail to secrete intrinsic factor because of atrophy, especially in the elderly.

Clinical and laboratory diagnosis. Vitamin B$_{12}$ is necessary for deoxyribonucleic acid (DNA) synthesis in all cells, for the synthesis of neurotransmitters, and for metabolism of homocysteine. Therefore B$_{12}$ deficiency leads to signs and symptoms involving many organ systems.[14,15] The most notable symptoms involve

- Gastrointestinal (GI) tract (e.g., loss of appetite, smooth and/or sore tongue, and diarrhea or constipation)
- Central nervous system (CNS) (e.g., paresthesias in fingers and toes, loss of coordination of legs and feet, tremors, irritability, somnolence, and abnormalities of taste and smell)
- Hematopoietic system (anemia)

Nuclear maturation retardation occurs in the developing cells in the bone marrow due to slowed DNA synthesis. The morphological result is cells with immature enlarged nuclei (megaloblasts) but cytoplasm that matures normally, resulting in mature cells larger than normal. The resulting anemia is called a *macrocytic, megaloblastic* (both morphological characteristics of nuclear maturation retardation) *anemia.*[15] Visual inspection of smears of both peripheral blood and bone marrow reveals characteristic megaloblastic changes in the appearance of erythrocytes (oval macrocytes) and WBCs. The development of neutrophils is also affected, resulting in large cells with hypersegmentation (>3 nuclear lobes). A mild pancytopenia—decreased numbers of all blood elements—also occurs. The usual laboratory test results found with vitamin B$_{12}$ deficiency are listed in Table 15-3.

Serum cobalamin (vitamin B$_{12}$) concentrations were in the past measured using a microbiologic assay and a cobalamin-dependent organism. This methodology assay has largely been replaced by a competitive displacement assay using radioactive cobalamin and intrinsic factor. Unfortunately, because of cross-reactivity with other cobamides, approximately 5% of patients will have cobalamin concentrations that appear to be within the normal range yet can be shown to have hematologic and/or neurologic signs of deficiency. There is increasing acceptance of the use of serum levels of the metabolic intermediates homocysteine and methylmalonate as more sensitive indicators of cobalamin deficiency. In the presence of inadequate cobalamin, these two compounds accumulate because of the cobalamin-dependence of their metabolizing enzymes, methionine synthase, and methylmalonyl-CoA-mutase, respectively. An elevated serum methylmalonate and plasma homocysteine concentration in the presence of normal RBC folate is strongly indicative of a pure deficiency of cobalamin.

Historically, the Schilling test was used to determine if impaired absorption is the reason for the cobalamin deficiency. In the Schilling test, cyano-(^{57}Co)-cobalamin is administered orally and is allowed to be absorbed, if possible. An unlabelled, intravenous (IV) injection of cobalamin follows and will displace some of the absorbed radioactive ^{57}Co-cobalamin from circulating transcobalamin, which is excreted and measured in the urine. If oral absorption is normal (e.g., the deficiency was caused by inadequate dietary intake), >8% of the radioactive cobalamin will be excreted in the urine. If abnormal, the test can be repeated at a later date (stage II test), adding exogenous intrinsic factor to the dose of oral labeled cyano(^{57}Co)-cobalamin to determine if inadequate urinary excretion secondary to poor absorption was due to a relative lack of the protein.[15] The availability of intramuscular injections of vitamin B$_{12}$ obviates the need to specify the defect in B$_{12}$ absorption and are favored in patients with impaired cobalamin absorption, regardless of the cause. Oral cobalamin can also be used in most patients with intrinsic factor deficiency, but regular monitoring is required to ensure efficacy and adherence to dosing. The availability of cobalamin supplementation and the complexity of the procurement and disposal of radioactive tracers discourage the use of the Schilling test.[15]

Folic Acid Deficiency

Folic acid is also called *pteroylglutamic acid.* Folates refer to folic acid or reduced forms of folic acid that may have variable numbers of glutamic acid residues attached to the folic acid molecule. The folates present in food are mainly in a polyglutamic acid form and must be hydrolyzed in the intestine to the monoglutamate form to be absorbed efficiently. The liver is the chief storage site. Adult daily requirements are approximately 50 mcg of folic acid, equivalent to about 400 mcg of food folates. Folate stores are limited, and anemia arising from a folate-deficient diet occurs in 4–5 months.[14]

Inadequate dietary intake is the major cause of deficiency. Folates are found in green, leafy vegetables such as spinach, lettuce, and broccoli. Inadequate intake can have numerous causes: alcoholics classically have poor nutritional intake of folic acid; certain physiological states such as pregnancy require an increase in folic acid; malabsorption syndromes (mentioned in the section on vitamin B$_{12}$) can also lead to defective absorption of folic acid; and celiac sprue can lead to folate malabsorption.[17]

TABLE 15-4. Examples of Causes of Drug-Induced Macrocytic Anemia[20]

Marrow toxicity and interference with folate metabolism
Alcohol
Marrow toxicity
Antineoplastic Agents
Zidovudine
Altered folate absorption
Phenytoin
Altered folate metabolism
Primidone, Phenobarbital
Methotrexate
Oral contraceptives
Pentamidine
Sulfasalazine
Sulfamethoxazole
Triamterene
Trimethoprim
Vitamin B$_{12}$ malabsorption
Proton pump inhibitors
Metformin
Colchicine
Neomycin
Para-aminosalicylic acid
Vitamin B$_{12}$ inactivation
Nitrous oxide

Certain medications (e.g., methotrexate, trimethoprim-sulfamethoxazole, and triamterene) can act as folic acid antagonists by interfering with the conversion of folic acid into its metabolically active form, tetrahydrofolic acid. Phenytoin and phenobarbital administration can interfere with the intestinal absorption or utilization of folic acid (see Table 15-4).[19]

Folic acid is required as the intermediate for one-carbon transfers in several biochemical pathways. After absorption, folate is reduced to tetrahydrofolate, and a carbon in one of several oxidation states is attached for transfer. Most transfer processes allow facile regeneration, but the majority of folate circulates as 5-methyl-tetrahydrofolate. Vitamin B$_{12}$ is required as a cofactor for the removal of the 5-methyl group to regenerate tetrahydrofolate, and in this step methionine is formed from homocysteine. A deficiency of vitamin B$_{12}$ will therefore lead to an accumulation of 5-methyl-tetrahydrofolate at the expense of other functional folate forms (the "folate trap"). Increased supplementation with folic acid cannot overcome the inability of a vitamin B$_{12}$-deficient human to form methionine from homocysteine, leading to neurologic and vascular toxicities from insufficient methionine and excessive homocysteine.

Clinical and laboratory diagnosis. Since folic acid is necessary for DNA synthesis, a deficiency causes maturation retardation in the bone marrow similar to that caused by vitamin B$_{12}$ deficiency. Folic acid deficiency is also characterized by a macrocytic, megaloblastic anemia.[20] (See Minicase 1.) However, with folic acid deficiency, pancytopenia does not develop as consistently as it does with vitamin B$_{12}$ deficiency.

Folate supplementation in patients with a folate deficiency will provide folate for the nonmethyl transfer steps that do not require vitamin B$_{12}$. These processes include RNA and DNA synthesis and can often, at least partially, reverse megaloblastic anemia. However, without adequate vitamin B$_{12}$, the lack of methionine synthesis will lead to potentially serious and irreversible neurological damage. It is not yet clear whether this damage is due to a deficiency in the methionine-dependent neurotransmitters and amino acids or to accumulation of homocysteine. Regardless, although folate deficiency is more common and easily treated, it is critical to correctly identify the cause of a megaloblastic anemia so that any vitamin B$_{12}$ deficiency is appropriately treated.

Folate Concentration

Normal range: serum folate: 5–25 mcg/L;
RBC folate: 166–640 mcg/L

Folate concentrations in both serum and in erythrocytes (RBCs) are used to assess folate homeostasis. A low serum folate indicates negative folate balance and can be expected to lead to folate deficiency when hepatic folate stores are depleted.

Microcytic Anemia

Iron Deficiency

Microcytic anemia, or anemia with abnormally small erythrocytes, is typically caused by iron deficiency. Decreased MCV is a late indicator of the deficiency (Figure 15-2). Daily requirements are approximately 1 mg of elemental iron for each 1 mL of RBCs produced, so daily requirements are approximately 20–25 mg for erythropoiesis.[21] Most of the iron needed within the body is obtained by recycling metabolized Hgb. Red blood cells have a lifespan of approximately 120 days. When old or damaged erythrocytes are taken up by macrophages in the liver, spleen, and bone marrow, the Hgb molecule is broken down and iron is extracted and stored with proteins. Only about 5% of the daily requirement (1 mg) is newly absorbed to compensate for losses due to fecal and urinary excretion, sweat, and desquamated skin.

Menstruating women require more iron because of increased losses. Iron requirements vary among women but averages 2 mg/day. Orally ingested iron is absorbed in the GI tract, which should permit just enough iron absorption to prevent excess or deficiency. Typically, 5% to 10% of oral intake is absorbed (normal daily dietary intake: 10–20 mg).[21]

Iron deficiency is usually due to inadequate dietary intake and/or increased iron requirements. Poor dietary intake, especially in situations that require increased iron (e.g., pregnancy), is a common cause. Other causes of iron deficiency include

- Blood loss due to excessive menstrual discharge
- Peptic ulcer disease
- Hiatal hernia
- Gastrectomy
- Gastritis due to the ingestion of alcohol, aspirin, and nonsteroidal anti-inflammatory drugs (NSAIDs)

- Bacterial overgrowth of the small bowel
- Inflammatory bowel disease
- Occult bleeding from GI carcinoma
- Starch or clay pica

Ionized, soluble iron is toxic because of its ability to mediate the formation of oxidative species. Iron is, therefore, bound to proteins both in and outside of cells. The iron–protein complex within the macrophage is known as *ferritin* (Figure 15-3). In the normal adult, approximately 500–1500 mg is stored as ferritin and 2500 mg of iron is contained in Hgb.[21] When the total quantity of extracted iron exceeds the amount that can be stored as ferritin, the excess iron is stored in an insoluble form called *hemosiderin*.

While ferritin is primarily stored in macrophages, small amounts can be found in plasma and can be measured. Therefore, a serum ferritin concentration reflects total body iron stores and is the most clinically useful method to evaluate patients for iron deficiency. Minicase 2 demonstrates this principle. Since the protein is an acute phase reactant, serum ferritin concentrations can be increased by chronic infections, fever, and inflammatory reactions.

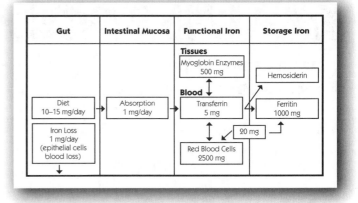

FIGURE 15-3. Intake, loss, and recycling of iron and iron storage forms.

The transport of iron in plasma and extracellular fluid occurs with two ferric ions bound to the protein transferrin, which when not binding iron or other metals is termed *apotransferrin*. Transferrin binds to specific membrane transferrin receptors where the complex enters the cell and releases the iron. Apotransferrin is released when the apotransferrin-receptor complex returns to the surface of the cell.

MINICASE 1

Anemia with Increased MCV

ANDREW B., A 45-YEAR-OLD MALE ALCOHOLIC, was admitted to the hospital because of pneumonia. His physical exam revealed an emaciated patient with ascites, dyspnea, fever, cough, and weakness. No cyanosis, jaundice, or peripheral edema was evident. His peripheral neurologic exam was within normal limits as were his serum electrolytes, urea nitrogen, creatinine, and glucose. The following CBC was obtained:

TEST NAME	RESULT	REFERENCE RANGE
RBC	3.0×10^6 cells/μL	$4.1–5.1 \times 10^6$ cells/μL for females
WBC	4.6×10^3 cells/μL	$4.4–11.0 \times 10^3$ cells/μL
Hgb	12.3 g/dL	12.3–15.3 g/dL for females
Hct	33.9%	36% to 45% for females
MCV	110.8 fL/cell	80–96 fL/cell
RDW	15.4%	11.5% to 14.5%
Platelet	174,000 cells/μL	150,000–450,000 cells/count μL
Neutrophils	68%	45% to 73%
Bands	6%	3% to 5%
Monocytes	11%	2% to 8%
Eosinophils	2%	0% to 4%
Basophils	2%	0% to 1%
Lymphocytes	11%	20% to 40%

Question: What abnormalities are present? What is the likely cause?

Discussion: Andrew B. has anemia, evidenced by the low RBC, Hgb, and Hct. The increased MCV identifies this as a macrocytic anemia. The RDW is elevated, indicating variability in the size of the erythrocytes. These findings are typical of folic acid deficiency, a common finding in alcoholics due to poor nutrition. Folic acid deficiency is more common than vitamin B_{12} deficiency because body stores are not durable. However, vitamin B_{12} deficiency must also be ruled out as it may arise with or without a concurrent folate deficiency. Hypovitaminosis B_{12} may arise from poor nutrition but is more commonly caused by pathologies such as pernicious anemia. It is critical that both serum folate and vitamin B_{12} concentrations be drawn in Andrew B. to guide appropriate supplementation. Replenishment of folate in a patient with hypovitaminosis B_{12} may temporarily improve the values of the hemogram, but failure to appropriately replenish vitamin B_{12} can lead to irreversible brain and nerve damage.

Pernicious anemia is a separate disease characterized by atrophic gastritis associated with antibodies against intrinsic factor and gastric parietal cells. Gastrectomy, removal of all or part of the stomach, can also lead to vitamin B_{12} deficiency because the procedure removes the production site of intrinsic factor. Achlorhydria from gastrectomy or drugs can decrease the release of cobalamin from meat. Defective or deficient absorption of the intrinsic factor vitamin B_{12} complex can be caused by inflammatory disease of the small bowel, ileal resection, and bacterial overgrowth in the small bowel.[17,18] Administration of colchicine, neomycin, and para-aminosalicylic acid can lead to impaired absorption of vitamin B_{12} (Table 15-4).

MINICASE 2

Anemia and Iron Stores

DENISE T. IS A 25-YEAR-OLD WOMAN seen in a community health clinic for a routine checkup. Her family history includes a sister with sickle cell disease. She has not been affected personally but has not been tested to determine her sickling genotype. She describes painful menstrual periods and takes aspirin for them. She also admits to a pica of ingesting cornstarch throughout the day. The following laboratory tests at right were done.

Question: What hematologic abnormalities are apparent from these results?

Discussion: Denise T. demonstrates an anemia as manifested by the decreased Hct, Hgb, and RBC. Her WBC count is normal. The RDW is elevated, indicating increased variability of erythrocyte size (anisocytosis). Because the MCV is low, we can presume that this microcytic, hypochromic form of anemia is most likely due to rather prolonged iron deficiency. This is corroborated by the iron studies, which indicate a low serum iron and transferrin saturation. Serum ferritin is also decreased, indicating that her iron stores are markedly reduced. The TIBC is increased both because of increased transferrin production and decreased iron available to bind to the protein. The platelet count is often mildly elevated in iron deficiency anemia reflecting stimulation of both erythropoiesis and megakaryopoiesis in the bone marrow as it responds to the anemia, albeit ineffectively, due to the inadequate availability of iron for Hgb synthesis.

There may be multiple causes of Denise T.'s iron deficiency. Most commonly, the combination of low dietary iron and blood loss from menstruation increases the frequency of iron deficiency anemia in women. An additional possibility is occult blood loss from GI ulcerations caused by aspirin. An exacerbating factor for this woman is her starch pica, or craving for unusual food. In addition to the high caloric intake associated with this particular pica, the starch decreases the bioavailability of ingested iron, decreasing the ability of Denise T. to absorb dietary or supplemental iron. Given the pica, parenteral iron may be considered.

TEST NAME	RESULT	REFERENCE RANGE
RBC	3.3×10^6 cells/μL	4.1–5.1×10^6 cells/μL for females
WBC	5.1×10^3 cells/μL	4.4–11.3×10^3 cells/μL
Hgb	8.3 g/dL	12.3–15.3 g/dL for females
Hct	26%	36% to 45% for females
MCV	78 fL/cell	80–96 fL/cell
RDW	16.1%	11.5% to 14.5%
Platelet count	475,000 cells/μL	150,000–450,000 cells/μL
Neutrophils	52%	45% to 73%
Bands	3%	3% to 5%
Monocytes	2%	2% to 8%
Eosinophils	1%	0% to 4%
Basophils	0%	0% to 1%
Lymphocytes	42%	20% to 40%
Serum iron	44 mcg/dL	50–150 mcg/dL
TIBC	451 mcg/dL	250–410 mcg/dL
Transferrin saturation	14%	30% to 50%
Serum ferritin	5.2 mcg/L	10–20 mcg/L

The tendency of ferritin to be falsely elevated with inflammatory processes has led to recent interest in using soluble transferrin receptor concentrations as an alternative marker of iron deficiency. The circulating receptor fragment is considered to reflect total body receptor expression and is elevated in times of increased erythropoiesis such as sickle cell anemia, thalassemias, and chronic hemolysis. If such causes of increased erythropoiesis can be excluded, elevated concentrations of circulating transferrin receptor are thought to reflect iron deficiency. The use of transferrin receptor concentrations may help determine if decreased ferritin concentrations are due to iron deficiency or to anemia of chronic (inflammatory) disease.

Clinical and laboratory diagnosis. The first change observed in the development of iron deficiency anemia is a loss of storage iron (hemosiderin). If the deficiency continues, a loss of plasma iron occurs. The decrease in plasma iron stimulates an increase in transferrin synthesis. When enough iron has been depleted such that supplies for erythropoiesis are inadequate, anemia develops. The RDW will rise, often before the MCV decreases to a notable degree. If the iron deficiency persists, the RBCs become smaller than usual (microcytic—low MCV) and not as heavily pigmented as normal RBCs (hypochromic) because they contain less Hgb than normal erythrocytes. Clinically, patients present with progressively worsening weakness, fatigue, pallor, shortness of breath, tachycardia, and palpitations. Numbness, tingling, and glossitis may exist.[10] Laboratory results for iron deficiency anemia are listed in Table 15-3. With adequate iron therapy, the maximal daily rate of Hgb regeneration is 0.3 g/dL.

Serum Ferritin

Normal range: >10–20 ng/mL or >10–20 mcg/L

Loss of storage iron (hemosiderin) was traditionally evaluated by iron-stained bone marrow aspirate. Serum ferritin has largely replaced these invasive tests as an indirect measure of iron stores. Serum ferritin concentrations are markedly reduced in iron deficiency anemia (3–6 mcg/L).

Serum Iron and Total Iron-Binding Capacity

Normal range: 60–150 mcg/dL or 10.7–26.9 μmol/L and total iron-binding capacity (TIBC) normal range: 250–400 mcg/dL or 45–72 μmol/L

The *serum iron* concentration measures iron bound to transferrin. This value represents about one-third of the *total iron-binding capacity (TIBC)* of transferrin.[21] The TIBC measures the iron-binding capacity of transferrin protein. In iron deficiency anemia, TIBC is increased due to a compensatory increase in transferrin synthesis.[22] This increase leads to a corresponding decrease in the percent transferrin saturation that can be calculated by dividing the serum iron by the TIBC, and then multiplying by 100. For example, a person with a serum iron concentration of 100 mcg/dL and a TIBC of 300 mcg/dL has a transferrin saturation of 33%. Iron deficient erythropoiesis exists whenever the percent saturation is 15% or less.

Other disease states besides iron deficiency that can alter serum iron and TIBC are infections, malignant tumors, and uremia.[9,10] Serum iron and TIBC both decrease in these disorders, unlike in iron deficiency anemia where serum iron decreases but TIBC increases. Anemia from these diseases is sometimes called anemia of chronic disease.

Normochromic, Normocytic Anemia

This classification encompasses numerous etiologies. Three causes are discussed: acute blood loss anemia, hemolytic anemia, and anemia of chronic disease.

Acute Blood Loss Anemia

Patients who suffer from acute hemorrhage may experience a dramatic drop in their whole blood volume. (See Minicase 3.) In this situation, the Hct is not a reliable indicator of the extent of anemia. It is a measure of the amount of packed red cells per unit volume of the blood, not the total body amount of red cells. The total whole blood volume may be markedly reduced, but in the acute phase of the hemorrhage the Hct may be normal or even slightly increased. Hemorrhage evokes vasoconstriction which initially prevents extravascular fluid from replacing intravascular fluid loss. Usually, both Hgb and Hct are decreased by the time that a CBC is obtained. This is most dramatically evident after the administration of crystalloid IV fluids by early medical responders to maintain intravascular volume, an example of iatrogenic replacement of intravascular fluid.

In patients with normal bone marrow, the production of RBCs increases in response to hemorrhage, resulting in reticulocytosis. If the patient is transfused, each unit of packed RBCs administered should increase the Hgb by 1 g/dL if the bleeding has stopped. Table 15-3 shows the usual laboratory findings in acute blood loss anemia.

Hemolytic Anemia

Hemolysis is the lysis of erythrocytes. Hemolysis often leads to irregularly shaped or fragmented erythrocytes, termed *poikilocytosis*. If hemolysis is rapid and extensive, severe anemia can develop, yet RBC indices (MCV and MCHC) remain unchanged in the short term. Patients with normal bone marrow respond with an increase in erythrocyte production to replace the lysed cells, and reticulocytosis is present. Specialized tests, called *antiglobulin tests*, can be useful in determining immune causes of hemolytic anemia.[22]

Plasma (free) Hgb measures the concentration of Hgb circulating in the plasma released from lysed RBCs. It is almost always elevated in the presence of intravascular hemolysis. Haptoglobin, an acute-phase reactant, binds free Hgb and carries it to the reticuloendothelial system. In the presence of intravascular hemolysis, haptoglobin is decreased. Concomitant corticosteroid therapy may confound interpretation because many diseases associated with in vivo hemolysis are treated with steroids. Serum haptoglobin may be normal or elevated in hemolysis if the patient is receiving steroids. If the increase in serum haptoglobin is from steroids, other acute-phase reactants such as prealbumin will often be elevated. Serum haptoglobin is also elevated in patients with biliary obstruction and nephrotic syndrome. It is variably decreased in folate deficiency, sickle cell anemia, thalassemia, hypersplenism, liver disease, and estrogen therapy or pregnancy.[8]

Immune hemolytic anemias are caused by the binding of antibodies and/or complement components to the erythrocyte cell membrane with subsequent lysis. The method used to detect autoantibodies already bound to erythrocytes is a direct antiglobulin test (DAT), sometimes referred to as the *direct Coombs test*. The method used to detect antibodies present in serum is an indirect antiglobulin test (IAT, indirect Coombs). The DAT is performed by combining a patient's RBCs with rabbit or goat antihuman globulin serum, which contains antibodies against human immunoglobulins and complement.[22] If the patient's RBCs are coated with antibody or complement, the antibodies in the antiglobulin serum bind to the immunoglobulins coating the RBCs, leading to the *agglutination* of the RBCs. The DAT is the only test that provides definitive evidence of immune hemolysis.[23] The DAT can also be used to investigate possible blood transfusion reactions.[22]

The IAT detects antibodies in the patient's serum. Patient serum is combined with several types of normal erythrocytes of known antigenic expression. Any antibodies able to bind to the antigens expressed on these sample RBCs will adhere after the serum is washed away. Antihuman immune globulin is then added and will bind to any of the patient's immune globulin that is present on the erythrocytes, followed by agglutination.[22,23]

The antiglobulin tests are very sensitive, but a negative result does not eliminate the possibility of antibodies bound to erythrocytes. An estimated 100–150 molecules of antibody must be bound to each erythrocyte for detection by the antiglobulin test.[22] Smaller numbers of antibodies give a false-negative reaction.

Numerous conditions and medications can be associated with immune hemolytic anemia (Table 15-5).[24] Medications can induce antibody formation by three mechanisms that result in a hemolytic anemia.

Autoimmune type. Methyldopa and procainamide are infrequently used cardiovascular drugs that may induce the formation of antibodies directed specifically against normal RBC proteins. This autoimmune state can persist for up to 1 month after drug administration has been discontinued. This mechanism is known as a true autoimmune type of antibody formation and is detected using the DAT.[24]

MINICASE 3

Anemia and Low Platelet Count

MICHAEL T., A 50-YEAR-OLD MALE with a long history of alcohol abuse, cirrhosis, and esophageal varices, was brought to the emergency department by concerned family members. The family said that he suddenly began coughing up bright red blood. As Michael T. was moved to a bed in the emergency department, he began coughing and vomiting large amounts of bright red blood. A stat CBC revealed the following:

TEST NAME	RESULT	REFERENCE RANGE
RBC	2.91×10^6 cells/µL	$4.5–5.9 \times 10^6$ cells/µL for males
WBC	6.6×10^3 cells/µL	$4.4–11.0 \times 10^3$ cells/µL
Hgb	8.0 g/dL	14–17.5 g/dL for males
Hct	28.2%	42% to 50% for males
MCV	92.4 fL/cell	80–96 fL/cell
RDW	14.1%	11.5% to 14.5%
Platelet	75,000 cells/µL	150,000–450,000 cells/count µL

Question: What does this CBC indicate?

Discussion: The presence of bright blood (as opposed to dark, "coffee ground" material) in the emesis indicates an acute and active bleed, either from a gastric ulcer or from esophageal varices. The CBC is consistent with acute blood loss. At the onset of bleeding, the RBC, Hgb, and Hct may show minimal changes. Here, the RBC, Hgb, and Hct are all moderately decreased, and the red cell indices are within normal limits, supporting a recent history of significant blood loss. The platelet count is also decreased, which may have led to the increasing blood loss. As could be anticipated from his history of alcohol abuse, the bleeding was found to arise from a ruptured esophageal varix secondary to liver cirrhosis as a result of alcoholic liver disease. Cirrhosis can also be associated with congestive splenomegaly which could have contributed to the moderate thrombocytopenia due to splenic sequestration of platelets.

Innocent bystander type. Antibodies to the drugs quinine and quinidine are examples of the immune complex (innocent bystander) mechanism.[19] Each drug forms a drug-protein complex with plasma proteins to which antibodies are formed. This drug–plasma, protein–antibody complex attaches to erythrocytes and fixes complement, which leads to lysis of the RBCs.[22] In this situation, the RBC is an innocent bystander. Examples of other drugs implicated in causing this type of hemolytic anemia are listed in Table 15-5.

Hapten type 1. The hapten (penicillin) type 1 mechanism is involved when a patient has produced antibodies to penicillin. If the patient receives penicillin at a future date, some penicillin can bind to the RBC membrane. The anti-penicillin antibodies, in turn, bind to the penicillin bound to the RBC, and hemolysis can result.

TABLE 15-5. Causes of Immune Hemolytic Anemia

Neoplasm

Chronic lymphocytic leukemia (CLL)
Lymphoma
Multiple myeloma

Collagen vascular disease

Systemic lupus erythematosus
Rheumatoid arthritis

Medication

Auto-immune type
Levodopa, mefenamic acid, methyldopa, procainamide
Innocent bystander type
Cefotaxime, ceftazidime, ceftriaxone, chlorpromazine, doxepin, fluorouracil, isoniazid, quinidine, quinine, rifampin, sulfonamides, thiazides
Hapten type 1
Cephalosporins, penicillins

Infections

Mycoplasma
Viruses

G6PD Deficiency Anemia

Glucose-6-phosphate dehydrogenase (G6PD) is an intracellular enzyme that forms the NADPH needed by the erythrocyte to synthesize the antioxidant glutathione. Variants of this enzyme are more commonly found in African Black (Gd^{A-}) and Mediterranean/Asian populations (Gd^{Med}) than in Caucasians. These variants have an impaired ability to resist the oxidizing effect of drugs and of collateral oxidative exposure to the granulocytic response to infections. Thus, exposure of patients with G6PD deficiency to oxidizing drugs or to an infection can lead to a dramatic, nonimmunologic hemolysis. Drug-induced hemolysis is less likely in the Gd^{A-} variant, but both variants are susceptible to infection-induced hemolysis.[26] Assessment of at-risk patients for signs of hemolysis (anemia, hemoglobinemia, dark urine, and back pain) is appropriate. Future, routine genotyping of patients will aid in drug selection and monitoring of at-risk populations.

Anemia of Chronic Disease

Mild-to-moderate anemia often accompanies renal failure, various infections, inflammatory traumatic illnesses, or neoplastic diseases that last over 1–2 months.[27] Chronic infections include pulmonary abscesses, tuberculosis (TB), endocarditis, pelvic inflammatory disease, and osteomyelitis. Chronic inflammatory illnesses (e.g., rheumatoid arthritis and systemic lupus erythematosus) and hematological malignancies (e.g., Hodgkin lymphoma, leukemia, and multiple myeloma) are also associated with anemia. Because these disorders as a group are common, anemia due to chronic disease is also quite common. While anemia of chronic disease is more commonly associated with normocytic, normochromic anemia, it can also cause microcytic anemia. Table 15-3 shows the usual laboratory results found in anemia of chronic disease.

MINICASE 4

Blast Crisis

DAVID D., A 46-YEAR-OLD MALE, presented to the emergency department with a temperature of 104°F (40°C), diarrhea, and abdominal pain. Urine and blood cultures were obtained, and he was given broad spectrum antibiotics. The CBC at right was obtained

Question: What does his CBC reveal?

Discussion: This CBC is grossly abnormal, showing marked leukocytosis with elevations in the absolute neutrophil count, neutrophil precursors, and blast cells. Due to the markedly abnormal populations of circulating WBCs, the automated hematology analyzer would not report a differential count. The reported differential is based on a manual differential count. Note although the percentage of neutrophils is decreased, a neutrophilia is revealed when the absolute number of neutrophils is calculated (e.g., $118.9 \times 10^3 \times 21\% = 25,000$ cells/μL; normal range 1800–7800 cells/μL). Bands and other precursor cells including blast cells can only be quantitated by the manual differential count. He has a normochromic, normocytic anemia and thrombocytopenia.

At first, one might expect that David D.'s condition could be consistent with an overwhelming infection. However, he has a marked number of immature WBC forms in the peripheral blood—metamyelocytes, myelocytes, promyelocytes, and particularly blasts. These forms are normally found only in the bone marrow and not in the circulation.

A bone marrow aspirate and biopsy reveals that he has chronic myelogenous leukemia (CML) with a blast (myeloblast) crisis. The anemia is likely myelophthisic, which occurs in part by the "crowding out" and suppressing of maturing red and white cells in the bone marrow by the neoplastic immature white cells including blast cells. This would also result in a normochromic, normocytic anemia.

TEST NAME	RESULT	REFERENCE RANGE
RBC	3.18×10^6 cells/μL	$4.5–5.9 \times 10^6$ cells/μL for males
WBC	118.9×10^3 cells/μL	$4.4–11.3 \times 10^3$ cells/μL
Hgb	9.9 g/dL	14–17.5 g/dL for males
Hct	29.5%	42% to 50% for males
MCV	92.8 fL/cell	80–96 fL/cell
RDW	14.1%	11.5% to 14.5%
Platelet	69,000 cells/μL	150,000–450,000 cells/count μL
Neutrophils	21%	45% to 73%
Bands	12%	3% to 5%
Metamyelocytes	5%	0%
Myelocytes	5%	0%
Promyelocytes	8%	0%
Lymphocytes	6%	20% to 40%
Atypical	0%	0% lymphocytes
Monocytes	2%	2% to 8%
Eosinophils	1%	0% to 4%
Basophils	10%	0% to 1%
Blasts	30%	0%

The pathogenesis of this anemia is not totally understood. Various investigations have found that the erythrocyte lifespan is shortened and that the bone marrow does not increase erythrocyte production to compensate for the decreased longevity. Iron utilization is also impaired. Although erythrocytes are frequently normal size, microcytosis can develop. One distinguishing feature between early iron deficiency anemia and a microcytic anemia of chronic disease is the normal serum ferritin that is present in the latter.[27]

In patients with anemia associated with chronic kidney disease, iron supplementation is recommended for those with ferritin concentrations less than 100 mcg/L. If anemia is present but ferritin concentrations are greater than 100 mcg/L, the need for iron is demonstrated by a transferrin saturation of <20%.[28] In the presence of sufficient iron stores, erythrocyte-stimulating agents (ESAs) such as recombinant erythropoietin and darbepoetin may be used to decrease a patient's need for blood cell transfusions. The FDA has recently modified recommendations for more conservative dosing of ESAs due to recent data suggesting ESAs increase the risk for serious adverse cardiovascular events. A target Hgb range is not provided in the recommendations. Instead, dosing should be individualized to use the lowest dose of ESA sufficient to reduce the need

for transfusion. Patients with chronic kidney disease (CKD) who are not on dialysis should consider starting ESA treatment only when the Hgb level is less than 10 g/dL and reduce or stop the ESA dose if the Hgb level exceeds 10 g/dL. For patients on dialysis, ESA treatment should be initiated when the Hgb level is less than 10 g/dL and reduce or interrupt the ESA dose if the Hgb level approaches or exceeds 11 g/dL. Monitoring of Hgb levels should be done at least weekly until stable and then monitored monthly.[29] Use of ESA therapy in patients with cancer has become controversial due to the increased risk of thromboembolism and shorter survival.[30] ESA therapy is only recommended in patients undergoing myelosuppressive chemotherapy who have a Hgb of less than 10 g/dL. As with CKD patients, dosing should be individualized to use the lowest dose of ESAs sufficient to reduce the need for transfusion. Use of ESAs is not recommended for cancer patients in any other circumstances. Due to the potential for adverse events from their use, the FDA has required participation of prescribers, pharmacies, and patients in a Risk Evaluation and Mitigation Strategy (REMS) for all erythropoietic agents.[31]

Hemoglobinopathies and Thalassemias

Hemoglobinopathies arise from synthesis of abnormal alpha-, or more commonly, beta-globin subunits of Hgb. The most common types of anemias related to hemoglobinopathies include *sickle cell trait/disease* and *hemoglobin C trait/disease.* Sickle cell trait is caused by the substitution of a valine amino acid for glutamate at position 6 on the beta-globin chain of producing Hgb S, while Hgb C results from a lysine substitution at the same position. The heterozygous carrier state for Hgb S or C is thought to provide a resistance to clinical manifestations and sequelae of malaria. Homozygous persons with both beta-globin chains carrying the valine substitution have sickle cell anemia and will have varying degrees of sickling of erythrocytes. This occurs most commonly under circumstances of hypoxia, infection, dehydration, or acidosis. Deoxygenated Hgb molecules polymerize into rod-like structures within the RBC, deforming the cell into a rigid, arched, sickled cell. These erythrocytes are not able to deform and pass through the capillaries or reticuloendothelial system. Hypoxia, ischemia, and even infarction occur in tissues downstream of these sites of impaired erythrocyte flow. Severe pain is usually present during these "sickle crises," and opiate analgesics are often needed in addition to hydration, transfusion, and other treatments. Diagnosis is made by inspection of the peripheral blood smear and by high-performance liquid chromatography (HPLC) hemoglobin analysis and electrophoresis of the patient's Hgb.[32,33]

Thalassemias are a more diverse group of hemoglobinopathies most commonly associated with persons of ancestry arising in the Mediterranean region. Unlike the qualitative change caused by the valine substitution in sickle cell patients, thalassemias are characterized by quantitative abnormalities in the alpha- or beta-globin subunits of Hgb. Since there are two alpha-globin and two beta-globin subunits in the normal Hgb tetramer, an inability to produce adequate amounts of one of the subunits would clearly lead to difficulty in synthesizing intact, complete Hgb molecules.[34]

Mild thalassemias are often diagnosed by a peripheral blood smear, which shows microcytic erythrocytes with minimal anemia. In more severe forms of thalassemia, some of the RBCs are nucleated, reflecting the intense pressure on erythropoiesis in the bone marrow to provide oxygen carrying capacity to the body even if it requires releasing immature, nucleated erythrocyte precursors. The type of thalassemia present is investigated using HPLC hemoglobin analysis and electrophoresis.

WHITE BLOOD CELL COUNT AND DIFFERENTIAL

White blood cells are divided into two general classifications:
1. Granulocytes or phagocytes (leukocytes that engulf and digest other cells)
2. Lymphocytes (leukocytes involved in the recognition of nonself cells or substances)

The functions of these general leukocyte classes are interrelated. For example, immunoglobulins produced by B

TABLE 15-6. Normal WBC Count and Differential

CELL TYPE	NORMAL RANGE (ADULT)	
Total WBC count	$4.4–11.0 \times 10^3$ cells/μL	
	Percentage	**Absolute Counts**
Polymorphonuclear neutrophils ("polys," "segs," PMN)	45% to 73%	1800–7800/μL
Band neutrophils ("bands," "stabs")	3% to 5%	0–700/μL
Lymphocytes	20% to 40%	1000–4800/μL
Monocytes	2% to 8%	200–1000/μL
Eosinophils	0% to 4%	0–450/μL

WBC = white blood cell.

lymphocytes are needed to coat or opsonize encapsulated bacteria so that neutrophils can more effectively identify, adhere, and engulf them for destruction.

When a CBC and differential is ordered for a patient, the resulting laboratory report will include a WBC count in a given volume of blood plus the relative percentage and absolute number of each cell type contributing to the total WBC. Therefore, the percentages of the WBC subtypes must add up to 100%. If one cell type increases, percentages of all other types will decrease. This decrease is not necessarily associated with any pathology. Table 15-6 is a general breakdown of the different types of WBCs and their usual percentages and absolute counts in peripheral blood.

The absolute segmented neutrophil count is the percentage of neutrophils and bands multiplied by the WBC count, a calculation performed by the automated hematology analyzer.

The CBC and differential is one of the most widely performed clinical laboratory tests. In the past, differentials were determined by a manual count of a standard number of cells. In addition to being labor-intensive and slow, this method is imprecise and inaccurate when compared to automated methods.[35] Clinical laboratories today commonly use automated methods for determining the WBC differential, but manual differential counts are still performed when abnormal WBCs are circulating in the peripheral blood. Automated instruments count thousands of cells and report not only the relative percentages of the various WBC types but also the absolute numbers, Hgb, RBC, platelets, and red cell indices. When reviewing a WBC differential, one must be aware of not only the relative percentages of cell types but also the absolute numbers. The percentages viewed in isolation can lead to incorrect conclusions. Minicase 4 demonstrates this principle.

Granulocytes

Granulocytes are phagocytes (eating cells) and derive their name from the presence of granules within the cytoplasm. The granules store lysozymes and other chemicals needed to oxidize and enzymatically destroy foreign cells. Granulocytic leukocytes include neutrophils, eosinophils, and basophils. Monocytes are phagocytic cells that mature into macrophages, which are predominantly found in tissue rather than in the circulation. When a peripheral smear of blood is prepared, three types of granulocytes are named by the staining characteristics of their cytoplasmic granules[8]:

1. Neutrophils retain neutral stains and appear light tan.
2. Eosinophils retain acidic dyes and appear red–orange.
3. Basophils retain basic dyes and appear dark blue to purple.

Granulocytes are formed in large numbers from the pluripotential stem cells in the bone marrow. They undergo numerous differentiation and proliferation steps in the marrow and are usually released into the peripheral blood in their mature form. A common exception is the appearance of band cells during an infection, as discussed below. Neutrophils, eosinophils, and basophils die in the course of destroying ingested organisms or particles, yielding pus. On the other hand, monocytes and macrophages do not usually need to sacrifice themselves when destroying target cells.

Neutrophils

Normal range: PMN leukocytes: 45% to 73%, 1800–7800/μL; bands: 3% to 5%, 0–700/μL

Neutrophils are also termed *segmented neutrophils* (or "segs") or *polymorphonuclear cells* (PMNs or "polys"). The less mature form of the neutrophil with a crescent-shaped nucleus is a band or stab cell. Bands derive their name from the morphology of their nucleus, which has not yet segmented into multiple lobes. Less mature forms of the neutrophil, such as the metamyelocyte and myelocyte, are normally not in the peripheral blood. The neutrophil is a phagocytic cell that exists to ingest and digest foreign proteins (e.g., bacteria and fungi).

Under normal conditions, about 90% of the neutrophils are stored in the bone marrow. When released, neutrophils will normally circulate rapidly for several hours before eventually marginating and rolling along the endothelium until finally stopping and adhering. This dynamic process of margination and demargination causes large shifts in the measured neutrophil count, since only the granulocytes that are circulating at the time are measured by a venipuncture. Neutrophils spend only about 6–8 hours in the circulation after which they move through the endothelium into the tissue. Unless used to engage a foreign body or sustained by the cytokine milieu, neutrophils then undergo programmed cell death, a noninflammatory process termed *apoptosis*.[36]

During an acute infection there is an increase in the percentage of neutrophils as they are released from the bone marrow and demarginate from the endothelium.[37,38] Less mature band forms may also be released, but these immature neutrophils are still considered to be active. The appearance of band cells in infections is termed a *left shift*. This may be due to the traditional order in which the differential was reported. It may also arise from the use of a left-to-right sequence in figures describing the process of neutrophil differentiation from the stem cell (see Figure 15-1).

When the neutrophils and/or bands are elevated, the percentage of lymphocytes usually decreases proportionately. Ratios of 10% to 15% lymphocytes may appear in these patients, but the relative *lymphopenia* arises from the concomitant increase in total WBCs. An exception is a neutrophilia caused by glucocorticoid treatment, which will cause a drop in the absolute lymphocyte count because of its lymphotoxic effect while increasing the absolute neutrophil count due to demargination.

Eosinophils and Basophils

Normal range: eosinophils: 0% to 4%, 0–450/μL; basophils: 0% to 1%, 0–200/μL

The functions of *eosinophils* and *basophils* are not completely known. Eosinophils are present in large numbers in the intestinal mucosa and lungs, two locations where foreign proteins enter the body.[11] Eosinophils can phagocytize, kill, and digest bacteria and yeast. Elevations of eosinophils counts can be seen in of parasitic infections, particularly those with parasitic migration through the tissues.

Basophils are present in small numbers in the peripheral blood and are the most long-lasting granulocyte in blood with a circulating lifespan of approximately 2 weeks.[2] They contain heparin, histamine, and leukotriene B_4.[39,40] Many signs and symptoms of allergic responses can be attributed to specific mast cell and basophil products.[39] Basophils are probably involved in immediate hypersensitivity reactions (e.g., extrinsic, or allergic, and asthmatic) in addition to delayed hypersensitivity reactions. Basophils may be increased in chronic inflammation and in some types of leukemia.

Monocytes/Macrophages

Normal range: monocytes: 2% to 8%, 200–1000/μL

Monocytes leave the circulation in 16–36 hours and enter the tissues where they complete their maturation into *macrophages*. Macrophages, present throughout the body, are concentrated in lymph nodes, alveoli of the lungs, spleen, liver, and bone marrow.[41] These tissue macrophages participate in the removal of foreign substances from the body. In addition to attacking foreign cells, they are involved in the destruction of old erythrocytes, denatured plasma proteins, and plasma lipids. Tissue macrophages also salvage iron from the Hgb of old erythrocytes and return the iron to transferrin for delivery to the bone marrow. Under appropriate stimuli, some monocytes/macrophages are transformed into antigen-presenting cells (APCs, also termed *dendritic cells*). These transformed macrophages are an important component of both cell-mediated (T lymphocytes) and soluble (B lymphocyte) immune activity against antigens.[41]

Lymphocytes and Plasma Cells

Normal range: lymphocytes: 20% to 40%, 1000–4800/μL

Lymphocytes make up the second major group of leukocytes. They are characterized by cytoplasm usually lacking granules and relatively round to oval, smooth nuclei. These cells give specificity and memory to the body's defense against foreign invaders.[42] The three subgroups of lymphocytes are

1. T lymphocytes (T cells)
2. B lymphocytes (B cells)
3. Natural killer cells (NK cells)

Lymphocytes are not phagocytic, but the NK and T cell subtypes are cytotoxic by virtue of complement activation and antibody-dependent cellular cytotoxicity (ADCC). Morphologic differentiation of lymphocytes is difficult; visual inspection of a blood smear cannot uniformly distinguish between T, B, and NK cells. Fortunately, lymphocytes can be distinguished by the presence of lineage-specific membrane markers, historically termed *clusters of differentiation (CD)*. Thus, mature T cells have CD3 and CD5, B cells have CD20, and NK cells have CD56 membrane markers.[40,43] Individual CD moieties may be surface proteins, enzymes, or adhesion molecules, to name a few. Labeled antibodies to specific CD molecules will identify the lineage of the lymphocyte, either in blood or in tissue.

Identification of the subtype of lymphocytes is not a routine clinical hematology test at present; they are reported simply as lymphocytes by automated cell counting instruments. However, in research applications and for the diagnosis of leukemias and lymphomas, subtypes can both be quantitated by *flow cytometry*. The blood is processed with the WBCs exposed to one or more CD-antibodies tagged with fluorescent dyes. The labeled cells flow individually past one or more lasers that induce the labeled cells to glow at wavelengths specific to the dye attached via the antibody to each cell. These fluorescing cells are counted and reported as percentage of the total number of cells analyzed. This method can be used to count virtually any cell that can be labeled with a fluorescent tag.[44] As discussed below, the identification of specific lymphocyte subtypes in this manner is increasingly used in determining the optimal treatment of various hematologic neoplasms.

With the help of T cells, B cells recognize foreign substances and are transformed into plasma cells, capable of producing antibodies (discussed later). Table 15-7 lists the types of disorders in which lymphocytes are increased or decreased.

T Lymphocytes

T lymphocytes are responsible for cell-mediated immunity and are the predominant lymphocytes in circulation and in tissue. They require partial maturation in the embryonic thymus, hence the name T cell. In addition to identifying infections, they oversee delayed hypersensitivity (seen with skin tests for TB, mumps, and *Candida*) and rejection of transplanted organs.[40] In order for a foreign antigen to be recognized by T cells, it must be "presented" by macrophages or dendritic cells on one of two complex, individualized molecules termed *major histocompatibility complexes (MHC1 and MHC2)*.

T cells can be further divided into helper and cytotoxic (or suppressor) cells, which, respectively, express the CD4 and CD8 markers. CD4 helper cells are not cytotoxic, but on recognizing an antigen will activate and produce cytokines such as IL-2, which stimulate nearby immune cells including macrophages and CD8 cytotoxic-suppressor T cells, B cells, and NK cells. CD4 helper T cells can again be divided into T_{H1} and T_{H2} subtypes. The T_{H1} subtype mediates the activation of macrophages and the delayed hypersensitivity response, while the T_{H2} subtype appears primarily responsible for B cell activation. The cellular specificity of these subtypes appears to arise primarily from their distinct pattern of cytokine production.

The HIV virus binds specifically to the CD4 receptor but does not elicit the desired antiviral response in most patients. This infection leads to destruction of this subset of T cells and a reversal of the CD4/CD8 ratio (normally >1). The CD4 lymphocyte count and viral burden measured by viral RNA are inversely related and seem to correlate with overall prognosis. Although the CD4 count remains a useful surrogate marker in monitoring the course and treatment of HIV-infected patients, viral loads are also increasingly measured. The lack of adequate numbers of active helper T cells that activate other immune cells leads to an increased susceptibility to numerous opportunistic infections and cancer, yielding a syndrome that is well-known as AIDS.[45,46] T cells are the primary mediator for host rejection of transplanted solid organs such as heart, lung, kidney, liver, and/or pancreas grafts. The peri- and postoperative treatment of solid organ graft recipients is directed toward minimizing the antigraft T cell response while not ablating the T cell population to the point of causing life-threatening infections. In practice, this is a narrow path plagued by viral and fungal infections that cause substantial morbidity and mortality in graft recipients.

Typically, T cell populations in graft recipients are not measured, and drug titration is based on biopsies of the transplanted organ, drug concentrations of the immunosuppressants, and blood counts. Anti-T cell treatments employed in transplant recipients include corticosteroids; muromonab, anti-CD3 antibody directed against the CD3 marker found on T cells; antihuman lymphocyte immunoglobulin; and inhibitors of T cell activation such as tacrolimus or mycophenolate. Since the immunoglobulins are typically obtained from nonhuman species, they can cause severe allergic reactions and are usually effective for only a short period.

Natural killer cells (NK) are derived from T cell lineage but are not as restricted in requiring MHC identification of the target cell. NK cells are thought to be particularly important for cytotoxic effects on virally-infected cells and cancer cells.

B Lymphocytes

B cells are named after similar avian lymphocytes that required maturation in an organ termed the *Bursa of Fabricius*. There is no equivalent organ in humans, and maturation of B lymphocytes occurs in the bone marrow. Quiescent, circulating B cells express one form of antibody, immunoglobulin M (IgM). When stimulated by activated T cells (APCs or dendritic cells), B cells are transformed into plasma cells that will produce one of five immunoglobulin types: IgA, IgD, IgE, IgG, or IgM.[40]

The two antibodies most commonly associated with the development of immunity to foreign proteins, viruses, and bacteria are IgM and IgG. IgE is associated with the development of allergic phenomena. IgA is secreted into the lumen of the GI tract and helps avoid sensitization to foodstuffs, and IgD is bound to the lymphocyte cell membrane.[40] Abnormal immunoglobulins can typically be detected using serum protein electrophoretic (SPEP) gels. Monoclonal hyperimmunoglobulinemias are identified by single peaks on SPEP gels and are

TABLE 15-7. Quantitative Disorders of White Blood Cells[18,19,21,22]

WBC ABNORMALITY	TYPICAL THRESHOLD (CELLS/µL)	POSSIBLE CAUSES
Neutrophilia	>12,000	Acute bacterial infection Trauma Myocardial infarction Chronic bacterial infection Labor and delivery Sickle cell crises Epinephrine, lithium, G-CSF, GM-CSF, glucocorticosteroids

Neutropenia	<1500	Radiation exposure
		Medications:
		    Antineoplastic cytotoxic agents
		    Captopril
		    Cephalosporins
		    Chloramphenicol
		    Ganciclovir
		    Methimazole
		    Penicillins
		    Phenothiazines
		    Procainamide
		    Ticlopidine
		    Tricyclic antidepressants
		    Vancomycin
		    Zidovudine
		Overwhelming acute bacterial infection
		Vitamin B_{12} or folate deficiency
		Salmonellosis
		Pertussis

Eosinophilia	>350	Allergic disorders/asthma Parasitic infections Leukemia Medications Angiotensin-converting enzyme inhibitors Antibiotics (or any allergic reaction to a drug)
Eosinopenia	<50	Acute infection
Basophilia	>300	Chronic inflammation Leukemia
Monocytosis	>800	Recovery state of acute bacterial infection Tuberculosis (disseminated) Endocarditis Protozoal or rickettsial infection Leukemia/lymphoma
Lymphocytosis	>4000	Infectious mononucleosis Viral infections (e.g., rubella, varicella, mumps, cytomegalovirus) Pertussis Tuberculosis Syphilis Lymphoma
Lymphopenia	<1000	HIV type 1 Radiation exposure Glucocorticosteroids Lymphoma (Hodgkin disease) Aplastic anemia

HIV = human immunodeficiency virus; G-CSF = granulocyte colony-stimulating factor; GM-CSF = granulocyte-macrophage colony-stimulating factor.

typically associated with plasma (B) cell neoplasms. Polyclonal hyperimmunoglobulinemias can be associated with infections and inflammatory reactions.

Lymphopenia and hypogammaglobulinemia (a decrease in the total quantity of immunoglobulin) are seen as a consequence of steroid treatment, transplant rejection prophylaxis, and anticancer treatment, but can also paradoxically arise from leukemias. In general, lymphopenia is more common in chemotherapy regimens that include high doses of glucocorticosteroids. Glucocorticosteroids bind to a receptor on lymphocytes and are lymphotoxic, even to the point of initiating cellular apoptosis.[43] Interestingly, although HIV-1 infections lead to lymphopenia, other viral infections (e.g., infectious mononucleosis, hepatitis, mumps, varicella, rubella, herpes simplex, herpes zoster, and influenza) often increase the number of circulating lymphocytes (lymphocytosis), which are primarily activated T cells looking for virally-infected cells to attack and destroy.[47,48]

Leukocyte Disorders

Patients can suffer from three major classes of *leukocyte disorders:* functional, quantitative, and myeloproliferative. *Functional disorders* involve defects in recognition, metabolism, cytotoxic effects, signaling, and other related activities. Routine laboratory values are not intended to evaluate these abnormalities and will not be discussed further here.

Quantitative disorders involve too few or too many leukocytes. Possible causes are listed in Table 15-7. Neutropenia is usually considered to exist when the neutrophil count is less than 1500 or 1800 cells/μL.[49] When the neutrophil count is less than 500 cells/μL, normal defense mechanisms are greatly impaired and the patient is at increased risk of spontaneous bacterial and fungal infections. A neutrophil count less than 100/μL is termed *agranulocytosis.* This is usually encountered after chemotherapy is administered, especially following regimens intended to ablate the bone marrow in preparation for a stem cell transplant. An infection is probable if agranulocytosis is prolonged, so patients at risk are often given prophylactic antibiotics. When infections do occur in such patients, they can be very difficult to successfully treat—even with normally effective antibiotics—because the number and phagocytic activity of the neutrophils are impaired.

Agranulocytosis may be caused by aplastic anemias that reflect inadequate myelopoiesis. Aplastic anemias (inadequate production of blood cells by the bone marrow) have multiple causes including drug, toxin, or radiation exposure; congenital defect; or age-related fatty or fibrotic bone marrow replacement. The *anemia* in this term is misleading since production of other blood cell types can also be decreased resulting in pancytopenia.

Myelodysplastic anemias are characterized by abnormal maturation of red cells and/or WBCs, usually manifesting a hypercellular bone marrow with peripheral blood cytopenias due to ineffective (abnormal) hematopoiesis. These are typically classified by the French-American-British (FAB) or the more recent World Health Organization (WHO) system based on the marrow morphology identified from a bone marrow aspirate. The usual treatment course is supportive care (i.e., transfusions or stem cell transplant in patients for whom this is feasible).[50]

Neutrophilia (increased circulating neutrophils) is caused by both increased release from the bone marrow and a shift of marginated cells into the circulation. This rapid rise in the number of circulating cells can be caused by acute infections, trauma, or administration of epinephrine or corticosteroids. Prolonged neutrophilia may be due to sustained overproduction caused by ongoing bacterial infections or tissue damage (e.g., cell death, infarction).

Leukemias

Neoplasms of the bone marrow cells usually involve a leukocyte line and are thus termed *leukemias.* Leukemias are broadly classified as being acute or chronic, and leukemias are either of myeloblastic/myelogenous lineage or lymphoblastic/lymphocytic lineage.[51] The clinical course and biology of various leukemias varies. Almost all leukemias fall within one of the four categories below:

- Acute myeloblastic leukemia (AML)
- Acute lymphoblastic leukemia (ALL)
- Chronic myelogenous leukemia (CML)
- Chronic lymphocytic leukemia (CLL)

Although the clinical course will vary among these neoplasms, a common denominator is the proliferation of the neoplastic cell line and suppression of normal hematopoiesis. The neoplastic cells may arise from cells of varying levels of differentiation of either a myeloblastic/myelogenous or lymphoblastic/lymphocytic lineage. Morphology and CD membrane markers will vary among individuals but be fairly uniform throughout the disease course in a given patient. The morphology and CD markers of cells obtained from the diagnostic bone marrow aspirate and flow cytometry respectively are used to assign an FAB classification of M0 through M7 to subtype AML or to diagnose ALL. Today cytogenetic analysis of leukemic cell populations has become a major determinate of therapy in acute leukemia. Other morphologic features and surface marker combinations are used to characterize the other leukemias.

Multiple (plasma cell) myeloma is notable in that it is a plasma cell neoplasm of the bone marrow. The monoclonal neoplastic plasma cells produce a single immunoglobulin isotype (IgG, IgA, light chain only, IgD, IgE, or rarely IgM). This single, monoclonal protein is referred to as the *M-protein.* The M-protein is usually identified using SPEP. The specific immunoglobulin type can be defined with a subsequent step of serum immunoglobulin-specific antibodies (e.g., anti-IgG). Other laboratory findings associated with multiple myeloma include Bence Jones protein (light chain) in urine, hypercalcemia, increased ESR, normochromic, normocytic anemia, and coagulopathy.[52]

Chronic *myeloproliferative* disorders involve an abnormal proliferation of more mature bone marrow cells. Excessive or uncontrolled proliferation of all cell lines leads to polycythemia vera, a malignancy of where erythrocyte overproduction is the most prominent abnormality. Chronic myelogenous leukemia is characterized by a chromosomal translocation [t(9:22), "Philadelphia chromosome"] that creates a fusion product (Bcr/Abl) resulting in autonomous tyrosine kinase activity, a growth signaling enzyme. Some patients without the Philadelphia chromosome have been thought to have CML in the past. However, new techniques suggest that the translocation is fundamental to the diagnosis of CML, and that in its absence these individuals are more likely to have some other myeloproliferative disorder.[53] Patients with CLL present with increased numbers of circulating mature B lymphocytes, which are monoclonal.

Patients with chronic leukemias may live for several years with minimal treatment because of the indolent nature of the disease. In the past, patients with CML would typically develop a transformation of their disease into a life-threatening accelerated phase or blast crisis. Fortunately with the development of tyrosine kinase inhibitor medications, this fatal complication is often avoided or substantially delayed today. Although the chronic leukemias are less aggressive than the acute leukemias, they are persistent and often not curable with chemotherapy; stem cell transplantation may be appropriate in selected patients.

Lymphomas. A lymphoma is a neoplasm of lymphocytic lineage, which typically predominates in lymph nodes forming tissue masses rather than being primarily located in the bone marrow. The lymphomas are classified into two main groups, non-Hodgkin lymphoma (NHL) and Hodgkin lymphoma. The pattern of tissue involvement—termed either *diffuse* or *follicular* (nodular)—and the cytology of the neoplastic lymphoid cells (primarily the size and appearance of the cell nucleus) are used to morphologically subclassify non-Hodgkin lymphoma.[54] The WHO classification of NHL also uses CD surface markers, cytogenetics, and molecular studies to further define subcategories of NHL. Non-Hodgkin lymphomas can also be practically divided into aggressive and indolent forms. The aggressive lymphomas grow and spread quickly but are generally more likely to be eradicated with current, intensive chemotherapy. In contrast, the slower-growing, indolent lymphomas are not as responsive and are more difficult to cure, but these often have a long disease course. Hodgkin lymphoma is generally a more treatable lymphoma. The neoplastic cellular element is termed the *Reed-Sternberg cell*. This is a very large cell with a lobulated nucleus and prominent nucleoli. It is typically surrounded by a nonneoplastic inflammatory background population of lymphocytes, eosinophils, neutrophils, plasma cells, and macrophages.

Non-Hodgkin lymphomas predictably involve lymphoid cells of B cell lineage more commonly than T cell lineage, and many express CD markers characteristic of mature lymphocytes. Identification of the CD20 marker on B cell lymphomas provides an opportunity to treat these patients with recombinant antibodies specific to this surface marker.

Leukocyte Phenotype-Guided Drug Therapy

Translational research is increasingly successful in identifying both gross and subtle differences between normal and cancerous cells. These differences can then be used to develop new diagnostic and therapeutic tools for the treatment of patients with hematogenous tumors. Patients with leukemias expressing the Bcr/Abl fusion protein are therefore likely to be treated with tyrosine kinase inhibitors such as imatinib, dasatinib, or nilotinib.[55]

Another example of targeted treatment of lymphocytes is the use of antibodies such as rituximab to CD20 to treat patients identified as having CD20+ B cell lymphomas. The Fab portion of the antibody binds to the CD20 antigen, and the Fc portion of the antibody activates T cell–mediated cytotoxicity to cause destruction of the bound cell.[56] The same CD20 epitope on the lymphomas is being used for the targeted immune and radioactive cytotoxicity of ibritumomab treatment. This treatment combines rituximab with ibritumomab, another CD20-directed antibody linked to indium-111 or to yttrium-90. Ibritumomab-111In is administered first, and the emitted gamma rays are imaged to assess appropriate distribution of the CD20 antibody. If acceptable, subsequent doses of ibritumomab-90Y are administered to irradiate the CD20+ lymphoma cells with beta particles.

Denileukin diftitox is another novel cytotoxic drug that is presently indicated for CD25+ cutaneous T cell lymphomas (mycosis fungoides and Sézary Syndrome), but that is also being explored for the treatment of other T cell–mediated disorders such as steroid-refractory graft-versus-host disease and systemic T cell lymphomas.[57] Denileukin diftitox is a fusion protein composed of human IL-2 fused with diphtheria toxin. The IL-2 moiety of the drug preferentially binds to cells that express the IL-2 receptor (e.g., T cells containing CD25/CD122/CD152). Once the IL-2 receptor and bound drug are internalized and the protein cleaved, the diphtheria toxin is activated and causes cell death due to protein inhibition.

SUMMARY

This chapter has presented a brief characterization of the lineage and function of red and WBCs. Normal laboratory values have been presented, but it is important to realize that normal ranges will vary slightly depending on the laboratory conducting the analysis and the population being studied.

In hematology, as in most medical sciences, it is important to consider the background and context of the tests used. For example, the Wintrobe RBC indices were characterized at a time when the iron-transporting proteins and vitamin needs of erythropoiesis were unknown. In most cases, abnormalities of the indices reflect a long-term inadequacy of iron, folate, or vitamin B_{12}. Biochemical markers such as circulating ferritin, transferrin receptors, folate, homocysteine, and methylmalonate are likely to be of increasing importance in the early detection of such deficiencies.

Similarly, the definition of lineage specific markers (CD phenotypes) on leukocytes has revolutionized our ability to diagnose and treat leukemias. General diagnoses such as AML will likely continue to be used, but increasingly specific characterization of the surface markers, biochemistry, and genetics of such cells will provide new opportunities to more effectively treat such diseases.

Although there is increasing precision and sophistication in identifying molecular changes associated with hematologic pathologies, the importance of understanding the fundamentals of clinical hematology cannot be discounted. Infections and chronic leukemias will continue to be diagnosed and monitored from an elevated WBC, and anemias will be identified and treated through routine blood examinations. Old and new technologies will increasingly complement one another in clinical hematology.

Learning Points

1. How do iron deficiency and nutrient deficiency (folate and/or vitamin B_{12}) differ in their presentation in a hemogram?

Answer: As expressed by the term *anemia* in each of these circumstances, the total RBC (erythrocyte) count will be low, as will the Hgb and Hct. Iron deficiency is characterized by small (microcytic, low MCV) and pale (hypochromic) erythrocytes. In contrast, both folate and vitamin B_{12} deficiency classically present with larger (macrocytic, elevated MCV) erythrocytes. Another difference often noted in the hemogram is an elevated reticulocyte count in patients with iron deficiency after treatment with supplemental iron.

2. What are the roles of transferrin, ferritin, and TIBC, and how are laboratory values for these substances interpreted?

Answer: Transferrin is a plasma protein with high avidity to highly reactive metal ions such as iron and chromium. Its primary role is to transport iron to the bone marrow for erythrocyte synthesis, while in the process protecting intervening tissue from the reactivity of the metal ion. Ferritin is another minor iron plasma transport protein, but differs from transferrin in that it enters cells of the reticuloendothelial system, where it serves its greater role as the storage form of iron. Ferritin protein not bound to iron is termed *apoferritin*. Most of the iron binding protein in the plasma is transferrin, and the serum TIBC is an indirect measure of the transferrin concentration. When iron stores are low (iron deficiency), the liver synthesizes more transferrin. Thus, the residual, unbound capacity of the transferrin (and thus TIBC) will be increased. In anemia of chronic disease, the plasma iron and transferrin concentrations are both low, so although the transferrin saturation may be decreased, it will often be within the normal range. Liver disease or malnutrition can also slow the production of transferrin, which may complicate the interpretation of the TIBC.

3. What are typical reasons why WBC counts are elevated, and how can the differential cell count help clarify the causality?

Answer: A sustained elevation of WBC count is typically due to infections, psychological stress, or leukemias. Infections, epinephrine and exercise cause a demargination of neutrophils from the endothelium, causing a transient, increased percentage of neutrophils, but a normal absolute lymphocyte count. In contrast, corticosteroids also cause neutrophil demargination but are also lymphotoxic, so the absolute lymphocyte count will decrease. Bacterial infections are associated with an increase in the percentage and absolute number of neutrophils and to the release of premature neutrophils (band cells) from the bone marrow. Very high or low WBC counts, or abnormal differential count percentages and unusual cell morphology increase the suspicion of leukemia.

REFERENCES

1. Gulati GL, Ashton JK, Hyun BH. Structure and function of the bone marrow and hematopoiesis. *Hematol Oncol Clin North Am.* 1988;2:495-511.

2. Finch CA, Harker LA, Cook JD. Kinetics of the formed elements of the human blood. *Blood.* 1977;50:699-707.

3. Kipps TJ. The cluster of differentiation antigens. In: Lichtman MA, Kipps TJ, Seligsohn U, et al., eds. *William's Hematology.* 8th ed. New York, NY: McGraw-Hill; 2010:193-229.

4. Kaushasky K. Hematopoietic stem cells, progenitors, and cytokines. In: Lichtman MA, Kipps TJ, Seligsohn U, et al., eds. *William's Hematology.* 8th ed. New York, NY: McGraw-Hill; 2010:231-245.

5. Ryan DH. Examination of the marrow. In: Lichtman MA, Kipps TJ, Seligsohn U, et al., eds. *William's Hematology.* 8th ed. New York, NY: McGraw-Hill; 2010:25-36.

6. Prchal JT. Production of erythrocytes. In: Lichtman MA, Kipps TJ, Seligsohn U, et al., eds. *William's Hematology.* 8th ed. New York, NY: McGraw-Hill; 2010:435-448.

7. Bull BS, Herrmann PC. Morphology of the erythron. In: Lichtman MA, Kipps TJ, Seligsohn U, et al., eds. *William's Hematology.* 8th ed. New York, NY: McGraw-Hill; 2010:409-428.

8. Perkins SL. Examination of the blood and bone marrow. In: Greer JP, Foerster J, Lukens J, et al., eds. *Wintrobe's Clinical Hematology.* 11th ed. Philadelphia PA: Lippincott Williams & Wilkins; 2004:3-25.

9. Vajpayee N, Graham SS, Bem S. Basic examination of the blood and bone marrow. In: McPherson RA, Pincus MR, ed. *Clinical Diagnosis and Management by Laboratory Methods.* 22nd ed. Philadelphia, PA: WB Saunders; 2011:510-535.

10. Massey AC. Microcytic anemia: differential diagnosis and management of iron deficiency anemia. *Med Clin North Am.* 1992;76:549-566.

11. Gulati GL, Hyun BH. The automated CBC. A current perspective. *Hematol Oncol Clin North Am.* 1994;8:593-603.

12. Sox HC, Liang MH. The erythrocyte sedimentation rate: guidelines for rational use. *Ann Intern Med.* 1986;104:515-523.

13. Bull BS, Brailsford JD. The zeta sedimentation ratio. *Am J Clin Pathol.* 1972;40:550-559.

14. Lee GR, Herbert V. Nutritional factors in the production and function of erythrocytes. In: Greer JP, Foerster J, Lukens J, et al., eds. *Wintrobe's Clinical Hematology.* 11th ed. Philadelphia PA: Lippincott Williams & Wilkins: 2004:228-266.

15. Green R. Folate, cobalamin, and megaloblastic anemias In: Lichtman MA, Kipps TJ, Seligsohn U, et al., eds. *William's Hematology.* 8th ed. New York, NY: McGraw-Hill; 2010:533-564.

16. Bunting RW, Bitzer AM, Kennedy RM, et al. Prevalence of intrinsic factor antibodies and vitamin B$_{12}$ malabsorption in older patients admitted to a rehabilitation hospital. *J Am Geriatr Soc.* 1990;38:743-747.

17. Phillips DL, Keeffe EB. Hematologic manifestations of gastrointestinal disease. *Hematol Oncol Clin North Am.* 1987;1:207-228.

18. Ravel R. Clinical laboratory medicine: Factor deficiency anemia. In: Ravel R, ed. *Clinical Laboratory Medicine: Clinical Application of Laboratory Data.* 6th ed. St Louis, MO: Mosby; 1995:22-34.

19. Sutphin SD. Drug-induced diseases. In: Anderson PO, Knoben JE, Troutman WG, eds. *Handbook of Clinical Drug Data.* 11th ed. New York, NY: McGraw-Hill; 2010:918-993.

20. Colon-Otero G, Menke D, Hook CC. A practical approach to the differential diagnosis and evaluation of the adult patient with macrocytic anemia. *Med Clin North Am.* 1992;76:581-597.

21. Erslev AJ, Gabuzda TG. *Pathophysiology of Blood.* Philadelphia, PA: WB Saunders; 1985.

22. Downs LT. Immunohematology. In: McPherson RA, Pincus MR, ed. *Clinical Diagnosis and Management by Laboratory Methods.* 22nd ed. Philadelphia, PA: WB Saunders; 2011:675-730.

23. Tabara IA. Hemolytic anemias. Diagnosis and treatment. *Med Clin North Am.* 1992;76:649-668.

24. Neff AT. Autoimmune hemolytic anemias. In: Greer JP, Foerster J, Lukens J, et al., eds. *Wintrobe's Clinical Hematology.* 11th ed. Philadelphia PA: Lippincott Williams & Wilkins: 2004:1157-1182.

25. Blum MD, Graham DJ, McCloskey CA. Temafloxacin syndrome: review of 95 cases. *Clin Infect Dis.* 1994;18:946-950.

26. Golan DE. Hemolytic anemias: red cell membranes and metabolic effects. In: Goldman L, Ausiello D, eds. *Cecil Textbook of Medicine.* 22nd ed. Philadelphia, PA: WB Saunders; 2004:1021-1030.

27. Means, RT Jr. Anemias secondary to chronic disease and systemic disorders. In: Greer JP, Foerster J, Lukens J, et al., eds. *Wintrobe's Clinical Hematology.* 11th ed. Philadelphia PA: Lippincott Williams & Wilkins: 2004:1445-1465.

28. Dubois RW, Goodnough LT, Ershler WB, et al. Identification, diagnosis, and management of anemia in adult ambulatory patients treated by primary care physicians: evidence-based and consensus recommendations. *Curr Med Res Opin.* 2006;22:385-395.

29. FDA Drug Safety Communication. Modified dosing recommendations to improve the safe use of erythropoiesis-stimulating agents (ESAs) in chronic kidney disease. http://www.fda.gov/Drugs/DrugSafety/ucm259639.htm. Accessed December 24, 2011.

30. Rizzo JD, Brouwers M, Hurley P, et al.; American Society of Clinical Oncology, American Society of Hematology. American Society of Clinical Oncology/American Society of Hematology clinical practice guideline update on the use of epoetin and darbepoetin in adult patients with cancer. *J Clin Oncol.* 2010;28(33):4996-5010.

31. FDA Drug Safety Communication. Erythropoiesis-Stimulating Agents (ESAs): Procrit, Epogen and Aranesp. http://www.fda.gov/Drugs/DrugSafety/PostmarketDrugSafetyInformationforPatientsandProviders/ucm200297.htm. Accessed December 31, 2011.

32. Fixler J, Styles L. Sickle cell disease. *Pediatr Clin North Am.* 2002;49:1193-1210.

33. Wang WC, Lukens JN. Sickle cell anemia and other sickling syndromes. In: Greer JP, Foerster J, Lukens J, et al., eds. *Wintrobe's Clinical Hematology.* 11th ed. Philadelphia PA: Lippincott Williams & Wilkins: 2004:1263-1312.

34. Lo L, Singer ST. Thalassemia: current approach to an old disease. *Pediatr Clin North Am.* 2002;49:1165-1191.

35. Krause JR. The automated white blood cell differential. A current perspective. *Hematol Oncol Clin North Am.* 1994;8:605-616.

36. Gottlieb R. Apoptosis. In: Lichtman MA, Kipps TJ, Seligsohn U, et al., eds. *William's Hematology.* 8th ed. New York, NY: McGraw-Hill; 2010:161-168.

37. Strausbaugh LJ. Hematologic manifestations of bacterial and fungal infections. *Hematol Oncol Clin North Am.* 1987;1:185-206.

38. McKenzie SB, Laudicina RJ. Hematologic changes associated with infection. *Clin Lab Sci.* 1998;11:239-251.

39. Serafin WE, Austen KF. Mediators of immediate hypersensitivity reactions. *N Engl J Med.* 1987;317:30-34.

40. Male D, Brostoff J, Roitt IM, et al. *Immunology.* 7th ed. New York, NY: Mosby; 2006:59-86.

41. Gordon S, Pluddermann A. Production, distribution, and fate of monocytes and macrophages. In: Lichtman MA, Kipps TJ, Seligsohn U, et al., eds. *William's Hematology.* 8th ed. New York, NY: McGraw-Hill; 2010:1021-1034.

42. Broom HE. Morphology of lymphocytes and plasma cells. In: Lichtman MA, Kipps TJ, Seligsohn U, et al., eds. *William's Hematology.* 8th ed. New York, NY: McGraw-Hill; 2010:1079-1086.

43. Kipps TJ. Composition and biochemistry of lymphocytes and plasma cells. In: Lichtman MA, Kipps TJ, Seligsohn U, et al., eds. *William's Hematology.* 8th ed. New York, NY: McGraw-Hill; 2010:1087-1094.

44. Paraskevas F. Clinical flow cytometry. In: Greer JP, Foerster J, Lukens J, et al., eds. *Wintrobe's Clinical Hematology.* 11th ed. Philadelphia PA: Lippincott Williams & Wilkins: 2004:99-130.

45. Ho DD, Pomerantz RJ, Kaplan JC. Pathogenesis of infection with human immunodeficiency virus. *N Engl J Med.* 1987;317:278-286.

46. Mindel A, Tenant-Flowers M. ABC of AIDS: natural history and management of early HIV infections. *BMJ.* 2001;322:1290-1293.

47. Baranski B, Young N. Hematologic consequences of viral infections. *Hematol Oncol Clin North Am.* 1987;1:167-183.

48. Friedman AD. Hematologic manifestations of viral infections. *Pediatric Ann.* 1996;25:555-560.

49. Dale DC. Neutropenia and neutrophilia. In: Lichtman MA, Kipps TJ, Seligsohn U, et al., eds. *William's Hematology.* 8th ed. New York, NY: McGraw-Hill; 2010:939-950.

50. Vardiman JW, Thiele J, Arber DA, et al., The 2008 revision of the World Health Organization (WHO) classification of myeloid neoplasms and acute leukemia: rationale and important changes. *Blood.*;114:937-951.

51. Wetzler M, Byrd JC, Bloomfield CD. Acute and chronic myeloid leukemia. In: Fauci AS, Braunwald E, Kasper DL, et al., eds. *Harrison's Principles of Internal Medicine.* 17th ed. New York, NY: McGraw-Hill; 2008:677-686.

52. Van Rhee F, Anaissie E, Angtucao E, et al. Myeloma. In: Lichtman MA, Kipps TJ, Seligsohn U, et al., eds. *William's Hematology.* 8th ed. New York, NY: McGraw-Hill; 2010:1645-1681.

53. Liesveld JL, Lichtman MA. Chronic myelogenous leukemia and related disorders. In: Lichtman MA, Kipps TJ, Seligsohn U, et al., eds. *William's Hematology.* 8th ed. New York, NY: McGraw-Hill; 2010:1331-1380.

54. Gascoyne R, Skinnider B. *Pathology* of malignant lymphoma. In: Lichtman MA, Kipps TJ, Seligsohn U, et al., eds. *William's Hematology.* 8th ed. New York, NY: McGraw-Hill; 2010:1511-1526.

55. Guilhot F, Apperley J, Kim DW, et al. Dasatinib induces significant hematologic and cytogenetic responses in patients with imatinib-resistant or -intolerant chronic myeloid leukemia in accelerated phase. *Blood.* 2007;109:4143-4150.

56. Maloney DG, Smith B, Rose A. Rituximab: mechanism of action and resistance. *Semin Oncol.* 2002;29(suppl):2-9.

57. Foss F, Clinical experience with denileukin diftitox (ONTAK). *Semin Oncol.* 2006;3(1 Suppl 3):S11-S16.

58. Tsimberidou AM, Giles FJ, Estey E, et al. The role of gemtuzumab ozogamicin in acute leukaemia therapy. *Br J Hematol.* 2006;132(4):398-409.

CHAPTER 16

HEMATOLOGY: BLOOD COAGULATION TESTS

LEA E. DELA PEÑA

The contribution of material written by James B. Groce III, Julie B. Lemus, and Sheila M. Allen in previous editions of this book is gratefully acknowledged.

Objectives

After completing this chapter, the reader should be able to

- Describe the role of platelets, the coagulation cascade, and fibrinolytic system in normal hemostasis

- List the laboratory tests used to assess platelets and discuss factors that may influence their results

- List the laboratory tests used to assess coagulation and explain their use in evaluating anticoagulant therapy

- List the laboratory tests used to assess clot degradation and disseminated intravascular coagulation (DIC) and discuss their limitations

- Interpret results and suggest followup action given results of laboratory tests used for evaluating coagulation and anticoagulant therapy in a case description

- Discuss the availability and use of point-of-care testing devices specifically for platelet and coagulation tests

Normal hemostasis involves a complex interaction among the vascular sub-endothelium, platelets, coagulation factors, and proteins that promote clot formation and subsequent clot degradation as well as inhibitors of these substances. Disruption in normal hemostasis can result in bleeding or excessive clotting. Bleeding can be caused by trauma or damage to vessels, acquired or inherited deficiencies of coagulation factors, or physiological disorders of platelets, whereas, excessive clotting can result from abnormalities of the vascular endothelium, alterations in blood flow, or deficiencies in clotting inhibitors.

Clinicians must monitor the hemostasis process in individual patients to ensure their safety from an imbalance in this complex system. For example, practitioners routinely order platelet tests in patients on certain antineoplastic medications to assess for thrombocytopenia. Likewise, clinicians closely monitor coagulation tests for patients receiving anticoagulants to prevent thromboembolic or hemorrhagic complications. Overall, the hemostatic process is intricate and requires a clinician knowledgeable in its dynamics for quality assessment.

This chapter reviews normal coagulation physiology, common tests used to assess coagulation and hypercoagulable states, and, finally, factors that alter coagulation tests.

PHYSIOLOGICAL PROCESS OF HEMOSTASIS

Normal hemostasis involves the complex relationship among participants that promote clot formation (platelets and the coagulation cascade), inhibit coagulation, and dissolve the formed clot. Each phase of the process is briefly reviewed.

Clot Formation

Numerous mechanisms promote and limit coagulation. Factors that promote coagulation include malignancy, estrogen therapy, pregnancy, obesity, immobilization, damage to the blood vessel wall, and areas of low blood flow or venous stasis. Normal blood flow dilutes activated clotting factors and results in their degradation in various tissues (e.g., liver) and by proteases. However, in areas of low flow or venous stasis, activated clotting factors may not be readily cleared.

Platelets

Platelets are non-nucleated, disk-shaped structures, 1–5 microns in diameter, which are formed in the extravascular spaces of bone marrow from megakaryocytes. Megakaryocyte production and maturation are promoted by the hormone thrombopoietin, which is synthesized in the bone marrow and liver. The lungs and other tissues can retain megakaryocytes and thus also produce platelets.[1] Two-thirds of the platelets are found in the circulation and one-third in the spleen; however, in splenectomized patients nearly 100% are in the circulation.

The average human adult makes approximately 100 billion platelets per day, with the average platelet circulating for 7–10 days; transfused platelets have a shorter lifespan of 4–5 days.[1] On aging, platelets are destroyed by the spleen, liver, and bone marrow. Throughout their lifespan, platelet function is affected by numerous factors such as medications, vitamins, foods, spices, and systemic conditions, including chronic renal disease and hematological disorders (e.g., myeloproliferative and lymphoproliferative diseases, dysproteinemias, and the presence of antiplatelet antibodies).

The primary function of platelets is to regulate hemostasis, but platelets also play a prominent role in the pathological formation of arterial thrombi. Three processes (platelet adhesion, activation, and aggregation) are essential for arterial thrombus formation. The surface of normal blood vessels does not stimulate platelet adhesion due to the presence of antithrombogenic and vasoactive substances.[2,3] However, endothelial injury to the vasculature is often caused by flow abnormalities, trauma, or the rupture of atherosclerotic plaque in the vessel wall. Subendothelial structures, such as collagen, basement membrane, and fibronectin, then become exposed (Figure 16-1), which can result in platelet adhesion. Platelet adhesion is enhanced by substances such as epinephrine, thrombin, adenosine diphosphate (ADP), serotonin, collagen, and von Willebrand factor (vWF).[4] Circulating vWF acts as a binding ligand between the subendothelium and glycoprotein Ib receptors on the platelet surface.

Once adhesion occurs, platelets change shape and activation occurs. Substances such as collagen, ADP, thrombin, and thromboxane A_2 (TxA$_2$) stimulate the change in platelet shape and cause platelets to release their contents including ADP, serotonin (5HT), platelet factor 3 (PF3), and platelet factor 4 (PF4).[2] Following platelet adhesion and activation, platelet aggregation completes the formation of the hemostatic plug. This process is mediated by glycoprotein IIb/IIIa receptors on the platelet surface with fibrinogen acting as the primary binding ligand bridging between platelets. Platelets have numerous Gp IIb/IIIa binding sites, which are an attractive option for antiplatelet drug therapy.[2,4]

ADP and TxA$_2$ recruit additional platelets, which aggregate to the platelets that are already bound to the subendothelial tissues. In addition to promoting aggregation, TxA$_2$, 5HT, and other substances are potent vasoconstrictors that limit blood flow to the damaged site. When vascular damage is minimal, the vasoconstriction and platelet aggregation (formation of a platelet plug) may be sufficient to limit bleeding.

However, the platelet plug is not stable and can be dislodged. To form a more permanent hemostatic plug, the clotting system must be stimulated. By releasing PF3, platelets initiate the clotting cascade and concentrate activated clotting factors at the site of vascular (endothelial) injury.

Prostaglandins (PGs) play an important role in platelet function. Figure 16-2 displays a simplified version of the complex arachidonic acid pathways that occur in platelets and on the vascular endothelium. Thromboxane A$_2$, a potent stimulator of platelet aggregation and vasoconstriction, is formed in platelets. In contrast, prostacyclin (PG2), produced by endothelial cells lining the vessel luminal surface, is a potent inhibitor of platelet aggregation and a potent vasodilator that limits excessive platelet aggregation.

Cyclooxygenase and PG2 are clinically important. An aspirin dose of 80 mg/day acetylates and irreversibly inhibits cyclooxygenase in the platelet. Platelets are rendered incapable of forming arachidonic acid and PGs. This effect of low-dose aspirin lasts for the lifespan of the exposed platelets (up to 12 days).

Vascular endothelial cells also contain cyclooxygenase, which converts arachidonic acid to PG2. Aspirin in high doses inhibits the production of PG2. However, because the vascular endothelium can regenerate PG2, aspirin's effect is much shorter here than on platelets. Thus, aspirin's effect at

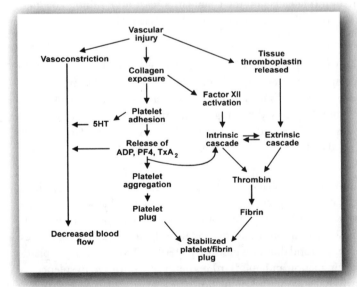

FIGURE 16-1. Relationship between platelets and the clotting cascade in the generation of a stabilized fibrin clot. 5HT = serotonin; ADP = adenosine diphosphate; PF4 = platelet factor 4; TxA$_2$ = thromboxane A$_2$.

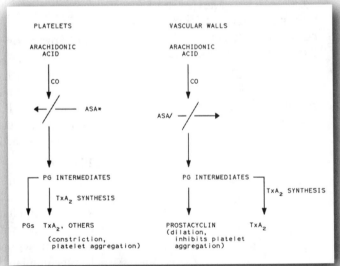

FIGURE 16-2. Formation of thromboxane A$_2$ (TxA$_2$), prostaglandins (PGs), and prostacyclin in platelets and vascular endothelial cells. CO = cyclooxygenase; ASA* = low-dose, irreversible, inactivation of platelet cyclooxygenase; ASA/ = high-dose inactivation of platelet cyclooxygenase.

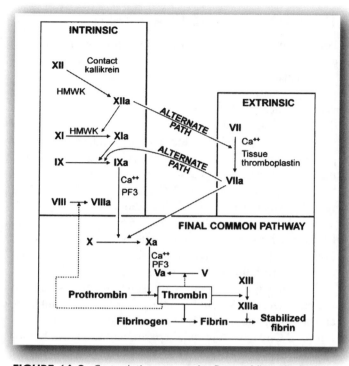

FIGURE 16-3. Coagulation cascade. Dotted lines indicate thrombin's feedback action, which modifies factors V and VIII. HMWK = high molecular weight kininogen. (Reproduced, with permission, from reference 5.)

TABLE 16-1. Characteristics of Coagulation Factors[1,6]

FACTOR	NAMES	APPROXIMATE HALF-LIFE (HR)
I	Fibrinogen	72–120
II	Prothrombin	72
III	Thromboplastin, tissue extract	
IV	Calcium	
V	Proaccelerin, labile factor, accelerator globulin	12
VI	Originally referred to as accelerin, but now recognized as activated factor V; this numeral is no longer used	N/A
VII	Proconvertin, serum prothrombin conversion accelerator, stable factor, autoprothrombin I	3–4
VIII	Antihemophilic factor, antihemophilic globulin, platelet cofactor I, antihemophilic factor A	8–12
IX	Plasma thromboplastin component, Christmas factor, antihemophilic factor B, platelet cofactor II, autoprothrombin II	24
X	Stuart-Prower factor	36
XI	Plasmin thromboplastin antecedent	72
XII	Hageman factor	48
XIII	Fibrin stabilizing factor, Laki-Lorand factor, and fibrinase	240–336

high doses may both inhibit platelet aggregation and block the aggregation inhibitor PG2. This phenomenon is the rationale for using low doses of aspirin 80–325 mg/day to help prevent myocardial infarction.

In summary, a complex interaction between the platelet and blood vessel wall maintains hemostasis. Once platelet adhesion occurs, the clotting cascade may become activated. After thrombin and fibrin are generated, the platelet plug becomes stabilized with insoluble fibrin at the site of vascular injury.

Coagulation Cascade

The ultimate goal of the coagulation cascade (Figure 16-3) is to generate fibrin from thrombin. Fibrin forms an insoluble mesh surrounding the platelet plug. Platelets concentrate activated clotting factors at the site of vascular injury.

The nomenclature and half-lives for the coagulation proteins are shown in Table 16-1. The coagulation cascade is typically divided into the intrinsic, extrinsic, and common pathways: the intrinsic and extrinsic pathways provide different routes to generate factor X while the common pathway results in thrombin formation. Coagulation is initiated by vascular injury or damage that exposes blood to tissue factor (TF), which then binds to factor VII at the start of the extrinsic pathway. The binding of TF to factor VII activates the latter to VIIa. The complex formed by TF and factor VIIa can then activate factor X to Xa at the start of the common pathway. Alternatively, the TF-factor VIIa complex can first convert factor IX to factor IXa, with factor VIIIa as a cofactor, which is part of the intrinsic pathway. Factor IXa can then activate factor X into Xa; thus, both the intrinsic and extrinsic pathways activate factor

X in the final common pathway. Factor Xa with factor Va as a cofactor activates prothrombin (factor II) into thrombin (factor IIa). In the clotting cascade, thrombin not only converts fibrinogen into fibrin, but it can also convert factor XIII to factor XIIIa, which stabilizes the fibrin clot.[4] In addition to the direct effects and feedback mechanisms of thrombin shown in Figure 16-3, thrombin also stimulates platelet aggregation and activates the fibrinolytic system.

Additional factors within the pathway. Factors such as calcium and vitamin K play an intricate role within the various pathways in the coagulation cascade. Calcium is essential for the platelet surface binding of several factors within the pathway. Vitamin K facilitates the calcium binding function of factors II, VII, IX, and X via carboxylation. These processes are critical in activating proteins within the pathway.

Inhibition of Coagulation

Mechanisms that limit *coagulation* include the natural inhibitors such as antithrombin (AT) and the vitamin K dependent proteins C and S, tissue factor pathway inhibitor (TFPI), and the fibrinolytic system. Endothelial cells produce several substances that have antithrombotic effects which may also activate the fibrinolytic system.[4] Platelet aggregation is prevented by substances such as PG2 and nitric oxide, both of which are generated by the vessel wall.[1,4] Generation of plasminogen activators also can limit platelet aggregation.[1] Several

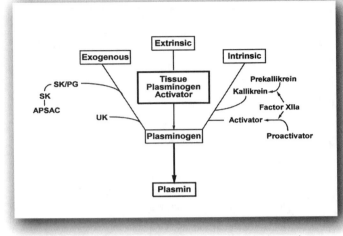

FIGURE 16-4. Exogenous, extrinsic, and intrinsic pathways for activation of plasminogen. APSAC = anistreplase; SK = streptokinase; SK/PG = streptokinase-plasminogen complex; UK = urokinase. (Reproduced, with permission, from reference 7.)

medications can also inhibit coagulation by acting on platelets (aspirin, clopidogrel, prasugrel) or one or more clotting factors (warfarin, low molecular weight heparins [LMWHs], unfractionated heparin [UFH], dabigatran, rivaroxaban, apixaban, and direct thrombin inhibitors [DTIs]).

High concentrations of thrombin, in conjunction with thrombomodulin, activate protein C, which can then inactivate cofactors Va and VIIIa; thus, there is a negative feedback mechanism that will block further thrombin generation and subsequent steps in the coagulation cascade.[8] Protein S serves as a cofactor for protein C. Antithrombin inactivates thrombin as well as factors IX, X, and XI, and this process can be hastened by heparin. Heparin and AT combine one-to-one, and the complex neutralizes the activated clotting factors and inhibits the coagulation cascade. Deficiencies in these natural inhibitors can result in increased generation of thrombin, which can lead to recurrent thromboembolic events often starting at a young age. Tissue factor pathway inhibitor impedes the binding of TF to factor VII, essentially inhibiting the extrinsic pathway (Figure 16-3). Unfractionated heparin and LMWHs can release TFPI from lipoproteins.[4] The complex mechanisms that limit thrombus formation are shown in Figure 16-4.

Clot Degradation

Fibrinolysis is the mechanism by which formed thrombi are lysed to prevent excessive clot formation and vascular occlusion. As discussed previously, fibrin is formed in the final common pathway of the clotting cascade. Tissue plasminogen activator (tPA) and urokinase plasminogen activator (uPA) activate plasminogen, which generates plasmin. *Plasmin* is the enzyme that eventually breaks down fibrin into fibrin degradation products (FDPs). Medications can either activate (e.g., streptokinase, alteplase, urokinase, reteplase, and tenecteplase) or inhibit (tranexamic acid, aminocaproic acid, and aprotinin) fibrinolysis.

TESTS TO EVALUATE HEMOSTASIS

For the purpose of discussion, bleeding and clotting disorders are organized by tests that assess

- Platelets
- Coagulation
- Clot degradation
- Hypercoagulable states

Tests to assess platelets include platelet count, volume (mean platelet volume [MPV]), function (e.g., bleeding time [BT] and platelet aggregation), and others. Thrombin time (TT), reptilase time, prothrombin time (PT)/international normalized ratio (INR), activated partial thromboplastin time (aPTT), activated clotting time (ACT), fibrinogen assay, and others are laboratory tests that assess coagulation. Clot degradation is assessed with tests for FDPs and D-dimer. Fibrinolysis also is monitored with the euglobulin lysis test.

A hypercoagulable state workup may include activated protein C (APC) resistance and the factor V Leiden mutation, anticardiolipin antibody, antiphospholipid antibody, antiplasmin, AT, C-reactive protein, heparin neutralization, homocystine, lipoprotein, plasminogen, plasminogen activator inhibitor 1 (PAI1), platelet hyperaggregation, proteins C and S, prothrombin G20210A mutation, reptilase time, and TT. These tests are often performed in panels since the presence of more than one predisposition to thrombosis further increases the risk for thrombosis.[8]

In addition, general hematological values such as hemoglobin (Hgb), hematocrit (Hct), red blood cell (RBC) count, and white blood cell (WBC) count, as well as urinalysis and stool guaiac tests may be important to obtain when evaluating blood and coagulation disorders; some of these tests are further discussed in Chapter 15: Hematology: Red and White Blood Cell Tests. Table 16-2 is a summary of common tests used to evaluate bleeding disorders and monitor anticoagulant therapy.

Platelet Tests

Platelet Count

Normal range: 150,000–450,000/μL

The only test to determine the number or concentration of platelets in a blood sample is the *platelet count,* through either manual (rarely done) or automated methods. Interferences with platelet counts include RBC fragments, platelet clumping, and platelet satellitism (platelet adherence to WBCs). Automated platelet counts are performed on anticoagulated whole blood. Most instrumentation that performs hematological profiles provides platelet counts. Platelets and RBCs are passed through an aperture generating an electric pulse with a magnitude related to the size of the cell/particle. The pulses are counted, and the platelets are separated from the RBCs by size providing the platelet count and MPV as well as the RBC count and mean corpuscular volume (MCV).

Thrombocythemia. An abnormal platelet count can have many causes. Thrombocythemia, also known as *thrombocytosis* or *elevated platelet count,* may be caused by several factors including

TABLE 16-2. Summary of Coagulation Tests for Hemorrhagic Disorders and Anticoagulant Drug Monitoring[a]

DISORDER OR DRUG	PLATELET COUNT	BT	PT/INR	APTT	COMMENTS
Thrombocytopenic purpura	Low	Prolonged	WNL	WNL	
Glanzmann thrombasthenia	WNL	WNL or prolonged	WNL	WNL	Platelets appear normal
von Willebrand disease	Low or WNL	WNL or prolonged	WNL	WNL or prolonged	Factor VIII levels low or WNL, vFW (antigen level and/or activity) low or WNL
Fibrinogen deficiency	WNL	WNL	Prolonged	Prolonged	BT prolonged if severe, fibrinogen levels decreased, TT prolonged
Warfarin therapy	WNL	WNL or prolonged	Prolonged	WNL or prolonged	BT prolonged if overdosed
Heparin therapy	WNL	WNL or prolonged	WNL or prolonged	Prolonged	Platelet count may decrease[b]
Vascular purpura	WNL	WNL	WNL	WNL	Normal platelet count distinguishes this from other forms of purpura such as TTP or ITP

aPTT= activated partial thromboplastin time; BT= bleeding time; ITP= idiopathic thrombocytopenic purpura; PT/INR= prothrombin time/international normalized ratio; TTP= thrombotic thrombocytopenic purpura; vWF= von Willebrand factor; WNL= within normal limits.
[a]Italic type indicates most useful diagnostic or therapeutic tests.
[b]Significant thrombocytopenia may occur as a heparin side effect in 1% to 5% of patients.

- Stress
- Infection
- Splenectomy
- Trauma
- Asphyxiation
- Rheumatoid arthritis
- Iron-deficiency anemia
- Posthemorrhagic anemia
- Cirrhosis
- Chronic pancreatitis
- Tuberculosis
- Occult malignancy
- Recovery from bone marrow suppression

Values of 500,000–800,000/µL are not uncommon. Thrombocythemia may be seen with any of the chronic myeloproliferative neoplasms, essential thrombocythemia, polycythemia vera, chronic myelogenous leukemia, or idiopathic myelofibrosis. Clinical consequences of thrombocythemia include thrombosis, hemorrhage, and microcirculatory disturbances. Thrombotic events may be either arterial or venous and include cerebrovascular accidents, myocardial infarction, deep venous thrombosis, pulmonary embolism, and intra-abdominal (portal and hepatic) vein thrombosis. Hemorrhagic complications usually involve the skin and/or mucous membranes, which include ecchymosis, epistaxis, and menorrhagia. Microcirculatory disturbances, such as headache, paresthesias, and erythromelalgia, may be due to microthrombi, which results in occlusion and ischemia. Additionally, patients with thrombocythemia may have abnormalities in platelet function studies, which can manifest as bleeding problems.

Thrombocytopenia. Mucosal and/or cutaneous bleeding is the most common clinical consequence of thrombocytopenia; however, patients with only modest decreases in platelet counts may be asymptomatic. (See Minicase 1.) When the platelet count falls below 20,000/µL, the patient is at risk of spontaneous bleeding. Therefore, platelet transfusions are often initiated. Bleeding may occur at higher platelet counts (e.g., 50,000/µL) if trauma occurs. The most common cause of death in a patient with severe thrombocytopenia is central nervous system (CNS) bleeding such as intracranial hemorrhage.

Numerous drugs have been associated with thrombocytopenia (Table 16-3). However, heparin and antineoplastics are the most common ones implicated. Thrombocytopenia is also common with radiation therapy. Many drugs associated with thrombocytopenia alter platelet antigens resulting in the formation of antibodies to platelets (e.g., heparin, penicillin, and gold). Several diseases, such as thrombotic thrombocytopenic purpura (TTP), idiopathic thrombocytopenic purpura (ITP), disseminated intravascular coagulation (DIC), and hemolytic-uremic syndrome, result in rapid destruction of platelets. Other causes of thrombocytopenia include viral infections; pernicious, aplastic, and folate/B_{12}-deficiency anemias; complications of pregnancy; massive blood transfusions; exposure to dichlorodiphenyltrichloroethane (DDT); and human immunodeficiency virus (HIV) infections.

Heparin-induced thrombocytopenia (HIT) is an antibody-mediated adverse reaction to heparin, occurring in 0.2% to 5% of all heparin-treated adults, which may cause venous and arterial thrombosis.[9] Specifically, this is due to the development of IgG antibodies that bind to the heparin PF4 complex.

TABLE 16-3. Partial List of Agents Associated with Thrombocytopenia[a]

Aldesleukin	Methimazole
Allopurinol	Nalidixic acid
Amphotericin B	Penicillamine
Amrinone	Penicillins
Antineoplastics	Pentamidine
Antiviral agents	Phenytoin
Azathioprine	Propylthiouracil
Carbamazepine	Quinacrine
Cephalosporins	Quinidine
Chloramphenicol	Quinine
Chlorpropamide	Radiation
Etretinate	Sulfonamides
Gold compounds	Tamoxifen
Griseofulvin	Thiazide diuretics
H2 antagonists	Tolbutamide
Heparin	Trimethoprim
Interferons	Valproic acid

[a]Some drugs listed cause an idiosyncratic, drug-induced thrombocytopenia while others induce formation of antiplatelet antibodies (gold, penicillins, and heparin). Exceptions include amrinone, antineoplastics, and possibly amphotericin B, which cause a direct toxic effect that may be dose related.

Patients receiving UFH are generally at a higher risk of developing HIT than patients receiving LMWH. Low molecular weight heparin does not bind as well as UFH to PF4, which is thought to be due to the smaller size of LMWH compared to UFH. Therefore, the heparin-PF4 complex is less likely to form with LMWH, and there are less IgG antibodies generated. The frequency or risk of HIT is influenced by certain factors such as heparin preparation, route, dose, and duration of heparin therapy, patient population, gender, and previous history of heparin exposure.[10,11] The animal source of heparin may also play a role in determining who develops HIT; bovine UFH seems to carry a higher risk compared to porcine UFH.[11]

The 4Ts score is a clinical prediction tool to help physicians determine the probability of their patient having HIT. This tool looks at thrombocytopenia, timing of platelet count fall or thrombosis, thrombosis or other clinical sequelae, and other causes for thrombocytopenia; a score of 0–2 is assigned for each of the four parts based on specific patient characteristics to determine the probability of HIT occurring in that particular patient.[10] Heparin-induced thrombocytopenia is manifested both by clinical and serological features, and diagnosis of HIT is usually made when antibody formation is detected by an in vitro assay plus one or more of the following: unexplained decrease in platelet count (usually ≥30%, even if the nadir remains above 150×10^9/L), venous or arterial thrombosis, limb gangrene, necrotizing skin lesions at the heparin injection site, or acute anaphylactoid reactions occurring after intravenous (IV) heparin bolus administration.[10]

There are two types of tests to help diagnose HIT: the enzyme-linked immunosorbent assay (ELISA), which identifies anti-PF4/heparin antibodies and functional assays, such as the C-serotonin release assay (SRA) or the heparin-induced platelet activation (HIPA) assay, both of which detect antibodies that induce heparin-dependent platelet activation.[9-11] The ELISA test has high sensitivity and wide availability, with a relatively rapid turnaround time compared to the functional assays, which makes it a good screening test. However, the ELISA test has limited specificity so there may be false-positive results, especially in patients with antiphospholipid syndrome or systemic lupus erythematosus.[9,11] In contrast, the functional assays have high specificity, which are useful for confirming a positive ELISA test but are technically difficult and require the use of radioactivity and/or donor platelets.[9,11]

The typical onset for HIT is 5–10 days following the start of heparin; however, onsets occurring either earlier or later than this have been reported. Rapid-onset HIT occurs when platelet counts fall within 24 hours of heparin initiation, which is typically due to repeated heparin exposure within the past 100 days, and thus patients still have circulating HIT antibodies. Delayed-onset HIT, where thrombocytopenia occurs several days after discontinuation of heparin, has also been reported and is associated with DIC.[9,12-17] Platelet counts should be checked in patients receiving UFH or LMWH if the clinician deems the risk of HIT >1%; in these cases, recommendations are for platelet counts to be done every 2–3 days from days 4–14, or when heparin is stopped.[10] If the risk of HIT is <1%, then platelet monitoring is not recommended.[10] For patients

TABLE 16-4. Incidence of HIT According to Patient Characteristics and Recommendations for Monitoring Platelets[10]

Risk of Developing HIT	>1%	<1%
Patient characteristics/examples	• Postoperative patients on prophylactic dose or therapeutic dose UFH ≥4 days • Cardiac surgery patients	• Medical patients on prophylactic or therapeutic-dose UFH or LMWH ≥4 days • Postoperative patients on prophylactic or therapeutic dose LMWH ≥4 days • Patients receiving UFH flushes • Obstetrics patients • Intensive care patients
Frequency of platelet counts	Every 2–3 days from days 4–14, or until heparin is discontinued, whichever occurs first	Routine monitoring is not recommended

HIT = heparin-induced thrombocytopenia; LMWH = low molecular weight heparin; UFH = unfractionated heparin.

who received heparin within the past 100 days, platelets should be checked at baseline and then within 24 hours of starting heparin.[10] Table 16-4 outlines the patient characteristics associated with the risk of developing HIT.

If HIT is suspected and/or confirmed, UFH and/or LMWH should be discontinued. Direct thrombin inhibitors, such as argatroban, lepirudin, or bivalirudin, can be used instead of UFH or LMWH and are FDA-approved for use in HIT. Fondaparinux is a synthetic, indirect inhibitor of factor Xa. Although it is not FDA-approved for use in patients with HIT, there have been reports of successfully using fondaparinux as an alternative anticoagulant in the HIT population; however, there are also reports of fondaparinux-associated HIT or complications from using fondaparinux in patients with HIT.[18-30,31-37] The 9th edition of the *American College of Chest Physicians Evidence-Based Clinical Practice Guidelines* recommends the use of fondaparinux in HIT as a second-line agent to other DTIs in hospitalized patients or as a first-line parenteral agent in patients who develop an acute thrombosis unrelated to HIT as a bridge until warfarin therapy can be used.[10] In patients who require warfarin for longer term anticoagulation, it is recommended to wait to start warfarin until platelets have recovered to at least 150 x 10⁹/L and to start at low doses.[10]

Mean Platelet Volume

Normal range: 7–11 fL (varies with laboratory)

Mean platelet volume (MPV), the relationship between platelet size and count, is most likely to be used by clinicians in assessing disturbances of platelet production. Mean platelet volume is useful in distinguishing between hypoproductive and hyperdestructive causes of thrombocytopenia (Figure 16-5). Despite the widespread availability of this platelet index, many clinicians do not use it in clinical decision-making. In the past, this disuse was attributed to difficulties with the laboratory measurement of indices.

Many laboratories routinely report the MPV as part of the complete blood count (CBC), especially if a differential is requested. In general, lower platelet counts are common with higher platelet volumes, as an inverse relationship exists between the platelet count and the MPV. This inverse relationship correlates with platelet production within the bone marrow. Although MPV is most valuable in distinguishing hypoproductive from hyperdestructive causes of thrombocytopenia, a definitive diagnosis cannot be made based on MPV alone. In thrombocytopenia, an elevated MPV suggests no problem with platelet production, when in fact, production is reflexively increased. Conversely, a normal or low MPV suggests impaired thrombopoiesis. Determination of MPV requires a blood collection tube containing an anticoagulant. Usually, such tubes contain the anticoagulant ethylenediamine tetraacetic acid (EDTA), which causes an inflation of the MPV.[38]

Currently, MPV is not widely used but may evolve into a valuable screening test for the disorders listed in Table 16-5. Interesting data relating MPV to these disorders continues to surface. For example, the MPV is often elevated at the time of myocardial infarction, although it is not specific enough to be of diagnostic value. Studies have suggested though that a high MPV at 6 months postinfarction may be a predictor of reinfarction. Mean platelet volume is altered in the presence of numerous other medical conditions (Table 16-5).[39,40] For example, a fall in MPV is common in patients with enlarged spleens (hypersplenism) due to preferential sequestering of larger platelets within the spleen. An increase in MPV is seen during the third trimester of pregnancy in preeclamptic patients, where an increase in platelet size results from increased platelet consumption.[41] The MPV is also elevated in hyperthyroid patients but declines to normal as they become euthyroid. In contrast, hypothyroid patients often have a high platelet count and a low MPV.[42,43]

The inverse relationship of a high MPV and a low platelet count is demonstrated in other conditions including respiratory disease, renal failure, and sepsis.[44-46] Unlike most other conditions that demonstrate the inverse relationship of MPV and platelet count, both are low in HIV infection. These decreases suggest an impairment of synthesis and maturation

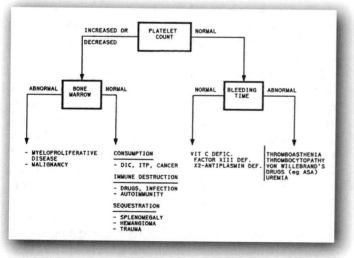

FIGURE 16-5. Assessment of abnormalities of homeostasis based on platelet count, bone marrow exam, and BT.

TABLE 16-5. Conditions That Alter MPV[a]

INCREASE IN MPV	DECREASE IN MPV
Diabetes mellitus	HIV infection
Hereditary	Host chemotherapy
Hyperthyroidism	Hypersplenism
Immune thrombocytopenic purpura	Hypothyroidism
Myocardial infarction	Marrow aplasia
Pregnancy-induced hypertension	Reactive thrombocytosis
Renal failure	
Respiratory disease	
Sepsis	

[a]Reference ranges for MPV vary among laboratories and are inversely proportional to the platelet count.

of megakaryocytes as well as enhanced platelet destruction in the bloodstream.[47] Administration of erythropoietin stimulates megakaryocyte cell line production that leads to an increase in MPV. Thrombopoietin probably causes the same effect.[48-51] The role of thrombopoietin has lead to advances in the treatment of thrombocytopenia caused by deficient production of platelets (e.g., in patients undergoing bone marrow transplantation or cancer chemotherapy).[51]

Platelet Function

Abnormalities of *platelet function* may be either inherited or acquired. Bleeding as a result of an inherited versus acquired abnormality may be difficult to prove. Common bleeding sites in patients with inherited disorders of platelet function include ecchymosis of the skin, epistaxis, gingival bleeding, and menorrhagia. Less common bleeding disorders are gastrointestinal hemorrhage and hematuria. Hematomas and hemarthroses (the predominant sites of bleeding in patients with inherited familial clotting disorders) are rare, except after trauma.[52]

Although the sites of bleeding are predictable, the severity is not predictable in patients with inherited disorders of platelet function.[52] Unfortunately, the risk of bleeding and bleeding patterns in patients with acquired platelet dysfunction are less predictable and more difficult to distinguish. Because both inherited and acquired etiologies increase the risk of bleeding, patients overtly bleeding without a clear cause or without an invasive procedure should be suspect for one of these platelet function disorders.[52]

Bleeding time (normal range: 2–9 minutes). The bleeding time (BT) is a measure of platelet function, but this test is neither specific, nor sensitive; thus, it does not help differentiate among the types of problems seen in disorders of primary hemostasis, such as von Willebrand disease and platelet function defects. This would account for its declining use and elimination by some institutional clinical laboratories. Additionally, the test is invasive and must be performed by a trained healthcare worker. To perform the test, small cuts are made on the forearm of the patient, and the time it takes to stop bleeding is measured.[1] Several factors can prolong the BT including thrombocytopenia, certain medications, and conditions such as uremia and macroglobulinemia. Most acquired disorders affecting BT are related to medications that decrease platelet numbers or reduce platelet function. These include aspirin, thienopyridines (ticlopidine, clopidogrel, prasugrel), GPIIb/IIIa inhibitors (abciximab, eptifibatide, tirofiban), and phosphodiesterase inhibitors (dipyridamole).

Aspirin irreversibly acetylates cyclooxygenase (Figure 16-2). Platelets cannot synthesize new cyclooxygenase, and the effect of aspirin persists for the lifespan of the exposed platelets. The prolongation of BT caused by aspirin is somewhat shorter than the platelet lifespan (8–12 days), because platelets formed after aspirin exposure are not affected. Heparin and warfarin may also prolong BT but not by affecting platelet aggregation. Other drugs that may prolong BT are listed in Table 16-6. While nonacetylated salicylates do not impair platelet aggregation or affect BT, all other nonsteroidal anti-inflammatory drugs (NSAIDs) reversibly inhibit platelet cyclooxygenase and

TABLE 16-6. Medications and Drug Classes That May Cause Abnormalities of Platelet Function

| MEDICATION | ABNORMALITY | |
	ABNORMAL BT	ABNORMAL PLATELET AGGREGATION
Aspirin	√	√
Beta-blocking agents		√
Calcium channel blockers	√	√
Cephalosporins	√	√
Chemotherapeutic agents	√	√
Clofibrate		√
Clopidogrel	√	√
Dextran	√	√
Ethanol	√	√
Heparin	√	√
Nitrofurantoin	√	√
Nitroglycerin	√	√
NSAIDs	√	√
Phenothiazines		√
Quinidine	√	
Thrombolytic agents	√	
Ticlopidine	√	√
Warfarin	√	

Source: Adapted from reference 53.

inhibit aggregation as long as the drug remains in the plasma. Therefore, the clinician can estimate the time it takes for BT to normalize after withdrawing these drugs by knowing their respective half-lives (i.e., 100% elimination of NSAIDs from the blood stream occurs after five half-lives have elapsed). Although BT is influenced by some drugs, it is not used to monitor drug therapy. The increase in BT caused by aspirin may have beneficial effects in the treatment and prevention of cardiovascular disease. The proven value of aspirin for acute treatment of myocardial infarction and secondary prevention of cardiovascular disease is well established; however, the use of aspirin for primary prevention of cardiovascular disease remains an individual clinical judgment.

Platelet aggregation. With the many drawbacks of the BT, there was a need for a test that could aid in the diagnosis of defects in platelet function. This is especially true when considering the interpatient variability seen when taking clopidogrel. Adverse events may occur if patients do not respond to this medication. The ability of platelets to aggregate is most commonly measured by preparing a specimen of platelet-rich plasma and warming it to 98.6°F (37°C) with constant stirring. This test is performed with an aggregometer that measures light transmission through a sample of platelets in suspension. After a baseline reading is obtained, a platelet-aggregating agonist (e.g., epinephrine, collagen, ADP, or arachidonic acid) is added. As platelets aggregate, more light passes through the sample. The change in optical density can be measured photometrically

MINICASE 1

Bleeding Disorders

HELEN M., A 56-YEAR-OLD FEMALE, was hospitalized with a long-standing history of cirrhosis. Physical examination revealed a cachectic-appearing female with distended abdomen, petechial hemorrhages, and asterixis. Helen M. was taking lisinopril, metoprolol, pravastatin, ranitidine, allopurinol, and MVI. She denied taking over-the-counter medications.

The following laboratory parameters were determined for Helen M.:

LABORATORY STUDY	NORMAL RESULTS	PATIENT'S TEST RESULTS
PT	10–13 sec	14.8 sec
INR	Varies around 0.9–1.1	1.49
aPTT	21–45 sec	54 sec
CBC		
Hgb	12.3–15.3 g/dL	11 g/dL
Hct	42% to 52%	33%
Platelet count	140,000–440,000/μL	87,000/μL
MPV	7–11 fL	14 fL
AST	8–42 International Units/L	85 International Units/L
ALT	3–30 International Units/L	25 International Units/L
Albumin	3.5–5 g/dL	1.4 g/dL

Question: What specific test(s) were performed to assess the pertinent patient findings from the history and physical examination? How might these tests relate to normal hemostasis?

Discussion: Preliminary screening was done using the PT/INR and aPTT; they were used as a preliminary screening for Helen M. Her elevations above baseline are consistent with coagulopathies common in patients with liver dysfunction. This increase occurs because of a diminished ability of the liver to manufacture clotting factors.

Platelet count determination and general hematologic values (Hgb and Hct) are consistent with physical examination findings (petechial hemorrhages), revealing Helen M. to be moderately thrombocytopenic and mildly anemic. As expected, the lowered platelet count and higher platelet volume demonstrate the inverse relationship that typically exists when thrombocytopenia occurs. The lowered platelet count could be due to splenic sequestration of platelets due to splenomegaly in association with liver cirrhosis. However, the physical examination did not describe splenomegaly, and the MPV would not be elevated in this situation. Liver function and albumin tests suggest that cirrhosis is the etiology of Helen M.'s petechial hemorrhages. There could be a consumptive component to the coagulopathy as well, which would explain the moderate thrombocytopenia with an increased MPV due to platelet destruction. Table 16-2 summarizes common tests to evaluate bleeding disorders and monitor anticoagulant therapy.

With Helen M., history is important. Both allopurinol and ranitidine have been associated with thrombocytopenia, which could also account for petechial hemorrhages. Helen M. denies using aspirin or NSAIDs, but many patients unknowingly ingest over-the-counter products, such as analgesics and cold preparations. Aspirin and NSAIDs interfere with platelet aggregation and can prolong BT.

and recorded as an aggregation curve, which is then printed on a plotter. Although this light transmittance aggregometry (LTA) is the gold standard in platelet function analysis, it is expensive and requires specially trained personnel to run the test.

Interpretation of platelet aggregation tests involves a comparison of the patient's curves with the corresponding curves of a normal control. To eliminate the optical problems of turbidity with lipemic plasma, the patient and the normal control should be fasting. Patients should not take medications that affect platelet aggregation (e.g., aspirin, NSAIDs, clopidogrel, prasugrel) for approximately 7–14 days prior to the test because they may interfere with test results.

Novel point-of-care technologies, including the Platelet Function Analyzer (PFA-100, DadeBehring) and the Rapid Platelet Function Assay (RPFA) (Verify Now™ Accumetrics, Inc.), allow for rapid and meaningful evaluation of platelet function, although major differences between different devices do exist. The PFA-100 is not as sensitive to clopidogrel while the RPFA is sensitive to the effects of GPIIB/IIIa antagonists.[54]

Other Platelet Tests

The measurement of platelet-specific substances, such as PF4 and beta-thromboglobulin, can now be performed by radioimmunoassay or enzyme immunoassay. High concentrations of these substances may be observed with CAD, acute myocardial infarction (AMI), and thrombosis, where platelet lifespan is reduced. Since numerous drugs can potentially cause thrombocytopenia, detection of antibodies directed by specific drugs against platelets may help to determine the culprit. Platelet survival can be measured by injecting radioisotopes that label the platelets. Serial samples can then determine platelet survival, which is normally 8–12 days.

Coagulation Tests

Coagulation tests are useful in the identification of deficiencies of coagulation factors responsible for bleeding as well as thrombotic disorders. The most commonly performed tests, including the PT, INR, aPTT, and ACT, also are used to monitor anticoagulant therapy. Numerous, high-precision automated laboratory methods are available to perform these tests. However, an overall lack of standardization across coagulation testing can lead to considerable variation in test results and their interpretation. Normal and therapeutic ranges established for one test method are not necessarily interchangeable with other methods, especially when differences in endpoint detection or reagents exist. Therefore, it is important to interpret test results based on the specific performance characteristics of the method used to analyze samples.

Careful attention to blood collection technique and sample processing—as well as laboratory quality control—is critical for reliable coagulation test results. Blood is collected in syringes or vacuum tubes that contain heparin, EDTA, or sodium citrate. Because heparin and EDTA interfere with several clotting factors, only sodium citrate is used for coagulation and platelet tests. Errors in coagulation can be large unless quality assurance is strict with specimen collection, reagents, controls, and equipment. Factors that promote clotting and interfere with coagulation studies include

- Tissue trauma (searching for a vein)
- Prolonged use of tourniquet
- Small-bore needles
- Vacuum tubes
- Heparin contamination from indwelling catheters
- Slow blood filling into collection tube

Coagulation studies may be used to assess certain bleeding disorders such as hemophilia A (factor VIII deficiency) or hemophilia B (factor IX deficiency). These deficiencies, which are inherited sex-linked recessive traits, primarily affect males and cause over 90% of hemophilia cases. Other bleeding disorders include von Willebrand disease, the most common hereditary bleeding disorder, and deficiencies in fibrinogen or factors II, V, VII, X, XI, XIII, and/or a combination of these factors.

Patients with thrombotic disorders may have their hypercoagulability evaluated with specific assays for

- Antithrombin
- Protein C
- Protein S
- Prothrombin G20210A mutation (factor V Leiden)
- APC resistance mutation

Normal reference ranges for AT and proteins C and S tests are often reported as a percent of normal activity, with 100% being the mean normal value. For AT, the normal activity level is 80% to 130%; for both proteins C and S, normal activity levels are 70% to 140%. As alluded to previously, deficiencies can result in frequent, recurrent thromboembolic events in patients with these disorders. Because these deficiencies are rare, their respective assays are not discussed here in detail. Acquired, transient deficiencies of any of these inhibitors may be observed during thrombotic states. Therefore, these parameters should not be assessed during the acute phase of thrombosis or while the patient is currently on anticoagulant therapy since a false-positive result may occur. It is recommended to test for AT, protein C, protein S, and APC resistance after the thrombosis has been resolved when the patient is off of heparin or warfarin for approximately 2 weeks; the test for prothrombin G20210A mutation is not affected by current anticoagulant therapy.[55]

Activated protein C resistance, due to the factor V Leiden mutation, is the most prevalent hereditary predisposition to venous thrombosis. It is present in 5% of the general Caucasian population and is less common or rare in other ethnic groups.[55-58] It accounts for 20% of unselected patients with a first deep vein thrombosis and 50% of familial cases of thrombosis.[59] Patients with the heterozygous form of factor V Leiden mutation are at four- to sevenfold higher risk of developing venous thromboembolism (VTE), while those with the homozygous form can be as high as 80-fold higher risk.[56] APC usually prolongs the aPTT more than twofold in controls (normal persons) and less than twofold in affected individuals. Presence of lupus anticoagulants, lepirudin, argatroban and bivalirudin may cause inaccurate results in the commonly used aPTT clotting-time based assay but do not affect DNA-based tests.[60,61]

Prothrombin G20210A mutation is the second most common hereditary predisposition to venous thrombosis. DNA-based methods, such as the polymerase chain reaction (PCR)-based assay, are used to determine the presence or absence of a specific mutation at nucleoside position 20210 in the prothrombin gene. A normal test would show absence of the G20210A mutation. The test identifies individuals who have the G20210A mutation and reveals whether the affected individual is heterozygous or homozygous for the mutation; patients with the heterozygous form are at a two- to fourfold higher risk of venous thrombosis, while those with the homozygous form are at even higher risk.[56]

Prothrombin Time/International Normalized Ratio

Normal range for PT: 10–13 sec but varies based on reagent-instrument combinations; therapeutic range for INR depends on indication for anticoagulation; most indications: 2.0–3.0

The *prothrombin time (PT)*, also called *ProTime*, test is used to assess the integrity of the extrinsic and common pathways (factors II, V, VII, X). The PT, based on Quick's method first described in 1935, is determined by adding calcium and an activator (thromboplastin) containing both the TF and the phospholipid necessary to promote the activation of factor X by factor VIIa in the patient's plasma.[62] The time it takes for clot formation to occur after the addition of the thromboplastin and calcium is the PT. Deficiencies or inhibitors of extrinsic and/or common pathway clotting factors would result in a prolonged PT; however, it should be noted that the PT is more sensitive to deficiencies in the extrinsic pathway (factor VII) compared to the common pathway (factors V, X, II, and fibrinogen).[63]

Assay performance characteristics, standardization, and reporting. The PT is dependent on the thromboplastin source and test method used to detect clotting. Thromboplastin reagents are derived from animal or human sources and include recombinant products. Factor sensitivity is highly dependent on the source of the thromboplastin, and can exhibit variability between different lots of the same reagent. Some thromboplastin reagents are less sensitive to changes in factor activity. This means that it takes a more significant decrease in factor activity to produce a prolongation of the PT. Differences in reagent sensitivity, combined with the influence of endpoint detection, affect clotting time results both in the normal and therapeutic ranges. Large differences in factor sensitivity between comparative methods can result in conflicting interpretation of results, both in the assessment of factor deficiencies and adequacy of anticoagulation therapy.

Since PT results can vary widely depending on the thromboplastin source, a standardized reporting method has been used, which is known as the *international normalized ratio (INR)*. The INR is calculated according to the following equation:

$$INR = (patient\ PT/mean\ normal\ PT)^{ISI}$$

The international sensitivity index (ISI) expresses the sensitivity of the thromboplastin reagent compared to the World Health Organization (WHO) reference standard. The more sensitive or responsive the reagent, the lower the ISI; reagents with ISI values of <1.7 are recommended for use when monitoring patients on oral anticoagulant therapy.[62] Theoretically, an INR result from one laboratory should be comparable to an INR result from a different laboratory, even though the PTs may be different. The citrate concentration also may affect the ISI determination of certain reagents, with higher citrate concentrations leading to higher INR results; using blood samples anticoagulated with 3.2% citrate, instead of higher concentrations, can help mitigate this problem

There are other factors that may influence the PT. If heparin-sensitive thromboplastin reagents are used, falsely elevated PT/INR values may result. These inaccurate values might suggest sufficient anticoagulation with oral anticoagulation therapy and result in the premature discontinuation of heparin.

Although the INR system has greatly improved the standardization of the PT, one can still expect differences in INRs reported with two different methods, particularly in the upper therapeutic and supratherapeutic ranges. The greater the differences in the ISI values for two comparative methods, the more likely differences will be noted in the INR. Laboratories and anticoagulation clinics should review the performance characteristics of the PT method used to evaluate their specific patient populations and report changes in methods to healthcare professionals, particularly those monitoring anticoagulant therapy.

Heparin may also prolong PT since it affects factor II in the common pathway; the addition of a heparin neutralizing agent to the blood sample can blunt this effect at heparin concentrations up to 2 units/mL.[63] However, at higher concentrations of heparin, whether due to higher doses of heparin or sample collection issues, the neutralizing agent may not be enough and the PT may be prolonged. These "crossover" effects may have to be considered when oral and parenteral anticoagulants are given concomitantly for several days to avoid premature discontinuation of the parenteral agent.

Monitoring warfarin therapy. Both the PT and INR may be reported when monitoring warfarin therapy, although clinically, only the INR is used to adjust therapy. Warfarin exerts its anticoagulant effects by interfering with the synthesis of vitamin K-dependent clotting factors (II, VII, IX, and X) and the natural anticoagulant proteins C, S, and Z. Specifically, warfarin inhibits vitamin K-reductase and vitamin K epoxide-reductase (VKOR), which blocks the activation of vitamin K to its reduced form. Reduced vitamin K is needed for the carboxylation of clotting precursors of factors II, VII, IX, and X. Noncarboxylated clotting factor precursors are nonfunctional,

and thus an anticoagulated state is achieved.[62] Warfarin is manufactured as a racemic mixture of (S)- and (R)-enantiomers; the S-enantiomer is more potent than the R-enantiomer at inhibiting VKOR, which is why the S-enantiomer is responsible for the majority of the anticoagulant effects of warfarin. The S-enantiomer is metabolized largely by CYP2C9 while the R-enantiomer is metabolized mostly by CYP1A2, and CYP3A4; other CYP enzymes are also involved in the metabolism of warfarin although to a lesser extent.

Current *Antithrombotic Therapy and Prevention of Thrombosis: American College of Chest Physicians Evidence-Based Clinical Practice Guidelines* recommend an INR of 2.0–3.0 for most indications; exceptions include, but are not limited to, patients with mechanical prosthetic heart valves in the mitral position and patients with recurrent thromboembolic events with a therapeutic INR, where an INR of 2.5–3.5 is recommended.[64-68] Results below the therapeutic range indicate that the patient is at increased risk for clotting, and warfarin doses may need to be increased. Results above the therapeutic range indicate the patient is at risk for bleeding and warfarin doses may need to be decreased. Numerous drugs, disease states, and other factors prolong the INR in patients receiving warfarin by various mechanisms of action (Table 16-7).

Pharmacogenomics and oral anticoagulant therapy. Genetic variability in the genes coding for CYP2C9, VKORC1 (vitamin K epoxide reductase complex subunit 1), and CYP4F2 can influence warfarin dosing by altering its pharmacokinetics and/or pharmacodynamics. CYP2C9 and VKORC1 have a larger influence compared to CYP4F2. Specifically, patients with CYP2C9*2 and CYP2C9*3 variations have a reduced clearance of the (S)-warfarin enantiomer, which results in lower maintenance dose requirements of warfarin, increased risk of bleeding, and a possible longer time to achieve a stable dosing regimen.[71] Two main haplotypes of VKORC1, low-dose haplotype group A, seen predominantly in Asian patients, and high-dose haplotype group B, seen predominantly in African-American patients, contribute to the interindividual variability of warfarin dosing. The specific single nucleotide polymorphisms (SNPs) involved are the -1639G>A and 1173C>T.

Patients with the AA genotype (predominately Asians) require lower doses of warfarin compared to Caucasians, while patients with the GG genotype (predominantly African-Americans) require higher doses compared to Caucasians.[71] The CYP4F2 enzyme normally plays a role in the conversion of vitamin K to vitamin KH_2, which is needed to carboxylate the clotting factor precursors; patients with a polymorphism in the 433Met allele of the CYP4F2 gene will have greater vitamin K availability leading to higher warfarin dose requirements.[71] Unlike CYP2C9 polymorphisms, neither VKORC1 nor CYP4F2 have been associated with increased bleeding risks or prolonged time to achieving a stable dose of warfarin. The Hispanic population is underrepresented in warfarin pharmacogenomic studies, so until further data becomes available, Hispanics and non-Hispanic Caucasians are likely considered similar in terms of pharmacogenetic outcomes related to warfarin.[71]

TABLE 16-7. Factors Altering Pharmacokinetics and Pharmacodynamics of Warfarin[69]

ANTICOAGULANT EFFECT POTENTIATED	ANTICOAGULANT EFFECT COUNTERACTED
Low vitamin K intake	Increased vitamin K intake
Reduced vitamin K absorption in fat malabsorption	
Drugs that slow hepatic catabolism of warfarin:	Drugs that increase hepatic catabolism of warfarin:
Amiodarone	Barbiturates
Anabolic steroids	Carbamazepine
Cimetidine	Griseofulvin
Clarithromycin	Rifampin
Clofibrate	
Disulfiram	Alcohol (chronic consumption)
Erythromycin	
Fluconazole	Reduced absorption of warfarin by cholestyramine
Isoniazid	
Ketoconazole	
Metronidazole	
Oral fluoroquinolones	
Phenylbutazone	
Phenytoin	
Piroxicam	
Quinidine	
Sulfinpyrazone	
Tamoxifen	
Thyroxine	
Trimethoprim–sulfamethoxazole	
Vitamin E (megadose)	
Liver disease	
Hypermetabolic states	
Pyrexia	
Thyrotoxicosis	
Alcohol (acute consumption or binge drinking)	
Displacement of warfarin from albumin binding sites	

Four manufacturers are currently marketing their warfarin pharmacogenomics testing devices; each one tests for the CYP2C9*2 and CYP2C9*3, as well as either the VKORC1 -1639G/A or the VKORC1 1173C/T SNPs.[71] The product labeling for Coumadin® (warfarin) has been updated to include information about the potential impact of pharmacogenomics on the dosing of this medication as well as a pharmacogenetics dosing table, which may help clinicians select an initial dose of warfarin if genetic information is known, specifically in regard to CYP2C9 and VKORC1.[72] For clinicians who do utilize genetic testing for their patients on warfarin, they can use either the dosing table provided in the package insert or a dosing algorithm to estimate a starting dose for their patient. Algorithms take into account not only the results of genetic testing, but also other factors such as age, body size, smoking status, use of other medications like amiodarone, other disease states, and vitamin K intake. Subsequent dosing changes should be made based on results of the INR test. There are several barriers to widespread adoption of pharmacogenetic testing and dosing[71]: unavailability of testing at many medical centers, which leads to outsourcing of tests and a long turnaround time for results; lack of reimbursement for testing leading to large out-of-pocket expenses for patients (estimates run from $200 to $500); lack of support of genetic testing by professional organizations; and lack of clinician acceptance and knowledge of interpreting and applying test results. The 9th edition of the *Antithrombotic Therapy and Prevention of Thrombosis: American College of Chest Physicians Evidence-Based Clinical Practice Guidelines* recommends against the routine use of pharmacogenetic testing when initiating a patient on warfarin.[65] Genetic testing, if utilized, should be used along with patient characteristics, clinical considerations, and continued INR monitoring for optimal outcomes associated with warfarin use.

Dabigatran and rivaroxaban are two novel oral anticoagulants recently approved in the United States. Although genetic variants have not been well studied regarding these medications, there are some potential genes that may influence a patient's response to these medications. The CYP enzymes are not important to the metabolism of dabigatran, although the CYP 3A4/5 and CYP2J2 do play a role in the metabolism of rivaroxaban and may serve as a cause of genetic variability in patients using rivaroxaban. Additionally, both dabigatran and rivaroxaban are P-glycoprotein substrates, which is encoded by the ABCB1 gene where several SNPs have been identified.[71] Thus, future studies may be directed at elucidating whether the ABCB1 genotype, the CYP enzymes, and/or polymorphisms at the drugs' target action site may serve as potential sources of variability in the dosing of these agents.

Activated Partial Thromboplastin Time
Normal range: varies by manufacturer, generally between 22–38 sec; therapeutic range for heparin-treated patients is 1.5–2.5 times control aPTT

The *activated partial thromboplastin time (aPTT)* is used to screen for deficiencies and inhibitors of the intrinsic pathway (factors VIII, IX, XI, and XII) as well as factors in the final common pathway (factors II, V, and X). The aPTT is also commonly used as a surrogate assay to monitor UFH and DTIs. The aPTT, reported as a clotting time in seconds, is determined by adding an aPTT reagent and calcium to the patient's blood sample. The reagent contains phospholipids from animal, human, vegetable, or recombinant sources, as well as surface activators including kaolin, silica, or elegiac acid.[73] Normal ranges vary depending on the reagent/instrument combination used to perform the test, but they generally are between 25–35 seconds.

Factor and heparin sensitivity as well as the precision of the aPTT test depend both on the reagents and instrumentation. In addition, some aPTT reagents are formulated for increased sensitivity to lupus anticoagulants. Despite numerous attempts to standardize the aPTT, very little progress has been made. The difficulty in part may reflect differences in opinion as to the appropriate heparin sensitivity, the need to have lupus anticoagulant sensitivity for targeted patient populations, and suitable factor sensitivity to identify deficiencies associated with increased bleeding risk. Normal and therapeutic ranges must be established for each reagent instrument combination, and ranges should be verified with changes in lots of the same reagent. Laboratory errors may cause either prolongation or shortening of the aPTT; these may include inappropriate amount and/or concentration of anticoagulant in the collection tube, time between collection of the blood specimen and performing the assay, inappropriate collection site (i.e., through a venous catheter, which contains heparin), and/or inappropriate timing of blood collection.[63]

Causes of aPTT prolongation. In addition to reagent specific issues impacting on aPTT responsiveness, hereditary diseases, or other acquired causes may prolong aPTT test results. Causes of aPTT prolongation include

- Hereditary
  - Deficiency of factor VIII, IX, XI, XII, prekallikrein, or high molecular weight kininogen (HMWK) (PT is normal)
  - Deficiency of fibrinogen or factor II, V, or X (PT is also prolonged)

It should be noted that aPTT reagents may respond differently if a patient has a single factor deficiency versus a multiple factor deficiency; patients with single factor deficiency have a more predictable aPTT prolongation compared to patients with multiple factor deficiencies.[74]

- Acquired
  - Lupus anticoagulant (PT usually normal)
  - Heparin (PT less affected than aPTT, PT may be normal)
  - Lepirudin, bivalirudin, or argatroban (PT usually also prolonged)
  - Liver dysfunction (PT affected earlier and more than aPTT) (Minicase 1)
  - Vitamin K deficiency (PT affected earlier and more than aPTT)
  - Warfarin (PT affected earlier and more than aPTT)
  - DIC (PT affected earlier and more than aPTT)
  - Specific factor inhibitors (PT normal except in the rare case of an inhibitor against fibrinogen, factor II, V, or X)
  - Decreased nutritional intake; malabsorption
  - Myeloproliferative disease

Though used to detect clotting factor deficiencies, today, the aPTT is used primarily for monitoring therapeutic heparin therapy. The generally accepted therapeutic range of heparin

is an aPTT ratio of 1.5–2.5 times control, though this has not been confirmed by randomized trials.[75] Given the inter- and intrapatient variability that can result from aPTT reagents, alternative means of monitoring heparin therapy are being scrutinized. This 1.5–2.5 aPTT ratio corresponds to[75]

- A plasma heparin concentration of 0.2–0.4 units/mL by assay using the protamine titration method
- A plasma heparin concentration of 0.3–0.7 units/mL by assay using the inhibition of factor Xa

Unfractionated heparin should be given by continuous IV infusion or subcutaneous injection, with exact dosing dependent on the indication. The aPTT should be drawn at baseline, 4–6 hours after continuous IV heparin is begun, and 4–6 hours after each subsequent dosage adjustment, since this interval approximates the time to achieve steady-state levels of heparin. Institutions may have their own specific heparin dosing nomogram or base their nomogram off one used in clinical studies; studies have shown several benefits to using a heparin nomogram, including decreased time to therapeutic anticoagulation, decreased time to achieving target aPTT levels, and decreased number of recurrent VTE thromboembolism episodes.[76-82] Nomograms also allow quick fine-tuning of anticoagulation by nurses without continuous physician input.

aPTT determinations obtained earlier than 6 hours, when a steady-state concentration of heparin has not been achieved, may be combined with heparin concentrations for dosage individualization using non-steady-state concentrations. This approach has been demonstrated to reduce the incidence of subtherapeutic aPTT ratios significantly during the first 24 hours of therapy.[83,84] This finding is important because the recurrence rate of thromboembolic disease increased when aPTT values were not maintained above 1.5 times the patient's baseline aPTT during the first 24 hours of treatment.[85,86]

Warfarin effect on aPTT. Although warfarin also elevates the aPTT, aPTT is not used to monitor warfarin therapy. Studies have shown a strong correlation between the increase in PT/INR and a corresponding increase in aPTT with warfarin therapy.[87,88] Therefore, if warfarin is started in a patient receiving heparin, the clinician should expect some elevation in aPTT.

Heparin concentration measurements may provide a target plasma therapeutic range, especially in unusual coagulation situations such as pregnancy, where the reliability of clotting studies is questionable. In this setting, shorter than expected aPTT results in relation to heparin concentration measurements may be indicative of increased circulating levels of factor VIII and increased fibrinogen levels.[89] Patients may have therapeutic heparin concentrations measured by whole blood protamine sulfate titration or by the plasma anti-Xa heparin assay. However, they may have aPTTs not significantly prolonged above baseline. This difference has been referred to as a dissociation between the aPTT and the heparin concentration.[90] Many of these patients have very short pretreatment aPTT values.

Decreased aPTT levels. While most attention has been focused on causes of prolonged aPTT levels, there is growing evidence of adverse events associated with decreased aPTT

MINICASE 2

A Patient on Anticoagulants

BRENDA C., A 56-YEAR-OLD FEMALE with atrial fibrillation and hypertension, presented to the emergency department with signs and symptoms of a new DVT. A routine heparin regimen was started. Brenda C. had the following laboratory determinations performed 6 hours after initiation of heparin:

LABORATORY RESULTS	NORMAL RESULTS	PRETREATMENT PATIENT RESULTS	POSTHEPARIN RESULTS
PT (sec)	10–13	11.1	12.3
INR	1+0.1	0.98	1.18
aPTT (sec)	21–45	19	23
ATIII (%)	80–120	57	50

Question: What might account for this Brenda C.'s postheparin elevation in PT? Why was the aPTT not prolonged? What long-term anticoagulation strategies are potential options for Brenda C.?

Discussion: Brenda C. was started on a continuous IV heparin infusion with plans to convert to long-term warfarin, per the institution's protocol. Subsequent postheparin laboratory determinations revealed a hypercoagulable state consistent with thromboembolic disease. Circulating procoagulants account for the patient's low pretreatment aPTT. ATIII—the cofactor with which heparin binds to exert its anticoagulant effect—is depressed, making the patient hypercoagulable. Subsequent to the initiation of heparin, the ATIII concentration declined further. This drop reflected the binding of ATIII to heparin.

Despite a normal dosing protocol for heparin, Brenda C.'s initial aPTT value (obtained 6 hours after the loading dose and continuous maintenance infusion of heparin) remained low. One might be suspicious of pseudoheparin resistance or dissociation of the aPTT responsiveness after adequate treatment with heparin. To assess the likelihood of this situation, a heparin concentration measurement could be obtained (discussed later) to demonstrate adequate heparinization despite a subtherapeutic aPTT determination.

Prior to initiation of concomitant warfarin therapy, Brenda C.'s PT increased slightly to 12.3 seconds. Minimal prolongation of the PT may be expected from heparin's influence. This degree of elevation is consistent with this observation. Brenda C.'s INR should be followed, with the desired endpoint of warfarin therapy being an INR of 2–3. After 3 months, Brenda C. should be reassessed to see if further warfarin therapy is needed; she may have a choice between staying on warfarin longterm due to the atrial fibrillation, or she could switch to either rivaroxaban or dabigatran.

Six weeks later, Brenda C. presents for her regular INR followup. Her INRs have remained fairly stable between 2–3 while on warfarin 5 mg PO daily. She reports that her physician prescribed amiodarone 200 mg PO daily for rhythm control 3 weeks ago. Today her INR is 6.2, but she has no signs or symptoms of bleeding or bruising.

Question: How should her INR results be interpreted? What should be done next? How could this be prevented in the future?

Discussion: Brenda C.'s INR is supratherapeutic likely due to a drug interaction between warfarin and amiodarone. The clinician should also assess whether Brenda C. has reduced her overall intake of vitamin K-rich foods or if she has taken any extra doses of warfarin since these two factors may also increase the INR value (Table 16-7). Brenda C.'s dose of warfarin should be held for a few days and then reduced appropriately due to concomitant longterm amiodarone therapy. Her INR levels should be closely monitored during this time and for awhile thereafter. In the future, she should be instructed to inform her healthcare provider of any medication changes as soon as possible. If she chooses to switch to either dabigatran or rivaroxaban in the future, this drug interaction is no longer clinically relevant.

---

levels, with frequencies ranging from 6% to 20% of all aPTT tests performed (not including errors related to inappropriate blood collection).[91,92] Several reports have stated that a shortened aPTT may indicate a risk factor for hypercoagulability.[93-99] Clotting factors of the intrinsic pathway as well as vWF levels and activity have been elevated in some patients presenting with decreased aPTT levels, which provides some evidence that patients with decreased aPTT levels are hypercoagulable.[92] However, it should also be noted that shortened aPTT levels may be associated with other conditions such as acute bleeding, increased in-hospital mortality, impaired fasting glucose, or diabetes, hyperthyroidism, and myocardial infarction.[73,100-104] There is no definitive answer whether a shortened aPTT is a cause, consequence, or just an association with these other conditions. To rule out whether a shortened aPTT is due to a laboratory error, such as inappropriate specimen collection, a repeat collection and repeat testing should be performed.[91]

Heparin alone has minimal anticoagulant effects; when it is combined with AT (normal range: 80% to 120%), the inhibitory action of AT on coagulation enzymes is magnified 1000-fold resulting in the inhibition of thrombus propagation. Patients who are AT deficient (<50%) may be difficult to anticoagulate, as seen with DIC (Minicase 3). The DIC syndrome is associated not only with obvious hemorrhage but also with occult diffuse thrombosis.

Another use for heparin concentrations is to demonstrate both efficacy and safety with LMWH, which have several indications for use: prophylaxis against deep vein thrombosis following hip or knee replacement or abdominal surgery or in acutely ill medical patients with restricted mobility; treatment of acute deep vein thrombosis (DVT) or pulmonary embolism (PE); prophylaxis of ischemic complications due to unstable angina and non-Q-wave myocardial infarction; and treatment of ST segment elevation myocardial infarction (STEMI) with or without percutaneous coronary intervention (PCI).[106-108] However, clinically, the anti-factor Xa levels are more routinely used for this class of medications. Low molecular weight heparin has a pharmacokinetic and pharmacodynamic profile, which makes routine monitoring unnecessary in most circumstances. Exceptions include special populations,

MINICASE 3

A Case of DIC

TERESA G., A 36-YEAR-OLD FEMALE in her third trimester of pregnancy, was hospitalized with clinical suspicion of DIC because of acute onset of respiratory failure, circulatory collapse, and shock. The following laboratory values for Teresa G. were obtained:

LABORATORY RESULTS	NORMAL RESULTS	PATIENT RESULTS
PT	10–13 sec	16 sec
aPTT	25–35 sec	59 sec
TT	25–35 sec	36 sec
CBC		
Hgb	12.3–15.3 g/dL	9.8 g/dL
Hct	36% to 45%	27.7%
Platelet count	150,000–450,000/μL	64,000/μL
MPV	7–11 fL	17 fL
FDP (latex)	<10 mcg/mL	120 mcg/mL
ATIII	80% to 120%	57%
D-dimer	<200 ng/mL	2040 ng/mL

Question: What laboratory tests are used to determine if a patient is experiencing DIC? What are the expected laboratory results for these tests?

Discussion: Laboratory findings of DIC may be highly variable, complex, and difficult to interpret. Both PT and aPTT should be prolonged (and they are prolonged in Teresa G.), but this may not always occur. Because of this, the usefulness of both PT and aPTT determinations may be helpful in making the diagnosis. TT is prolonged as expected. The platelet count is typically and dramatically decreased. Teresa G.'s MPV is inversely related to her decreased platelet count as expected, suggesting a hyperdestructive phenomenon versus a hypoproliferative state. Although FDPs are elevated, this rise is not solely pathognomonic for DIC. Increased D-dimer levels are strongly suggestive of DIC. ATIII determination reveals a considerable decrease consistent with DIC. Decreased ATIII is useful and reliable for diagnosis of DIC in the absence of D-dimer testing ability.

Current recommendations for patients with decreased aPTT results on heparin are that such patients be managed by monitoring heparin concentrations using a heparin assay to avoid unnecessary dosage escalation without compromising efficacy.[90,105] These patients, referred to as *pseudoheparin resistant,* may be identified as having a poor aPTT response (to an adequate heparin concentration >0.3 units/mL via plasma anti-Xa assay) despite high doses of heparin (>50,000 units/24 hr; usual dose is 20,000–30,000 units/24 hr) (Minicase 2).[105] When higher doses of heparin (>1500 units/hr) are required to maintain therapeutic aPTT values, high concentrations of heparin-binding protein or phase reactant proteins bind and neutralize heparin. Additionally, thrombocytosis, or AT deficiency may exist.[90]

such as those patients with renal failure or severe obesity who are at risk of being overdosed when weight-adjusted regimens are used. Both PT and aPTT times are not significantly prolonged at recommended doses of LMWHs.[89,109] However, both efficacy and safety can be demonstrated by assaying anti-factor Xa levels. This assay is recommended to be drawn 4 hours after administration of a therapeutic weight-adjusted dose of LMWH, when anti-factor Xa activity has peaked. An effective plasma concentration range is approximately 0.5–1.1 plasma anti-Xa units/mL for twice daily subcutaneous dosing of LMWH. The effective plasma concentration for once daily dosing of LMWH is less certain but has been recommended to be approximately 1–2 plasma anti-Xa units/mL.[110]

Bleeding risk and test results. The major determinants of bleeding are the

- Intensity of the anticoagulant effect
- Underlying patient characteristics
- Use of drugs that interfere with hemostasis (see Tables 16-3 and 16-6)
- Length of anticoagulant therapy

When evaluating anticoagulation treatment, one must weigh the potential for decreased thrombosis risk versus the increased bleeding risk. The risk of bleeding associated with continuous IV heparin in patients with acute thromboembolic disease is approximately 5%. Some evidence suggests that this bleeding increases with an increase in heparin concentration.

However, evidence also suggests that serious bleeding can occur in patients prone to bleeding even when the anticoagulant response is in the therapeutic range. The risk of bleeding is usually higher earlier in therapy, when both heparin and warfarin are given together, which may be related to excessive anticoagulation. Also, patients who have a coexisting disease that elevates the PT, aPTT, or both (e.g., liver disease) are often at much higher risk of bleeding. In these patients, the use and intensity of anticoagulation that should be employed are controversial.

Activated Clotting Time

Normal range: 70–180 sec but varies

Activated clotting time (ACT), also known as *activated coagulation time,* is frequently used to monitor heparin or DTIs when very high doses are required, such as during invasive procedures like cardiopulmonary bypass surgery, PTCA, extracorporeal membrane oxygenation (ECMO), valve replacements, or carotid endarterectomy.[111,112] The ACT can also be used to monitor heparin neutralization using protamine, although a return to baseline ACT does not indicate full neutralization.[113] Most ACTs are run using a point-of-care testing apparatus using whole blood; thus, it may be run directly in the operating room as well as at the bedside when a rapid heparinization is required (e.g., hemodialysis unit, operating room, and cardiac catheterization laboratories).

ACT responsiveness remains linear in proportion to an increasing dose of heparin, whereas the aPTT has a log-linear relationship to heparin concentration. The latter should result in stricter control of dose-response changes when using the ACT compared to the aPTT.[111] Corresponding ACT values up to 400 seconds demonstrate this dose-response relationship, but ACT lacks reproducibility for values in excess of 600 seconds as well as low concentrations of heparin. ACT test results can be influenced by factors such as[114]

- Testing device
- Testing technique
- Sample temperature
- Hemodilution
- Platelet count and/or function
- Factor deficiencies
- Hypothermia
- Lupus anticoagulants

There is a wide correlation when comparing results of the aPTT and ACT, which suggests that these tests are not equivalent and may result in dissimilar clinical decisions.[115] In view of the lack of advantages over the aPTT for monitoring heparin for treatment of venous thromboembolism, the ACT is not highly recommended for use in this setting. The main indication to use the ACT over the aPTT is for a patient receiving high dose heparin or DTIs.

Anti-Xa

Normal range: varies based on specific anticoagulant used for treatment of existing VTE
- *Heparin: 0.3–0.7 units/mL*
- *LMWH: 0.5–1 units/mL (twice daily dosing);*
  1–2 units/mL (once daily dosing)
- *Fondaparinux, rivaroxaban: not established*

The *anti-Xa* level may be used to monitor LMWH when given in therapeutic doses; however, routine monitoring is not usually done since LMWH has a more predictable dose-response relationship than UFH. Monitoring anti-Xa levels can be considered in patients with poor renal function, pregnant patients, and patients with extremes in body weight.[75] Levels should be drawn 4 hours after the LMWH injection, otherwise sub- or supratherapeutic levels may occur. When ordering an anti-Xa test, it is imperative that the correct calibrator is used to ensure correct results; for example, the LMWH calibrator cannot be used to measure anti-Xa activity of fondaparinux.

Fibrinogen Assay

Normal range: 200–400 mg/dL

While the PT and aPTT are used to screen for deficiencies in the intrinsic, extrinsic, and common pathways, the *fibrinogen assay* is most commonly used to assess fibrinogen concentration. Fibrinogen assays are performed by adding a known amount of thrombin to a dilution of patient plasma. The fibrinogen concentration is determined by extrapolating the patient's clotting time to a standard curve. Elevated fibrinogen levels may be due to pregnancy or acute phase reactions, and may be associated with an increased risk of cardiovascular disease.[116] Decreased fibrinogen is associated with DIC and hepatic

cirrhosis; PT and aPTT levels may also be increased, and patients may have symptomatic bleeding. Additionally, supratherapeutic heparin concentrations >1 unit/mL may result in falsely low fibrinogen concentration measurements. Thrombin time (discussed below) is the most sensitive test for fibrinogen deficiency, and it is prolonged when fibrinogen concentrations are below 100 mg/dL. However, the actual fibrinogen concentration occasionally must be determined. Fibrinogen levels are usually drawn as part of a DIC panel, when further exploring the reasons for an elevated PT or aPTT level, or to further evaluate unexplained bleeding in a patient.

Thrombin Time

Normal range: 17–25 sec but varies according to thrombin concentration and reaction conditions

Also known as *thrombin clotting time,* the *thrombin time (TT)* measures the time required for a plasma sample to clot after the addition of bovine or human thrombin and is compared to that of a normal plasma control. Deficiencies in both the intrinsic and extrinsic systems do not affect TT, which assesses only the final phase of the common pathway or essentially the ability to convert fibrinogen to fibrin.

Prolongation of TT may be caused by hypofibrinogenemia, dysfibrinogenemia, heparin, DTIs, or the presence of FDPs.[4] The TT is ultrasensitive to heparin; therefore, it is only useful to show whether or not heparin is present in the blood sample, not as a monitoring test. In thrombolytic therapy, laboratory monitoring may not prevent bleeding or ensure thrombolysis. However, some clinicians recommend measuring TT, fibrinogen, plasminogen activation, or FDPs to document that a lytic state has been achieved. Typically, TT is >120 seconds 4–6 hours after "adequate" thrombolytic therapy.

Reptilase Time

Normal range: 16–24 sec

The *reptilase time* is a variation of the TT test in which venom from the pit viper is mixed with the patient's plasma sample instead of thrombin. Like the TT, reptilase time measures the clotting time in seconds during the conversion of fibrinogen to fibrin. However, unlike the TT, heparin will not cause a prolongation of the reptilase time, so if heparin is the only cause of a prolonged TT, reptilase time will be normal. Therefore, reptilase time can be used to evaluate fibrinogen status in heparinized patients.

Ecarin Clotting Time

The *ecarin clotting time (ECT)* test is a specific assay for thrombin generation. It is used to monitor parenteral DTIs and has been postulated as a way to monitor the new oral DTIs like dabigatran. Ecarin is added to the patient's plasma, which cleaves prothrombin to meizothrombin, a serine protease similar to thrombin.[117] Direct thrombin inhibitors inhibit meizothrombin so the ECT can quantify the amount of DTI in the body by measuring the time for meizothrombin to convert fibrinogen into fibrin. Thus, a longer ECT corresponds to larger drug concentrations. ECT is not affected by other anticoagulants such as warfarin or heparin so it is more specific for DTI activity than aPTT, PT, or TT.[117] Currently the ECT is not used

MINICASE 4

A Patient on Thrombolytic Therapy

ALFRED F., A 44-YEAR-OLD MALE, had clinical signs and symptoms and electrocardiogram findings consistent with acute anterior-wall myocardial infarction requiring emergent angioplasty. He received urokinase without successful opening of the coronary artery. Subsequently, Alfred F. was heparinized. The following pre- and post-therapy coagulation lab studies were obtained:

LABORATORY STUDY	NORMAL RESULTS	PRETHERAPY	POST-THERAPY
PT	10–13 sec	12.2 sec	17 sec
aPTT	25–35 sec	35 sec	69 sec
Fibrinogen	200–400 mg/dL	300 ng/mL	22 ng/mL
FDP (latex)	<10 mcg/mL	<10 mcg/mL	>160 mcg/mL
D-dimer	<200 ng/mL	<200 ng/mL	300 ng/mL
Plasminogen	80% to 120%	70%	22%

Question: What might explain the elevated FDP? What accounts for the fall in the plasminogen level on completion of the lytic therapy? Finally, why is the D-dimer concentration not elevated in proportion to the greatly elevated FDP concentration?

Discussion: The elevated post-therapy PT and aPTT are consistent with heparinization after intracoronary thrombolytic therapy. The FDP concentration is elevated because urokinase resulted in fibrinogenolysis. Many FDPs are generated in this setting. By the nature of thrombolytic therapy, plasminogen is converted to plasmin, accounting for the decline in the plasminogen percentage. Because thrombolytic therapy was unsuccessful in full clot lysis (with predominate fibrinogenolysis), the D-dimer concentration is not greatly elevated. For this assay to have been more elevated, degradation products arising from cross-linked fibrin (fibrinolysis) would have had to be present. Fibrinogen concentrations should be followed periodically in patients receiving thrombolytic agents.

Diagnostic followup: If TT, PT, or aPTT is prolonged and if circulating inhibitors or bleeding disorders are suspected, further tests are usually performed. These may include assays for specific clotting factors to determine if a specific deficiency exists. For example, hemophilia or autoimmune diseases may be associated with inhibitors such as antifactor VIII and the lupus anticoagulant.

---

to monitor quantitative levels of oral DTIs since there is no "standard" with which to calibrate the test; rather it simply can tell the clinician whether or not any medication is present in the patient's blood.[118]

Clot Degradation Tests

Clot degradation tests are useful in assessing the process of fibrinolysis. These tests include fibrin FDPs and D-dimer, which can be used in the diagnosis of DIC or thrombosis and in monitoring the safety and efficacy during thrombolytic therapy.

Thrombolytics (e.g., streptokinase, anistreplase, alteplase, urokinase, reteplase, and tenecteplase) are exogenous agents that lyse clots already formed. They are used in the treatment of myocardial infarction, venous thromboembolism, and peripheral arterial occlusion. The mechanism by which they activate fibrinolysis can variably impact circulating proteins, hence the necessity for close monitoring to minimize bleeding complications and ensure efficacy. Numerous laboratory parameters have been evaluated for this purpose, which include PT, aPTT, BT, fibrinogen, FDPs, and D-dimer. These laboratory parameters are discussed throughout this chapter and Minicase 4.

Fibrin Degradation Products

Normal range: <10 mcg/mL but varies with assay
Excessive activation of thrombin leads to overactivation of the fibrinolytic system and increased production of *fibrin degradation products (FDPs)*. Excessive degradation of fibrin and fibrinogen also increases FDPs. This increase can be observed with DIC or thrombolytic drugs. Fibrin degradation products can be monitored during thrombolytic therapy, but they may not be predictive of clot lysis. Under normal conditions, FDPs should be below 2 mcg/mL of plasma when using the

semiquantitative Thrombo-Wellco test. However, this test is labor intensive and subject to observer variability.[119] A quantitative, automated assay for FDPs has been described in which the 95% confidence interval for normal subjects consisted of values between 2 and 7 mcg/mL.[120] False-positive reactions may occur in healthy women immediately before and during menstruation and in patients with advanced cirrhosis or metastatic cancer.

D-Dimer

Normal range: <0.5 mcg/mL or <200 ng/mL but varies with specific assay
D-dimer is a neoantigen formed when thrombin initiates the transition of fibrinogen to fibrin and activates factor XIII to cross link the fibrin formed. This neoantigen is formed as a result of plasmin digestion of cross-linked fibrin. The D-dimer test is specific for FDPs, whereas the formation of fibrinolysis (discussed previously) may be either fibrinogen or fibrin derived following plasmin digestion (Figure 16-6).

The D-dimer is often used to diagnose or rule out thrombosis in the initial assessment of a patient suspected of having acute thromboembolism; results are typically elevated if a patient is positive for VTE. However, D-dimer is a sensitive, but nonspecific, marker for VTE because other causes such as malignancy, DIC, infection, inflammation, and pregnancy can also elevate the D-dimer levels; thus, a positive result does not necessarily confirm a diagnosis of VTE, but a negative result can help rule out a VTE. Clinical correlation is essential, and further diagnostic workup is warranted with a positive test result to rule out other disorders as causes for abnormal levels. The 9th edition of the *Antithrombotic Therapy and Prevention of Thrombosis:*

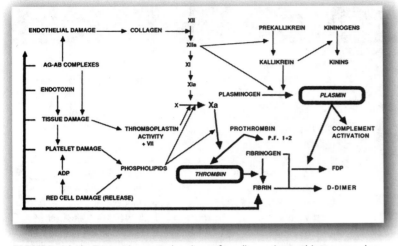

FIGURE 16-6. Triggering mechanisms for disseminated intravascular coagulation. (Reproduced, with permission, from reference 70.)

TABLE 16-8. Laboratory Differential Diagnosis of DIC

MONITORING PARAMETER	DIC	PRIMARY FIBRINOLYSIS	TTP	CHRONIC LIVER DISEASE
FDP	↑	↑	WNL to ↑	WNL to ↑
D-dimer	↑	↑	WNL	WNL
PT	↑	↑	WNL	↑
aPTT	↑	↑	WNL	WNL to ↑
Fibrinogen	↓	↓	WNL	Variable
Platelet count	↓	WNL	WNL to ↓	↓
LFTs	WNL	WNL	WNL	↑
Blood urea nitrogen	↑	WNL	↑	WNL

↓ = decreased; ↑ = increased; WNL = within normal limits;
LFTs = liver function tests; TTP = thrombotic thrombocytopenic purpura.

American College of Chest Physicians Evidence-Based Clinical Practice Guidelines recommends that a D-dimer test may be used as one possible diagnostic aid in patients with low or moderate probability for first-event VTE.[121]

In addition to diagnose or rule out VTE, D-dimer has been used for its predictive value for recurrent thromboembolism in patients treated for first event idiopathic VTE. Studies have shown that patients with normal levels of D-dimer after treatment for first event idiopathic VTE have a low risk for VTE recurrence, whereas abnormal levels of D-dimer are predictive of VTE recurrence.[122-123] Thus, in patients with abnormal levels of D-dimer, an extended duration of anticoagulation therapy could be considered.

D-dimer is also a common test used to diagnose and evaluate patients with DIC. The International Society on Thrombosis and Hemostasis as well as the Japanese Ministry of Health have devised scoring systems for DIC based on clinical and laboratory data; specific laboratory measurements include platelet counts, PT, fibrinogen, and FDPs.[124] The clinical and laboratory results are given specific scores, and when added up, indicate

whether a patient is likely to have DIC. Although a D-dimer test is not specifically mentioned in either scoring system, it is often used as a fibrin degradation marker, and it is a simple and quick test to perform. Table 16-8 provides a list of the laboratory parameters, including the D-dimer, used to diagnose DIC (Mini-cases 3 and 4).

Near-Patient or Point-of-Care Testing Devices

Several point-of-care testing devices are available for different coagulation tests such as PT/INR, ACT, D-dimer, and platelet function tests. By design, point-of-care coagulation testing methods are easy to use by multiple healthcare professionals, adaptable to a number of patient care environments, require minimal to no sample processing, and are an extension of central laboratory testing when rapid turnaround is required. Like central laboratory testing, none of the PT, aPTT, and ACT methods are standardized and users are required to verify performance characteristics for normal and therapeutic ranges and should have an understanding of the potential limitations due to sample type, sample stability, and volume. Although some instruments perform only one assay, a number of devices are capable of performing multiple tests. These devices typically are used in hospital settings and may be more cost effective than single assay platforms because hospitals can standardize all point-of-care coagulation testing using one system. Generally, point-of-care testing is not as precise as a fully automated central laboratory system that requires minimal user intervention, although in most cases the imprecision is an acceptable compromise for rapid turnaround.

Clinicians should have quality control measures in place to ensure the reliability of results; this includes ensuring that the testing device and components are properly working, personnel operating the device have adequate training, and results obtained via point-of-care testing are verified to be similar to those obtained via traditional venipuncture and analyzed in a laboratory.[125] Point-of-care testing uses whole blood, a sample that may be more physiologically relevant and result in a more accurate assessment of true coagulation potential. Many of these devices have some type of data management system that can interface with the health system's information system. The more advanced systems can restrict operator access, store a lot of specific information, manage quality control functions, and flag out-of-range results. These systems are usually reliable, but system performance and accuracy of results are reliant on routine maintenance and adherence to manufacturers' guidelines on test procedures and operational environment. A quality assurance program that utilizes recommended quality control materials and troubleshooting measures is essential to all clinical programs using point-of-care devices.

Point-of-care coagulation testing offers specific clinical advantages, especially when used to monitor antithrombotic therapy because test results can be combined with clinical presentation to make more timely decisions regarding therapeutic intervention. This is especially significant in cardiac intervention laboratories, surgical settings, and critical care units where immediate turnaround time is essential to patient care decisions. These technologies will become increasingly relevant as new antithrombotic strategies become standard of care in critical care environments. While many of the newer drugs do not require routine monitoring, the availability of rapid interventional testing may be critical to the selection of certain therapies for target patient populations, particularly when these drugs have a long half-life or cannot be completely reversed. Concomitant therapy is being used increasingly in cardiac patients, especially during cardiac intervention and so the potential for thrombotic or hemorrhagic problems may be increased without the ability to rapidly confirm coagulation potential, both at the initiation of therapy and at the conclusion of a procedure.

In outpatient settings, point-of-care testing may not only be clinically beneficial, but also more cost effective and convenient than central laboratory testing, particularly in oral anticoagulation clinics and home healthcare settings. Patients can be informed of their INR results and subsequent dosing instructions within minutes, which is an obvious time-saving element. Certain patient variables may limit the accuracy of results obtained from the currently available point-of-care devices for INR monitoring. These include concurrent use of LMWH or UFH, presence of antiphospholipid antibodies, and Hct levels above or below device-specific boundaries.

Patient self-testing (PST) and patient self-management (PSM) for INR are newer options for properly selected and trained patients on long-term warfarin therapy. Patient self-testing is when a patient tests their own INR but relies on a clinician for interpretation of results and any modifications to the current regimen. Patient self-management is when the patients test their own INR and adjust their own therapy, usually based off an algorithm, which offers more patient autonomy and control over their own dosages. One pooled analysis showed that patients utilizing PST and/or PSM had a reduction in thromboembolic events, but not hemorrhagic events or death.[126] Another meta-analysis showed a lower thromboembolic risk, lower total mortality, and no increased risk for major bleeding in patients using PST and PSM; both of these meta-analyses compared PST/PSM to usual laboratory-based INR monitoring.[127] Improvements in patient satisfaction and quality of life were seen in studies comparing PST/PSM to usual care as well.[127,128] While there are benefits to a PST/PSM model of care, including increased convenience to the patient, there are also issues that limit the widespread use of PST and/or PSM in the United States. These include reimbursement from insurance companies, lack of large scale randomized trials utilizing a U.S. population, low levels of awareness or understanding among healthcare practitioners and patients about these options, and inability to operate the testing device.[129] Additionally, the cost-effectiveness of PST/PSM is not well defined. Higher costs are associated with the cost of the test strip as well as increased testing frequency, but this may be offset by the convenience of PST/PSM, especially for patients who live far away from testing facilities, those who

have difficulty with scheduled appointments, or those who frequently travel.[65,129] Appropriate patient selection is essential for PST/PSM to be effective; ideal patient candidates, or their caregivers, should have manual dexterity, visual acuity, mental ability to perform the test, confidence and ability to responsibly participate in self-care, and the ability to complete a structured training course.[129]

SUMMARY

Many factors contribute to normal hemostasis, including interactions among vascular subendothelium, platelets, coagulation factors, natural anticoagulant proteins C and S, and substances that promote clot degradation such as tPA. In the clinical setting, the impact of these and other considerations must be evaluated. Disorders of platelets or clotting factors can result in bleeding, which may necessitate the monitoring of specific clotting tests. The MPV test is useful in distinguishing between hypoproductive versus hyperdestructive causes of thrombocytopenia.

Coagulation tests such as aPTT, ACT, and PT/INR are used to monitor heparin and warfarin therapies. In general, coagulation tests are used for patients receiving anticoagulants, thrombolytics, and antiplatelet agents. The availability of rapid diagnostic tests to manage LMWH, DTIs, and platelet inhibitor drugs may influence the adoption of these newer therapies. When fibrinolysis occurs, monitoring of FDPs is necessary. Other indications for routine use of these tests include primary coagulopathies and monitoring of drugs that may cause bleeding abnormalities. Finally, other available tests (e.g., D-dimer and AT level determinations) might improve diagnostic assessment of patients and ensure appropriate treatment selection.

Learning Points

1. What is the INR in relation to PT?

Answer: Prothrombin time results are not standardized as various reagent sources and test methods are used when performing this test among differing laboratories. The INR is a calibration method developed to standardize the reported PT results. The method considers the sensitivity of individual reagents as well as the clot detection instrument used, designated as ISI. Although INR reporting has improved the standardization of the PT, there still remains potential problems (e.g., ISI calibration, sample citrate concentration, etc.). Thus, laboratories should review the performance of their individual methods used in reporting PT/INRs and inform clinicians who are interpreting these results of any changes.

2. How often should one monitor platelets after the initiation of UFH in the prevention of HIT?

Answer: HIT is an antibody-mediated adverse reaction to heparin, which can cause arterial and venous thrombosis. It is estimated to occur in 1% to 5% of patients receiving UFH. Platelet counts should be checked often in patients receiving UFH; the exact frequency depends on several factors. For patients receiving therapeutic doses of UFH for treatment of venous or arterial thrombosis, platelets should be monitored at least every other day until day 14 or until UFH is stopped. In those patients receiving UFH for postoperative prophylaxis, platelets should be monitored at least every other day between day 4 and 14 or until UFH is stopped. For patients who have received heparin within the past 100 days or in whom exposure history is uncertain, platelets should be checked at baseline and then within 24 hours of starting UFH.

3. How long after the discontinuation of aspirin (ASA) or nonsteroidal NSAIDs will it take for the BT to normalize?

Answer: Bleeding time is an indirect test of platelet aggregation. Aspirin irreversibly acetylates cyclooxygenase. As platelets cannot synthesize new cyclooxygenase, the effect of ASA persists for the lifespan of the exposed platelets. The prolongation of BT by ASA is shorter than the platelet lifespan of 8–12 days because platelets formed after ASA exposure are not affected. Nonsteroidal anti-inflammatory drugs reversibly inhibit platelet cyclooxygenase and aggregation as long as the drug remains in the plasma. Thus, the clinician can estimate the time it takes for BT to normalize after withdrawing these drugs by knowing their respective half-lives. The consideration of BT is important to clinicians who are managing patients on either ASA or NSAIDs perioperatively (i.e., prior to gastroscopy or bronchoscopy with biopsies) to decrease bleeding complications. The clinician must also consider the cardiovascular risks of withdrawing ASA perioperatively versus the potential for bleeding complications and the need for alternative analgesics in patients who have withdrawn from NSAIDs.

REFERENCES

1. Hoffman R, Benz EJ, Shattill SJ, et al. *Hematology: Basic Principles and Practice.* Philadelphia, PA: Churchill Livingston Elsevier; 2009.

2. Steinhubl SR, Moliterno DJ. The role of the platelet in the pathogenesis of atherothrombosis. *Am J Cardiovasc Drugs.* 2005;5:399-408

3. Furie B, Furie BC. Mechanisms of thrombus formation. *N Engl J Med.* 2008;359:938-949.

4. Konkle B. Chapter 58. Bleeding and thrombosis. In: Longo DL, Kasper DL, Jameson JL, et al., eds. *Harrison's Principles of Internal Medicine.* 18th ed. New York: McGraw-Hill; 2012. http://0-www.accesspharmacy.com.millennium.midwestern.edu/content.aspx?aID=9113485. Accessed January 21, 2012.

5. Corriveau DM. Plasma proteins: factors of the hemostatic mechanism. In: Corriveau DM, Fritsma GA, eds. *Hemostasis and Thrombosis in the Clinical Laboratory.* Philadelphia, PA: JB Lippincott; 1988:34-66.

6. Giangrande P. Six characters in search of an author: the history of the nomenclature of coagulation factors. *Br J Haematol.* 2003;121:703-712.

7. Crabbe SJ, Cloninger CC. Tissue plasminogen activator: a new thrombolytic agent. *Clin Pharm.* 1987;6:33-86.

8. Khan S, Dickerman JD. Hereditary thrombophilia. *Thromb J.* 2006;4:15-32.

9. Cuker A, Cines DB. How I treat heparin-induced thrombocytopenia (HIT). *Blood.* 2012 Jan 13 [Epub ahead of print]. Accessed January 28, 2012.

10. Linkins LA, Dans AL, Moores LK, et al. Treatment and prevention of heparin-induced thrombocytopenia. Antithrombotic Therapy and Prevention of Thrombosis, 9th ed: American College of Chest Physicians Evidence-Based Clinical Practice Guidelines. *Chest.* 2012;141:e495S-e530S.

11. Cuker A. Recent advances in heparin-induced thrombocytopenia. *Curr Opin Hematol.* 2011;18:315-322.

12. Warkentin TE, Kelton JG. Delayed-onset heparin-induced thrombocytopenia and thrombosis. *Ann Intern Med.* 2001;135:502-506.

13. Rice L, Attisha WK, Drexler A, et al. Delayed-onset heparin induced thrombocytopenia. *Ann Intern Med.* 2002;136:210-215.

14. Jackson MR, Neilson WJ, Lary M. Delayed-onset heparin induced thrombocytopenia and thrombosis after intraoperative heparin anticoagulation four case reports. *Vasc Endovasc Surg.* 2006;40:67-70.

15. Aoki J, Iguchi Y, Kimura K, et al. A pulmonary embolism caused by delayed-onset heparin-induced thrombocytopenia in a patient with ischemic stroke. *Inter Med.* 2009;48:921-924.

16. Omran AS, Karimi A, Ahmadi H, et al. Delayed-onset heparin-induced thrombocytopenia presenting with multiple arteriovenous thromboses: case report. *J Med Case Reports.* 2007;1:131-135.

17. Refaai MA, Warkentin TE, Axelson M, et al. Delayed-onset heparin-induced thrombocytopenia, venous thromboembolism, and cerebral venous thrombosis: a consequence of heparin "flushes." *Thromb Haemost.* 2007;98:1139-1140.

18. Papadopoulos S, Flynn JD, Lewis DA. Fondaparinux as a treatment option for heparin-induced thrombocytopenia. *Pharmacotherapy.* 2007;27:921-926.

19. Grouzi E, Kyriakou E, Panagou I, et al. Fondaparinux for the treatment of acute heparin-induced thrombocytopenia: a single-center experience. *Clin Appl Thromb Hemost.* 2010;16:663-667.

20. Badger NO. Fondaparinux (Arixtra®), a safe alternative for the treatment of patients with heparin-induced thrombocytopenia? *J Pharm Pract.* 2010;23:235-238.

21. Spyropoulos AC, Magnuson S, Koh SK. The use of fondaparinux for the treatment of venous thromboembolism in a patient with heparin-induced thrombocytopenia and thrombosis caused by heparin flushes. *Ther Clin Risk Manag.* 2008;4:653-657.

22. Wellborn-Kim JJ, Mitchell GA, Terneus WF, et al. Fondaparinux therapy in a hemodialysis patient with heparin-induced thrombocytopenia type II. *Am J Health-Syst Pharm.* 2010;67:1075-1079.

23. Wester JPJ, Leyte A, Oudemans-van Straaten HM, Bosman RJ, et al. Low-dose fondaparinux in suspected heparin-induced thrombocytopenia in the critically ill. *Neth J Med.* 2007;65:101-108.

24. Efird LE, Kockler DR. Fondaparinux for thromboembolic treatment and prophylaxis of heparin-induced thrombocytopenia. *Ann Pharmacother.* 2006;40:1383-1387.

25. Filis K, Lagoudianakis EE, Pappas A, et al. Heparin-induced thrombocytopenia and phlegmasia cerulean dolens of the upper limb successfully treated with fondaparinux. *Acta Haematol.* 2008;120:190-191.

26. Pappalardo F, Scandroglio A, Maj G, et al. Treatment of heparin-induced thrombocytopenia after cardiac surgery: preliminary experience with fondaparinux. *J Thorac Cardiovasc Surg.* 2010;139:790-792.

27. Kovacs MJ. Successful treatment of heparin induced thrombocytopenia (HIT) with fondaparinux. *Thromb Haemost.* 2005;93:999-1000.

28. Corbett TL, Elher KS, Garwood CL. Successful use of fondaparinux in a patient with a mechanical heart valve replacement and a history of heparin-induced thrombocytopenia. *J Thromb Thrombolysis.* 2010;30:375-377.

29. Al-Rossaies A, Alkharfy KM, Al-Ayoubi F, et al. Heparin-induced thrombocytopenia: comparison between response to fondaparinux and lepirudin. *Int J Clin Pharm.* 2011;33:997-1001.

30. Ciurzynski M, Jankowski K, Pietrzak B, et al. Use of fondaparinux in a pregnant woman with pulmonary embolism and heparin-induced thrombocytopenia. *Med Sci Monit.* 2011;17:CS56-CS59.

31. Modi C, Satani D, Cervellione KL, et al. Delayed-onset heparin-induced thrombocytopenia type-2 during fondiparinux (Arixtra*) therapy. *Proc West Pharmacol Soc.* 2009;52:5-7

32. Burch M, Cooper B. Fondaparinux-associated heparin-induced thrombocytopenia. *Proc (Bayl Univ Med Cent).* 2012;25:13-15.

33. Warkentin TE, Maurer BT, Aster RH. Heparin-induced thrombocytopenia associated with fondaparinux. *N Engl J Med.* 2007;356:2653-2655.

34. Ratuapli SK, Bobba B, Zafar H. Heparin-induced thrombocytopenia in a patient treated with fondaparinux. *Clin Adv Hematol Oncol.* 2010;8:61-65.

35. Pistulli R, Oberle V, Figulla HR, et al. Fondaparinux cross-reacts with heparin antibodies in vitro in a patient with fondaparinux-related thrombocytopenia. *Blood Coagul Fibrinolysis.* 2011;22:76-78.

36. Miranda AC, Donovan JL, Tran MT, et al. A case of unsuccessful treatment of heparin-induced thrombocytopenia (HIT) with fondaparinux. *J Thromb Thrombolysis.* 2012;33:133-135.

37. Salem M, Elrefai S, Shrit MA, et al. Fondaparinux thromboprophylaxis-associated heparin-induced thrombocytopenia syndrome complicated by arterial thrombotic stroke. *Thromb Haemost.* 2010;104:1071-1072.

38. Bath PMW, Butterworth RJ. Platelet size: measurement, physiology and vascular disease. *Blood Coagul Fibrinolysis.* 1996;7:157-161.

39. Martin JF, Bath DM, Burr ML. Influence of platelet size on outcome after myocardial infarction. *Lancet.* 1991;338:1409-1411.

40. Burr ML, Holliday RM, Fehily AM, et al. Hematological prognostic indices after myocardial infarction: evidence from the diet and reinfarction trial (PART). *Eur Heart J.* 1992;13:166-170.

41. Singer CRJ, Walker JJ, Cameron A, et al. Platelet studies in normal pregnancy and pregnancy induced hypertension. *Clin Lab Haematol.* 1986;8:27-32.

42. Haubenstock A, Panzer S, Vierhapper H. Reversal of hyperthyroidism to euthyroidism leads to increased numbers of small size platelets. *Thromb Haemost.* 1988;60:346-347.

43. Panzer S, Haubenstock A, Minar E. Platelets in hyperthyroidism: studies on platelet counts, mean platelet volume, 111-indium labeled platelet kinetics and platelet associated immunoglobulins G and M. *J Clin Endocrinol Metab.* 1990;70:491-496.

44. Wedzicha JA, Cotter FE, Empey DW. Platelet size in patients with chronic airflow obstruction with and without hypoxemia. *Thorax.* 1988;43:61-64.

45. Michalak E, Walkowiak B, Paradowski M, et al. The decreased circulating platelet mass and its relation to bleeding time in chronic renal failure. *Thromb Haemost.* 1991;65:11-14.

46. Bessman JD, Gardner FH. Platelet size in thrombocytopenia due to sepsis. *Surg Gynecol Obstet.* 1983;156:177-180.

47. Koenig C, Sidhu G, Schoentag RA. The platelet volume-number relationship in patients infected with the human immunodeficiency virus. *Am J Clin Pathol.* 1991;96:500-503.

48. de Sauvage FJ, Hass PE, Spencer SD, et al. Stimulation of megakaryocytopoiesis and thrombopoiesis by the c-Mpl ligand. *Nature.* 1994;369:533-538.

49. Lok S, Kaushansky K, Holly RD, et al. Cloning and expression of murine thrombopoietin cDNA and stimulation of platelet production in vivo. *Nature.* 1994;369:565-568.

50. Kaushansky K, Lok S, Holly RD, et al. Promotion of megakaryocyte progenitor expansion and differentiation by the c-Mpl ligand thrombopoietin. *Nature.* 1994;369:568-571.

51. Wendling F, Maraskovsky E, Debili N, et al. c-Mpl ligand is a humoral regulator of megakaryocytopoiesis. *Nature.* 1994;369:571-574.

52. George JN, Caen JP, Nurden AT. Glanzmann's thrombasthenia: the spectrum of clinical disease. *Blood.* 1990;75:1383-1395.

53. George JN, Shattil SJ. The clinical importance of acquired abnormalities of platelet function. *N Engl J Med.* 1991;324:27-39.

54. Harle CC. Point-of-care platelet function testing. *Semin Cardiothorac Vasc Anesth.* 2007;11:247-251.

55. Margetic S. Diagnostic algorithm for thrombophilia screening. *Clin Chem Lab Med.* 2010;48(suppl 1):S27-S39.

56. Pajic T. Factor V Leiden and FII 20210 testing in thromboembolic disorders. *Clin Chem Lab Med.* 2010;48(suppl 1):S79-S87.

57. Rees DC, Cox M, Clegg JB. World distribution of factor V Leiden. *Lancet.* 1995;346:1133-1134.

58. Ridker PM, Miletich JP, Hennekens CH, et al. Ethnic distribution of factor V Leiden in 4047 men and women. *J Am Med Assoc.* 1997;277:1305-1307.

59. Svensson PJ, Dahlback B. Resistance to activated protein C as a basis for venous thrombosis. *N Engl J Med.* 1994;330:517-522.

60. Akthar MS, Blair AJ, King TC, et al. Whole blood screening test for factor V Leiden using a Russell Viper Venom time-based assay. *Am J Clin Pathol.* 1998;109:387-391.

61. Martorell JR, Munoz-Castillo R, Gil JL. False-positive activated Protein C resistance due to antiphospholipid antibodies is corrected by platelet extract. *Thromb Haemost.* 1995;74:796-797.

62. Ageno W, Gallus AS, Wittkowsky A, et al. Oral anticoagulant therapy: antithrombotic therapy and prevention of thrombosis, 9th ed: American College of Chest Physicians Evidence-Based Clinical Practice Guidelines. *Chest.* 2012;141(suppl):e44S-e88S.

63. Kamal AH, Teferi A, Pruthi RK. How to interpret and pursue an abnormal prothrombin time, activated partial thromboplastin time, and bleeding time in adults. *Mayo Clin Proc.* 2007;82:864-873.

64. You JJ, Singer DE, Howard PA, et al. Antithrombotic therapy for atrial fibrillation: antithrombotic therapy and prevention of thrombosis, 9th ed: American College of Chest Physicians Evidence-Based Clinical Practice Guidelines. *Chest.* 2012;141(suppl):e531S-e575S.

65. Holbrook A, Schulman S, Witt DM, et al. Evidence-based management of anticoagulant therapy: antithrombotic therapy and prevention of thrombosis, 9th ed: American College of Chest Physicians Evidence-Based Clinical Practice Guidelines. *Chest.* 2012;141(suppl):e152S-e184S.

66. Kearon C, Akl EA, Comerota AJ, et al. Antithrombotic therapy for VTE disease: antithrombotic therapy and prevention of thrombosis, 9th ed: American College of Chest Physicians Evidence-Based Clinical Practice Guidelines. *Chest.* 2012;141(suppl):e419S-e494S.

67. Lansberg MG, O'Donnell MJ, Khatri P, et al. Antithrombotic and thrombolytic therapy for ischemic stroke: antithrombotic therapy and prevention of thrombosis, 9th ed: American College of Chest Physicians Evidence-Based Clinical Practice Guidelines. *Chest.* 2012;141(suppl):e601S-e636S.

68. Whitlock RP, Sun JC, Fremes SE, et al. Antithrombotic and thrombolytic therapy for valvular disease: antithrombotic therapy and prevention of thrombosis, 9th ed: American College of Chest Physicians Evidence-Based Clinical Practice Guidelines. *Chest.* 2012;141(suppl):e576S-e600S.

69. McKernan A. The reliability of international normalized ratios during short-term oral anticoagulant treatment. *Clin Lab Haematol.* 1988;10:63-71.

70. Bick RL. Disseminated intravascular coagulation: objective criteria for clinical and laboratory diagnosis and assessment of therapeutic response. *Clin Appl Thrombosis/Hemostasis.* 1995;1(1):3-25.

71. Cavallari LH, Shin J, Perera MA. Role of pharmacogenomics in the management of traditional and novel oral anticoagulants. *Pharmacotherapy.* 2011;31:1192-1207.

72. Coumadin [package insert]. Princeton, NJ: Bristol-Myers Squibb Company; 2011.

73. Lippi G, Favaloro EJ. Activated partial thromboplastin time: new tricks for an old dogma. *Semin Thromb Hemost.* 2008;34:604-611.

74. Ng VL. Prothrombin time and partial thromboplastin time assay considerations. *Clin Lab Med.* 2009;253-263.

75. Garcia DA, Baglin TP, Weitz JI, et al. Parenteral anticoagulants: antithrombotic therapy and prevention of thrombosis, 9th ed: American College of Chest Physicians Evidence-Based Clinical Practice Guidelines. *Chest.* 2012;141(suppl):e24S-43S.

76. The Global Use of Strategies to Open Occluded Coronary Arteries (GUSTO III) Investigators. A comparison of reteplase with alteplase for acute myocardial infarction. *N Eng J Med.* 1997;337:1118-1123.

77. Granger CB, Hirsh J, Califf RM, et al. Activated partial thromboplastin time and outcome after thrombolytic therapy for acute myocardial infarction. *Circulation.* 1996;93:870-878.

78. The global use of strategies to open occluded coronary arteries (GUSTO) IIa investigators. Randomized trial of intravenous heparin vs. recombinant hirudin for acute coronary syndromes. *Circulation.* 1994;90:1631-1637.

79. Antman EM, for the TIMI 9A investigators. Hirudin in acute myocardial infarction: safety report from the thrombolysis and thrombin inhibition in myocardial infarction (TIMI) 9A trial. *Circulation.* 1994;90:1624-1630.

80. Raschke RA, Reilly BM, Guidry JR, et al. The weight-based heparin dosing nomogram compared with a "standard care" nomogram: a randomized controlled trial. *Arch Intern Med.* 1993;119:874-881.

81. Cruickshank MK, Levine MN, Hirsh J, et al. A standard heparin nomogram for the management of heparin therapy. *Arch Intern Med.* 1991;151:333-337.

82. Gunnarsson PS, Sawyer WT, Montague D, et al. Appropriate use of heparin: empiric vs. nomogram-based dosing. *Arch Intern Med.* 1995;155:526-532.

83. Groce JB, Gal P, Douglas JB, et al. Heparin dosage adjustment in patients with deep-vein thrombosis using heparin concentrations rather than activated partial thromboplastin time. *Clin Pharm.* 1987;6:216-222.

84. Kandrotas RJ, Gal P, Douglas JB, et al. Rapid determination of maintenance heparin infusion rates with the use of nonsteady-state heparin concentrations. *Ann Pharmacother.* 1993;27:1429-1433.

85. Basu D, Gallus A, Hirsh J, et al. A prospective study of the value of monitoring heparin treatment with the activated partial thromboplastin time. *N Engl J Med.* 1972;287:324-327.

86. Hull RD, Raskob GE, Hirsh J, et al. Continuous intravenous heparin compared with intermittent subcutaneous heparin in the initial treatment of proximal-vein thrombosis. *N Engl J Med.* 1986;315:1109-1114.

87. Hauser VM, Rozek SL. Effect of warfarin on the activated partial thromboplastin time. *Drug Intell Clin Pharm.* 1986; 20:964-967.

88. Kearon C, Johnston M, Moffat K, et al. Effect of warfarin on activated partial thromboplastin time in patients receiving heparin. *Arch Intern Med.* 1998;158:1140-1143.

89. Groce JB. Heparin and low molecular weight heparin. In: Murphy JE, ed. *Clinical Pharmacokinetics.* 2nd ed. Bethesda, MD: American Society of Health-System Pharmacists; 2001:165-198.

90. Levine MN, Hirsh J, Gent M, et al. A randomized trial comparing activated partial thromboplastin time with heparin assay in patients with acute venous thromboembolism requiring large doses of heparin. *Arch Intern Med.* 1994;154:49-56.

91. Lippi G, Salvagno GL, Ippolito L, et al. Shortened activated partial thromboplastin time: causes and management. *Blood Coagul Fibrinolysis.* 2010;21:459-463.

92. Mina A, Favaloro E, Mohammed S, et al. A laboratory evaluation into the short activated partial thromboplastin time. *Blood Coagul Fibrinolysis.* 2010;21:152-157.

93. Legnani C, Mattarozzi S, Cini M, et al. Abnormally short activated partial thromboplastin time values are associated with increased risk of recurrence of venous thromboembolism after oral anticoagulation withdrawal. *Br J Haematol.* 2006;134:227-232.

94. Hron G, Eichinger S, Weltermann A, et al. Prediction of recurrent venous thromboembolism by the activated partial thromboplastin time. *J Thromb Haemost.* 2006;4:752-756.

95. Tripodi A, Chantarangkul V, Martinelli I, et al. A shortened activated partial thromboplastin time is associated with the risk of venous thromboembolism. *Blood.* 2004;104:3631-3634.

96. Korte W, Clarke S, Lefkowitz JB. Short activated partial thromboplastin times are related to increased thrombin generation and an increased risk for thromboembolism. *Am J Clin Pathol.* 2000;113:123-127.

97. Reddy NM, Hall SW, MacKintosh FR. Partial thromboplastin time: prediction of adverse events and poor prognosis by low abnormal values. *Arch Intern Med.* 1999;159:2706-2710.

98. Zakai NA, Ohira T, White R, et al. Activated partial thromboplastin time and risk of future venous thromboembolism. *Am J Med.* 2008;121:231-238.

99. Aboud MR, Ma DDF. Increased incidence of venous thrombosis in patients with shortened activated partial thromboplastin times and low ratios for activated protein C resistance. *Clin Lab Haem.* 2001;23:411-416.

100. Ten Boekel E, de Kieviet W, Bartels PC. Subjects with shortened activated partial thromboplastin time show increased in-hospital mortality associated with elevated D-dimer, C-reactive protein and glucose levels. *Scand J Clin Lab Invest.* 2003;63:441-448.

101. Lippi G, Franchini M, Targher G, et al. Epidemiological association between fasting plasma glucose and shortened APTT. *Clin Biochem.* 2009;42:118-120.

102. Zhao Y, Zhang J, Zhang J, et al. Diabetes mellitus is associated with shortened activated partial thromboplastin time and increased fibrinogen values. *PLoS One.* 2011;6:e16470.

103. Lippi G, Franchini M, Targher G. Hyperthyroidism is associated with shortened APTT and increased fibrinogen values in a general population of unselected outpatients. *J Thromb Thrombolysis.* 2009;28:362-365.

104. Madi AM, Greci LS, Nawaz H, et al. The activated partial thromboplastin time in early diagnosis of myocardial infarction. *Blood Coagul Fibrinolysis.* 2001;12:495-499.

105. Hirsh J, Hull RD. Treatment of venous thromboembolism. *Chest.* 1986;89(suppl 5):426S-433S.

106. Lovenox [package insert]. Bridgewater, NJ: Sanofi-Aventis US LLC; 2011.

107. Fragmin [package insert]. Woodcliff Lake, NJ: Eisai Inc; 2010.

108. Innohep [package insert]. Boulder, CO: Pharmion Corporation; 2010.

109. Colwell CW, Spiro TE, Trowbridge AA, et al. Use of enoxaparin, a low-molecular-weight heparin, and unfractionated heparin for the prevention of deep venous thrombosis after elective hip replacement. *J Bone Joint Surg.* 1994;76-A:3-14.

110. Laposta M, Green D, Van Cott EM, et al. College of American Pathologists Conference XXXI on Laboratory Monitoring of Anticoagulant Therapy. The clinical use and laboratory monitoring of low-molecular-weight heparin, danaparoid, hirudin and related compounds, and argatroban. *Arch Pathol Lab Med.* 1998;122:799-807.

111. 111.Simko RJ, Tsung FFW, Stanek EJ. Activated clotting time versus activated partial thromboplastin time for therapeutic monitoring of heparin. *Ann Pharmacother.* 1995;29:1015-1021.

112. SpinlerSA, Wittkowsky AK, Nutescu EA, et al. Anticoagulation monitoring part 2: unfractionated heparin and low-molecular-weight heparin. *Ann Pharmacother.* 2005;39:1275-1285.

113. Perry DJ, Fitzmaurice DA, Kitchen S, et al. Point-of-care testing in haemostasis. *Br J Haematol.* 2010;150:501-514.

114. Van Cott EM. Point-of-care testing in coagulation. *Clin Lab Med.* 2009;29:543-553.

115. Smythe MA, Koerber JM, Nowak SN, et al. Correlation between activated clotting time and activated partial thromboplastin times. *Ann Pharmacother.* 2002;36:7-11.

116. Kakafika AI, Liberopoulos EN, Mikhailidis DP. Fibrinogen: a predictor of vascular disease. *Curr Pharm Des.* 2007;13:1647-1659.

117. Wilcox R, Pendleton RC, Smock KJ. Hospital-based clinical implications of the novel oral anticoagulant, dabigatran etexilate, in daily practice. *Hosp Pract* (Minneap). 2011;39:23-34.

118. Favaloro E, Lippi G, Koutts J. Laboratory testing of anticoagulants: the present and the future. *Pathology.* 2011;43:682-692.

119. Sigal SH, Cembrowski GS, Shattil SJ, et al. Prototype quantitative assay for fibrinogen/fibrin degradation products: clinical evaluation. *Arch Intern Med.* 1987;147:1790-1793.

120. Conrad J, Samama MM. Theoretic and practical considerations on laboratory monitoring of thrombolytic therapy. *Semin Thromb Hemost.* 1987;13:212-222.

121. Bates SM, Jaeschke R, Stevens SM, et al. Diagnosis of DVT: antithrombotic therapy and prevention of thrombosis, 9th ed: American College of Chest Physicians Evidence-Based Clinical Practice Guidelines. *Chest.* 2012;141:e351s-e418s.

122. Verhovsek M, Douketis JD, Yi Q, et al. Systematic review: D-dimer to predict recurrent disease after stopping anticoagulant therapy for unprovoked venous thromboembolism. *Ann Intern Med.* 2008;149:481-490.

123. Palareti G, Cosmi B, Legnani C, et al. D-dimer testing to determine the duration of anticoagulation therapy. *N Engl J Med.* 2006;355(17):1780-1789.

124. Tripodi A. D-dimer testing in laboratory practice. *Clin Chem.* 2011;57:1256-1262.

125. Perry DJ, Fitzmaurice DA, Kitchen S, et al. Point-of-care testing in haemostasis. *Br J Haematol.* 2010;150:501-

126. Heneghan C, Ward A, Perera R, et al. Self-monitoring of oral anticoagulation: systematic review and meta-analysis of individual patient data. *Lancet.* 2012;379:322-334.

127. Bloomfield HE, Krause A, Greer N, et al. Meta-analysis: effect of patient self-testing and self-management of long-term anticoagulation on major clinical outcomes. *Ann Intern Med.* 2011;154:472-482.

128. Matchar DB, Jacobson A, Dolor R, et al. Effect of home testing of international normalized ratio on clinical events. *N Engl J Med.* 2010;363:1608-1620.

129. Nutescu EA, Bathija S, Sharp LK, et al. Anticoagulation patient self-monitoring in the United States: considerations for clinical practice adoption. *Pharmacotherapy.* 2011;31:1161-1174.

QUICKVIEW | Platelet Count

PARAMETER	DESCRIPTION	COMMENTS
Common reference ranges		
Adults	150,000–450,000/µL	
Critical value	>800,000 or <20,000	
Inherent activity?	Determines the number or concentration of platelets in a blood sample	
Location		
Production	Bone marrow	Also can be produced by lungs and other tissues
Storage	Not stored	$2/3$ found in circulation, $1/3$ found in spleen
Secretion/excretion	Destroyed by spleen, liver, bone marrow	
Causes of abnormal values		
High	Acute hemorrhage	
	Iron deficiency anemia	
	Diseases: splenectomy, rheumatoid arthritis, occult malignancy, myeloproliferative neoplasms	
Low	Hypersplenism	
	Severe B$_{12}$, folate deficiency	
	Diseases: TTP, ITP, DIC, aplastic anemia, myelodysplasia, leukemia	Table 16-3
	Drugs	
Signs and symptoms		
High	Thrombosis: CVA, DVT, PE, portal vein thrombosis	
Low	Bleeding: mucosal, cutaneous	CNS bleeding (i.e., intracranial hemorrhage) is the most common cause of death in patients with severe thrombocytopenia
After event, time to...		
Initial elevation	Days to weeks	
Peak values	Days to weeks	
Normalization	Weeks to months	
Causes of spurious results	Values outside 50,000–500,000/µL Hct <20 or >50%	Need to review the peripheral blood smear to confirm automated platelet counts in these instances

CNS = central nervous system; CVA = cerebrovascular accident; DIC = disseminated intravascular coagulation; DVT = deep vein thrombosis; PE = pulmonary embolism; TTP = thrombotic thrombocytopenic purpura; ITP = idiopathic thrombocytopenic purpura.

QUICKVIEW | PT and INR

PARAMETER	DESCRIPTION	COMMENTS
Common reference ranges		
Adults	PT 10–13 sec INR 1+0.1	INR therapeutic ranges will vary if patient is on warfarin and depending on indication for warfarin; usual therapeutic ranges are either 2–3 or 2.5–3.5
Pediatrics	PT <16 sec	PT levels in the newborn are generally prolonged compared to adults; however, by 6 months of age, levels are comparable to adults
Critical value	PT >15 sec INR—depends on indication, but >5 is commonly used as a critical value	Unless on warfarin
Inherent activity	Indirect measure of coagulation factors, particularly factor VII, which has the shortest half-life and thus is affected most rapidly by warfarin	
Location		
Production	Coagulation factors produced in liver	
Storage	Not stored	
Secretion/excretion	None	
Causes of abnormal values		
High	Diseases: liver disease Malabsorption/malnutrition Drug: warfarin	Table 16-7
Low	None	
Signs and symptoms		
High	Increased risk of bleeding and ecchymosis	Risk increases as PT or INR value increases
Low	Potential thrombosis if on vitamin K antagonist	
After event, time to...		
Initial elevation	6–12 hr	
Peak values	Days to weeks	
Normalization	Hours–days	Depends, if reversed with vitamin K
Causes of spurious results	Improper laboratory collection	
Additional info	Used to monitor warfarin	Target levels depend on indication for warfarin

INR = international normalized ratio; PT = prothrombin time.

QUICKVIEW | aPTT

PARAMETER	DESCRIPTION	COMMENTS
Common reference ranges		
Adults	25–35 sec	May vary by reagent/instrument used
Critical value	>100 sec	
Inherent activity?	Used to monitor unfractionated heparin activity	If patient is on unfractionated heparin for treatment of deep venous thrombosis or pulmonary embolism, aim for 1.5–2.5 times control aPTT
Location		
Production	Coagulation factors produced in liver	
Storage	Not stored	$2/3$ found in circulation, $1/3$ found in spleen
Secretion/excretion	None	
Causes of abnormal values		
High	Hereditary: deficiency of factors II, V, VIII, IX, X, XI, XII, HMWK, prekallikrein, fibrinogen	
	Acquired: lupus anticoagulant, heparin, DTIs, liver dysfunction, vitamin K deficiency, warfarin, DIC	aPTT not used to monitor warfarin therapy
Low	Labs drawn before 6 hr if on heparin	
Signs and symptoms		
High	Increased risk of hemorrhage	Risk increases as aPTT increases
Low	Thrombosis	
After event, time to...		
Initial elevation	6–12 hr	
Peak values	Hours to days	
Normalization	Hours to days	
Causes of spurious results	Improper laboratory collection	Need to do manual counts in these instances
Additional info	Used to monitor heparin	Dosing nomograms vary by institution

aPTT = activated partial thromboplastin time; DIC = disseminated intravascular coagulation; DTIs = direct thrombin inhibitors.

QUICKVIEW | anti-Xa

PARAMETER	DESCRIPTION	COMMENTS
Common reference ranges		
Adults	0.3–0.7 units/mL	For establishment of therapeutic heparin range using blood samples from heparinized patients
		For once daily therapeutic dosing of LMWH
		Values may vary depending on LMWH preparation used
Inherent activity?	Used to establish therapeutic heparin range and monitor LMWH activity	
Location		
Production	Coagulation factors produced in liver	
Storage	Not stored	
Secretion/excretion	None	
Causes of abnormal values		
High	Overdosage of LMWH	
	Poor renal function	
Low	Labs drawn prior to 4 hr after dose is administered	
	Underdosage of LMWH	
Signs and symptoms		
High	Increased risk of bleeding and bruising	
Low	Potential thrombosis	
After event, time to...		
Initial elevation	0–4 hr	
Peak values	4 hr	
Normalization	Hours to days	
Causes of spurious results	Improper timing of collection	Should be drawn 4 hr after dose is administered
Additional info	Used to monitor LMWH	

LMWH = low molecular weight heparin.

CHAPTER 17

INFECTIOUS DISEASES

SHARON M. ERDMAN, RODRIGO M. BURGOS, KEITH A. RODVOLD

(continued on 402)

Objectives

After completing this chapter, the reader should be able to

- List the common tests utilized by the microbiology laboratory for the identification of bacteria

- Describe the types of clinical specimens that may be submitted for Gram stain and culture

- Discuss the processes involved in staining and culturing a specimen for bacteria, including the time required to obtain a result from either method; describe the clinical utility of the information obtained from a Gram stain or a culture

- Identify bacteria according to Gram stain results (Gram-positive versus Gram-negative), morphology (cocci versus bacilli), and growth characteristics (aerobic versus anaerobic)

- Define normal flora; identify anatomic sites of the human body where normal flora are commonly present and those sites that are typically considered sterile; identify bacteria that are considered normal flora in each of those sites

- Describe the most common causative pathogens based on infection type or anatomic site of infection

- Describe the common methods used for determining antimicrobial susceptibility including technique, type of result derived, clinical implications, and limitations of each method; demonstrate the ability to use susceptibility information to make clinical decisions with regard to choosing an appropriate antimicrobial regimen for a patient

The assessment, diagnosis, and treatment of a patient with an infection may appear to be an overwhelming task to some clinicians. This may be partly due to the nonspecific presentation of many infectious processes; the continuously changing taxonomy, diagnostic procedures, and antimicrobial susceptibility patterns of infecting organisms; and the continuous, albeit diminishing, introduction of new antimicrobials to the existing large collection of anti-infective agents. This chapter focuses on the laboratory tests that may be utilized for the diagnosis of infectious diseases. It is important to note that diagnostic tests for many infectious diseases, particularly the diagnosis of human immunodeficiency virus (HIV) infection, are continuously being modified to reflect technological advances in laboratory procedures.

This chapter describes some of the laboratory tests that are utilized in the diagnosis of the most common infections due to bacteria, fungi, mycobacteria, viruses, and other organisms. Information regarding white blood cells (WBCs) and their role in infection is discussed in Chapter 15: Hematology: Red and White Blood Cell Tests. Laboratory tests utilized in the diagnosis of viral hepatitis, *Helicobacter pylori* gastrointestinal infection, and *Clostridium difficile* pseudomembranous colitis are addressed in Chapter 12: Liver and Gastroenterology Tests. Lastly, the background, normal ranges, and clinical utility of the erythrocyte sedimentation rate (ESR) and C-reactive protein (CRP) as they relate to inflammatory diseases are addressed in Chapter 18: Rheumatic Diseases; however, this chapter will provide a brief discussion regarding their clinical utility in the diagnosis and management of infectious diseases.

BACTERIA

Bacteria are small, unicellular, prokaryotic organisms that contain a cell wall but lack a well-defined nucleus. They are a diverse group of microorganisms that exist in different shapes and morphologies with varying rates of pathogenicity. Bacteria are a common cause of infection in both the community and hospital setting and can cause infection in patients with normal or suppressed immune systems. Bacteria must be considered potential causative pathogens in any patient presenting with signs and symptoms of infection.

The Identification of Bacteria

Several factors should be considered when choosing an appropriate antimicrobial regimen for the treatment of infection, including patient characteristics (e.g., immune status, age, end-organ function, drug allergies, and severity of illness), drug characteristics (e.g., spectrum of activity, pharmacokinetics, penetration to the site of infection, and proven clinical efficacy), and infection characteristics including the site/type of infection (suspected or known) and potential causative organism(s). Therefore, appropriate diagnosis is a key factor in selecting appropriate empiric and definitive antibiotic therapy for the treatment of an infection. In the case of a suspected infection, appropriate culture specimens should be obtained for laboratory testing from the suspected site of infection *before* antibiotics are initiated, if possible, in an attempt to isolate and identify the causative pathogen. Special attention should be placed on specimen collection and timely transport to the laboratory

Objectives

- Define minimum inhibitory concentration (MIC), MIC_{50}, MIC_{90}, MIC susceptibility breakpoints, and minimum bactericidal concentration (MBC)

- Describe the information that is utilized to construct an antibiogram; discuss the clinical utility of the antibiogram when choosing empiric antibiotic therapy for the treatment of a patient's infection

- Understand the basic methods that may be utilized in the diagnosis of systemic fungal infections

- Discuss the laboratory tests that are commonly utilized in the diagnosis of infections due to *Mycobacterium tuberculosis* and nontuberculous mycobacteria

- Discuss the laboratory tests that are commonly utilized in the diagnosis of common viral infections such as influenza, herpes simplex virus (HSV), cytomegalovirus (CMV), and respiratory syncytial virus (RSV)

- Discuss the laboratory tests that are commonly utilized in the diagnosis of human immunodeficiency virus (HIV); describe the laboratory tests that are commonly utilized in the assessment and monitoring of patients with HIV infection

- Understand the laboratory tests that may be performed for the diagnosis of infections due to miscellaneous or uncommon organisms such as *Borrelia burgdorferi*, *Treponema pallidum*, *Legionella pneumophila*, and *Pneumocystis (carinii) jirovecii*

- Understand the clinical utility of laboratory tests routinely performed for the diagnosis of infection in:
  - Cerebrospinal fluid (CSF) when meningitis is suspected
  - Respiratory secretions when upper or lower respiratory tract infections are suspected
  - Urine, prostatic secretions, or genital secretions when a genitourinary tract infection is suspected
  - Otherwise sterile fluid when infection is suspected (e.g., synovial fluid and peritoneal fluid)

since the accuracy of the results will be limited by the quality and condition of the submitted specimen.[1-4] Table 17-1 lists common biologic specimens that are often submitted to the microbiology laboratory for bacteriologic analysis.[1-4]

When a specimen from the suspected site of infection is submitted to the microbiology laboratory, a number of different microbiologic tests are performed to aid in identification of the infecting bacteria. The most common laboratory tests utilized for the identification of bacteria include direct microscopic examination using specialized stains (Gram stain) and growth of the microorganism using culture techniques. When bacteria grow in culture, tests are performed to identify the infecting organism and to determine the susceptibility of the bacteria to various antimicrobial agents.

The Gram Stain

The *Gram stain* is the most common staining method utilized for the microscopic examination of bacteria and is most appropriate for evaluation of fluids (cerebrospinal fluid [CSF], pleural, synovial, etc.), respiratory tract secretions, and wound/abscess swabs or aspirates.[4] The Gram stain classifies bacteria into one of two groups, namely Gram-positive or Gram-negative, based on their reaction to an established series of dyes and decolorizers. The difference in stain uptake between

TABLE 17-1. Common Biologic Specimens Submitted for Culture[1-4]

Abscess, lesion, wound, pustule—swab or aspirate

Blood

Bone marrow

Body fluids—amniotic, abdominal, bile, pericardial, peritoneal, pleural, or synovial by needle aspiration

Bone—biopsy of infected area

CSF—by lumbar puncture or directly from shunt

Cutaneous—hair and nail clippings, skin scrapings, aspiration of leading edge of skin infection

Ear—middle ear specimen by myringotomy; outer ear specimen by swab or biopsy

Eye—swab of conjunctiva, corneal scrapings, vitreal or anterior chamber fluid

Foreign bodies—intravenous catheter tip by roll plate method; prosthetic heart valve, prosthetic joint material, intrauterine device, etc.

Gastrointestinal—gastric aspirate for AFB; gastric biopsy for *H. pylori*, rectal swab for VRE, stool cultures

Genital tract—cervical, endometrial, urethral, vaginal, or prostatic secretions

Respiratory tract—sputum, tracheal aspirate, BAL, pharyngeal or nasopharyngeal swab, sinus aspirate

Tissue—biopsy specimen

Urine—clean catch midstream specimen, catheterized specimen, suprapubic aspirate

AFB = acid-fast bacilli; BAL = bronchoalveolar lavage; CSF = cerebrospinal fluid; VRE = vancomycin-resistant enterococci.

Gram-positive and Gram-negative bacteria is primarily due to differences in their bacterial cell wall composition and permeability.[2,5-8] While the Gram stain does not provide an exact identification of the infecting organism (e.g., *Klebsiella pneumoniae* versus *Serratia marcescens*), it does provide rapid (within minutes), preliminary information about the potential infecting organism that can be used to guide empiric antibiotic therapy while waiting for the culture results, which may take 24–48 hours or more. The Gram stain is useful for characterizing most clinically-relevant bacteria, but is unable to detect intracellular bacteria (e.g., *Chlamydophila*), bacteria without cell walls (e.g., *Mycoplasma*), and organisms that are too small to be visualized with light microscopy (e.g., spirochetes).[6-8]

The current Gram stain methodology is a slight modification of the original process developed by Hans Christian Gram in the late 19th century.[2,5-8] The Gram stain procedure involves a number of staining and rinsing steps that can all be performed within a few minutes. The first step involves applying, drying, and heat-fixing a thin smear of a biological specimen to a clean glass slide. Once the slide has cooled, it is then rinsed with crystal or gentian violet (a purple dye) followed by Gram's iodine, decolorized with an ethanol or acetone rinse, and then counterstained with safranin (a pink or red dye) with a gentle, tap water rinse performed between each of these steps. The slide is then blotted dry and examined under a microscope using the oil immersion lens. If bacteria are present, they are examined for stain uptake, morphology (round = coccus, rod = bacillus), and organization (e.g., pairs, clusters, etc.). Gram-positive bacteria stain purple due to retention of the crystal violet-iodine complex in their cell walls, while Gram-negative bacteria stain red because they do not retain crystal violet and are counterstained by safranin.[2,5,6,9] The results of the Gram stain (e.g., Gram-positive cocci in pairs or Gram-negative rods) are utilized to provide information about the possible infecting organism before the culture results become available. Table 17-2 lists the most likely bacteria based on Gram stain results.[2,10,11] A clinician can use the information from the Gram stain to select an empiric antibiotic regimen directed against the most likely pathogen causing the patient's infection before the final culture and susceptibility results are available (which may take days). Once the culture and susceptibility results are known, the initial empiric antibiotic regimen can be deescalated, if necessary, to target the infecting bacteria (directed therapy).

Besides providing a clue regarding the potential infecting organism, the Gram stain also helps to determine the **presence** of bacteria in biological specimens obtained from normally sterile body fluids (e.g., CSF, pleural fluid, synovial fluid, and urine directly from the bladder) and from specimens where infection is suspected (e.g., abscess fluid, wound swabs, sputum, and tissue); the number or relative quantity of infecting bacteria; the presence of WBCs; and the adequacy of the submitted specimen (e.g., large numbers of epithelial cells in a sputum or urine sample may signify contamination).[1,2,4,6,7,9,11]

Culture and Identification

The results from the Gram stain provide preliminary information regarding the potential infecting bacteria. In order for the bacteria to be definitively identified, the clinical specimen is also processed to facilitate bacterial growth in culture and then observed for growth characteristics (e.g., type of media, aerobic versus anaerobic, and shape and color of colonies) and reactions to biochemical testing. Under normal circumstances, the results of bacterial culture are typically available within 24–48 hours of specimen setup and processing.

In order for a bacteria to be grown successfully in culture, the specific nutritional and environmental growth requirements of the bacteria must be taken into consideration.[2-4,8,12,13] There are several clinical microbiology textbooks and reference manuals available that can assist the microbiology laboratory with the selection of appropriate culture media and environmental conditions to facilitate the optimal growth of bacteria based on specimen type and suspected bacteria.[2-4,8,12,13]

Several types of primary culture media are available that enhance or optimize bacterial growth including nutritive media (blood or chocolate agar), differential media, selective media, and supplemental broth.[1-3,8,12] The most commonly utilized bacterial growth media are listed in Table 17-3. Blood and chocolate agar plates are *nutritive* or *enrichment* media because they support the growth of many different types of aerobic and anaerobic bacteria. Blood agar is also considered to be *differential* media because it can distinguish between organisms based on certain growth characteristics, such as between the different streptococci based on hemolysis patterns. MacConkey (Mac), eosin methylene blue (EMB), colistin-nalidixic acid (CNA), and phenylethyl alcohol (PEA) agar plates are all *selective* media because they preferentially support the growth of specific organisms from a sample (e.g., Gram-negative or Gram-positive bacteria) through the use of antimicrobials, dyes, or alcohol incorporated into their media. Trypticase soy broth (TSB) and thioglycollate broth are considered *supplemental* media since they are used for subculturing bacteria detected on agar plates, or as back-up cultures to agar plates for the detection of small quantities of bacteria in biological specimens.

Once a clinical specimen is processed using the appropriate media, the plates must be incubated in the appropriate environment to support bacterial growth. The environmental factors that should be controlled during incubation include oxygen or carbon dioxide content, temperature, pH, and moisture content of the medium and atmosphere.[1,12] The oxygen requirements for growth differ among organisms. Strict *aerobic* bacteria, such as *Pseudomonas aeruginosa* and *Staphylococcus aureus*, grow best in ambient air containing 21% oxygen and a small amount of carbon dioxide.[1] Strict *anaerobes*, such as *Bacteroides* spp., are unable to grow in an oxygen-containing environment and require a controlled environment containing 5% to 10% carbon dioxide for optimal growth. Facultative anaerobes, such as *Escherichia coli* and some streptococci, can grow in the presence or absence of oxygen. Overall, most clinically-relevant bacteria grow best at 35°C to 37°C (the temperature

TABLE 17-2. Preliminary Identification of Medically Important Bacteria Using Gram Stain Results[2,10,11]

GRAM STAIN RESULT	LIKELY BACTERIAL PATHOGEN
Gram-positive (stain purple)	
Gram-positive cocci in clusters	***Staphylococcus* spp.** Coagulase-positive: *S. aureus* Coagulase-negative: *S. epidermidis, S. hominis, S. saprophyticus, S. haemolyticus, etc.*
Gram-positive cocci in pairs	***Streptococcus pneumoniae***
Gram-positive cocci in chains	**Viridans (α-hemolytic) Streptococci** (*S. milleri, S. mutans, S. salivarius, S. mitis*) **Group (β-hemolytic) Streptococci** (*S. pyogenes, S. agalactiae*, Groups C, F, and G streptococci) ***Peptostreptococcus* spp.**
Gram-positive cocci in pairs and chains	*Enterococcus* spp. (*E. faecalis, E. faecium, E. durans, E. gallinarum, E. avium, E casseliflavus, E. raffinosus*)
Gram-positive bacilli	
Nonspore-forming	***Corynebacterium* spp.** (*C. diphtheriae, C. jeikeium, C. striatum, etc.*) ***Lactobacillus* spp.** ***Listeria monocytogenes*** ***Propionibacterium* spp.** (*P. acnes*)
Spore-forming	***Bacillus* spp.** (*B. anthracis, B. cereus, etc.*) ***Clostridium* spp.** (*C. perfringens, C. difficile, C. tetani*) ***Streptomyces* spp.**
Branching, filamentous	***Actinomyces* spp.** (*A. israelii*) ***Erysipelothrix rhusiopathiae*** ***Nocardia* spp.** (*N. asteroides*)
Gram-negative (stain red)	
Gram-negative cocci	***Neisseria* spp.** (*N. gonorrhoeae, N. meningitidis, etc.*) ***Veillonella* spp.** (*V. parvula*)
Gram-negative coccobacilli	***Haemophilus* spp.** (*H. influenzae, H. parainfluenzae, H. ducreyi, etc.*) ***Moraxella catarrhalis***
Gram-negative bacilli	
Lactose-fermenting	***Aeromonas hydrophila*** ***Citrobacter* spp.** (*C. freundii, C. koseri*) ***Enterobacter* spp.** (*E. cloacae, E. aerogenes*) ***Escherichia coli*** ***Klebsiella pneumoniae*** ***Pasteurella multocida*** ***Vibrio cholerae***
Non-lactose-fermenting	***Acinetobacter* spp.** ***Alcaligenes* spp.** ***Burkholderia cepacia*** ***Morganella morganii*** ***Proteus* spp.** (*P. mirabilis, P. vulgaris*) ***Pseudomonas* spp.** (*P. aeruginosa, P. putida, P. fluorescens*) ***Salmonella* spp.** (*S. typhi, S. paratyphi, S. enteritidis, S. typhimurium*) ***Serratia marcescens*** ***Shigella* spp.** (*S. dysenteriae, S. sonnei*) ***Stenotrophomonas maltophilia***
Other Gram-negative bacilli	***Bacteroides* spp.** (*B. fragilis, B. thetaiotamicron, B. ovatus, B. distastonis*) ***Brucella* spp.** ***Bordetella* spp.** ***Campylobacter jejuni*** ***Francisella tularensis*** ***Helicobacter pylori*** ***Legionella* spp.**
Gram-variable (stain both Gram-positive and Gram-negative in the same smear)	
Gram-variable bacilli	***Gardnerella vaginalis***

TABLE 17-3. Some Commonly Used Bacterial Growth Media[1-3,8,12]

GROWTH MEDIUM	COMPOSITION	USES
Agars		
SBA	5% sheep blood	The most commonly used all-purpose medium with ability to grow most bacteria, fungi, and some mycobacteria; also used for determination of hemolytic activity of streptococci
Chocolate agar, enriched	2% hemoglobin or Iso-VitaleX in peptone base	All-purpose medium that supports growth of most bacteria; especially useful for growth of *Haemophilus* spp. and pathogenic *Neisseria* spp.
EMB or Mac agar	Peptone base with sugars and dyes that yield differentiating biochemical characteristics	Included in primary setup of nonsterile specimens; selective isolation of Gram-negative bacteria; differentiates between lactose- and nonlactose-fermenting enteric bacteria
PEA or CNA agar	Nutrient agar bases with supplemental agents to inhibit growth of aerobic Gram-negative bacteria	Included in primary setup of nonsterile specimens; selective isolation of Gram-positive cocci and anaerobic Gram-negative bacilli
Broths		
TSB	All purpose enrichment broth	Used for subculturing bacteria from primary agar plates; supports the growth of many fastidious and nonfastidious bacteria
Thioglycollate broth	Pancreatic digest of casein, soy broth, and glucose	Supports the growth of aerobic, anaerobic, microaerophilic, and fastidious bacteria

CNA = colistin-nalidixic acid; EMB = eosin methylene blue; Mac = MacConkey; PEA = phenylethyl alcohol; SBA = sheep blood agar; TSB = trypticase soy broth.

of the human body), a pH of 6.5 to 7.5, and in an atmosphere rich in moisture, which is the reason why agar plates are sealed (to trap moisture).[12]

Bacteria grown successfully in culture appear as colonies on the agar plates. Identification of the bacteria are based on evaluation of colony characteristics (size, pigmentation, shape, and surface appearance); the assessment of culture media and environmental conditions that supported the growth of the bacteria; the changes that occurred to the culture media as a result of bacterial growth; the aroma of the bacteria; the Gram stain result of individual colonies; and metabolic properties.[3,12] Biochemical tests are either enzyme-based, where the presence of a specific enzyme is measured (e.g., catalase, oxidase, indole, or urease tests), or based on the presence and measurement of metabolic pathways or byproducts (e.g., oxidative and fermentation tests or amino acid degradation).[3,12] Examples of biochemical tests include the presence of catalase in the organism or the ability of a bacteria to ferment glucose. Most biochemical tests are performed using manual or automated commercial identification systems.[12,14,15] Some of the commercial identification systems consist of multicompartment biochemical tests in a single microtiter tray so that several biochemical tests can be performed simultaneously.[12,14,15] The information derived from the macroscopic examination of the bacteria and the results of biochemical tests are then combined to determine the specific identity of the bacteria.

Colonization, Contamination, or Infection

The growth of an organism from a submitted biologic specimen does not always indicate the presence of infection; it may represent the presence of bacterial contamination or colonization.[9,11] Table 17-4 lists the anatomic sites, fluids, and tissues of the human body that are sterile and include the bloodstream, the CSF, internal organs and tissues, bone, synovial fluid, peritoneal fluid, pleural fluid, pericardial fluid, and urine taken directly from the bladder or kidney. Other body sites, particularly those with a connection to the outside environment, have microorganisms called *normal flora* that naturally *colonize* their surfaces. Normal bacterial flora can be found on the skin and in the respiratory, gastrointestinal, and genitourinary tracts; the bacteria that typically colonize these body sites are listed in Table 17-5.[11,16] Typically, normal flora are harmless bacteria that rarely cause infection. They are often located in the same areas of the body as pathogenic bacteria and are thought to be protective by inhibiting the growth of pathogenic organisms through competition for nutrients and stimulating the production of cross-protective antibodies.[11,16] However, normal flora bacteria may potentially become pathogenic and cause infection in patients with suppressed immune systems or after translocation to normally sterile body sites and tissues during

TABLE 17-4. Normally Sterile Body Sites

Bloodstream

CSF

Pericardial fluid

Pleural fluid

Peritoneal fluid

Synovial fluid

Bone

Urine (directly from the bladder or kidney)

CSF = cerebrospinal fluid.

TABLE 17-5. Body Sites with Normal Colonizing Bacterial Flora[11,16]

Skin	Respiratory tract
Corynebacterium spp.	Viridans streptococci
Propionibacterium spp.	Anaerobic streptococci
Staphylococcus spp. (especially coagulase-negative staphylococci)	*Haemophilus* spp.
	Neisseria spp.
Streptococcus spp.	

Gastrointestinal tract	Genitourinary tract
Bacteroides spp.	*Lactobacillus* spp.
Clostridium spp.	*Streptococcus* spp.
Escherichia coli	*Staphylococcus* spp.
Klebsiella pneumoniae	*Mycoplasma hominis*
Enterococcus spp.	*Corynebacterium* spp.
Anaerobic streptococci	*Bacteroides* spp.
	Prevotella spp.
	Enterobacteriaceae

trauma, intravascular line insertion, or surgical procedures, especially when the skin is not adequately cleansed in the latter situations. In addition, pathogenic bacteria may colonize body sites when they are present but do not invade host tissue or cause the signs and symptoms of infection that are listed in Table 17-6.

Contamination occurs when an organism is accidentally introduced into a biologic specimen during specimen collection, transport, or processing. Bacteria that cause contamination typically originate from the skin of the patient (especially if not cleansed adequately before specimen acquisition), the clinician, or the laboratory technician, but may also come from the environment. A common biologic specimen contaminant is *Staphylococcus epidermidis,* which is an organism that can normally colonize the skin. In addition, the presence of normal vaginal or perirectal flora in the urine culture of a patient without evidence of a urinary tract infection (UTI) (absence of symptoms or WBCs) may also be indicative of contamination.

Infection occurs when an organism invades and damages host tissues eliciting a host response and symptoms consistent with an infectious process. When determining the presence of infection in an individual patient, several factors should be considered such as the clinical condition of the patient (e.g., fever and purulent discharge), the presence of laboratory signs of infection (e.g., high WBC count), the results of microbiologic stains and cultures, and the results from radiographic tests.[9] Table 17-6 describes some of the local and systemic clinical signs and symptoms, laboratory findings, and radiographic findings that may be present in a patient with infection. The exact clinical, laboratory, and radiographic signs of infection vary based on the site of infection, the age of the patient, and the severity of illness of the patient. For example, a patient with pneumonia may have a fever, productive cough, shortness of breath, tachypnea, leukocytosis, and an infiltrate on chest x-ray, while a patient with a lower UTI will have symptoms such as urinary frequency, urgency, and dysuria. In addition, the typical signs and symptoms of infection may not be present in the elderly or in patients who are immunocompromised

TABLE 17-6. Clinical, Laboratory, and Radiographic Signs of Infection

CLINICAL

Localized

Pain and inflammation at site of infection—erythema, swelling, warmth (wound, skin lesion, abscess, cellulitis)

Purulent discharge (wound, vaginal, urethral discharge)

Sputum production and cough (pneumonia)

Diarrhea

Dysuria, frequency, urgency, suprapubic tenderness, costovertebral angle tenderness (UTI)

Headache, stiff neck, photophobia (meningitis)

Systemic

Fever

Chills, rigors

Malaise

Tachycardia

Tachypnea

Hypotension

Mental status changes

LABORATORY

Increased WBC count—peripherally or at the site of infection

Increased neutrophil percentage, including an increase in immature neutrophils (bands or stabs) in the WBC differential called a "shift to the left"

Hypoxemia (lung infections)

Elevated lactate

Positive Gram stain and/or culture from site of infection

Elevated ESR and CRP

Elevated procalcitonin levels

Positive antigen test or antibody titers

RADIOGRAPHIC

Chest x-ray with consolidation, infiltrate, effusion, or cavitary nodules in patients with lung infections

Bone x-ray or MRI—periosteal elevation or bony destruction in patients with osteomyelitis

Head CT/MRI—ring-enhancing lesions in patients with brain abscesses

CRP = C-reactive protein; CT = computed tomography; ESR = erythrocyte sedimentation rate; MRI = magnetic resonance imaging; UTI = urinary tract infection; WBC = white blood cell.

(e.g., neutropenic patients and patients with acquired immunodeficiency syndrome [AIDS]).

The diagnosis of infection is usually suspected in a patient with a positive culture accompanied by clinical, laboratory, and radiographic findings suggestive of infection. In clinical practice, there are several situations that will warrant a thorough investigation to determine if the patient with a positive culture from a biologic specimen is truly infected. Since false-positive cultures can be associated with the use of additional laboratory tests, radiographic tests, unnecessary antibiotics, increased length of hospitalization and patient costs, every positive culture should warrant an evaluation for clinical significance.[17] Certain bacteria have a propensity to commonly cause infection in particular body sites and fluids, as demonstrated in Table 17-7.[4,16,18,19] This information can help the clinician determine if the bacteria isolated in the culture is a commonly encountered pathogen at the particular site of infection.[16,18] For instance, the growth of *Streptococcus pneumoniae* from the sputum of a patient with signs and symptoms of community-acquired pneumonia (CAP) is a significant finding since *S. pneumoniae* is the most common cause of CAP and the patient is exhibiting symptoms of pneumonia. However, the growth of *Staphylococcus epidermidis* from a blood or wound culture from an asymptomatic patient should be evaluated for clinical significance since it may represent contamination of the submitted specimen.[11] The information in Table 17-7 regarding the most common causative organism by infection site can also be used to select empiric antibiotic therapy before culture results are available by guiding the selection of an antibiotic regimen with activity against the most common causative bacteria at the suspected site of infection, as illustrated in Minicase 1.

Occasionally, patients with infection may have negative cultures, particularly in the setting of previous antibiotic use, improper culture collection methods, or the submission of inadequate specimens. In this setting, the clinical condition of the patient may establish the presence of infection despite negative cultures, where the suspected site of infection should help guide antibiotic therapy based on most likely causative organisms that cause infection at that site.[9]

Antimicrobial Susceptibility Testing

Once an organism has been cultured from a biologic specimen, further testing is performed in the microbiology laboratory to determine the antibiotic susceptibility of the infecting organism to help direct and streamline antimicrobial therapy. Due to the continual emergence of resistance in many organisms, bacterial susceptibility testing is imperative for determining the antimicrobial agents that could potentially be used for the treatment of the patient's infection. There are a number of different methods that can be utilized to determine the antibiotic susceptibility of a particular organism, and these methods can either (1) directly measure the activity of an antibiotic against the organism or (2) detect the presence of a specific resistance mechanism in the organism, as described in Table 17-8.[9,11,20-25] Microbiology labs often utilize several different methods for susceptibility testing in order to accurately

TABLE 17-7. Common Pathogens by Site of Infection[4,16,18,19]

MOUTH	SKIN AND SOFT TISSUE	BONE AND JOINT
Anaerobic streptococci	*Staphylococcus aureus*	*Staphylococcus aureus*
Peptococcus spp.	*Streptococcus pyogenes*	*Streptococcus pyogenes*
Peptostreptococcus spp.	*Staphylococcus epidermidis*	*Streptococcus* spp.
Actinomyces israelii	*Pasteurella multocida*	*Staphylococcus epidermidis*
	Clostridium spp.	*Neisseria gonorrhoeae*
		Gram-negative bacilli

INTRA-ABDOMINAL	URINARY TRACT	UPPER RESPIRATORY TRACT
Escherichia coli	*Escherichia coli*	*Streptococcus pneumoniae*
Proteus mirabilis	*Proteus mirabilis*	*Haemophilus influenzae*
Klebsiella spp.	*Klebsiella* spp.	*Moraxella catarrhalis*
Enterococcus spp.	*Enterococcus* spp.	*Streptococcus pyogenes*
Bacteroides spp.	*Staphylococcus saprophyticus*	
Clostridium spp.		

LOWER RESPIRATORY TRACT COMMUNITY-ACQUIRED	LOWER RESPIRATORY TRACT HOSPITAL-ACQUIRED	MENINGITIS
Streptococcus pneumoniae	**Early-Onset (within 4 days of hospitalization)**	*Streptococcus pneumoniae*
Haemophilus influenzae	*Klebsiella pneumoniae*	*Neisseria meningitidis*
Moraxella catarrhalis	*Escherichia coli*	*Haemophilus influenzae*
Klebsiella pneumoniae	*Enterobacter* spp.	Group B streptococcus
Legionella pneumophila	*Proteus* spp.	*Escherichia coli*
Mycoplasma pneumoniae	*Serratia marcescens*	*Listeria monocytogenes*
Chlamydophila pneumoniae	*Haemophilus influenzae*	
	Streptococcus pneumoniae	
	MSSA	
	Late Onset (>4 days after hospitalization)	
	Pathogens above plus MDR organisms:	
	Acinetobacter spp.	
	Pseudomonas aeruginosa	
	MRSA	
	Legionella pneumophila	

MDR = multidrug resistant; MRSA = methicillin-resistant *Staphylococcus aureus*; MSSA = methicillin-susceptible *Staphylococcus aureus*.

MINICASE 1

Using Lab Test Results to Guide the Choice of an Empiric Antibiotic Regimen for Hospital-Acquired Pneumonia

MARIE A., A 68-YEAR-OLD FEMALE, was admitted to the University Hospital 4 days ago for management of a right cerebral vascular accident (CVA). Prior to this admission, she had been living at home with her husband and had been previously healthy without recent hospitalizations or antibiotic therapy within the past few years. Marie A. initially required ICU admission for management of her CVA and was recently transferred to the medical floor after stabilization. She continues to have L-sided hemiparesis, and has been deemed to be an aspiration risk by physical therapy/occupational therapy. On hospital day 4, Marie A. developed a temperature of 102.3°F, chills, tachypnea, a productive cough, and shortness of breath requiring supplemental oxygen via nasal cannula. Her physical exam is significant for an increased respiratory rate of 24 breaths/min and decreased breath sounds in the right middle lobe on lung exam. Her laboratory results reveal a total WBC count of 18,000 cells/mm³ (4800–10,800 cells/mm³) with 70% neutrophils (45% to 73%), 19% bands (3% to 5%), 7% lymphs (20% to 40%), and 4% monos (3% to 8%). Her chest x-ray displays right middle lobe consolidation consistent with pneumonia. The differential diagnosis includes bacterial pneumonia, so an expectorated sputum sample is obtained for Gram stain and culture. The Gram stain reveals >25 WBC/hpf, <10 epi/hpf, and many Gram-negative rods. The physician taking care of Marie A. asks you to recommend empiric antibiotic therapy to treat her pneumonia before the final culture results are available.

Question: What is the most likely causative organism of Marie A.'s pneumonia, and which empiric antibiotic therapy would you choose based on the Gram stain results?

Discussion: Marie A. most likely has early-onset (within 4 days of hospitalization) hospital-acquired pneumonia (HAP), where the most common causative organisms (Table 17-7) in early-onset HAP include *Streptococcus pneumoniae; Haemophilus influenzae;* Gram-negative bacteria such as *Klebsiella pneumoniae, Escherichia coli, Enterobacter* spp., *Serratia marcescens, Proteus* spp.; *Staphylococcus aureus* (methicillin-susceptible *Staphylococcus aureus* [MSSA]); and atypical bacteria such as *Legionella pneumophila* (especially in patients with diabetes mellitus, underlying lung disease, renal failure, or suppressed immune systems). Based on the Gram stain results demonstrating the presence of Gram-negative rods (Table 17-2), Marie A. most likely has HAP due to *Klebsiella pneumoniae, Escherichia coli, Enterobacter* spp., *Serratia marcescens,* or *Proteus* spp., which is not unexpected since Gram-negative bacteria are the most common cause of HAP overall. Based on the most recent Infectious Diseases Society of America (IDSA) guidelines for the management of HAP, Marie A. should receive empiric therapy with either ceftriaxone, ertapenem, or a fluoroquinolone (levofloxacin, ciprofloxacin, or moxifloxacin) based on her lack of risk factors for a multidrug-resistant (MDR) organism.[19] The antibiotic regimen can be modified to more directed therapy, if possible, once the results of the culture and susceptibility are available.

TABLE 17-8. Antimicrobial Susceptibility Testing Methods[9,11,20-25]

Methods that directly measure antibiotic activity

Dilution susceptibility tests: broth macrodilution (tube dilution), broth microdilution, agar dilution

Disk diffusion: Kirby Bauer

Antibiotic concentration gradient methods: Etest®, SGE

Other specialized tests:

> Measure bactericidal activity—MBC testing, time-kill studies, SBT

> Susceptibility testing of antibiotic combinations (synergy testing)—checkerboard technique, time-kill curve technique, disk diffusion, Etest®

Methods that detect the presence of antibiotic resistance mechanisms

β-lactamase detection

Detection of HLAR

Agar screens for detection of MRSA or VRE

Chloramphenicol acetyltransferase detection

Molecular methods involving NA hybridization and amplification

---

Etest® = epsilometer test; HLAR = high-level aminoglycoside resistance; MBC = minimum bactericidal concentration; MRSA = methicillin-resistant *Staphylococcus aureus;* NA = nucleic acid; SBT = serum bactericidal test; SGE = spiral gradient endpoint; VRE = vancomycin-resistant enterococci.

determine the activity of antibiotics against many different types of bacteria (e.g., aerobic, anaerobic, and fastidious). The Clinical and Laboratory Standards Institute (CLSI) continuously updates and publishes standards and guidelines for the susceptibility testing of aerobic and anaerobic bacteria to assist microbiology labs in determining the specific antibiotics and test methods that should be utilized based on the particular organism or the particular clinical situation/infection.[3,20,21,26–28]

Methods That Directly Measure Antibiotic Activity

There are a number of different tests that measure the activity of an antibiotic against a particular organism. *Quantitative* tests measure the exact concentration of an antibiotic necessary for inhibiting the growth of the bacteria, and *qualitative* tests measure the comparative activity of antibiotics against the organism. It is important to note that the test results and interpretation of susceptibility from each of these methods will be reported by the laboratory based on the methodology that was utilized. The advantages and disadvantages of the different antimicrobial susceptibility testing methods are listed in Table 17-9.[9,11,20,25,29,30]

Dilution Methods (Macrodilution and Microdilution)

Several dilution methods exist that measure the activity of an antibiotic against a particular organism. Both broth dilution and agar dilution methods quantitatively measure the in vitro

TABLE 17-9. Advantages and Disadvantages of Antimicrobial Susceptibility Testing Methods[9,11,20,25,29,30]

METHOD	ADVANTAGES	DISADVANTAGES
Broth macrodilution (tube dilution)	An exact MIC is generated	Each antibiotic is tested individually
	The MBC can also be determined, if desired	Method is labor and resource intensive
Broth microdilution (automated)	Simultaneously tests several antibiotics	MIC range (rather than exact MIC) is typically reported
	Utilizes less labor and resources	The number of antibiotics and concentrations that are tested are predetermined and limited
	Commercially-prepared trays or cards can be used	
Agar dilution	An exact MIC is generated	Very time-consuming
	Several isolates can be tested simultaneously on the same plate at a relatively low cost	Antibiotic plates need to be prepared manually when needed and can be stored only for short periods of time
	Able to test susceptibility of fastidious bacteria since agar supports their growth	Plates are not commercially available; must be prepared by the lab
Disk diffusion (Kirby-Bauer)	Simultaneously tests several antibiotics	Exact MICs cannot be determined
		Cannot be used for fastidious or slow-growing bacteria
SGE test	An exact MIC is generated	Relatively expensive
	Easy to perform	Can test only one antibiotic at a time
		Plates are not commercially available; must be prepared by the lab
Etest®	An exact MIC is generated	Relatively expensive
	Easy to perform	Only certain antibiotics are available as Etest® strips
	Several antibiotics can be tested on the same plate	

Etest® = epsilometer test; MBC = minimum bactericidal concentration; MIC = minimum inhibitory concentration; SGE = spiral gradient endpoint.

activity of antibiotics against a particular organism. Broth dilution can be performed using *macrodilution* or *microdilution*, where the main differences between the methods include the volume of broth utilized, the number of antibiotics that can be simultaneously tested, and the manner in which the test results are generated and reported. The agar dilution method differs in that it is performed using solid growth media.

Broth macrodilution. Broth macrodilution, or the tube-dilution method, is one of the oldest methods of antimicrobial susceptibility testing and is often considered the gold standard. This method is performed in test tubes in which twofold serial dilutions of the antibiotic being tested (with concentrations tested based on clinically-achievable serum or site concentrations of the antibiotic in mcg/mL) are placed in a liquid growth media (1 mL of broth or greater) to which a standard inoculum (5×10^5 cfu/mL) of the infecting bacteria is added.[20,25-27,29] The tests tubes are incubated for 16–24 hours at 35°C and then examined macroscopically for the presence of turbidity or cloudiness, which is an indication of bacterial growth.[11,20,25,27,29] The test tube containing the lowest antibiotic concentration that completely inhibits visible growth (the broth in the tube appears clear to the unaided eye) represents the minimum inhibitory concentration (MIC) in mcg/mL (Figure 17-1).[20,25,27,29]

The CLSI has established interpretive criteria for the MIC results of each antibiotic against each bacteria as *Susceptible (S)*, *Intermediate (I)*, and *Resistant (R)*. The exact MICs that

separate or define these three categories for an antibiotic are known as their *MIC breakpoints*.[20,21,25] Minimum inhibitory concentrations have been categorized as S, I, and R to help predict the probable response of a patient's infection to a particular antibiotic.[9,21,25] Bacteria that are categorized as "susceptible" to a given antibiotic will, most likely, be eradicated during treatment of the infection since concentrations of the antibiotic represented by the MIC are easily achieved using standard doses of the antibiotic. "Intermediately" susceptible bacteria display higher MICs, where successful treatment may be achieved if higher than normal doses of an antibiotic are utilized or the antibiotic concentrates at the site of infection.[25] In clinical practice, antibiotics displaying intermediate susceptibility against an organism are rarely used for treatment of the infection since clinical response is unpredictable. One of the only clinical scenarios where intermediately-susceptible antibiotics are used is when the organism displays resistance to all other agents tested. Lastly, organisms that are "resistant" to an antibiotic display extremely high MICs that exceed the normal achievable serum concentrations of the antibiotic, even if maximal doses are utilized, so that a poor clinical response would be expected.

Minimum inhibitory concentration breakpoints for each antibiotic against each bacteria are based on a number of factors including achievable serum concentrations of the antibiotic after normal dosing; the inherent susceptibility of the organism to the antibiotic; the site of infection and ability of the

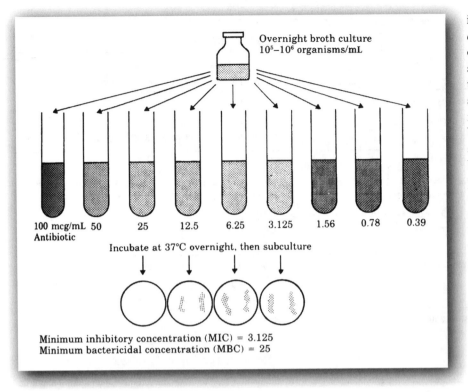

Overnight broth culture
10^5–10^6 organisms/mL

100 mcg/mL 50   25   12.5   6.25   3.125   1.56   0.78   0.39
Antibiotic

Incubate at 37°C overnight, then subculture

Minimum inhibitory concentration (MIC) = 3.125
Minimum bactericidal concentration (MBC) = 25

FIGURE 17-1. Broth macrodilution susceptibility testing for MIC and MBC. (Reprinted, with permission, from reference 9.)

antibiotic to obtain adequate concentrations at that site; pharmacodynamic analysis with Monte Carlo simulations to predict efficacy; and the results of clinical efficacy trials of the antibiotic against infections due to the specific organism.[20,21,26,27,30] The safe and effective dose of each antibiotic is typically determined using pharmacokinetic, safety, and efficacy data gathered during preclinical stages of drug development. Since each antibiotic has its own unique pharmacokinetic profile and recommended dosage range, it is not surprising that each antibiotic achieves different serum concentrations after standard dosing. For example, intravenously-administered piperacillin/tazobactam achieves much higher serum concentrations and area under the serum concentration time curve (AUC) than intravenously-administered levofloxacin. Therefore, the MIC breakpoint for susceptibility for piperacillin/tazobactam against Enterobacteriaceae is higher (≤16 mcg/mL) than levofloxacin (≤2 mcg/mL). Another factor that is considered in the determination of MIC breakpoints is the inherent in vitro activity of the antibiotic against the organism. Some antibiotics are inherently more active against an organism than others; this is reflected by a lower MIC required to inhibit bacterial growth. The site of infection should also be considered, as this may predict the potential usefulness of the antibiotic depending on its ability to achieve adequate concentrations at the site of infection. An antibiotic might be very active against a particular organism in vitro, but may be ineffective in vivo due to poor penetration to the site of infection. In fact, there are a few clinical situations where the site of infection is directly incorporated into the MIC interpretation of an antibiotic, such as

in the case of meningitis due to *Streptococcus pneumoniae*, where the interpretation of ceftriaxone and penicillin susceptibility should be determined utilizing meningitis breakpoints of both drugs. Monte Carlo analysis, using population pharmacokinetic data of the antibiotic and MIC distribution data from susceptibility studies of an organism, are also performed in MIC breakpoint determination to evaluate the percentage of time the particular antibiotic being evaluated will achieve adequate serum concentrations or particular pharmacodynamic indices for the treatment of that organism in a simulated population. Lastly, the results from clinical trials evaluating the efficacy of an individual antibiotic are also considered in MIC breakpoint determination where a correlation is made between the individual MIC value of the infecting organism and clinical efficacy or failure (e.g., what was the MIC of the organisms associated with clinical failure of the antibiotic?). In general, it is the responsibility of the clinician to determine if a drug listed as "susceptible" from an individual isolate susceptibility report is useful for the treatment of a particular infection based on the pharmacokinetic parameters (site penetration) and clinical efficacy studies of the antibiotic for that infection type.

An additional step can be added to the broth macrodilution test to determine the actual antibiotic concentration that kills 99.9% of the bacterial inoculum, which is also known as the *minimum bactericidal concentration (MBC)*.[20,22,24] Samples from all of the test tubes from the original broth macrodilution test that did not exhibit visible growth are subcultured on agar plates and incubated at 35°C for 18–24 hours (Figure 17-1).[9,22] The plate representing the lowest antibiotic concentration that does not support the growth of any bacterial colonies is defined as the MBC. Because a higher concentration of an antibiotic may be necessary to kill the organism rather than just inhibit its growth, the MIC is always equal to or lower than the MBC. The determination of the MBC is not routinely performed in clinical practice, and is only considered useful in rare clinical circumstances such as in suspected treatment failure during the treatment of severe or life-threatening infections including endocarditis, meningitis, osteomyelitis, or sepsis in immunocompromised patients.[9,20,22–24]

Broth macrodilution is useful because an exact MIC (and, if needed, an MBC) of the infecting organism can be derived. The results of broth macrodilution are reported as the MIC of the antibiotic against the infecting organism with its corresponding interpretive category (S, I, and R). However, broth macrodilution is rarely utilized in microbiology laboratories since the methodology is resource and labor intensive, making it impractical for everyday use.

Broth microdilution. Broth microdilution susceptibility testing was developed to overcome some of the limitations of the broth macrodilution method and has become the most commonly used method for susceptibility testing of bacteria in microbiology labs.[11,20,25,27,29] Instead of utilizing standard test tubes with twofold serial dilutions of antibiotics, this method utilizes manually- or commercially-prepared disposable microtiter cassettes or trays containing up to 96 wells that can simultaneously test the susceptibility of up to 12 antibiotics depending on the product used.[11,20,25,27,29] Several examples of microtiter trays are shown in Figures 17-2 (a) and 17-2 (b). The wells in the broth microdilution trays contain a smaller volume of broth (0.05–0.1 mL) to support bacterial growth than broth macrodilution (1.0 mL or more). The microtiter tray is inoculated with a standardized inoculum of the infecting organism and incubated for 16–20 hours. The tray is then examined for bacterial growth by direct visualization utilizing light boxes or reflecting mirrors, or by automated, computer-assisted readers. The MIC represents the microdilution well containing the lowest antibiotic concentration that completely inhibits visible bacterial growth (e.g., did not produce turbidity). A number of companies commercially supply broth microdilution panels that contain broth with appropriate antibiotic concentrations according to guidelines for conventional broth dilution methods. Depending on the product or system, the results can either be read manually/semiautomated or automated. Some examples of the manual/semiautomated systems include BBL Sceptor (BD Microbiology Systems; no longer available), Sensititre Vizion® System (Trek Diagnostics Systems, Inc.), and MicroScan autoSCAN®-4 (Siemens Healthcare Diagnostics, Inc.). Examples of the automated systems include Vitek®-2 (bioMérieux Diagnostics, Inc.), MicroScan WalkAway® Plus System (Siemens Healthcare Diagnostics, Inc.), Sensititre ARIS® 2X and AIM® (Trek Diagnostics Systems, Inc.), and the Phoenix™ Automated Microbiology System (BD Microbiology Systems). The automated systems have also been engineered to aid with bacterial identification, and are able to provide more rapid susceptibility results (within 8 hours) due to shortened incubation times.[30]

Because of the size constraints of microtiter cassettes, only a limited number of antibiotics and concentrations can be incorporated into the trays. Typically, drugs that have inherent activity against the class of bacteria being tested (e.g., Gram-positive versus Gram-negative) are included in the trays. For example, when determining the susceptibility of Enterobacteriaceae, it is impractical to include antibiotics in the microtiter trays that do not have activity against these organisms, such as penicillin, nafcillin, or vancomycin. The same holds true for susceptibility testing of Gram-positive organisms, where it would be impractical to test the susceptibility of piperacillin or ceftazidime against *Staphylococcus aureus* because these agents have limited antistaphylococcal activity. In addition, the trays are not large enough to incorporate the full range of antibiotic concentrations usually tested using broth macrodilution. Therefore, the concentrations incorporated into the wells for each antibiotic often reflect the CLSI interpretive category

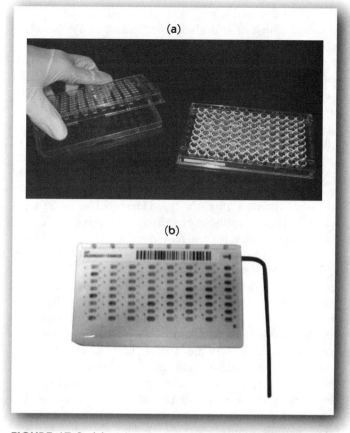

FIGURE 17-2. (a). A broth microdilution susceptibility panel containing 98 reagent wells and a disposable tray inoculator. (Reprinted, with permission, from reference 25.) (b). Example of microtiter cassette used in automated systems that test for bacterial susceptibilities to various antimicrobials. (Reprinted, with permission, Vitek 2 systems card, bioMérieux, 2008.)

breakpoints of S, I, and R for the particular group of organisms. Most microbiology laboratories utilize CLSI guidelines and standards to guide appropriate testing and reporting of antimicrobial susceptibilities.

The test results of broth microdilution occasionally include an exact MIC but more often are expressed as an MIC range because of the limited antibiotic concentrations tested for each antibiotic. For example, if bacterial growth is not detected in the lowest concentration tested of a particular antibiotic using broth microdilution, the MIC would be reported as less than or equal to that concentration tested. The MIC could be much lower, but the exact MIC could not be determined because lower concentrations of the antibiotic were not tested due to the size constraints of the cassettes. As in broth macrodilution, the test results for broth microdilution are often reported to the clinician as the MIC (or MIC range) of the antibiotic against the infecting bacteria with its corresponding CLSI interpretive category (S, I, and R).

The advantages of broth microdilution include the ability to test the susceptibility of multiple antibiotics simultaneously; ease of use when commercially-prepared microtiter trays are utilized; rapid results with the automated methods; and decreased cost and labor.[20,25,27,30] The disadvantages of broth microdilution include the lack of flexibility of antibiotics available in commercially-prepared microtiter cassettes; the limitation on the number of concentrations that can be tested for each antibiotic due to size constraints of the trays; and the reporting of an MIC range rather than the true MIC against an infecting organism.[20,25,30]

Agar dilution. Agar dilution is another quantitative susceptibility testing method that utilizes twofold serial dilutions of an antibiotic incorporated into agar growth medium, which is then placed into individual Petri dishes.[20,25,29,30] The surface of each plate is inoculated with a droplet of standardized bacterial suspension (1×10^4 cfu/mL) and incubated for 18–20 hours at 35°C. The susceptibility of several different bacteria can be evaluated simultaneously on the plates. The MIC is represented by the plate with the lowest concentration of antibiotic that does not support visible growth of the bacteria. The advantages of agar dilution include the ability to simultaneously test the susceptibility of a number of different bacteria; the ability to perform susceptibility testing of fastidious organisms since the agar is able to adequately support their growth; and generation of an exact MIC of the infecting bacteria. However, agar dilution is not commonly utilized in most microbiology labs because it is resource and labor intensive. In addition, the antibiotic plates are not commercially available and need to be prepared before each test since they can be only stored for short periods of time.[20,25,29,30]

Disk Diffusion Method (Kirby-Bauer)

The *disk diffusion method* is a well-standardized and highly reproducible qualitative method of antimicrobial susceptibility testing that was developed by Kirby and Bauer in 1966, before broth microdilution, in response to the need for a more practical susceptibility test capable of measuring the susceptibility of multiple antibiotics simultaneously.[20,25,28–30] Commercially-prepared, filter paper disks containing a fixed concentration of an antibiotic are placed on solid media agar plates inoculated with a standardized inoculum of the infecting organism ($1–2 \times 10^8$ cfu/mL). The plates are large enough to accommodate up to 12 different antibiotic disks at the same time (see Figure 17-3). The plate is inverted to avoid moisture on the agar surface, and then incubated for 16–18 hours in ambient air at 35°C. During this incubation time, the antibiotic diffuses out of the disk into the surrounding media, with the highest concentration closest to the disk, as the bacteria multiply on the surface of the plates.[20,25,29] The bacteria will only grow in areas on the plate where the concentrations of the antibiotic are too low to inhibit bacterial growth. At the end of incubation period, the plates are examined for the inhibition of bacterial growth by measuring the diameter (in millimeters) of the clear zone of inhibition surrounding each filter paper disk. In general, the larger the zone size, the more active the antibiotic is against the organism.

The diameter of the zone of inhibition is correlated to the MIC of the antibiotic from broth or agar dilution against the infecting organism using regression analysis.[20,25,28–30] The CLSI has established interpretive criteria based on this relationship

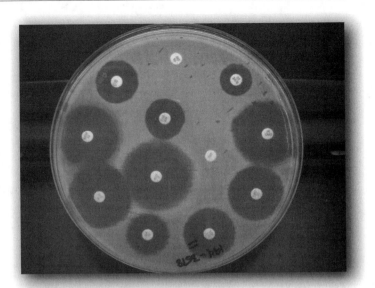

FIGURE 17-3. A disk diffusion test with an isolate of *Escherichia coli* from a urine culture. The diameters of all zones of inhibition are measured and those values translated to categories of susceptible, intermediate, or resistant using the latest tables published by the CLSI. (Reprinted, with permission, from reference 25.)

to categorize zone diameters as S, I, and R for each antibiotic against each organism.[2,25,28,29] Subsequently, the results of the disk diffusion test are considered qualitative because the results only reveal the zone of inhibition and category of susceptibility of the antibiotic against the infecting organism rather than an MIC.

The disk diffusion susceptibility test allows the simultaneous testing of a number of antibiotics in a relatively easy and inexpensive manner, and also provides flexibility in determining the antibiotics that will be tested for susceptibility, providing a filter paper disk for that antibiotic is available. However, the major disadvantages of disk diffusion include the inability to generate an exact MIC and the difficulty in determining the susceptibility of fastidious or slow-growing organisms.

Antibiotic Concentration Gradient Methods

Epsilometer test. The Epsilometer test or Etest® (bioMérieux Diagnostics, Inc.) combines the benefits of broth microdilution with the ease of disk diffusion.[11] The Etest® method simultaneously evaluates numerous concentrations of an antibiotic using a single plastic strip impregnated on one side with a known, predefined concentration gradient of an antibiotic. The other side of the Etest® strip is marked with a numeric scale that depicts the concentration of antibiotic at that location on the reverse side of the test strip.[2,9,20,25] Like disk diffusion, the Etest® strip is applied onto a solid media agar plate that has been inoculated with a standardized concentration of the infecting bacteria. Several Etest® strips can be placed on the same agar plate providing simultaneous susceptibility testing of several antibiotics.[9,20,25] During overnight incubation, bacteria multiply on the agar plates as the antibiotic diffuses out of the Etest® strip according to the concentration gradient. Bacterial growth will occur only in areas on the agar plate where drug concentrations

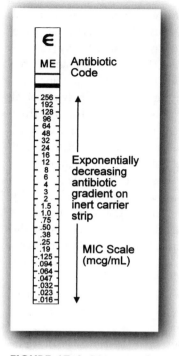

FIGURE 17-4. Diagram of Etest® strip and gradient.

are below those required to inhibit growth. An elliptical zone of growth inhibition will form around the Etest® strip, and the MIC is read as the drug concentration where the ellipse intersects the plastic strip (see Figures 17-4 and 17-5).[2,20,25]

The results from the Etest® are reported as the MIC of the infecting bacteria with the corresponding CLSI susceptibility interpretation. The MIC results derived from the Etest® correlate well with the results obtained using other susceptibility testing methods.[9,20,25,30] The advantages of the Etest® method include its ease of use, the ability to evaluate the susceptibility of several antibiotics simultaneously; the exact MIC of the infecting bacteria can be determined; and the laboratory can choose the antibiotics to be tested. However, the Etest® method is considerably more expensive than disk diffusion or broth microdilution methods, the results may be reader-dependent, and testing is limited to only those antibiotics for which an Etest® strip is commercially available.

The Etest® is currently used in some labs for the susceptibility testing of fastidious bacteria, such as *Streptococcus pneumoniae*, *Haemophilus influenzae*, and anaerobes, as well as for those bacteria in which a routine susceptibility test is not available and an MIC result is preferred.[9,25,30]

Spiral gradient endpoint test. The spiral gradient endpoint (SGE) test (Spiral Biotech, Inc., Bethesda, MD) is an antibiotic gradient diffusion test that utilizes agar plates containing a continuous radial concentration gradient of antibiotic in the agar from the center of the plate, where the concentration is the highest, to the edge of the plate, where the concentration is the lowest.[9,30] The plates are not commercially available but can be made by individual labs with specialized equipment. The infecting bacteria is deposited onto the agar as a radial streak and incubated. Up to 15 bacteria can be tested using a single plate. The MIC is determined by measuring the radial distance between growth at the edge of the plate and where growth is inhibited toward the center of the plate. This measurement is used to compute the concentration of antibiotic at that particular location, which is the MIC.[9,30] This method is relatively easy to perform and generates an exact MIC of the infecting bacteria. However, it is relatively expensive, can only test the susceptibility of one antibiotic per plate, and requires the use of specialized equipment. Therefore, it is not routinely used by most microbiology labs.

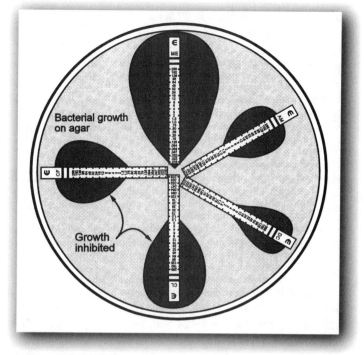

FIGURE 17-5. Etest® strips on agar showing inhibition of bacterial growth.

Specialized Susceptibility Tests

Additional tests may be performed in the microbiology lab to provide further information on the activity of an antibiotic against an organism. These specialty susceptibility tests may measure the bactericidal activity of the antibiotic (e.g., MBC testing, serum bactericidal tests [SBTs], and time-kill curves), or the activity of antimicrobials in combination against an infecting organism (e.g., synergy testing using the checkerboard technique or time-kill studies). These tests are not routinely performed in most microbiology labs due to both biological and technical difficulties, complexity in the interpretation of the results, and uncertain clinical applicability.[20,22–24,31]

Testing methods for determining bactericidal activity. Several methods measure the direct killing activity of an antibiotic against an organism and, if used, should only be performed for antibiotics that are generally considered to be bactericidal. As noted earlier, there are only a limited number of clinical circumstances where this information may be useful. The determination of bactericidal activity likely has the best clinical utility in the treatment of infections at anatomic sites where host defenses are minimal or absent such as endocarditis, meningitis, and osteomyelitis; as well as in the treatment of severe and life-threatening infections in immunocompromised patients.[9,20,22–24,31] Testing methods that determine the bactericidal activity of an antibiotic include the MBC test, time-kill assays, and SBTs.[20,22–24,31]

The MBC is the lowest concentration of an antibacterial agent that kills 99.9% of the bacterial inoculum, which represents a ≥3 log reduction in the original inoculum.[11,23] The methodology for determination of the MBC has been previously described in detail in the section on Broth Macrodilution since it is an extension of that test. CLSI has developed guidelines to standardize the methodology for MBC testing.[31] If the MBC exceeds the achievable serum concentrations of the antibiotic, "tolerance" or treatment failure may be observed.[20] Tolerance occurs when a normally bactericidal antibiotic can only inhibit the growth of bacteria based on MBC testing. Minimum bactericidal concentration testing is not routinely performed by most labs because it is labor intensive with limited clinical utility.[20,22,31]

Time-kill studies, also known as *time-kill curves,* measure the rate of bacterial killing over a specified period of time, which is in contrast to the MBC, which measures the bactericidal activity of the antibiotic at a single point in time following an incubation period.[20,24,31] For time-kill studies, a standardized bacterial inoculum is inserted into test tubes containing broth with several different concentrations of an antibiotic (usually the MIC and multiples of the MIC in separate tubes). Samples of the antibiotic-broth solutions are obtained at predetermined time intervals to evaluate the number of viable bacterial colonies present over the 24-hour incubation period.[11,20,24,31] The number of viable bacteria present at each time point are plotted over time to determine the rate and extent of bacterial killing of the antibiotic against the organism. A ≥3 log reduction in viable bacterial counts is representative of bactericidal activity.[11,20,24,31] Because of the labor and resources involved, this test is not routinely performed in clinical microbiology labs, but is often used in the research setting.

The SBT or Schlichter's test is similar to MIC and MBC testing, except the SBT testing method measures the bacterial killing activity of the *patient's serum* against their own infecting organism after they have received a dose of an antibiotic.[9,20,23,24,31-33] The methodology is very similar to determining the MIC using broth macrodilution, but dilutions of the patient's serum are utilized instead of two-fold serial dilutions of an antibiotic.[9,20,24,31-33] The patient's serum is obtained at predefined intervals before and after a dose of an antibiotic, specifically at the time of expected peak concentration and at the time of expected trough concentration. The patient's serum is then serially diluted and inoculated with a standardized concentration of the infecting organism. The SBT is the highest dilution of the patient's serum that reduces the original standardized bacterial inoculum by ≥99.9%. The results of the SBT are reported as a titer, which represents the number of twofold serial dilutions of the patient's serum that led to bacterial killing (e.g., SBT = 1:16), with a higher titer indicating better activity against the organism.[20,22,24,31-33] The CLSI has developed methodology standards for performance of the SBT.[31,33] However, this test is not routinely performed by most microbiology labs due to technical difficulties; limited data available regarding the clinical usefulness of SBTs in guiding therapy (only in endocarditis, osteomyelitis, and serious infections in febrile neutropenia); the inability of results to directly predict the response to therapy; and limited clinical applicability.[22-24,31-33]

Antimicrobial combination testing (synergy testing). In the treatment of bacterial infections, there are clinical situations where combination antimicrobial therapy will be utilized, with the decision to use combination therapy primarily based on the severity of infection, the causative organism, and/or the particular type of infection.[11] The potential benefits of combination antibiotic therapy include (1) expanding the antimicrobial spectrum of activity, especially for empiric therapy for a life-threatening infection or for the treatment of polymicrobial infections; (2) producing synergistic bactericidal activity from the combination that is not achieved with each agent alone, such as the use of ampicillin and gentamicin for the treatment of enterococcal endocarditis; and (3) decreasing the emergence of resistant organisms, most notably in the treatment of tuberculosis (TB).[19,24] Routine antimicrobial susceptibility tests measure the activity of one antibiotic against a particular organism. There are several tests, however, that evaluate the effects of combination antimicrobial therapy against an infecting organism, with the results being expressed as one of three types of activity[11,20]:

- **Synergy:** The activity of the antimicrobial agents in combination is significantly greater than the additive effects of each agent alone.
- **Indifference:** The activity of the antimicrobial agents in combination is similar to the additive effects of each agent alone.
- **Antagonism:** The activity of the antimicrobial agents in combination is less than the additive effects of each agent alone.

Therefore, before an antibiotic combination is utilized, it may be useful to determine the effects of the antimicrobial combination against the infecting organism, especially since some antibacterial combinations may produce suboptimal effects.

Synergy testing of an antimicrobial combination is performed using the checkerboard technique, the time-kill curve technique, the disk diffusion assay, or the Etest® method.[11,20,24] The checkerboard and time-kill curve techniques are the tests used most often. The checkerboard technique is performed in macrodilution tubes or microtiter plates containing serial dilutions of the antibiotics alone and in combination. The tubes or plates are incubated for 24 hours with a standardized inoculum of the infecting bacteria. The effect of the antibiotic combination is determined by comparing the MICs of the agents when used in combination with the MICs of each agent alone. A synergistic combination displays lower MICs than when each agent is used alone. The time-kill curve method for combination therapy is similar to the time-kill curve method used to determine the rate of bacterial killing of a single agent, except that two antibiotics are added to the tubes in fixed concentrations. The effect of the antibiotic combination is determined by comparing the time-kill rates of combination therapy with the time-kill rates of each agent alone. A synergistic combination displays 100-fold or more greater killing activity than the most potent agent tested alone.[11,20] In the clinical setting, synergy testing methods are not routinely performed due to their tedious, time-consuming methodologies; their expense; and their limited clinical applicability in predicting clinical outcome.[11,20,24]

Methods Detecting the Presence of Antibiotic Resistance Mechanisms

Detection of Beta-Lactamase Activity

To date, over 890 different beta-lactamase enzymes have been characterized.[34] Beta-lactamase enzymes can be chromosomally-, plasmid-, or transposon-mediated, and may be produced constitutively or inducibly. These enzymes cause hydrolysis of the cyclic amide bond in the beta-lactam ring and, depending on the type of enzyme, may result in inactivation of one or numerous beta-lactam antibiotics. It is important to understand the consequences of detecting a particular beta-lactamase enzyme in an organism because certain enzymes produce resistance only to certain antimicrobials.[20,23,34,35]

There are a number of methods that detect the presence of a beta-lactamase enzyme depending on the organism and type of beta-lactamase enzyme suspected. Some tests directly detect the presence of beta-lactamase activity, while other beta-lactamase enzymes (such as the inducible or extended spectrum beta-lactamases) can be suspected based on resistance patterns and MICs derived from routine susceptibility tests.

The assays that directly detect beta-lactamase activity include the acidimetric, iodometric, and chromogenic tests. All of these tests directly measure the presence of beta-lactamase enzyme by observing a color change based on reactions to different substrates, and can be performed in a short period of time with results available within minutes to hours.[2,22] The chromogenic test is the most common direct test utilized by microbiology laboratories due to its reliability in detecting beta-lactamase enzymes produced by many different bacteria.[23] The chromogenic tests utilize chromogenic cephalosporins (nitrocefin, cefesone, or cefinase) incorporated into filter paper disks or strips that produce a colorimetric change if they are hydrolyzed by beta-lactamase enzymes present when a sample of the clinical specimen is inoculated onto the disk or strip. Test tube assays utilizing chromogenic cephalosporins can also be also utilized. A positive reaction using one of these direct beta-lactamase tests for *Haemophilus influenzae, Moraxella catarrhalis,* and *Neisseria gonorrhoeae* predicts resistance to only penicillin, ampicillin, and amoxicillin, but not to other beta-lactam antibiotics that are more stable to hydrolysis by beta-lactamase enzymes.[2] A positive beta-lactamase test for *Staphylococcus* spp. predicts resistance to penicillin, ampicillin, amoxicillin, carbenicillin, ticarcillin, and piperacillin.

Extended-spectrum beta-lactamases (ESBLs) are plasmid-encoded, beta-lactamase enzymes that can hydrolyze penicillins, first-, second-, and third-generation cephalosporins, and aztreonam, and can be inhibited by beta-lactamase-inhibitors such as clavulanic acid.[34,35] For some organisms, such as the Enterobacteriaceae and *Pseudomonas* spp., the production of ESBL enzyme may be inducible so that the detection of beta-lactamase enzyme cannot fully predict the antibiotic susceptibility (or resistance) of the organism.[2,23,36] Therefore, direct beta-lactamase testing for these organisms is not recommended since it may produce misleading results. In the recent past, routine susceptibility tests using CLSI breakpoints did not always detect ESBL-producing organisms. The detection of ESBLs in these organisms was improved by the introduction of CLSI guidelines outlining the use of confirmatory tests, which involved MIC and disk diffusion screening breakpoints for particular antibiotics using beta-lactamase inhibitors.[21,23,26–28,34–37] In addition, several automated systems, such as Vitek®-2 and the Phoenix™ System, contain ESBL detection tests that, when used with expert system software, are able to accurately detect ESBLs, including some ESBLs not detected by the CLSI confirmatory methods.[37]

AmpC beta-lactamases are chromosomally- or plasmid-mediated beta-lactamase enzymes that hydrolyze first-, second-, and third-generation cephalosporins and cephamycins, and also display resistance to currently available beta-lactamase-inhibitors such as clavulanic acid, sulbactam, and tazobactam. Many Gram-negative bacteria, such as *Serratia marcescens, *P*seudomonas aeruginosa,* indole-positive *Proteus* spp., *A*cinetobacter spp., *C*itrobacter freundii spp., and *E*ntero-bacter spp. (often referred to as the SPICE or SPACE bacteria) contain chromosomally-mediated, inducible AmpC enzymes that, when hyperproduced, can also hydrolyze penicillins and aztreonam in addition to the cephalosporins and cephamycins listed above.[34,37] AmpC hyperproduction can occur during the treatment of infection due to one of these organisms, especially when a strong inducer is used such as ceftazidime or clavulanic acid.[34] Plasmid-mediated AmpC enzymes have been reported in *Klebsiella* spp., *Proteus mirabilis, Citrobacter koseri,* and *Salmonella* spp., and often display an antibiotic susceptibility profile similar to that of chromosomally-mediated AmpC hyperproducers.[34,37] All SPICE and SPACE bacteria should be assumed to be AmpC producers, so that specific tests to detect AmpC production are not essential.[37] Plasmid-mediated AmpC beta-lactamases can be detected by demonstrating cephamycin hydrolysis using the AmpC disk test, the Modified Hodge test, or the three-dimensional test.[37]

There are several types of carbapenemase enzymes that have been characterized (metallo-beta-lactamases, serine carbapenemases such as *Klebsiella pneumoniae* carbapenemase or KPC), which are able to hydrolyze carbapenems and other beta-lactam antibiotics.[34,37] Carbapenemase enzymes may be chromosomally- (*Stenotrophomonas maltophilia*) or plasmid-mediated (KPCs, *Pseudomonas aeruginosa, Acinetobacter* spp.), with plasmid-mediated strains often displaying resistance to multiple other drug classes.[37] The modified Hodge test can be used for carbapenemase detection on isolates with elevated carbapenem MICs; however, it cannot differentiate between carbapenemase types.[23,37]

In 2010, the CLSI lowered the cephalosporin and carbapenem breakpoints for Enterobacteriaceae in an attempt to better identify antibiotic agents with predictable efficacy against these bacteria with potentially multiple resistance mechanisms and eliminated the recommendation to perform specialized testing to detect ESBL-, AmpC-, or carbapenemase-mediated resistance. However, this recommendation has gained considerable criticism from many clinicians and microbiologists since detection of the exact mechanism of resistance is thought to be important for both treatment and epidemiologic purposes.[37]

High-Level Aminoglycoside Resistance

The aminoglycoside antibiotics have relatively poor activity against *Enterococcus* spp. due to poor intracellular uptake, so they cannot be utilized as monotherapy in the treatment of infections due to enterococci. However, they may be combined with ampicillin, penicillin, or vancomycin in order to achieve synergistic bactericidal activity, as in the treatment of entero-coccal endocarditis or enterococcal osteomyelitis. Gentamicin and streptomycin are the two most commonly used amino-glycosides in this situation and are, therefore, the agents most commonly tested for synergistic activity. Supplemental testing can be performed to detect the presence of high-level amino-glycoside resistance (HLAR), which predicts the lack of syner-gism between gentamicin or streptomycin and cell-wall active agents against *Enterococcus* spp.[2,23,30,36]

The presence of HLAR can be evaluated using the agar dilution screening method utilizing agar plates containing high concentrations of gentamicin (500 mcg/mL) and strep-tomycin (2000 mcg/mL) or the broth dilution method where the well contains BHI broth containing high concentrations of gentamicin (500 mcg/mL) and streptomycin (1000 mcg/mL).[2,23] The plates or wells are inoculated with a standardized suspension of the infecting *Enterococcus* spp. and incubated for 24 hours in ambient air.[23] The growth of one or more *Enterococ-cus* spp. colonies on the agar plate or in the well demonstrates the presence of HLAR, and the corresponding aminoglycoside cannot be used with a cell-wall active agent to achieve syner-gistic bactericidal activity. High-level aminoglycoside resis-tance can also be detected utilizing a disk diffusion method where disks containing high concentrations of gentamicin (120 mcg) and streptomycin (300 mcg) are utilized.[2,23] High-level aminoglycoside resistance to gentamicin also confers resis-tance to tobramycin, netilmicin, and amikacin, but not neces-sarily streptomycin, which should be tested independently.[2,23] A modified test using kanamycin may be used to predict HLAR to amikacin for strains of *Enterococcus faecalis*; however, this test is not generally available in most labs.[2,23] Testing for HLAR is usually performed only on enterococcal isolates from infec-tions that require combination bactericidal activity, such as bacteremia, endocarditis, osteomyelitis, or meningitis.[23,30]

Tests for the Detection of MRSA, VISA, VRSA, and VRE

Several tests can quickly detect or confirm the presence of meth-icillin-resistant *Staphylococcus aureus* (MRSA) or vancomycin-resistant enterococci (VRE). For the detection or confirmation of MRSA, the cefoxitin disk diffusion test, oxacillin-salt agar screening tests, culture-based chromogenic media, rapid latex agglutination (LA) tests, or molecular methods utilizing real-time polymerase chain reaction (PCR) can be utilized.[23,38-41] The cefoxitin disk diffusion test is performed using routine CLSI procedures, with modified interpretive criteria utilized to detect MRSA, where MRSA is reported for *S. aureus* strains with a zone size of ≤21 mm.[23,28] This test has also been useful in detecting methicillin-resistance in coagulase-negative staphylococci.[23]

The oxacillin-salt agar screening tests have been widely used for the detection of MRSA, but they appear to lack sensitivity for the detection of strains that exhibit heteroresistance.[23] A standard inoculum of *S. aureus* is inoculated onto an agar plate containing Mueller-Hinton agar (MHA) supplemented with 4% sodium chloride and 6 mcg/mL of oxacillin, and incu-bated in ambient air for 24 hours.[2,23,36] The growth of more than one colony indicates MRSA, which also confers resistance to nafcillin, oxacillin, cloxacillin, dicloxacillin, and all cephalo-sporins excluding ceftaroline. However, this test is not recom-mended for the detection of methicillin-resistance in other *Staphylococcus* spp.[23,36]

Culture-based chromogenic media, some of which include MRSA*Select* (Bio-Rad Laboratories, Redmond, WA), Spectra MRSA (Remel Laboratories, Lenexa, KS), and CHROMagar (BD Sparks, MD), lead to the production of a characteristic pigment in the presence of MRSA.[23] These tests are typically utilized for MRSA screening rather than diagnosis of infection, and are less sensitive and slower than molecular methods.[23] There are numerous rapid commercial LA tests for the detec-tion of MRSA (MRSA Screen Test [Denka-Seikin Co., Ltd., Tokyo, Japan], the PBP 2' Test [Oxoid Limited, Basingstroke, UK], the Mastalex test [Mast Diagnostics, Booth, UK], and the Slidex MRSA Detection test [bioMérieux]) that utilize LA to directly detect the presence of penicillin-binding protein (PBP) 2a, the protein encoded by the *mecA* gene in MRSA.[23,40] These tests can be performed within 10–15 minutes from bacterial colonies cultured on blood agar plates, decreasing the overall MRSA detection time by approximately 24 hours when compared to standard methods, and are highly sensitive and specific for the detection of MRSA.[40]

The GeneOhm™ MRSA Assay (BD, Franklin Lakes, NJ) the Xpert MRSA (Cepheid, Sunnyvale, CA), and the LightCycler MRSA Advanced test (Roche Diagnostics, Indianapolis, IN) are approved real-time PCR assays for the rapid, direct detec-tion of nasal colonization by MRSA for the prevention and control of MRSA infection in healthcare institutions.[23,38,39] These assays can detect the presence of MRSA directly from nasal swab specimens within 2 hours using real-time PCR that couples primers specific for *mecA* and the *S. aureus*-specific gene *orfX* (sensitivity 93%, specificity 96%).[38,39] A PCR-based test also exists for the detection of *Staphylococcus aureus* and MRSA from blood cultures positive for Gram positive cocci in clusters (XPert MRSA/SA BC test, Cepheid, Sunnyvale, CA), with results typically available within 1 hour of culture positiv-ity.[41] The manufacturer has recently suspended availability of the product due to invalid results and is currently performing product improvements.

The CLSI reference broth microdilution method can accu-rately detect vancomycin intermediate *Staphylococcus aureus* (VISA, MIC 4–8 mcg/mL) and vancomycin-resistant *Staphy-lococcus aureus* (VRSA, MIC ≥16 mcg/mL).[23] The use of BHI plates with 6 mcg/mL of vancomycin (VRE screening plates described below) can be considered for the detection of *Staphy-lococcus aureus* strains with an MIC of 8 mcg/mL, but is not useful for VISA strains with an MIC of 4 mcg/mL. Lastly, the disk diffusion test is unable to accurately detect VISA strains, but will detect VRSA strains mediated by *vanA*.[23]

Current automated susceptibility testing methods, including Vitek 2 and the Phoenix system, are now able to accurately detect the presence of VRE.[23] However, VRE can also be detected utilizing the vancomycin agar screen test, which is most often performed on rectal swab specimens to detect carriers of VRE. A standard inoculum of the infecting *Enterococcus* spp. is inoculated onto an agar plate supplemented with brain heart infusion broth (BHI) containing vancomycin 6 mcg/mL and incubated in ambient air for 24 hours.[2,23,36] The presence of any growth demonstrates the presence of VRE. This test is most useful for detecting acquired vancomycin resistance in *E. faecalis* and *E. faecium*, but is not useful for strains that display intrinsic resistance to vancomycin, such as *E. gallinarum* and *E. casseliflavus*. The vancomycin agar screening method test is also useful to detect the presence of a newly emerging resistant pathogen, namely vancomycin-intermediate *Staphylococcus aureus* (VISA).[11,23,30,36]

D Test for Detecting Inducible Clindamycin Resistance

Resistance to clindamycin in staphylococci and beta-hemolytic streptococci is typically mediated by expression of the *erm* gene conferring resistance to macrolides, lincosamides, streptogramin b, or MLSb-type resistance, which can be constitutive or inducible.[20,23] Staphylococcal or beta-hemolytic streptococcal isolates that are macrolide resistant but clindamycin susceptible should be evaluated for inducible clindamycin resistance using the "D" test.[20,23] The D test is a disk diffusion procedure where a 15-mcg erythromycin disk is placed 15–26 mm apart from a 2-mcg clindamycin disk on an agar plate inoculated with the infecting organism.[20,23] If inducible clindamycin resistance is present in the organism, the clindamycin zone of inhibition will be flattened on the side nearest the erythromycin disk, demonstrating the letter "D" in appearance. Organisms that display a flattening of the clindamycin zone are D test positive and will be reported resistant to clindamycin in the final laboratory report.

Special Considerations for Fastidious or Anaerobic Bacteria

The susceptibility testing of fastidious bacteria (e.g., *Haemophilus influenzae, N. gonorrhoeae,* and *Streptococcus pneumoniae*) and anaerobes cannot be performed utilizing standard broth microdilution, disk diffusion, or automated susceptibility testing methods since these organisms require more complex growth media and environmental conditions to support bacterial growth.[36,42–45] The cultivation of fastidious bacteria or anaerobes may require media with supplemental nutrients, prolonged incubation times, and/or incubation in atmospheres with higher CO_2 concentrations.[45] Microbiology reference texts and CLSI standards have been developed to outline specific methodologies (broth dilution, disk diffusion, and automated methods), quality control guidelines, and interpretive breakpoint criteria that should be utilized for the susceptibility testing of these bacteria.[21,25–29,36,42–45]

The clinical significance of anaerobes as a cause of infection is more widely appreciated, and the susceptibility of anaerobes to various anti-infective agents is no longer predictable.[9,42–44,46,47] The handling and processing of biologic specimens for anaerobic culture and susceptibility testing are extremely crucial to the validity of the results since most anaerobic bacteria of clinical importance are intolerant to oxygen.[2,9,42] Specimens should be collected in appropriate anaerobic transport systems (commercially-available vials or tubes) that contain specialized media and atmospheric conditions to support the growth of the anaerobic bacteria until the specimen is processed in the lab.[2,42] Once collected, the specimens should be transported to the lab within minutes to hours of collection, set up for culture in anaerobic jars or chambers in the appropriate growth media, and incubated in anaerobic atmospheric conditions. The clinical specimens that provide the best yield for anaerobic culture include aspirated or tissue biopsy specimens.[2,42,47]

The identification of anaerobic bacteria by an individual hospital laboratory may be performed using one of three methods: (1) presumptive identification based on information from the primary growth plates including the Gram stain results, patterns of growth on selective or differential media, plate and cell morphology, and results of various rapid spot and disk tests; (2) definitive identification based on the results of individual biochemical tests that detect the presence of preformed enzymes found in certain anaerobes; and (3) rapid identification of anaerobes using commercially-available detection panels, which also rapidly detect the presence of preformed enzymes such as the BBL Crystal Anaerobe ID (Becton Dickinson and Company), the RapID-ANA II (Remel, Inc.), the Rapid Anaerobe Identification Panel (Siemens Healthcare Diagnostics, Inc.), or the Vitek®-2 ANC (bioMérieux Diagnostics, Inc.).[2,43] Many hospital laboratories do not have the resources for commercially-available, anaerobic bacteria identification systems, and rely on the first two methods for presumptive identification of anaerobic bacteria. If necessary, clinical isolates can be sent to a reference lab for further testing.

Most clinical microbiology labs do not currently offer routine susceptibility testing of anaerobic bacteria because of the uncommon occurrence of pure anaerobic infections, the uncertain role of anaerobes in mixed infections, the previous predictable susceptibility of anaerobic bacteria to antibiotics, the previous lack of standardization of antimicrobial susceptibility testing of anaerobes, and the technical difficulties in performing the tests.[30,43,44,46,47] However, it is becoming apparent that routine antimicrobial susceptibility testing of anaerobic bacteria is necessary due to the increasing incidence of serious infections caused by anaerobic bacteria, the emerging resistance of anaerobic bacteria to multiple antibiotic agents, and the poor clinical outcomes observed when ineffective antibiotics are utilized for the treatment of infections due to anaerobes.[30,43,44,46,47]

The susceptibility testing of anaerobic bacteria has undergone numerous methodological modifications and standardization over the past several years.[9,44,46,47] The CLSI has recently published a standard outlining when anaerobic susceptibility testing should be considered, which methods of susceptibility testing should be utilized, when and how surveillance susceptibility reporting should be performed, and which antibiotic agents should be tested for susceptibility.[46]

Susceptibility testing for anaerobes should be performed in patients with serious or life-threatening infections such as endocarditis, brain abscess, osteomyelitis, joint infection, refractory or recurrent bacteremia, and infection of prosthetic devices or vascular graft infections.[9,43,44,46] Susceptibility testing should also be performed in patients with persistent or recurring anaerobic infections despite appropriate antibiotic therapy.[9,44,46] Lastly, susceptibility testing of anaerobic bacteria should be periodically performed within geographic areas or individual institutions to monitor regional susceptibility patterns of anaerobic bacteria over time.[43,44,46]

The recommended anaerobic susceptibility testing methods include agar dilution and broth microdilution using supplemented *Brucella* broth, both of which can be reliably performed by most clinical microbiology labs.[9,43,44,46,47] The agar dilution method is the gold standard reference method that can be utilized to test the susceptibility of any anaerobic bacteria, while the broth microdilution method has only been validated for antimicrobial susceptibility testing of *Bacteroides fragilis* group organisms.[44,46] In contrast to agar dilution, the broth microdilution method can evaluate the susceptibility of multiple antibiotics simultaneously. Otherwise, the general methodology for each of these tests is similar to those described above for aerobic bacteria. Other methods that are utilized for susceptibility testing of anaerobes include agar dilution, broth microdilution, and the Etest®. Broth disk elution and disk diffusion are not recommended since their results do not correlate with the agar dilution reference method.[43,44,46,47] Beta-lactamase testing of anaerobes can be performed according to CLSI guidelines using chromogenic disks.[44,46]

Since routine antimicrobial susceptibility of anaerobes is not performed by all hospital microbiology laboratories or for all anaerobic isolates, antibiotic therapy for infections due to anaerobes is usually selected empirically based on susceptibility reports published by reference labs.[44] However, if susceptibility testing is performed on an individual anaerobic isolate, the results should be used to guide the anti-infective therapy for the patient.

Methods for Reporting Susceptibility Results

Individual Isolate Susceptibility Reports

When a bacterial isolate is recovered from a clinical specimen, the identification and susceptibility results are compiled in a report that is available electronically or via a hard copy and placed into the patient's chart. The bacterial identification and antibiotic susceptibility report often contains the following information: the patient's name, medical record number, the date and time of specimen collection, the source of specimen collection (e.g., blood, wound, urine, etc.), the bacteria that were identified (if any), and the list of antibiotics tested for susceptibility along with their MIC or disk diffusion results and CLSI interpretive category, as shown in Figure 17-6.[20,48]

In some hospitals, the susceptibility report may also contain information regarding the usual daily doses and costs of the antibiotics that were tested.

Once the culture and susceptibility results are available, this information should be utilized, if necessary, to change the patient's empiric antibiotic regimen, which usually covers a broad-spectrum of bacteria, to a more *directed* antibiotic regimen targeted at the infecting bacteria and susceptibility. The directed antibiotic regimen should be chosen based on clinical and economic factors, some of which include the severity of infection, the site of infection, the activity of the antibiotic against the infecting organism, the proven efficacy of the antibiotic in the treatment of the particular infection, the overall spectrum of activity of the antibiotic (a narrow spectrum agent is preferred), the end-organ function of the patient, the presence of drug allergies, the route of administration required (oral versus parenteral), and the daily cost of the antibiotic, etc. The susceptibility report provides some of the information required for the antibiotic decision-making process, namely, the site of infection, the identification of the infecting organism(s), and the susceptibility of the infecting organism(s).

As seen in the sample susceptibility report in Figure 17-6, there may be a number of antibiotics to which the infecting organism is susceptible, often with differing MICs. It is not always advantageous to choose the antibiotic with the lowest MIC against a particular organism on a susceptibility report. As discussed earlier in this chapter, each antibiotic has different MIC breakpoints corresponding to S, I, and R for each bacteria based on a number of factors. Some drugs, such as the parenteral piperacillin-tazobactam, are assigned higher MIC breakpoint values for susceptibility since they achieve higher serum and/or site concentrations than other antibiotics. Because of this, a simple number comparison of the MIC between antibiotics should not be performed. The choice of antibiotic should be based on the knowledge of the MICs that are acceptable for a particular drug-bacteria combination, the site of infection, the penetration of the antibiotic to the site of infection, as well

Patient Name: Jane Doe
Medical Record Number: 1111111
Specimen Collection Date and Time: April 20, 2013, 0730
Specimen Type: Blood
Organism Identification: Staphylococcus aureus

ANTIMICROBIAL SUSCEPTIBILITY

Antibiotic	MIC (mcg/mL)	Interpretive Category
Penicillin	≥16	Resistant
Ampicillin/Sulbactam	≤4	Susceptible
Cefazolin	≤8	Susceptible
Oxacillin	0.5	Susceptible
Trimethoprim/Sulfa	≤10	Susceptible
Vancomycin	≤0.5	Susceptible
Clindamycin	≤0.5	Susceptible
Erythromycin	≤0.5	Susceptible

FIGURE 17-6. Example of microbiology laboratory report with bacterial identification and antibiotic susceptibility.

as the clinical and economic parameters listed above. In the sample report in Figure 17-6, oxacillin (nafcillin) or cefazolin would be an acceptable choice for the treatment of *Staphylococcus aureus* bacteremia in a patient without drug allergies since these agents are active against the infecting organism, have been demonstrated to be effective in the treatment of systemic staphylococcal infections, are relatively narrow-spectrum antibiotics, and are inexpensive. Minicase 2 is an example illustrating the use of a culture and susceptibility report in the antibiotic decision-making process.

The decision regarding the antibiotics that will be reported on an individual susceptibility report for a bacterial isolate is typically based on input from a multidisciplinary committee (e.g., Antimicrobial Subcommittee, Infectious Diseases Subcommittee, Antimicrobial Stewardship Team) comprised of infectious diseases physicians, the infectious diseases pharmacists, the Infection Control Committee, and the microbiology laboratory of a given hospital.[2] These decisions are often based on the antibiotics that are available on the hospital formulary, the level of control of antibiotic use that is desired, and the tests that are utilized by the microbiology laboratory for susceptibility testing. Tables that outline the antibiotics that should be routinely tested and reported for certain organisms can be found in the CLSI Performance Standards and Guidelines for susceptibility testing of bacteria.[21,26-28]

The methods utilized for reporting antibiotic susceptibility of bacteria for individual isolates include general reporting, selective reporting, and cascade reporting. *General reporting* involves reporting all antibiotics that were tested for susceptibility against the organism without any restrictions or analysis. *Selective reporting* strategies include information on the susceptibility of antibiotics available for routine use on the hospital formulary or only those antibiotics that are useful for the treatment of a particular organism or infection type. An example of selective reporting would be the exclusion of cefazolin from the susceptibility report of a CSF sample growing *E. coli* since

---

MINICASE 2

Using Lab Test Results to Guide Choice of an Antibiotic Regimen for Urosepsis/ Pyelonephritis

DIANA J., A 27-YEAR-OLD FEMALE, presents to the Urgent Visit Center with complaints of urinary frequency and urgency, pain on urination, and hematuria for the past 2 days. The patient also states that she recently developed a fever to 101.6°F and has experienced intractable nausea and vomiting for the past 24 hours. Upon presentation in clinic, she is febrile (102.3°F), hypotensive (90/60), and lethargic; physical exam reveals right costovertebral angle and suprapubic tenderness. A urine dipstick performed in clinic is leukocyte esterase positive, and a urine pregnancy test is negative. Because she is so ill-appearing, the clinic physician admits the patient to the hospital. Her past medical history is significant for recurrent UTIs, with three episodes over the past 6 months that have required antibiotic therapy including trimethoprim–sulfamethoxazole and ciprofloxacin. Diana J. reports no known drug allergies. Upon admission, a urinalysis, urine culture, and blood cultures are performed. The results of her urinalysis and cultures are at the right.

Question: What is an appropriate recommendation for antibiotic therapy for this patient?

Discussion: Diana J. is presenting with pyelonephritis and urosepsis (complicated UTI), making the acquisition of a urinalysis, urine culture, and blood culture useful in guiding antimicrobial treatment since her past UTIs and subsequent antibiotic treatment put her at risk for acquiring an infection with a resistant bacteria. Based on her presenting symptoms and the findings on her physical examination, Diana J. most likely has acute, pyelonephritis. Because she is hypotensive on admission and is experiencing significant nausea and vomiting, she should initially be treated with a parenteral antibiotic that displays activity against the infecting organism and has been proven clinically to display efficacy against complicated UTIs. Based on lack of antibiotic allergies and the results of her urine culture and susceptibility, Diana J. can be treated with parenteral cefazolin or ceftriaxone.

Urinalysis: Yellow, cloudy; pH 7.0, specific gravity 1.015, protein negative, RBC trace, WBC 50–100/hpf, leukocyte esterase positive, nitrite positive

Midstream Urine Culture/Susceptibility: >100,000 cfu/mL of *Escherichia coli*

ANTIBIOTIC TESTED	MIC RESULT	INTERPRETATION
Ampicillin	>32 mcg/mL	R
Ampicillin–sulbactam	8 mcg/mL	S
Cefazolin	1 mcg/mL	S
Ceftriaxone	1 mcg/mL	S
Imipenem	1 mcg/mL	S
Gentamicin	0.5 mcg/mL	S
Ciprofloxacin	4 mcg/mL	R
Trimethoprim–sulfamethoxazole	>80 mcg/mL	R

Blood culture/susceptibility: *Escherichia coli*

ANTIBIOTIC TESTED	MIC RESULT	INTERPRETATION
Ampicillin	>32 mcg/mL	R
Ampicillin–sulbactam	8 mcg/mL	S
Cefazolin	1 mcg/mL	S
Ceftriaxone	1 mcg/mL	S
Imipenem	1 mcg/mL	S
Gentamicin	0.5 mcg/mL	S
Ciprofloxacin	4 mcg/mL	R
Trimethoprim–sulfamethoxazole	>80 mcg/mL	R

R = resistant; S = susceptible.

cefazolin is not a suitable treatment option for meningitis. *Cascade reporting* strategies include information on the susceptibility of antibiotics that the hospital/committee considers to be first-line choices for the treatment of a particular organism or infection, with reporting of second-line agents if the first-line agents are inappropriate for the treatment of the particular infection, or if the first-line agents are inactive against the infecting organism. This process is utilized as a method to control the inappropriate use of broad-spectrum or expensive antibiotics.[2,48] An example of cascade reporting is the reporting of the susceptibility result of amikacin against *Pseudomonas aeruginosa* only if the organism is resistant to gentamicin and/or tobramycin, which are less expensive aminoglycoside agents.

ANTIBIOTIC SUSCEPTIBILITIES Jan.–Dec. 1993
Numbers are percent susceptible (# isolates)

Antibiotic Formulary Status — Bold = FORMULARY, Upper/Lower = RESERVED

Antibiotic	Acinetobacter calcoaceticus (11)	Enterobacter aerogenes (12)	Enterobacter cloacae (30)	Escherichia coli (271)	Haemophilus influenzae (53)	Klebsiella pneumoniae (63)	Proteus mirabilis (37)	Pseudomonas aeruginosa (101)	Staphylococcus aureus (153)	Enterococci (gp D strep) (97)	Enterococcus faecium (12)	Usual dose	Cost/day (includes administration costs)	Pharmacy (x2549) / Microbiology (x5529)
AMPICILLIN				73	73		100			97		1–2 g IV q 6 hr	$4–5	
AMOXICILLIN-CLAVULANATE					95							250–500 mg PO TID	$4–6	
CEFAZOLIN				97		97	100		87			500 mg IV q 8 hr	$6	
CEFOTETAN			63	100		100	100					1–2 g IV q12 hr	$18–35	
Ceftazidime	100	92						98				1–2 g IV q 8 hr	$31–61	
Ceftriaxone		92	86	100	100	100	100					1–2 g IV q 24 hr	$25–50	
Cefuroxime		92	72	99	97	98	100					750 mg IV q 8 hr	$14	
Ciprofloxacin	100	100	100	100		100	100	95	90	78		250–750 mg PO BID	$4–9 (only oral form available)	
CLINDAMYCIN									91			600 mg q 8 hr	IV - $9 PO - $8	
ERYTHROMYCIN									72			500 mg q 6 hr	IV - $7 PO - $0.20	
GENTAMICIN	91	100	100	100		100	100	92				80 mg IV q 8 hr	$5	
Imipenem	100	100	100					91				500 mg IV q 8-6 hr	$60–79	
METRONIDAZOLE												500 mg q 6 hr	IV - $7 PO - $.50	
OXACILLIN									87			2 g IV q 6 hr	$10	
NITROFURANTOIN			100	99						99	95	50–100 mg PO q 6 hr for urine isolates only	$2–3	
PENICILLIN G												1 million units IV q 4 hr	$9	
TETRACYCLINE			85	85		92			92			250–500 mg PO q 6 hr	$0.20	
TICARCILLIN	100	83	63	74			100	89				3 g IV q 4	$48	
Ticarcillin-clavulanate	Activity superior to ticarcillin versus staph, most gram neg. rods and anaerobes (including B. fragilis). Activity same as ticarcillin versus Pseudomonas, Acinetobacter, Enterobacter.											3.1 g IV q 6 hr	$43	
Tobramycin	100	100						100				80 mg IV q 8 hr	$18	
TRIMETHOPRIM-SULFAMETHOXAZOLE	91	100	97	92	92	90	97		94			20 mL IV q 12 hr / 1 DS Tab PO BID	IV - $3 PO - $0.15	
Vancomycin									99	100	92	1 g IV q 12 hr	$15	

FIGURE 17-7. Example of a hospital antibiogram.

Hospital Susceptibility Reports (Hospital Antibiograms)

Many hospitals prepare and publish an annual cumulative report of the antimicrobial susceptibility profiles of the organisms that have been isolated from the patients within their hospital, healthcare system, or institution, called a *cumulative antibiogram*. The cumulative antibiogram usually reflects the antibiotic susceptibility patterns of isolates obtained from patients in the hospital who were admitted with an infection or developed an infection in the hospital (nosocomially-acquired); although, some hospitals with a large outpatient population may also include isolates from patients in the surrounding community, usually in a separate outpatient table. Antibiotic therapy must often be initiated at the suspicion of infection since many infectious diseases are often acute where a delay in treatment may result in significant morbidity or mortality (e.g., meningitis and pneumonia). Therefore, the cumulative antibiogram is a useful tool for selecting the most appropriate *empiric* antibiotic therapy based on the susceptibility of the organism that is most likely causing the patient's infection (Table 17-7) while waiting for the culture and susceptibility results.[48] During empiric therapy selection, an antibiotic is typically chosen based on the local susceptibility patterns of the most likely infecting organism, as described in Minicase 3. However, once the culture and susceptibility results of the infecting bacteria are known, antibiotic therapy should be streamlined, if necessary, to an agent with more targeted activity against the organism. In order for the cumulative antibiogram to be clinically useful, the susceptibility data from patient isolates should be appropriately collected, analyzed, and reported according to the CLSI guidelines, which are outlined in Table 17-10.[48]

The cumulative antibiogram contains information on the percent of isolated organisms that were susceptible to antibiotics tested over the time frame of the antibiogram, as illustrated in Figure 17-7.[48] The information is derived by dividing the number of organisms susceptible to a particular antibiotic by the total number of single-patient isolates collected and reported (with duplicate patient isolates removed). The calculations can be performed either manually or using automated systems that have been programmed using appropriate definitions to remove duplicate patient isolates. The data published in the cumulative antibiogram should be based on input from infectious diseases physicians, infectious disease pharmacists, the Infection Control Committee, the Pharmacy and Therapeutics Committee, and the microbiology laboratory of a given hospital or healthcare system. Cumulative antibiograms may contain separate data tables for reporting the susceptibility of Gram-positive, Gram-negative, and anaerobic bacteria; as well as separate data tables reporting the antibiotic susceptibility patterns of organisms isolated from patients in key patient care units (e.g., Burn Unit, Medical ICU, Pediatric Unit, Med-Surg Unit, outpatient clinic, nursing home, etc.), with particular infection types (e.g., susceptibility of bloodstream isolates or urinary tract isolates), with specific medical conditions (e.g., cystic fibrosis, transplant patients, etc.), or by organism (e.g., susceptibility of *Staphylococcus aureus*). For some organisms, the cumulative antibiogram will only contain information regarding the presence of bacterial resistance mechanisms,

MINICASE 3

Using Lab Test Results to Guide Choice of an Antibiotic Regimen for Bacteremia

DAVID M. IS A 45-YEAR-OLD MALE who sustained multiple traumatic injuries after a motorcycle accident. He has required multiple surgeries over the past 10 days for fracture stabilization. In the last 12 hours, he has spiked a temperature to 39°C and has developed shaking chills. His other vital signs are stable, and his physical exam does not demonstrate any significant findings. Urinalysis, urine culture, and blood cultures are performed to determine the potential etiology for his new fever. In addition, a chest x-ray is performed, which did not demonstrate any pulmonary infiltrates. The lab calls the surgical floor later that day to report that the blood cultures are positive for Gram-negative rods. The patient is allergic to penicillin (nonurticarial rash), and the hospital antibiogram is pictured in Figure 17-7.

Question: What empiric antibiotic regimen should be used to treat David M.'s Gram-negative rod bacteremia?

Discussion: Nosocomial Gram-negative bacteremia is a potentially life-threatening infection, which requires aggressive antibiotic therapy for treatment. The choice of whether to use monotherapy or combination therapy while waiting for culture and susceptibility results in this setting will often depend on the clinical condition of the patient and local susceptibility patterns. Combination antibiotic therapy might provide some antibacterial synergy, as well as provide coverage against a wide range of potential infecting bacteria. Based on the hospital antibiogram in Figure 17-7, it is desirable to choose antibiotics that retain good activity (>85% susceptible) against Gram-negative bacteria isolated at the institution, namely, *Pseudomonas aeruginosa, E. coli, Klebsiella pneumoniae, Serratia marcescens,* and *Enterobacter cloacae,* as well as choose agents that have demonstrated efficacy in the treatment of bacteremia. Since David M. is clinically stable and displays only a rash to penicillin therapy, some useful therapeutic options include imipenem, meropenem, ceftazidime, cefepime, or ciprofloxacin monotherapy. If he begins to clinically deteriorate, an aminoglycoside, such as tobramycin, or a fluoroquinolone, may be added to the carbapenem or cephalosporin while waiting for the results of the culture and susceptibility. The antibiotic regimen can be modified to more directed therapy, if possible, once the results of the culture and susceptibility are available.

particularly when routine susceptibility testing is difficult to perform, such as in the case of *Haemophilus influenzae* where the percentage of isolates that produce beta-lactamase enzyme during the time period of the cumulative antibiogram will be reported. Other information may be incorporated into a cumulative antibiogram including antibiotic dosing guidelines, recommended empiric antibiotic choices based on infection type, antibiotic cost data, etc.[48]

Surveillance Susceptibility Testing of Large Numbers of Isolates

Surveillance susceptibility testing is a useful method to monitor the susceptibility of bacteria to antimicrobial agents over time, and can be performed in an individual hospital or within a geographic location (e.g., regionally, nationally, and internationally).[20] Surveillance studies typically report the overall susceptibility of the bacteria to particular anti-microbial agents using CLSI breakpoints, along with other susceptibility parameters such as the MIC_{50} and the MIC_{90}. To determine the MIC_{50} or MIC_{90}, the MIC values from the bacteria studied are arranged in ascending order where the MIC_{50} is the MIC value representing 50% of the bacterial population (the MIC value of the isolate that represents 50% of the bacterial population studied) and the MIC_{90} is the MIC that represents 90% of the bacterial population (the MIC value of the isolate that represents 90% of the bacterial population studied). The MIC_{90} value is usually higher than the MIC_{50} value. This information

TABLE 17-10. CLSI Recommendations for Cumulative Antibiogram Development[48]

1. In order to serve as a continuously useful tool to guide appropriate empiric antibiotic therapy, the cumulative antibiogram should be compiled, analyzed, and reported at least annually.

2. Only the first clinical isolate of a given species of bacteria per patient per analysis period (yearly if that is the time frame of the antibiogram) should be included in the cumulative susceptibility report regardless of site of isolation, susceptibility pattern of the bacteria, or other phenotypic characteristics. The inclusion of duplicate clinical isolates from the same patient will lead to incorrect reporting of actual bacterial resistance patterns.

3. To provide a reasonable statistical estimated of susceptibility, only species of bacteria where at least 30 isolates have been collected, tested, and reported during the time period of the antibiogram should be included.

4. Data from isolates recovered during surveillance cultures (e.g., MRSA and VRE), environmental cultures, or other nonpatient sources should not be included in the antibiogram.

5. The cumulative susceptibility report should include all antibiotics that were tested for susceptibility, regardless if they were reported in the final susceptibility report for the individual patient.

6. Only bacterial isolates where all routine antibiotics have been tested for susceptibility should be included. Results of agents selectively tested or supplemental tested should not be included in the cumulative susceptibility report. For example, if only isolates resistant to primary agents were then analyzed for susceptibility to secondary agents, this will bias the resistance results toward higher levels of resistance to the secondary agents.

7. Data may be stratified and reported by age, unit in which the isolate was collected (e.g., MICU, SICU, outpatient clinic), or by site of collection (e.g., blood isolates, CSF isolates, and urine isolates) as long as duplicate patient isolates are removed and there are a sufficient number of isolates collected (>30) during the time frame of the antibiogram.

is useful for detecting the emergence of subclinical antibiotic resistance where the MIC_{50} and MIC_{90} of a particular agent may be increasing over time but are still below the MIC susceptibility breakpoint.

Additional Considerations When Interpreting Susceptibility Results

The successful treatment of a patient's infection involves an understanding of the interactions among the patient, the infecting organism, and the antibiotic. It is important to note that antimicrobial susceptibility testing only measures one of these factors, namely, the activity of the antibiotic against the infecting organism in a laboratory setting. The current methodologies for antibiotic susceptibility testing are unable to reproduce the interaction between the antibiotic and the bacteria at the site of infection where a multitude of host factors (e.g., immune system function, concomitant disease states and drugs) and drug factors (e.g., pharmacokinetic parameters including concentration of free drug at the site of infection and protein binding) play an integral role.

FUNGI

Fungi are classified as one of the six kingdoms of life. There are approximately 500 named species of fungi that are known to cause infection in humans and other vertebrate animals.[49] Approximately 50 fungal species are associated with infections in healthy subjects and the majority of fungal infections occur in immunocompromised or debilitated patients by organisms that are part of the normal human flora. However, an increasing number of serious and life-threatening opportunistic infections are being caused by ubiquitous environmental molds.

One of the most challenging and frustrating aspects of diagnostic medical mycology is the terminology, taxonomy, classification, and nomenclature of fungi. For example, the correct name for a species of fungi is that which was published earliest and met the requirements in the International Code of Botanical Nomenclature (http://www.bgbm.org/iapt/nomenclature/code/default.htm). All subsequent names are considered synonyms; however, exceptions do exist, particularly when a later name is more commonly used than the earlier name or if research requires a species to be transferred to a different genus. Changes have occurred between kingdoms as well. For example, members of the genus *Pneumocystis*, which were originally placed in the kingdom Protozoa, are now reclassified as fungi and placed in the phylum Ascomycota. The common human pathogen from this genus is *Pneumocystis jirovecii* (formerly *Pneumocystis carinii*). Because of these issues, the reader is referred to the latest editions of standard microbiology textbooks and reference manuals (e.g., *Manual of Clinical Microbiology*, American Society for Microbiology Press) for more detailed information on taxonomy and classifications of fungi. In addition, a glossary of common mycological terms is often included.[49]

Fungi are eukaryotic and can be either unicellular or multicellular organisms. Fungi have cell walls composed mainly of chitins, glucan, and mannam with a membrane-bound cell nucleus with chromosomes. The dominant sterol in the cytoplasmic membrane of fungi is ergosterol, compared to cholesterol in mammalian cells. These organisms are heterotropic (e.g., require exogenous energy sources) and can reproduce by either asexual (involving mitosis) or sexual (involving meiosis) cell division. Fungi may exist in a morphologic form that results from sexual reproduction (teleomorph, or perfect state) and/or a form that results from asexual reproduction (anamorph or imperfect state), where each of the forms has its own name (e.g., the sexual form of *Scedosporium apiospermum* complex is *Pseudallescheria boydii*).

Fungi have traditionally been categorized into mold, yeast, or dimorphic fungi based on morphological and structural features (Table 17-11).[49-53] *Molds* (or moulds) are long, cylindrical, and threadlike (filamentous) fungi that form multicellular mycelium or thallas, an intertwined mass of branching hyphae [tube-like extensions or filament-like cells], with septa (having cross walls; being septate) or pauciseptate. An asexual spore (conidium) is produced on conidiophores, a specialized hyphal structure that serves as a stalk, and macroconidia and/or microconidia may be present. Thermally, monomorphic molds can be divided into four groups: (1) Zygomycetes; (2) dematiaceous fungi; (3) dermatophytes; and (4) hyaline hyphomycetes. Zygomycetes have broad hyphae that are almost nonseptate with asexual spores (sporangiospores) formed by cleavage in a saclike structure (sporangium). The most common Zygomycetes observed in the clinical laboratory are from the order Mucorales, which are associated with severe fungal infections referred to as *mucormycosis*. Two genera from the order Entomophthorales, *Basidiobolus* and *Conidiobolus*, are less commonly observed Zygomycetes but are responsible for subcutaneous infections in otherwise healthy individuals. Dematiaceous fungi produce dark colored colonies of olive, brown, gray or black due to melanin pigment in the cell walls. Some of the common infections associated with dematiaceous fungi include chromoblastomycosis, phaeohyphomycosis, and mycetoma. Dematiaceous fungi also cause tinea nigra and black piedra. Dermatophytes are most often associated with superficial fungal infections (tinea or ringworm) of the skin, hair, and nails. These filamentous fungi colonize the outermost layer of the skin and digest keratin as a source of nutrients. The three genera (*Microsporum*, *Trichophyton*, and *Epidermophyton*) are differentiated by their conidium formation (macroconidia or microconidia). Hyaline hyphomycetes are colorless, septate hyphae molds that produce conidia that may be either colorless or pigmented. *Coccidioides immitis* and *Coccidioides posadasii* are known pathogens from this group while most other organisms cause opportunistic infections in immunocompromised patients.

Yeasts (and yeast-like organisms) appear as round or oval cells that are unicellular and generally reproduce at their surface by budding (blastoconidia). Some produce pseudohyphae (an elongated chain of cells, like a chains of sausages, resembling hyphae; however, borders between cells are delineated by marked constrictions) while others have true hyphae (tend to be straighter and without constrictions at the septa),

TABLE 17-11. Categorization of Selected Medically Important Fungi[53,a]

YEASTS AND YEAST-LIKE ORGANISMS		DIMORPHIC FUNGI[b]	
Candida spp.	Saccharomyces cerevisiae	Histoplasma capsulatum	Penicillium marneffei
Cryptococcus spp.	Trichosporon spp.	Blastomyces dermatitidis	Sporothrix schenckii complex[d]
Rhodotorula spp.	Blastoschizomyces capitatus	Paracoccidioides brasiliensis	

MOLDS

Zygomycetes[c]	Dematiaceous Fungi	Dermatophytes	Hyaline Hyphomycetes
Rhizopus spp.	Fonsecaea pedrosoi	Microsporum spp.	Coccidioides spp.[b]
Mucor spp.	Fonsecaea compacta	Trichophyton spp.	Hormographiella aspergillata
Rhizomucor spp.	Rhinocladiella spp.	Epidermophyton floccosum	Emmonsia spp.
Lichtheimia corymbifera complex	Phialophora verrucosa		Aspergillus spp.
Apophysomyces elegans	Pleurostomophora richardsiae		Penicillum spp.
Saksenaea vasiformis	Phaeoacremonium parasiticum		Paecilomyces spp.
Cunninghamella bertholletiae	Phialemonium spp.		Scopulariopsis spp.
Basidiobolus spp.	Cladophialophora spp.		Acremonium spp.
Conidiobolus coronatus	Pseudallescheria boydii		Fusarium spp.
	(sexual state)		Lechythophora spp.
	Scedosporium apiospermum		
	(asexual state)		
	Scedosporium prolificans		
	Ochroconis gallopava		
	Exophiala jeanselmei complex		
	Exophiala dermatitidis		
	Hortaea werneckii		
	Stachybotrys chartarium		
	Curvularia spp.		
	Bipolaris spp.		
	Exserohilum spp.		
	Alternaria spp.		

[a]Refer to reference 53 for further details and other organisms not listed.

[b]*Coccidioides immitis* is often placed with dimorphic fungi (listed in this table under hyaline hyphomycetes since it does not produce yeast-like colonies or cells at 35°C to 37°C on routine mycology agar).

[c]Results from molecular studies have recommended that the phylum Zygomycota be divided among a new phylum, Glomeromycota and four subphyla, changing the class Zygomycetes to glomeromycetes. Many textbooks continue to Zygomycetes until the taxonomy is definitively resolved. Among the subphylum Mucormycotina, the order Mucorales includes the genera *Rhizopus*, *Mucor*, *Rhizomucor*, and *Lichtheimia* (formerly *Absidia*). The subphylum Entomophthoromycotina contains the order Entomophthorales, which includes genera *Basidiobolus* and *Conidiobolus*.

[d]*Sporothrix schenckii* grows as a dematiaceous mold when incubated at 25°C to 30°C but is yeast-like at 35°C to 37°C. It is commonly categorized among dimorphic fungi but is often considered as a dematiaceous mold.

which may be septate or without septate (aseptate). Ascospores (a sexual spore in a saclike structure [ascus]) are produced by only some yeast. Yeasts are the most frequent encountered fungi in the clinical microbiology laboratory and are considered opportunistic pathogens. *Candida* spp. and *Cryptococcus* spp. are among the most common yeasts causing fungal infections. Yeasts are not considered as a formal taxonomic group but as a growth form of unrelated fungi (members of the phyla Basidiomycota and Ascomycota).

Dimorphic fungi have two distinct morphological forms where their growth forms can change from a multicellular mold (in their natural environment or when cultured at 25°C to 30°C) to budding, unicellular yeasts (during tissue invasion or when cultured at 35°C to 37°C). Medically important dimorphic fungi include *Histoplasma capsulatum*, *Blastomyces dermatitidis*, *Paracoccidioides brasiliensis*, *Penicillium marneffei*, and *Sporothrix schenckii*. All of these fungi are considered pathogenic and must be handled with caution in the clinical laboratory.

The Identification of Fungi

The following section provides a brief summary of the common methods currently used in diagnostic testing of medically important fungi.[50-53] Fungal identification has traditionally been based on morphological characteristics such as the color of the colonies, the size and shape of cells, the presence of a capsule, and the production of hyphae, pseudohyphae, or chlamydospores; however, culture remains the "gold standard" in most clinical microbiology laboratories. Deoxyribonucleic acid (DNA) sequence analysis and molecular characteristics are being rapidly explored and gaining a larger role in fungal identification, particularly when morphology-based identification is atypical, confusing, or not helpful (e.g., organisms that fail to sporulate) and in cases where precise identification is required (e.g., epidemiological studies).

Laboratory diagnosis of fungal infections includes direct microscopic examination, isolation in culture, morphologic identification, biochemical, serologic, and molecular diagnostic testing. As with all types of infections, appropriate biological specimens need to be selected, collected, and transported to the laboratory for immediate processing.[50] Since different fungi are capable to causing infection at a number of anatomical sites, specimens from the site of infection as well as peripheral blood specimens should be considered and submitted for culture and microscopic examination. Communication with the laboratory regarding the clinical infection and suspected fungi is important, and may be useful for determining how best to process specimens safely and efficiently, including pretreatment and staining procedures, selection and incubation of media, and choice of additional diagnostic testing. Early identification of the infecting fungal pathogen may have direct diagnostic, epidemiologic, prognostic, and therapeutic implications.

The first step is usually identifying yeast-like fungi (pasty, opaque colonies) from molds (large, filamentous, colonies that vary in texture, color, and topography). Drawings, color plates, and brief descriptions found in standard textbooks can serve as a guide and assist in the preliminary identification of fungi seen on direct microscopic examination of clinical specimens.[52,53] Microscopic examination of the clinical specimen can delineate morphologic features (Table 17-12) and often provides preliminary identification of many fungi (e.g., *Aspergillus* spp., Zygomycetes, dematiaceous molds). Microscopic morphology can often provide definitive identification of a mold whereas the addition of biochemical tests, serology, and/or nucleic acid (NA)–based molecular testing are usually needed for identifying the genus and species of most yeast and yeast-like fungi. Direct microscopic examination of properly stained clinical specimens and tissue sections is usually the most rapid (within a few minutes or hours) and cost-effective method for a preliminary diagnosis of fungal infection. In addition, microscopic detection of fungi can assist the laboratory in the selection of media and interpretation of culture results.

The Gram stain that is typically used for bacterial processing may also allow the detection of most fungi, especially *Candida* spp., since the size of the smallest fungi is similar in size to large bacteria; the presence of budding cells can also be observed. A wide range of stains are available (Table 17-13) to assist in the rapid detection of fungal elements.[51-53] A common approach to wet preparations of specimens or smeared dried material is to use a 10% solution of potassium hydroxide (KOH) with or without fluorescent calcofluor white (CFW) stain. The strong alkaline KOH solution digests tissue elements in order to allow better visualization of the fungi, while the CFW stain binds to chitin and polysaccharides in the fungal cell wall allowing it to appear white under ultraviolet light. Specific staining techniques are often used to outline morphologic features that are diagnostic and distinctive of the suspected fungal organism (e.g., India ink stain for detection of a polysaccharide capsule of *Cryptococcus neoformans*). In suspected cases of histoplasmosis, the Giemsa or Wright stain is useful for detecting intracellular yeast cells within macrophages from blood or bone marrow specimens.

Histopathologic stains are extremely valuable for identifying fungal elements in tissues and host tissue reactions to fungal infection. Histology laboratories commonly use stains such as hematoxylin and eosin (H&E) for these general purposes. Periodic acid-Schiff (PAS) and Gridley fungus (GF) stains can also assist in visualization of fungal elements, especially if debris is present in the tissue background. Special stains such as Gomori methenamine silver (GMS), mucicarmine, and Fontana-Masson (FM) are useful for enhancing the detection of specific fungal elements (see Table 17-13).[51-53]

Culture remains the gold standard for isolation and identification of fungi suspected of causing infection. Petri plates are preferred over screw-cap tubes because of the larger surface area and dilution of inhibitory substances in the specimens. However, for laboratory safety reasons, most thermally dimorphic fungi (e.g., *Histoplasma*, *Blastomyces*, *Paracoccidioides*, *Penicillium marneffei*) and *Coccidioides* spp. are pathogenic and should be grown on slants (i.e., avoid the use of Petri plates and slide culture). A variety of media are available for the isolation and cultivation of yeasts and molds (Table 17-14).[51,53] Sabouraud dextrose and brain heart infusion (SDBHI) or BHI agar are enriched media commonly recommended to permit the growth of yeasts and molds. Several media, with (selective) and without (nonselective) inhibitory agents, should be used since no one media is adequate for all the different types of specimens or organisms. Antibiotics such as chloramphenicol or gentamicin are included as inhibitory substances of most bacterial contaminants whereas cycloheximide is used to inhibit saprophytic fungi and prevent the overgrowth of contaminating molds. Nonselective media (without inhibitory agents) should be used with specimens from sterile sites and when suspected fungi are likely to be inhibited by cycloheximide (e.g., *Aspergillus fumigatus*, *Fusarium*, *Scopulariopsis*, *Cryptococcus neoformans/gattii*, some *Candida* spp., most Zygomycetes) or by antibiotics (e.g., *Nocardia* or other filamentous bacteria). Direct microbiological examination (outlined above) of clinical specimens can assist in the selection of media based on specimen type and suspected pathogen. In addition, the choice of media will be influenced by the patient population, local endemic pathogens, cost, availability, and laboratory preferences.

Proper incubation temperature and sufficient incubation time are also needed to optimize the recovery of medically important fungi from clinical specimens. Inoculated media should be incubated aerobically at 30°C. If an incubator at that temperature is not available, then 25°C (room temperature) can be considered. Other temperatures (e.g., 35°C to 37°C for thermally dimorphic organisms) should be reserved for selected fungi that prefer a higher temperature. In general, yeasts are detected within 5 days or less, dermatophytes within 1 week, and dematiaceous and dimorphic fungi between 2–4 weeks. Cultures should be regularly reviewed (e.g., every day the first week, every 2–3 days the second week, twice during the third week, once weekly thereafter) to account for the growth rates and identification of fungi. Incubating cultures for 4 weeks is usually necessary before no growth of fungus should be considered. Several factors influence the length of incubation including the choice of media (e.g., yeasts on chromogenic [48

TABLE 17-12. Laboratory Testing and Characteristic Features Used in the Diagnosis of Selected Opportunistic and Pathogenic Fungi[52,53]

| FUNGAL ORGANISM | MICROSCOPIC MORPHOLOGIC FEATURES OF CLINICAL SPECIMENS | MORPHOLOGIC FEATURES IN CULTURE | | SEROLOGIC TESTS | | ADDITIONAL TESTS FOR IDENTIFICATION |
		MACROSCOPIC	MICROSCOPIC	ANTIGEN	ANTIBODY	
Candida spp.	Blood; bone marrow; catheter sites; eye; respiratory sites; skin, nails, mucous membrane; urine; vaginal, urethral, prostatic secretions or discharge; multiple systemic sites	Round to oval budding yeasts (3–6 μm in diameter), singly, in chains, or in small loose clusters; true hyphae (no or slight constrictions at the septa) and pseudohyphae (5–10 μm in diameter; chains of elongated blastoconidia) when invading tissues; blastoconidia develop along the sides of either type of hyphae

Candida glabrata slightly smaller (2–5 μm in diameter) than other species and does not produce any hyphal forms | Variable morphology; colonies usually pasty, white to tan and opaque; may have smooth or wrinkled morphology | Clusters of blastoconidia, pseudohyphae and/or terminal chlamydospores in some species | Part of (1→3)-β-D-glucan panfungal detection | | Germ tube production by *Candida albicans*, *Candida dubliniensis*, and *Candida stellatoidea*

PNA-FISH

Carbohydrate assimilation

Morphology on corn meal agar |
| *Cryptococcus neoformans* | Most commonly in CSF and blood; bone marrow; catheter sites; respiratory sites; skin, mucous membrane; urine; multiple systemic sites | Spherical (football shaped) or round, budding yeasts of variable size (2–15 μm) with thin dark walls; thick capsule may or may not be present; no hyphae or pseudohyphae | Colonies are shiny, mucoid, dome-shaped, and cream to tan in color | Budding spherical cells of varying size; capsule present; no pseudohyphae; cells may have multiple narrow-based buds | Latex antigen detection or EIA test | | India ink can demonstrate capsule in ~50% of cases on smeared specimens

Tests for urease (+), phenoloxidase (+), and nitrate reductase (-)

Mucicarmine and melanin stains in tissue |

TABLE 17-12. Laboratory Testing and Characteristic Features Used in the Diagnosis of Selected Opportunistic and Pathogenic Fungi (cont'd) [52,53]

FUNGAL ORGANISM	POTENTIAL CLINICAL SPECIMENS	MICROSCOPIC MORPHOLOGIC FEATURES OF CLINICAL SPECIMENS	MORPHOLOGIC FEATURES IN CULTURE		SEROLOGIC TESTS		ADDITIONAL TESTS FOR IDENTIFICATION
			MACROSCOPIC	MICROSCOPIC	ANTIGEN	ANTIBODY	
Aspergillus spp.	CSF; eye; respiratory sites; skin; mucous membrane; urine; multiple systemic sites	Septate with uniform diameter (3–6 μm); dichotomously branched hyphae at 45° angles; tend to grow in radial fashion (like spokes on a wheel)	Varies with species; Aspergillus fumigates: blue-green to gray; Aspergillus flavus: yellow to green; Aspergillus niger: black with white margins and yellow surface mycelium	Varies with species; conidiophores with enlarged vesicles covered with flask-shaped metulae or phialides; hyphae are hyaline and septate	Galactomannan detection is useful tool in the diagnosis of invasive aspergillosis Part of (1→3)-β-D-glucan panfungal detection	Useful for chronic and allergic aspergillosis	Molecular techniques are attractive as alternative methods but are mainly in-house systems without standardization being available
Zygomycetes	CSF; eye; respiratory sites; skin; mucous membrane; multiple systemic sites	Broad, thin-walled, pauciseptate hyphae (6–25 μm) with nonparallel sides and branching irregularly, nondichotomous, and at various angles; hyphae stain poorly with GMS stain and often stain well with H&E stain	Colonies are rapid growing, wooly or fluffy colonies (cotton candy-like), and gray-black in color	Differentiation of various genera based on presence and location (or absence) of rhizoids, nature of sporangio-phores, shape of columella, appearance of an apophysis, and size and shape of the sporangia			
Dematiaceous molds	CSF; eye; respiratory sites; skin; mucous membrane; multiple systemic sites	Pigmented (brown, tan, or black) polymorphous hyphae (2–6 μm in diameter) with single septa and in chains of swollen rounded cells	Colonies are usually rapidly growing, wooly, and gray, olive, black, or brown in color	Varies depending on genus and species; hyphae are pigmented; conidia may be single or in chains, smooth or rough, and dematiaceous			

TABLE 17-12. Laboratory Testing and Characteristic Features Used in the Diagnosis of Selected Opportunistic and Pathogenic Fungi (cont'd) [52,53]

| FUNGAL ORGANISM | MICROSCOPIC MORPHOLOGIC FEATURES OF CLINICAL SPECIMENS | MORPHOLOGIC FEATURES IN CULTURE | | SEROLOGIC TESTS | | ADDITIONAL TESTS FOR IDENTIFICATION |
	POTENTIAL CLINICAL SPECIMENS	MACROSCOPIC	MICROSCOPIC	ANTIGEN	ANTIBODY	
Histoplasma capsulatum	Blood; bone marrow; CSF; eye; respiratory sites; skin, mucous membrane; urine; multiple systemic sites	Small (2–4 μm in diameter), oval to round budding cells; often clustered within histiocytes or intracellular (macrophages, monocytes) Can be difficult to differentiate *Histoplasma* from other small yeasts (e.g., *Candida* spp.) or some parasites	Colonies are slow growing and white or buff brown in color (25°C); yeast phase colonies (37°C) are smooth, white, and pasty	Thin, septate hyphae that produce tuberculate macroconidia and smooth wall microconidia (25°C); small, oval, budding yeasts produced at 37°C	Various methods for initial antigen screening	Antigen screening test should be validated with antibody testing	AccuProbe may be useful for confirming identification Exoantigen test kit is available for confirming identification
Blastomyces dermatitidis	CSF; respiratory sites; skin, mucous membrane; urine; multiple systemic sites	Large (8–15 μm in diameter) and spherical, thick-walled (commonly referred to as "double contoured") cell; each yeast cell produces a single bud, attached to parent cell on a broad base	At 25°C to 30°C, colonies vary from cottony or fluffy white with aerial mycelium (first 2–3 days) then to a glabrous, tan, nonconidiating colony. When grown at 35°C to 37°C, cream to tan color, wrinkled, folded, and glabrous (waxy in appearance)	On a wet mount at 25°C to 30°C, septate hyphae with one-celled smooth conidia (lollipop-like appearance); at 37°C, large, thick walled and double contoured yeast-like cell, budded on a broad base	Sandwich EIA available to detect antigenuria and antigenemia in disseminated blastomycosis	Immunodiffusion test is the most useful method	AccuProbe may be useful for confirming identification Exoantigen test kit is available for confirming identification

TABLE 17-12. Laboratory Testing and Characteristic Features Used in the Diagnosis of Selected Opportunistic and Pathogenic Fungi (cont'd) [52,53]

FUNGAL ORGANISM	POTENTIAL CLINICAL SPECIMENS	MICROSCOPIC MORPHOLOGY — FEATURES OF CLINICAL SPECIMENS	MORPHOLOGIC FEATURES IN CULTURE — MACROSCOPIC	MORPHOLOGIC FEATURES IN CULTURE — MICROSCOPIC	SEROLOGIC TESTS — ANTIGEN	SEROLOGIC TESTS — ANTIBODY	ADDITIONAL TESTS FOR IDENTIFICATION
Coccidioides immitis/posadasii	Blood; bone marrow; CSF; eye; respiratory sites; skin, mucous membrane; urine; multiple systemic sites	Round, thick-walled spherules that vary in size (20–200 μm in length); mature spherules contain small (2–15 μm in diameter) endospores; septate hyphae, barrel-shaped arthroconidia may be seen in cavitary and necrotic lesions	Great variation in morphology; at 25°C or 37°C, colonies initially appear moist and glabrous, rapidly develops a white, cottony aerial mycelium, which becomes gray-white to a tan or brownish	Hyaline hyphae with rectangular (barrel-shaped) arthroconidia separated by empty disjunctor cells	EIA using antibodies against *Coccidioides* galactomannan	Various methods (ID, complement-fixation most reliable) for initial antibody screening (principle antigen used in these test is coccidioidin)	AccuProbe may be useful for confirmation of unknown isolates as *Coccidioides* species (but does not distinguish between two species of *Coccidioides*) Immunodiffusion test for exoantigen to identify the organism
Sporothrix schenckii	Blood; CSF; respiratory sites; skin, mucous membrane; multiple systemic sites	Small (2–6 μm in diameter) yeast-like cells of varying sizes and shapes (oval or round or cigar shaped); single or multiple elongated "pipe stem;" bud is on a narrow base	At 25°C to 30°C, colonies are initially small, smooth, moist and white to pale orange to orange-gray with no cottony aerial hyphae; later, colonies become moist, wrinkled, leathery, or velvety and darken to brown or black; at 35°C to 37°C, colonies are white to tan, dry, smooth and yeast-like	At 25°C to 30°C, thin or narrow, septate, and branching, with slender, tapering conidiophores rising at right angles; conidia borne in rosette-shaped clusters at the end of the conidiophores; at 35°C to 37°C, variable-sized round, oval, and fuisform budding yeasts (cigar bodies)		LA test is commercially available (particularly for disseminated cases)	

TABLE 17-12. Laboratory Testing and Characteristic Features Used in the Diagnosis of Selected Opportunistic and Pathogenic Fungi (cont'd) [52,53]

FUNGAL ORGANISM	POTENTIAL CLINICAL SPECIMENS	MICROSCOPIC MORPHOLOGIC FEATURES OF CLINICAL SPECIMENS	MORPHOLOGIC FEATURES IN CULTURE		SEROLOGIC TESTS		ADDITIONAL TESTS FOR IDENTIFICATION
			MACROSCOPIC	MICROSCOPIC	ANTIGEN	ANTIBODY	
Penicillium marneffei	Blood; bone marrow; CSF; respiratory sites; skin, mucous membrane; urine; multiple systemic sites	Oval (2.5–5 μm in length) or elongated or cylindrical, curved yeast-like cells; found within histiocytes (intracellular); has visible septa and budding does not occur (reproduces by fission [arthroconidium-like])	Colonies are flat, powdery to velvet, and tan, and then produce diffusible red–yellow pigment at 25°C to 30°C; at 35°C to 37°C, colony is soft, white to tan, dry, yeast-like	At 25°C to 30°C, smooth conidiophores with 4–5 terminal metulae bearing phialides; chains of short, narrow extensions connect the round to oval conidia in a "paint brush" distribution; at 35°C to 37°C, arthroconidial yeast cells divide by fission and may elongate			
Pneumocystis jirovecii	Respiratory sites; multiple systemic sites	Cysts are round, ovoid, or collapsed crescent shaped (4–7 μm in diameter); stains should be used to visualize cyst forms for diagnosis; trophozoites are small (1–4 μm in diameter), pleomorphic forms	Not applicable	Not applicable		Useful for epidemiology studies but not for diagnosis	Immunospecific stain commercially available

CSF = cerebrospinal fluid; EIA = enzyme immunoassay; ID = immunodiffusion; LA = latex agglutination.

TABLE 17-13. Stains Used to Enhance the Direct Microscopic Detection of Fungi[51-53]

STAIN (ABBREVIATION)	DETECTION	CHARACTERISTICS/COMMENTS
Alcian blue	*Cryptococcus neoformans* (in CSF)	Histopathologic stain for mucin
Brown and Brenn (B&B)	*Nocardia, Actinomadura,* etc. (demonstrates the bacterial filaments of the actinomycetes)	Stains fungi blue
Calcofluor white (CFW)	Most fungi including *Pneumocystis jirovecii* (cysts)	Binds to chitin in fungal cell wall and fluoresces bluish white against dark background; requires fluorescent microscope; mixed with KOH for easier and rapid observation of fungi
Fontana-Masson (FM)	Dematiaceous fungi, *Cryptococcus neoformans* and *Cryptococcus gattii;* may also be useful for *Aspergillus fumigates, Aspergillus flavus, Trichosporon* spp., and some Zygomycetes	Stains fungi brown to black against reddish background; demonstration of melanin or melanin-like substances in the lightly pigmented agents of phaeohyphomycosis
Giemsa or Wright stain	Visualization of intracellular *Histoplasma capsulatum;* trophic forms of *Pneumocystis jirovecii;* fission yeast cells of *Penicillium marneffei*	Stains blue-purple (fungi and bacteria); examination of bone marrow or peripheral blood smears for disseminated disease
Gomori methenamine silver (GMS)	Most fungi in histopathologic sections; *Pneumocystis jirovecii* (respiratory specimens)	Detects fungi elements; however, requires specialized staining method; stains hyphae and yeast forms gray to black against a pale green or yellow background
Gram stain	Yeast and pseudohyphae appear Gram-positive and hyphae (septate and aseptate) appear Gram-negative	Commonly performed on clinical specimens; some fungi stain poorly (e.g., *Cryptococcus* spp., *Nocardia*)
Gridley fungus (GF)	Most fungi in histopathologic sections	Fungi stain purplish red; filaments of actinomycetes are not stained
Hematoxylin and eosin (H&E)	General purpose histopathologic stain; best method for visualizing host tissue reactions to infecting fungus	Stains some fungal elements violet to bluish purple in contrast to lighter background; *Aspergillus* spp. and Zygomycetes stain well; some fungi difficult to differentiate from background
Immunohistochemical stains	*Aspergillus* spp., *Candida albicans, Pneumocystis jirovecii*	Commercial antibodies used in the immunohistochemical diagnosis of fungal infections, especially to distinguish fungal elements on atypical appearing tissue sections
India ink, nigrosin	*Cryptococcus neoformans* (in CSF)	Sensitivity is <50% of meningitis cases
Modified acid-fast	*Nocardia* (filaments are partially acid-fast and stain pink) and some isolates of *Blastomyces dermatitidis*	*Actinomyces* and other actinomycetes are negative
Mucicarmine	*Cryptococcus neoformans* (capsular material); cell walls of *Blastomyces dermatitidis* and *Rhinosporidium seeberi*	Histopathologic stain for mucin; capsular material stains deep rose to red; tissue elements stain yellow
Papanicolaou stain		Fungal elements stain pink to blue
Periodic acid-Schiff (PAS)	Histopathologic stain for fungi, especially yeast cells and hyphae in tissue; commonly used stain by dermatopathologists	Fungal elements stain bright pink–magenta or purple against orange background (picric acid counterstain) or green background (if light green used); hyphae of molds and yeast can be readily distinguished; demonstrates double-contoured refractile wall of *Blastomyces dermatitidis; Nocardia* do not stain well
Potassium hydroxide (KOH)	Most fungi (more readily visible)	Used to dissolve tissue material allowing more visible fungal elements
Toluidine blue	*Pneumocystis jirovecii* (respiratory specimens: biopsy or BAL)	Stains cysts of *Pneumocystis jirovecii* reddish blue or dark purple against light blue background

BAL = bronchoalveolar lavage; CSF = cerebrospinal fluid.

TABLE 17-14. Examples of Various Media Used for the Recovery of Fungi from Clinical Specimens[51,53]

GROWTH MEDIUM	COMMENTS AND USES
Primary Media Without Antibacterials or Antifungals	
Brain heart infusion (BHI) agar	Enriched media used for cultivation and isolation of all fungi; designed to enhance the recovery of fastidious dimorphic fungi than does SDA
Littman Oxgall agar	General purpose selective medium for isolation of all fungi. Restricts the spreading of fungal colonies; contains crystal violet and streptomycin to inhibit bacteria growth
Sabouraud dextrose agar (SDA)	Supports primary growth or sporulation and provides classic pigment and morphology
SDA, Emmons modification	Compared to SDA, Emmons Modification contains 2% (versus 4%) glucose and has a pH of 6.9 (versus pH 5.6 [slightly acidic])
SADHI medium	Enriched media using combined ingredients of BHI and SDA; supports growth of all fungi; designed for better recovery of fastidious dimorphic fungi than does SDA
Primary Media with Antibacterials or Antifungals	
Any of the above media	Usually with chloramphenicol (inhibits Gram-negative and Gram-positive bacteria) with or without gentamicin (inhibits Gram-negative bacteria); cycloheximide added to inhibit sensitive fast-growing saprophytic fungi
Inhibitory mold agar (IMA)	Enriched media providing better recovery of fastidious fungi than does SDA; usually contains chloramphenicol; some formulations contain gentamicin
Mycosel or mycobiotic	Selective medium containing chloramphenicol or cycloheximide primarily used for isolation of dermatophytes; can also be used for isolation of other pathogenic fungi from contaminant specimens
Selective/Differential Media	
Dermatophyte test medium (DTM) or dermatophyte identification medium (DIM)	Screening medium for the recovery, selection, and differentiation of dermatophytes (e.g., *Microsporum, Trichophyton, Epidermophyton*) from hair, skin, and nail (cutaneous) specimens; contains chloramphenicol, gentamicin, and cycloheximide; other saprophytic fungi and *Aspergillus* spp. can grow on this medium (thus, it is only recommended as a screening medium)
Yeast extract phosphate	Used for isolation and sporulation of slowly growing dimorphic fungi (i.e., *Histoplasma capsulatum* and *Blastomyces dermatitidis*) from contaminated specimens; contains chloramphenicol and ammonium hydroxide to suppress bacteria, moulds, and yeasts and further permit detection of dimorphic fungi
CHROMagar candida	Chromogenic media used for direct and rapid differentiation of many clinically important yeast spp; contains chloramphenicol to inhibit bacteria and is available with or without fluconazole (selection of fluconazole-resistant *Candida krusei*); CHROMagar differentiates more *Candida* spp. than CAN2; useful in identifying mixed cultures of yeasts
ChromID candida agar (CAN2)	Chromogenic media used for direct and rapid identification of *Candida albicans* versus other species of yeasts; useful in identifying mixed cultures of yeasts
Specialized Media	
Cornmeal agar (CMA)	CMA with 1% dextrose used for the cultivation of fungi and differentiation of *Trichophyton mentagrophytes* from *Trichophyton rubrum* (based on pigment production); CMA with Tween 80 used for the cultivation and differentiation of *Candida* spp. (based on mycelial characteristics); Tween 80 promotes growth and production of red pigment by *Trichophyton rubrum*
Potato dextrose agar (PDA) or potato flake agar (PFA)	PDA is used to stimulate conidium production by fungi and enhance pigment production by some dermatophytes; PDA is most commonly used with slide culture technique to view morphological characteristics; PFA used for the simulation of conidia of fungi; PFA may include cycloheximide and chloramphenicol
Rapid sporulation agar (RSA)	Cultivation of ascosporogenous yeasts (e.g., *Saccharomyces cerevisiae*); contains chloramphenicol and chlortetracycline to inhibit bacteria and cycloheximide to inhibit saprobic fungi
Niger seed or bird seed and esculin base medium (EBM)	Selective and differential medium for isolation of *Cryptococcus* spp., especially *Cryptococcus neoformans* and *Cryptococcus gattii*

hours] versus routine media [5–7 days]) and type of fungus suspected (e.g., slow growing dimorphic systemic fungi may need 8 weeks).

Once the organism has been cultured and isolated, the following approach has usually been conducted: (1) determine the morphology of the unknown fungus and determine if it is consistent with any of the groups listed in Table 17-11 or filamentous bacterium (some of the aerobic actinomycetes [e.g., *Nocardia*] resemble fungi and must be ruled out); and (2) note the rate of growth, colony (macroscopic) and microscopic morphologies of the possible organism(s) (Table 17-12) and refer to necessary textbooks to compare descriptions, drawings, color plates, discussions of characteristics, and other test results to assist in differentiating the likely organism.[52,53] In the case of yeasts and yeast-like organisms, additional testing such as the germ tube test, biochemical testing using commercially-available systems, or the urease test may allow species identification of isolates from various body sites.

Antigen Detection

Cell wall components of various invasive fungi have been used as diagnostic markers for antigen testing. Galactomannan is a polysaccharide component of the *Aspergillus* cell wall that is released by growing hyphae. A commercial enzyme-linked immunosorbent assay (ELISA) (Platelia Aspergillus [Bio-Rad], Marens-La-Coquette, France) is available to detect circulating galactomannan antigen in blood and has been shown to be an earlier diagnostic marker for invasive aspergillosis in neutropenic patients with hematologic malignancies.[52] The monitoring of antigen titers has also been shown to correlate with the response to antifungal therapy, patient survival, and autopsy findings in neutropenic patients.

Latex antigen detection and enzyme immunoassay (EIA) are sensitive (93% to 100%) and specific (93% to 100%) diagnostic tests for the detection and quantitation of circulating *Cryptococcus neoformans* (capsular galactoxylomannan) polysaccharide antigen in serum and CSF.[52] Antigen testing is considered to be the primary diagnostic test for screening CSF for suspected cases of cryptococcal meningitis since the India ink procedure has a low sensitivity. The reported titer determinations of the two testing methods (e.g., EIA versus latex testing) or from different commercial latex kits are not numerically similar. Thus, the same testing method and latex kit should be used to monitor serial samples for a patient. False-negative and false-positive (e.g., rheumatoid factor) results have been reported for each testing method.

Enzyme immunoassay can be used to detect *Histoplasma capsulatum* antigen in body fluids (e.g., blood, urine, CSF or bronchoalveolar lavage [BAL] fluid). It has been recommended that the antigen screening test be validated by antibody testing (e.g., immunodiffusion [ID] and/or complement fixation [CF]).[52] The diagnosis of histoplasmosis should be based on a combination of diagnostic test results since antigen testing is associated with cross-reactivity to other fungal infections and the test sensitivity varies with disease presentation (e.g., 77% for acute pulmonary histoplasmosis, 34% for subacute

pulmonary histoplasmosis, 21% for chronic pulmonary histoplasmosis, 92% for progressively disseminated histoplasmosis) and specimen type (80% to 95% in urine, 25% to 50% in CSF, 93.5% in BAL). Antigen detection is generally not used as a diagnostic tool for blastomycosis and has a limited role for coccidioidomycosis due to low levels of detection in antigenemia and antigenuria, cross-reactions, and false-positive reactions. Antigen detection tests for *Histoplasma capsulatum*, *Blastomyces dermatitidis*, and *Coccidioides* species are performed by MiraVista Diagnostics (Indianapolis, Indiana) on a fee-for-service basis.

Commercial assays for the detection of (1→3)-beta-D-glucan, a major cell wall component of common pathogenic yeasts, have been used as a panfungal diagnostic tool for invasive fungal infections such as aspergillosis, *Fusarium* infection, trichosporonosis, and candidiasis.[52] In the United States, Fungitell (Glucatell) serum detection test is the only available EIA for detecting (1→3)-beta-D-glucan. The manufacturer's recommended guidelines for a positive (1→3)-beta-D-glucan value is ≥80 pg/mL. False-positive results have been observed in hemodialysis patients (with cellulose membranes), patients treated with certain blood products (e.g., albumin, immunoglobulins), and patients with bacterial infections or have been exposed to glucan-containing materials (e.g., gauze). Concurrent beta-lactam therapy, such as piperacillin–tazobactam or amoxicillin–clavulanate, and antitumoral polysaccharides have been associated with cross-reactions. This assay is nonspecific and should be used in conjunction with clinical examination of the patient and other diagnostic tests and procedures in order to make a conclusive diagnosis of invasive fungal infection. This diagnostic assay is not useful for mucoraceous molds (e.g., Zygomycetes, *Rhizopus*), which do not produce (1→3)-beta-D-glucan), or *Cryptococcus* species and *Blastomyces* dermatitidis because they produce only low levels of (1→3)-beta-D-glucan).

Antigen detection methods and serology for *Candida* spp. in blood cultures have not been reliable in distinguishing between colonization, candidemia, and disseminated candidiasis.[52] Extreme variability has been observed in both sensitivity and specificity, making the currently available tests unreliable for establishing a diagnosis. Several commercial kits are available for the detection of capsular galactoxylomannan (cryptococcal antigen) and are able to detect *Cryptococcus neoformans* and *Cryptococcus gattii*. The combination of antigen detection test and an India ink stain of the CSF are recommended for the primary evaluations of suspected cases of cryptococcal meningitis. False-positive and false-negative results have been reported with the various methodologies.

Serology

Several different methodologies for antibody testing (e.g., tube precipitin [TP], CF assays, ID, LA, and EIA) have been investigated for the detection of specific fungal pathogens.[52] Interpretation of *serology* results for most fungal infections requires knowledge of the laboratory technique used to perform the antibody testing. Serologic assays are most useful as diagnostic testing of fungal infections in the immunocompetent host since a poor antibody response is common in immunosuppressed patients resulting in a false-negative result.

The presence of antibody has assisted in the diagnosis of invasive infections such as coccidioidomycosis, histoplasmosis, and paracoccidiodomycosis.[52] The most reliable serological tests for diagnosing coccidioidomycosis have been ID and CF, where heated and/or unheated coccidioidin is used as the principal antigen in these tests. Serologic tests (ID, CF, and LA) for the clinical diagnosis of infections caused by *Histoplasma capsulatum* are commercially available. These tests have been the most useful in patients with chronic pulmonary or disseminated histoplasmosis. Immunodiffusion and CF are the most common serologic methods used for the diagnosis of para-coccidioidomycosis. No commercial kits for either method are available (fee-for-service, Cerodex Laboratories, Washington, OK). Finally, serology testing has been useful for the diagnosis of noninvasive diseases such as allergic bronchopulmonary aspergillosis and aspergilloma.[52]

Molecular Diagnosis

Currently there are a limited number of molecular diagnostic tests available for the detection and identification of fungi in the clinical laboratory.[52,53] For fungal isolates grown in pure culture, NA hybridization probes, DNA sequencing, peptide NA fluorescence in situ hybridization probes, and laboratory-developed PCR tests are available. Molecular methods used in the direct detection and identification of fungi from patient specimens are limited to a few laboratory-developed PCR tests targeting specific fungal agents. A commercially-available platform (Luminex xMAP, Luminex, Austin, TX) with PCR amplification, flow cytometry, and dual-laser system is available for high throughput and species-specific identification with user-designed (or outside vendor) probes. For laboratory-developed methods, proper validation of NA tests is needed before routine use can occur in the clinical laboratory. Clinicians will need to contact their laboratory to determine which tests are available and which molecular diagnostic tests may need to be sent to a reference laboratory. At this time, a combination of morphologic and molecular testing methods is best used for species identification.

Several probe-based assays have become commercially available for the identification of dimorphic fungi and *Candida* spp.[52,53] AccuProbe (Gen-Probe, San Diego, CA) uses hybridization to target rRNA present in a fungal culture, which is detected by a labeled single-stranded DNA probe. Three separate probes, with high sensitivity and specificity, are approved by the Food and Drug Administration (FDA) and available for the identification of *Blastomyces dermatitidis*, *Coccidioides immitis*, and *Histoplasma capsulatum*. The *Blastomyces dermatitidis* probe has the potential to cross-react with other fungi including *Emmonsia* species, *Paracoccidiodes brasiliensis*, and *Gymnascella* spp. In addition, the *Coccidioides* probe is unable to distinguish between species, namely *Coccidioides immitis* and *Coccidioides posadasii*.

Peptide nucleic acid-fluorescence in situ hybridization (PNA FISH Yeast Traffic Light Probe, AdvanDx, Woburn, MA) is available for the direct identification of *Candida* spp. on blood smears from cultures that are Gram stain positive for yeasts.[53] After the Gram stain and the hybridization process is completed, *Candida albicans* and *Candida parapsilosis* are identified microscopically as bright green fluorescing cells, while *Candida tropicalis* fluoresces bright yellow, and *Candida glabrata* and *Candida krusei* fluoresce bright red. Other yeasts do not fluoresce. The colors of the light probes also provides an indication about the potential use of fluconazole in these patients since *Candida albicans* and *Candida parapsilosis* are generally susceptible to fluconazole (green light for go), *Candida glabrata* can be resistant to fluconazole and *Candida krusei* is intrinsically resistant to fluconazole (red light for stop). The yellow signal produced by *Candida tropicalis* indicates that caution should be used since fluconazole susceptibility is variable for this organism. This method has a significant impact over traditional identification methods, which could take up to three or more days for identification of *Candida* spp., as well as guiding the most effective antifungal drug therapy.

MALDI-TOF Mass Spectrometry

Matrix-assisted laser desorption ionization time-of-flight (MALDI-TOF) mass spectrometry (MS) has been shown to be a rapid and accurate method for identifying yeasts and molds recovered on culture media.[52–54] Reports on the use of MALDI-TOF MS for routine rapid identification have focused on clinically important yeasts (e.g., *Candida* spp., *Cryptococcus neoformans*) and dermatophyte species. Filamentous fungi have been more difficult because of different developmental forms on agar media and the influences of the phenotype. MALDI-TOF MS is likely to become the primary diagnostic method for rapid identification of fungus isolates in the clinical microbiology laboratory. This technology is ideal for genus and species identification, and has the potential for accurate strain typing and identification for fungi, bacteria, and mycobacterium.

The advantages of the MALDI-TOF MS for fungal identification is the low cost of materials (a few cents) for each organism identification and the rapidity to results (approximately 11 minutes if just one isolate is tested; 2.5 minutes per isolate in a batch of 96 isolates, with the average time per isolate in published reports being 4–6 minutes). However, the current limitations include the initial costs of instrumentation for the system, lack of sample preparation techniques, inadequate fungal spectra in the database and software of commercial systems (e.g., Bruker and Shimadzu), and lack of FDA approval of any currently available system. Expansion of database libraries and developments in sample preparation are rapidly occurring to establish validated and routine procedures for a large number of clinically important fungal strains and species. Evidence from several studies also suggests that MALDI-TOF MS could be developed for performing rapid antifungal susceptibility testing.

Antifungal Susceptibility Testing

The importance of antifungal susceptibility testing has become increasingly recognized as a useful component in the treatment optimization of invasive infections caused by *Candida* spp. because of the increasing number of available antifungal agents, emerging resistance issues to standard therapy, and the changing epidemiology of invasive fungal disease. The CLSI has developed standardized reference methods for macrodilution and microdilution susceptibility testing of yeasts and molds, as well as disk diffusion methods of yeasts and nondermatophyte filamentous fungi.[55-58] The commercial availability of simplified and/or automated testing methods (e.g., Etest strip; Vitek 2; Sensititre YeastOne) consistent with CLSI reference methods is allowing an increasing number of clinical laboratories to routinely perform antifungal susceptibility testing.

Interpretive MIC breakpoints based on CLSI-recommended in vitro susceptibility testing methods have been recommended for *Candida* spp.[58] The results of several recent comprehensive reviews regarding the microbiological, molecular, pharmacodynamic, and clinical antifungal data for *Candida* spp. has been recently reviewed, and species-specific interpretive clinical breakpoints have been proposed for fluconazole, voriconazole, and the echinocandins (Table 17-15).[59-61] These recent reports have also been useful for the establishment of epidemiologic cutoff values, detection of emerging resistance among *Candida* spp., and harmonization of antifungal susceptibility testing standards by CLSI and European Committee on Antimicrobial Susceptibility Testing (EUCAST).[59-61] Interpretive breakpoint criteria for other fungal pathogens remain to be standardized.

TABLE 17-15. Proposed Species-Specific Interpretative MIC Breakpoints for In Vitro Susceptibility Testing of *Candida* spp.[59-61]

| ANTIFUNGAL AGENT | *CANDIDA* SPP. | MIC BREAKPOINT (mcg/mL) | | | |
		SUSCEPTIBLE	SUSCEPTIBLE-DOSE DEPENDENT	I	R
Fluconazole	C. albicans, C. tropicalis, C. parapsilosis	≤2	4		≥8
	C. glabrata		≤32		≥64
Voriconazole	C. albicans, C. tropicalis, C. parapsilosis	≤0.125		0.25–0.5	≥1
	C. krusei	≤0.5		1	≥2
Anidulafungin, caspofungin, micafungin	C. albicans, C. tropicalis, C. krusei	≤0.25		0.5	≥1
	C. parapsilosis, C. guilliermondii	≤2		4	≥8
Anidulafungin, caspofungin	C. glabrata	≤0.12		0.25	≥0.5
Micafungin	C. glabrata	≤0.06		0.12	≥0.25

I = intermediate; R = resistant.

VIRUSES

There are approximately 650 viruses that are known to cause infection in humans and other vertebrate animals.[62] The three major properties that classify viruses into families include (1) the NA core (either DNA or ribonucleic acid [RNA], but not both); (2) whether the viral NA is single- or double-stranded; and (3) the presence or absence of a lipoprotein envelope (Tables 17-16 and 17-17).[62-64] Virus families can be further categorized on the basis of morphology (e.g., size, shape, and substructure), mode of replication, and molecular and genomic characteristics. The most recent information on the rapidly changing classification and taxonomy of viruses can be obtained from the website database (www.ncbi.nlm.nih.gov/ICTVdb/) that has been established by The International Committee on Taxonomy of Viruses (ICTV). The 2011 ICTV report now recognizes five hierarchical ranks consisting of six orders, 94 families, 22 subfamilies, 395 genera, and 2475 species of viruses; however, over 3000 viruses remain unclassified.

The Identification of Viruses

The ability to detect and accurately identify viruses in the clinical laboratory has increased during the last 30 years as a result of wider applicability of diagnostic laboratory techniques with increased sensitivity and decreased turnaround time, the availability of newer reagents and rapid commercial diagnostic kits, and the addition of new antiviral drugs for specific viral infections.[64-66] In addition, the improvements in cell cultures and increased availability of viral antigen and nucleic-acid hybridization and amplification-based tests (including

TABLE 17-16. Characteristics and Laboratory Diagnosis of Selected DNA Viruses of Medical Importance to Humans[62-64]

FAMILY	NATURE	ENVELOPE	SHAPE	NUCLEOCAPSID, SYMMETRY	EXAMPLES OF SPECIES COMMONLY INFECTING HUMANS	METHODS COMMONLY USED FOR DETECTION OF VIRUS[a]
Adenoviridae	dsDNA, linear	No	Isometric	Icosahedral	Human adenovirus A to G	Cell culture, IA, NA, histology (myocarditis, pericarditis)
						IA, EM (fecal specimens)
Anelloviridae	ssDNA (-), circular	No	Isometric	Icosahedral	Torque teno virus 1	Cell culture
Hepadnaviridae	dsDNA, circular	Yes	Spherical	Icosahedral	HBV	IA, NA, serology
Herpesviridae	dsDNA, linear	Yes	Spherical	Icosahedral	Human herpesvirus 1 and 2 (HSV-1 HSV-2)	Cell culture, IA, NA
					Human herpesvirus 3 (VZV)	Cell culture, IA, NA
					Human herpesvirus 4 (EBV)	Serology, NA, histology (lymphoid disorders)
					Human herpesvirus 5 (human CMV)	Cell culture, NA, histology (diarrhea or hepatitis), serology (pharyngitis)
					Human herpesvirus 6 (HHV-6) and 7 (HHV-7)	NA, serology (parotitis)
					Human herpesvirus 8 (Kaposi sarcoma–associated herpesvirus)	Serology, histology, NA
Papillomaviridae	dsDNA, circular	No	Isometric	Icosahedral	Human papillomavirus (HPV 1, 4, 5, 32, 41)	NA, cytopathology
Parvoviridae	ssDNA, linear	No	Isometric	Icosahedral	Human parvovirus B19 (exanthema in children)	NA, serology
Polyomaviridae	dsDNA, circular	No	Isometric	Icosahedral	JC polyomavirus (JCV)	NA, histology
					BK polyomavirus (BKV)	NA, cytology
Poxviridae	dsDNA, linear	Yes	Brick-shaped or oval	Complex	Variola virus (Smallpox virus); Vaccinia virus; Cowpox virus; Monkeypox virus	EM, NA, serology, cell culture[b]
					Molluscum contagiosum virus	Histology

(-) = negative stranded; CMV = cytomegalovirus; EBV = Epstein-Barr virus, EM = electron microscopy; dsDNA, double-stranded DNA; HAV = hepatitis A virus; HBV = hepatitis B virus; HPV = human papillomavirus; HSV = herpes simplex virus; IA = immunoassay; NA = nucleic acid; ssDNA = single-stranded DNA; VZV = varicella-zoster virus.

[a]Commonly used methods in clinical laboratories: Immunoassays (including immunofluorescence assay (IFA); enzyme-linked immunosorbent assay (ELISA), and immunochromatographic assay (ICA).

[b]The isolation of some pathogens (e.g., Smallpox) requires biosafety level (BSL) 3 or 4 facilities, usually only in specialized centers collaborating with World Health Organization. The isolation of Vaccinia virus requires BSL-2 (grows readily in cell culture).

TABLE 17-17. Characteristics and Laboratory Diagnosis of Selected RNA Viruses of Medical Importance to Humans[62-64]

FAMILY	NATURE	ENVELOPE	SHAPE	NUCLEOCAPSID, SYMMETRY	EXAMPLES OF SPECIES INFECTING HUMANS	METHODS COMMONLY USED FOR DETECTION OF VIRUS[a]
Arenaviridae	ssRNA , circular	Yes	Spherical	Helical	Lassa virus	Serology, NA; BSL 4
					Lymphocytic choriomeningitis virus (LCMV)	Serology, NA
					Guanarito virus	Serology; BSL 4
					Junin virus	Serology; BSL 4
					Machupo virus	Serology; BSL 4
					Sabia virus	Serology; BSL 4
Astroviridae	ssRNA (+), linear	No	Isometric	Icosahedral	Human astrovirus	EM, NA, IA
Bornaviridae	ssRNA (-), linear	Yes	Spherical	Helical	Borna disease virus	Serology, IA, NA
Bunyaviridae	ssRNA, linear	Yes	Spherical, pleomorphic	Helical	California encephalitis virus	Serology, antibody detection in CSF
					La Crosse virus	Serology, antibody detection
					Hantaan virus	Serology, EM, NA
Caliciviridae	ssRNA (+), linear	No	Isometric	Icosahedral	Norovirus	IA, NA
					Sapporo virus	EM, IA, NA
Coronaviridae	ssRNA (+), linear	Yes	Spherical, pleomorphic	Helical	Human coronavirus 229E, NL63, HKU1	EM, NA (rhinitis), Serology (pneumonia)
Deltavirus	ssRNA, circular	Yes	Spherical	Helical	HDV	Serology, histology
Filoviridae	ssRNA (-), linear	Yes	Filamentous, pleomorphic	Helical	Cote d'Ivoire ebolavirus; Sudan ebolavirus; Zaire ebolavirus	IA, NA, cell culture; BSL 4
					Lake Victoria marburgvirus	EM, cell culture; BSL 4
Flaviviridae	ssRNA (+), linear	Yes	Spherical	Icosahedral	Tick-borne encephalitis virus	Serology, antibody detection (CSF)
					Dengue virus	Serology, NA, antibody detection (CSF)
					Japanese encephalitis virus	Serology, antibody detection (CSF)
					Murray Valley encephalitis virus	Serology, antibody detection (CSF), NA
					St. Louis encephalitis virus	Serology, antibody detection (CSF)
					West Nile virus	Serology, antibody detection (CSF)
					Yellow fever virus	Serology, NA, histology
					Yellow fever virus	Serology, NA
Hepeviridae	ssRNA (+), linear	No	Isometric	Icosahedral	HEV	Serology
Orthomyxoviridae	ssRNA (-), linear	Yes	Pleomorphic	Helical	Influenza virus A, B, C	Rapid culture, IA; NA is an emerging test

TABLE 17-17. Characteristics and Laboratory Diagnosis of Selected RNA Viruses of Medical Importance to Humans (cont'd)[62-64]

FAMILY	NATURE	ENVELOPE	SHAPE	NUCLEOCAPSID, SYMMETRY	EXAMPLES OF SPECIES INFECTING HUMANS	METHODS COMMONLY USED FOR DETECTION OF VIRUS[a]
Paramyxoviridae	ssRNA (-), linear	Yes	Pleomorphic	Helical	Mumps virus	Cell culture, NA, serology
					Measles virus	Serology, NA, histology
					Parainfluenza virus 1,2,3,4	Cell culture, IA, NA
					Human RSV	Cell culture, IA, NA, rapid antigen tests
					Human metapneumovirus	Cell culture, NA
Picobirnaviridae	dsRNA, linear	No	Isometric	Icosahedral	Human picobirnavirus	Cell culture, NA
Picornaviridae	ssRNA (+), linear	No	Isometric	Icosahedral	Human enterovirus A, B, C, D	Cell culture, NA
					Human rhinovirus A, B, C	Cell culture (usually not necessary), NA
					HAV	Serology
					Human parechovirus	Cell culture, NA
Reoviridae	dsRNA, linear	No	Isometric	Icosahedral	Rotavirus A, B, C	IA, LA
Retroviridae	ssRNA (+), linear	Yes	Spherical	Icosahedral	Human immunodeficiency viruses types 1 (HIV-1) and 2 (HIV-2)	Serology, NA
					Primate T-lymphotropic viruses, (HTLV-1 and HTLV-2)	Serology, NA
					Simian foamy virus	Serology, NA
Rhabdoviridae	ssRNA (-), linear	Yes	Bullet shaped	Helical	Rabies virus	Histology, IA, NA
					Arboviruses including alphaviruses	Serology, NA
Togaviridae	ssRNA (+), linear	Yes	Spherical	Icosahedral	Rubella virus	Serology, cell culture

(+) = positive stranded; (-) = negative stranded; BSL = biosafety level; CSF = cerebrospinal fluid; dsRNA = double-stranded RNA; EM = electron microscopy; HAV = hepatitis A virus; HCV = hepatitis C virus; HDV = hepatitis D virus; HEV = hepatitis E virus; HIV = human immunodeficiency virus; IA = immunoassay; LA = latex agglutination; NA = nucleic acid; ssRNA = single-stranded RNA; RSV = respiratory syncytial virus.
[a]Commonly used methods in clinical laboratories: Immunoassays, including immunofluorescence assay (IFA); enzyme-linked immunosorbent assay (ELISA); and immunochromatographic assay (ICA).

real-time PCR) are allowing diagnostic virology laboratories to provide clinical services for the increasing frequency of infectious diseases that depend on viral diagnosis.[66,67]

It is important to note that all diagnostic tests for the identification of viruses are not available at each institution, and the clinician will need to establish a relationship with the laboratory that will be performing viral testing. In certain clinical situations, samples may need to be sent out for diagnostic testing at either large reference or public health laboratories since they are able to provide the necessary methods that are difficult or impossible to routinely perform in the clinical virology laboratory. In addition, certain viruses (e.g., arboviruses, arenaviruses, filiviruses, Variola virus, and rabies virus) require testing

at biosafety level (BSL) 3 or 4 facilities and are often sent to the Centers for Disease Control and Prevention (CDC) or the CDC's Division of Vector-Borne Infectious Diseases.[64]

The ability to accurately diagnose a viral infection is highly dependent on appropriate selection, timing, collection, and handling of biological specimens.[63,65] In general, the highest titers of viruses are present early in the course of illness and decrease as the duration of illness increases. Therefore, it is very important to collect specimens for the detection of viruses early in the course of an infection. In most cases, identification of viruses is a specimen-driven process. Since collection procedures are highly dependent on viruses being suspected, attention needs to be taken regarding collection containers and devices as well as transport systems (e.g., whether a viral transport medium is needed). The different types of clinical specimens that can be collected for viral culture and antigen detection include respiratory specimens (e.g., nasopharyngeal swabs, aspirates, and washes; throat swabs; BAL and bronchial washes), blood, bone marrow, CSF, stool, biopsy tissue, urine, ocular specimens, vesicles and other skin lesions, and amniotic fluid. In addition, specimens for molecular diagnostic testing (e.g., PCR and other nucleic amplification techniques) must be obtained following specific guidelines so that the stability and amplifiability of the nucleic acids are ensured.

Once the sample is collected, it should be promptly transported to the laboratory in a sterile, leak-proof container using the appropriate viral transport media to maximize viral recovery. Every effort should be made to prevent delay between the time of specimen collection and its arrival to the laboratory. When delays are expected, viral samples should be refrigerated at 4°C or frozen at –70°C. Subsequently, the laboratory will need to follow specific processing procedures for each specimen and the different diagnostic viral test methodologies.

The laboratory techniques used in the diagnosis of viral infections include cell culture, cytology and histology, electron microscopy (EM), antigen detection, NA detection, and serologic testing.[64-67] The choice of test(s) will vary depending on the clinical syndrome or disease, virus(es) involved, patient characteristics, collection site, purposes of the test (e.g., screening, diagnosis, confirmation or monitoring), time to result, laboratory capabilities/staff expertise, and cost. The following section, as well as Tables 17-16 and 17-17, provide a brief summary of the common methods currently used in diagnostic testing of common viruses.[64-67] For more detailed information, the reader is referred to current published literature, standard reference books, and the latest edition of reference manuals (e.g., *Manual of Clinical Microbiology*, American Society for Microbiology Press).

Cell Culture

The use of *cell culture* rapidly expanded the knowledge about the epidemiology, clinical characteristics, and diagnosis of common viral infections in the 1950s and 1960s. Subsequently, the use of cell cultures to isolate a virus became the gold standard method for the diagnosis of viral infections in most clinical virology laboratories.[64,67] The advantages of cell culture include good specificity and sensitivity, the capability of detecting multiple viruses if present, and the cultivation of the virus for further laboratory testing (e.g., susceptibility testing, serologic strain typing), if needed. Cell cultures can be useful when combined with highly specific monoclonal antibodies (MAbs), if the cost of other testing methods are greater than cell cultures or when the clinical laboratory does not have the ability and/or equipment to perform molecular detection methods. The disadvantages of cell culture include the long time needed for the detection of viruses using conventional cell culture (e.g., days to weeks), the need for cell culture facilities, the expense of performing cell culture, and the methodology is not applicable to all viruses (e.g., some viruses have not been successfully grown in cultures). The technical demand that cell

cultures place on the diagnostic virology laboratory is being challenged by the rapid evolution of antigen screening assays and NA amplification tests.

There are several different types of cell culture that are available to grow clinically important viruses.[65,67] A cell line can be established once a cell culture has been subcultured in vitro. The different types of cell lines can be divided into three categories: primary, diploid (also called *low passage cell lines*), and heteroploid. Primary cell lines (e.g., rhesus monkey kidney [RhMK] cells or human amnion cells) are prepared from animal or human tissues and can withstand only one or two passages until the cells die. Diploid cell lines are usually derived from fetal or newborn cells (e.g., human embryonic lung fibroblast lines such as WI-38 or MRC-5) and can undergo 20 to 50 passages before cells are unable to survive. Continuous cell lines can undergo an indefinite number of passages without reducing the sensitivity to virus infection. Heteroploid cell lines are characteristically derived from human or animal cancers (e.g., human epidermoid lung carcinoma [HEp-2, HeLa]) or are cells transformed in vitro (e.g., LLC-MK$_2$). Heteroploid cell lines can also include genetically engineered cells (e.g., ELVIS cell mixture for the detection of HSV types 1 and 2). Most specimens are inoculated onto two or more cell lines (e.g., RhMK, MRC-5, HEp-2) based on the most likely viruses associated with the type of clinical specimen that was submitted.

The growth of a virus from a clinical specimen provides direct evidence that the patient was infected with a virus. The main method for detecting growth from the cell culture method is by microscopic examination of the unstained cell cultured monolayers for morphological changes or cytopathic effect (CPE).[65-67] The characteristics of the CPE (e.g., which cell culture types were affected; what is the resultant shape of the cells; whether the effect is focal or diffuse; the time of its appearance and progression) can be used for primary and/or definitive identification of the virus. Subsequently, fluorescent antibody (FA) staining of cells with virus-specific MAbs harvested from the culture is often used to confirm the identification of the virus. Molecular or ancillary traditional testing can alternatively be used for viral identification.

Some viruses, such as influenza, parainfluenza, and mumps virus, will grow in cell cultures without producing CPE so that other methods are used to identify and detect these viruses, including hemadsorption and interference.[65-67] Hemadsorption is used to detect these viruses, which can grow rapidly and reach high titers in cell cultures without producing CPE. Hemadsorption involves the removal of the culture medium from the inoculated cell culture, adding a suspension of erythrocytes and examining for hemadsorption with a low-power microscope as manifested by adherence of the red cells to the cell culture monolayer due to the presence of a hemadsorbing virus. Used to detect viruses such as rubella, interference involves growing a virus that yields a cell culture resistant to other viruses (to which it is normally susceptible). The viruses that produce hemadsorption or interference subsequently can be identified by staining with virus-specific monoclonal antibodies or antiserum.

Shell vial with centrifugation and pre-CPE detection are used to decrease the amount of time required to grow a virus by conventional cell cultures. [65–67] This technique makes use of cells grown on microscope coverslips that are placed within shell vials and covered with culture media. After cultures are incubated for 1–3 days, FA staining is performed on the cells on the coverslips to recognize an antigen in the nucleus of infected cells. Shell vial cultures have been commonly applied for the detection of cytomegalovirus (CMV), HSV, varicella-zoster virus (VZV), enteroviruses, and the human respiratory viruses. Centrifugation-enhanced rapid cell cultures can also be used with co-cultivated cells (e.g., mixture of two cell lines together) or genetically engineered cells (e.g., ELVIS [enzyme-linked virus-inducible system], BGMK-hDAF [buffalo green monkey kidney cell line]) for the rapid identification (e.g., 16 to 72 hours) and blind staining of multiple viruses from a single shell vial or tray well. [66,67]

Cytology and Histology

Cytologic examination can be performed on smears prepared from samples that are applied to a microscope slide or "touch preps" of unfixed tissues. [65] Cytologic findings are suggestive of a viral infection and provide identification of cell morphologies (e.g., "owl's eye" nuclear inclusions consistent with CMV). The specific virus cannot be identified unless virus-specific immunostaining techniques are used. Applications of *cytology* to viral diagnosis include the Tzanck smear with Giemsa reagent for demonstrating the presence of HSV or VZV infection, Papanicolaou staining of cells obtained from the uterine cervix (Pap smear) for providing evidence of human papillomavirus (HPV) infection, and cytologic staining of urinary sediments for screening the presence of either CMV or polyomaviruses JCV and BKV.

Similar to cytology, histologic examination of tissue provides evidence to suggest a group of viruses that may be causing infection, but it does not identify a specific virus. [64,66] Despite this shortcoming, histopathology has been useful in differentiating between asymptomatic viral shedding and clinically important infections of CMV and has been used for the diagnosis of CMV infections in tissue samples obtained from biopsy or at autopsy. In addition, detection of specific viral antigens by immunohistochemistry (IHC) and detection of specific viral nucleic acids by in situ hybridization (ISH) has allowed specific viruses to be identified by histopathology.

Electron Microscopy

Viruses are the smallest infectious pathogens that range in diameter from 18–300 nm. [65] Direct visualization of a virus with a light microscope can only be performed on pathogens with a diameter greater than 200 nm. The *electron microscopy (EM)* allows visualization of characteristic viral morphology, and unlike direct detection or molecular methodologies, is capable of detecting the distinctive appearances of multiple viruses, if present. [65] Electron microscopy is considered the most useful routine test for poxviruses. [66] Diagnostic virology laboratories also commonly use EM for detection of viruses that are not detected with cell cultures or other methods (e.g.,

gastroenteritis viruses such as noroviruses, coronaviruses, astroviruses, enteric adenovirus, and calicivirus). [64,66]

Several techniques have been incorporated to allow the visualization of viruses with EM from various types of clinical specimens. Negative staining is a technique for identification of viruses in fluid samples, stool samples, and blister fluid. Thin sectioning can be performed on tissue samples that have been fixed with specific fixatives for EM study, and it can be used to visualize the herpesviruses, respiratory viruses, and rabies virus.

More sensitive methods are replacing the routine use of EM for detecting clinically significant viruses. [64,66] The advantages of EM include its economical, quick (e.g., same day), adaptable, and straightforward approach for detecting viruses. The major disadvantages of EM include poor sensitivity, initial equipment expenses, and the need of highly skilled laboratory staff.

Direct Antigen Detection

Antigen detection methods involve the use of virus-specific antibodies directed toward viral antigens in a clinical specimen. [59] Examples of viruses that can be identified by direct antigen detection include respiratory syncytial virus (RSV), influenza virus, parainfluenza virus, adenovirus, HSV, VZV, CMV, rotavirus, hepatitis B virus (HBV), and measles virus. [64,66] The advantages of direct antigen detection include the rapidity of diagnosis (e.g., hours to 1 day), the usefulness for the identification of viruses that are difficult to culture, and the detection of viral specific antigens even if viable virus is not present in the clinical specimen. The disadvantages include the potential for false-positive and false-negative results, the difficulty of performing batch testing, and the lack of sensitivity necessary for diagnostic applications for all viruses (e.g., not applicable for rhinoviruses since there are more than 90 serotypes and cross-reacting antibodies).

The techniques commonly used for antigen detection include immunofluorescence assay (IFA; direct and indirect), EIA (including ELISA), chemiluminescent and fluorescence-based immunoassay, and particle agglutination assays. Several membrane immunochromatographic assays (ICAs; dipstick tests) are available as influenza diagnostic tests (e.g., Directigen Flu A or A+B Test, QuickVue influenza, Directigen Flu A+B). These viral antigen tests have become simple to use and allow rapid detection (within minutes) of specific antigens from a single specimen in the clinical laboratory and at the point of care (e.g., outpatient facilities, physician offices, patient's bedside). A recent systematic review found rapid influenza diagnostic tests (RIDTs) to have high specificity but moderate and variable sensitivity (higher in children and for detecting influenza A). [68] The need for improved sensitivity of RIDTs was also observed during the 2009 pandemic of H1N1 influenza.

Serology

Serologic tests are designed to detect an antibody response in serum samples after exposure to viral antigens has occurred. [65] The major uses of *serology* for the detection of viral infections include the demonstration of immunity or exposure to a virus, the diagnosis of postinfectious sequelae, and the screening of blood products. In several clinical situations, serologic testing remains the primary means for the laboratory diagnosis of viruses that are difficult to culture or detect by direct methods (e.g., rubella virus, Epstein-Barr virus [EBV], hepatitis viruses, HIV, arboviruses).[64,66] Serologic testing may also serve as a supportive or adjunctive role in clinical situations where viral cultures or direct detection methods are available.

For viral infections, serologic testing can (1) identify the virus; (2) distinguish the strain or serotype; (3) differentiate between primary infection and reinfection; and (4) determine if the infection is in an acute or convalescent phase. Virus-specific immunoglobulin antibodies (e.g., IgM or IgG) are produced during the time course of a viral infection. In general, virus-specific IgM is detected in serum sooner than virus-specific IgG. The results measure the relative concentration of antibody in the body as a titer, with the titer representing the lowest antibody concentration (or inverse of the greatest dilution; a dilution of 1:128 is expressed as a titer of 128) that demonstrates activity in a patient's serum. The exact value for a titer varies with each testing method, the specific virus involved, the timing of specimen collection, and the presence of active disease.

For most viral infections, virus-specific IgM can be detected as soon as 3–7 days after the onset of infection. The presence of virus-specific IgM in a single serum sample shortly after the onset of symptoms (acute phase) is usually indicative of a very recent or current primary infection. Titers of virus-specific IgM usually decline to near undetectable amounts within 1–4 months after the onset of infection. Virus-specific IgG can be detected during the acute phase of infection (e.g., 1–2 weeks) and will continue to increase for several months before reaching a maximal titer. Thereafter, the IgG titer will decline, but it usually remains detectable in serum for the remainder of a person's life. Seroconversion has occurred when at least a fourfold increase in IgG titer has occurred between serum samples collected in the acute and convalescent (2–4 weeks afterward) phases. The presence of virus-specific IgG is also indicative of a past infection.

Serologic tests are also used to assess the immunity or exposure to a virus. The presence of antibody can detect which patients have been previously infected by or vaccinated for a specific virus. For example, a positive result (presence of antibody) for rubella in a woman of childbearing age implies that congenital infection will not occur during subsequent pregnancies. A negative result (absence of antibody) implies susceptibility to infection, and the woman should receive rubella vaccination if she is not pregnant. Some other examples of viruses for which serologic determination of immune status is useful include hepatitis A and B (HAV, HBV), measles, mumps, parvovirus B19, and VZV.[65,66]

The techniques commonly used for serologic assays include CF, EIA, IFA, anticomplement immunofluorescence, and Western immunoblotting. In the diagnosis of certain viral syndromes (e.g., central nervous system [CNS] infections), a serology panel may be helpful so that a battery of antigens is tested for antibody to several viruses. The advantages of viral serology include the assessment of immunity or response of a virus isolated from a nonsterile site, serum specimens are easy to obtain and store, and it can be used to identify viruses that are difficult to culture or detect by immunoassay. The disadvantages include the time to results (e.g., few days to weeks), the potential for cross-reactions between different viruses, and the need for both acute and convalescent specimens.

Molecular Diagnosis

The detection of specific viral nucleic acids (NAs) by molecular diagnostic techniques is revolutionizing the field of diagnostic virology.[64-67] Molecular methods are rapidly becoming the "gold standard" in clinical virology laboratories and will likely replace older techniques such as cell cultures for detecting clinically significant viruses. The techniques used in viral NA detection include direct hybridization assays, target (template) amplification (e.g., PCR, self-sustained sequence replication [3SR] method, strand displacement amplification [SDA]), and signal amplification (e.g., branched-chain DNA [bDNA] assay and hybrid capture assay). Among these, PCR has been the most important technique in diagnostic virology because of its versatility in detecting DNA or RNA, as well as being able to provide qualitative and quantitative information on specific viral nucleic acids.

The use of NA detection has become the standard of care (e.g., HCV and HIV) or the test of choice for routine diagnosis of many viral infections (e.g., bocaviruses, HSV CNS infections, human HVS 6 and 7, human metapneumovirus, HPV).[64,66] The FDA has cleared or approved commercial molecular detection assays, several viruses including hepatitis B and C viruses (HBV, HCV), HIV, HSV, CMV, adenovirus, avian flu, enteroviruses, influenza, and HPV. An FDA-approved multiplex PCR kit (e.g., xTAG Respiratory Viral Panel) is also available for rapidly screening 12 common respiratory viruses (e.g., RSV, influenza A and B, adenovirus) or subtypes. An up-to-date listing of FDA-cleared/approved molecular diagnostics tests is available on the website of the Association of Molecular Pathology (www.amp.org).

The advantages of viral NA detection methods include the rapidity of results (e.g., hours for real-time PCR and one to several days for other methods), maximal sensitivity for virus-specific detection and identification, adequate to excellent specificity, increasing availability of commercial assays, the ability to detect viruses that are difficult to culture, and the ability to detect nucleic acids without viable virus present in the clinical specimen. The disadvantages of these techniques include the need for molecular facilities for selected tests, labor-intense methodology, and a potential for PCR contamination that may lead to false-positive results. Molecular assays are rapidly becoming the standard of care for diagnosing viral infections as well as monitoring antiviral therapy and patient outcomes.[64,66]

Antiviral Susceptibility Testing

The emergence of drug-resistant strains of viruses to antiviral agents is an increasing problem, especially in immunocompromised hosts. Unlike antibiotics, in vitro susceptibility testing of viruses has not been routinely available. The major variables that have limited the standardization of antiviral susceptibility testing include cell lines, inoculums titer, incubation period, testing range of antiviral drug concentrations, reference strains, assay methodology, and criteria, calculation, and interpretation of end-points.[69]

Susceptibility testing has been performed by phenotypic and/or genotypic assays for HIV-1, HBV, HSV, VZV, CMV, and influenza viruses.[69] The CLSI has published an approved standard for phenotypic susceptibility testing of HSV.[70] This standard outlines the use of a plaque reduction assay and denotes resistance to acyclovir and foscarnet when IC_{50} values are ≥2 mcg/mL and ≥100 mcg/mL, respectively. Interpretation of these values must be carefully made in conjunction with the clinical response of the individual patient. Other consensus documents for antiviral susceptibility testing are needed.

HUMAN IMMUNODEFICIENCY VIRUS

Human immunodeficiency virus (HIV) is the causative agent of AIDS. The HIV virus is an enveloped, positively-stranded RNA virus that belongs to the Retroviridae (retrovirus) family and *Lentivirus* genus. The mature virus measures approximately 100 nm in diameter and has a characteristic conical core containing proteins, enzymes, and two identical copies of single-stranded RNA. Viral proteins within the core and the lipid envelope play a significant role in the detection, diagnosis, and treatment of HIV.[71,72] The replication process of HIV involves transcription of viral RNA into proviral DNA using the reverse transcriptase (RT) enzyme. The proviral DNA is then integrated into the host's genome using the integrase enzyme, resulting in lifelong latent infection. The virus is transmitted to humans by the exchange of blood or other body fluids containing the virus through sexual contact; exposure to contaminated blood; transfusion of contaminated blood and/or blood products; or via contaminated needles (e.g., intravenous drug abusers or accidental needle sticks). In addition, infants can acquire HIV from an infected mother in utero, during labor or delivery, or during breast-feeding.[71,73]

There are two distinct serotypes of HIV, namely HIV-1 and HIV-2; while HIV-1 is the most prevalent serotype of HIV infections worldwide, HIV-2 infection is most commonly distributed in Western Africa and other limited geographic locations.[71–73] Routine diagnostic testing of HIV-2 is not recommended in the United States since its prevalence is extremely low. Thus, the following discussion will focus mainly on laboratory tests used for the diagnosis and management of HIV-1 infection. However, HIV-2 testing may be indicated in persons at risk for HIV-2 infection or for those who have symptoms suggestive of HIV infection with negative or indeterminate test results for HIV-1. In addition, all blood donations in the United States are tested for both HIV-1 and HIV-2.[71–73]

Laboratory Tests for HIV-1 Infection

Several laboratory tests are available for the diagnosis and monitoring of patients with HIV-1 infection. The most common virologic testing methods include HIV-1 antibody assays, HIV-1 p24 antigen assays, DNA-PCR, plasma HIV-1 RNA (viral load) assays, and viral phenotypic and genotypic assays. In addition, the absolute number of CD4+ lymphocytes and the ratio of helper (CD4+) to suppressor (CD8+) lymphocytes (CD4+:CD8+ ratios) are routinely measured to evaluate the patient's immune status and response to antiretroviral therapy, since HIV primarily infects and depletes CD4+ T helper lymphocytes. Viral cultures for HIV are not typically performed beyond clinical research studies due to the labor-intensive nature of the testing methods as well as the extensive time required to obtain results.[63–65]

Laboratory tests for HIV-1 infection are clinically utilized for (1) diagnosing HIV-1 infection; (2) monitoring progression of HIV infection and the response to antiretroviral therapy; and (3) screening blood donors. The selection of these tests is highly dependent on the clinical situation, the patient population, and the specified purpose for the testing, as described in Table 17-18.[73–77] (See Minicase 4.) The following section briefly reviews each of the specific tests. Detailed descriptions of the various commercial assays and their clinical applications have been recently reviewed elsewhere.[71,73,74,78]

HIV Antibody Tests

Infection with HIV affects both humoral and cell-mediated immune function. The humoral immune response results in the production of antibodies directed against HIV-specific proteins and glycoproteins. For most patients, antibodies to

---

MINICASE 4

Testing for HIV After Occupational Exposure

JAMES D. IS A NURSE IN THE EMERGENCY DEPARTMENT who is currently finishing up his overnight shift. He is drawing blood from an unresponsive patient during an emergency and he accidentally sticks himself with a used large bore needle before the patient is transported to a different hospital. Because of this exposure, James D. is instructed to immediately seek attention at Employee Health to obtain testing for HIV and HCV. The HIV and hepatitis C status of the patient is unknown. James D. is advised by the physician at Employee Health to submit a blood sample for immediate testing, as well as to return at regular intervals during the next 6 months for additional testing.

Question: How long will James D. have to wait before he can be certain that he did not acquire HIV from the exposure?

Discussion: The hallmark tests for diagnosing HIV infection include the ELISA (or EIA) and a confirmatory western blot. The ELISA test detects the presence of anti-HIV antibodies, which may take several weeks to months before they appear in the blood of a newly infected patient. The HIV status of the source patient is unknown. Therefore, if possible, the source patient should be questioned regarding risk factors that may predispose to HIV infection, as well as undergo HIV testing (rapid screen and ELISA). Even if the source patient is currently HIV negative by ELISA, James D. will need to undergo testing for at least 6 months before HIV infection can be ruled out.

TABLE 17-18. Recommended Laboratory Tests for the Diagnosis, Monitoring, and Blood Donor Screening for HIV[73–77]

CLINICAL SITUATION	RECOMMENDED TEST(S)	COMMENTS
Diagnosis of HIV infection (excluding infants and acute infection)	Antibody ELISA and confirmatory WB	The combination of ELISA and WB testing has a positive predictive value of ~100%
Diagnosis of acute HIV infection	Antibody ELISA, confirmatory WB, plasma HIV RNA viral load, p24 antigen assay	Plasma HIV RNA is generally very high (>100,000 copies/mL)
Diagnosis of HIV in infants (<18 months of age) born to HIV-infected mother	HIV DNA PCR or plasma HIV RNA viral	Initial testing recommended between 14 and 21 days of life, 1–2 months, and 3–6 months; diagnosis of HIV by two positive virologic tests; HIV antibody testing not recommended due to persistence of maternal antibody
Indeterminate HIV-1 WB result	Repeat HIV-1 antibody ELISA and WB; plasma HIV RNA viral load	Careful patient history to assess the risks for HIV-1 or HIV-2 infection; consider testing for HIV-2; perform more sensitive diagnostic tests; repeat HIV-1 antibody testing in 3–6 months
Prognosis	Plasma HIV RNA viral load and CD4+ T cell count	Risk of disease progression greater with HIV RNA >100,000 copies/mL
Response to antiretroviral therapy	Plasma HIV RNA viral load and CD4+ T cell count	Decision to start therapy should be based on laboratory results as well as clinical findings, patient interests, adherence issues, and risks of toxicity and drug interactions
Antiretroviral drug resistance testing	Phenotypic and/or genotypic resistance assays	Recommended for acute and chronic HIV infection on entry into care, treatment naïve patients, pregnant patients, and cases of virologic failure (testing recommended within 4 weeks of treatment discontinuation); not recommended for patients with HIV RNA <1000 copies/mL
Blood donor screening	Antibody ELISA and WB; p24 antigen; plasma HIV RNA viral load	In the United States, the blood from all donors is tested for HIV-1 and HIV-2 antibodies as well as p24 antigens

DNA = deoxyribonucleic acid; ELISA = enzyme-linked immunosorbent assay; HIV = human immunodeficiency virus; RNA = ribonucleic acid; PCR = polymerase chain reaction; WB = western blot.

HIV-1 can be detected in the blood by 4–8 weeks after exposure to the virus; however, it may take up to 6–12 months in some patients. There are a number of tests currently available for the detection of HIV-antibody in infected patients.

The methodology of EIA (commonly referred to as ELISA) is widely used as the *initial* screening test to detect HIV-specific antibodies.[71,73,74,79] Like all immunoassays, ELISA is based on the concept of antigen and antibody reaction to form a measurable precipitate. The ability of ELISA to detect HIV antibodies during earlier infection has improved over recent years. Although less specific, first-generation ELISA tests introduced in 1985 were capable of detecting HIV-1 antibodies as soon as 40 days after exposure. Second-generation ELISA, introduced in 1987, incorporated recombinant antigens that increased specificity, sensitivity, and the ability to detect antibodies as soon as 34 days after infection. With the introduction of antigens from HIV-2, and the addition of antigens from HIV-1 groups M, N, and O and group M subtypes in the 1990s, specificity and sensitivity were improved. Third-generation ELISA, introduced in the mid 1990s, were redesigned as an antigen-antibody-antigen format, which dramatically improved sensitivity and specificity, and are able to detect immunoglobulin M

(IgM) and non-IgG antibodies as soon as 22 days after infection. Fourth-generation ELISA detects the presence of both HIV antibodies and p24 antigen, which has reduced the detection period to 15 days after infection, similar to the period of detection of p24 antigen. Commercial ELISA kits utilized by most diagnostic laboratories can detect both HIV-1 and HIV-2, and have a sensitivity and specificity of greater than 99%; however, false-positive and false-negative results can occur. False-positive results have been reported with improper specimen handling (e.g., heating) and in patients with autoimmune diseases, recent influenza vaccination, acute viral infection, alcoholic liver disease, chronic renal failure requiring hemodialysis, lymphoma, hematologic malignancies, and positive rapid plasma reagin (RPR) tests due to reactivity of the antibodies used for testing. Thus, ELISA should not be used alone in making a diagnosis of HIV infection, and positive results *must be confirmed* with a more specific test such as the western blot (WB). Several causes have been identified for false-negative ELISA results and include the concomitant use of immunosuppressive therapy, the presence of severe hypogammaglobulinemia, and testing for HIV infection shortly after infection [acute HIV infection] or too late in the course of HIV infection.[71,73]

The results of the ELISA test are reported as reactive (positive) or nonreactive (negative). If the initial result is nonreactive, no further testing for HIV antibodies is performed and the person is considered uninfected unless they are suspected of having acute HIV infection. When the initial result is reported as reactive, the same test should be repeated in duplicate. If the repeated result is nonreactive, then it can be assumed that an assay or laboratory error occurred during the first test and the patient is considered uninfected. If the duplicate test is also reactive, the results should be reported as "repeatedly reactive" and a more specific supplemental test for confirming the presence of antibodies specific to HIV-1 must be performed in order to confirm the diagnosis of HIV infection.[73,80]

The WB is the confirmatory test of choice for detecting HIV-specific antibody.[71,73,79,80] The WB is a protein electrophoretic immunoblot technique that detects specific antibodies to HIV protein and glycoprotein antigens. The proteins and glycoproteins are detected by WB as "bands" and can be divided into Env (envelope) glycoproteins (gp41, gp120, gp160), Gag or nuclear proteins (p17, p24/25, p55), and Pol or endonuclease-polymerase proteins (p34, p40, p52, p68). The WB test is reported as positive, indeterminate, or negative based on the presence or absence of bands representing HIV antibodies. Criteria for the interpretation of WB results have been published by different health organizations and may vary depending on the issuing body. For example, according to the World Health Organization (WHO), a WB is considered positive if any two Env bands are found, whereas the Centers for Disease Control and Prevention (CDC) considers a WB as positive if bands are present for two of three HIV-specific proteins including p24, gp41, and gp120/160. An indeterminate result represents the presence of bands associated with HIV, but do not meet the criteria for a positive result. A WB result without bands for HIV antibodies is considered negative, and it can be assumed that the ELISA results were a false positive. The WB characteristically has a lower level of sensitivity but is highly specific. The WB test is not considered a suitable initial screening test for detecting the presence of HIV antibodies because it is technically difficult to perform, expensive, associated with a relatively high rate of indeterminate results (4 to 20%), and has a long turnaround time (results are available in 1–2 weeks).[71,73,74] Indeterminate WB results can occur because of testing too early or too late in the course of HIV infection, cross-reactivity with HIV-2 infection, cross-reactivity with HIV-1 subtype O, or the production of nonspecific antibody reactions. If the WB result is indeterminate, then repeat testing with the ELISA and WB is necessary. In addition, specific antibody testing for HIV-2 or other diagnostic test methods may need to be considered (see Table 17-18).

Rapid HIV screening tests. Recent technological advances have allowed for the development of rapid (e.g., 30 minutes) screening tests for the detection of HIV antibodies. The methodology of the rapid HIV antibody assays involves typically either membrane EIA or ICA. Currently, seven rapid HIV-1

screening tests have been approved by the FDA for use in the United States: OraQuick Advance Rapid HIV-1/2 Antibody Test (OraSure Technologies, Inc., Bethlehem, PA), Uni-Gold Recombigen (Trinity Biotech, Bray, Ireland), Reveal G3 (MedMira, Halifax, Nova Scotia), Multispot HIV-1/HIV-2 (Bio-Rad Laboratories, Redmond, WA), Clearview HIV 1/2 Stat Pak and Clearview Complete HIV 1/2 (Chembio Diagnostic Systems, Medford, NY), and INSTI Rapid HIV-1 Antibody Test (bioLytical Laboratories, Inc., Richmond, BC).[71,78] The study and development of new rapid HIV tests continues, while an older testing method, Abbott's Single Use Diagnostic System HIV-1 (SUDS), has been removed from the market. All seven currently approved tests display specificity and sensitivity similar to ELISA, require only basic training in test performance and interpretation, can be stored at room temperature, and require minimal specialized laboratory equipment.[71,78] The OraQuick Advance Rapid HIV-1/2 Antibody Test, UniGold Recombigen, Clearview HIV 1/2 Stat Pak, and Clearview HIV 1/2 Complete tests have received waivers under the Clinical Laboratory Improvement Amendments (CLIA), which allow point-of-care testing where dedicated laboratories are not available as they are less complex to perform and have minimal chance for error.[71,78,81]

The OraQuick Rapid test is a lateral flow immunochromatographic strip (e.g., similar to dipsticks for pregnancy testing) designed as a point-of-care test that can be performed using an oral fluid sample or whole blood sample obtained from a finger stick. A small drop of blood is placed onto a collection loop device, which is then inserted into a vial containing developer solution and stirred. When using an oral specimen, patients are instructed to swab their gums with the collection device, which is then inserted into the developer solution vial. The test device should be inserted into the vial until the results are directly read from the device at no less than 20 minutes (however not greater than 60 minutes). The appearance of two reddish bands is indicative of a reactive (or positive) test for HIV-1 antibodies while the presence of a single reddish band at the control location of the device signifies a negative test.[71,78,82]

The Uni-Gold Recombigen test is a qualitative immunoassay used for the rapid detection of HIV antibodies outside the clinical laboratory using whole blood obtained from a finger stick or venipuncture. The testing procedure involves filling a pipette with blood and placing one drop onto the sample port of the test cartridge. Four drops of a washing reagent are then applied to the sample port, with results read no sooner than 10 minutes and no later than 12 minutes following the application of the washing reagent. A positive result is indicated by the appearance of a line in the test area on the device as well as a line in the control area, while the appearance of only one line in the control area represents a negative test.[71,78,82]

The Clearview HIV 1/2 Stat-Pak is a single-use, ICA designed as a point-of-care test for the diagnosis of HIV-1 or HIV-2 infection. A small drop of whole blood from a finger stick or venipuncture is applied to the sample well on a test cartridge followed by the application of three drops of buffer solution. Results should be read within 15–20 minutes but not later than 20 minutes. A positive test will show two lines, one in the control area and one in the test area while a negative result will have one line in the control area. Similarly, Clearview HIV 1/2 Complete is approved for point-of-care testing for the diagnosis of HIV-1 and HIV-2 infection. It is a closed system test that resembles a syringe with a sampler tip, a test strip enclosed in the barrel, and a single-use vial with buffer at the base of the barrel. It requires less blood volume and reduces biohazard exposure risks. The INSTI Rapid HIV-1 Antibody Test has not yet been waived by CLIA, but employs a simple methodology with results in 60 seconds. After collecting a small amount of blood from a finger stick, the sample is added to vial number 1, the sample diluent. The entire contents of vial number 1 is subsequently poured into the center of a membrane unit, which captures any HIV antibodies present in the sample. A color developer in vial number 2 is poured into the center of the membrane unit, which generates a blue control spot and a second spot if antibodies against HIV are present. The contents of vial number 3, a clarifying solution, are added to the membrane unit to produce more distinct test and control spots.

Rapid HIV testing has proven useful for the detection of HIV infection in a number of clinical settings such as during the labor and delivery of pregnant women at high-risk of HIV infection with unknown serostatus for the purposes of preventing perinatal transmission, facilities where return rates for HIV test results are low, and following occupational exposure to potentially HIV-infected body fluids (e.g., through a needle stick) where immediate decisions regarding postexposure prophylaxis are needed.[71,78,80,83] As with other screening tests for HIV-1 antibodies (including ELISA), a positive result from a rapid HIV test must be confirmed with an alternative method of testing such as WB before the final diagnosis of HIV infection can be established. If the results of a rapid HIV test are negative, a person is considered uninfected. However, retesting should be considered in persons with possible exposure to HIV within the previous 3 months since the testing may have been performed too early in the infection to detect antibodies to the virus.[71,75,78]

Noninvasive HIV-1 tests. Several tests have been developed for testing HIV antibodies from oral fluid or urine.[71,73,80,83] The Orasure Western Blot Kit (OraSure Technologies, Bethlehem, PA) is a supplemental confirmatory test for the OraSure HIV-1 Oral Specimen Collection Device, which uses a cotton fiber pad that is placed between the cheek and lower gum for 2 minutes to collect oral mucosal transudate containing IgG. The Orasure HIV-1 oral device is FDA-approved and has a specificity of 99.4% (similar to EIA). The OraQuick ADVANCE Rapid HIV-1/2 Antibody Test (OraSure Technologies, Bethlehem, PA) detects antibodies against HIV-1 and HIV-2 by swabbing a flat pad against the upper and lower outer gums once, and inserting the sample collection pad into the developer solution vial. After 20 minutes, the results window will indicate whether HIV antibodies have been detected. Two urine-based HIV-1 tests (ELISA and WB) have also been FDA-approved for use, but are associated with lower sensitivity and specificity than

the oral fluid testing. As with ELISA testing of blood samples, confirmatory testing is required for both types of tests if the initial results are positive. Noninvasive HIV-1 testing should be considered in persons unable to access healthcare facilities, have poor venous access, or are reluctant to have their blood drawn. The advantages of these tests include avoidance of blood drawing for sample collection, ease of use, low cost, and stability of samples for up to 3 weeks at room temperature.[71,73]

Home sample collection tests. Several home sample collection tests for the detection of HIV infection are available over-the-counter.[73,80,83] A few drops of whole blood are obtained using a finger stick and placed on a blood specimen card. The dried blood spot is mailed to a designated laboratory that uses ELISA to detect HIV-1 antibodies. The person calls the designated lab for the results (positive or negative for HIV antibodies) over the next 3–7 business days. A telephone counselor provides the test results, telephone support, information, guidance about repeat testing, and referral as needed. The advantages of home sample collection tests include ready access to HIV-1 testing, convenience, lower costs, anonymity, and privacy.[73]

p24 Antigen Tests

A main structural core protein of HIV is *p24*, with levels of p24 antigen being elevated during the early stages of HIV infection. Testing for p24 antigen has diagnostic utility during early infection when low levels of HIV antibody are present.[71,74] The direct detection of HIV-1 p24 antigen can be performed using a plasma or serum EIA assay.[73,80] Similar to antibody testing, positive results of the initial testing for HIV-1 p24 antigen must be retested in duplicate using the same EIA method. In addition, these results need to be confirmed with a neutralization assay due to the potential for p24 antigen testing to produce false-positive reactions resulting from interfering substances.[71,73]

The p24 antigen test may be used for screening blood donors, detecting growth in viral cultures, and as an alternative diagnostic test for HIV-1 in patients suspected of having acute HIV infection or infants less than 18 months of age born to HIV-infected mothers (Table 17-18).[71,73,80] The advantages of the p24 antigen test include the earlier detection of HIV infection compared to antibody testing (16 days versus 22 days); it is easier to perform; has a low cost; and has a specificity that approaches 100%. However, the DNA PCR assays and plasma HIV-RNA concentrations demonstrate greater sensitivity and have replaced the p24 antigen tests in many clinical situations.

HIV DNA PCR

Human immunodeficiency virus DNA polymerase chain reaction (PCR) is used for early detection of proviral HIV-1 DNA in a patient's peripheral blood mononuclear cells (PBMCs). Human immunodeficiency virus DNA PCR is currently recommended for the diagnosis of HIV infection in infants (<18 months of age) born to HIV-infected mothers, and any clinical situations where antibody tests are inconclusive or undetectable (Table 17-18).[71,75] Antibody tests are not useful for diagnosing HIV infection in infants since maternal HIV antibodies can persist in the infant for up to 18 months after birth. Therefore, infants should be tested with the HIV DNA PCR or HIV RNA viral load test initially between 14 and 21 days of age, then at 1–2 months, and age 3–6 months.[75] Negative tests at birth can be repeated at 14 days of life since the assay sensitivity is increased by 2 weeks of life. In order to confirm the diagnosis of HIV infection, a positive result at any sampling time needs to be confirmed by a second HIV virologic test. HIV infection may be excluded in infants with two or more negative HIV virologic results when initial testing occurred at age ≥1 month and the second testing occurred at age ≥4 months.[75]

The advantages of the HIV DNA PCR test include a high level of sensitivity and specificity (96 and 99% at ~1 month of age, respectively), the requirement for only a small volume of blood (e.g., 200 μl), and the rapid turnaround time. The disadvantages include the expense, the high level of interlaboratory variability, and the availability of only one commercial assay (Roche Amplicor HIV DNA assay; Roche Diagnostics, Indianapolis, IN) that is not currently FDA-approved.[71,75]

HIV-RNA Concentration (HIV RNA Viral Load)

The accurate measurement of plasma HIV-RNA concentrations (also known as the *HIV viral load*) in conjunction with CD4+ T lymphocyte count has become an essential component in the management of patients with HIV-1 infection.[71,75,76] These two laboratory tests provide the clinician with information regarding a patient's virologic and immunologic status, which is needed to make decisions regarding the initiation or changing of antiretroviral therapy and to predict the risk of disease progression from HIV infection to AIDS. In addition, plasma HIV-RNA concentrations can assist in the diagnosis of HIV infection in selected clinical situations (see Table 17-18).[75,76]

Current methods that measure the amount of HIV-RNA in plasma include coupling reverse transcription (RT) to a DNA polymerase chain reaction (RT-PCR), identification of HIV-RNA with signal amplification by bDNA and nucleic acid sequence-based amplification (NASBA). Currently, there are five commercial assays approved by the FDA for clinical use: Amplicor HIV-1 Monitor version 1.5 (Roche Diagnostics, Indianapolis, IN), VERSANT HIV-1 RNA 3.0 Assay (Siemens Healthcare Diagnostics, Tarrytown, NY), NucliSens HIV-1 RNA QT (bioMérieux, Inc., Durham, NC), Cobas AmpliPrep/Cobas TaqMan HIV-1 versions 1 and 2 (Roche Diagnostics, Indianapolis, IN), and RealTime TaqMan HIV-1 (Abbott Molecular, DesPlaines, IL).[71,76] The results of these tests are expressed as the number of HIV copies/mL. Higher HIV-RNA levels (e.g., >100,000 copies/mL) represent a substantial risk for disease progression. These assays differ in their dynamic ranges and lower limits of detection of HIV viral copies/mL of plasma. For example, the VERSANT assay has a lower limit of detection of <75 copies/mL while the Cobas AmpliPrep/ Cobas TaqMan version 2 assay detection limit is <20 copies/ mL. Some of these assays have different versions according to the degree of automation and simplicity. For instance, the Amplicor HIV-1 Monitor version 1.5 is a manual test; the Cobas Amplicor HIV-1 Monitor is semi-automated, and the Cobas AmpliPrep/Cobas Amplicor HIV-1 Monitor is automated. Additionally, the Amplicor HIV-1 Monitor and its variants exists as two FDA-approved assays; standard and ultrasensitive, due to its limited dynamic range. The standard assay has a lower limit of detection of 400 copies/mL compared to the ultrasensitive assay which has a limit of 50 copies/mL. It is recommended to utilize both assays concurrently when testing samples that fall outside of the dynamic range. Therefore, if a viral load is reported as "undetectable," it signifies that the plasma HIV-RNA concentrations are below the lower limits of detection of the assay utilized.[71,76] When performing plasma HIV-RNA viral load levels for each patient, the same laboratory and method should be utilized to minimize variation.

Once the diagnosis of HIV-1 infection has been confirmed, a plasma HIV-RNA level should be measured to assist in the decision to start or defer therapy. Ideally, a plasma HIV-RNA level (and CD4+ T lymphocyte count) is measured on two separate occasions as the baseline measurement. The decision to start antiretroviral therapy will depend on the clinical findings and symptoms of the patient, the results of the plasma HIV-RNA levels and CD4+ T lymphocyte count, the willingness of the patient to adhere to therapy, and the potential risks associated with therapy. When initiating antiretroviral therapy, current guidelines recommend monitoring plasma HIV-RNA levels at the following time intervals: immediately before treatment initiation and 2–8 weeks after starting or changing antiretroviral drug therapy; 3–4 months following therapy initiation and every 3–4 months while on therapy; and anytime when clinically indicated, including those patients who experience a significant decline in CD4+ T lymphocyte count. HIV-RNA testing is not recommended during the period of an acute illness (e.g., bacterial or *Pneumocystis jirovecii* pneumonia) or in patients who have been recently vaccinated as these circumstances may increase the viral load for 2–4 weeks. For patients receiving antiretroviral therapy, the goals of therapy include specific reductions in the HIV viral load measured in log reductions over a given time frame as well as achieving a viral load "below the limits of detection." Changes in the amount of plasma HIV-RNA and are often reported in log base 10 values. For example, a change from 10,000 to 1000 copies/mL in a patient on antiretroviral therapy would be considered a 1-log decrease in viral load. With optimal therapy, plasma HIV-RNA levels should decrease by ≥1 $\log_{10}$ during the first 2–8 weeks after initiation of therapy, and should continue to decline over subsequent weeks, with the ultimate goal of achieving an undetectable viral load (e.g., <50 copies/mL) in 16–24 weeks after initiation of therapy.[76] However, every patient responds differently. For patients who are not on therapy, plasma HIV-RNA levels should be monitored every 3–4 months to assess the patient's risk of disease progression and to determine the need for antiretroviral therapy. The reader is encouraged to review the most recent HIV diagnostic and treatment guidelines since recommendations for different patient populations are continuously being modified as newer data becomes available.[75–77]

CD4+ T Lymphocyte Count

The cell-mediated immune function effects of HIV infection are demonstrated by reductions in the CD4+ *lymphocyte count.* Flow cytometry can be used to identify the various subsets of lymphocytes by their cluster of differentiation (CD) of specific monoclonal antibodies to surface antigens. The CD4+ T lymphocytes are the helper-inducer T cells, whereas the CD8+ T lymphocytes are the cytotoxic-suppressor T cells. HIV infection causes a decrease in the total number of lymphocytes (particularly the CD4+ T lymphocytes) as well as changes in the ratios of the different types of lymphocytes. CD4+ T lymphocyte counts of <200 cells/mm³ (normal count 800–1100 cells/mm³) or a CD4+ T lymphocyte percentage of <14% of the total lymphocyte count (normal 40% of total lymphocytes) are indicative of severe immunosuppression, placing the patient at risk for the development of opportunistic infections.[76]

As stated earlier, the CD4+ T lymphocyte count is utilized in conjunction with the plasma HIV-RNA level to provide essential information regarding a patient's virologic and immunologic status, risk of disease progression from HIV infection to AIDS, and whether to initiate or change antiretroviral therapy.[75-77] Due to the significant impact on disease progression and survival, most guidelines recommend monitoring CD4+ T lymphocyte counts at baseline and every 3–6 months to aid in the decision to initiate antiretroviral therapy, assess the immunologic response to treatment, and determine the need for any opportunistic infection chemoprophylaxis.[76] Current HIV treatment guidelines recommend initiation of antiretroviral therapy in all HIV-infected patients with a CD4+ T lymphocyte count <350 cells/mm³ regardless of the plasma HIV RNA viral load. Also, treatment should be offered to patients with CD4+ T lymphocyte counts between 350 and 500 cells/mm³. When the CD4+ T lymphocyte count is >500 cells/mm³, the decision to start therapy in asymptomatic patients is less clear and should be individualized. Therapy may need to be considered in patients with a high rate of decline in CD4+ T lymphocyte (defined as >100 cell/mm³ per annum), even when the current count is 500 cells/mm³ or greater. Additionally, antiretroviral therapy is recommended in patients with HIV-associated nephropathy, HBV co-infection when treatment for HBV is indicated, and patients who are pregnant regardless of CD4+ T lymphocyte count. However, since HIV treatment recommendations are constantly evolving based on new data, the reader is referred to the most recent HIV treatment guidelines for specific details on when antiretroviral therapy should be initiated in an individual patient based on clinical and laboratory parameters.

Phenotypic and Genotypic Assays for Antiretroviral Drug Resistance

Resistance of HIV-1 to antiretroviral drugs is an important cause for treatment failure. *Genotypic assays* utilize gene sequencing or probes to detect resistance mutations known to confer drug resistance in the RT or protease genes of HIV-1. Two genotypic assays have been approved by the FDA: TruGene (Siemens Healthcare Diagnostics, Tarrytown, NY) and ViroSeq (Abbott Molecular, DesPlaines, IL).[72] *Phenotypic*

assays measure the quantity of viral replication in the presence of various concentrations of antiretroviral agents. Sequences from the RT and protease genes of the patient's HIV virus are inserted into a wild-type virus in the laboratory. The concentration of the drug needed to inhibit 50% of viral replication (inhibitory concentration 50% [IC50]) is reported. The ratio of IC values for the test and reference viruses is calculated and used to report the fold-increase in resistance of each antiretroviral agent. The interpretation of results from both assays is complex and requires expert knowledge and consultation.[73,76]

The current guidelines recommend drug resistance testing for patients with acute and chronic HIV infection when they enter into care, regardless of the decision to initiate antiretroviral therapy; pregnant women prior to antiretroviral therapy initiation; women contemplating or entering pregnancy with a detectable HIV-RNA level during treatment; patients with virologic failure while receiving antiretroviral therapy; and patients with suboptimal suppression of plasma HIV-RNA level after the initiation of antiretroviral therapy.[76] Genotypic assays are typically recommended for resistance testing in treatment naïve patients and pregnant women. In the setting of virologic failure, current guidelines recommend performing resistance testing immediately after or within 4 weeks of the discontinuation of antiretroviral therapy for optimal results. Resistance testing is not recommended in patients with plasma HIV-RNA levels <1000 copies/mL.

The advantages and disadvantages of genotypic and phenotypic assays for the detection of HIV-1 resistance have been previously described.[73] The genotypic assay may be preferred over the phenotypic assay because of availability, clinical utility, faster turnaround time (1–2 weeks versus 2–3 weeks), and lower cost.[72] However, both assays are complex, technically demanding, and expensive, and are not routinely performed in most clinical laboratories.

Additional Laboratory Testing for HIV Patients

Coreceptor tropism assays. Following attachment of HIV to the CD4+ T lymphocytes, fusion of the virus and CD4+ cell membranes involves binding to a coreceptor molecule. The two coreceptors utilized by HIV are chemokine coreceptor 5 (CCR5) and/or CXC coreceptor (CXCR4). The recently-approved antiretroviral agent, maraviroc, is a CCR5-coreceptor antagonist that prevents the entry of HIV into the CD4+ cell by binding to the CCR5 receptor. Most acutely or recently infected patients harbor the CCR5-tropic virus, while untreated patients with advanced disease and/or those with disease progression shift from CCR5-tropic to CXCR4-tropic or both (dual- or mixed-tropic). Treatment-experienced patients with high levels of drug resistance are more likely to harbor dual- or mixed-tropic virus. Current HIV treatment guidelines recommend performing a coreceptor tropism assay when considering the use of a CCR5-coreceptor antagonist, or in the event of virologic failure during maraviroc therapy.[76] Currently, two phenotypic assays measure viral tropism; *Phenoscript* assay (VIRalliance, Paris, France) and *Trofile* assay (Monogram Biosciences, Inc., South San Francisco, CA), and one genotypic tropism assay is available in the United States (Genotypic Coreceptor Tropism

Test, Quest Diagnostics), although it has a lower predictive value compared to the traditional phenotypic assay.[84]

HLA-B*5701 screening. Abacavir, a nucleoside reverse transcriptase inhibitor (NRTI), is associated with a potentially life-threatening hypersensitivity reaction reported in 5% to 8% of patients in clinical trials. The hypersensitivity reaction appears to occur more frequently in white patients (5% to 8%) than black patients (2% to 3%), and is associated with the presence of MHC class I allele HLA-B*5701. Human immunodeficiency virus treatment guidelines recommend screening patients for the presence of HLA-B*5701 prior to the initiation of abacavir-containing regimens in areas where the screening test is available, and those patients with a positive result should not receive abacavir. However, the HLA-B*5701 screening test may not be available in many clinical laboratories, therefore; the initiation of abacavir therapy can be reasonably considered using clinical judgment with appropriate monitoring and extensive patient education about the signs and symptoms of the hypersensitivity reaction.[76]

MYCOBACTERIA

Mycobacteria are nonmotile, nonspore-forming, aerobic bacilli that continue to cause infection as well as significant morbidity and mortality, especially in developing countries.[85–92] Currently, over 100 species of mycobacteria have been identified, with only a number of species causing infection in humans including *M. tuberculosis*, *M. leprae*, *M. avium complex*, *M. kansasii*, *M. fortuitum*, *M. chelonae*, *M. marinum*, and *M. abscessus*.[85–88] Depending on the species, mycobacteria can be nonpathogenic, pathogenic, or opportunistic and, therefore, may cause infection in both normal and immunocompromised hosts. Table 17-19 lists the most common pathogenic mycobacteria

species with their typical associated infections and environmental sources.[85–91]

Mycobacteria are generally divided into two groups based on epidemiology and spectrum of disease: (1) the *M. tuberculosis* complex including the species *M. tuberculosis*, *M. bovis*, *M. bovis* bacille Calmette-Guerin (BCG), *M. africanum*, and *M. microti*; and (2) nontuberculous mycobacteria (NTM, or also referred to as mycobacteria other than tuberculosis [MOTT]), which include all other species of mycobacteria.[87,88]

Mycobacterium tuberculosis is the most clinically significant mycobacteria, and is the causative organism of tuberculosis (TB). The incidence of TB in the United States had been declining between 1953 (when it became a notifiable disease) and 1985 as a result of improved diagnostic methods, enhanced public health efforts to isolate patients infected with TB, and the introduction of effective antimycobacterial agents.[86,88,93] This decline in TB cases led experts to predict the elimination of the disease by 2010. However, between 1986 and 1992, an increase in the incidence of TB was observed in the United States due to deterioration of the TB public health programs, the emergence of the HIV epidemic, the increase in immigration to the United States, and the emergence of MDR TB.[86,93] Since 1992, the number of cases of TB in the United States has steadily declined due to improved public health control strategies.[82] Despite the advances in medical care and treatment, TB continues to be one of the most common infectious diseases worldwide. The World Health Organization (WHO) estimated that over 12 million persons were infected with TB worldwide in 2010, including over 8 million new cases and 1.6 million deaths that year.[94] Since TB can be transmitted from person-to-person, rapid diagnosis is necessary to decrease the spread of infection.[93]

TABLE 17-19. Pathogenic Mycobacteria and Associated Infections[85–91]

MYCOBACTERIUM SPECIES	ASSOCIATED INFECTIONS	ENVIRONMENTAL SOURCES
Mycobacterium tuberculosis complex (tuberculosis [TB])	Pulmonary infection, lymphadenitis, musculoskeletal infection, gastrointestinal infection, peritonitis, hepatitis, pericarditis	Humans
Mycobacterium bovis	Soft tissue infection, gastrointestinal infection	Humans, cattle
Mycobacterium leprae (Leprosy, Hansen disease)	Skin and soft tissue infections	Humans, armadillos
Mycobacterium avium complex (MAC)	Pulmonary infection, cutaneous ulcers, lymphadenitis, disseminated infection	Soil, water, swine, cattle, birds
Mycobacterium kansasii	Pulmonary infection, musculoskeletal infection, disseminated infection, cervical lymphadenitis	Water, cattle
Mycobacterium fortuitum	Skin and soft tissue infections, disseminated infection	Soil, water, animals, marine life
Mycobacterium chelonae	Skin and soft tissue infections, osteomyelitis, disseminated infection	Soil, water, animals, marine life
Mycobacterium abscessus	Skin and soft tissue infections, osteomyelitis, disseminated infection	Soil, water, animals, marine life
Mycobacterium marinum	Skin and soft tissue infections, bacteremia	Fish, fresh water, salt water
Mycobacterium ulcerans	Skin and soft tissue infections, osteomyelitis	Soil, stagnant water

The Identification of Mycobacteria

Mycobacteria possess a number of unique characteristics that contribute to the difficulties with the growth, identification, and treatment of these organisms. The cell wall of mycobacteria is complex and composed of peptidoglycan, polypeptides, and a lipid-rich hydrophobic layer.[87,88] This cell wall structure confers a number of distinguishing properties in the mycobacteria including (1) resistance to disinfectants and detergents; (2) the inability to be stained by many common laboratory identification stains; (3) the inability of mycobacteria to be decolorized by acid solutions (a characteristic that has given them the name of acid-fast bacilli [AFB]); (4) the ability of mycobacteria to grow slowly; and (5) resistance to common anti-infective agents.[85,87,88] These characteristics have led to the continuous modification and improvement of laboratory practices used in the identification and diagnosis of mycobacterial infections. Many of these laboratory practices involve specialized staining techniques, growth media, identification techniques, environmental conditions (BSL-3 facilities for *M. tuberculosis*), and susceptibility testing methods that may be unavailable in some clinical laboratories.[88,90]

The ability to accurately cultivate mycobacteria is highly dependent upon the appropriate selection and collection of biologic specimens for staining and culture.[3,88] Since different mycobacteria are capable of causing a number of infections (as listed in Table 17-19), the following biologic specimens may be submitted for mycobacterial culture based on the site of infection: respiratory tract secretions (e.g., expectorated or induced sputum and bronchial washings) or gastric lavage specimens for the diagnosis of pulmonary TB; CSF for the diagnosis of tuberculous meningitis; blood for the diagnosis of disseminated *Mycobacterium avium* complex (MAC) infection; stool for the diagnosis of disseminated MAC infection; and urine, tissue, exudate or wound drainage, bone marrow, sterile body fluids, lymph node tissue, and skin specimens for infection due to any mycobacteria.[86-90] For the diagnosis of pulmonary TB, several early morning expectorated or induced sputum specimens are recommended to enhance diagnostic accuracy. Biologic specimens for mycobacterial culture should be immediately processed according to specified guidelines to prevent the overgrowth of bacteria that may also be present in the specimen, and should be concentrated to enhance diagnostic capability.[86,88,90]

Similar to the processing of specimens for bacterial culture, biologic specimens submitted for mycobacterial culture should be stained for microscopic examination and plated for culture. The staining techniques and culture media, however, are somewhat different since mycobacteria are poorly visualized in the Gram stain (they do not reliably take up the dyes and are referred to as *acid-fast*) and take longer to grow than conventional bacteria.

Staining with subsequent microscopic examination for mycobacteria is a rapid diagnostic test that involves the use of stains that are taken up by the lipid and mycolic acid components in the mycobacterial cell wall.[87,88] Several acid-fast stains are available for the microscopic examination of mycobacteria,

including carbolfuchsin-based stains that are viewed using light microscopy (Ziehl-Neelsen or Kinyoun method) and fluorochrome stains (auramine-rhodamine) examined under fluorescence microscopy that are thought to be more sensitive tests, especially on direct specimens.[3,87-89,95] The sensitivity of the staining method is highly dependent on the type of clinical specimen, the species of mycobacteria present, the technique utilized in specimen processing, the thickness of the smear, and the experience of the laboratory technologist.[3,86-88] The staining methods can detect the presence of mycobacteria in a clinical specimen but cannot differentiate between species of mycobacteria. Therefore, several molecular techniques have been commercially developed to augment identification, which utilize NA amplification (PCR) to detect *M. tuberculosis* complex in acid-fast smear positive respiratory specimens (Amplicor *Mycobacterium tuberculosis* Test by Roche Diagnostic Systems and the Amplified *Mycobacterium tuberculosis* Direct Test by Gen-Probe) or acid-fast smear negative respiratory samples (Amplified *Mycobacterium tuberculosis* Direct Test by Gen-Probe).[3,85-88,90,92,95] Both of these tests display high sensitivity in detecting the presence of *M. tuberculosis* complex in smear-positive respiratory specimens (>97%).[3,88,95] Because of their high specificity and the rapid availability of results, the CDC recommends performing NA amplification tests on respiratory specimens of patients suspected of having pulmonary TB.[96,97] However, none of these assays are currently FDA-approved for the detection of *Mycobacterium* from nonrespiratory specimens.[96,97]

For optimal cultivation and identification of mycobacteria, a combination of culture media, including at least one solid growth medium and one liquid growth medium, should be utilized during specimen processing to facilitate growth and optimize pigment production of the organism.[3,87-89,91,93,95] The preferred commercially-available solid growth media for the cultivation of mycobacteria include an agar-based medium such as Middlebrook 7H10, or an egg-based medium such as Lowenstein-Jensen. There are several liquid growth media systems that are available for culture of mycobacteria, some of which employ continuous automated monitoring systems for the detection of mycobacterial growth.[3,87-89,91,92] The liquid growth media systems often provide more rapid isolation of AFB compared to conventional solid media, with results within 10 days as compared to 17 days or longer using solid growth media.[86,88-90,95] The most commonly used semiautomated systems with liquid growth media include the MB Redox (Heipha Diagnostica Biotest), BACTEC 460TB system (Becton Dickinson), the Septi-Chek AFB System (Becton Dickinson), and the Mycobacteria Growth Indicator Tube (MGIT, Becton Dickinson).[3,87,88,91,95] The most commonly used automated, continuous monitoring systems with liquid growth media include the ESP Culture System II (Trek Diagnostics), the BACTEC 9000 MB System (Becton Dickinson), the MB BacT/Alert System (bioMérieux), and the BACTEC MGIT 960 (Becton Dickinson).[3,87,88,91,95] Once growth is detected in the liquid media systems, an acid-fast stain is performed on the specimen to confirm the presence of mycobacteria, with subsequent subculture onto solid media.

The optimal growth conditions of mycobacteria depend on the species; therefore, the clinical laboratory should follow a standardized procedure outlining the process that should be used to enhance cultivation of the suspected *Mycobacterium* from the submitted clinical specimen based on the suspected site of infection. The optimal conditions for incubation of mycobacterial cultures are 28°C to 37°C in 5% to 10% CO_2 for 6–8 weeks, depending on the organism.[3,88,90,91] Cultures for mycobacteria typically require prolonged incubation periods, sometimes up to 8 weeks, since most of the more common pathogens grow rather slowly. Rapidly growing mycobacteria such as *M. fortuitum*, *M. chelonae*, and *M. abscessus* typically grow within 7 days on solid media, while slow growing mycobacteria such as *M. tuberculosis* complex, *M. avium* complex, *M. kansasii*, and *M. marinum* require 7 days to 7 weeks for growth.[87,89,91] Therefore, culture tubes or plates are examined weekly during the incubation period for the presence of mycobacterial growth.

Colonies grown in culture are examined microscopically for characteristic colonial morphologic features, pigmentation, and growth rate; are subjected to biochemical tests; and are evaluated using rapid molecular detection methods such as PCR methods mentioned earlier, DNA hybridization using DNA probes, and/or chromatographic methods (such as high-performance liquid chromatography [HPLC] or gas liquid chromatography [GLC] to detect mycobacterial lipids) for definitive identification.[3,88–92] The DNA probes can only be utilized with mycobacteria grown in culture (not directly on patient specimens); are highly sensitive and specific; and are commercially available for the rapid identification of *M. tuberculosis* complex, *M. gordonae*, *M. kansasii*, and *M. avium* complex.[3,88–91] The molecular methods have replaced the use of biochemical tests in many laboratories since they provide more accurate identification in a significantly shorter time frame, within 14–21 days of specimen receipt as compared to several weeks or months using traditional identification methods.[86,92]

Susceptibility Testing of Mycobacteria

The choice of antibiotic or antimycobacterial agent to utilize in the treatment of mycobacterial infection depends on the species of mycobacteria involved. It is important for the clinician to have an understanding of the typical susceptibility patterns of specific mycobacterial species, the current treatment guidelines outlining which and how many drugs to use, and the methodology available for drug susceptibility testing for the particular mycobacterial species being treated.

Standardized guidelines have been published for the susceptibility testing of *M. tuberculosis* complex.[98] Susceptibility testing is currently recommended on the initial isolate of all patients with *M. tuberculosis* complex infection, on isolates from patients who remain culture positive after 3 months of appropriate therapy, and on isolates from patients who are not clinically responding to therapy.[3,88,93,98] Susceptibility testing of *M. tuberculosis* complex is initially performed with primary antituberculous agents such as isoniazid (using 2 concentrations,

0.2 and 1.0 mcg/mL), rifampin, ethambutol, and pyrazinamide. However, if resistance to any of these first-line drugs is detected, susceptibility testing should be subsequently performed using second-line drugs including streptomycin, a higher concentration of ethambutol (10 mcg/mL), ethionamide, capreomycin, ciprofloxacin, ofloxacin or levofloxacin, kanamycin, p-aminosalicylic acid, and rifabutin.[88,90,98]

Susceptibility testing of *M. tuberculosis* complex can be performed directly using mycobacteria from a smear-positive specimen (direct method) or using mycobacteria isolated from culture (indirect method).[88,90] The direct method of mycobacterial susceptibility testing produces faster results but is less standardized, so that susceptibility testing is usually performed using isolates grown in culture.[88,90] Four conventional methods are utilized worldwide for determining the susceptibility of *M. tuberculosis* isolates to antituberculous agents including the absolute concentration method, the resistance ratio method, the agar proportion method, and the agar proportion method using liquid medium (commercial radiometric, nonradiometric, or broth systems including the BACTEC 460TB System [Becton Dickinson]; BACTEC MGIT 960 [Becton Dickinson]; ESP Culture System II [Trek Diagnostics]; MB/BacT-Alert 3D [bioMérieux]). The agar proportion method and the commercial broth systems are the methods most commonly used for mycobacterial susceptibility testing in the United States.

The agar proportion method is a modified agar dilution test that evaluates the extent of growth of a standardized inoculum of *M. tuberculosis* in control and drug-containing agar medium. The organism is considered resistant if growth is greater than 1% on the agar plate containing critical concentrations of the antituberculous drug.[98] The critical concentration for each drug represents the lowest concentration of the drug that inhibits 95% of "wild type" *M. tuberculosis* strains that have never been exposed to the drug.[88,98] Susceptibility results using the agar proportion method are typically available 21 days after the plates have been inoculated.

The commercial susceptibility testing systems utilize liquid growth medium where the growth of the organism is measured in the presence and absence of antituberculous drugs.[86,88–91,95,98] These systems provide rapid susceptibility results for the primary antituberculous agents, but cannot be used for susceptibility testing of second-line agents. Commercial susceptibility tests are recommended over agar proportion methods since the results are often available within 5–7 days after inoculation and can help guide appropriate therapy without the unnecessary delay of the agar proportion method.[86,90,91,98]

There are a number of other susceptibility testing methods that are currently being evaluated for drug susceptibility testing of *M. tuberculosis*. Many antimycobacterial drugs are now available in Etest® strips, including streptomycin, ethambutol, isoniazid, and ethionamide.[92,95,98] Several studies have evaluated their performance as compared to the commercial methods; however, further studies are needed to validate the use of the Etest® as a suitable, alternative susceptibility testing method.

In addition, newer molecular methods for drug susceptibility testing of *M. tuberculosis* are currently being evaluated that are easier to perform and produce more reliable results in a shorter period of time.[88–92] These methods include PCR amplification, DNA sequencing line probe assays, or reverse hybridization-based probe assays for the detection of specific drug-resistance mutations. Further study, however, is warranted before newer susceptibility testing methods can replace conventional methods.

Guidelines for susceptibility testing of NTM have recently been published by the CLSI, where testing is only recommended on the initial isolate for clinically significant isolates (blood, tissue, etc.) that display variability in susceptibility to antituberculous drugs or for organisms that may be associated with acquired resistance.[98] The guidelines contain protocols for the susceptibility testing of rapidly growing NTM (*M. fortuitum, M. chelonae,* and *M. abscessus*) and slow-growing NTM (*M. avium* complex, *M. kansasii,* and *M. marinum*), including the recommended methodology and drugs to be tested for each organism.[87,88,90,98] Standard broth microdilution should be utilized to evaluate the susceptibility of any clinically significant, rapidly-growing NTM.[89,98] Drugs that may be considered for susceptibility testing include amikacin, cefoxitin, ciprofloxacin, clarithromycin, doxycycline, imipenem, sulfamethoxazole, trimethoprim–sulfamethoxazole, and tobramycin (for *M. chelonae* only).[89,98] Susceptibility testing of *M. avium* complex is recommended for clarithromycin only using a broth-based method (macrodilution or micro-dilution) for initial blood or tissue isolates in patients with disseminated infection; for clinically significant isolates from patients receiving previous or current macrolide therapy; for isolates from patients who develop bacteremia while receiving macrolide prophylaxis; and for isolates from patients who relapse while receiving macrolide therapy.[89,98] Regarding the other slow-growing NTM, susceptibility testing of *M. kansasii* should only be routinely performed on rifampin using the commercial radiometric systems, broth microdilution, or the modified proportion method; while routine susceptibility testing of *M. marinum* is not recommended.[89,98]

Skin Testing

The *Mantoux test* or *tuberculin skin test (TST)* is one test available for the detection of latent TB, and involves the intradermal injection of a purified protein derivative (PPD) of the tubercle bacilli, which is obtained from a culture filtrate derived by protein precipitation.[90,99] Injection of the PPD into individuals previously exposed to TB will elicit a delayed hypersensitivity reaction involving T cells that migrate to the area of intradermal injection (usually the dorsal aspect of the forearm), inducing the release of lymphokines that produce induration and edema within 48–72 hours after injection. The diameter of induration is measured between 48–72 hours after injection by a healthcare professional.[90,99] Published guidelines are available for interpretation of the TST reaction based on the size of the induration and clinical and demographic characteristics of the patient. An induration of ≥5 mm is considered positive in persons at high risk of developing tuberculous disease

including HIV infected patients; patients receiving immunosuppressive therapy; patients who have been recently exposed to a person with TB; and patients with an abnormal chest radiographic consistent with prior TB.[85,90,99] An induration of ≥10 mm is considered positive in patients who are not immunocompromised and possess no other identified risk factors for developing tuberculous disease such as recent immigrants from high prevalence countries; injection drug users; residents and employees of high-risk settings (e.g., prisons, healthcare facilities, and mycobacteria lab personnel); persons with chronic medical conditions of high risk (e.g., diabetes, silicosis, and chronic renal failure), and children younger than 4 years of age.[85,90,99] An induration of ≥15 mm is considered positive in persons at low risk for developing active infection with TB.[85,90,99]

A two-step TST is recommended by the CDC in certain populations (*initial* skin testing of newly hired healthcare workers without a documented negative TST within the past 12 months and persons expected to undergo serial screening for TB, such as residents and staff of long-term care facilities) to identify those individuals with past TB infection whose delayed-type hypersensitivity to tuberculin has diminished over time.[100,101] The first TST is administered as described above, with a second TST administered following the same procedure 1–3 weeks later in persons with a negative initial test.[100] The premise behind the administration of two TSTs in these settings is to delineate between past TB infection or BCG vaccination from recent conversion/infection. That is, the first injection will stimulate (boost) the delayed hypersensitivity response in a patient with previous TB infection or BCG vaccination and that the second TST will then elicit a positive reaction.[100,101]

Blood Assay for *Mycobacterium Tuberculosis*

Two in vitro diagnostic tests using whole blood have become recently available in the United States for the detection of latent *Mycobacterium tuberculosis* infection (blood assay for *Mycobacterium tuberculosis* [BAMT]; QuantiFERON®-TB Gold In-Tube test, [Cellestis, Inc., Chadstone, Victoria, Australia], and T-SPOT.TB [Oxford Immunotec, Oxoford, United Kingdom]).[86,88] These tests utilize ELISA to measure the amount of interferon gamma (IFN-γ) released from sensitized lymphocytes from prior exposure to *M. tuberculosis* following overnight incubation with PPD from *Mycobacterium tuberculosis* and control antigens.[100,102] Because the tests utilize peptide antigens from *M. tuberculosis*, they have more specificity than the TST for the diagnosis of latent *M. tuberculosis* infection, and will not produce false-positive results in patients with previous BCG vaccination or infection due to NTM.[100,102] The results of BAMT testing are stratified according to risk for TB infection (like the TST), but are not influenced by the subjectivity of reader bias or error, as may be seen with the TST. Since these tests are unable to distinguish between active or latent infection, the exact role of the BAMT and/or the TST in the diagnosis of latent TB infection is unclear and currently under investigation. However, the BAMT test can be used to assist in the diagnosis of latent TB infection in high-risk populations such as recent immigrants from high prevalence countries, injection drug users, inmates, prison employees, and healthcare workers at high risk for exposure to TB.[100,102] The BAMT test can also be considered as the initial and serial screening test for latent TB infection in healthcare workers and military personnel.[100,102] It is important to note that the FDA has approved these tests as aids in the diagnosis of *M. tuberculosis* infection, and are intended to be used in conjunction with other diagnostic techiques.[102]

LABORATORY TESTS UTILIZED FOR THE IDENTIFICATION OF UNCOMMON OR MISCELLANEOUS ORGANISMS

There are a number of pathogenic organisms that are difficult to detect or cultivate using the standard microbiologic procedures outlined above. These organisms often pose a diagnostic dilemma since they often require specialized testing for identification. It is beyond the scope of this chapter to describe all of the specialized testing methods that are available to detect these organisms; however, an abbreviated list can be found in Table 17-20.[43,103-130]

TABLE 17-20. Specialized Laboratory Tests for the Detection of Specific Organisms[43,103–130]

ORGANISM	TYPE OF ORGANISM	CLINICAL FINDINGS AND INFECTIONS	DIAGNOSTIC METHOD	POSITIVE RESULT	REFERENCES
Bordetella pertussis (Whooping cough)	Bacteria	Upper respiratory tract symptoms, characteristic whooping cough, pneumonia	Culture	Growth within 3–4 days; best when performed early in course of infection	103–105
			DFA	Detection of *B. pertussis* antigen	
			PCR	Direct detection in 1–2 days	
Borrelia burgdorferi (Lyme disease)	Spirochete	Erythema migrans, pericarditis, arthritis, neurologic disease	Culture	Hold cultures for up to 12 weeks	106, 107
			IFA or ELISA (screen)	Measures IgG and IgM antibodies against *B. burgdorferi*	
			WB (confirm)	Measures IgG and IgM antibodies against *B. burgdorferi*	
			PCR	Can detect low numbers of spirochetes	
Brucella spp.	Bacteria	Systemic infection (can involve any organ); spondylitis, arthritis, endocarditis	Culture	Growth within 7 days, but cultures should be held for 30 days	108, 109
			SAT	Detects antibodies to most *Brucella* spp.; titer of ≥1:160 is diagnostic	
			ELISA	Useful for detection of chronic or past brucellosis	
			PCR	Detection of *Brucella*-specific DNA sequences	
Chlamydophila pneumoniae	Atypical bacteria	Upper respiratory tract infections, pharyngitis, pneumonia	Culture	Monoclonal antibodies detect organism in culture	103, 110, 111
			CF	Fourfold rise in antibody titer between paired sera (acute and convalescent samples)	
			MIF	Fourfold rise in antibody titer between paired sera (acute and convalescent samples) or a single serum sample with an IgM titer of 1:16 or an IgG titer 1:512	
			EIA	Detection of IgG, IgM, or IgA against *C. pneumoniae*	
			PCR	Detection of *C. pneumoniae* DNA	

TABLE 17-20. Specialized Laboratory Tests for the Detection of Specific Organisms (cont'd)[43,103–130]

ORGANISM	TYPE OF ORGANISM	CLINICAL FINDINGS AND INFECTIONS	DIAGNOSTIC METHOD	POSITIVE RESULT	REFERENCES
Clostridium difficile (Pseudomembranous colitis)	Anaerobic bacteria	Pseudomembranous colitis, diarrhea	Culture using CCFA growth media	Growth within 48 hr; most sensitive test	43, 112, 113
			CCNA or EIA toxin test	Detection of toxin A or B activity; cell cytotoxicity test more sensitive than EIA	
			PCR	Rapid sensitive and specific detection of *C. difficile tcdB* gene	
Coxiella burnetti (Q fever)	Bacteria	Acute or chronic systemic illness, pneumonia, hepatitis, endocarditis	Culture with DFA	Growth in 6–14 days, organism detected by DFA	103, 110
			IFA, EIA, CF	IgM titer of 1:50 or an IgG titer of 1:200	
Cryptosporidium parvum	Protozoa	Acute diarrhea (self-limiting to severe), abdominal pain, dehydration	Modified acid fast staining	Detection of oocysts in stool or intestinal scrapings	114, 115
			IFA using a monoclonal antibody against oocyst	Detection of oocysts in stool or intestinal scrapings	
			EIA	Detection of *C. parvum* antigen in stool or intestinal scrapings	
			PCR	Detection of differentiation of *Cryptosporidium* spp.	
Ehrlichia spp.	Bacteria	HME and HGA—fever, myalgia, headache, malaise, leukopenia, thrombocytopenia, and elevated AST and ALT; may be life-threatening	Indirect immunofluorescence serology	Single sample IgG titer of >1:128 or a fourfold rise in antibody titer between paired sera (acute and convalescent samples)	116, 117
			Peripheral blood smear Wright stain	Intracytoplasmic inclusions	
			PCR	Detection of *E. chaffeensis* or *E. phagocytophilum* DNA sequences	
Entamoeba histolytica	Protozoa	Amebiasis: intestinal (colitis, diarrhea) and extraintestinal (liver abscess)	Stool exam for ova and parasites (O & P)	Detection of trophozoites and/or cysts	114, 118, 119
			Culture using axenic or xenic methods	Growth of *E. histolytica*	
			Serology (indirect FA, LA, ID, CF, ELISA)	Detection of *E. histolytica* antibodies	
			Antigen detection on fresh stool samples	Detection of *E. histolytica* or *E. dispar* specific antigen	
Giardia lamblia	Protozoa	Acute diarrhea (self-limiting to severe), malabsorption syndromes, low-grade fever, chills, abdominal pain	Stool exam for ova and parasites (O & P)	Detection of trophozoites and/or cysts	114, 118
			Wet preps or stains of duodenal material	Detection of trophozoites and/or cysts	
			EIA, DFA, or ICA antigen detection assays	Detection of trophozoite and/or cyst antigens	

TABLE 17-20. Specialized Laboratory Tests for the Detection of Specific Organisms (cont'd)[43,103–130]

ORGANISM	TYPE OF ORGANISM	CLINICAL FINDINGS AND INFECTIONS	DIAGNOSTIC METHOD	POSITIVE RESULT	REFERENCES
Helicobacter pylori	Bacteria	Peptic ulcer disease	Urea breath test	Positive test indicative of the presence of organism	120, 121
			Serologic tests	Detect IgG antibodies against *H. pylori*	
			Stool antigen assays (EIA)	Detection of *H. pylori* antigen	
			Urease test on antral biopsy specimen	Positive test indicative of the presence of organism	
			FISH, PCR	Detection of *H. pylori* DNA	
Legionella pneumophila	Atypical bacteria	Pneumonia	Culture (using specialized media)	Growth in 3–5 days	103, 122, 123
			DFA staining	Binds to *L. pneumophila* antigen to produce fluorescence	
			IFA serology	Fourfold rise in antibody titer between paired sera (acute and convalescent samples)	
			Urinary antigen detection (EIA, RIA, ICA)	Detects *Legionella pneumophila* serogroup 1 antigen only	
			PCR	Detection of *Legionella* spp. DNA	
Leishmania spp.	Protozoa	Cutaneous, mucocutaneous, or visceral (VL, kala-azar) infection; can infect reticuloendothelial system	Giemsa staining and light microscopy	Amastigotes within the specimen	114, 124
			Culture	Growth of promastigotes	
			IFA, DAT, ELISA (VL)	Detection of anti-leishmanial antibodies in blood or serum	
			LA (VL)	Detection of leishmanial antigen in urine	
			PCR (VL)	Detection of *Leishmania* DNA	
Leptospira spp.	Spirochetes	Leptospirosis (self-limiting with fevers, chills, myalgia, headache, aseptic meningitis); icteric leptospirosis (severe form associated with jaundice, bleeding, and renal failure)	Dark-field microscopy or immunofluorescence	Detection of motile leptospires	125
			Culture	Growth within 6 weeks	
			Serology using MAT	Fourfold or greater rise in agglutinating antibody titer between paired sera (acute and convalescent samples)	
			ELISA	Detection of leptospiral antibodies	
			PCR	Detection of leptospiral DNA	
Mycoplasma hominis	Atypical bacteria	Urogenital tract infections including prostatitis, PID, bacterial vaginosis, urethritis; systemic infection in neonates and immunocompromised patients	Culture using selective media	Growth within 5 days	126, 127
Mycoplasma pneumoniae	Atypical bacteria	Pneumonia, tracheobronchitis	EIA serology	Fourfold or greater rise in antibody titer between paired sera (acute and convalescent samples)	103, 126, 127
			NAAT, PCR	Detection of *M. pneumoniae* DNA	

TABLE 17-20. Specialized Laboratory Tests for the Detection of Specific Organisms (cont'd)[43,103–130]

ORGANISM	TYPE OF ORGANISM	CLINICAL FINDINGS AND INFECTIONS	DIAGNOSTIC METHOD	POSITIVE RESULT	REFERENCES
Plasmodium falciparum, P. vivax, P. ovale, P. malariae (Malaria)	Protozoa	Symptoms include high fever (cyclic with *P. vivax, P. ovale, P. malariae*), chills, nausea, vomiting, severe headache, anemia, abdominal pain; life-threatening with *P. falciparum*	Thick and thin blood films stained with Giemsa stain (gold standard)	Presence of malarial parasites	114, 128
			Fluorescent-assisted microscopy	Detection of fluorescence when dyes are taken up by the nucleus of the parasite	
			PCR (only in well-equipped labs)	Detection of malaria-specific DNA sequences	
			ICA antigen assays	Detection of malaria-specific antigens	
Pneumocystis carinii (jirovecii)	Fungus with protozoal characteristics	Pneumonia, extrapulmonary infection	Microscopic exam after stain of induced sputum, BAL specimen or tissue biopsy	Detection of trophic or cystic forms	129
			DFA or IFA	Detection of cysts or trophozoites	
			PCR (not routinely used)	Detection of *P. jirovecii*-specific DNA	
Rickettsia rickettsii (Rocky Mountain spotted fever [RMSF])	Rickettsia	Fever, chills, headache and rash in patient with recent tick bite; myalgias, malaise, nausea, vomiting, abdominal pain, focal neurologic findings; small vessel vasculitis may result in life-threatening complications	IFA (gold standard)	Fourfold or greater rise in IgM or IgG antibody titers between paired sera (acute and convalescent samples)	117
			EIA or LA	Detection of IgM or IgG antibodies	
Taenia solium	Tapeworm	Neurocysticercosis (infection within brain tissue) causing seizures, headache, focal neurologic deficits; muscular and subcutaneous abscesses	Serology by EITB	Detection of antibodies to *T. solium* glycoprotein antigens	114
			ELISA on CSF	Detection of anticysticercal antibodies or cysticercal antigens	
Toxoplasma gondii (Toxoplasmosis)	Protozoa	Encephalitis, myocarditis, lymphadenitis, polymyositis, chorioretinitis, toxoplasmosis during pregnancy, congenital toxoplasmosis	Serology testing by Sabin-Feldman Dye test, IFA, ELISA, IgG avidity test, agglutination	Positive IgG antibody	114, 130
			Analysis of CSF or body fluid/tissue	Demonstration of tachyzoites	
			PCR	Detection of *T. gondii*-specific DNA	

TABLE 17-20. Specialized Laboratory Tests for the Detection of Specific Organisms (cont'd)[43,103–130]

ORGANISM	TYPE OF ORGANISM	CLINICAL FINDINGS AND INFECTIONS	DIAGNOSTIC METHOD	POSITIVE RESULT	REFERENCES
Ureaplasma urealyticum	Atypical bacteria	Urogenital tract infections including prostatitis, PID, bacterial vaginosis, urethritis; systemic infection in neonates and immunocompromised	Culture using selective media	Growth within 5 days	126, 127
			PCR	Detection of NA or gene targets	

ALT = alanine aminotransferase; AST = aspartate aminotransferase; BAL = bronchoalveolar lavage; CCFA = cycloserine cefoxitin fructose agar; CCNA = cell cytotoxicity neutralization assay; CF = complement fixation; CSF = cerebrospinal fluid; DAT = direct agglutination test; DFA = direct fluorescent antibody; DNA = deoxyribonucleic acid; EIA = enzyme immunoassay; ELISA = enzyme-linked immunosorbent assay; EITB = enzyme-linked immunoelectrotransfer blot; FISH = fluorescent in situ hybridization; HGA = human granulocytic anaplasmosis; HME = human monocytic ehrlichiosis; ICA = immunochromatographic assay; ID = immunodiffusion; IgG = Immunoglobulin G; IgM = immunoglobulin M; IFA = immunofluorescent assay/indirect fluorescent antibody; LA = latex agglutination; MAT = microscopic agglutination; MIF = microimmunofluorescence; NA = nucleic acid; NAAT = nucleic acid amplification test; PCR = polymerase chain reaction; PID = pelvic inflammatory disease; RIA = radioimmunoassay; SAT = serum agglutination test; VL = visceral leishmaniasis; WB = western blot.

LABORATORY TESTS UTILIZED FOR THE DIAGNOSIS OF SPECIFIC INFECTIONS

Meningitis

Meningitis is considered to be an infectious disease medical emergency requiring prompt, accurate diagnosis and treatment. Meningitis may be caused by bacteria, viruses, fungi, or mycobacteria, and produce a resulting clinical presentation of acute or chronic meningitis depending on the causative organism. In a patient with suspected meningitis, a lumbar puncture is performed to obtain CSF for laboratory analysis to aid in the diagnosis of the infection, including the potential causative organism.[131–137] In patients who present with papilledema, altered consciousness, new onset seizures, or focal neurologic findings, a head computed tomography (CT) may be performed prior to the lumbar puncture to exclude the presence of a space-occupying lesion, which may put the patient at risk for brain herniation after lumbar puncture.[132]

A lumbar puncture involves the aseptic insertion of a spinal needle into the subarachnoid space at the lumbar spine level for the aspiration of 5–20 mL of CSF for analysis.[131,133] When initiating the lumber puncture, the opening pressure may be measured (normal opening pressure = 50–195 mm H_2O in adults), and is often elevated in patients with meningitis and concomitant cerebral edema or an intracranial focus of infection.[132,135] The CSF should be placed in three to four separate sterile screw-cap tubes and immediately transported to the laboratory for rapid processing. The first two tubes of CSF are processed for microbiologic (e.g., Gram stain, fungal stains, AFB stain, culture, and antigen detection) and chemical studies (e.g., general appearance, glucose, and protein), while the last two tubes are processed for determination of the WBC count with differential as described below. The typical CSF chemistry, hematology, and microbiologic findings in patients with meningitis caused by different pathogens are listed in Table 17-21.[132–137]

TABLE 17-21. Typical CSF Findings in Patients with Meningitis[132–137]

	NORMAL	BACTERIAL MENINGITIS	VIRAL INFECTION	FUNGAL MENINGITIS	TUBERCULOUS MENINGITIS
Opening pressure (mm H_2O)	<180	>195			
WBCs (count/mm³)	0–5	400–20,000 (mean 800)	5–2000 (mean 80)	20–2000 (mean 100)	5–2000 (mean 200)
WBC differential	No predominance	≥80% PMNs	>50% lymphs, 20% PMNs	>50% lymphs	>80% lymphs
Protein (mg/dL)	<50	>100	30–150	40–150	>50
Glucose (mg/dL)	45–100 (²/₃ of serum)	<45 (<½ of serum)	45–70	30–70	<40
Gram stain (% positive)	—	60–90	Negative	Negative	37–87 (AFB smear)

AFB = acid-fast bacilli; CSF = cerebrospinal fluid; PMNs = polymorphonuclear leukocytes; lymphs = lymphocytes; WBCs = white blood cells.

Chemistry and Hematology

In patients with meningitis, the CSF often appears cloudy due to the presence of WBCs, protein, and bacteria.[132] The chemistry and hematology results from the CSF analysis correlate directly with the probability of infection, so that negative findings exclude the likelihood of meningitis in almost all cases.[132,133,135,136] Patients with acute bacterial meningitis often demonstrate marked abnormalities in the chemistry analysis of the CSF, with protein concentrations of >100 mg/dL and glucose concentrations <45 mg/dL (or a CSF:blood glucose ratio of <0.5) due, in part, to disruption of the blood brain barrier.[132,135,136]

Hematologic analysis of the CSF involves a determination of the WBC count with corresponding WBC differential, the results of which may suggest the potential causative organism of the meningitis. Patients with acute bacterial meningitis often demonstrate an elevated CSF WBC count (>400 cells/mm³), with a neutrophilic predominance (>80% neutrophils). In contrast, patients with viral, fungal, or mycobacterial meningitis often display lower CSF WBC counts (5–200 cells/mm³), with a predominance of lymphocytes.

CSF Stain and Culture

For patients with suspected bacterial meningitis, a Gram stain and culture should be performed on CSF. The Gram stain will demonstrate an organism in 60% to 90% of patients with bacterial meningitis and is helpful in selecting appropriate empiric antibiotic therapy.[132,134–136] However, the sensitivity of the CSF Gram stain diminishes to 40% to 60% in patients who have received antibiotics prior to the lumber puncture (as known as *partially-treated meningitis*).[134] In patients with meningitis due to viruses, fungi, or mycobacteria, the Gram stain is usually negative and specialized tests should be used, such as the India ink stain or *Cryptococcus* antigen test for the detection of *Cryptococcus neoformans* or the acid-fast stain for the detection of *Mycobacterium tuberculosis*.

All CSF specimens should be processed for culture based on the type of meningitis (acute versus chronic) and the organism suspected of causing the infection. In patients with bacterial meningitis, the cultures are often positive within 24–48 hours. In patients with nonbacterial meningitis, culture specimens should be incubated for longer periods of time (up to 2–6 weeks), since these organisms often take longer to grow.

Other Specialized Tests

Several specialized tests may be performed on CSF specimens to aid in the detection of the causative organism. These tests include bacterial antigen detection using LA, latex fixation, or EIA; fungal antigen detection; antibody detection; and bacterial, viral, or mycobacterial PCR assay.[132–137]

Bacterial antigen testing on CSF specimens is considered a rapid diagnostic test since the results are available well before the results of the CSF culture. The commercially-available tests utilize antibody-coated particles that bind to specific capsular antigens of the most common bacterial pathogens that cause acute meningitis, including *S. pneumoniae, Neisseria meningitidis, H. influenzae* type B, and group B streptococci. The tests are performed by combining CSF (although it can also be performed using urine or serum) with antibody-coated particles and observing for agglutination, which signifies the presence of the bacterial antigen in the specimen. If visible agglutination does not occur, either the antigen is not present or it is present in insufficient amounts to cause detectable agglutination. Routine bacterial antigen detection of CSF specimens is not recommended because they are not more sensitive than the traditional Gram stain, the results lack high specificity or sensitivity, the results rarely impact patient treatment, and their use has not been shown to be cost-effective.[3,132] However, bacterial antigen testing may be useful in patients with negative Gram stains or in patients that have received previous antimicrobial therapy.[132–134,136] The Binax NOW® *Streptococcus pneumoniae* antigen test is a noninvasive test that has recently been approved by the FDA to aid in the diagnosis of meningitis due to *Streptococcus pneumoniae*.[138] It is a rapid ICA that detects the C-polysaccharide antigen of the *S. pneumoniae* cell wall in CSF of patients suspected of having pneumococcal meningitis.[138] The test is highly sensitive and specific, with results available within 15 minutes.[138] In addition, the test is not influenced by previous antibiotic therapy. The results of the antigen test are considered presumptive and should be utilized with the results of culture when making the diagnosis of pneumococcal meningitis.

Fungal antigen testing is available for *Histoplasma capsulatum* and *Cryptococcus neoformans*.[133,137] The antigen testing for *Cryptococcus neoformans* has become an important diagnostic tool that has become useful in predicting the course of infection and for monitoring the response to antifungal therapy.

For some organisms, diagnostic tests that detect the presence of antibody in the CSF are available, including syphilis (*Treponema pallidum*), Lyme disease (*Borrelia burgdorferi*), and *Coccidioides immitis*.[137]

Polymerase chain reaction assays are the most useful test for the diagnosis of viral infections of the CNS, and they can be used to detect the presence of HSV, CMV, VZV, EBV, and enterovirus in the CSF.[64,67,132] The PCR assay involves the amplification of small amounts of specific DNA of the target organism followed by subsequent identification and verification. PCR is also available for the detection of *S. pneumoniae, N. meningitidis, Listeria monocytogenes,* and *Mycobacterium tuberculosis*; however, the time and expense of performing PCR assays for these organisms has limited their routine clinical use.[132]

Streptococcal Pharyngitis

Acute pharyngitis is one of the most common infections encountered in medicine and can occur in both children and adults. Acute pharyngitis can be caused by a number of organisms (e.g., bacteria and viruses), which produce similar signs and symptoms of infection. Antibiotic therapy is only recommended for patients with pharyngitis due to bacteria, especially group A streptococci (*Streptococcus pyogenes*).[139] Since group A strep pharyngitis comprises only a small percentage of patients with acute pharyngitis, it is important that a rapid, reliable diagnostic test be available to avoid unnecessary antibiotic use in patients with acute viral pharyngitis.

The gold standard diagnostic test for acute pharyngitis due to group A streptococcus is the throat culture, which often takes one to two days for results. Therefore, rapid antigen detection tests (RADTs) have been developed to expedite and confirm the diagnosis of group A streptococcal pharyngitis, with most tests yielding results within 15 minutes.[139,140] Positive RADT tests expedite the initiation of antibiotic treatment in the appropriate patient. There are several RADT tests that are commercially available, with the newer tests employing EIA, optical immunoassay, or chemiluminescent DNA probes to produce >95% specificity and ≥90% sensitivity.[139,140] However, since there is limited data comparing the performance of the different RADT tests to throat culture (the gold standard), it is recommended that a negative RADT test in children and adolescents be confirmed with a throat culture to rule out group A streptococcal pharyngitis.[139,140]

Pneumonia

There are a number of obstacles that make the diagnosis of bacterial *pneumonia* quite difficult. First, the respiratory tract is colonized with bacteria that may or may not be contributing to the infectious process. When obtaining a sample for culture, lower respiratory tract secretions can become contaminated with secretions or bacteria colonizing the upper respiratory tract; therefore, expectorated sputum samples should be evaluated to determine if contamination with saliva or upper respiratory tract flora has occurred (assessment of the adequacy of the sample).[131,141,142] If bacteria other than normal respiratory flora are isolated, the clinician must determine the relative importance and significance of the organism(s) isolated as a potential cause of pneumonia by assessing the presence of signs and symptoms of respiratory tract infection in the patient. In some patients, adequate sputum specimens are difficult to obtain without invasive procedures such as BAL or protected specimen brush (PSB). Invasive procedures are occasionally utilized to aid in the diagnosis of pneumonia in patients who are not able to expectorate an adequate sputum sample, in immunocompromised patients, and in patients with HAP or ventilator-associated pneumonia (VAP).[19,141,143] Despite the best efforts at obtaining a lower respiratory tract sputum specimen for culture, as many as 50% of patients with pneumonia have negative cultures.[141,142]

In order to obtain an adequate expectorated sputum sample, the patient should be instructed to provide sputum generated from a deep cough. All expectorated sputum samples should be screened to ensure that the specimen is adequate and has not been contaminated by saliva or upper respiratory tract flora prior to processing for culture.[131,141,142] Information utilized to assess the adequacy of an expectorated sputum sample is derived from visualization of the Gram stain of the specimen. Expectorated sputum specimens that contain greater than 25 WBCs/hpf and less than 10 squamous epithelial cells/hpf are considered adequate for further processing and culture.[141,142] Samples with greater than 10 epithelial cells/

hpf are representative of upper respiratory tract contamination (saliva) and should not be processed for culture. The sputum Gram stain from an adequate sputum specimen may be used to guide empiric antibiotic therapy when the specimen is purulent and contains a predominant organism. Antibiotic therapy should be modified based on the culture results, especially if they reveal an infecting organism.

A noninvasive test, called the Binax NOW® *Streptococcus pneumoniae* antigen test, is available to aid in the diagnosis of pneumonia due to *Streptococcus pneumoniae*.[3,138,141,143] This test is a rapid ICA that detects the C-polysaccharide antigen of the *S. pneumoniae* cell wall in the urine of patients suspected of having pneumococcal pneumonia.[138,141,143] The results of the test are available within 15 minutes, are not influenced by previous antibiotic therapy, and display 86% sensitivity and 94% specificity in detecting *S. pneumoniae* antigen in the urine.[138,141–143] The *S. pneumoniae* urinary antigen test should be considered in patients when a sputum sample for culture cannot be obtained in a timely fashion, in patients with severe pneumonia requiring ICU admission, in patients at risk for pneumococcal pneumonia (asplenic, alcohol abuse, liver disease), in patients with pneumonia and concomitant pleural effusion, in patients who failed previous outpatient antibiotic therapy, and in patients who have received antibiotics before a specimen for culture has been obtained.[142,143] Results of the urinary antigen test are presumptive and should be utilized with the results of the sputum culture when establishing the diagnosis of pneumococcal pneumonia.

In the case of pneumonia caused by atypical bacteria such as *Legionella pneumophila*, *Mycoplasma pneumoniae*, or *Chlamydophila pneumoniae*, antigen detection tests (*Legionella* urinary antigen test for the detection of *Legionella* serogroup 1) or serologic tests may be utilized to aid in the diagnosis of infection due to these organisms since they are difficult to culture in the lab (see Table 17-20).[3,141–143] In addition, the diagnosis of infection due to *Bordetella pertussis* (pertussis or whooping cough) can be established utilizing culture (more sensitive if performed within 2 weeks of the onset of symptoms), serology (not useful in infants and the elderly; utilized late in course of illness), and/or PCR (useful for diagnosis in patients with symptoms >2 weeks).[103–105]

In patients with HAP or VAP, semiquantitative analysis of tracheal aspirates or sputum cultures or a quantitative analysis from specimens obtained during BAL may be performed to differentiate between infection and colonization based on the history of prior antibiotic use in the patient and the number of organisms recovered in the sputum specimen.[19] Diagnostic thresholds for pneumonia based on colony counts recovered from a quantitative BAL specimen may differ among institutions. Studies evaluating quantitative BAL or PSB specimens for the diagnosis of HAP or VAP utilize a diagnostic threshold between 10^3 to 10^5 cfu/mL of an organism for the diagnosis of pneumonia.[19,141]

Genitourinary Tract Infections

Urinary Tract Infections

Urinary tract infections are among the most common community-acquired and nosocomially-acquired bacterial infections, prompting more than 8 million office visits and over 100,000 hospitalizations per year.[144–147] Urinary tract infections are especially common in females due to the close proximity of the urethra (which is shorter than males) to the perirectal and vaginal regions, which are both colonized with bacteria. Because of this anatomic difference, bacteria are able to easily ascend the urethra in females and potentially cause infection in the bladder (cystitis) and upper urinary tract (pyelonephritis). In addition, hospitalized patients (male and female) with indwelling urinary catheters are at increased risk for developing UTIs, with approximately 20% of catheterized patients developing a UTI even with only short-term catheterization.[145]

Under normal circumstances, urine within the bladder is sterile since all anatomic sites above the urethra within the urinary tract are not colonized with bacteria. However, the urethra is colonized with bacteria. If noninvasive urine collection methods are utilized for specimen collection, the urine will travel through the urethra and may inadvertently collect bacteria as it passes through the nonsterile environment. Therefore, diagnostic criteria have been developed to discriminate between infection, bacterial colonization, or bacterial contamination based on quantitative colony counts from urine cultures as well as the presence of inflammatory cells and epithelial cells in the urinalysis.[144–146]

Urine samples for urinalysis and culture can be collected a number of ways. The most common method involves the collection of a clean-catch, midstream urine sample. Before obtaining the sample, the patient should be instructed to clean and rinse the periurethral area with a mild detergent, and then retract the labial folds or penile foreskin when beginning to urinate. The patient should attempt to collect the urine in a sterile cup at the midpoint of the urine stream, collecting urine a few seconds after the start of urination, which is why it is also called a *midstream urine sample.*

Other methods for urine collection involve invasive procedures such as straight catheterized urine and suprapubic bladder aspiration. Both of these methods avoid the potential contamination of the urine specimen by the urethra since the urine is collected directly from the bladder. In hospitalized patients with indwelling urinary catheters, urine specimens should be collected directly from the urinary catheter by aspirating the catheter port or tubing (representing freshly voided urine) rather than obtaining the specimen from the collection bag (urine collected over a period of time).[144,145,148]

In all cases, urine samples should be immediately transported to the laboratory for processing. The exact processing of the urine sample will typically depend on the infection type. Urine samples from patients with uncomplicated cystitis may only be analyzed using screening tests such as reagent strip testing (dipsticks), while samples from other patients with UTIs (e.g., recurrent UTIs, pyelonephritis, and UTIs in patients with indwelling catheters) may be analyzed using microscopic examination and culture.

The urine from women with uncomplicated cystitis is usually only evaluated using screening tests since the results are rapidly available and most useful at excluding the presence of a UTI.[144] The most common rapid screening tests include commercially-available reagent test strips, or urine dipsticks, that contain the leukocyte esterase test and the nitrate reductase test, and provide a negative predictive value of 98%.[144,145] The leukocyte esterase test detects the presence of leukocyte esterase, which is an enzyme found in neutrophils. The nitrate reductase test detects the presence of urinary nitrite produced by the reduction of nitrate by nitrate-reducing enzymes of common urinary tract pathogens.[144–146] Positive results from either the leukocyte esterase test or nitrate reductase test warrant treatment for a UTI without the need for urine culture in women with uncomplicated cystitis.

The urine from patients with recurrent UTIs, complicated UTIs, or catheter-associated UTIs is typically evaluated using a urinalysis (microscopic examination) and urine culture. The urinalysis is a rapid test that involves the macroscopic and microscopic examination of the urine sample for color, clarity, specific gravity, and the presence of protein, glucose, red blood cells (RBCs), WBCs, bacteria, and epithelial cells. The urinalysis is performed either manually or through the use of automated instruments. Urinalysis findings that suggest a UTI include specimen cloudiness and the presence of pyuria (>10 WBC/hpf).[144–146] The detection of pyuria, hematuria, proteinuria, or bacteriuria in the urinalysis may be an indication of infection, but none of these alone is specific for infection. The presence of squamous epithelial cells (>2–5 epithelial cells/hpf) in the urine sample suggests poor specimen collection and possible contamination.

The urine culture remains the hallmark lab test for the diagnosis of UTIs, with quantitative cultures providing the most useful data for determining the clinical significance of isolated bacteria. To establish the diagnosis of a UTI, urine cultures from midstream urine samples should display $>10^5$ cfu/mL of a single potential uropathogen with concomitant pyuria on urinalysis; however, some women with symptomatic cystitis may have lower colony counts of bacteria. Colony counts of $>10^3$ cfu/mL with pyuria are considered clinically relevant in urine specimens from patients with indwelling urethral or suprapubic catheters, intermittent catheterization, men, or children.[144,147] Urine specimens obtained by suprapubic aspiration that display $>10^2$ cfu/mL with pyuria are indicative of the presence of infection.[144-146,148]

Prostatitis

Bacterial *prostatitis* can present as an acute or chronic infection that typically occurs in males over the age of 30 years.[146] The diagnosis of acute bacterial prostatitis is often based on the clinical presentation of the patient as well as the presence of bacteria in a urine specimen. Digital palpation of the prostate and prostatic massage to express purulent secretions are not recommended for the diagnosis of acute bacterial prostatitis since they may induce bacteremia. However, the diagnosis of chronic bacterial prostatitis often cannot be established based on clinical grounds alone since the symptoms are nonspecific and the prostate is often not acutely inflamed. Therefore, chronic prostatitis is classically established through the analysis of sequential urine and prostatic fluid cultures.[146,149] Initially, two samples of urine are obtained for culture—one sample on initiation of urination (VB-1) and one sample obtained at midstream (VB-2). Next, prostate fluid is obtained for culture by massaging the prostate to produce expressed prostatic secretions (EPS). Lastly, a urine sample (VB-3) is obtained after prostatic secretions have been obtained and sent for culture. The diagnosis of chronic bacterial prostatitis is made when the EPS sample contains greater than 10 times the quantity of bacteria cultured from VB-1 or VB-2, or if the VB-3 contains 10 times the quantity of bacteria cultured from VB-1 or VB-2.[146,149] An abbreviated 2-glass specimen method is commonly used in clinical practice and is described in Chapter 22: Common Medical Disorders of Aging Males—Clinical and Laboratory Test Monitoring.

Sexually Transmitted Diseases

Gonorrhea

Infection due to *Neisseria gonorrhoeae* is the second most common sexually transmitted disease (STD) reported in the United States, with most infections involving the mucosa of the cervix, the urethra, the rectum, and the pharynx.[150,151] Infections caused by *N. gonorrhoeae* include localized, uncomplicated, or complicated genital infections (e.g., urethritis, cervicitis, endometritis, pelvic inflammatory disease [PID] in women, and urethritis or epididymitis in men), pharyngitis, anorectal infections, and disseminated infection (e.g., septic arthritis and meningitis) in both men and women.[150,151] Women with genital tract infection and patients with pharyngeal infection are often asymptomatic, while men with urethritis often display symptoms of dysuria and urethral discharge. In addition, patients with *N. gonorrhoeae* are often coinfected with other STDs, such as *Chlamydia trachomatis,* syphilis, or *Trichomonas vaginalis;* therefore, the diagnosis and treatment of all possible STDs in the patient and their sexual partners are important considerations in the control of STDs.[151]

The diagnosis of infection due to *N. gonorrhoeae* can be established using stained clinical smears, culture, or nonculture techniques (EIA, DNA probe techniques, or nucleic acid amplification tests [NAATs]) of urethral, endocervical or urine specimens (NAATs only) that detect cellular components of *N. gonorrhoeae*.[4,150-153] Urethral, endocervical, and vaginal specimens for the detection of gonorrhea using culture or hybridization techniques should be obtained using a urogenital swab and transported to the laboratory in modified Stuart's or Amie's charcoal transport media.[4,150,152]

Culture on selective media remains the diagnostic standard for the identification of *N. gonorrhoeae*.[150,153] Culture is recommended for the diagnosis of gonorrhea from urethral, endocervical, vaginal, pharyngeal, or rectal swabs specimens and should be performed on specimens from all patients (and sexual partners) with suspected gonococcal infections.[150]

Culture is also used as a confirmatory test in patients who have suspected gonorrhea based on positive-stained smears or nonculture tests if the specimen has been adequately maintained. Occasionally, susceptibility testing is performed on *N. gonorrhoeae* isolates, especially in patients failing apparent appropriate therapy, to guide the choice of antibiotic therapy, as well as for epidemiologic purposes. In either case, patients are typically treated empirically with an antibiotic that demonstrates excellent activity against gonorrhea, keeping in mind that the incidence of beta-lactamase-producing, penicillin-resistant gonococci is increasing.

A presumptive diagnosis of gonorrhea can be made using direct microscopic examination of a clinical specimen using a Gram stain and oxidase test, where Gram-negative, oxidase-positive diplococci are demonstrated.[150-153] In addition, the presence of neutrophils on a Gram stain of a urethral specimen is also helpful in establishing the presumptive diagnosis of urethritis.[151] The Gram stain is both sensitive and specific for the presumptive diagnosis of *N. gonorrhoeae* as a point-of-care test for men with urethral discharge, but is not as useful as a single diagnostic test when evaluating endocervical or pharyngeal specimens. Additional tests, such as culture, should be performed to confirm the identification of the organism.

Nonculture tests available for the detection of *N. gonorrhoeae* (even in nonviable organisms) include NAATs, which are able to amplify organism-specific DNA sequences, and the NA hybridization (probe) test, which hybridizes any complementary rRNA that is present in the specimen (cannot differentiate organisms).[150,151] Several NAATs for the detection of *N. gonorrhoeae* are commercially available, and have been designed to detect RNA or DNA sequences using amplification techniques. These tests have been FDA-approved for the detection of *N. gonorrhoeae* in endocervical and vaginal swabs from women, urethral swabs from men, and urine samples from men and women.[150,151] These tests are also useful for the detection of *N. gonorrhoeae* from clinical specimens that have not been adequately maintained during transport or collection for culture methods to be utilized.

Chlamydia

Chlamydia trachomatis is the most common STD in the United States, with 3–4 million infections occurring annually in sexually active adolescents and adults.[150,152] Infection with *C. trachomatis* is now a reportable communicable disease in all 50 states of the United States, with a significant increase in reported cases observed from 1987–2001. *C. trachomatis* can cause a number of infections including cervicitis, endometritis, and PID in women; and urethritis, epididymoorchitis, prostatitis, and proctitis (via receptive anal intercourse) in men.[150] Infection with *C. trachomatis* is also thought to contribute to female infertility and ectopic pregnancies. It is estimated that over $2.4 billion is spent annually on the direct and indirect costs associated with the management of *C. trachomatis* infections.

The majority of patients with chlamydial infections are asymptomatic, so that screening is necessary to detect the presence of the organism.[151] Because of the asymptomatic nature of chlamydia, it is thought that the current rates of reporting underestimate the true incidence of infection due to this organism. Screening for the presence of *C. trachomatis* is typically performed on specimens obtained from patients presenting with other STDs since chlamydia often coexists with other STD pathogens.

Culture and nonculture methods are available for the detection of chlamydia. Culture involves the inoculation of the biologic specimen onto a confluent monolayer of susceptible cells that develop characteristic intracellular inclusions within 48–72 hours when infected by *C. trachomatis* that can be detected using a fluorescent monoclonal antibody stain.[150] Cell culture is not routinely utilized due to lack of standardization, technical difficulty, cost, and length of time to yield results (at least 48 hours). Therefore, other nonculture approaches for the laboratory diagnosis of chlamydia have been developed, including the direct fluorescent antibody (DFA) test and NAATs.

The DFA test involves the staining of a biologic specimen with a fluorescein-labeled monoclonal antibody that binds to *C. trachomatis*-specific antigens (elementary bodies). If the patient is infected with *C. trachomatis*, the antibodies will react with the elementary bodies of the chlamydia in the secretions to produce fluorescence.

The other nonculture test used for the detection of *Chlamydia trachomatis* is the NAAT, which has largely replaced tissue culture and DFA tests because of greater sensitivity and specificity.[150,151,153] There are a number of commercially-available NAATs for the detection of *C. trachomatis* that have been designed to detect RNA or DNA sequences using PCR, ligase chain reaction (LCR), and various amplification techniques. These tests have been FDA-approved for the detection of *C. trachomatis* in endocervical or vaginal swabs from women, urethral swabs from men, and rectal swab or urine samples from men and women.[151]

Syphilis

The spirochete, *Treponema pallidum*, is the causative pathogen of an STD known as *syphilis*. There are a number of clinical manifestations and stages of syphilis that are based primarily on presenting symptoms and natural history of the infection[151,153,154]:

- **Primary syphilis**—characterized by painless ulcers called *chancres* that are typically located at the site of inoculation or initial infection (usually in genital area) and spontaneously resolve over 1–8 weeks.
- **Secondary syphilis**—characterized by systemic symptoms including fever, weight loss, malaise, headache, lymphadenopathy, and a mucocutaneous skin rash (generalized or localized, often involving the palms or the soles of the feet) resulting from hematogenous or lymphatic spread of the organism; if untreated, the manifestations resolve within 4–10 weeks.
- **Latent syphilis**—occurs after secondary syphilis where the organism is still present, but the patient is without symptoms; this subclinical infection can only be detected by serologic tests.
- **Late/tertiary syphilis**—occurs in approximately 35%

of untreated patients up to 10–25 years after initial infection; manifested as progressive disease involving the ascending aorta and/or CNS (neurosyphilis).

Treponema pallidum cannot be grown in culture; therefore, the diagnosis of syphilis involves the direct detection of the spirochete in biologic specimens by microscopy or the detection of treponemal-specific antibodies using serologic testing.

Direct detection methods can be performed on an appropriate clinical specimen obtained from suspicious genital or skin lesions, including lesion exudate or tissue. The direct detection of *Treponema pallidum* using dark-field microscopy involves the immediate examination (within 20 minutes of collection) of the biologic specimen under a microscope with a dark-field condenser, looking for the presence of motile spirochetes, where *T. pallidum* can be visualized as 8–10 µm, spiral-shaped organisms.[4,153,154] Another test for the direct detection of *Treponema pallidum* is the direct fluorescent antibody (DFA-TP) test where the biologic specimen is combined with fluorescein-labeled monoclonal or polyclonal antibodies specific for *T. pallidum*, and examined by fluorescence microscopy. The interaction between the antibodies and treponemal-specific antigens will produce fluorescence that can be visualized using microscopy.

There are two types of serologic tests that are utilized for the diagnosis of syphilis. The first type of serologic test measures the presence of *nontreponemal* or reaginic antibodies, such as the Venereal Disease Research Laboratory (VDRL) test and the RPR test. The other type of serologic test measures the presence of *treponemal* antibodies, such as the fluorescent treponemal antibody absorption (FTA-ABS) test and the microhemagglutination *Treponema pallidum* (MHA-TP) test.[151,153,154]

The nontreponemal antibody tests (VDRL, RPR) measure the presence of reagin, an antibody-like protein produced in patients with syphilis. However, reagin is also produced in patients with other illnesses including autoimmune diseases, leprosy, TB, malaria, and injection drug use, so false-positive RPR results may occur.[133] Both the RPR and VDRL tests are flocculation tests in which visible clumps are produced in the presence of the reagin antibody (*T. pallidum*) in the submitted specimen. For the VDRL test, the biologic specimen (serum, CSF) is combined with cardiolipin-lecithin coated cholesterol particles on a glass slide and examined microscopically.[154] If the reagin antibody is present in the biologic specimen, visual clumping will occur and be reported as reactive (medium and large clumps). This test can also be quantified by evaluating dilutions of the biologic specimen for reactivity, with the dilution that produces a fully reactive result being reported as the VDRL titer (e.g., 1:8 or 1:32). Therefore, the VDRL titer is also utilized to monitor a patient's response to therapy. The high titers present in untreated disease (e.g., 1:32) traditionally decrease fourfold by 6–12 months and become undetectable in 1–2 years.

The RPR test is a modification of the VDRL test and is commercially available as a reaction card. Sera from the patient is placed on the reaction card and observed for clumping. The RPR result is quantified by evaluating dilutions of the biologic specimen for reactivity, with the dilution that produces a fully reactive result being reported as the RPR titer (e.g., 1:8 or 1:32). The RPR titer is also utilized to monitor a patient's response to therapy, where a fourfold decline in titer 6–12 months after therapy would be suggestive of response. The RPR is easier to perform than the VDRL and is used by many laboratories and blood banks for routine syphilis screening. However, the RPR should not be used for the analysis of CSF specimens.

Because the nontreponemal antibody detection tests are nonspecific, false-positive (up to 1% to 2%) results can occur. Because they are relatively nonspecific, they are most useful for *screening* for the presence of syphilis.[153] In addition, since it takes several weeks for the development of reagin antibodies, false-negative results (up to 25% of patients with primary syphilis) can occur in the early stages of the disease. A positive result from the RPR or VDRL test should be confirmed with the FTA-ABS or the MHA-TP test, which both measure the presence of treponemal-specific antibody.

In the FTA-ABS test, the patient's serum or CSF is initially absorbed with non-*T. pallidum* antigens to reduce cross-reactivity and then applied to a slide on which *T. pallidum* organisms have been fixed followed by addition of a fluorescein-conjugated antihuman antibody for detection of specific antitreponemal antibodies. The amount of fluorescence is subjectively measured by the laboratory technician and reported as reactive, minimally reactive, or nonreactive. Therefore, this test is difficult to standardize among different laboratories. Because this test is also fairly expensive, it is primarily used to verify the results of a positive VDRL or RPR, rather than as a routine screening tool.[154] The FTA-ABS test can detect antibodies earlier in the course of syphilis than nontreponemal tests and, once positive, will remain positive for the life of the patient.

The MHA-TP test is performed utilizing erythrocytes from a turkey, sheep, or other mammal that have been coated with treponemal antigens. These erythrocytes are then mixed with the patient's serum and observed for agglutination, which signifies the presence of antibodies directed against *T. pallidum*. The results are reported as reactive (positive) or nonreactive (negative).

Lastly, EIA tests and PCR-based tests for the detection of *T. pallidum* are being evaluated as screening or confirmatory tests for the diagnosis of syphilis, especially for patients where serologic testing is not reliable.[151,153]

Trichomonas

Infection caused by the protozoan, *Trichomonas vaginalis,* is one of the most common and treatable STDs in the world.[154] *Trichomonas vaginalis* is typically diagnosed through detection of actively motile organisms during microscopic examination of wet preparations of vaginal secretions, urethral discharge, prostatic fluid, or urine sediment.[114,118,153] Because the sensitivity of the wet preparation is 50% to 70%, other diagnostic tests have been developed for the detection of *Trichomonas vaginalis* to enhance diagnostic yield, sensitivity, and specificity.[118,151,153] Culture using Diamond's medium is considered the diagnostic gold standard and is associated with >80% sensitivity; however, culture methods require proper collection and rapid

inoculation for best results, so it is not routinely performed by most labs.[118] Several rapid antigen detection methods are commercially available for the diagnosis of infection due to *Trichomonas vaginalis* that are easy to perform and employ different assays (IFA and capillary flow ICA).[114,118] Lastly, NA detection methods can also be utilized to diagnose *Trichomonas,* including direct DNA probe (Affirm VPIII, Becton Dickinson and Company) and PCR (Amplicor, Roche Diagnostic Corp.).[118,151]

Herpes Simplex Virus

Herpes simplex virus (HSV) is the most common cause of genital ulceration in the United States.[153] There are two serotypes of HSV that cause infection: HSV type 1 (HSV-1), most often associated with oropharyngeal infection (cold sores), and HSV type 2 (HSV-2), most commonly associated with genital tract infection. Some patients with genital herpes are asymptomatic, while others experience recurrent vesicular and ulcerative genital lesions, typically at the site of initial infection. In either case, HSV can be transmitted to others by direct contact with virus in secretions from lesions during primary infection or during reactivation of the infection.

In many patients, the diagnosis of HSV is made based on characteristic findings during physical examination, which may include painful vesicles, vesicles that have evolved into pustules, and/or shallow ulcers with an erythematous base. If lesions compatible with HSV infection are present, the diagnosis can be confirmed by performing a Tzanck smear of a specimen obtained by scraping the base of an active lesion, and visualizing the specimen for characteristic viral intranuclear inclusions using microscopy (cytology and histology).[65,155] Viral culture is the gold standard for the diagnosis of HSV and can also be performed on the specimen from the active lesion; however, it may take up to 5–7 days for the virus to grow and be identified.[151]

Other tests that can be used for the diagnosis of HSV infection include HSV antigen detection (e.g., DFA, indirect fluorescent antibody [IFA], immunoperoxidase staining, and EIA); HSV DNA detection by in situ hybridization; and HSV DNA-PCR.[65,151,155] The results from these tests are often available sooner than traditional cell culture and are most useful when rapid detection of HSV is necessary, such as for the diagnosis of encephalitis or before an impending birth.[153] In addition, there are also commercially-available, FDA-approved serology kits for the diagnosis of HSV-1 and HSV-2 that detect antibody produced against specific HSV antigens. Herpes simplex virus serologic tests are primarily used in research; for the diagnosis of genital herpes in patients with suspected genital lesions; for patients with known or suspected exposure to HSV; and for determining the serostatus of pregnant women or patients undergoing organ or bone marrow transplantation.[156]

Assessing Sterile Body Fluids for the Presence of Infection

Sterile body fluids such as pericardial fluid (pericarditis), pleural fluid (empyema), synovial fluid (septic arthritis), and peritoneal fluid (peritonitis) can be analyzed for the presence

TABLE 17-22. Pleural Fluid Findings and Interpretation[158-160]

	TRANSUDATIVE (SUGGESTIVE OF CHF, CIRRHOSIS)	EXUDATIVE (SUGGESTIVE OF INFECTION SUCH AS EMPYEMA, MALIGNANCY, PANCREATITIS WITH ESOPHAGEAL PERFORATION, SLE)
Appearance	Clear, serous	Cloudy
pH	>7.2	<7.2
LDH (International Units/L)	<200	≥200
Pleural fluid LDH to serum LDH ratio	<0.6	>0.6
Protein (g/dL)	<3.0	>3.0
Pleural fluid to serum protein ratio	<0.5	>0.5
Glucose (mg/dL)	>60 (same as serum)	<40–60
WBCs (count/mm^3)	<10,000	>10,000
WBC differential	<50% PMNs	If infectious, depends on pathogen

CHF = congestive heart failure; LDH = lactate dehydrogenase; PMNs =polymorphonuclear leukocytes; SLE = systemic lupus erythematosus; WBC = white blood cell.

of infection. The specimens should be aseptically obtained by needle aspiration, placed in sterile collection tubes, and immediately transported to the lab for fluid analysis and culture. Approximately 1–5 mL of fluid should be obtained when analyzing pericardial, pleural, or synovial fluid, while up to 10 mL of peritoneal fluid is required for the diagnosis of peritonitis.[157] All sterile fluids should be processed for cell count (establishing the presence of WBCs with differential), chemistry (protein and glucose), direct microscopic examination including Gram stain (presence of bacteria), and culture. For pleural and synovial fluids, specific criteria are available to aid in the diagnosis of infection (see Tables 17-22 and 17-23).[158-163] Peritoneal fluid characteristics that may be suggestive of peritonitis include a WBC of >250 cells/mm^3, a lactate concentration >25 mg/dL, a pH <7.35, a fluid:blood glucose ratio of <0.7 (in tuberculous peritonitis), and an elevated protein concentration (except in cirrhotic patients).[164] The diagnosis of infection in each of these sites should be established based on the presence of WBCs and other characteristic chemistry abnormalities in the sterile fluid specimen, the growth of a pathogenic organism from the cultured material, and the characteristic signs and symptoms of infection at the infection site.

ACUTE PHASE REACTANTS AND INFECTION

Chapter 18: Rheumatic Diseases provides information on the background, normal range, and clinical utility of acute phase reactants such as the ESR and the CRP as they relate to the diagnosis of inflammatory diseases. The ESR and CRP may also be elevated in the presence of infection.[165-171] Elevations in the ESR and CRP do not differentiate between inflammatory or infectious processes since they increase in response to tissue injury of any cause. However, the ESR and CRP are often elevated in the presence of infection—with increased levels reported in bacterial otitis media, osteomyelitis, endocarditis, PID, and infections in transplant patients—and may serve as an adjunctive modality to aid in the diagnosis of these infections.[165-171] Serial measurement of the ESR, and especially the CRP, may also be useful in assessing the response to antibiotic therapy in the treatment of deep-seated infections such as endocarditis or osteomyelitis.[165-171]

Procalcitonin is the precursor of calcitonin, a calcium regulatory hormone, which is also an acute phase reactant that increases in response to systemic inflammation since it is thought to represent the activation of innate immunity in response to invasion by bacteria, malaria, and some fungi (not viruses).[165,172-174] It was originally believed that procalcitonin levels increased in response to tissue injury or sepsis induced only by infection; however, levels of procalcitonin may

TABLE 17-23. Synovial Fluid Findings and Interpretation[161-163]

	NORMAL	NONINFLAMMATORY (OSTEOARTHRITIS, TRAUMA, AVASCULAR NECROSIS, SLE, EARLY RHEUMATOID ARTHRITIS)	INFLAMMATORY (RHEUMATOID ARTHRITIS, SPONDYLOARTHROPATHIES, VIRAL ARTHRITIS, CRYSTAL-INDUCED ARTHRITIS)	PURULENT (BACTERIAL INFECTION, TUBERCULOUS INFECTION, FUNGAL INFECTION)
WBCs (count/mm^3)	<150	<3000	3000–50,000	>50,000
WBC differential	No predominance	<25% PMNs	>70% PMNs, variable	>75% to 90% PMNs
Protein (g/dL)	1.3–1.8	3–3.5	>3.5	>3.5
Glucose (mg/dL)	Normal	Normal	70–90	<40–50

PMNs = polymorphonuclear leukocytes; SLE = systemic lupus erythematosus; WBC = white blood cell.

be elevated in other inflammatory diseases or situations such as autoimmune diseases, severe trauma, cirrhosis, pancreatitis, and hypotension during surgery.[165,173,174] Current research suggests that the level of procalcitonin elevation may provide useful diagnostic information, with levels ≥10 mcg/mL indicative of sepsis/systemic bacterial infection, levels between 2 and 10 mcg/mL suggestive of sepsis, and levels between 0.25 and 2 mcg/mL suggestive of other conditions or localized infection.[173] In addition, the procalcitonin level may be useful for assessing the efficacy of empiric antibiotic therapy as well as for determining when antibiotic therapy can be discontinued during the treatment of an infection. However, further research is needed to define the exact role of procalcitonin in the diagnosis and management of infections.[174]

SUMMARY

Although infectious disease is a rapidly changing field because of new challenges and technological advances, the diagnosis of many infectious illnesses depends on proper performance and interpretation of numerous basic laboratory tests. For example, the Gram stain is a readily available, invaluable tool for examining clinical specimens for the presence of bacteria. Culture of clinical specimens using appropriate growth media allows the cultivation of many infecting bacteria in the clinical laboratory. Because empiric antimicrobial therapy is based on the patient's history and clinical condition, information from a Gram stain and culture are useful in targeting antibiotic therapy toward the infecting organism.

Susceptibility tests for rapidly growing aerobic bacteria are commonly performed using an automated microdilution or a manual disk diffusion method. Bacterial susceptibilities to various antimicrobial agents are reported as S, I, and R. National standards for susceptibility testing are available and help guide the performance of the tests, the choice of antimicrobial agents to evaluate for susceptibility, and the reporting procedures of susceptibility tests by the clinical microbiology laboratory. Moreover, susceptibility information should be considered in conjunction with patient-specific data (e.g., clinical condition, site of infection, drug allergies, and renal function) to design an appropriate antimicrobial drug regimen for a patient.

New testing methods and guidelines have recently become available for the recovery, identification, and susceptibility testing of fungi, mycobacteria, and viruses. These processes may challenge the clinical microbiology laboratory due to their requirements for specialized staining, culturing, and susceptibility testing procedures.

Lastly, several infection types (e.g., meningitis, UTIs, etc.) and certain pathogens (e.g., *Borrelia burgdorferi* and *Legionella pneumophila*) often require specialized laboratory testing to aid in the identification of the infecting organism. The clinician should be aware of the diagnostic tests currently available for these infections.

Learning Points

1. What methods do most microbiology laboratories in the United States use to perform antimicrobial susceptibility testing, and how is this information conveyed to the clinician?

Answer: Microbiology labs often utilize several methods for antimicrobial susceptibility testing in order to accurately determine the activity of antibiotics against many different types of bacteria (e.g., aerobic, anaerobic, and fastidious). However, most laboratories predominantly utilize automated broth microdilution methods (Vitek, Vitek-2, MicroScan) that utilize commercially-prepared, disposable microtiter trays/cassettes for antimicrobial susceptibility testing that can test the susceptibility of multiple antibiotics simultaneously, while decreasing cost and labor. The antimicrobial susceptibility results for each bacteria are compiled in a report that contains the following information: antibiotic tested, MIC or MIC range (especially with automated broth microdilution methods), and CLSI interpretive criteria (S, I, and R). These reports are usually located in the patient's medical chart (electronic or paper) and in the hospital/laboratory information system. The reader is referred to Minicase 2 for a specific example of an antimicrobial susceptibility report.

2. What laboratory tests are utilized in the diagnosis of HIV infection? What surrogate laboratory markers are used to assess the immunocompetence of patients infected with HIV?

Answer: There are several laboratory tests that are available for the diagnosis and monitoring of patients with HIV-1 infection. The hallmark tests for diagnosing HIV infection include the ELISA or EIA and WB. The ELISA is widely used as the initial screening test to detect HIV-specific antibodies. Because false-positive ELISA tests may occur in some patients, a more specific supplemental test such as the WB must be performed to confirm the presence of antibodies specific to HIV-1. The CD4 cell count and the plasma HIV viral load are the two surrogate laboratory markers that are routinely used throughout the course of HIV infection to assess the immunocompetence of patients infected with HIV, and are often used to determine the indications for antiretroviral treatment as well as to monitor the effectiveness of antiretroviral therapy.

3. What are the major laboratory tests that are used in the diagnosis of the UTIs, meningitis, pneumonia, and septic arthritis?

Answer: In patients with signs and symptoms suggestive of a UTI, a urine sample (clean-catch midstream, catheterized specimen, suprapubic aspiration) is usually sent to the lab for microscopic analysis (urinalysis) and culture. In patients with signs and symptoms suggestive of meningitis, a lumbar puncture is performed to obtain CSF that is evaluated for general appearance, glucose concentration, protein concentration, WBC count, WBC differential, Gram stain, and culture.

In addition, depending on the medical history of the patient, specialized tests may also be performed on the CSF. In patients with signs and symptoms suggestive of pneumonia, a sputum sample (expectorated, BAL, protected specimen brush) is submitted to the lab for adequacy evaluation, Gram stain and culture, and, occasionally, *Streptococcus pneumoniae* urinary antigen. In patients with suspected septic arthritis, a synovial fluid aspirate is analyzed for cell count (presence of WBCs with differential), chemistry (protein and glucose), direct microscopic examination including Gram stain (presence of bacteria), and culture. Patients with septic arthritis may also have an elevated ESR or CRP. Also, in all of the above infections, patients may also exhibit leukocytosis and/or a left shift, which would be demonstrated on a CBC.

REFERENCES

1. Specimen management. In: Forbes BA, Sahm DF, Weissfeld AS, eds. *Diagnostic Microbiology*. 12th ed. St Louis, MO: Mosby Inc; 2007:62-77.

2. Garcia LS, Isenberg HD, eds. *Clinical Microbiology Procedures Handbook*. 3rd ed. Washington DC: American Society for Microbiology Press; 2010.

3. Murray PR, Witebsky FG. The clinician and the microbiology laboratory. In: Mandell GL, Bennett JE, Dolin R, eds. *Principles and Practice of Infectious Diseases*. 7th ed. Philadelphia, PA: Elsevier Churchill Livingstone; 2010:233-265.

4. Baron EJ, Thomson RB. Specimen collection, transport, and processing: Bacteriology. In: Versalovic J, Carroll KC, Funke G, Jorgensen JH, et al., eds. *Manual of Clinical Microbiology*. 10th ed. Washington DC: American Society for Microbiology Press; 2011:228-271.

5. Popescu A, Doyle RJ. The Gram stain after more than a century. *Biotech Histochem*.1996;71(3):145-151.

6. Role of microscopy. In: Forbes BA, Sahm DF, Weissfeld AS, eds. *Diagnostic Microbiology*. 12th ed. St Louis, MO: Mosby Inc; 2007:78-92.

7. Woods GL, Walker DH. Detection of infection and infectious agents by use of cytologic and histologic stains. *Clin Microbiol Rev*. 1996;9(3):382-404.

8. Atlas RM, Snyder JW. Reagents, stains and media: Bacteriology. In: Versalovic J, Carroll KC, Funke G, et al., eds. *Manual of Clinical Microbiology*. 10th ed. Washington DC: American Society for Microbiology Press; 2011:272-303.

9. Graman PS, Menegus MA. Microbiology laboratory tests. In: Reese RE, Betts RF, eds. *A Practical Approach to Infectious Diseases*. 4th ed. New York, NY: Little, Brown and Company; 1996:935-966.

10. Bacteria. In: Wilborn JW. *Microbiology*. Springhouse, PA: Springhouse Corporation; 1993:36-50.

11. Rybak MJ, Aeschlimann JR, LaPlante KL. Laboratory tests to direct antimicrobial pharmacotherapy. In: DiPiro JT, Talbert RL, Yee GC, et al., eds. *Pharmacotherapy: A Pathophysiologic Approach*. 8th ed. New York, NY: McGraw-Hill Companies Inc; 2011:1797-1812.

12. Traditional cultivation and identification. In: Forbes BA, Sahm DF, Weissfeld AS, eds. *Diagnostic Microbiology*. 12th ed. St Louis, MO: Mosby Inc; 2007:93-119.

13. Busse HJ, Denner EBM, Lubitz W. Classification and identification of bacteria: current approaches to an old problem. Overview of methods used in bacteria systematics. *J Biotechnol*. 1996;47:3-38.

14. Overview of bacterial identification methods and strategies. In: Forbes BA, Sahm DF, Weissfeld AS, eds. *Diagnostic Microbiology*. 12th ed. St Louis, MO: Mosby Inc; 2007:216-247.

15. Stager CE, Davis JR. Automated systems for identification of microorganisms. *Clin Microbiol Rev*. 1992;5:302-327.

16. Highlander SK, Versalovic J, Petrosino JF. The human microbiome. In: Versalovic J, Carroll KC, Funke G, et al., eds. *Manual of Clinical Microbiology*. 10th ed. Washington DC: American Society for Microbiology Press; 2011:188-198.

17. Bates DW, Goldman L, Lee TH. Contaminant blood cultures and resource utilization: the true consequences of false-positive results. *JAMA*. 1991;265:365-369.

18. Reese RE, Betts RF. Principles of antibiotic use. In: Reese RE, Betts RF, eds. *A Practical Approach to Infectious Diseases*. 4th ed. New York, NY: Little, Brown and Company; 1996:1059-1097.

19. American Thoracic Society and Infectious Diseases Society of America. Guidelines for the management of adults with hospital-acquired, ventilator-associated, and healthcare-associated pneumonia. *Am J Respir Crit Care Med*. 2005;171:388-416.

20. Laboratory methods and strategies for antimicrobial susceptibility testing. In: Forbes BA, Sahm DF, Weissfeld AS, eds. *Diagnostic Microbiology*. 12th ed. St Louis, MO: Mosby Inc; 2007:187-214.

21. Clinical and Laboratory Standards Institute (CLSI). *Development of In Vitro Susceptibility Testing Criteria and Quality Control Parameters; Approved Guideline*. 3rd ed. CLSI document M23-A3. Wayne, PA: Clinical and Laboratory Standards Institute; 2008.

22. Peterson LR, Shanholtzer CJ. Tests for bactericidal effects of antimicrobial agents: technical performance and clinical relevance. *Clin Microbiol Rev*. 1992;5:420-432.

23. Swenson JM, Patel JB, Jorgensen JH. Special phenotypic methods for detecting antibacterial resistance. In: Versalovic J, Carroll KC, Funke G, et al., eds. *Manual of Clinical Microbiology*. 10th ed. Washington DC: American Society for Microbiology Press; 2011:1155-1179.

24. DeGirolami PC, Eliopoulos G. Antimicrobial susceptibility tests and their role in therapeutic drug monitoring. *Clin Lab Medicine*. 1987;7:499-512.

25. Jorgensen JH, Ferraro MJ. Antimicrobial susceptibility testing: A review of general principles and contemporary practices. *Clin Infect Dis*. 2009;49:1749-1755.

26. Clinical and Laboratory Standards Institute (CLSI). *Performance Standards for Antimicrobial Susceptibility Testing: Twenty-Second Informational Supplement*. CLSI document M100-S22.Wayne, PA: Clinical and Laboratory Standards Institute; 2012.

27. Clinical and Laboratory Standards Institute (CLSI). *Methods for Dilution Antimicrobial Susceptibility Tests for Bacteria That Grow Aerobically; Approved Standard*. 9th ed. CLSI document M07-A9. Wayne, PA: Clinical and Laboratory Standards Institute; 2012.

28. Clinical and Laboratory Standards Institute (CLSI). *Performance Standards for Antimicrobial Disk Susceptibility Tests; Approved Standard*. 9th ed. CLSI document M2-A11. Wayne, PA: Clinical and Laboratory Standards Institute; 2012.

29. Patel JB, Tenover FC, Turnidge JD, et al. Susceptibility test methods: dilution and disk diffusion methods. In: Versalovic J, Carroll KC, Funke G, et al., eds. *Manual of Clinical Microbiology*. 10th ed. Washington DC: American Society for Microbiology Press; 2011:1122-1143.

30. Louie M, Cockerill FR. Susceptibility testing: phenotypic and genotypic tests for bacteria and mycobacteria. *Infect Dis Clin North Am*. 2001;15(4):1205-1226.

31. Clinical and Laboratory Standards Institute (CLSI)/National Committee for Clinical Laboratory Standards. *Methods for Determining Bactericidal Activity of Antimicrobial Agents*. CLSI/NCCLS document M26-A. Wayne, PA: Clinical and Laboratory Standards Institute; 1999.

32. Reller LB. The serum bactericidal test. *Rev Infect Dis*. 1986;8:803-808.

33. Clinical and Laboratory Standards Institute (CLSI)/National Committee for Clinical Laboratory Standards. *Methodology for the Serum Bactericidal Test*. CLSI/NCCLS document M21-A. Wayne, PA: Clinical and Laboratory Standards Institute; 1999.

34. Bush K. Bench-to-bedside review: The role of β-lactamases in antibiotic-resistant Gram-negative infections. *Critical Care*. 2010;14:224.

35. Paterson DL, Bonomo RA. Extended-spectrum β-lactamases: A clinical update. *Clin Microbiol Rev*. 2005:18:657-686.

36. Jorgensen JH, Ferraro MJ. Antimicrobial susceptibility testing: special needs for fastidious organisms and difficult-to-detect resistance mechanisms. *Clin Infect Dis*. 2000;30:799-808.

37. Thomson KS. Extended-spectrum- β-lactamases, AmpC, and carbapenemase issues. *J Clin Microbiol*. 2010;48:1019-1025.

38. Tenover FC. Rapid detection and identification of bacterial pathogens using novel molecular technologies: infection control and beyond. *Clin Infect Dis*. 2007;44:418-423.

39. BD GeneOhm™ MRSA Assay [package insert]. Ste Foy Qc, Canada: BD Diagnostics; 2006.

40. MRSA Latex Test [product information]. Tokyo, Japan: Denka-Seiken.

41. Cepheid Xpert® MRSA/SA BC [product brochure]. Sunnyvale, CA: Cepheid; 2012.

42. Anaerobic bacteriology: overview and general considerations. In: Forbes BA, Sahm DF, Weissfeld AS, eds. *Diagnostic Microbiology*. 12th ed. St Louis, MO: Mosby Inc; 2007:455-462.

43. Anaerobic bacteriology: laboratory considerations. In: Forbes BA, Sahm DF, Weissfeld AS, eds. *Diagnostic Microbiology*. 12th ed. St Louis, MO: Mosby Inc; 2007:463-477.

44. Citron DM, Hecht DW. Susceptibility test methods: anaerobic bacteria. In: Versalovic J, Carroll KC, Funke G, et al., eds. *Manual of Clinical Microbiology*. 10th ed. Washington DC: American Society for Microbiology Press; 2011:1204-1214.

45. Hindler JA, Jorgensen JH. Susceptibility tests methods: fastidious bacteria. In: Versalovic J, Carroll KC, Funke G, et al., eds. *Manual of Clinical Microbiology*. 10th ed. Washington DC: American Society for Microbiology Press; 2011:1180-1203.

46. Clinical and Laboratory Standards Institute (CLSI). *Methods for Antimicrobial Susceptibility Testing of Anaerobic Bacteria; Approved Standard*. 8th ed. CLSI document M11-A8. Wayne, PA: Clinical and Laboratory Standards Institute; 2012.

47. Hecht DW. Evolution of anaerobe susceptibility testing in the United States. *Clin Infect Dis*. 2002;35(suppl 1):S28-S35.

48. Clinical and Laboratory Standards Institute (CLSI). *Analysis and Presentation of Cumulative Antimicrobial Susceptibility Test Data; Approved Guideline*. 3rd ed. CLSI document M39-A3. Wayne, PA: Clinical and Laboratory Standards Institute; 2009.

49. Brandt ME, Warnock DW. Taxonomy and classification of fungi. In: Versalovic J, Caroll KC, Jorgensen JH, et al. *Manual of Clinical Microbiology*. 10th ed. Washington DC: ASM Press; 2011:1747-1755.

50. McGowan KL. Specimen collection, transport, and processing: mycology. In: Versalovic J, Caroll KC, Jorgensen JH, et al. *Manual of Clinical Microbiology*. 10th ed. Washington DC: ASM Press; 2011:1756-1766.

51. Snyder JW, Atlas RM, LaRocco MT. Reagents, stains, and media: mycology. In: Versalovic J, Caroll KC, Jorgensen JH, et al. *Manual of Clinical Microbiology*. 10th ed. Washington DC: ASM Press; 2011:1767-1775.

52. Shea YR. General approaches for direct detection of fungi. In: Versalovic J, Caroll KC, Jorgensen JH, et al., eds. *Manual of Clinical Microbiology*. 9th ed. Washington DC: American Society for Microbiology Press; 2011:1776-1792.

53. Larone DH. *Medically Important Fungi: A Guide to Identification*. 5th ed. Washington DC: ASM Press; 2011.

54. Croxatto A, Prod'hom G, Greub G. Applications of MALDI-TOF mass spectrometry in clinical diagnostic microbiology. *FEMS Microbiol Rev*. 2012;36:380-407.

55. Clinical and Laboratory Standards Institute (CLSI). *Reference Method for Broth Dilution Antifungal Susceptibility Testing of Yeasts; Approved Standard*. 3rd ed. CLSI document M27-A3. Wayne, PA: Clinical and Laboratory Standards Institute; 2008.

56. Clinical and Laboratory Standards Institute (CLSI). *Reference Method for Broth Dilution Antifungal Susceptibility Testing of Filamentous Fungi; Approved Standard*. 2nd ed. CLSI document M38-A2. Wayne, PA: Clinical and Laboratory Standards Institute; 2008.

57. Clinical and Laboratory Standards Institute (CLSI). *Method for Antifungal Disk Diffusion Susceptibility Testing of Yeasts; Approved Guideline*. 2nd ed. CLSI document M44-A2. Wayne, PA: Clinical and Laboratory Standards Institute; 2009.

58. Johnson EM, Espinel-Ingroff AV, Pfaller MA. Susceptibility test methods: yeast and filamentous fungi. In: Versalovic J, Carroll KC, Jorgensen JH, et al., eds. *Manual of Clinical Microbiology*. 10th ed, Washington DC: ASM Press; 2011:2020-2037.

59. Pfaller MA, Diekema DJ, Andes D, et al. Wild-type MIC distributions, epidemiological cutoff values and species-specific clinical breakpoints for fluconazole and *Candida*: time for harmonization of CLSI and EUCAST broth microdilution methods. *Drug Resist Updates* 2010;13:180-195.

60. Pfaller MA, Andes D, Arendrup MC, et al. Clinical breakpoints for voriconazole and *Candida* spp. revisited: review of microbiologic, molecular, pharmacodynamic, and clinical data as they pertain to the development of species-specific interpretive criteria. *Diagn Microbiol Infect Dis* 2011;70:330-343.

61. Pfaller MA, Diekema DJ, Andes D, et al. Clinical breakpoints for the echinocandins and *Candida* revisited: integration of molecular, clinical, and microbiological data to arrive at species-specific interpretive criteria. *Drug Resist Updates*. 2011;14:164-176.

62. Lefkowitz EJ. Taxonomy and classification of viruses. In: Versalovic J, Carroll KC, Funke G, et al. *Manual of Clinical Microbiology*. 10th ed. Washington, DC: ASM Press; 2011:1265-1275.

63. Forman MS, Valsamakis A. Specimen collection, transport, and processing: virology. In: Versalovic J, Carroll KC, Funke G, et al., eds. *Manual of Clinical Microbiology*. 10th ed. Washington, DC: ASM Press; 2011:1276-1288.

64. Landry ML, Caliendo AM, Ginocchio CC, et al. Algorithms for detection and identification of viruses. In: Versalovic J, Carroll KC, Funke G, et al. *Manual of Clinical Microbiology*. 10th ed. Washington, DC: ASM Press; 2011:1297-1301.

65. Laboratory methods in basic virology. In: Forbes BA, Sahm DF, Weissfeld AS, eds. *Diagnostic Microbiology*. 12th ed. St Louis, MO: Mosby Inc; 2007:718-776.

66. Ginocchio CC, Harris PC. Reagents, stains, media, and cell cultures: virology. In: Versalovic J, Carroll KC, Funke G, et al., eds. *Manual of Clinical Microbiology*. 10th ed. Washington, DC: ASM Press; 2011:1289-1296.

67. Leland DS, Ginocchio CC. Role of cell culture for virus detection in the age of technology. *Clin Microbiol Rev* 2007;20:49-78.

68. Chartrand C, Leeflang MMG, Minion J, Brewer T, Pai M. Accuracy of rapid influenza diagnostic tests: a meta-analysis. *Ann Intern Med*. 2012;156:500-511.

69. Arens MQ, Swierkosz EM. Susceptibility test methods: viruses. In: Versalovic J, Carroll KC, Funke G, et al., eds. *Manual of Clinical Microbiology*. 10th ed. Washington, DC: ASM Press; 2011:1729-1743.

70. Clinical and Laboratory Standards Institute (CLSI). *Antiviral Susceptibility Testing: Herpes Simplex Virus by Plaque Reduction Assay*. CLSI document M33-A. Wayne, PA: Clinical and Laboratory Standards Institute; 2004.

71. Griffith BP, Campbell S, Caliendo AM. In: Human immunodeficiency viruses. In: Murray PR, Baron EJ, Jorgensen JH, et al., eds. *Manual of Clinical Microbiology*. 10th ed. Washington DC: ASM Press; 2011:1302-1322.

72. Scosyrev E. An overview of the human immunodeficiency virus featuring laboratory testing for drug resistance. *Clin Lab Sci*. 2006;19(4):231-248.

73. Hodinka RL. Human immunodeficiency virus. In: Truant AL, ed. *Manual of Commercial Methods in Clinical Microbiology*. Washington, DC: ASM Press; 2002:100-127.

74. Dax EM, Arnott A. Advances in laboratory testing for HIV. *Pathology*. 2004;36(6):551-560.

75. Panel on Antiretroviral Therapy and Medical Management of HIV-Infected Children. Guidelines for the use of antiretroviral agents in pediatric HIV infection. 2011(August 11):1–268. Available at www.aidsinfo.nih.gov/ContentFiles/Pediatric Guidelines.pdf. Accessed January 6, 2012.

76. Panel on Antiretroviral Guidelines for Adults and Adolescents. Guidelines for the use of antiretroviral agents in HIV-infected adults and adolescents. Department of Health and Human Services. 2012(March 27):1-239. Available at http://aidsinfo.nih.gov/ContentFiles/AdultandAdolescentGL.pdf. Accessed March 27, 2012.

77. Panel on Treatment of HIV-Infected Pregnant Women and Prevention of Perinatal Transmission. Recommendations for the use of antiretroviral drugs in pregnant HIV-1 infected women for maternal health and interventions to reduce perinatal HIV-1 transmission in the United States. 2011(September 14):1–207. Available at http://aidsinfo.nih.gov/ContentFiles/PerinatalGL.pdf. Accessed January 6, 2012.

78. Franco-Paredes C, Tellez I, del Rio C. Rapid HIV testing: a review of the literature and implications for the clinician. *Current HIV/AIDS Reports*. 2006;3:159-165.

79. Butto S, Suligoi B, Fanales-Belasio E, et al. Laboratory diagnostics for HIV infection. *Ann Ist Super Sanita*. 2010;46:24-33.

80. Mylonakis E, Paliou M, Lally M, et al. Laboratory testing for infection with the human immunodeficiency virus: established and novel approaches. *Am J Med*. 2000;109:568-576.

81. Branson BM. State of the art for diagnosis of HIV infection. *Clin Infect Dis*. 2007;45(suppl):221S-225S.

82. Rapid HIV test kits. *Health Devices*. 2006(May):157-177.

83. Revised recommendations for HIV testing of adults, adolescents, and pregnant women in health-care settings. *MMWR*. 2006;55(RR-14):1-17.

84. Wilkin TJ, Su Z, Kagan R, et al. Comparison of Quest Diagnostics to Trofile and Trofile ES coreceptor tropism assays for predicting virologic response to maraviroc (MVC), a CCR5 antagonist. Program and abstracts of the 50th Interscience Conference on Antimicrobial Agents and Chemotherapy; September 12–15, 2010; Boston, Massachusetts. Abstract A-932.

85. Mycobacterium. In: Murray PR, Rosenthal KS, Kobayashi GS, et al., eds. *Medical Microbiology*. 4th ed. St Louis, MO: Mosby Inc; 2002:366-377.

86. Woods GL. Mycobacteria. In: Henry JB, ed. *Clinical Diagnosis and Management by Laboratory Methods*. 20th ed. Philadelphia, PA: WB Saunders Company; 2001:1144-1157.

87. Pfyffer GE. *Mycobacterium*: general characteristics laboratory detection, and staining procedures. In: Murray PR, Baron EJ, Jorgensen JH, et al., eds. *Manual of Clinical Microbiology*. 9th ed. Washington DC: American Society for Microbiology Press; 2007:543-572.

88. Mycobacteria. In: Forbes BA, Sahm DF, Weissfeld AS, eds. *Diagnostic Microbiology*. 12th ed. St Louis, MO: Mosby Inc; 2007:478-509.

89. American Thoracic Society and Infectious Diseases Society of America. Diagnosis, treatment and prevention of nontuberculous mycobacterial diseases. *Am J Respir Crit Care Med*. 2007;175:367-416.

90. American Thoracic Society Committee on Microbiology, Tuberculosis and Pulmonary Infections. Diagnostic standards and classification of tuberculosis in adults and children. *Am J Respir Crit Care Med*. 2000;161:1376-1395.

91. Hale YM, Pfyffer GE, Salfinger M. Laboratory diagnosis of mycobacterial infections: new tools and lessons to be learned. *Clin Infect Dis*. 2001;33:834-846.

92. Pfyffer GE, Palicova F. *Mycobacterium*: General characteristics, laboratory detection, and staining procedures. In: Murray PR, Baron EJ, Jorgensen JH, et al., eds. *Manual of Clinical Microbiology*. 10th ed. Washington DC: ASM Press; 2011:472-502.

93. American Thoracic Society/ Center for Disease Control and Prevention/Infectious Diseases Society of America: Controlling tuberculosis in the United States. *Am J Respir Crit Care Med*. 2005:172:1169-1227.

94. World Health Organization. *Global Tuberculosis Control: WHO Report 2011*. Geneva, Switzerland: World Health Organization; 2011.

95. Palomino JC. Nonconventional and new methods in the diagnosis of tuberculosis: feasibility and applicability in the field. *Eur Respir J*. 2005;26(2):339-350.

96. Richter E, Brown-Elliot BA, et al. *Mycobacterium*: Laboratory characteristics of slowly growing mycobacteria. In: Murray PR, Baron EJ, Jorgensen JH, et al., eds. *Manual of Clinical Microbiology*. 10th ed. Washington DC: ASM Press; 2011:503-524.

97. Centers for Disease Control and Prevention. Updated guidelines for the use of nucleic acid amplification tests in the diagnosis of tuberculosis, 2009. *MMWR*. 2009;58(01):7-10.

98. Clinical and Laboratory Standards Institute (CLSI). *Susceptibility Testing of Mycobacteria, Nocardiae, and Other Aerobic Actinomycetes; Approved Standard*. 2nd ed. CLSI document M24-A2. Wayne, PA: Clinical and Laboratory Standards Institute; 2011.

99. American Thoracic Society and Center for Disease Control and Prevention. Targeted tuberculin testing and treatment of latent tuberculosis infection. *MMWR*. 2000;49(RR6):1-54.

100. Centers for Disease Control and Prevention. Guidelines for preventing the transmission of *Mycobacterium tuberculosis* in health-care settings, 2005. *MMWR*. 2005;54(RR17):1-141.

101. Frenzel EC, Thomas GA, Hanna HA. The importance of two-step tuberculin skin testing for newly employed healthcare workers. *Infect Control Hosp Epidemiol*. 2006;27:512-514.

102. Centers for Disease Control and Prevention. Updated Guidelines for using the interferon Gamma release assays to detect *Mycobacterium tuberculosis* infection. *MMWR*. 2010;59(RR-5):1-26.

103. Hindiyeh M, Carroll KC. Laboratory diagnosis of atypical pneumonia. *Semin Resp Infect*. 2000;15:101-103.

104. *Bordetella pertussis and Bordetella parapertussis*. In: Forbes BA, Sahm DF, Weissfeld AS, eds. *Diagnostic Microbiology*. 12th ed. St Louis, MO: Mosby Inc; 2007:435-439.

105. Wood N, McIntyre P. Pertussis: Review of epidemiology, diagnosis, management and prevention. *Paediatr Respir Rev*. 2008;9:201-212.

106. Dam AP. Recent advances in the diagnosis of Lyme disease. *Expert Rev Mol Diagn*. 2001;1:413-427.

107. American College of Physicians. Guidelines for the laboratory evaluation and diagnosis of Lyme disease. *Ann Intern Med*. 1997;127(12):1106-1108.

108. Brucella. In: Forbes BA, Sahm DF, Weissfeld AS, eds. *Diagnostic Microbiology*. 12th ed. St Louis, MO: Mosby Inc; 2007:430-434.

109. Al Dahouk S, Nockler k. Implications of laboratory diagnosis on brucellosis therapy. *Expert Rev Anti Infect Ther* 2011;9:833-845.

110. Obligate intracellular and nonculturable bacterial agents. In: Forbes BA, Sahm DF, Weissfeld AS, eds. *Diagnostic Microbiology*. 12th ed. St Louis, MO: Mosby Inc; 2007:510-524.

111. Burillo A, Bouza E. *Chlamydophila pneumoniae. Infect Dis Clin N Am.* 2010;24:61-71.

112. Cohen SH, Gerding, DN, et al. Clinical practice guidelines for *Clostridium difficile* infection in adults: 2010 update by the Society for Healthcare Epidemiology of America (SHEA) and the Infectious Diseases Society of America (IDSA). *Infect Control Hosp Epidemiol.* 2010;31:431-455.

113. Kufelnicka AM, Kirn TJ. Effective utilization of evolving methods for the laboratory diagnosis of *Clostridium difficile* infection. *Clin Infect Dis* 2011;52:1451-1457.

114. Laboratory methods for the diagnosis of parasitic infections. In: Forbes BA, Sahm DF, Weissfeld AS, eds. *Diagnostic Microbiology.* 12th ed. St. Louis; Mosby Inc; 2007:543-627.

115. Xiao L, Cama V. Cryptosporidium. In: Versalovic J, Carroll KC, Funke G, et al., eds. *Manual of Clinical Microbiology.* 10th ed. Washington DC: American Society for Microbiology Press; 2011:2180-2189.

116. Dumler SJ, Madigan JE, Pusteria N, et al. Ehrlichiosis in humans: epidemiology, clinical presentation, diagnosis, and treatment. *Clin Infect Dis.* 2007;45(suppl 1):S45-S51.

117. Diagnosis and management of tickborne rickettsial diseases: Rocky Mountain spotted fever, ehrlichiosis, and anaplasmosis—United States. *MMWR.* 2006;55(RR04):1-27.

118. Leber AL, Novak-Weekley SN. Intestinal and urogenital amebae, flagellates, and ciliates. In: Versalovic J, Carroll KC, Funke G, et al., eds. *Manual of Clinical Microbiology.* 10th ed. Washington DC: American Society for Microbiology Press; 2011:2149-2171.

119. Fotedar R, Stark D, Beehe N, et al. Laboratory diagnostic techniques for *Entamoeba* species. *Clin Microbiol Rev.* 2007;20(3):511-532.

120. Suerbaum S, Michetti P. *Helicobacter pylori* infection. *N Engl J Med.* 2002;347:1175-1186.

121. McNulty CAM, Lehours P, Megraud F. Diagnosis of *Helicobacter pylori* infection. *Helicobacter.* 2011;16(Suppl 1):10-18.

122. Cunha BA. The atypical pneumonias: clinical diagnosis and importance. *Clin Microbiol Infect.* 2006;12(suppl 3):12-24.

123. Tronel H, Hartemann P. Overview of diagnostic and detection methods for legionellosis and *Legionella* spp. *Lett Appl Microbiol.* 2009;48:653-656.

124. Mondal S, Bhattacharya P, Ali N. Current diagnosis and treatment of visceral leishmaniasis. *Expert Rev Anti infect Ther.* 2010;8:919-944.

125. Toyokawa T, Ohnishi M, Koizumi N. Diagnosis of acute leptospirosis. *Expert Rev Anti Infect Ther.* 2011;9:111-121.

126. Cell-wall deficient bacteria: *Mycoplasma* and *ureaplasma.* In: Forbes BA, Sahm DF, Weissfeld AS, eds. *Diagnostic Microbiology.* 11th ed. St Louis, MO: Mosby Inc; 2002:587-594.

127. Waites KB, Taylor-Robinson D. Mycoplasma and ureaplasma. In: Versalovic J, Carroll KC, Funke G, et al., eds. *Manual of Clinical Microbiology.* 10th ed. Washington DC: American Society for Microbiology Press; 2011:970-985.

128. The Malaria Eradication Research Agenda (malERA) Consultative Group on Diagnoses and Diagnostics. A research agenda for malaria eradication: Diagnoses and diagnostics. *PLoS Medicine.* 2011;8:1-10.

129. Cushion MT. Pneumocystis. In: Versalovic J, Carroll KC, Funke G, et al., eds. *Manual of Clinical Microbiology.* 10th ed. Washington DC: American Society for Microbiology Press; 2011:1822-1835.

130. Montoya JG, Liesenfeld O. Toxoplasmosis. *Lancet.* 2004;363:1965-1976.

131. Wilson ML. Clinically relevant cost-effective clinical microbiology. *Am J Clin Pathol.* 1997;107:154-167.

132. Tunkel AR, Hartman BJ, Kaplan SL, et al. Practice guidelines for the management of bacterial meningitis. *Clin Infect Dis.* 2004;39:1267-1284.

133. Meningitis and other infections of the central nervous system. In: Forbes BA, Sahm DF, Weissfeld AS, eds. *Diagnostic Microbiology.* 12th ed. St Louis, MO: Mosby Inc; 2007:822-831.

134. Mitropoulos IF, Hermsen ED, Rotschafer JC. Central nervous system infections. In: DiPiro JT, Talbert RL, Yee GC, et al., eds. *Pharmacotherapy: A Pathophysiologic Approach.* 8th ed. New York, NY: McGraw-Hill Companies Inc; 2011:1825-1844.

135. Tunkel AR, van de Beek D, Scheld WM. Acute meningitis. In: Mandell GL, Bennett JE, Dolin R, eds. *Principles and Practice of Infectious Diseases.* 7th ed. Philadelphia, PA: Elsevier Churchill Livingstone; 2010:1189-1229.

136. Thomson RB, Bertram H. Laboratory diagnosis of central nervous system infections. *Infect Dis Clin North Am.* 2001;15:1047-1071.

137. Zunt JR, Marra CM. Cerebrospinal fluid testing for the diagnosis of central nervous system infections. *Neurol Clin North Am.* 1999;17:675-689.

138. Binax NOW® *Streptococcus pneumoniae* Antigen Test [product information]. Scarborough, ME: Binax Inc; March 2005.

139. Bisno AL, Gerber MA, Gwaltney JM, et al. Practice guidelines for the diagnosis and management of Group A streptococcal pharyngitis. *Clin Infect Dis.* 2002;35:113-125.

140. Leung AK, Newman R, Kumar A, et al. Rapid antigen detection testing in diagnosing group A beta-hemolytic streptococcal pharyngitis. *Expert Rev Mol Diagn.* 2006;6(5):761-766.

141. Infections of the lower respiratory tract. In: Forbes BA, Sahm DF, Weissfeld AS, eds. *Diagnostic Microbiology.* 12th ed. St Louis, MO: Mosby Inc; 2007:798-813.

142. Bartlett JG. Diagnostic tests for agents of community-acquired pneumonia. *Clin Infect Dis.* 2011;52(suppl 4):S296-S304.

143. Mandell LA, Wunderink RG, Anzueto A, et al. Infectious Diseases Society of America/American Thoracic Society consensus guidelines on the management of community-acquired pneumonia in adults. *Clin Infect Dis.* 2007;44:S27-S72.

144. Graham JC, Galloway A. The laboratory diagnosis of urinary tract infections. *J Clin Pathol.* 2001;54:911-919.

145. Infections of the urinary tract. In: Forbes BA, Sahm DF, Weissfeld AS, eds. *Diagnostic Microbiology.* 12th ed. St Louis, MO: Mosby Inc; 2007:842-855.

146. Coyle EA, Prince RA. Urinary tract infections and prostatitis. In: DiPiro JT, Talbert RL, Yee GC, et al., eds. *Pharmacotherapy: A Pathophysiologic Approach.* 8th ed. New York, NY: McGraw-Hill Companies Inc; 2011:1995-2010.

147. Gupta K, Hooton TM, et al. International clinical practice guidelines for the treatment of acute uncomplicated cystitis and pyelonephritis in women: A 2010 update by the Infectious Diseases Society of America and the European Society for Microbiology and Infectious Diseases. *Clin Infect Dis.* 2011;52:103-120.

148. Hooton TM, Bradley SF, et al. Diagnosis, prevention and treatment of catheter-associated urinary tract infections in adults: 2009 international clinical practice guidelines from the Infectious Diseases Society of America. *Clin Infect Dis.* 2010;50:625-663.

149. Meares EM, Stamey TA. Bacteriologic localization patterns in bacterial prostatitis and urethritis. *Invest Urol.* 1968;5:492-518.

150. Center for Disease Control and Prevention (CDC). Screening tests to detect *Chlamydia trachomatis* and *Neisseria gonorrhoeae* infections—2002. *MMWR.* 2002;51:1-27.

151. Center for Disease Control and Prevention (CDC). Sexually transmitted diseases treatment guidelines—2010. *MMWR.* 2010;59 (R12):1-110.

152. Genital tract infections. In: Forbes BA, Sahm DF, Weissfeld AS, eds. *Diagnostic Microbiology.* 12th ed. St Louis, MO: Mosby Inc; 2007:856-872.

153. Knodel LC. Sexually transmitted diseases. In: DiPiro JT, Talbert RL, Yee GC, et al., eds. *Pharmacotherapy: A Pathophysiologic Approach.* 8th ed. New York, NY: McGraw-Hill Companies Inc; 2011:2011-2028.

154. The spirochetes. In: Forbes BA, Sahm DF, Weissfeld AS, eds. *Diagnostic Microbiology*. 12th ed. St Louis, MO: Mosby Inc; 2007:533-541.

155. Jerome KR, Morrow RA. Herpes simplex viruses and Herpes B virus. In: Versalovic J, Carroll KC, Funke G, et al., eds. *Manual of Clinical Microbiology*. 10th ed. Washington DC: American Society for Microbiology Press; 2011:1530-1544.

156. Ashley RL. Performance and use of HSV type-specific serology test kits. *Herpes*. 2002;9:38-45.

157. Normally sterile body fluids, bone and bone marrow, and solid tissues. In: Forbes BA, Sahm DF, Weissfeld AS, eds. *Diagnostic Microbiology*. 12th ed. St Louis, MO: Mosby Inc; 2007:904-913.

158. Pierson DJ. Disorders of the pleura, mediastinum, and diaphragm. In: Wilson JD, Braunwald E, Isselbacher KJ, et al., eds. *Harrison's Principles of Internal Medicine*. 12th ed. New York, NY: McGraw Hill Inc; 1991:1111-1116.

159. Penn RL, Betts RF. Lower respiratory tract infections (including tuberculosis). In: Reese RE, Betts RF, eds. *A Practical Approach to Infectious Diseases*. 4th ed. New York, NY: Little Brown and Company; 1996:258-349.

160. Septimus E. Pleural effusion and empyema. In: Mandell GL, Bennett JE, Dolin R, eds. *Principles and Practice of Infectious Diseases*. 7th ed. Philadelphia, PA: Elsevier Churchill Livingstone; 2010:917-924.

161. Shmerling RH. Synovial fluid analysis: A critical reappraisal. *Rheum Infect Dis Clin North Am*. 1994;20:503-512.

162. Ohl CA. Infectious arthritis of native joints. In: Mandell GL, Bennett JE, Dolin R, eds. *Principles and Practice of Infectious Diseases*. 7th ed. Philadelphia, PA: Elsevier Churchill Livingstone; 2010:1443-1456.

163. Armstrong EP, Friedman AD. Bone and joint infections. In: DiPiro JT, Talbert RL, Yee GC, et al., eds. *Pharmacotherapy: A Pathophysiologic Approach*. 8th ed. New York, NY: McGraw-Hill Companies Inc; 2011:2029-2040.

164. Levison ME, Bush LM. Peritonitis and intraperitoneal abscesses. In: Mandell GL, Bennett JE, Dolin R, eds. *Principles and Practice of Infectious Diseases*. 7th ed. Philadelphia, PA: Elsevier Churchill Livingstone; 2010:1011-1034.

165. Dayer E, Dayer JM, Roux-Lombard P. Primer: the practical use of biological markers of rheumatic and systemic inflammatory diseases. *Nat Clin Pract Rheumatol*. 2007;3(9):512-520.

166. Saadeh C. The erythrocyte sedimentation rate: old and new clinical applications. *South Med J*. 1998;91(3):220-225.

167. Johnson HL, Chiou CC, Cho CT. Applications of acute phase reactants in infectious diseases. *J Microbiol Immunol Infect*. 1999;32(2):73-82.

168. Young B, Gleeson M, Cripps AW. C-reactive protein: a critical review. *Pathology*. 1991;23(2):118-124.

169. Hogevik H, Olaison L, Andersson R, Alestig K. C-reactive protein is more sensitive than erythrocyte sedimentation rate for diagnosis of infective endocarditis. *Infection*. 1997;25(2):82-85.

170. Olaison L, Hogevik H, Alestig K. Fever, C-reactive protein, and other acute-phase reactants during treatment of infective endocarditis. *Arch Intern Med*. 1997;157(8):885-892.

171. Heiro M, Helenius H, Sundell J, et al. Utility of serum C-reactive protein in assessing the outcome of infective endocarditis. *Eur Heart J*. 2005;26(18):1873-1881.

172. Whicher J, Bienvenu J, Monneret G. Procalcitonin as an acute phase marker. *Ann Clin Biochem*. 2001;38:483-493.

173. Schneider HG, Lam QT. Procalcitonin for the clinical laboratory: a review. *Pathology*. 2007;39(4):383-390.

174. Gilbert DN. Use of plasma procalcitonin levels as an adjunct to clinical microbiology. *J Clin Microbiol*. 2010:48:2325-2329.

CHAPTER 18

RHEUMATIC DISEASES

TERRY L. SCHWINGHAMMER

Objectives

After completing this chapter, the reader should be able to

- Describe the physiologic basis for rheumatologic laboratory tests and the pathophysiologic processes that result in abnormal test results

- Understand the appropriate clinical applications for laboratory tests used to diagnose or assess the activity of individual rheumatic diseases

- Interpret the results of laboratory tests used to diagnose or manage common rheumatic diseases

- Use the results of rheumatologic laboratory tests to make decisions about the effectiveness of pharmacotherapy

- Employ laboratory tests to identify and prevent adverse reactions to drugs used to treat rheumatic diseases

The diagnosis and management of most rheumatic diseases depend primarily on patient medical history, symptoms, and physical examination findings. A variety of laboratory tests are used to assist in the diagnosis of rheumatologic disorders, but many are nonspecific tests that are not pathognomonic for any single disease. However, the results of some specific laboratory tests may be essential for confirming the diagnosis of some diseases. Consequently, laboratory tests are important diagnostic tools when used in concert with the medical history and other subjective and objective findings. Some laboratory test results are also used to assess disease severity and to monitor the beneficial and adverse effects of pharmacotherapy.

The diagnostic utility of a laboratory test depends on its sensitivity, specificity, and predictive value (Chapter 1: Definitions and Concepts). Tests that are highly sensitive and specific for certain rheumatic diseases often have low predictive values because the prevalence of the suspected rheumatic disease is low. The most important determinant of a laboratory test's diagnostic usefulness is the pretest probability of disease, or a clinician's estimated likelihood that a certain disease is present based on history and clinical findings. As the number of disease-specific signs and symptoms increases and approaches diagnostic confirmation, the pretest probability also increases.

After briefly reviewing pertinent physiology of immunoglobulins, this chapter discusses various tests used to diagnose and assess rheumatic diseases, followed by interpretation of these test results in common rheumatic disorders. Tests used to monitor antirheumatic pharmacotherapy are also described.

STRUCTURE AND PHYSIOLOGY OF IMMUNOGLOBULINS

Many rheumatologic laboratory tests involve detection of immunoglobulins (antibodies) that are directed against normal cellular components. The structure and functions of immunoglobulins are reviewed briefly here to facilitate understanding of these tests.

When the immune system is challenged by a foreign substance (antigen), activated B lymphocytes differentiate into immunoglobulin-producing plasma cells. Immunoglobulins are Y-shaped proteins with an identical antigen-binding site (called *Fab* or *fraction antigen-binding*) on each arm of the Y (Figure 18-1). Each arm is composed of a light (L) amino acid chain covalently linked to a heavy (H) amino acid chain. The terms *light* and *heavy* refer to the number of amino acids in each chain. Because the heavy chain has more amino acids than the light chain, it is longer and has a higher molecular weight.

Both types of chains have a variable region (VL and VH) and a constant region (C_L and C_H). The variable regions contain the antigen-binding sites and vary in amino acid sequence. The sequences differ to allow immunoglobulins to recognize and bind specifically to thousands of different antigens. Within the variable regions, there are four framework regions (FWR) and three complementarity-determining regions (CDR); together these make up the antigen-binding pocket. The constant region of the light chain (CL) is a single section. Immunoglobulins that have identical constant regions in their heavy chains (e.g., C_H1, C_H2, and C_H3) are of the same class.

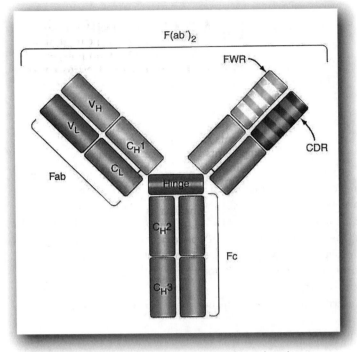

FIGURE 18-1. Schematic of the antibody molecule. (Reproduced, with permission, from Diamond B, Grimaldi C. B cells. In: Firestein GS, Budd RC, Harris ED Jr, et al., eds. *Kelley's Textbook of Rheumatology.* 8th ed. Philadelphia, PA: Saunders Elsevier; 2009:178.)

The five classes of immunoglobulins are IgA, IgD, IgE, IgG, and IgM. Depending on the immunoglobulin, the constant region of the heavy chain has either three domains and a hinge region (IgA, IgD, and IgG) that promotes flexibility, or four domains without a hinge region (IgE and IgM). Thus, the immunoglobulin's heavy chain determines its class (alpha heavy chains, IgA; delta heavy chains, IgD; epsilon heavy chains, IgE; gamma heavy chains, IgG; and mu heavy chains, IgM). Tests are available to measure the serum concentrations of the general types of immunoglobulins as well as immunoglobulins directed against specific antigens (viruses, other infectious agents, other allergens).

In Figure 18-1, the second and third domains (C_H2 and C_H3) of the heavy chain are part of the Fc (fraction crystallizable) portion of the immunoglobulin. This portion has two important functions: (1) activation of the complement cascade (discussed later); and (2) binding of immunoglobulins (which react with and bind antigen) to cell surface receptors of effector cells such as monocytes, macrophages, neutrophils, and natural killer (NK) cells.[1]

TESTS TO DIAGNOSE AND ASSESS RHEUMATIC DISEASES

Blood tests that are relatively specific for certain rheumatic diseases include rheumatoid factors (RFs), anticyclic citrullinated peptide (anti-CCP) antibodies, antinuclear antibodies (ANAs), antineutrophil cytoplasmic antibodies (ANCAs), and complement. Nonspecific blood and other types of tests include erythrocyte sedimentation rate (ESR), C-reactive protein (CRP), analysis of synovial fluid, and others.

Where applicable, the sections that follow discuss quantitative assay results (where normal values are reported as a range of concentrations), qualitative assay results (where assay results are reported as only positive or negative), and their use in common rheumatic and nonrheumatic diseases.

Rheumatoid Factor

Rheumatoid factors (RFs) are immunoglobulins that are abnormally directed against the Fc portion of IgG. These immunoglobulins do not recognize the IgG as being "self." Therefore, the presence of RFs in the blood indicates an autoimmune process. The RF measured in most laboratories is IgM-anti-IgG (an IgM antibody that specifically binds IgG). Like all IgM antibodies, IgM RF is composed of five subunits whose Fc portions are attached to the same base. The variable regions of each IgM antibody can bind up to five IgG molecules at its multiple binding sites, making IgM RF the most stable and easiest to quantify.

Rheumatoid factors are most commonly associated with rheumatoid arthritis (RA) but are not specific for that disease. Other rheumatic diseases in which circulating RFs have been identified include systemic lupus erythematosus (SLE), systemic sclerosis (scleroderma), mixed connective tissue disease (MCTD), and Sjögren syndrome.[2] The significance of RFs in these diseases is unknown.

The presence of RF is not conclusive evidence that a rheumatic disease exists. Patients with various acute and chronic inflammatory diseases as well as healthy individuals may be RF positive. Nonrheumatic diseases associated with RFs include mononucleosis, hepatitis, malaria, tuberculosis, syphilis, subacute bacterial endocarditis, cancers after chemotherapy or irradiation, chronic liver disease, hyperglobulinemia, and cryoglobulinemia.

The percentage of individuals with positive RF concentrations and the mean RF concentration of the population increase with advancing age. Although RFs are associated with several rheumatic and many nonrheumatic diseases, the concentrations of RFs in these diseases are lower than those observed in patients with RA.

Quantitative Assay Results

Normal values: <1:80 or less than 40–60 International Units/mL
When a quantitative RF test is performed, results are reported as either a dilutional titer or a concentration in International Units per milliliter. Rheumatoid factor titers are reported positive as a specific serum dilution. That is, serum is diluted serially (e.g., 1:20, 1:40, 1:80, 1:160, 1:320); the ability to detect RF is tested at each dilution. The greatest dilution that results in a positive test is reported as the endpoint. A titer of >1:80 or a concentration >40–60 International Units/mL is generally considered to be positive.

Qualitative Assay Results

The dilutional titer chosen to indicate a positive RF excludes 95% of the normal population. Stated another way, at a serum dilution at which 95% of the normal population is RF negative,

70% to 90% of RA patients will have a positive RF test. The remaining RA patients who have RF titers within the normal range may be described as seronegative.

Anticyclic Citrullinated Peptide (anti-CCP) Antibodies

The anti-CCP test is also known as *anticitrullinated protein antibody (ACPA)* or *citrulline antibody*. This antibody binds to the nonstandard amino acid citrulline that is formed from removal of amino groups from arginine. Nonstandard amino acids are generally not found in proteins and often occur as intermediates in the metabolic pathways of standard amino acids. In the joints of RA patients, proteins may be transformed to citrulline during the process that leads to joint inflammation. The anti-CCP antibody is present in most patients with RA but is found much less often in patients with other diseases. The test is highly specific for RA; when these antibodies are present, there is a 90% to 95% likelihood that the patient has RA. The combination of both positive RF and positive anti-CCP antibody has 99.5% specificity for RA.

The anti-CCP test is most useful in helping to identify the etiology of inflammatory arthritis in patients with negative RF titers. Anti-CCP antibodies are detected in about 50% to 60% of patients with early RA, usually after 3–6 months of symptoms.[3] It has been theorized that citrulline antibodies represent the earlier stages of RA in this situation. The presence of anti-CCP antibodies has also been associated with more erosive forms of RA. Therefore, research is needed to determine whether anti-CCP–positive patients with early stage RA disease benefit from aggressive treatment at an early stage of disease.

Quantitative and Qualitative Assay Results

Normal values: <20 EU/mL (assay dependent)

Quantitative anti-CCP antibodies are tested by enzyme-linked immunosorbent assay (ELISA) and are reported in ELISA units (EU). The relationship between these values and qualitative results are generally reported as (1) <20 EU: negative; (2) 20–39 EU: weakly positive; (3) 40–59 EU: moderately positive; and (4) >60 EU: strongly positive.

Antinuclear Antibodies

Antinuclear antibodies (ANAs) are a heterogeneous group of autoantibodies directed against nucleic acids and nucleoproteins within the nucleus and cytoplasm. Intracellular targets of these autoantibodies include deoxyribonucleic acid (DNA), ribonucleic acid (RNA), individual nuclear histones, acidic nuclear proteins, and complexes of these molecular elements (Table 18-1).[4-7]

The ANA test is included in the diagnostic criteria for idiopathic SLE, drug-induced lupus, and MCTD because of its high rate of positivity in these disorders. However, its low specificity makes it unsuitable for use as a screening test for rheumatic or nonrheumatic diseases in asymptomatic individuals. A positive ANA can also be found in otherwise healthy individuals. Antinuclear antibodies are also associated with various genetic and environmental factors (e.g., intravenous drug abuse), hormonal factors, and increased age. They also are associated with nonrheumatic diseases, both immunologically

mediated (e.g., Hashimoto thyroiditis, idiopathic pulmonary fibrosis, primary pulmonary hypertension, idiopathic thrombocytopenic purpura, and hemolytic anemia) and nonimmunologically mediated (e.g., acute or chronic bacterial, viral, or parasitic infections; and neoplasm).

Antibody tests that have clinical utility for diagnosis of SLE, drug-induced lupus, and other diseases include the following:

1. **Double-stranded DNA (dsDNA) antibodies**—These antibodies are relatively specific for SLE, which makes them useful for diagnosis of the disorder. In some patients with SLE, the titers tend to rise with a disease flare and fall (usually into the normal range) when the flare subsides. Thus, dsDNA titers may be helpful in managing disease activity in some SLE patients. The dsDNA antibodies have been found in low titers in many other autoimmune diseases (e.g., RA, Sjögren syndrome, systemic sclerosis, Raynaud disease, MCTD, discoid lupus, juvenile rheumatoid arthritis (JRA), and autoimmune hepatitis).[6] Presence of dsDNA antibodies has also been reported in patients receiving some drugs used to treat rheumatic diseases (e.g., minocycline, etanercept, infliximab, and penicillamine).

2. **Single-stranded DNA (ssDNA) antibodies**—These antibodies identify and react primarily with purine and pyrimidine bases within the beta helix of dsDNA. They may also bind with nucleosides and nucleotides. They are much less specific for SLE than dsDNA antibodies. Therefore, ssDNA antibodies are of limited usefulness for diagnosing SLE.[6] They also do not correlate well with disease activity and are not helpful for managing ongoing disease.

3. **Smith (Sm) antibodies**—These antibodies bind to a series of nuclear proteins complexed with small nuclear RNAs. These complexes are known as *small nuclear ribonucleoprotein particles (snRNPs)* and are important in the processing of RNA transcribed from DNA.[6] The Sm antibody test has low sensitivity (10% to 50% depending on assay methodology) but high specificity (55% to 100%) for SLE. Titers usually remain positive after disease activity has subsided and titers of anti-DNA antibodies have declined to the normal range. Thus, the Sm antibody titer may be a useful diagnostic tool, especially when anti-DNA antibodies are undetectable. There is currently no evidence that monitoring Sm antibodies is useful for following the disease course or predicting disease activity.[6]

4. **Ribonucleoprotein (RNP) or uridine-rich ribonuclear protein (U_1RNP) antibodies**—This antibody system reacts to antigens that are related to Sm antigens. However, these antibodies bind only to the U_1 particle, which is involved in splicing nuclear RNA into messenger RNA. Ribonucleoprotein antibodies are found in many patients with SLE (3% to 69%) and low titers may be detected in other rheumatic diseases (e.g., Raynaud disease, RA, systemic sclerosis).[6] Importantly, RNP antibodies are a hallmark feature of MCTD. A positive

TABLE 18-1. Laboratory and Clinical Characteristics of Antibodies to Nuclear/Cytoplasmic Antigens

ANA	TARGETED CELLULAR MATERIAL	SENSITIVITY	SPECIFICITY
dsDNA	dsDNA	SLE: 70% RA: 1% Systemic sclerosis: <1%	SLE: high (>95%) Drug-induced lupus: low (1% to 5%) RA: low (1%) Systemic sclerosis: low (<1%) Sjögren syndrome: low (1% to 5%)
Sm[a]	Nuclear ribonucleoproteins	SLE: 25% Drug-induced lupus: 1% RA: 1% Systemic sclerosis: <1% Sjögren syndrome: 1% to 5%	SLE: high (97%)
ssDNA	ssDNA	SLE: 80% Drug-induced lupus: 80% RA: 60%	SLE: low Drug-induced lupus: low RA: moderate
Histone	Chromatin and DNA-packing protein	SLE: 70% Drug-induced lupus: 95% RA: 15% to 20% Systemic sclerosis: <1%	SLE: moderate Drug-induced lupus: high RA: low Systemic sclerosis: low
RNP (or U_1RNP)	Nuclear ribonucleoproteins	MCTD: 100% SLE: 40% Systemic sclerosis: <1% RA: 25% Polymyositis: <1%	MCTD: low SLE: low Systemic sclerosis: low RA: low Polymyositis: low
Ro[a]/SSA[b]	Nuclear ribonucleoproteins	Sjögren syndrome: 10% to 60% SLE: 40% Polymyositis: 18% RA: 5% Systemic sclerosis: 5%	Sjögren syndrome: moderate SLE: low Polymyositis: low RA: low Systemic sclerosis: low
La[a]/SSB[b]	Nuclear ribonucleoproteins	Sjögren syndrome: 70% to 95% SLE: 10% to 35%	Sjögren syndrome: high (94%) SLE: low
Centromere (ACA)	Chromatin and centromere	Systemic sclerosis: 25% to 30% CREST: 50% to 90% Raynaud disease: 15% to 30%	Systemic sclerosis: high CREST, Raynaud disease: high (>95%)
DNA topoisomerase I (Scl_{70})	Chromatin and DNA-catalyzing protein	Systemic sclerosis: 15% to 20%	Systemic sclerosis: high (>95%)
Jo-1	Cytoplasm and histidyl tRNA synthetase	SLE: low Drug-induced lupus: low RA: low Systemic sclerosis: low Sjögren syndrome: low Polymyositis: 30% Jo-1 syndrome: 50%	SLE: low Drug-induced lupus: low RA: low Systemic sclerosis: low Sjögren syndrome: low Polymyositis with interstitial lung disease: high Jo-1 syndrome: high

ACA = anticentromere antibody; ANA = antinuclear antibody; CREST = syndrome characterized by calcinosis, Raynaud disease, esophageal motility disorder, sclerodactyly, and telangiectasias; DNA = deoxyribonucleic acid; dsDNA = double-stranded DNA; La/SSB = La/Sjögren syndrome B antibody; MCTD = mixed connective tissue disease; RA = rheumatoid arthritis; RNP = ribonucleoprotein; Ro/SSA = Ro/Sjögren syndrome A antibody; SLE = systemic lupus erythematosus; Scl_{70} = scleroderma-70 or DNA topoisomerase I antibody; Sm = Smith antibody; ssDNA = single-stranded DNA; U_1RNP = uridine-rich ribonuclear protein.

[a]Represents the first two letters of the surname of the patient whose serum was used to identify the reaction in agar diffusion.

[b]Sjögren syndrome A and B.

Source: From references 4–7.

test in a patient with suspected MCTD increases the probability that this diagnosis is correct, even though the test is nonspecific. On the other hand, a negative anti-RNP in a patient with possible MCTD virtually excludes this diagnosis.

5. **Histone (nucleosome) antibodies**—These antibodies target the protein portions of nucleosomes, which are DNA-protein complexes comprising part of chromatin. These antibodies are present in virtually all cases of drug-induced lupus. In fact, the diagnosis of drug-induced lupus should be questioned in their absence. Most cases of drug-induced lupus are readily diagnosed because a commonly implicated drug (e.g., hydralazine, isoniazid, procainamide) is being taken or a strong temporal relationship exists between drug initiation and the onset of SLE signs and symptoms. However, in some cases of potential drug-induced lupus, histone autoantibody testing can be helpful. Histone antibodies appear less commonly in other diseases, including adult RA, juvenile RA, autoimmune hepatitis, scleroderma, and others. There is some evidence that histone antibodies correlate with disease activity in SLE.

Two closely-related ANA tests are detected frequently in patients with Sjögren syndrome, but they are nonspecific; they may also be helpful for diagnosis of SLE.

1. Ro/Sjögren syndrome A (Ro/SSA) antibody
2. La/Sjögren syndrome B (La/SSB) antibody

The presence of either antibody in patients with suspected Sjögren syndrome strongly supports the diagnosis. It is unusual to detect the La/SSB antibody in patients with SLE or Sjögren syndrome in the absence of the Ro/SSA antibody. In women of childbearing age who have a known connective-tissue disease (e.g., SLE, MCTD), a positive Ro/SSA antibody is associated with an infrequent but definite risk of bearing a child with neonatal SLE and congenital heart block. Presence of the Ro/SSA antibody also correlates with late-onset SLE and secondary Sjögren syndrome. In patients who are ANA negative but have clinical signs of SLE, a positive Ro/SSA antibody may be useful in establishing a diagnosis of SLE.

It has been recommended that the Ro/SSA antibody test be ordered in the following situations[7]: (1) pregnant women with SLE; (2) women with a history of giving birth to children with heart block or myocarditis; (3) individuals with a history of unexplained photosensitive skin eruptions; (4) patients suspected of having a systemic connective tissue disease with a negative ANA screening test; (5) patients with xerostomia, keratoconjunctivitis sicca, and/or salivary and lacrimal gland

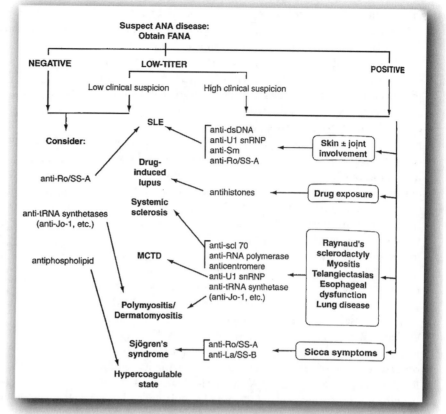

FIGURE 18-2. Algorithm for the use of ANAs in the diagnosis of connective tissue disorders. (Reproduced, with permission, from Peng ST, Craft JE. Antinuclear antibodies. In: Firestein GS, Budd RC, Harris ED Jr, et al., eds. *Kelley's Textbook of Rheumatology.* 8th ed. Philadelphia, PA: Saunders Elsevier; 2009:752.)

enlargement; and (6) patients with unexplained small vessel vasculitis or atypical multiple sclerosis.

Two ANAs are highly specific for systemic sclerosis (scleroderma), but the tests have low sensitivity:

1. Anticentromere antibody (ACA)
2. DNA topoisomerase I (ScI$_{70}$) antibody—These two antibodies are highly specific for systemic sclerosis and related diseases such as CREST syndrome (associated with **c**alcinosis, **R**aynaud disease, **e**sophageal dysmotility, **s**clerodactyly, and **t**elangiectasias), Raynaud disease, and occasionally SLE. When systemic sclerosis is suspected on clinical grounds, antibody testing for ACA and ScI$_{70}$ can be useful in making the diagnosis. However, negative results do not exclude the disease because of low test sensitivity.

The *Jo-1 antibody (anti-Jo)* is highly specific for idiopathic inflammatory myopathy (IIM) including polymyositis and dermatomyositis, or myositis associated with another rheumatic disease or interstitial lung disease.

Figure 18-2 provides guidelines for the use of the ANA test in diagnosing rheumatic disorders. The titer or quantitative value should be considered when evaluating the clinical significance of ANA test results.

Quantitative Antinuclear Antibody Assay Results

Normal: Negative at 1:20 dilution (varies among laboratories)
The indirect immunofluorescence antinuclear antibody test (FANA) is a rapid and highly sensitive method for detecting the presence of ANAs.[4] Although the FANA is positive in >95% of patients with SLE, it is also positive in some normal individuals and patients with drug-induced lupus and other autoimmune diseases. An ELISA also provides a rapid and highly sensitive method for detecting the presence of ANA. Many laboratories perform screening ANA tests by the ELISA technique because it can be automated and is less labor intensive; FANA testing is performed only in specimens testing positive by ELISA.[5]

Laboratories usually report the ANA titer, which is the highest serum dilution that remains positive for ANAs. A very high concentration (titer >1:640) should raise suspicion for an autoimmune disorder but is not in itself diagnostic of any disease. In the absence of clinical findings, these individuals should be monitored closely for the overt development of an autoimmune disorder. On the other hand, a high ANA titer is less useful in a patient who already has definite clinical evidence of a systemic autoimmune disease. The finding of a low antibody titer (<1:80) in the absence of signs or symptoms of disease is not of great concern, and such patients require less frequent followup than those with very high titers. False-positive ANAs are common in the normal population and tend to be associated with low titers (<1:40). The positive antibody titers in healthy persons tend to remain fairly constant over time; this finding can also be seen in patients with known disease.

Qualitative Antinuclear Antibody Assay Results

The pattern of nuclear fluorescence after staining may reflect the presence of antibodies to one or more nuclear antigens. The nuclear staining pattern was used commonly in the past, but pattern type is now recognized to have relatively low sensitivity and specificity for individual autoimmune diseases. For this reason, specific antibody tests have largely replaced use of patterns.[5] The common immunofluorescent patterns are as follows:

1. **Homogeneous**—This pattern is seen most frequently in patients with SLE but can also be observed in patients with drug-induced lupus, RA, vasculitis, and polymyositis. This pattern reflects antibodies to the DNA-histone complex.
2. **Speckled**—This pattern is also seen most frequently in SLE but can appear in patients with MCTD, Sjögren syndrome, progressive systemic sclerosis, polymyositis, and RA. This pattern is produced by antibodies to Sm, Ro/SSA, La/SSB, DNA topoisomerase I (ScI$_{70}$), and other antigens.
3. **Nucleolar**—This pattern is infrequently observed in patients with SLE but is more frequently seen in patients with polymyositis, progressive systemic sclerosis, and vasculitis. It is produced by antibodies to RNA polymerase I and a number of other antigens.
4. **Peripheral or nuclear rim**—This is the only pattern that is highly specific for any rheumatic disease and is

observed predominantly (98%) in SLE patients. It is produced by antibodies to DNA (dsDNA, ssDNA) and nuclear envelope antigens (antibodies to components of the nuclear envelope, such as certain glycoproteins).

Table 18-1 summarizes the most frequently identified ANAs, their corresponding targeted cellular material, and disease sensitivities and specificities.[4–7]

Antineutrophil Cytoplasmic Antibodies

As the name implies, *antineutrophil cytoplasmic antibodies (ANCAs)* are antibodies directed against neutrophil cytoplasmic antigens. Testing for ANCAs is important for the diagnosis and classification of various forms of vasculitis. In these disorders, the target antigens are proteinase 3 (PR3) and myeloperoxidase (MPO). Both antigens are located in the azurophilic granules of neutrophils and the peroxidase-positive lysosomes of monocytes. Antibodies that target PR3 and MPO are known as *PR3-ANCA* and *MPO-ANCA*.[8] There is an association between ANCA and several major vasculitic syndromes: Wegener granulomatosis, microscopic polyangiitis, Churg-Strauss syndrome, and certain drug-induced vasculitis syndromes.[8]

Wegener granulomatosis is a vasculitis of unknown origin that can damage organs by restricting blood flow and destroying normal tissue. Although any organ system may be involved, the disorder primarily affects the respiratory tract (sinuses, nose, trachea, and lungs) and the kidneys. Approximately 90% of patients with active generalized Wegener granulomatosis have ANCAs. In patients with limited disease presentations, up to 40% may be ANCA-negative. Thus, although a positive ANCA test is useful to support a suspected diagnosis, a negative ANCA test does not exclude it. For this reason, the ANCA test is usually not used alone to diagnose this disorder.

In patients with vasculitis, immunofluorescence after ethanol fixation reveals two characteristic patterns: cytoplasmic (cANCA) and perinuclear (pANCA). With cANCA, there is diffuse staining throughout the cytoplasm, which is usually caused by antibodies against PR3. The pANCA pattern is characterized by staining around the nucleus and perinuclear fluorescence. In vasculitis patients, the antibody causing this pattern is generally directed against MPO.

Although detection and identification of ANCAs is most useful in diagnosing various vasculitides, ANCAs have been reported in connective tissue diseases (e.g., RA, SLE, and myositis), chronic infections (e.g., cystic fibrosis, endocarditis, and HIV), and gastrointestinal diseases (e.g., inflammatory bowel disease, sclerosing cholangitis, and autoimmune hepatitis). Some medications may induce vasculitis associated with positive ANCA (usually MPO-ANCA).[9] The drugs most strongly associated with ANCA-associated vasculitis are propylthiouracil and methimazole. Hydralazine, minocycline, penicillamine, allopurinol, procainamide, clozapine, phenytoin, rifampin, cefotaxime, isoniazid, and indomethacin are less commonly associated with the disorder.[8]

TABLE 18-2. Disease Associations of Antinuclear Cytoplasmic Antibodies (ANCAs)

ANCA	SENSITIVITY	SPECIFICITY
cANCA	Extended Wegener granulomatosis: >90% Limited Wegener granulomatosis: 70% to 85% Microscopic polyarteritis: 50% Polyangiitis overlap syndrome: 40% Idiopathic crescentic glomerulonephritis: 30% Churg-Strauss syndrome: 10% Classic polyarteritis nodosa: 10%	Wegener granulomatosis disease spectrum: 98% (extended Wegener granulomatosis; limited Wegener granulomatosis-microscopic polyarteritis; polyangiitis overlap syndrome; and idiopathic crescentic glomerulonephritis)
pANCA	Ulcerative colitis: 60% to 75% Crohn disease: 10% to 20% Autoimmune chronic active hepatitis: 60% to 70% Primary biliary cirrhosis: 30% to 40% Primary sclerosing cholangitis: 60% to 85% RA with Felty syndrome: 90% to 100% RA with vasculitis: 50% to 75% RA: 20% to 40%	Ulcerative colitis: >90%; all others low
Anti-MPO	Idiopathic crescentic glomerulonephritis: 70% Churg-Strauss syndrome: 70% Microscopic polyarteritis: 50% Wegener granulomatosis: 20% Classic polyarteritis nodosa: 20% Polyangiitis overlap syndrome: 20%	Systemic vasculitis and/or idiopathic crescentic glomerulonephritis: 94% to 99%

cANCA = cytoplasmic antineutrophil cytoplasmic antibody; MPO = myeloperoxidase; pANCA = perinuclear antineutrophil cytoplasmic antibody; RA = rheumatoid arthritis.

Quantitative Assay Results

When used in the diagnosis of Wegener granulomatosis, the specificity of PR3-ANCA is approximately 90%. The sensitivity of the test is about 90% when the disease is active and 40% when the disease is in remission. Thus, the sensitivity of PR3-ANCA is related to the extent, severity, and activity of the disease at the time of testing.

The utility of obtaining serial PR3-ANCA tests in assessing disease activity is controversial. Some data suggest that a rise in titers predicts clinical exacerbations and justifies increasing immunosuppressive therapy. However, other studies have shown that disease flares cannot be predicted in a timely fashion by elevations in ANCA titers. Further, the immunosuppressive and cytotoxic therapies used are associated with substantial adverse effects. For these reasons, an elevation in ANCA should not be used as the sole justification for initiating immunosuppressive therapy. Rather, patients with rising ANCA titers should be monitored closely with therapy withheld unless there are clear clinical signs of active disease.[8]

Qualitative Assay Results

The sensitivity and specificity of cANCA, pANCA, and anti-MPO tests for various diseases are listed in Table 18-2. The presence of cANCAs denotes a spectrum of diseases ranging from idiopathic pauci-immune, necrotizing glomerulonephritis to extended Wegener granulomatosis.[10] In most cases of vasculitis, renal disorder, and granulomatous disease, patient sera are negative for cANCAs.

The pANCA test has limited diagnostic value. A positive pANCA test should be followed by antigen-specific assays such as anti-MPO. In ulcerative colitis, the specificity of the pANCA

test has been reported to be as high as 94%. However, with only moderate sensitivity and inconsistent correlation between titers and disease activity, pANCA screening may be of little value. Although sensitivity can reach 85% in primary sclerosing cholangitis, the pANCA test lacks specificity in the differential diagnosis of autoimmune hepatic diseases. In RA, pANCA may be related to aggressive, erosive disease. The sensitivity of the test increases in RA complicated by vasculitis, but its specificity remains low.

Complement

The complement system consists of at least 17 different plasma proteins that provide a defense mechanism against microbial invaders and serve as an adjunct or "complement" to humoral immunity. The system works by depositing complement components on pathologic targets and by the interaction of plasma proteins in a cascading sequence to mediate inflammatory effects such as opsonization of particles for phagocytosis, leukocyte activation, and assembly of the membrane attack complex (MAC).[11] Six plasma control proteins and five integral membrane control proteins regulate this cascade. These proteins circulate normally in a precursor (inactive) form (e.g., C3 and C4). When the initial protein of a given pathway is activated, it activates the next protein (e.g., C3a and C4a) in a cascading fashion similar to that seen with coagulation factors.

Activation of this system can occur through any one of three proteolytic pathways:

1. **Classical pathway**—This pathway is activated when IgM or IgG antibodies bind to antigens such as viruses or bacteria.

2. **Alternative pathway**—This is an evolutionary surveil-

lance system that does not require the presence of specific antibodies.

3. **Lectin pathway**—This pathway is activated similarly to the classical pathway, but instead of antibody binding, mannose-binding protein (MBP) binds to sugar residues on the surface of pathogens.

Activation by any of the three pathways generates enzymes that cleave the third and fifth complement components (C3 and C5). A final common (or terminal) sequence culminates in the assembly of the MAC. Five proteins (C5 through C9) interact to form the MAC, which creates transmembrane channels or pores that displace lipid molecules and other elements, resulting in disruption of cell membranes and cell lysis.

Because the complement system is an important part of immune system regulation, complement deficiency predisposes an individual to infections and autoimmune syndromes. In disorders associated with autoantibodies and the formation of immune complexes, the complement system can contribute to tissue damage.

Serum complement levels reflect a balance between synthesis and catabolism. Hypocomplementemia occurs when the C3 or C4 concentration falls below its reference range. Most cases of hypocomplementemia are associated with hypercatabolism (complement depletion) due to activation of the immune system rather than decreased production of complement components (hyposynthesis). Most diseases associated with the formation of IgG- or IgM-containing circulating immune complexes can cause hypocomplementemia. Rheumatic diseases included in this category are SLE, RA with extra-articular disease, and systemic vasculitis. Nonrheumatic diseases associated with hypocomplementemia include subacute bacterial endocarditis, hepatitis B surface antigenemia, pneumococcal infection, gram-negative sepsis, viral infections (e.g., measles), recurrent parasitic infections (e.g., malaria), and mixed cryoglobulinemia.[11]

Because errors in interpretation of complement study results can occur, three important aspects should be considered when interpreting these results:

1. Reference ranges are relatively wide. Therefore, new test results should be compared with previous test results rather than with a reference range. It is most useful to examine serial test results and correlate changes with a patient's clinical picture.

2. Normal results should be compared with previous results, if available. Inflammatory states may increase the rate of synthesis and elevate serum complement protein levels. For example, some SLE patients have concentrations of specific complement components that are 2–3 times the upper limit of normal (ULN) when their disease is clinically inactive. When the disease activity increases to the point that increased catabolism of complement proteins occurs, levels may then fall into the reference range. It would be a misinterpretation to conclude that these "normal" concentrations represent an inactive complement system. Consequently, serial determinations of complement levels may be more informative than measurements at a single point.

3. Complement responses do not correlate consistently with disease activity. In some patients, the increase and decrease of the complement system should not be used to assess disease activity.

Assessment of the complement system should include measurement of the total hemolytic complement activity by the complement hemolytic 50% (CH_{50}) test and determination of the levels of C3 and C4.

Complement Hemolytic 50%

Reference range: 100–250 International Units/mL

The *complement hemolytic (CH_{50})* measures the ability of a patient's serum to lyse 50% of a standard suspension of sheep erythrocytes coated with rabbit antibody. All nine components of the classical pathway are required to produce a normal reaction. The CH_{50} screening test may be useful when a complement deficiency is suspected or a body fluid other than serum is involved. For patients with SLE and lupus nephritis, serial monitoring of CH_{50} may be useful for guiding drug therapy.

C3 and C4

Reference ranges: C3, 72–156 mg/dL or 0.72–1.56 g/L; C4, 20–50 mg/dL or 0.2–0.5 g/L

Because C3 is the most abundant complement protein, it was the first to be purified and measured by immunoassay. However, C4 concentrations appear to be more sensitive to smaller changes in complement activation and more specific for identifying complement activation by the classic pathway. Results of C3 and C4 testing are helpful in following patients who initially present with low levels and then undergo treatment, such as those with SLE.

Acute-Phase Reactants

The concentration of a heterogeneous group of plasma proteins, called *acute-phase proteins* or *acute-phase reactants*, increases in response to inflammatory stimuli such as tissue injury and infection. Concentrations of CRP, serum amyloid A protein, alpha$_1$-acid glycoprotein, alpha$_1$-antitrypsin, fibrinogen, haptoglobin, prealbumin, ferritin, and complement characteristically increase, whereas serum transferrin, albumin, and transthyretin concentrations decrease. Their collective change is referred to as the *acute-phase response*.

In general, if the inflammatory stimulus is acute and of short duration, these proteins return to normal within days to weeks. However, if tissue injury or infection is persistent, acute-phase changes may also persist. Additionally, white blood cell (WBC) and platelet counts may be elevated significantly.

Rheumatic diseases are chronic and associated with varying severities of inflammation. The ESR and CRP are two tests that can be helpful in three ways: (1) estimating the extent or severity of inflammation; (2) monitoring disease activity over time; and (3) assessing prognosis.[12] Unfortunately, both tests are nonspecific and cannot be used to confirm or exclude any particular diagnosis.

Erythrocyte Sedimentation Rate

Reference range (Westergren method): 0–15 mm/hr for males; 0–20 mm/hr for females

The *erythrocyte sedimentation rate (ESR)* has been used widely as a reflection of the acute-phase response and inflammation for many years. The test is performed by placing anticoagulated blood in a vertical tube and measuring the rate of fall of erythrocytes in mm/hr. In rheumatic diseases, the ESR is an indirect screen for elevated concentrations of acute-phase plasma proteins, especially fibrinogen.[12] An elevated ESR occurs when higher protein concentrations (especially fibrinogen) cause aggregation of erythrocytes, causing them to fall faster.

A number of factors unrelated to inflammation may result in an increased ESR, including obesity, increasing age, and some drugs. The ESR also responds slowly to an inflammatory stimulus. Despite these limitations, the test remains in wide use because it is inexpensive and easy to perform, and a tremendous amount of data is available about its clinical significance in numerous diseases. The Westergren method of performing an ESR test is preferred over the Wintrobe method because of the relative ease of performing the former method in clinical or laboratory settings.

Correlation of serial Westergren ESR results with patient data may influence therapeutic decisions. Two rheumatic diseases, polymyalgia rheumatica and temporal arteritis (giant cell arteritis), are almost always associated with an elevated Westergren ESR. The ESR is usually >60 mm/hr and frequently >100 mm/hr in these disorders. During initial therapy or treatment initiated after a disease flare, a significant decrease or a return to a normal ESR usually indicates that systemic inflammation has decreased substantially. In the absence of clinical symptoms, an increased ESR may indicate that more aggressive therapy is needed. Disease activity can then be monitored by ESR results. Of course, if symptoms are present, they should not be ignored.

C-Reactive Protein

Reference range: 0–0.5 mg/dL or 0–0.005 g/L
C-reactive protein (CRP) is a plasma protein of the acute-phase response. In response to a stimulus such as injury or infection, CRP can increase up to 1000 times its baseline concentration. The precise physiologic function of CRP is unknown, but it is known to participate in activation of the classical complement pathway and interact with cells in the immune system.

Serum CRP levels can be quantitated accurately and inexpensively by immunoassay or laser nephelometry. Most healthy adults have concentrations of <0.3 mg/dL, although concentrations of 1 mg/dL are sometimes seen. Moderate increases range from 1–10 mg/dL, and marked increases are >10 mg/dL.[12] Values above 15–20 mg/dL are usually associated with bacterial infections. In general, concentrations >1 mg/dL reflect the presence of a significant inflammatory process. As with the Westergren ESR, serial measurements of CRP are the most valuable, especially in chronic inflammatory diseases.

Currently, the routine use of CRP for the assessment of rheumatic diseases is limited. As with the ESR, CRP concentrations generally increase and decrease with worsening and improving signs and symptoms, respectively. Nevertheless, CRP concentrations are not disease specific, nor are they part of the diagnostic criteria for any rheumatic disease.

Using an assay method called *high-sensitivity CRP (hs-CRP)*, several studies have shown a correlation between elevated levels and cardiovascular events including myocardial infarction. Although controversial, recent research suggests that CRP is simply a marker for atherosclerosis and cardiovascular disease rather than a cause.[13] The American Heart Association recommends obtaining hs-CRP levels in patients at intermediate risk of a cardiovascular event (i.e., those whose Framingham multiple risk factor scoring projects a 10-year CHD risk in the range of 10% to 20%).[14] In these patients, an elevated CRP (>3 mg/L) is considered to confer high risk. A level of 1–3 mg/L is average risk, and <1 mg/L is low risk. Levels >10 mg/L should be disregarded for coronary risk prediction purposes and the patient should be evaluated for clear sources of systemic inflammation or infection.

It is important to note that the units of measurement for the hs-CRP (mg/L) are different from those of the conventional CRP test (mg/dL). Because CRP levels fluctuate over time, the hs-CRP should be measured twice at least 2 weeks apart and the two values averaged. At the time of this writing, no clinical trials had been conducted to determine whether treating patients on the basis of elevated hs-CRP levels alone is beneficial or cost-effective. Thus, the precise role of hs-CRP testing as a predictor of cardiovascular disease awaits the results of further clinical studies.

Human Leukocyte Antigen B27 (HLA-B27)

Human leukocyte antigen B27 is an antigen on the surface of WBCs encoded by the B locus in the major histocompatibility complex (MHC) on chromosome 6. The HLA-B27 test is qualitative and will be either present or absent. Its presence is associated with autoimmune diseases known as *seronegative spondyloarthropathies*. An HLA-B27 test may be ordered when a patient has pain and inflammation in the spine, neck, chest, eyes, or joints and an autoimmune disorder associated with the presence of HLA-B27 is the suspected cause. The test may be obtained to confirm a suspected diagnosis of ankylosing spondylitis, Reiter syndrome, or anterior uveitis. However, a positive test cannot distinguish among these diseases and cannot be used to predict progression, severity, prognosis, or the degree of organ involvement. Some patients with these disorders may have a negative HLA-B27 test. Further, the test cannot definitively diagnose or exclude any rheumatologic disease. It is frequently ordered in concert with other rheumatologic tests (e.g., RF, ESR, CRP), based on the clinical presentation.

A positive HLA-B27 in a person without symptoms or a family history of HLA-B27 associated disease is not clinically significant. For example, it does not help predict the likelihood of developing an autoimmune disease. The presence or absence of HLA antigens is genetically determined. If a family member has an HLA-B27 related rheumatologic disease, other family members who share the HLA-B27 antigen have a higher risk of developing a similar disease.

New genetic testing methods permit separation of HLA-B27 into subtypes. Approximately 15 subtypes have been identified; the most common are HLA-B27*05 and HLA-B27*02. The precise clinical significance of individual subtypes is an area of continuing investigation.

Synovial Fluid Analysis

Synovial fluid is essentially an ultrafiltrate of plasma to which synovial cells add hyaluronate. This fluid lubricates and nourishes the avascular articular cartilage. Normally, synovial fluid is present in small amounts and is clear and acellular (<200 cells/mm³) with a high viscosity because of the hyaluronic acid concentration. Normal fluid does not clot because fibrinogen and clotting factors do not enter the joint space from the vascular space. Protein concentration is approximately one-third that of plasma, and glucose concentration is similar to that of plasma.

When performing arthrocentesis (joint aspiration), a needle is introduced into the joint space of a diarthrodial joint. With a syringe, all easily removed synovial fluid is drained from the joint space. Arthrocentesis is indicated as a diagnostic procedure when septic arthritis, hemarthrosis (blood within a joint), or crystal-induced arthritis is suspected. Furthermore, arthrocentesis may be indicated in any clinical situation, rheumatic or nonrheumatic, if the cause of new or increased joint inflammation is unknown. Arthrocentesis is also performed to administer intra-articular corticosteroids.

When arthrocentesis is performed, the synovium may be inflamed, allowing fibrinogen, clotting factors, and other proteins to diffuse into the joint. Therefore, the collected synovial fluid should be placed in heparinized tubes to prevent clotting and to allow determination of cell type and cell number.

If diagnostic arthrocentesis is indicated, the aspirated joint fluid should be analyzed for volume, clarity, color, viscosity, cell count, culture, glucose, and protein. Synovial fluid is subsequently reported as normal, noninflammatory, inflammatory, or septic.[15] Table 18-3 presents the characteristics of normal and three pathological types of synovial fluid. The presence and type of crystals in the fluid should be determined. The presence of crystals identified by polarized light microscopy with red compensation can be diagnostic (Table 18-4). (See Minicase 1.)

Nonrheumatic Tests

The three most commonly performed groups of nonrheumatic tests performed in rheumatology are the *complete blood count (CBC)*, *serum chemistry panel*, and *urinalysis*. These tests are not specific for any rheumatologic disorder, and abnormal results may occur in association with many rheumatic and

TABLE 18-3. Synovial Fluid Characteristics and Classification

CHARACTERISTIC	NORMAL	NON-INFLAMMATORY	INFLAMMATORY	SEPTIC
Viscosity	High	High	Low	Variable
Color	Colorless to straw	Straw to yellow	Yellow	Variable
Clarity	Transparent	Transparent	Translucent–opaque	Opaque
WBC (/mm³)	<200	200–3000	3000–50,000	>50,000
PMN	<25%	<25%	Often >50%	>75%
Culture	Negative	Negative	Negative	Often positive
Glucose (a.m. fasting)	≅ Blood	≅ Blood	>25 mg/dL but lower than blood	<25 mg/dL (much lower than blood)
Protein (g/dL)	1–2	1–3	3–5	3–5

PMN = polymorphonuclear leukocyte; WBC = white blood cell.

TABLE 18-4. Morphology of Synovial Fluid Crystals Associated with Joint Disease

CRYSTALS	SIZE (MM)	MORPHOLOGY	BIREFRINGENCE[a]	DISEASES
Monosodium urate	2–10	Needles, rods	Negative	Gout
CPPD	2–10	Rhomboids, rods	Positive (weak)	CPPD crystal deposition disease (pseudogout), OA
Calcium oxalate	2–10	Polymorphic, dipyramidal shapes	Positive	Renal failure
Cholesterol	10–80	Rectangles with notched corners; needles	Negative or positive	Chronic rheumatoid or osteoarthritic effusions
Depot corticosteroids	4–15	Irregular rods, rhomboids	Negative or positive	Iatrogenic postinjection flare

CPPD = calcium pyrophosphate dihydrate; OA = osteoarthritis.
[a]The property of birefringence is the ability of crystals to pass light in a particular plane. When viewed under polarized light, the crystals are brightly visible in one plane (birefringent), but are dark in a plane turned 90°. Birefringence observed under polarized light can be categorized as "positive" and "negative" based on the speed at which rays of light travel through the crystals in perpendicular planes (at right angles).

nonrheumatic diseases. These tests are discussed from a more general perspective in other chapters.

The CBC includes hemoglobin, hematocrit, red blood cell (RBC) indices (MCV, MCH, and MCHC), WBC count, WBC differential, and platelet count. Chronic inflammatory diseases such as RA and SLE are commonly associated with anemia (low hemoglobin and hematocrit). The RBC indices often indicate that the anemia is normochromic and normocytic; this is often referred to as *anemia of chronic disease*. Anemia may also be associated with a low MCV (microcytic anemia). Microcytic anemia accompanies chronic blood loss, which may occur as a result of drug therapy for rheumatic diseases (e.g., gastroduodenal hemorrhage from nonsteroidal anti-inflammatory drugs [NSAIDs]). Additional tests may be necessary to rule out iron deficiency anemia (e.g., stool guaiac, serum iron, and total iron binding capacity). The platelet count may be elevated in some disorders (thrombocytosis) and decreased in others (thrombocytopenia). Leukopenia may be present, and the WBC differential may reflect either increases or decreases in various cell elements. Leukopenia may be associated with Felty syndrome and may also be caused by therapy with immunosuppressive agents used to treat rheumatic diseases.

The chemistry panel may include baseline measurements of electrolytes (e.g., sodium, potassium, chloride, and carbon dioxide) and tests of hepatic and renal function. Systemic lupus erythematosus may be associated with hepatic dysfunction, which can be assessed by determination of hepatic transaminases (aspartate aminotransferase [AST], alanine aminotransferase [ALT]), total and direct bilirubin, alkaline phosphatase, and gamma glutamyl transferase (GGT). Some drugs used in the treatment of rheumatologic disease may also cause hepatic injury. Chronically poor nutrition may result in low serum albumin and total protein levels. Renal function tests (usually the serum creatinine (SCr) and blood urea nitrogen [BUN]) may provide evidence of renal involvement in patients with lupus nephritis. The urinalysis with microscopic evaluation is useful in detecting proteinuria, hematuria, and pyuria, which may be seen in SLE and with use of drugs to treat rheumatologic disorders.

INTERPRETATION OF LABORATORY TESTS IN SELECTED RHEUMATIC DISEASES

Rheumatoid Arthritis in Adults

In 2010, the American College of Rheumatology (ACR) and the European League Against Rheumatism published new classification criteria for rheumatoid arthritis (RA) (summarized in Table 18-5).[16] The criteria were developed to help define homogeneous treatment populations for research trials, not for clinical diagnosis. In practice, the clinician must establish the diagnosis for an individual patient using many more aspects

---

MINICASE 1

Assessment of Crystal-Induced Arthropathy

NORMAN S., AN 85-YEAR-OLD MAN, presented to the emergency department unable to bear weight on his right leg. Physical examination revealed a swollen, inflamed, and painful right knee without systemic signs or symptoms of infection. Norman S. was otherwise in good health except for several gout attacks over the past 10 years.

The right knee was aspirated and drained. Several drops of slightly cloudy, light yellow aspirate were placed on a slide and sent to pathology. The remaining aspirate was sent in heparinized tubes to the laboratory for Gram stain, bacterial culture, cell count, and chemistry panel.

Examination of the slide revealed a mixture of needle-shaped, rhomboid or rod, and variably shaped crystals. The slide was then viewed under a polarizing light microscope with a first-order red plate compensator. Most crystals demonstrated weak positive birefringence.

After receiving the pathology report, the emergency department physician reviewed the preliminary laboratory results of the knee aspirate (see Table 18-3 for reference values):

- 25,000 WBCs/mm³
- 55% PMNs
- 4.5 g/dL protein
- No bacteria or other organisms were seen on Gram stain

Question: What is the likely diagnosis in Norman S.? What additional laboratory studies should be performed?

Discussion: When Norman S. presented initially, septic arthritis would be high on the list of differential diagnoses. The absence of systemic signs and symptoms of infection does not rule out this condition. The aspiration of cloudy, yellow fluid from a red, swollen, and painful knee is consistent with infection and/or inflammation. Therefore, appropriate diagnostic tests were performed on the synovial fluid.

His history of gout may have suggested a recurrent acute gouty attack as the most likely diagnosis. However, microscopic examination revealed a mixture of crystal shapes, and polarizing light microscopy distinguished their most likely chemical composition. Based on the weak positive birefringence findings and variable crystal shapes, the crystals were probably composed of calcium pyrophosphate dihydrate (CPPD). Thus, the most likely diagnosis is calcium pyrophosphate deposition disease (pseudogout). In gouty arthritis, the monosodium urate crystals are needle-shaped and demonstrate bright negative birefringence. In both gout and pseudogout, phagocytosed crystals within polymorphonuclear leukocytes (PMNs) are usually observed in inflamed joints. The total synovial fluid leukocyte concentration is usually 15,000–30,000 cells/mm³, often with up to 90% neutrophils.

Additional laboratory studies that should be obtained include a serum uric acid level to rule out gout and SCr and BUN concentrations to assess kidney function. If the serum uric acid is elevated, consideration could be given to obtaining a 24-hour urine collection to determine if Norman S. is an overproducer or underexcretor of uric acid. These results could assist in the selection of prophylactic antihyperuricemic therapy, should that be considered desirable.

(including perhaps some additional laboratory tests) based on the clinical presentation. Nevertheless, the formal classification criteria are useful as a general guide to making a clinical diagnosis. The previous 1987 ACR criteria were designed to distinguish patients with established RA from patients with other rheumatic disorders.[17] In contrast, the 2010 criteria are aimed at diagnosing RA earlier in newly-presenting patients so patients can be started on treatment sooner, with the goal of preventing erosive joint damage and improving long-term outcomes.[18] Patients with erosive disease typical of RA and those with longstanding disease (including patients whose disease is inactive with or without treatment) should also be classified as having RA if they previously fulfilled the 2010 criteria.[16]

Two mandatory criteria must be met before the classification criteria can be applied to an individual patient. First, there must be evidence of definite clinical synovitis in at least one joint as determined by an expert assessor; the distal interphalangeal (IP) joints, first carpometacarpal joints, and first metatarsophalangeal (MTP) joints are *excluded* from consideration because these joints are usually involved in osteoarthritis (OA). Second, the synovitis cannot be better explained by another disease such as SLE, psoriatic arthritis, or gout. The score-based algorithm shown in Table 18-5 is then applied to patients who meet the two target population criteria. The scores of categories A through D are added; a score of at least 6 out of 10 is needed

TABLE 18-5. 2010 ACR and EULAR Classification Criteria for Rheumatoid Arthritis

JOINT DISTRIBUTION (0–5)	POINTS
1 large joint (shoulder, elbow, hip, knee, ankle)	0
2–10 large joints	1
1–3 small joints (MCP joints, PIP joints, 2nd–5th MTP joints, thumb IP joints, wrists)	2
4–10 small joints	3
>10 joints (with at least one small joint)	5
SEROLOGY (0–3)	
Negative RF AND negative ACPA	0
Low-positive RF OR low-positive ACPA	2
High-positive RF OR high-positive ACPA	3
ACUTE PHASE REACTANTS (0–1)	
Normal CRP AND normal ESR	0
Abnormal CRP OR abnormal ESR	1
SYMPTOM DURATION (0–1) (by patient report)	
<6 weeks	0
≥6 weeks	1

ACPA = anticitrullinated protein antibody; ACR = American College of Rheumatology; CRP = C-reactive protein; ESR = erythrocyte sedimentation rate; EULAR = European League Against Rheumatism; IP = interphalangeal; MCP = metacarpophalangeal; MTP = metatarsophalangeal; PIP = proximal interphalangeal; RF = rheumatoid factor.
Source: Adapted from reference 16.

for classifying a patient as having definite RA. Patients with lower scores can be reassessed subsequently, as they may meet the criteria cumulatively over time.

Rheumatoid Factor

In patients with RA, affected diarthrodial joints have an inflamed and proliferating synovium infiltrated with T lymphocytes and plasma cells. Plasma cells in the synovial fluid generate large amounts of IgG RF and abnormally low amounts of normal IgG. However, plasma cells in the bloodstream of patients with RA produce IgM RF predominantly.[2]

From 75% to 80% of adults with RA have a positive RF titer, and most of those who are positive have titers of at least 1:320. A positive RF is not specific for the diagnosis of RA. Some connective diseases, such as SLE and Sjögren syndrome, are also associated with positive RF titers. Rheumatoid factor levels may also be increased in some infections (e.g., malaria, rubella, hepatitis C). Further, up to 5% of the normal healthy population may be RF positive. Patients with RA generally have higher RF titers than individuals with other nonrheumatic conditions. In RA patients with a positive RF, the titer generally increases as disease activity (inflammation) increases. Consequently, as the serum RF titer increases, the specificity of the test for the diagnosis of RA also increases.[2] Higher titers or serum concentrations suggest the presence of more severe disease than with lower levels and are associated with a worse prognosis.

Rheumatoid factor is one of the two serologic tests (along with anti-CCP antibodies/ACPA) included in the 2010 ACR/EULAR classification criteria for RA (Table 18-5). Based on the reporting of RF levels in International units/mL, a *negative* RF is considered to be less than or equal to the ULN for the laboratory and assay. A *low-positive* test is higher than the ULN but less than or equal to 3 times the ULN. A *high-positive* test is more than 3 times the ULN for the assay. When the RF is reported as only positive or negative by the laboratory, patients reported as having a positive RF should be scored as "low-positive" for RF scoring purposes.[16]

Although RFs are usually identified and quantified from serum samples, RA is a systemic, extravascular, autoimmune disease affecting the synovium. As a result, some RFs may be present in sites other than peripheral blood. IgG RFs are found in the synovial fluid of many patients with severe RA. IgA RF may be detected in the saliva of patients with RA or Sjögren syndrome. The presence of IgE RF is correlated with extra-articular findings of RA.[2]

Although the majority of patients with RA are seropositive for RF, some patients have negative titers. However, some of these patients may have non-IgM RF, predominantly IgG RF. Also, some seronegative patients convert to seropositive on repeat testing. A small percentage of adult RA patients (<10%) are considered to be truly seronegative. When compared with RF-positive patients, seronegative patients usually have milder arthritis and are less likely to develop extra-articular manifestations (e.g., rheumatoid nodules, lung disease, and vasculitis).

Because current treatment guidelines call for aggressive early treatment of RA—before end-organ damage—clinicians must be aware of the relationship between disease onset and

RF development. Unfortunately, the RF test is least likely to be positive at the onset of RA, when it might be of the most help. After RA has been diagnosed, RF titers are not routinely used to assess a patient's current clinical status or modify a therapeutic regimen. A specific titer or a change in titers for an individual does not correlate reliably with disease activity.

In summary, RF is not sensitive or specific enough to use as the sole laboratory test to diagnose RA. Although it is present in the majority of patients with RA, it is negative in some patients with the disease. RF may be useful as a prognostic indicator, as RA patients with high RF titers generally have a more severe disease course.

Anti-CCP Antibodies

Patients with established RA are typically treated aggressively early in the disease course because most damage from bone erosions occurs within the first 2 years in 90% of patients. For this reason, an accurate early diagnosis is critical. Many patients with early RA have mild, nonspecific symptoms; in these cases, the ability to detect a disease-specific antibody such as anti-CCP could be of crucial diagnostic and therapeutic importance.

The *anti-CCP antibody* test has several useful characteristics as a marker for RA diagnosis and prognosis: (1) it is as sensitive as RF and more specific than RF for RA in patients with early as well as fully established disease; (2) it may be detectable in seemingly healthy persons years before the onset of clinical RA findings; (3) it may predict the future development of RA in patients with undifferentiated arthritis; and (4) it may be a predictor for the eventual development of erosive disease. As stated previously, anti-CCP antibodies can be detected in about 50% to 60% of patients with early RA, usually after having nonspecific symptoms for 3–6 months prior to seeing a physician.

In some patients with nonspecific arthritis, it is difficult to make a definitive diagnosis of RA because of the lack of disease-specific serum markers for other conditions in the differential diagnosis. In some situations, the presence of anti-CCP antibodies may help differentiate RA from polymyalgia rheumatica or erosive forms of SLE.[3] However, the anti-CCP test is not 100% specific for RA; positive tests have also been reported in some patients with other autoimmune rheumatic diseases (SLE, Sjögren syndrome, psoriatic arthritis), tuberculosis, and chronic lung disease.[19]

Several reports suggest that patients with early RA who are anti-CCP positive go on to develop more erosive disease than those who are antibody-negative.[3] Early identification of patients who are at risk for a more severe disease course could lead to more rapid and aggressive institution of disease-modifying therapies. However, clinical trials are needed to determine whether this diagnostic and therapeutic approach is indeed beneficial.

Antinuclear Antibodies

Antinuclear antibodies are usually negative in patients with RA. The frequency of positive ANAs in patients with RA is highly variable. As determined by indirect immunofluorescence, this frequency varies from 10% to 70%, depending on the substrate used and the titer considered positive. In patients with a positive ANA, tests for dsDNA and Sm antibodies should be performed because these tests are highly specific for SLE.

Complement

The serum *complement* level is usually normal or elevated in RA. Complement elevations often occur as part of the acute-phase response. These increases parallel changes in other acute-phase proteins (e.g., CRP). Elevations of total hemolytic activity (CH_{50}), C3, and C4 are usually observed during active stages of most rheumatic diseases, including RA. The presence of circulating immune complexes in RA may lead to hypercatabolism of complement and acquired hypocomplementemia.

Acute Phase Reactants

As in other inflammatory diseases, the nonspecific ESR test is usually elevated in active RA. The degree of elevation is directly related to the severity of inflammation; the Westergren ESR can be 50–80 mm/hr or more in patients with severely active RA. It usually decreases or normalizes when systemic inflammation decreases during initial treatment or after treatment for a disease flare. However, there is a large variability in response to treatment among individuals. Subsequent increases in disease activity will be mirrored by corresponding increases in ESR.

C-reactive protein levels may be elevated (approximately 2–3 mg/dL) in adult RA patients with moderate disease activity. However, there is substantial individual variability, and 5% to 10% of such patients have normal values. Some patients with severe disease activity have levels of 14 mg/dL or higher.

Because of their nonspecificity, the ESR and CRP are of little use in distinguishing between RA and other rheumatic diseases such as OA or mild SLE. These tests are more appropriate for monitoring disease activity in RA. Elevations of ESR and CRP are individually associated with radiologic damage in RA as assessed by the number of joint erosions. Elevation of both ESR and CRP is a stronger predictor of radiologic progression than an elevation in CRP alone.[19]

Synovial Fluid Analysis

Arthrocentesis and *synovial fluid analysis* are performed to exclude gout, pseudogout, or infectious arthritis if a joint effusion is present and the diagnosis is uncertain.[20] Synovial fluid analysis should include WBC count with differential, analysis for crystals, and Gram stain and culture. In early RA, the analysis typically reveals straw-colored, turbid fluid with fibrin fragments.[15] A clot will form if the fluid is left standing at room temperature. There are usually 5000–25,000 WBC/mm³, at least 85% of which are PMNs. Complement C4 and C2 levels are usually slightly decreased, but the C3 level is generally normal. The glucose level is decreased, sometimes to <25 mg/dL. No crystals should be present, and cultures should be negative.

Nonrheumatic Tests

The CBC may reveal an anemia that is either normochromic-normocytic (anemia of chronic disease) or hypochromic-microcytic (MCV <80 μm³). Anemia of chronic disease is not associated with erythropoietin deficiency. Microcytic anemia is due to iron deficiency that may result from gastrointestinal blood loss associated with drug use (e.g., NSAIDs) or other causes. Further testing must be performed to identify the source of bleeding (e.g., stool guaiac testing and endoscopy).

The WBC count may show a slight leukocytosis with a normal differential. Eosinophilia (>5% of the total WBC count) may be associated with RF-positive severe RA. Felty syndrome may be associated with granulocytopenia.

Thrombocytosis may be present in clinically active RA as part of the acute-phase response. As the disease improves spontaneously or as a result of drug therapy, the platelet count returns toward normal.

Serum chemistries may reveal low serum albumin and total protein levels because of poor nutrition and loss of appetite. Renal function, hepatic injury tests, and urinalysis should be normal. Abnormalities in renal or liver function caused by comorbid conditions are important because they may affect choice of pharmacotherapy or drug dosing.

Juvenile Idiopathic Arthritis

The term *juvenile idiopathic arthritis (JIA)* encompasses a heterogeneous group of childhood arthritis conditions of unknown cause. Because JIA includes a variety of arthritis categories that differ from adult-onset RA, the term JIA has replaced the name *juvenile rheumatoid arthritis (JRA)*.[21] Juvenile idiopathic arthritis begins before the 16th birthday and persists for at least 6 weeks; other known causes must be excluded before the diagnosis of JIA can be made. Juvenile idiopathic arthritis is divided into categories based on presenting clinical and laboratory findings: (1) systemic arthritis; (2) oligoarthritis; (3) polyarthritis (RF negative); (4) polyarthritis (RF positive); (5) psoriatic arthritis; (6) enthesitis-related arthritis; and (7) undifferentiated arthritis.[21,22]

The diagnosis of JIA is made primarily on clinical grounds. There is no single laboratory test or combination of tests that can confirm the diagnosis. However, laboratory tests can be useful in providing evidence of inflammation, supporting the clinical diagnosis, and monitoring toxicity from therapy.

Rheumatoid Factor

Rheumatoid factor-positive polyarthritis constitutes 5% to 10% of JIA cases. It is defined as arthritis affecting five or more joints in the first 6 months of disease with a positive RF test on two occasions at least 3 months apart.[21] Rheumatoid factor-positive polyarthritis is 6–12 times more common in girls than boys. As in adult RA, the RF test usually detects IgM-anti-IgG. Rheumatoid factor-negative polyarthritis constitutes 20% to 30% of new JIA cases. It also includes arthritis in five or more joints during the first 6 months, but the RF test is negative.

Oligoarthritis is the most common form of JIA; it is 4 times more common in girls than boys and has a peak onset before the age of 6 years. Oligoarthritis affects four or fewer joints in the first 6 months; the RF test is usually negative. The RF is negative in systemic arthritis, psoriatic arthritis, enthesitis-related arthritis, and undifferentiated arthritis.

Anti-CCP Antibodies

Only about 8% of patients with JIA have positive anti-CCP antibodies.[23] This is consistent with the fact that JIA is a heterogeneous group of disorders, most of which are different from adult RA. Similar to RA in adults, positive anti-CCP antibodies in JIA have been associated with RF-positive disease and erosive arthritis.[21] In JIA patients with RF-positive polyarthritis, anti-CCP antibodies may be more specific than RF. Overall, measurement of anti-CCP antibodies is not often helpful in diagnosing JIA.

Antinuclear Antibodies

In oligoarthritis, 50% to 70% of children have positive ANA tests, typically 1:40 to 1:320. The highest prevalence of ANA seropositivity (65% to 85%) is seen in young girls with oligoarticular onset JIA and uveitis. The ANA test is positive in 40% of patients with RF-negative polyarthritis and occasionally positive in patients with RF-positive polyarthritis. The ANA is positive in about 50% of children with psoriatic arthritis. It may be positive in some patients with enthesitis-related arthritis. The test is seldom positive (<10%) in children with systemic JIA.

Complement

As with adult-onset RA, serum complement components (especially C3) are usually elevated in systemic JIA.

Acute Phase Reactants

In systemic arthritis, the ESR and CRP are typically very high during an acute flare. In oligoarthritis, there is little systemic inflammation, and the ESR and CRP are usually normal. Some cases of oligoarthritis may be associated with mildly or moderately elevated ESR or CRP; however, elevated acute phase reactants in this category should raise suspicion for other conditions, such as subclinical inflammatory bowel disease associated with arthropathy. Acute phase reactants may be elevated in either RF-positive or RF-negative polyarthritis and in psoriatic arthritis. The ESR may be elevated in enthesitis-related arthritis, but this abnormality should raise suspicion for subclinical inflammatory bowel disease.

Synovial Fluid Analysis

Arthrocentesis in JIA is typically consistent with inflammatory fluid. As in adult RA, synovial fluid glucose levels are low.

Nonrheumatic Tests

Children with systemic arthritis may have anemia, leukocytosis with neutrophilia, and thrombocytosis. The anemia is normochromic-normocytic (anemia of chronic disease); hemoglobin values may be in the range of 7–10 g/dL. White blood cell counts in the range of 20,000–30,000 cells/mm³ are not uncommon, and counts may exceed 60,000–80,000 cells/mm³. In severe cases, liver enzymes, ferritin, and coagulation screen may also be abnormal. Patients with enthesitis-related or psoriatic arthritis may have a mild anemia of chronic disease.

Systemic Lupus Erythematosus

Criteria for the classification of *systemic lupus erythematosus (SLE)* were developed by the ACR in 1971 and revised in

TABLE 18-6. ACR Revised Classification Criteria for SLE[a]

CRITERION	DEFINITION
1. Malar rash	Fixed erythema, flat or raised, over the malar eminences, tending to spare the nasolabial folds
2. Discoid rash	Erythematous raised patches with adherent keratotic scaling and follicular plugging; atrophic scarring may occur in older lesions
3. Photosensitivity	Skin rash as a result of unusual reaction to sunlight, by patient history or physician observation
4. Oral ulcers	Oral or nasopharyngeal ulceration, usually painless, observed by a physician
5. Arthritis	Nonerosive arthritis involving two or more peripheral joints, characterized by tenderness, swelling, or effusion
6. Serositis	a) Pleuritis—convincing history of pleuritic pain or rub heard by a physician or evidence of pleural effusion OR b) Pericarditis—documented by electrocardiogram or rub or with evidence of pericardial effusion
7. Renal disorder	a) Persistent proteinuria >0.5 g/day or >3+ if quantitation not performed OR b) Cellular casts—may be red cell, hemoglobin, granular, tubular, or mixed
8. Neurologic disorder	a) Seizures—in the absence of offending drugs or known metabolic derangements (e.g., uremia, ketoacidosis, or electrolyte imbalance) OR b) Psychosis—in the absence of offending drugs or known metabolic derangements (e.g., uremia, ketoacidosis, or electrolyte imbalance)
9. Hematologic disorder	a) Hemolytic anemia—with reticulocytosis OR b) Leukopenia—<4000/mm³ total on two or more occasions OR c) Lymphopenia—<1500/mm³ on two or more occasions OR d) Thrombocytopenia—<100,000/mm³ in the absence of offending drugs
10. Immunologic disorder	a) Anti-DNA: antibody to native DNA in abnormal titer OR b) Anti-Sm: presence of antibody to Sm nuclear antigen OR c) Positive finding of antiphospholipid antibodies based on (1) an abnormal serum level of IgG or IgM anticardiolipin antibodies, (2) a positive test result for lupus anticoagulant using a standard method, or (3) a false-positive serologic test for syphilis known to be positive for at least 6 months and confirmed by Treponema pallidum immobilization or fluorescent treponemal antibody absorption test
11. ANA	Abnormal titer of ANA by immunofluorescence or an equivalent assay at any point in time and in the absence of drugs known to be associated with drug-induced lupus syndrome

ANA = antinuclear antibody; DNA = deoxyribonucleic acid; IgG = immunoglobulin G; IgM = immunoglobulin M.

[a]For the purpose of identifying patients in clinical studies, a person shall be said to have SLE if any four or more of the 11 criteria are present, serially or simultaneously, during any interval of observation.

Source: Adapted from references 24 and 25.

1982 and 1997 (Table 18-6).[24,25] The criteria were developed for research purposes to ensure that SLE patients reported in the literature actually have the disease.[26] The wide variety of manifestations and unpredictable course often make SLE difficult to diagnose. The classification criteria can be helpful in establishing the diagnosis, especially for patients with longstanding, established disease. Because SLE tends to involve organ systems sequentially over a period of years, the classification system lacks sensitivity for patients early in the disease course.

The diagnosis of SLE may be made if any four of the 11 classification criteria are present, serially or simultaneously, during any observation period. However, even if four criteria are fulfilled a clinician may elect not to diagnose SLE because of contradictory history and physical examination findings. Likewise, patients with only three classification criteria may

have their signs and symptoms diagnosed as SLE when strong clinical suspicion is present.[6]

Antinuclear Antibodies

Antinuclear antibody testing is usually performed initially if SLE is suspected because of its high sensitivity and ease of use. At least 95% of active, untreated patients with SLE have a positive ANA, usually at a titer of 1:160 or higher.[27] For patients presenting with rheumatic signs and symptoms (e.g., joint pain, joint swelling, and morning stiffness) and signs suggestive of SLE (e.g., butterfly rash, photosensitivity, oral ulcers, and discoid rash), a positive ANA test is one of the 11 possible SLE classification criteria established by the ACR (Table 18-6).[24,25] On the other hand, a negative ANA test does not exclude the diagnosis in patients with typical features of the disease.

MINICASE 2

Evaluation of Systemic Lupus Erythematosus

JOHN A., A 50-YEAR-OLD MAN, presents to his family physician complaining of fever, sore throat, and "feeling run down" for 5 days. Even though he had stayed home from work for the past 5 days, his skin appeared to be slightly sunburned in sun-exposed areas.

His past medical history is significant for hypertension and a myocardial infarction 6 months ago complicated by arrhythmias afterward. He has a 20 pack-per-year smoking history. His family physician had referred him to a rheumatologist 11 months ago because of intermittent joint pain that was not characteristic of OA. No diagnosis was made at that visit. The results of laboratory tests at that time indicated a low-titer RF (1:80) and a positive ANA rim pattern at a titer of 1:160.

His current medications (stable for the past 6 months) include enalapril, ibuprofen, procainamide, and one aspirin a day. He is allergic to penicillin and intolerant to erythromycin (stomach upset).

After her examination, the physician performed a rapid strep test (results negative) and throat culture and prescribed tetracycline. John A. continued to take tetracycline after his physician's office notified him of a positive throat culture for *Streptococcus pyogenes*.

Five days after starting tetracycline, John A. returned to his physician's office because of continued fever and malaise. His sore throat had resolved. Physical examination revealed a continued fever; slightly labored breathing without productive cough, signs of pneumonia, bronchitis, or congestive heart failure; and sunburned arms and neck. John A. mentioned that he had done light yard work, having forgotten that his antibiotic could make his skin sensitive to the sun.

When asked about his breathing, John A. indicated that he could not breathe deeply when he exerted himself because of chest pain. However, the pain was not like what he had during his heart attack. He stated that he had started taking more ibuprofen because his fingers and knees hurt.

Reluctant to put John A. on steroids, the physician asked him to stop taking tetracycline. She gave him a prescription for enough trimethoprim–sulfamethoxazole to complete 7 days of antibiotic therapy. Furthermore, she had blood drawn for a CBC with differential, chemistry panel, RF, and ANAs. In addition, a second appointment was made with the rheumatologist.

John A. had completed his antibiotic course by the date of the rheumatology visit. His fever was still present, and all other signs and symptoms were unchanged except that his breathing was slightly more painful and labored and his sunburn was improved. Laboratory results obtained by the rheumatologist:

- WBCs 2000 cells/mm³ (reference range 4.4–11.0 cells/mm³) with 71% neutrophils (45% to 74%), 3% bands (3% to 5%), 20% lymphocytes (20% to 40%), 5% monocytes (2% to 8%), 1% eosinophils (0% to 4%), 0% basophils (0% to 1%), and 0% metamyelocytes (0%)
- An unchanged RF titer (1:80)
- A high-titer ANA (1:320) rim pattern
- A urine dipstick that was significantly positive for protein
- Absence of antihistone antibodies

Blood was drawn to identify the specific ANAs present; the results subsequently reported the presence of anti-dsDNA antibodies.

Question: What are two likely diagnoses, which one is most likely, and what data support that diagnosis?

Discussion: This case demonstrates that it is often difficult to diagnose SLE. John A.'s initial presentation was typical of an ongoing viral or bacterial infection. As a result of documented drug allergies and intolerances, tetracycline was a reasonable choice for his bacterial infection. Moreover, his reaction to sunlight was not unexpected because of the concurrent antibiotic use. However, both fever and photosensitivity are potential presenting symptoms for SLE and drug-induced SLE, which are often recognized weeks to months after nonacute presentations.

John A.'s previous arthritic symptoms occurred before procainamide was started, making drug-induced SLE less likely. Furthermore, antihistone antibodies were absent. These antibodies are present in >95% of cases of drug-induced SLE, particularly those taking procainamide (or hydralazine, chlorpromazine, or quinidine). Other autoantibodies are not usually seen in this situation. Although antihistone antibodies are seen in as many as 80% of patients with idiopathic SLE, these patients also have other autoantibodies, such as those against DNA.

Even though the first RF and ANA tests were positive, John A. was febrile, and photosensitivity was present prior to tetracycline ingestion. Systemic lupus erythematosus was not diagnosed at that time. However, after completion of antibacterial therapy, symptoms continued and evidence of pleuritis occurred. Therefore, the family physician referred him to a rheumatologist.

With additional evidence of a lupus-like syndrome (leukopenia and proteinuria), a specific ANA test was ordered and anti-dsDNA antibodies were detected. Based on John A.'s symptoms, their time of presentation, and highly specific anti-dsDNA antibodies, the diagnosis of idiopathic SLE was made.

Although drug-induced SLE was unequivocally ruled out, discontinuing procainamide (and changing to an alternative antidysrhythmic) may help alleviate some of his symptoms. Additional studies needed to fully evaluate John A. include a chest x-ray to assess the nature and severity of the pleuritis (or possible pericarditis) and perhaps complement levels and an ESR.

The ANA test has low specificity for SLE; many other conditions are associated with a positive test (e.g., systemic sclerosis, polymyositis, dermatomyositis, RA, autoimmune thyroiditis or hepatitis, infections, malignancies, and many drugs). Some healthy persons may also have a positive ANA test. Consequently, results of an ANA test are always interpreted in light of a patient's clinical presentation.

Anti-dsDNA and Anti-ssDNS Antibodies

The *antidouble-stranded DNA (anti-dsDNA)* test is positive in 70% of patients with SLE at some point in the disease course, and the test is 95% specific for SLE. (See Minicase 2.) In contrast, testing for antibodies to single-stranded DNA (anti-ssDNA) has poor specificity for SLE but is more sensitive (90%). Although the anti-ssDNA antibody appears to be important in the immunopathogenesis of SLE, the test has little diagnostic utility because of poor specificity.

There is evidence that anti-dsDNA and anti-ssDNA antibodies are important in the pathogenesis of lupus nephritis because they appear to correlate with its presence and severity. Titers of these antibodies tend to fall with successful treatment, frequently becoming undetectable during sustained remission.

Anti-Sm, Anti-Ro/SSA, and Anti-La/SSB Antibodies
The *anti-Sm* antibody is an immunoglobulin specific against Sm, a ribonucleoprotein found in the cell nucleus. The anti-Sm antibody test is positive in 10% to 30% of SLE patients, and presence of these antibodies is pathognomonic for SLE.[26] *Anti-Ro/SSA* and *anti-La/SSB* antibodies are present in 10% to 50% and 10% to 20% of patients with SLE, respectively, but they are not specific for the disease.

Complement
Total CH_{50} levels are decreased at some point in most patients with SLE. Complement levels decrease in SLE because of deposition of immune complexes in active disease (hypercatabolism). Complement depletion has been associated with increased disease severity, particularly renal disease. Analysis of various complement components has revealed low levels of C1, C4, C2, and C3. Serial determinations have demonstrated that decreased levels may precede clinical exacerbations.[11] As acute episodes subside, levels return toward normal. Some authorities consider it helpful to follow complement measurements in SLE patients receiving treatment, especially if C4 and C3 were low at the time of diagnosis.[11]

Acute Phase Reactants
Serum ESR and CRP concentrations are elevated in many patients with active SLE, but many individuals have normal CRP levels. Those with acute serositis or chronic synovitis are most likely to have markedly elevated CRP levels. Patients with other findings of SLE, such as lupus nephritis, may have modest or no elevations.

Several studies have examined the hypothesis that elevations in CRP during the course of SLE result from superimposed infection rather than activation of SLE. In hospitalized patients, substantially elevated serum CRP levels occur most frequently in the setting of bacterial infection. Consequently, CRP elevations >6–8 mg/dL in patients with SLE (as well as other diseases) should signal the need to exclude the possibility of infection. Such CRP increases should not be considered proof of infection, because CRP elevation can be related to active SLE in the absence of infection.

Nonrheumatic Tests
Antiphosopholipid antibodies (i.e., *anticardiolipin antibodies* and the so-called *lupus anticoagulant*) can occur as an idiopathic disorder and in patients with autoimmune and connective tissue diseases such as SLE.[28] Anticardiolipin antibody and the lupus anticoagulant are closely related but different antibodies. Consequently, an individual can have one antibody and not the other. These antibodies react with proteins in the blood that are bound to phospholipid, a type of fat molecule that is part of normal cell membranes. Antiphospholipid antibodies interfere

with the normal function of blood vessels by causing narrowing and irregularity of the vessel (vasculopathy), thrombocytopenia, and thrombosis. These changes can lead to complications such as recurrent deep venous thrombosis, stroke, myocardial infarction, and fetal loss. The presence of these antibodies may increase the risk of future thrombotic events. This clinical situation is referred to as the *antiphospholipid syndrome (APS)*. The diagnosis of APS is made when an individual has an antiphospholipid antibody documented either by a solid-phase assay (anticardiolipin) or by a test for an inhibitor of phospholipid-dependent clotting (lupus anticoagulant) along with a clinical event.[28] When APS occurs in patients with no other diagnosis, it is referred to as *primary APS*. Patients who also have SLE or another rheumatic disease are said to have secondary APS.

Anemia is present in many patients with SLE. The CBC may reveal a normochromic-normocytic anemia (anemia of chronic disease) that is not associated with erythropoietin deficiency. Hemolytic anemia with a compensatory reticulocytosis may also occur due to antierythrocyte antibodies. This is one of 11 diagnostic criteria for SLE (Table 18-6) and occurs in approximately 10% of patients. The majority of patients also have a positive Coombs test. Anemia in SLE can also result from blood loss, renal insufficiency, medications, infection, hypersplenism, and other reasons.[26]

Leukopenia, also one of the SLE classification criteria, is common but usually mild. It results primarily from decreased numbers of lymphocytes, which may be caused by the disease or its treatment. If the patient is not being treated with corticosteroids or immunosuppressive agents, ongoing immunologic activity should be suspected. Neutropenia in SLE may occur from immune mechanisms, medications, bone marrow suppression, or hypersplenism.[26]

Mild thrombocytopenia (100,000–150,000/mm³) occurs in 25% to 50% of patients with SLE and is usually due to immune-mediated platelet destruction. Increased platelet consumption and impaired platelet production may also be contributing factors.[26] Also, liver function tests may reveal increased hepatic aminotransferases (AST, ALT), lactate dehydrogenase, and alkaline phosphatase in patients with active SLE. These elevations usually decrease as the disease improves with treatment. The urinalysis with microscopic analysis may show proteinuria (>500 mg/24 hr) in about 50% of patients. Hematuria and pyuria may also occur. However, renal disease may exist in the presence of a normal urinalysis.

Osteoarthritis
Osteoarthritis (OA) results from the complex interplay of numerous factors, such as joint integrity, genetics, mechanical forces, local inflammation, and biochemical processes.[29] It is not generally considered to be an autoimmune disease. The synovium is normal, and the synovial fluid usually lacks inflammatory cells. While affected joints are painful, they are frequently not inflamed. The primary use of laboratory tests when OA is suspected is to rule out other disorders in the differential diagnosis.

TABLE 18-7. Routine Laboratory Tests to Monitor Patients Receiving Selected Drugs for Treatment of Rheumatoid Arthritis or Systemic Lupus Erythematosus

DRUG	DISEASE	LABORATORY TEST	ADVERSE DRUG REACTION	INCIDENCE (%)
Methotrexate	RA	CBC with differential and platelet count Hepatic aminotransferases, bilirubin, serum albumin Monitor for infection	Leukopenia Pancytopenia Hepatotoxicity Infection, sepsis	0–3 0–2 4–21 Rare
Leflunomide	RA	CBC with differential and platelet count Hepatic aminotransferases, bilirubin	Pancytopenia Elevated aminotransferases Hepatic necrosis	<1 5–10 Rare
Hydroxychloroquine	RA	CBC with differential and platelet count Urinalysis	Thrombocytopenia Proteinuria	0–6 0–6
Sulfasalazine	RA	CBC with differential and platelet count Hepatic aminotransferases	Leukopenia Hepatotoxicity	0–3 1–6
Anti-TNF Agents	RA	Baseline tuberculin skin test CBC with differential and platelet count Monitor for infection	Activation of tuberculosis Infection, sepsis	Rare Rare
Abatacept	RA	Baseline tuberculin skin test CBC with differential and platelet count Monitor for infection	Infection, sepsis	Rare
Anakinra	RA	CBC with differential and platelet count Monitor for infection	Neutropenia	8 Rare
Rituximab	RA	CBC with differential and platelet count Monitor for infection	Infection, sepsis	Rare
Tocilizumab	RA	CBC with differential and platelet count Monitor for infection Hepatic transaminases Fasting lipid panel	Infection, sepsis Hepatic enzyme elevations Dyslipidemia	Rare Rare Variable
Cyclosporine	RA	BUN, SCr, cyclosporine trough blood concentrations Serum potassium, uric acid Hepatic aminotransferases, bilirubin	Nephrotoxicity Hyperkalemia, hyperuricemia Hepatotoxicity	25–38 Variable 4–7
Tacrolimus		BUN, SCr, tacrolimus trough blood concentrations Serum potassium, magnesium, phosphorus Hepatic aminotransferases, bilirubin	Nephrotoxicity Hyperkalemia, hypomagnesemia, hypophosphatemia Hepatotoxicity	Variable Variable Variable
Mycophenolate mofetil	SLE	CBC with differential and platelet count Monitor for infection	Neutropenia, red cell aplasia Opportunistic infections, sepsis	23–45 Variable
Belimumab	SLE	Monitor for infection	Infection, sepsis	Variable
Cyclophosphamide	RA	CBC with differential and platelet count Urinalysis Monitor for infection	Leukopenia Proteinuria, hematuria Infection, sepsis	5–40 (dose dependent) 8, 15–26 Rare
Azathioprine	RA	CBC with differential and platelet count Hepatic aminotransferases Urinalysis Monitor for infection	Leukopenia Hepatotoxicity Proteinuria Infection, sepsis	0–32 0–5 2 Rare
NSAIDs, including aspirin	RA, OA, SLE	CBC with differential and platelet count Hepatic aminotransferases BUN, SCr; sodium, potassium Urinalysis	Anemia (due to gastroduodenal ulceration and blood loss) Hepatotoxicity Nephrotoxicity; electrolyte disturbances Proteinuria, hematuria, pyuria	Variable Rare Rare Rare

TABLE 18-7. (continued)

DRUG	DISEASE	LABORATORY TEST	ADVERSE DRUG REACTION	INCIDENCE (%)
Corticosteroids	RA, SLE	CBC with differential and platelet count	Anemia due to peptic ulceration and blood loss	Rare
		Serum sodium, potassium, bicarbonate	Electrolyte disturbances	Variable
		Serum calcium	Osteoporosis	Variable
		Blood glucose	Hyperglycemia	Variable
		Fasting lipid panel	Dyslipidemia	Variable
		Urinalysis	Glycosuria	Variable

BUN = blood urea nitrogen; CBC = complete blood count; NSAIDs = nonsteroidal anti-inflammatory drugs; OA = osteoarthritis; RA = rheumatoid arthritis; SLE = systemic lupus erythematosus; TNF = tumor necrosis factor.
[a]Adalimumab, certolizumab, etanercept, golimumab, and infliximab.
Source: Adapted from references 32–35.

There are no clinical laboratory tests that are specific for the diagnosis of OA. Laboratory tests that may be performed in patients suspected of having OA include ESR, RF titers, and evaluation of synovial fluid.[29] The ESR (and CRP) is usually normal but may be slightly increased if inflammation is present. The RF test is negative, and serum chemistries, hematology tests, and urinalysis are normal.

Synovial fluid analysis may be undertaken, especially in patients with severe, acute joint pain. Findings generally reveal either a noninflammatory process or mild inflammation (WBC <2000 cells/mm³). Crystals are absent when the synovial fluid is examined using compensated polarized light microscopy.

Fibromyalgia

Fibromyalgia is a common syndrome associated with pain, fatigue, sleep disturbances, and other medical problems.[30] According to the criteria for fibromyalgia established by an ACR committee in 1990, an individual must have both a history of chronic widespread pain and tenderness at 11 or more of 18 specific tender point sites on physical examination.[31] However, many people who carry the clinical diagnosis of fibromyalgia do not meet these precise criteria. In fact, some authorities contend that a formal diagnosis of fibromyalgia is unnecessary provided that fibromyalgia symptoms are recognized.[30]

Laboratory testing should be used prudently when evaluating patients with clinical features suggestive of fibromyalgia. A satisfactory patient assessment is usually obtained by a careful medical history and physical examination and perhaps performance of routine laboratory tests, such as CBC and serum chemistry to rule out other disorders. Serologic tests such as ANA titers are not usually necessary unless there is strong evidence of an autoimmune disorder.

If the results of laboratory testing suggest a diagnosis other than fibromyalgia, a more directed evaluation is required. Individuals who actually have fibromyalgia are sometimes misdiagnosed with autoimmune disorders. This may be due to the common complaints of arthralgias, myalgias, fatigue, morning joint stiffness, and a history of swelling of the hands and feet. Conversely, patients with existing autoimmune diseases may suffer from symptoms suggestive of fibromyalgia.

TESTS TO MONITOR ANTIRHEUMATIC DRUG THERAPY

Antirheumatic therapies can cause significant adverse reactions that are reflected in laboratory test results.[32–35] Abnormal test results may necessitate dose reduction, temporary discontinuation, or permanent withdrawal of the offending drug. The laboratory tests most commonly affected are the WBC count, platelet count, hepatic aminotransferases, total bilirubin, SCr, BUN, and urinalysis (Table 18-7).

A decrease in WBC count (leukopenia) is considered to be clinically significant when the total count is 3000–3500 cells/mm³ (3.0–3.5 × 10⁹/L) or lower, because immune defenses are compromised. Leukopenia is due primarily to a relative and absolute decrease of neutrophils (neutropenia). Pancytopenia indicates a suppression of all cell lines, including WBCs, RBCs, (anemia), and platelets (thrombocytopenia). Aplastic anemia indicates a complete arrest of blood cell production in the bone marrow. Increases in hepatic aminotransferases of 2–3 times baseline may be clinically important. In the urinalysis, the most common abnormalities identified are proteinuria, hematuria, pyuria, and casts.

TESTS TO GUIDE MANAGEMENT OF GOUT AND HYPERURICEMIA

The serum uric acid and urine uric acid concentrations are the two most commonly used tests to diagnose gout and assess the effectiveness of its treatment. The BUN and SCr should also be monitored as appropriate.

Serum Uric Acid

Reference range:
4.0–8.5 mg/dL or 237–506 mmol/L for males >17 years old;
2.7–7.3 mg/dL or 161–434 mmol/L for females >17 years old
Uric acid is the metabolic end-product of the purine bases of DNA. In humans, uric acid is not metabolized further and is eliminated unchanged by renal excretion. It is completely filtered at the renal glomerulus and is almost completely reabsorbed. Most excreted uric acid (80% to 86%) is the result of active tubular secretion at the distal end of the proximal convoluted tubule.[36]

As urine becomes more alkaline, more uric acid is excreted because the percentage of ionized uric acid molecules increases. Conversely, reabsorption of uric acid within the proximal tubule is enhanced and uric acid excretion is suppressed as urine becomes more acidic.

In plasma at normal body temperature, the physicochemical saturation concentration for urate is 7 mg/dL. However, plasma can become supersaturated, with the concentration exceeding 12 mg/dL. In nongouty subjects with normal renal function, urine uric acid excretion abruptly increases when the *serum uric acid* concentration approaches or exceeds 11 mg/dL. At this concentration, urine uric acid excretion usually exceeds 1000 mg/24 hr.

Hyperuricemia

When serum uric acid exceeds the upper limit of the reference range, the biochemical diagnosis of *hyperuricemia* can be made. Hyperuricemia can result from an overproduction of purines and/or reduced renal clearance of uric acid. When specific factors affecting the normal disposition of uric acid cannot be identified, the problem is diagnosed as *primary* hyperuricemia. When specific factors can be identified (e.g., another disease or drug therapy), the problem is referred to as *secondary* hyperuricemia.

As the serum urate concentration increases above the upper limit of the reference range, the risk of developing clinical signs and symptoms of gouty arthritis, renal stones, uric acid nephropathy, and subcutaneous tophaceous deposits increases. However, many hyperuricemic patients are asymptomatic. If a patient is hyperuricemic, it is important to determine if there are potential causes of false laboratory test elevation and contributing extrinsic factors. In general, clinical studies have not shown that impaired renal function is caused by chronic hyperuricemia (unless there are other renal risk factors and excluding acute uric acid nephropathy resulting from tumor lysis syndrome). However, long-term, very high serum uric acid levels (e.g., $\geq$13 mg/dL in men and 10 mg/dL in women) may predispose individuals to renal dysfunction. This level of hyperuricemia is uncommon, and a conclusive link to renal insufficiency has not been established. Also, renal disease accompanying hyperuricemia is often related to uncontrolled hypertension. Correction of hyperuricemia has no measurable effect on renal function.[37]

Exogenous causes. Medications are the most common exogenous causes of hyperuricemia. The two primary mechanisms whereby drugs increase serum uric acid concentrations are (1) decreased renal excretion resulting from drug-induced renal dysfunction or competition with uric acid for secretion within the kidney tubules, and (2) rapid destruction of large numbers of cells from antineoplastic therapy for leukemias and lymphomas.

The reduction in glomerular filtration rate accompanying renal impairment decreases the filtered load of uric acid and causes hyperuricemia. A number of drugs cause hyperuricemia by renal mechanisms that may include interference with renal clearance of uric acid. These agents include low-dose aspirin, pyrazinamide, nicotinic acid, ethambutol, ethanol, cyclosporine, acetazolamide, hydralazine, ethacrynic acid, furosemide, and thiazide diuretics. Diuretic-induced volume depletion results in enhanced tubular reabsorption of uric acid and a decreased filtered load of uric acid. Salicylates, including aspirin, taken in low doses (1–2 g/day) may decrease urate renal excretion. Moderate doses (2–3 g/day) usually do not alter urate excretion. Large doses (>3 g/day) generally increase urate renal excretion, thereby lowering serum urate concentrations.

Many cancer chemotherapeutic agents (e.g., methotrexate, nitrogen mustards, vincristine, 6-mercaptopurine, and azathioprine) increase the turnover rate of nucleic acids and the production of uric acid. Drug-induced hyperuricemia after cancer chemotherapy, especially high-dose regimens, can lead to acute renal failure. Allopurinol is routinely administered prophylactically to decrease uric acid formation. In other clinical situations, drug-induced hyperuricemia may not be clinically significant.

The decision to continue or discontinue a drug that may be causing hyperuricemia is dependent on three factors: (1) the risk of precipitating gouty symptoms, based on the patient's past history and current clinical status; (2) the feasibility of substituting another drug that is less likely to affect uric acid disposition; and (3) the plausibility of temporarily or permanently discontinuing the drug. If the regimen of the causative drug must remain unchanged, pharmacologic treatment of hyperuricemia may be instituted.

Diet is another exogenous cause of hyperuricemia. High-protein weight-reduction programs can greatly increase the amount of ingested purines and subsequent uric acid production. If the average daily diet contains a high proportion of meats, the excess nucleoprotein intake can lead to increased uric acid production. Fasting or starvation also can cause hyperuricemia because of increased muscle catabolism. Furthermore, lead poisoning from paint, batteries, or "moonshine," in addition to recent alcohol ingestion, obesity, diabetes mellitus, and hypertriglyceridemia, is associated with increases in serum uric acid concentration. (See Minicase 3.)

Endogenous causes. Endogenous causes of hyperuricemia include diseases, abnormal physiological conditions that may or may not be disease related, and genetic abnormalities. Diseases include (1) renal diseases (e.g., renal failure); (2) disorders associated with increased destruction of nucleoproteins (e.g., leukemia, lymphoma, polycythemia, hemolytic anemia, sickle cell anemia, toxemia of pregnancy, and psoriasis); and (3) endocrine abnormalities (e.g., hypothyroidism, hypoparathyroidism, pseudohypoparathyroidism, nephrogenic diabetes insipidus, and Addison disease).

Predisposing abnormal physiological conditions include shock, hypoxia, lactic acidosis, diabetic ketoacidosis, alcoholic ketosis, and strenuous muscular exercise. In addition, males and females are at risk of developing asymptomatic hyperuricemia at puberty and menopause, respectively.

Genetic abnormalities include Lesch-Nyhan syndrome, gout with partial absence of the enzyme hypoxanthine guanine phosphoribosyltransferase, increased phosphoribosyl

MINICASE 3

Hyperuricemia and Gout

MATTHEW B., A 45-YEAR-OLD OBESE MAN, recently began a daily exercise program in an attempt to lose 50 pounds. In addition, he began a high-protein liquid diet because he knew that "fatty foods are not healthy."

Two weeks later, he went to his family physician for his first complete physical examination in approximately 7 years. He told his physician not to tell him that he had to lose weight because he was already walking briskly for 1 hour 3 times a week and was watching his diet carefully. The only abnormal finding on physical examination was a high blood pressure (BP) of 150/95 mm Hg. After drawing blood for a CBC with differential and a full chemistry panel and obtaining a urine sample for urinalysis, the physician prescribed hydrochlorothiazide 25 mg once daily for hypertension. Three days later, Matthew B. was notified that his laboratory results, including serum uric acid, were normal.

Two weeks later, Matthew B. returned on crutches to see his physician. He explained that he had injured his right foot 3 days prior. When taking his daily walk before sunrise, he had accidentally stubbed his right foot on a rock. Two nights ago, he had awakened with a fever and felt as if his right great toe was "in a vise while an ice-cold knife was being pushed into the joint."

Examination of Matthew B.'s right foot revealed abrasions on all five toes. The skin of the great toe appeared shiny, and the toe was swollen and warm to the touch. Matthew B. was also in obvious pain. Whitish fluid was oozing from a small wound on the dorsal aspect of the great toe. After anesthetizing the joint, the physician aspirated several drops of whitish fluid. He then performed a Gram stain and examined the fluid on a slide, finding needle-shaped crystals but no bacteria. He also ordered a serum uric acid level.

Question: What is Matthew B.'s likely diagnosis? What would constitute appropriate therapy?

Discussion: Matthew B. probably experienced his first acute gout attack. Although his previous serum uric acid concentration was described as normal, one endogenous and two exogenous factors may have precipitated this attack. Hypertension is frequently associated with hyperuricemia. Also, the sudden change to a high-protein diet greatly increased his ingestion of purines, which are metabolized to uric acid. Finally, Matthew B. was also started on hydrochlorothiazide, which is an inhibitor of the renal clearance of uric acid. The abrupt change in physical exertion probably did not contribute to the attack because it was low in intensity.

Although Matthew B. attributed the condition to his traumatic toe-stubbing event, his physician noted that none of his other abraded toes appeared to be "infected." Examination of the synovial fluid using a polarizing-light microscope revealed monosodium urate crystals without bacteria (Table 18-4).

Treatment with a short course of anti-inflammatory doses of an NSAID would be appropriate therapy in this case. Although indomethacin in doses of approximately 50 mg 3 times a day for 5 days is a common regimen, other NSAIDs are also effective and may be associated with fewer adverse effects. Colchicine and oral corticosteroids are useful alternatives in certain situations. It may be advisable for Matthew B. to discontinue hydrochlorothiazide for 2 weeks until the acute episode resolves.

Matthew B. was told that his foot symptoms should greatly improve within 24–48 hours. After explaining the health risks of a high-protein diet, the physician convinced Matthew B. to begin a more balanced diet. The physician also informed Matthew B. that if the serum uric acid concentration he ordered was highly elevated, he probably would add a drug to reduce the level.

Four days later, Matthew B. received a call from his physician and was told that his serum uric acid concentration was high at 9.8 mg/dL (4.0–8.5 mg/dL). His physician stated that he would not prescribe any additional treatment at this time but asked the patient to return in 2 weeks for a repeat blood test and re-evaluation of his BP.

Question: Why did the physician decide to take this action? Why did he delay antihyperuricemic therapy?

Discussion: After discontinuing Matthew B.'s hydrochlorothiazide and recommending a balanced low-fat diet, the physician decided to wait and see if the elevated serum uric acid concentration would decline without antihyperuricemic therapy (e.g., allopurinol, probenecid). In 2 weeks, he would consider starting such treatment if the repeat serum uric acid concentration was not near normal. Alternative therapy would also be considered for Matthew B.'s hypertension.

Some clinicians recommend only observation after the first attack of acute gouty arthritis, especially if the episode was mild and responded quickly to treatment, the serum uric acid concentration was only minimally elevated, and a 24-hour urine collection for measurement of uric acid concentration was not excessive (e.g., <1000 mg/24 hr on a regular diet). Patients who meet these criteria may never have a second attack or only experience a subsequent attack months or even years later.

On the other hand, patients with a severe first attack associated with a high serum uric acid level (>10 mg/dL), or a 24-hour urinary uric acid excretion >1000 mg, should probably receive prophylactic treatment immediately after resolution of the acute attack. The results of a 24-hour urine collection would be useful in determining whether the patient is an overproducer or underexcretor of uric acid and help to guide therapy with either allopurinol or probenecid, respectively.

---

pyrophosphate P-ribose-PP synthetase, and glycogen storage disease type I.

Hypouricemia

Hypouricemia is not important pathophysiologically, but it may be associated with low-protein diets, renal tubular defects, xanthine oxidase deficiency, and drugs (e.g., high-dose aspirin, allopurinol, probenecid, and megadose vitamin C).

Assays and Interferences with Serum Uric Acid Measurements

In the laboratory, the concentration of uric acid is measured by either the phosphotungstate colorimetric method or the more specific uricase method. With the colorimetric method, ascorbic acid, caffeine, theophylline, levodopa, propylthiouracil, and methyldopa can all falsely elevate uric acid concentrations. With the uricase method, purines and total bilirubin

>10 mg/dL can cause a false depression of uric acid concentrations. False elevations may occur if ascorbic acid concentrations exceed 5 mg/dL or if plasma hemoglobin exceeds 300 mg/dL (in hemolysis).

Urine Uric Acid Concentration

Reference range: 250–750 mg/24 hr or 1.48–4.46 mol/24 hr
In hyperuricemic individuals who excrete an abnormal amount of uric acid in the urine (hyperuricaciduria), the risk of uric acid and calcium oxalate nephrolithiasis increases. However, the prevalence of stone formation is only twice that observed in the normouricemic population. When a stone does form, it rarely produces serious complications. Furthermore, treatment can reverse stone disease related to hyperuricemia and hyperuricaciduria.

Pathologically, uric acid nephropathy—a form of acute renal failure—is a direct result of uric acid precipitation in the lumen of collecting ducts and ureters. Uric acid nephropathy most commonly occurs in two clinical situations: (1) patients with marked overproduction of uric acid secondary to chemotherapy-induced tumor lysis (leukemia or lymphoma), and (2) patients with gout and profound hyperuricaciduria. Uric acid nephropathy also has developed after strenuous exercise or convulsions.[36]

In hyperuricemia unrelated to increased uric acid production, quantification of urine uric acid excreted in 24 hours can help to direct prophylaxis or treatment. Patients at higher risk of developing renal calculi or uric acid nephropathy (patients with gout or malignancies) excrete 1100 mg or more of uric acid per 24 hours. Prophylaxis may be recommended for these patients; allopurinol should be used instead of uricosuric agents (e.g., probenecid) to minimize the risk of nephrolithiasis. Prophylactic therapy may be started at the onset of gouty symptoms.[36]

SUMMARY

Most specific rheumatologic laboratory tests are used in the diagnosis or management of patients with RA or SLE. When used alone, none of these tests is diagnostic for any particular disease. Positive results of RF testing are most commonly seen in patients with RA. Although higher concentrations of RF are associated with more severe disease, RF titers or concentrations are not used to assess disease severity or clinical response to treatment.

Antinuclear antibody testing is most frequently performed in SLE diagnosis. A positive ANA occurs in the majority of patients diagnosed with drug-induced lupus or MCTD. Anti-double-stranded DNA and anti-Sm are disease-specific for SLE.

The cANCA antibody is highly specific for the disease spectrum of Wegener granulomatosis, and anti-MPO antibodies are highly specific for systemic vasculitis and/or idiopathic crescentic glomerulonephritis. The most complete screen of complement activation includes measurements of C3, C4, and CH_{50}.

The degree of general systemic inflammation can be estimated with the Westergren ESR and CRP tests. In RA, polymyalgia rheumatica, and temporal arteritis, elevated ESRs may indicate the need for more aggressive drug therapy. Unlike the ESR, CRP does not appear to increase with age and may be useful in assessing potential infection in SLE patients.

Rheumatoid arthritis may be associated with anemia of chronic disease and thrombocytosis, and SLE is normally associated with anemia of chronic disease and thrombocytopenia and occasionally with hemolytic anemia. Proteinuria, hematuria, and pyuria are often seen on urinalysis in SLE patients with active disease. When RA or SLE patients begin antirheumatic drug therapy, laboratory tests must be performed regularly to monitor for adverse drug effects.

Patients with hyperuricemia are usually asymptomatic. Prophylaxis or treatment of gout, if initiated, is begun after the first attack. The severity and frequency of the attacks guide the decision. Allopurinol prophylaxis is recommended for patients at risk of forming renal calculi.

Learning Points

1. How are laboratory tests used in patients with RA compared to those with OA?

Answer: Rheumatoid arthritis is a chronic, usually progressive, inflammatory disorder of unknown etiology characterized by polyarticular, symmetrical joint involvement and systemic manifestations. Because it is a systemic disorder, laboratory findings in RA may include (1) positive serum RF; (2) anti-CCP antibodies; (3) increased ESR; (4) increased CRP; (5) anemia (normocytic, normochromic type); (6) increased or decreased platelet count (thrombocytosis or thrombocytopenia); and (7) synovial fluid leukocytosis (WBCs >2000 cells/mm^3). Osteoarthritis is a chronic disorder usually affecting one or more weight-bearing joints (spine, knees, hips) resulting in pain, deformity, and limited joint function but without systemic manifestations. Because OA is limited to the affected joints, there are no systemic laboratory findings that are specific for the diagnosis. Laboratory testing is used primarily to exclude other disorders in the differential diagnosis. The ESR is usually normal but may be increased if there is substantial inflammation in affected joints. The synovial fluid usually lacks inflammatory cells.

2. How important are the sensitivity and specificity of laboratory tests for diagnosing or assessing rheumatologic diseases?

Answer: Sensitivity is defined as the ability of a test to show positive results in patients who actually have the disease. If a test is 100% sensitive, all patients with the disease will have a positive result. Low sensitivity leads to a high rate of *false-negative* results. For example, if a new test to diagnose RA is only 75% sensitive, this means that 25% of patients who actually have the disease will show a negative result. Specificity is defined as the ability of a test to show negative results in patients who do not actually have the disease. If a test is 100% specific, all patients who test positive actually have the disease. Lack of specificity leads to a high rate of *false-positive* results. If a new test to diagnose RA is only 75% specific, 25% of people tested who have a positive result do *not* actually have RA. For some laboratory tests, poor specificity is due to substances not associated with the disease that cross-react with the target compound.

3. What issues should be considered before ordering a laboratory test for a patient with a rheumatologic disorder?

Answer: Laboratory testing can be expensive and may be inconvenient to perform. Consequently, a number of questions should be posed before ordering another test. First, are the results of other tests already available that provide the same information? If a test was performed previously, are there important reasons to repeat the test now? Has enough time elapsed since the previous test to make new results meaningful? Will the results of this test change the diagnosis, prognosis, or therapeutic interventions I might make? In

other words, will knowing this result change what I do? Are the benefits to the patient worth the possible discomfort, inconvenience, and extra cost? The results of laboratory tests should always be interpreted in light of the clinical picture (i.e., the patient's signs and symptoms).

REFERENCES

1. Diamond B, Grimaldi C. B cells. In: Firestein GS, Budd RC, Harris ED Jr, et al., eds. *Kelley's Textbook of Rheumatology.* 8th ed. Philadelphia, PA: Saunders Elsevier; 2009:177-199.

2. Goodyear CS, Tighe H, McInnes IB. Rheumatoid factors and other autoantibodies in rheumatoid arthritis. In: Firestein GS, Budd RC, Harris ED Jr, et al., eds. *Kelley's Textbook of Rheumatology.* 8th ed. Philadelphia, PA: Saunders Elsevier; 2009:755-775.

3. Khosla P, Shankar S, Duggal L. Anti CCP antibodies in rheumatoid arthritis. *J Indian Rheumatol Assoc.* 2004;12:143-146.

4. Peng ST, Craft JE. Antinuclear antibodies. In: Firestein GS, Budd RC, Harris ED Jr, et al., eds. *Kelley's Textbook of Rheumatology.* 8th ed. Philadelphia, PA: Saunders Elsevier; 2009:741-754.

5. Reichlin M. Measurement and clinical significance of antinuclear antibodies. In: Rose BD, ed. *UpToDate.* Wellesley, MA: UpToDate; 2012.

6. Reichlin M. Antibodies to DNA, Sm, and RNP. In: Rose BD, ed. *UpToDate.* Wellesley, MA: UpToDate; 2012.

7. Reichlin M. Clinical significance of anti-Ro/SSA and anti-La/SSB antibodies. In: Rose BD, ed. *UpToDate.* Wellesley, MA: UpToDate; 2012.

8. Stone JH. Clinical spectrum of antineutrophil cytoplasmic antibodies. In: Rose BD, ed. *UpToDate.* Wellesley, MA: UpToDate; 2012.

9. Calabrese LH, Molloy ES, Duna G. Antineutrophil cytoplasmic antibody-associated vasculitis. In: Firestein GS, Budd RC, Harris ED Jr, et al., eds. *Kelley's Textbook of Rheumatology.* 8th ed. Philadelphia, PA: Saunders Elsevier; 2009:1429-1451.

10. Kerr GS, Fleischer TA, Hallahan CW, et al. Limited prognostic value of changes in antineutrophil cytoplasmic antibody titer in patients with Wegener's granulomatosis. *Arthritis Rheum.* 1993;36:365-371.

11. Atkinson JP. Complement system. In: Firestein GS, Budd RC, Harris ED Jr, et al., eds. *Kelley's Textbook of Rheumatology.* 8th ed. Philadelphia, PA: Saunders Elsevier; 2009:323-336.

12. Kushner I, Ballou SP. Acute phase reactants and the concept of inflammation. In: Firestein GS, Budd RC, Harris ED Jr, et al., eds. *Kelley's Textbook of Rheumatology.* 8th ed. Philadelphia, PA: Saunders Elsevier; 2009:767-775.

13. Schunkert H, Samani NJ. Elevated C-reactive protein in atherosclerosis–chicken or egg? *N Engl J Med.* 2008;359:1953-1955.

14. Pearson TA, Mensah GA, Alexander RW, et al. Markers of inflammation and cardiovascular disease: application to clinical and public health practice: a statement for healthcare professionals from the Centers for Disease Control and Prevention and the American Heart Association. *Circulation.* 2003;107:499-511.

15. El-Gabalawy HS. Synovial fluid analyses, synovial biopsy, and synovial pathology. In: Firestein GS, Budd RC, Harris ED Jr, et al., eds. *Kelley's Textbook of Rheumatology.* 8th ed. Philadelphia, PA: Saunders Elsevier; 2009:703-719.

16. Aletaha D, Neogi T, Silman AJ, et al. 2010 rheumatoid arthritis classification criteria: an American College of Rheumatology/European League Against Rheumatism collaborative initiative. *Arthritis Rheum.* 2010; 62:2569-2581.

17. Arnett FC. Revised criteria for the classification of rheumatoid arthritis. *Bull Rheum Dis.* 1989;38(5):1-6.

18. Cohen S, Emery P. The 2010 American College of Rheumatology/European League Against Rheumatism classification criteria for rheumatoid arthritis: a game changer. *Arthritis Rheum.* 2010;62:2592-2594.

19. Venables PJW, Maini RN. Diagnosis and differential diagnosis of rheumatoid arthritis. In: Rose BD, ed. *UpToDate*. Wellesley, MA: UpToDate; 2012.

20. Taylor PC, O'Dell JR, Maini RN. Clinically useful biologic markers in the diagnosis and assessment of outcome in rheumatoid arthritis. In: Rose BD, ed. *UpToDate*. Wellesley, MA: UpToDate; 2012.

21. Nistala K, Woo P, Wedderburn LR. Juvenile idiopathic arthritis. In: Firestein GS, Budd RC, Harris ED Jr, et al., eds. *Kelley's Textbook of Rheumatology*. 8th ed. Philadelphia, PA: Saunders Elsevier; 2009:1657-1675.

22. Petty RE, Southwood TR, Manners P, et al. International League of Associations for rheumatology classification of juvenile idiopathic arthritis: Second revision, Edmonton, 2001. *J Rheumatol*. 2004;31:390-392.

23. Aggarwal R, Liao K, Nair R. Anti-Citrullinated Peptide Antibody (ACPA) Assays and their Role in the Diagnosis of Rheumatoid Arthritis. *Arthritis Rheum*. 2009;61:1474-1483.

24. Tan EM, Cohen AS, Fries JF, et al. The 1982 revised criteria for the classification of systemic lupus erythematosus. *Arthritis Rheum*. 1982;25:1271-1277.

25. Hochberg MC. Updating the American College of Rheumatology revised criteria for the classification of systemic lupus erythematosus. *Arthritis Rheum*. 1997;40:1725.

26. Tassiulas IO, Boumpas DT. Clinical features and treatment of systemic lupus erythematosus. In: Firestein GS, Budd RC, Harris ED Jr, et al., eds. *Kelley's Textbook of Rheumatology*. 8th ed. Philadelphia, PA: Saunders Elsevier; 2009:1263-1300.

27. Schur PH, Wallace DJ. Diagnosis and differential diagnosis of systemic lupus erythematosus in adults. In: Rose BD, ed. *UpToDate*. Wellesley, MA: UpToDate; 2012.

28. Erkman D, Salmon JE, Lockshin MD. Antiphospholipid syndrome. In: Firestein GS, Budd RC, Harris ED Jr, et al., eds. *Kelley's Textbook of Rheumatology*. 8th ed. Philadelphia, PA: Saunders Elsevier; 2009:1301-1310.

29. Kalunian KC. Diagnosis and classification of osteoarthritis. In: Rose BD, ed. *UpToDate*. Wellesley, MA: UpToDate; 2012.

30. Wolfe F, Rasker JJ. Fibromyalgia. In: Firestein GS, Budd RC, Harris ED Jr, et al., eds. *Kelley's Textbook of Rheumatology*. 8th ed. Philadelphia, PA: Saunders Elsevier; 2009:555-569.

31. Wolfe F, Smythe HA, Yunus MB, et al. The American College of Rheumatology 1990 Criteria for the Classification of Fibromyalgia. Report of the Multicenter Criteria Committee. *Arthritis Rheum*. 1990;33:160-172.

32. Saag KG, Teng GG, Patkar NM, et al. American College of Rheumatology 2008 recommendations for the use of nonbiolgoic and biologic disease-modifying antirheumatic drugs in rheumatoid arthritis. *Arthritis Rheum*. 2008;59:762-784.

33. Schuna AS. Rheumatoid arthritis. In: DiPiro JT, Talbert RL, Yee GC, et al., eds. *Pharmacotherapy: A Pathophysiologic Approach*. 8th ed. New York, NY: McGraw-Hill; 2011:1583-1597.

34. American College of Rheumatology Ad Hoc Committee on Clinical Guidelines. Guidelines for monitoring drug therapy in rheumatoid arthritis. *Arthritis Rheum*. 1996;39:723-731.

35. Louie SG, Park B, Yoon H. Biological response modifiers in the management of rheumatoid arthritis. *Am J Health-Syst Pharm*. 2003;60:346-355.

36. Ernst ME, Clark EC. Gout and hyperuricemia. In: DiPiro JT, Talbert RL, Yee GC, et al., eds. *Pharmacotherapy: A Pathophysiologic Approach*. 8th ed. New York, NY: McGraw-Hill; 2011:1621-1632.

37. Wortmann RL. Gout and hyperuricemia. In: Firestein GS, Budd RC, Harris ED Jr, et al., eds. *Kelley's Textbook of Rheumatology*. 8th ed. Philadelphia, PA: Saunders Elsevier; 2009:1481-1506.

CHAPTER 19

CANCERS AND TUMOR MARKERS

PATRICK J. MEDINA, VAL ADAMS

Objectives

After completing this chapter, the reader should be able to

- Define tumor markers, describe the characteristics of an ideal tumor marker, and discuss the usefulness of tumor markers in the diagnosis, staging, and treatment of malignant diseases

- List malignant and nonmalignant conditions that may increase carcinoembryonic antigen (CEA) levels and define the role of CEA in the management of colon cancer

- Describe how CA-125 may be used to diagnose and monitor ovarian cancer

- Describe how human chorionic gonadotropin (HCG) and alpha fetoprotein (AFP) are used to diagnose and monitor germ cell tumors

- Discuss the role of estrogen and progesterone receptors (ERs, PRs) and human epidermal growth factor receptor 2 (HER2) in determining treatment decisions for breast cancer

- Outline the role of the BCR-ABL gene in the diagnosis and as a target for treatment in patients with chronic myelogenous leukemia (CML)

- Describe how mutations in epidermal growth factor receptor (EGFR), V-Ki-ras2 Kirsten rat sarcoma viral oncogene homolog (KRas), v-Raf murine sarcoma viral oncogene homolog B1 (BRAF), or anaplastic lymphoma kinase (ALK) are used in determining treatment decisions for melanoma, lung, and colorectal cancer

For most types of cancer, treatment is likely to be most successful if the diagnosis is made while the tumor mass is relatively small. Unfortunately, many common types of cancer (e.g., carcinomas of the lung, breast, and colon) are frequently not diagnosed until the tumor burden is relatively large and the patient has developed symptoms related to the disease. As the search for more effective treatments for cancer has intensified, much effort and many resources have also been dedicated to elucidating new methods of detecting cancers earlier while the tumor burden is low and the patient is asymptomatic. These efforts have led to improved radiologic and other diagnostic imaging, and the identification of biologic substances, which occur in relation to the tumor and can be detected even at very low concentrations in the blood or other body fluids.

The term *tumor marker* is used to describe a wide range of proteins that are associated with various malignancies. Typically, these markers are either proteins that are produced by or in response to a specific type of tumor, or they may be other physiologic proteins that are produced by malignant cells in excess of the normal concentrations. In either case, the concentration of the marker usually correlates with the volume of tumor cells (e.g., as the tumor grows or the number of malignant cells increases, the concentration of the marker also increases). In other cases the presence of a biologic marker may be used to predict response to treatment (e.g., the estrogen receptor [ER] or progesterone receptor [PR] in breast cancer) or to monitor the effects of treatment. More recently, some tumor markers have been shown to be essential to the viability of tumor cells, and specific therapies have been developed that target these markers of disease. These tumor markers are often identified by genetic mutations, translocations, or amplification of genetic material.

This chapter describes tumor markers that are used clinically to detect cancers, monitor cancer burden, and help choose drug therapy as well as the laboratory methods used to assess them. In addition the sensitivity, specificity, and factors that may interfere with evaluation of these tests are briefly discussed. For tumor markers that are widely used to screen for cancers, to confirm a cancer diagnosis, or to assess response to treatment, the clinical applications are described.

TUMOR MARKERS

Tumor markers may be found in the blood or other body fluids or may be measured directly in tumor tissues or lymph nodes. They can be grouped into three broad categories: (1) tumor-specific proteins are markers that are produced only by tumor cells—these proteins usually occur as a result of translocation of an oncogene and may contribute to the proliferation of the tumor; (2) nonspecific proteins related to the malignant cells including proteins that are expressed only during embryonic development and by cancer cells; and (3) proteins that are normally found in the body but are expressed or secreted at a much higher rate by malignant cells than normal cells.[1] In addition to the laboratory tests that are described in this chapter, it should also be remembered that abnormalities in other commonly used laboratory tests may provide some evidence that a malignancy exists. However, they are not related to specific tumors. For example, suppression of blood counts may represent infiltration of the bone marrow by tumor cells. Increased uric acid and/or lactate dehydrogenase (LDH) are frequently associated with large tumor burdens.

TABLE 19-1. Serum Tumor Markers in Clinical Use

TUMOR MARKER	MALIGNANT DISEASE	SCREENING	DIAGNOSIS	STAGING OR PROGNOSIS	MONITORING TREATMENT (OUTCOME OR DISEASE RECURRENCE)	COMMENTS
PSA	Prostate carcinoma	X		X	X	Must be combined with digital rectal examination of the prostate for screening; inflammatory disorders of the prostate and instrumentation of the genitourinary tract may increase PSA
CEA	Colon and breast carcinoma			X (in colon)	X	Hepatic cirrhosis, hepatitis, pancreatitis, peptic ulcer disease, hypothyroidism, ulcerative colitis, or Crohn disease may elevate CEA
CA 15-3, CA 27.29	Breast carcinoma			X	X	Other cancers (e.g., gastric, colorectal, lung), benign breast disease, and liver disease may all elevate levels
CA-125	Ovarian carcinoma			X	X	Endometriosis, ovarian cysts, liver disease, or pregnancy may elevate CA-125; in certain high-risk groups (strong family history) CA-125 in combination with ultrasound technology may be used to screen asymptomatic patients
HCG	Germ cell tumors of ovaries and testes; hydatidiform mole		X	X	X	Pregnancy, other types of cancer, or marijuana use may elevate HCG
CA 19-9	Pancreatic carcinoma			X	X	Pancreatitis, cirrhosis, gastric, and colon cancer may elevate CA 19-9
AFP	Hepatocellular carcinoma Testicular (nonseminomatous germ cell tumors)	X (hepato-cellular)	X	X	X	Pregnancy; hepatitis; cirrhosis; and pancreatic, gastric, lung, and colon cancers all can elevate AFP; some high-risk countries use AFP to screen for hepatocellular cancer
B_2M	Multiple (plasma cell) myeloma Chronic lymphocytic leukemia			X	X	Lymphomas, leukemia, and renal failure may elevate

AFP = alpha fetoprotein; B_2M = beta-2 microglobulin; CEA = carcinoembryonic antigen; HCG = human chorionic gonadotropin; PSA = prostate specific antigen.

Alkaline phosphatase is frequently elevated in patients with tumors of the biliary tract or bone. Occasionally, tumors may also produce hormones in excessive amounts, such as calcitonin or adrenocorticotropin.

Clinical Uses

Tumor markers are used for several purposes including detection of occult cancers in asymptomatic individuals (e.g., cancer screening and early detection), determining the relative extent or volume of disease (staging), estimating prognosis, predicting and assessing responsiveness to treatment, and monitoring for disease recurrence or progression.[1] Table 19-1 lists many of the commonly used tumor markers found in blood and their clinical applications. Table 19-2 lists tumor markers found on

tumor cells or genetic abnormalities found in tumor cells and their clinical applications. Table 19-3 lists genetic mutations or translocations that help determine the best therapy. The characteristics of an ideal tumor marker are somewhat dependent on the specific application. Normal values are provided though laboratory reference ranges (normal values) may slightly differ, as will the interpretation of the laboratory value in an individual patient. For example, rising levels of a tumor marker that are still in the normal range may indicate early tumor recurrence.

Sensitivity and Specificity

In order for a tumor marker to be clinically useful, it must have a high degree of *sensitivity* and *specificity*. That is, the presence of the marker should correlate with the presence of the tumor,

TABLE 19-2. Tumor Markers Found on/in Tumor Cells in Clinical Use

TUMOR MARKER	MALIGNANT DISEASE	SCREENING	DIAGNOSIS	STAGING OR PROGNOSIS	MONITORING TREATMENT (OUTCOME OR DISEASE RECURRENCE)	COMMENTS
ER/PR	Breast carcinoma			X		Used to determine benefit of hormonal therapies
HER2	Breast carcinoma			X		Used to determine benefit of anti-HER2 therapies
BCR-ABL gene	CML		X		X	Can be elevated in acute lymphoblastic leukemia and rarely in acute myeloid leukemia

CML = chronic myeloid leukemia; ER = estrogen receptor; HER2 = human epidermal growth factor receptor 2; PR = progesterone receptor.

TABLE 19-3. Tumor Markers Found on/in Tumor Cells in Clinical Use to Individualize Treatment

TUMOR MARKER	MALIGNANT DISEASE	TEST OUTCOME OF INTEREST	IMPACT ON DRUG SELECTION
EGFR	Lung	Mutation in exon 19 or 21	Mutation predictive of responding to erlotinib
KRas	Colorectal cancer	Mutation verus wild type	EGFR antibodies (cetuximab and panitumumab) only work with wild type
BRAF	Melanoma	BRAF V600E mutation	BRAF mutation predicts response to vemurafenib
ALK	Lung cancer	ALK rearrangement	ALK rearrangement predicts response to crizotinib

ALK = anaplastic lymphoma kinase; BRAF = v-Raf murine sarcoma viral oncogene homolog B1; EGFR = epidermal growth factor receptor; KRas = V-Ki-ras2 Kirsten rat sarcoma viral oncogene homolog.

and a negative test should indicate, with some certainty, that the patient does not have the cancer. Chapter 1: Definitions and Concepts describes the methodology in determining sensitivity and specificity and should be reviewed prior to reading this chapter. Knowledge of the sensitivity, specificity, and predictive values of tumor marker tests are particularly important when they are used to screen asymptomatic patients. If the tumor marker test is positive only in a portion of the patients that actually have the cancer or if the test is negative in patients who do have the disease, then diagnoses would be missed. In the case of malignant diseases, delay of the diagnosis until symptoms or other clinical findings appear may mean the difference between curable and incurable disease.

Outcomes studies evaluating the usefulness of tumor marker testing in asymptomatic individuals must result in decreased mortality rates due to the disease, not just establishment of a diagnosis. On the other hand, false-positive tests not only cause a high level of anxiety, they also typically result in the performance of very costly and sometimes invasive, additional diagnostic tests. Due to these limitations, the only tumor marker routinely used to screen for malignancies is prostate specific antigen (PSA). Although this is the single example, the use of PSA alone for prostate cancer screening is declining because it does not appear to reduce mortality.[2]

Sensitivity and specificity are also important when tumor marker tests are used to monitor for recurrent disease in patients who have previously been treated for the cancer. A negative tumor marker test that is known to have a high degree of specificity will give the patient, their family, and their clinicians a great deal of comfort and sense of security that the disease has been eliminated. If the test has a lower degree of sensitivity, then it is likely that other screening and diagnostic tests will need to be performed at regular intervals to monitor for disease recurrence. In some cases, the presence of a positive tumor marker may be indication enough to resume cancer treatment. A decision to initiate or resume treatment should be made when there is a high degree of certainty that there is actual disease present because most cancer treatments are associated with significant toxicity and a small, but appreciable, mortality risk. When tumor markers are used to assess the extent of disease or the presence of specific tumor characteristics (e.g., HER2/neu), the quantitative sensitivity may also be important in determining prognosis, appropriate diagnostic tests, and treatment options. Genetic mutational testing is a dichotomous endpoint that is present or not present; however, depending on the quality of tissue and type of testing the sensitivity (false negatives) can be affected.

Accessibility

If a tumor marker test is to be used to screen asymptomatic individuals for cancer, both the individuals and their clinicians are more likely to include them if they do not necessitate painful, risky, or lengthy procedures to obtain the necessary fluid or tissue. Most clinicians request and patients willingly provide samples of blood, urine, or sputum in the course of regular physical examinations. However, if a test requires biopsy of other tissues or involves procedures that are associated with a significant risk of morbidity, patients and clinicians are likely only to consent to or include them in physical examinations if there is a high likelihood—or other evidence that supports the presence—of the disease. Tumor markers that are obtained from tumor tissue directly are obtained at the time of diagnosis with the original tissue.

Cost-Effectiveness

Widespread screening of asymptomatic individuals with a tumor marker test can be quite expensive. It is not surprising that insurance companies, health plans, and health policy decision-makers are also more likely to support the inclusion of these tests during routine physical examinations or other screening programs if health economic evaluations demonstrate that they may result in lower overall treatment costs and a positive benefit to society, such as prolongation of the patient's productivity.

Prostate Specific Antigen

Standard reference range: 0–4.0 ng/mL
Prostate specific antigen (PSA) is a protein produced by both malignant and normal (benign) prostate tissue that is secreted into the blood. The role of PSA in the screening, diagnosis, and monitoring of treatment response of patients with prostate cancer is reviewed in Chapter 22: Common Medical Disorders of Aging Males—Clinical and Laboratory Test Monitoring.

Carcinoembryonic Antigen

Normal range: <2.5 ng/mL nonsmokers; <5.0 ng/mL smokers
Carcinoembryonic antigen (CEA) is a protein that is found in fetal intestine, pancreas, and liver. In healthy adults, the level of this protein is usually less than 2.5 ng/mL. Serum CEA levels are frequently elevated in patients with colon, breast, gastric, thyroid, or pancreatic carcinomas and a variety of nonmalignant conditions including hepatic cirrhosis, hepatitis, pancreatitis, peptic ulcer disease, hypothyroidism, ulcerative colitis and Crohn disease. Occasionally, CEA is also elevated in patients with lung cancer. Carcinoembryonic antigen levels are usually modestly increased in individuals who smoke, and the normal serum level in these individuals is usually considered to be less than 5.0 ng/mL. Nonmalignant conditions are usually not associated with CEA levels greater than 10 ng/mL. However, many patients with malignant conditions will have CEA levels that greatly exceed 10 ng/mL.

Blood samples for CEA testing preferably should be obtained in a red top tube. Following separation of the serum (or plasma), the specimen can be refrigerated if it is to be assayed within 24 hours or frozen at −20°C if the specimen is to be assayed later. Immunoassays from different manufacturers may provide different values, and, therefore, the same laboratory and assay method should be used whenever possible for repeat testing in an individual patient.

Carcinoembryonic antigen is most commonly used in the assessment of colon cancer. Unfortunately, this test does not have adequate sensitivity or specificity to make it a useful screening test for asymptomatic individuals. It may be elevated in a wide variety of conditions as noted above and may be negative in patients with widely metastatic disease. It is most commonly used in monitoring patients with a known history of colon cancer.[2] Following detection of early stage colon cancer by screening tests such as fecal occult blood and colonoscopy or sigmoidoscopy with biopsy confirmation of suspicious areas, a baseline serum CEA level is usually measured to assess if the tumor produces excessive amounts of CEA. If the CEA level is grossly increased, then the CEA level may be used to monitor the success of treatment or for evidence of tumor recurrence following successful treatment.

The CEA level also may provide some information on a patient's prognosis.[3,4] The elevation of CEA level may relate to the extent of disease (stage), which often correlates with overall survival. Following surgical removal of a colon cancer, the CEA level should return to normal (less than 2.5 ng/mL) within 4–6 weeks.[5] If the CEA level remains elevated beyond this point, it may indicate that either residual primary tumor or metastases are still present.

In early stage colon cancer (stages II and III), CEA levels should be followed every 3 months for at least 3 years after diagnosis once the adjuvant chemotherapy regimen ends.[6] The CEA level should decline to below the 5 ng/mL level within 1 month following surgery if all tumor was successfully removed.[5] If the CEA remains elevated, there is a high likelihood that the tumor will recur, and many surgeons would even consider a second-look surgery at that time for identification and removal of residual disease.[7] Rising CEA levels mandate evaluation of the patient for metastatic disease. In patients with metastatic disease CEA levels should be monitored at the start of therapy and then every 1–3 months during therapy.[8] Rising levels may indicate therapy failure, though increasing levels may result from chemotherapy at the beginning of treatment and require careful evaluation.[8,9] When CEA levels are monitored in conjunction with other followup tests including CT scans of the liver and colonoscopy, several studies have reported improved overall survival and other benefits, including cost-effectiveness, that are attributable to earlier detection of recurrent disease.[8,10]

Carcinoembryonic antigen may also be used to monitor breast cancer patients with metastatic disease. The American Society of Clinical Oncology (ASCO) guidelines for use of tumor markers in breast cancer state that CEA levels in combination with imaging, medical history, and physical exam may indicate treatment failure and prompt evaluation for worsening of disease.[11] Rising CEA levels alone should not be used to monitor treatment efficacy. Unlike colon cancer, monitoring of CEA levels in early stage breast cancer (stages I to III) is not recommended after a patient has received primary therapy. (See Minicase 1.)

CA 15-3 Antigen

Normal range: <30 units/mL
CA 15-3 (cancer antigen 15-3) is defined by an assay using monoclonal antibodies directed against circulating mucin antigen shed from human breast cancer. In addition to elevation in the serum of many women with breast cancer, it may

MINICASE 1

A Case of Elevated CEA Levels

PHIL L., A 64-YEAR-OLD WHITE MALE, presents to the clinic with a 6-week history of worsening diarrhea (five to six stools a day), pain in his right upper quadrant, and general gastrointestinal discomfort. Additional past medical history includes hypercholesterolemia for the past 5 years. Medications include simvastatin 20 mg daily. He drinks one to two glasses of wine a day and has a 30 pack/year history of smoking.

A review of systems revealed lethargy and slight confusion but no apparent distress. Vital signs showed a sitting BP of 125/75 mm Hg (standing BP not measured), a regular heart rate of 86 beats per minute, and a rapid and shallow respiratory rate of 36 breaths per minute. Phil L.'s physical examination was pertinent for signs of dehydration (poor skin turgor). Laboratory values are drawn. They are unremarkable, except for serum sodium 153 mEq/L (136–142 mEq/L), serum creatinine 1.7 mg/dL (0.6–1.2 mg/dL); and BUN 45 mg/dL (8–23 mg/dL). The decision is made to admit Phil L. based on his dehydration and worsening diarrhea. Additional laboratory values are drawn in the hospital and include a CEA level of 27 ng/mL.

Question: What is the most likely cause of Phil L.'s fluid status? How is the CEA level interpreted in relation to colon cancer? Should any other laboratory or imaging tests be obtained to further assess his cancer status?

Discussion: Phil L. most likely has a malignant tumor in his colon. Common signs and symptoms of colon cancer include pain and a change in bowel habits, which result from the tumor blocking part of the colonic lumen and interfering with normal colonic function. This can lead to the severe diarrhea and dehydration as seen in Phil L.

Although other nonmalignant conditions and smoking are also associated with increased CEA levels, levels greater than 10 ng/mL indicate a high likelihood of cancer. An elevated CEA level alone is not enough to make a diagnosis of colon cancer and a complete workup including CT scans and a tissue diagnosis will need to be obtained prior to therapy. Additional laboratory values that may be useful would be CA 19-9 levels and a complete hepatic panel to assess for metastatic disease.

The CEA level may be used in Phil L. to monitor the success of treatment, to check for evidence of tumor recurrence following primary treatment, and to provide some indication of his prognosis. Following successful surgery the CEA level should return to normal (less than 2.5 ng/mL) within 4–6 weeks. Depending on the stage of disease, Phil L. will have his CEA levels followed periodically to assess for disease recurrence or progression of metastatic disease.

---

also be elevated in lung cancer and other nonmalignant conditions including liver and breast disorders. Elevated CA 15-3 has been demonstrated to be a poor prognostic factor in early stage breast cancer, but the test is not sensitive enough to use as a screening test for early stage breast cancer.[12] This test is used in combination with imaging studies, physical examination, and medical history to monitor response to treatment in women with metastatic disease where no other reasonable measure of disease is feasible.[11] (See Minicase 2.)

CA 27.29 Antigen

Normal range <38 units/mL

CA 27.29 (cancer antigen 27.29) is also defined by an assay using a monoclonal antibody that detects circulating mucin antigen in blood.[11] It is a newer test than CA 15-3 but has the same clinical indications. CA 27.29 is used only in combination with other clinical factors such as imaging studies, physical examination, and medical history to monitor response to treatment in patients with metastatic breast cancer but is not useful as a screening test or for the detection of recurrence after primary therapy in early stage disease.[11]

CA 125 Antigen

Normal range: <35 units/mL

The *CA 125 antigen (cancer antigen 125)* is a protein, which is usually found on cells that line the pelvic organs and peritoneum. It may also be detected in the blood of women with ovarian cancer and those with adenocarcinoma of the cervix or fallopian tubes. It may be elevated in nonmalignant conditions including endometriosis, ovarian cysts, liver disease, and pregnancy, and occasionally in many other types of cancer.[13] It

is not, however, elevated by mucinous epithelial carcinomas of the ovaries. Levels of CA 125 also increase during menstruation and are lower at the luteal phase of the cycle.[14] Levels are lower in women who use systemic contraceptives and also decline following menopause.[15]

CA 125 is assessed using a blood sample collected in a red top tube. The sample should be refrigerated within 2 hours of collection. The level of CA 125 in the serum has been reported to correlate with the likelihood of malignancy, with levels greater than 65 units/mL strongly associated with the presence of a malignancy. However, they should not be considered diagnostic.[16,17] Several studies evaluating serial levels of CA 125 in healthy women have shown that serum levels may start to rise 1–5 years before the detection of ovarian cancer.[16,18] It does not, however, have sufficient sensitivity to be recommended as a routine screening test for ovarian cancer in asymptomatic women. The sensitivity in early stage ovarian cancer (before symptoms are usually evident) is believed to be less than 60%; thus, many cases would not be detected.[19] Using CA 125 levels with other tests such as transvaginal ultrasound has been investigated to increase the utility of CA 125. However, using transvaginal ultrasound in patients with elevated CA 125 levels does not appear to increase the detection of early tumors and the routine use of the combination is not recommended.[20] Some advocate that rising serial CA 125 levels could be used as a trigger to do more extensive (and often costly) screening tests in high-risk women; this approach has not proven beneficial and may result in unacceptable morbidity in women at average risk for ovarian cancer.[20]

MINICASE 2

A Case of Utilizing Tumor Markers for Breast Cancer

SARAH H., A 41-YEAR-OLD WHITE FEMALE, is recently diagnosed with breast cancer. She presented for her first scheduled routine mammogram, and a small lump was detected in her left breast. A fine-needle biopsy was done, and the lump was found to be positive for breast cancer. A complete workup determines that this is local disease and, she is diagnosed with stage II breast cancer. Additional medical history is unremarkable, and she only takes seasonal allergy medicine and drospirenone/ethinyl estradiol oral contraceptives.

A review of systems is noncontributory. Her physical examination was pertinent for a small lump palpable on the left breast near her nipple. Her cancer is evaluated for the presence of tumor markers, and the pathology shows ER/PR = positive and HER2 = 2+ on IHC.

Question: How will these markers be evaluated and used to make treatment decisions in Sarah H.? Are there any other tumor markers or tests you would recommend to be performed on Sarah H.?

Discussion: The two most important tumor markers in determining prognosis and treatment decisions are ER/PR status and HER2 status and both were performed on Sarah H.

Her ER/PR receptors were found to be positive. There are many ways to report ER/PR status with most being determined by IHC. Since the presence of even small amounts of ER/PR have been correlated with prognosis and the need for hormonal therapy, ER/PR status is commonly reported as either positive or negative. Since Sarah H.'s ER/PR status is positive, she will benefit from hormonal therapy that targets the ER receptor and likely be offered 5 years of tamoxifen based on her premenopausal status. The use of RT-PCR in determining ER/PR status could be done to confirm her ER/PR status.

Sarah H. also has her HER2 status reported. Her value was 2+ as determined by IHC. This value is in the inconclusive range. Since HER2 status is critical in determining the benefit from anti-HER2 therapies (e.g., trastuzumab and lapatinib), inconclusive values require further workup. The confirmatory test that should be performed is a FISH assay. This test measures both the number of HER2 gene copies and provides a ratio of HER2/CEP 17 (also called FISH ratio). A positive test for HER2 gene amplification is a gene copy number greater than 6 or a FISH ratio >2.2.

Sarah H. will need to have this test performed. If positive, she will be offered trastuzumab as part of her adjuvant therapy. A positive result may also dictate part of her chemotherapy regimen; anthracyclines generally are recommended in HER2 positive patients. If Sarah H. has a negative FISH test for HER2, then she will not receive adjuvant therapy and will instead receive a standard chemotherapy regimen followed by hormonal therapy.

Additional markers such as CEA, CA 15-3, and CA 27.29 would not be useful in following Sarah H. since she does not have metastatic disease and these markers are only useful for determining progressive disease during treatment for metastatic breast cancer.

Most often CA 125 is measured to monitor for evidence of disease recurrence or residual disease in women who have undergone surgical resection of ovarian cancer.[13] This use is efficacious in women whose tumors expressed CA 125 prior to surgery. For women who have undergone a tumor debulking operation prior to chemotherapy, a level measured approximately 3 weeks after surgery correlates with the amount of residual tumor mass and is predictive of overall survival.[21] Serial levels during and following chemotherapy are used to monitor response to treatment, disease progression, and prognosis. However, many women, with CA 125 levels that have returned to the normal reference range during treatment still have residual disease if a second-look laparotomy is done to pathologically evaluate the disease.[22] A more rapid decline of serum CA 125 during treatment has been associated with a more favorable prognosis.[13,23,24] Nadir values less than 10 units/mL predict improved survival and increases in CA 125 from the nadir (even when below 35 units/mL) may be used to predict disease progression.[22,25] Failure of the CA 125 level to decline may also be used to identify tumors that are not responding to chemotherapy and an increase usually indicates progression.[25] However, a large European trial in over 1400 women failed to demonstrate an improvement in survival in treating women based on rising CA 125 levels alone.[26] Additional trials are ongoing to confirm these results. Subsequently, rising CA 125 levels, without any other evidence of disease, requires careful clinical interpretation to determine if patients require treatment interventions.

Human Chorionic Gonadotropin

Normal range: serum <5 million International Units/mL
Human chorionic gonadotropin (HCG) is a glycoprotein consisting of alpha and beta subunits that is normally produced by the placenta during pregnancy.[27] Elevations in nonpregnant females and in males requires workup for malignant conditions. The beta subunit is most commonly used as the determinant in both serum as a tumor marker and in urine tests for pregnancy. Human chorionic gonadotropin is also commonly produced by tumors of germ cell origin including mixed germ cell or pure choriocarcinoma, tumors of the ovaries and testis, extragonadal tumors of germ cell origin, and gestational trophoblastic disease (e.g., hydatidiform mole). Occasionally islet cell tumors and gastric, colon, pancreas, liver, and breast carcinomas also produce HCG. Patients with trophoblastic disease often produce irregular forms of HCG that may or may not be recognized by the various automated assays and false-positive HCG immunoreactivity has also been reported. Newer highly specific and highly sensitive immunoassays have improved the reliability of this test. Radioimmunoassays and the DPC Immulite® HCG test have been reported to have the greatest accuracy.

In patients with testicular cancer, elevated levels of HCG may be present with either seminomatous (1% to 25%) or nonseminomatous disease (10% to 70%), depending on the stage of disease, so the test is not sensitive enough to be used as a screening tool for asymptomatic patients.[28] Human chorionic gonadotropin has an important prognostic role with levels greater than 50,000 million International Units/mL indicating a poor prognosis in nonseminomatous disease.[29] Most frequently, HCG is used to monitor response to therapy (i.e., an elevated level is evidence of residual disease following surgery) and to monitor for evidence of disease progression or recurrence during or after treatment.[30] Human chorionic gonadotropin has a half-life of only 18–36 hours, so serum levels decline rapidly following therapeutic interventions and failure to do so may indicate residual disease.[27,28,31]

CA 19-9 Antigen

Normal range: <37 units/mL

CA 19-9 (cancer antigen 19-9) is an oncofetal antigen expressed by several cancers including pancreatic (71% to 93% of cases), gastric (21% to 42% of cases), and colon (20% to 40% of cases) carcinomas. Serum for this test is collected in a red top tube, and the sample is frozen for shipping for analysis. The sensitivity of the test is insufficient to be useful as a screening test for early stage diseases. It was originally developed for colon cancer monitoring but is no longer recommended.[6] It is primarily used in pancreatic cancer to help discriminate benign pancreatic disease from cancer, to monitor for disease recurrence, and to assess the response to treatment interventions.[6,31] CA 19-9 levels have been used to evaluate the effectiveness of a chemotherapy regimen with rising values indicating a shorter patient survival and the possible need to change chemotherapy regimens.[32] An elevated CA 19-9 level is a poor prognostic factor in patients with inoperable pancreatic cancer.[33]

Alpha Fetoprotein

Normal range: <20 ng/mL

Alpha fetoprotein (AFP) is a glycoprotein made in the liver, gastrointestinal tract, and fetal yolk sac. It is found in high concentrations in the serum during fetal development (~3 mg/mL), and following birth it declines rapidly to <20 ng/mL. Serum for AFP evaluation should be collected in a red top tube and refrigerated until assayed using radioimmunoassay. It is elevated in about 70% of patients with hepatocellular carcinoma, 50% to 70% of patients with testicular nonseminomatous germ cell tumors, and occasionally in patients with other tumors such as pancreatic, gastric, lung, and colon cancers.[29] Nonmalignant conditions that may be associated with increased levels of AFP include pregnancy, hepatitis, and cirrhosis. In patients with nonseminomatous germ cell tumors, the level of AFP serum concentrations seems to correlate with the stage of the disease.[27,29] In some parts of the world, AFP is used as a screening test for hepatocellular carcinoma in patients who are positive for HBsAg, and, therefore, are at increased risk for hepatocellular carcinoma. In the United States, however, AFP is used primarily to assist in the diagnosis of hepatocellular carcinoma. Alpha fetoprotein levels greater than 1000 ng/mL are common in patients with hepatocellular carcinoma.[34,35]

Alpha fetoprotein levels are also used to monitor patients with both hepatocellular carcinoma and germ cell tumors for disease progression or recurrence and to assess the impact of treatment interventions. The serum half-life of AFP is 5–7 days, and usually an elevation of the serum level for more than 7 days following surgery is an indication that residual disease was left behind.[27,31] Following successful treatment for nonseminomatous germ cell tumors of the testis, HCG, and AFP are repeated every 1 or 2 months during the first year, every 2 or 3 months during the second year, and less frequently thereafter along with physical exams and chest x-rays.[27,29] Increases in these serum tests are considered an indication for further treatment such as chemotherapy. Rising levels in patients receiving chemotherapy indicate that therapy should be changed, whereas declining levels predict a more favorable outcome.[27,29]

Beta-2 Microglobulin

Normal range <2.5 mcg/mL

Beta-2 microglobulin (B_2M) is a protein found on the surface of lymphocytes as well as in small quantities in the blood and urine. Elevations of B_2M may be seen in lymphoproliferative disorders including multiple (plasma cell) myeloma and lymphoma. B_2M is renally excreted and may be elevated in nonmalignant conditions such as renal failure.[36]

Measurement of serum B_2M is most commonly done in the workup of multiple myeloma and is an important part of the staging and prognosis for that disease. Additionally, B_2M will be used to follow multiple myeloma patients for treatment efficacy with increases in B_2M potentially indicating progressive disease.[36] Patients with serum B_2M levels ≥5.5 mcg/mL are diagnosed as stage III patients and have a median survival of 29 months.[37]

Estrogen and Progesterone Receptor Assays

The levels of *estrogen receptor (ER)* and *progesterone receptor (PR)* in biopsy tissue from breast cancers predict both the natural history of the disease and the likelihood that the tumor will respond to hormonal manipulations. This test is not a blood test but requires tissue from the cancer obtained by a relatively noninvasive biopsy. Estrogen receptor status is also a prognostic factor with ER-negative tumors having a worse prognosis than ER-positive ones. For over 30 years, it has been the standard of practice to evaluate breast cancer tissue for these protein receptors and to use that information in directing therapeutic interventions. The relative concentration of hormone receptors can be determined using very small amounts of tumor tissue.

The current standard of practice is to measure each protein using immunohistochemistry (IHC); this method detects protein expression through an antibody-antigen interaction.[38] Although the method (e.g., antibody) used can vary, the biopsy is read by pathologists with the results reported as a percent positive cells. If greater than or equal to 1% of cells are positive, one is considered to have ER- or PR-positive disease.[38] Biopsies scored 1% to 10% may be considered "weakly" positive, and risks and benefits of hormonal therapy should be discussed with patients. Because of the variety of methods to evaluate IHC staining and the intra-/inter-observer variability, newer methods of measuring ER and PR status are under investigation including the use of reverse-transcriptase polymerase chain reaction (RT-PCR), which measures gene expression of ERs in tissue. Classification of ER- and PR- positive tumors are based on cutoff points of 6.5 and 5.5 units, respectively.[39] This test has demonstrated statistically significant superiority over IHC in predicting relapse in tamoxifen-treated, ER-positive patients in one retrospective trial.[39] Further validation of the test is needed before it becomes routinely used in clinical practice.[11]

Positive ER levels correlate with response to hormonal therapies including removal of the ovaries in premenopausal women or administration of an antiestrogen, such as tamoxifen, or an aromatase inhibitor such as anastrozole.[38] In addition, ER content in tumor biopsies correlates with benefit from adjuvant hormonal therapy following surgical removal of the tumor. After 15 years of followup in ER-positive breast cancer patients, tamoxifen decreased mortality by 9% in women who received 5 years of therapy.[40]

Human Epidermal Growth Factor Receptor 2

Human epidermal growth factor receptor 2, HER2/neu, (HER2) is a transmembrane glycoprotein member of the epidermal growth factor receptor (EGFR) family with intracellular tyrosine kinase activity.[41] This group of receptors functions in the growth and control of many normal cells as well as malignant cells. The gene that encodes for HER2 is c-erb B2.[41] About 20% of samples from human breast cancers exhibit amplification of c-erb B2 or overexpression of HER2.[42]

There are many potential clinical applications based on HER2 status in breast cancer: (1) studies have described the role of HER2 in the prognosis of patients with breast cancer, with poor prognosis seen in overexpressers; (2) HER2 status may predict responsiveness to certain chemotherapy (e.g., anthracycline, taxanes); (3) HER2 status may be used to predict resistance to other therapies (e.g., tamoxifen); and (4) HER2 status will predict benefit from anti-HER2 therapies such as trastuzumab and lapatinib.[43–47]

However, the considerable variability in study design and the well-recognized heterogeneity of the disease itself have made interpretation difficult, and HER-status alone should not determine whether or not a woman should receive specific adjuvant therapy or whether endocrine therapy should be used. [11] The authors did conclude that the benefit of anthracycline therapy in the adjuvant setting is greatest in HER2 positive tumors and that determining the benefit of taxane-based therapy is inconclusive at this time.[11]

It is well-established that HER2 overexpression is predictive of a response to treatment with trastuzumab (Herceptin®), a monoclonal antibody against HER2, and lapatinib (Tykerb®), a tyrosine kinase inhibitor of human epidermal growth factor receptor 1 (HER1) and HER2.[44,45] Therefore, it is necessary to evaluate all invasive breast cancers for HER2 status in order to select appropriate patients for these anti-HER2 therapies.[48]

Though a portion of the HER2 receptor can dissociate from the cell and be detected in the serum, biopsies of the tumor are routinely used to evaluate HER2 status. It can be measured for overexpression of the protein by IHC or by gene amplification,

most commonly by using fluorescence in situ hybridization (FISH) assays.[48] Several commercial assays have been recommended to aid in the selection of patients for anti-HER2 therapy. Immunohistochemistry assays assess for the overexpression of the HER2 protein and a score of 0, 1+, 2+, or 3+ is reported. Clinical trials have demonstrated that those with a score of 0 or 1+ should be considered HER2 negative and do not benefit from anti-HER2 therapy, and those that are 3+ are HER2 positive and benefit from therapy.[44,48] A score of 2+ should be considered inconclusive and requires further evaluation with a FISH assay.

The FISH assay can be used as the initial test for HER2 positivity and is preferred by some groups due to decreased variability and increased ability to predict efficacy of therapies aimed at the HER2 receptor.[48] The FISH assay measures both the number of gene copies of HER2 gene as well as provides a ratio of HER2/CEP 17 (also called *FISH ratio*). A positive test for HER2 gene amplification is a gene copy number greater than 4 or a FISH ratio greater than 2.0. HER2 negative tumors are defined as a gene copy number less than 4 or FISH ratio less than 2.0, and FISH ratios between 1.8–2.2 are inconclusive. Additional cells should be scored and the results compared.[48] Only patients with FISH-positive tumors derive benefit from anti-HER2 therapy.[48]

In summary, the routine testing for HER2 with either IHC or FISH is recommended in all patients with invasive breast cancer, with FISH as the preferred method.[11,48] Patients who are HER2 positive benefit from trastuzumab in the adjuvant setting and both trastuzumab and lapatinib in the metastatic setting.[44,45,49] The use of HER2 testing to determine benefit of additional therapies (e.g., tamoxifen, anthracyclines, taxanes) is inconclusive at this time.[11,48]

BCR-ABL

The identification of tumor markers in the pathogenesis of malignancy has led to the development of therapeutic strategies that specifically target the cause of the malignancy. By definition patients with chronic myelogenous leukemia (CML) possess the Philadelphia (Ph) chromosome that indicates the presence of the BCR-ABL fusion gene.[50,51] The BCR-ABL fusion gene can also be found in acute lymphoblastic leukemia and rarely in acute myeloid leukemia. ABL and BCR are normally found on chromosomes 9 and 22, respectively. The translocation of ABL and BCR t(9;22) in which both genes are truncated forming the characteristic BCR-ABL fusion gene on the Ph chromosome is diagnostic for CML and is present in all patients with the disease by definition.[50,51] The BCR-ABL gene encodes a protein with deregulated tyrosine kinase activity that has become the primary target for treating CML.

The Ph chromosome can be tested by the following three methods[50,51]: (1) conventional cytogenetic testing, in which bone marrow cells are aspirated and the individual chromosomes are examined for the presence of the Ph chromosome (the term *cytogenetic remission* has been developed to describe the elimination of the Ph chromosome on testing by

TABLE 19-4. Criteria for Cytogenetic and Molecular Response in Patients with Chronic Myelogenous Leukemia

CYTOGENETIC RESPONSE	MOLECULAR RESPONSE
Complete: Ph +0% Partial: Ph +1% to 35%	Complete response indicates BCR-ABL transcript nonquantifiable and nondetectable
Minor: Ph +36% to 65% Minimal: Ph +66% to 95% None: Ph + >95%	Major molecular response defined as reduction of BCR-ABL:ABL ratio to 0.1% or less

this method after treatment); (2) FISH testing, which can be done on either blood or bone marrow cells (genetic probes are utilized to look for abnormal cells that contain the BCR-ABL gene); and (3) RT-PCR testing, which is the most sensitive test for monitoring response to therapy and counts the number of cells that contain the BCR-ABL gene (it can be done on either blood or bone marrow cells). Testing with RT-PCR is referred to as *molecular monitoring* and responses are called *molecular responses*. Table 19-4 lists the response criteria for CML using cytogenetic and molecular monitoring.[50,51]

Therapies (e.g., imatinib, nilotinib, dasatinib) have been developed that target the abnormal tyrosine kinase activity of the BCR-ABL gene.[52] As mentioned, efficacy is monitored by the elimination of the Ph chromosome (cytogenetic or molecular) and detection of increasing amounts of the BCR-ABL fusion gene often require adjustments in therapy.

Several mutations in the BCR-ABL gene have been identified that may predict response to the currently available tyrosine kinase inhibitors. All CML patients should be tested for a threonine-to-isoleucine mutation at codon 315 (T315I) and may be referred for a stem cell transplantation since all three currently approved agents are inactive against this BCR-ABL mutation.[51] In patients who do not respond or relapse on initial therapy, additional BCR-ABL mutations should be tested for and may be useful in selecting the best second-line treatment options.[51]

Epidermal Growth Factor Receptor

Epidermal growth factor receptor (EGFR) (human epidermal growth factor receptor, HER1, c-erb B1) is a transmembrane glycoprotein member of the EGFR family with intracellular tyrosine kinase activity (TK) (same family as HER2). When EGFR receptors are activated, they support tumor growth by influencing cell motility, adhesion, invasion, survival, and angiogenesis. The gene that encodes for EGFR can have activating mutations in exon 18 through 21, but the ones of most interest influence the sensitivity or resistance to erlotinib (an EGFR tyrosine kinase inhibitor [TKi]). Class I mutations in exon 19 account for approximately 44% of all EGFR TK-activating mutations and a point mutation in exon 21 accounts for approximately 41% of EGFR TK-activating mutations. These mutations are most commonly found in adenocarcinoma of the lung from nonsmokers. They are also more common in Asians and females, which matches patient subset analysis

from clinical trials with erlotinib. Approximately 15% of all U.S. patients with adenocarcinoma of the lung have one of these activating mutations. A secondary mutation in exon 20 (T790M) has been found to convey resistance to the current EGFR TKi treatments. Recent recommendations state that all patients who are being considered for first-line therapy with an EGFR TKi should have mutational analysis run on their tumor tissue.[53] Epidermal growth factor receptor mutational analysis can be performed with a number of different assays; however, standard testing for patient care includes PCR amplification and genetic sequencing of exon 18 through 21.[54]

V-Ki-Ras2 Kirsten Rat Sarcoma Viral Oncogene Homolog

V-Ki-ras2 Kirsten rat sarcoma viral oncogene homolog (KRas) is an intracellular GTPase that plays an important role in signal transduction. Functionally, it works like an on/off switch that is downstream of a number of cell surface receptors including EGFR. When turned on, it conveys proliferative, growth, and survival signals; in the normal setting it turns off after conveying the activation signal. Mutated or oncogenic Ras performs the same function, but mutations in exon 1 (codons 12 and 13) lead to a permanently active Ras. Oncogenic Ras is found in 20% to 25% of all human tumors and in up to 90% of pancreatic cancers. This is obviously a target for drug development, but as of today no therapy has reached the market that inhibits this signal. It is, however, routinely used to select drug therapy, with patients having wild type (WT) (nonmutated) tumors more likely to respond to therapy. Mutated KRas is present in approximately 40% of colorectal tumors, where it conveys resistance to cetuximab and panitumumab. Current national guidelines and many payers require KRas mutational testing before giving either of these anti-EGFR monoclonal antibodies for colorectal cancer. Real-time PCR methods with fluorescent probes to common mutations in codon 12 and 13 are commonly used to determine if a KRas mutation exists; however, there are other methods including direct gene sequencing that can be used.[55]

V-Raf Murine Sarcoma Viral Oncogene Homolog B1

V-Raf murine sarcoma viral oncogene homolog B1 (BRAF) is a serine/threonine-specific protein kinase that plays an important role in signal transduction. It has activating mutations in 7% to 8% of all cancers and 40% to 60% of melanomas. The most common mutation (approximately 90%) is a glutamic acid for valine substitution at amino acid 600, which is known as the *V600E mutation.*[56] This mutation means that the kinase is always turned, signaling downstream partners in the mitogen-activated protein (MAP) kinase pathway. Vemurafenib, a drug specifically designed to inhibit the mutated BRAF, is now available to treat melanoma in patients whose tumor contains this mutation. Concurrent with the approval of vemurafenib, the cobas® 4800 BRAF V600 mutation test was introduced, which utilizes real-time PCR to identify the V600E mutation in tumors. The prescribing information requires that the test be performed and the result be positive for the mutation before using the drug.[56]

Anaplastic Lymphoma Kinase

Anaplastic lymphoma kinase (ALK) (EML4-ALK) is a fusion gene formed when the echinoderm microtubule-associated, protein-like 4 (EML4) is fused to ALK. The abnormal fusion protein promotes malignant cancer cell growth. This has recently become clinically relevant because a new drug, crizotinib, is highly effective for patients with lung cancer whose tumors contain this translocation. The mutation most commonly occurs in nonsmokers with lung adenocarcinoma, and it rarely occurs in combination with KRas or EGFR mutations. Though the mutation is found only in 2% to 7% of non-small-cell lung cancer patients, it should be routinely tested for due to significant improvement in outcomes with crizotinib treatment that targets this mutation. The rearrangement/fusion is usually detected with FISH; however, PCR and IHC can be used to identify the fusion gene or its protein product respectively.[57,58]

SUMMARY

In order to be clinically useful as a screening tool in asymptomatic individuals, tumor markers should be both sensitive and specific. Unfortunately, most of the tumor markers identified to date lack the sensitivity to be used in this capacity. In addition, many nonmalignant conditions cause elevations of these markers. Currently, only PSA is in widespread use as a screening tool when used along with the results of a digital rectal exam. Tumor markers are valuable to monitor for disease recurrence in patients who have undergone definitive surgery for cancers or to assess a patient's response to chemotherapy or other treatment interventions. In these situations, serial measurements of tests such as PSA for prostate cancer, CEA for colon cancer, HCG and AFP for testicular cancer, and CA 125 for ovarian cancer are considered standards in the followup care of patients with these malignancies. Increasingly tumor markers are being used to choose appropriate therapeutic strategies. Some tumor markers such as HER2 and ER are used as indicators of tumor sensitivity to therapies that target those receptors. Others such as the BCR-ABL gene, found in CML patients, provide a specific target in which therapeutic strategies have been developed to inhibit the actual pathogenesis of the cancer.

Learning Points

1. Are there any concerns with using tumor markers to screen for cancer?

Answer: At this time most tumor markers are neither sensitive nor specific enough to screen for cancer. The main issue with using tumor markers to screen for cancer is that the blood concentration of many of them can be increased in nonmalignant factors and by environmental conditions such as smoking. Thus, most tumor markers are used as prognostic factors, part of the staging of the cancer, and to monitor treatment effectiveness.

2. If a patient with CML has a complete cytogenetic response, are they considered cured of their leukemia and can they stop therapy?

Answer: Obtaining a complete cytogenetic response to therapies demonstrates that the patient is responding to treatment. However, molecular responses, in particular complete molecular responses, are the most sensitive test to determine if the Ph chromosome is still present. Unfortunately, reaching undetectable levels of BCR-ABL transcripts in a patient is not common and does not indicate cure and they should continue on therapy.

3. A patient with testicular cancer has his serum AFP level drawn 2 days after his surgery, and it is still elevated (250 ng/mL). Is this cause for concern?

Answer: Using serum tumor markers after surgery in testicular cancer is common, and the rate by which they decline has prognostic implications. However, since the serum half-life of AFP is 5–7 days, a level drawn so close to the surgery is of little value. In contrast, HCG has a half-life of only 18–36 hours. If HCG does not decrease within 2 days after surgery, this should be cause for concern.

REFERENCES

1. Duffy MJ. Role of tumor markers in patients with solid cancers: a critical review. *Eur J Intern Med.* 2007;18(3):175-184.

2. Slomski A. USPSTF finds little evidence to support advising PSA screening in any man. *JAMA.* 2011;306(23):2549-2551.

3. Harrison LE, Guillem JG, Paty P, et al. Preoperative carcinoembryonic antigen predicts outcomes in node-negative colon cancer patients: a multivariate analysis of 572 patients. *J Am Coll Surg.* 1997;185(1):55-59.

4. Wiratkapun S, Kraemer M, Seow-Choen F, et al. High preoperative serum carcinoembryonic antigen predicts metastatic recurrence in potentially curative colonic cancer: results of a five-year study. *Dis Colon Rectum.* 2001;44(2):231-235.

5. Minton JP, Martin EW, Jr. The use of serial CEA determinations to predict recurrence of colon cancer and when to do a second-look operation. *Cancer.* 1978;42(3 Suppl):1422-1427.

6. Locker GY, Hamilton S, Harris J, et al. ASCO 2006 update of recommendations for the use of tumor markers in gastrointestinal cancer. *J Clin Oncol.* 2006;24(33):5313-5327.

7. Graham RA, Wang S, Catalano PJ, et al. Postsurgical surveillance of colon cancer: preliminary cost analysis of physician examination, carcinoembryonic antigen testing, chest x-ray, and colonoscopy. *Ann Surg.* 1998;228(1):59-63.

8. Desch CE, Benson AB III, Somerfield MR, et al. Colorectal cancer surveillance: 2005 update of an American Society of Clinical Oncology practice guideline. *J Clin Oncol.* 2005;23(33):8512-8519.

9. Hine KR, Dykes PW. Prospective randomised trial of early cytotoxic therapy for recurrent colorectal carcinoma detected by serum CEA. *Gut.* 1984;25(6):682-688.

10. Barillari P, Ramacciato G, Manetti G, et al. Surveillance of colorectal cancer: effectiveness of early detection of intraluminal recurrences on prognosis and survival of patients treated for cure. *Dis Colon Rectum.* 1996;39(4):388-393.

11. Harris L, Fritsche H, Mennel R, et al. American Society of Clinical Oncology 2007 update of recommendations for the use of tumor markers in breast cancer. *J Clin Oncol.* 2007;25(33):5287-5312.

12. Martin A, Corte MD, Alvarez AM, et al. Prognostic value of pre-operative serum CA 15.3 levels in breast cancer. *Anticancer Res.* 2006;26(5B):3965-3971.

13. Karam AK, Karlan BY. Ovarian cancer: the duplicity of CA125 measurement. *Nat Rev Clin Oncol.* 2010;7(6):335-339.

14. Clarke-Pearson DL. Clinical practice. Screening for ovarian cancer. *N Engl J Med.* 2009;361(2):170-177.

15. Einhorn N, Sjovall K, Knapp RC, et al. Prospective evaluation of serum CA 125 levels for early detection of ovarian cancer. *Obstet Gynecol.* 1992;80(1):14-18.

16. Bast RC, Jr, Siegal FP, Runowicz C, et al. Elevation of serum CA 125 prior to diagnosis of an epithelial ovarian carcinoma. *Gynecol Oncol.* 1985;22(1):115-120.

17. Eltabbakh GH, Belinson JL, Kennedy AW, et al. Serum CA-125 measurements >65 U/mL. Clinical value. *J Reprod Med.* 1997;42(10):617-624.

18. Zurawski VR, Jr., Orjaseter H, Andersen A, et al. Elevated serum CA 125 levels prior to diagnosis of ovarian neoplasia: relevance for early detection of ovarian cancer. *Int J Cancer.* 1988;42(5):677-680.

19. Helzlsouer KJ, Bush TL, Alberg AJ, et al. Prospective study of serum CA-125 levels as markers of ovarian cancer. *JAMA.* 1993;269(9):1123-1126.

20. Buys SS, Partridge E, Black A, et al. Effect of screening on ovarian cancer mortality: the Prostate, Lung, Colorectal and Ovarian (PLCO) Cancer Screening Randomized Controlled Trial. *JAMA.* 2011;305(22):2295-2303.

21. Markman M, Liu PY, Rothenberg ML, et al. Pretreatment CA-125 and risk of relapse in advanced ovarian cancer. *J Clin Oncol.* 2006;24(9):1454-1458.

22. Prat A, Parera M, Peralta S, et al. Nadir CA-125 concentration in the normal range as an independent prognostic factor for optimally treated advanced epithelial ovarian cancer. *Ann Oncol.* 2008;19(2):327-331.

23. Juretzka MM, Barakat RR, Chi DS, et al. CA125 level as a predictor of progression-free survival and overall survival in ovarian cancer patients with surgically defined disease status prior to the initiation of intraperitoneal consolidation therapy. *Gynecol Oncol.* 2007;104(1):176-180.

24. Markmann S, Gerber B, Briese V. Prognostic value of Ca 125 levels during primary therapy. *Anticancer Res.* 2007;27(4A):1837-1839.

25. Liu PY, Alberts DS, Monk BJ, et al. An early signal of CA-125 progression for ovarian cancer patients receiving maintenance treatment after complete clinical response to primary therapy. *J Clin Oncol.* 2007;25(24):3615-3620.

26. Rustin GJ, van der Burg ME, Griffin CL, et al. Early versus delayed treatment of relapsed ovarian cancer (MRC OV05/EORTC 55955): a randomised trial. *Lancet.* 2010;376(9747):1155-1163.

27. Bosl GJ, Feldman DR, Bajorin DF. Cancer of the testis. In: DeVita VT, Lawrence TS, Rosenberg SA, eds. *Cancer: Principles and Practice of Oncology. 9th ed.* Philadelphia, PA: Lippincott Williams & Wilkins; 2011.

28. Cole LA, Shahabi S, Butler SA, et al. Utility of commonly used commercial human chorionic gonadotropin immunoassays in the diagnosis and management of trophoblastic diseases. *Clin Chem.* 2001;47(2):308-315.

29. Gilligan TD, Seidenfeld J, Basch EM, et al. American Society of Clinical Oncology Clinical Practice Guideline on uses of serum tumor markers in adult males with germ cell tumors. *J Clin Oncol.* 2010;28(20):3388-3404.

30. Toner GC, Geller NL, Tan C, et al. Serum tumor marker half-life during chemotherapy allows early prediction of complete response and survival in nonseminomatous germ cell tumors. *Cancer Res.* 1990;50(18):5904-5910.

31. Safi F, Schlosser W, Falkenreck S, et al. CA 19-9 serum course and prognosis of pancreatic cancer. *Int J Pancreatol.* 1996;20(3):155-161.

32. Ziske C, Schlie C, Gorschluter M, et al. Prognostic value of CA 19-9 levels in patients with inoperable adenocarcinoma of the pancreas treated with gemcitabine. *Br J Cancer.* 2003;89(8):1413-1417.

33. Maisey NR, Norman AR, Hill A, et al. CA19-9 as a prognostic factor in inoperable pancreatic cancer: the implication for clinical trials. *Br J Cancer.* 2005;93(7):740-743.

34. Soresi M, Magliarisi C, Campagna P, et al. Usefulness of alpha-fetoprotein in the diagnosis of hepatocellular carcinoma. *Anticancer Res.* 2003;23(2C):1747-1753.

35. Zhang BH, Yang BH, Tang ZY. Randomized controlled trial of screening for hepatocellular carcinoma. *J Cancer Res Clin Oncol.* 2004;130(7):417-422.

36. Munshi NC, Anderson KC. Plasma cell neoplasms. In: DeVita VT, Lawrence TS, Rosenberg SA, eds. *Cancer: Principles and Practice of Oncology. 9th ed.* Philadelphia, PA: Lippincott Williams & Wilkins; 2011.

37. Greipp PR, San Miguel J, Durie BG, et al. International staging system for multiple myeloma. *J Clin Oncol.* 2005;23(15):3412-3420.

38. Hammond ME, Hayes DF, Dowsett M, et al. American Society of Clinical Oncology/College Of American Pathologists guideline recommendations for immunohistochemical testing of estrogen and progesterone receptors in breast cancer. *J Clin Oncol.* 2010;28(16):2784-2795.

39. Badve SS, Baehner FL, Gray RP, et al. Estrogen- and progesterone-receptor status in ECOG 2197: comparison of immunohistochemistry by local and central laboratories and quantitative reverse transcription polymerase chain reaction by central laboratory. *J Clin Oncol.* 2008;26(15):2473-2481.

40. Effects of chemotherapy and hormonal therapy for early breast cancer on recurrence and 15-year survival: an overview of the randomised trials. *Lancet.* 2005;365(9472):1687-1717.

41. Citri A, Yarden Y. EGF-ERBB signalling: towards the systems level. *Nat Rev Mol Cell Biol.* 2006;7(7):505-516.

42. Slamon DJ, Clark GM, Wong SG, et al. Human breast cancer: correlation of relapse and survival with amplification of the HER2/neu oncogene. *Science.* 1987;235(4785):177-182.

43. Carlomagno C, Perrone F, Gallo C, et al. c-erb B2 overexpression decreases the benefit of adjuvant tamoxifen in early-stage breast cancer without axillary lymph node metastases. *J Clin Oncol.* 1996;14(10):2702-2708.

44. Cobleigh MA, Vogel CL, Tripathy D, et al. Multinational study of the efficacy and safety of humanized anti-HER2 monoclonal antibody in women who have HER2-overexpressing metastatic breast cancer that has progressed after chemotherapy for metastatic disease. *J Clin Oncol.* 1999;17(9):2639-2648.

45. Geyer CE, Forster J, Lindquist D, et al. Lapatinib plus capecitabine for HER2-positive advanced breast cancer. *N Engl J Med.* 2006;355(26):2733-2743.

46. Hayes DF, Thor AD, Dressler LG, et al. HER2 and response to paclitaxel in node-positive breast cancer. *N Engl J Med.* 2007;357(15):1496-1506.

47. Pritchard KI, Shepherd LE, O'Malley FP, et al. HER2 and responsiveness of breast cancer to adjuvant chemotherapy. *N Engl J Med.* 2006;354(20):2103-2111.

48. Sauter G, Lee J, Bartlett JM, et al. Guidelines for human epidermal growth factor receptor 2 testing: biologic and methodologic considerations. *J Clin Oncol.* 2009;27(8):1323-1333.

49. Romond EH, Perez EA, Bryant J, et al. Trastuzumab plus adjuvant chemotherapy for operable HER2-positive breast cancer. *N Engl J Med.* 2005;353(16):1673-1684.

50. Baccarani M, Cortes J, Pane F, et al. Chronic myeloid leukemia: an update of concepts and management recommendations of European LeukemiaNet. *J Clin Oncol.* 2009;27(35):6041-6051.

51. Radich JP. Measuring response to BCR-ABL inhibitors in chronic myeloid leukemia. *Cancer.* 2012;118(2):300-311.

52. Shami PJ, Deininger M. Evolving treatment strategies for patients newly diagnosed with chronic myeloid leukemia: the role of second-generation BCR-ABL inhibitors as first-line therapy. *Leukemia.* 2012;26(2):214-224.

53. Keedy VL, Temin S, Somerfield MR, et al. American Society of Clinical Oncology provisional clinical opinion: epidermal growth factor receptor (EGFR) Mutation testing for patients with advanced non-small-cell lung cancer considering first-line EGFR tyrosine kinase inhibitor therapy. *J Clin Oncol.* 2011;29(15):2121-2127.

54. Raman G, Wallace B, Patel K, et al. Update on Horizon scans of genetic tests currently available for clinical use in cancers. *AHRQ Technology Assessment Program.* 2011.

55. Allegra CJ, Jessup JM, Somerfield MR, et al. American Society of Clinical Oncology provisional clinical opinion: testing for KRas gene mutations in patients with metastatic colorectal carcinoma to predict response to anti-epidermal growth factor receptor monoclonal antibody therapy. *J Clin Oncol.* 2009;27(12):2091-2096.

56. Arkenau HT, Kefford R, Long GV. Targeting BRAF for patients with melanoma. *Br J Cancer.* 2011;104(3):392-398.

57. Just PA, Cazes A, Audebourg A, et al. Histologic subtypes, immunohistochemistry, FISH or molecular screening for the accurate diagnosis of ALK-rearrangement in lung cancer: A comprehensive study of Caucasian non-smokers. *Lung Cancer.* 2012;76(3):309-315.

58. Shaw AT, Solomon B, Kenudson MM. Crizotinib and testing for ALK. *J Natl Compr Canc Netw.* 2011;9(12):1335-1341.

QUICKVIEW | Carcinoembryonic Antigen (CEA)

PARAMETER	DESCRIPTION	COMMENTS
Common reference range		
Adults	<2.5 ng/mL	
Pediatrics	Unknown	
Critical value	Yes, levels >10 ng/mL generally indicate cancerous process	
Inherent activity	Unknown	
Location		
Production	Intestine, pancreas, liver	Normally found during fetal development only; detected in serum of patients
Storage	Unknown	
Secretion/excretion	Unknown	
Causes of abnormal values		
High	Cancer (mainly colon), smoking, hepatitis, pancreatitis, peptic ulcer disease, hypothyroidism, ulcerative colitis, Crohn disease	
Low	Not applicable	Usually less than 10 ng/mL in nonmalignant conditions
Signs and symptoms		
High level	Not applicable	
Low level	Not applicable	
After event, time to....		
Initial elevation	Not applicable	
Peak values		
Normalization		
Causes of spurious results	Not applicable	
Additional info	Not reliable to screen for cancers since elevated in other conditions; can be used to monitor effectiveness of therapy in patients with cancer	

QUICKVIEW | CA 125

PARAMETER	DESCRIPTION	COMMENTS
Common reference range		
Adults	<2.5 ng/mL	
Pediatrics	Unknown	
Critical value	Not applicable	
Inherent activity	Unknown	
Location		
Production	Protein found on cells of the pelvic peritoneum	Detected in serum of patients
Storage	Unknown	
Secretion/excretion	Unknown	
Causes of abnormal values		
High	Cancer (mainly ovarian, cervical, and fallopian tube carcinomas), endometriosis, ovarian cysts, liver disease, pregnancy, menstruation	
Low	Luteal phase of cycle, patients on oral contraceptives, menopausal women	
Signs and symptoms		
High level	Not applicable	
Low level	Not applicable	
After event, time to....		
Initial elevation	Not applicable	
Peak values		
Normalization		
Causes of spurious results	Not applicable	
Additional info	Not reliable to screen for cancers since elevated in other conditions; can be used to monitor effectiveness of therapy in patients with cancer; rate of rise and fall of levels may indicate prognosis and effectiveness of therapy	

QUICKVIEW | CA 15-3

PARAMETER	DESCRIPTION	COMMENTS
Common reference range		
Adults	<30 units/mL	
Pediatrics	Unknown	
Critical value	Not applicable	
Inherent activity	Unknown	
Location	Serum	
Production	Unknown	Antibody detects circulating mucin antigen secreted
Storage	Unknown	
Secretion/excretion	Secreted from breast tissue	
Causes of abnormal values		
High	Breast cancer, may be elevated in other cancers of lung, colon, ovary and pancreas origin and benign breast disorders	
Low	Not applicable	
Signs and symptoms		
High level	Not applicable	
Low level	Not applicable	
After event, time to….		
Initial elevation	Not applicable	
Peak values		
Normalization		
Causes of spurious results	Not applicable	
Additional info	Mainly used in combination with other markers or in clinical trials	

QUICKVIEW | CA 27.29

PARAMETER	DESCRIPTION	COMMENTS
Common reference range		
Adults	<38 units/mL	
Pediatrics	Unknown	
Critical value	Not applicable	
Inherent activity	Unknown	
Location	Serum	
Production	Unknown	Antibody detects circulating mucin antigen secreted
Storage	Unknown	
Secretion/excretion	Secreted from breast tissue	
Causes of abnormal values		
High	Breast carcinoma, may be elevated in benign breast disorders	
Low	Not applicable	
Signs and symptoms		
High level	Not applicable	
Low level	Not applicable	
After event, time to....		
Initial elevation	Not applicable	
Peak values		
Normalization		
Causes of spurious results	Not applicable	
Additional info	Mainly used in combination with other markers or in clinical trials	

QUICKVIEW | Human Chorionic Gonadotropin (HCG)

PARAMETER	DESCRIPTION	COMMENTS
Common reference range		
Adults	<5 million International Units/mL	Beta subunit commonly measured, serum levels drawn when used as a tumor marker
Pediatrics	Unknown	
Critical value	Not applicable	
Inherent activity	Unknown	
Location		
Production	Made by cells that make up the placenta	Detected in patient serum and urine
Storage	Unknown	
Secretion/excretion	Secreted from the placenta or malignant germ cells	
Causes of abnormal values		
High	Pregnancy, mixed germ cell tumors, or choriocarcinoma of the testes or ovary, increased in other rare tumors	If elevated in males or in nonpregnant females, cancer is suspected
Low	Not applicable	
Signs and symptoms		
High level	Not applicable	
Low level	Not applicable	
After event, time to....		
Initial elevation	Not applicable	
Peak values		
Normalization		
Causes of spurious results	Not applicable	
Additional info	Most commonly used in testicular cancer as a prognostic factor as well as to monitor effects of treatment; levels >50 million International Units/mL indicate a poor prognosis	

QUICKVIEW | CA 19-9

PARAMETER	DESCRIPTION	COMMENTS
Common reference range		
Adults	<37 units/mL	
Pediatrics	Unknown	
Critical value	Not applicable	
Inherent activity	Unknown	
Location		
Production	Pancreas, gastric cells, colon	Detected in patient serum
Storage	Unknown	
Secretion/excretion	Secreted from breast tissue	
Causes of abnormal values		
High	Pancreatic, gastric, and colon carcinomas; also in benign pancreatic disorders	
Low	Not applicable	
Signs and symptoms		
High level	Not applicable	
Low level	Not applicable	
After event, time to....		
Initial elevation	Not applicable	
Peak values		
Normalization		
Causes of spurious results	Not applicable	
Additional info	Only recommended to evaluate treatment response and recurrence in patients with pancreatic cancer	

QUICKVIEW | Alphafetoprotein (AFP)

PARAMETER	DESCRIPTION	COMMENTS
Common reference range		
Adults	<20 ng/mL	
Pediatrics	Unknown	
Critical value	Not applicable	
Inherent activity	Unknown	
Location		
Production	Protein made normally during fetal and neonatal stages by liver and yolk sac cells	Detected in patient serum; levels should decline after birth
Storage	Unknown	
Secretion/excretion	Unknown	
Causes of abnormal values		
High	Cancer (mainly liver and testicular); can be elevated in other cancers such as pancreatic, gastric, lung, and colon carcinomas; elevated in nonmalignant conditions including pregnancy, hepatitis, and cirrhosis	High results may be used to screen for liver cancer in parts of the world at increased risk for this malignancy
Low	Not applicable	
Signs and symptoms		
High level	Not applicable	
Low level	Not applicable	
After event, time to....		
Initial elevation	Not applicable	
Peak values		
Normalization		
Causes of spurious results	Not applicable	
Additional info	Only recommended to evaluate treatment response and recurrence in patients with testicular cancer	

QUICKVIEW | Beta-2 Microglobulin (B$_2$M)

PARAMETER	DESCRIPTION	COMMENTS
Common reference range		
Adults	<2.5 mcg/mL	
Pediatrics	Unknown	
Critical value	Not applicable	
Inherent activity	Unknown	
Location	Protein found on surface of lymphocytes and other MHC I molecules	Also present in small amounts in urine and blood; level should decline after birth
Production	Unknown	
Storage	Unknown	
Secretion/excretion	Unknown	
Causes of abnormal values		
High	Multiple (plasma cell) myeloma, lymphoma, and in patients with renal failure	Renally excreted so elevated levels may indicate renal failure
Low	Not applicable	
Signs and symptoms		
High level	May see signs of renal failure	
Low level	Not applicable	
After event, time to....		
Initial elevation	Not applicable	
Peak values		
Normalization		
Causes of spurious results	Not applicable	
Additional info	Used in patients with multiple myeloma to assist in determining prognosis	

MHC = major histocompatibility complex.

QUICKVIEW | Estrogen and Progesterone Receptors

PARAMETER	DESCRIPTION	COMMENTS
Common reference range		
Adults	Not applicable	Not a normal serum laboratory value, only determined in breast biopsies; if greater than 1% of cells are positive for the receptor, it is considered ER- or PR-positive
Pediatrics	Not applicable	
Critical value	Not applicable	
Inherent activity	Growth of breast and other hormone sensitive cells	
Location	Throughout the body (e.g., breast tissue, ovaries, bone)	Also present in small amounts in urine and blood; level should decline after birth
Production	Unknown	
Storage	Not applicable	
Secretion/excretion	Not applicable	
Causes of abnormal values		
High	Not applicable	It is unknown if the levels are higher in cancer, but they are checked to determine if blocking them with hormonal therapy will be useful
Low	Not applicable	
Signs and symptoms		
High level	May see signs of renal failure	
Low level	Not applicable	
After event, time to....		
Initial elevation	Not applicable	
Peak values		
Normalization		
Causes of spurious results	Not applicable	
Additional info	Antiestrogens (e.g., tamoxifen) and aromatase inhibitors (e.g., anastrozole) often given if these receptors are positive in women with breast cancer	

ER = estrogen receptor; PR = progesterone receptor.

QUICKVIEW | Human Epidermal Growth Factor Receptor 2 (HER2)

PARAMETER	DESCRIPTION	COMMENTS
Common reference range		
Adults	Considered positive by IHC if 3+ cells stain for HER2 or by FISH if HER2 gene copy number >4 or FISH ratio >2.0	Not a normal serum laboratory value, only determined in breast biopsies; FISH preferred
Pediatrics	Not applicable	
Critical value	Not applicable	
Inherent activity	Protein involved in normal growth and development of cells by activating intracellular pathways that send growth signals to the nucleus	In cancer the growth signal is abnormal and amplified leading to uncontrolled proliferation of the cancerous cells
Location	Surface of many epidermal cells	Also present in small amounts in urine and blood; level should decline after birth
Production	Not applicable	
Storage	Not applicable	
Secretion/excretion	Not applicable	
Causes of abnormal values		
High	Cancer	Either number of receptors may be higher or there may be an increase in HER2 gene copies indicating increased function of the gene
Low	Not applicable	
Signs and symptoms		
High level	Not applicable	
Low level	Not applicable	
After event, time to....		
Initial elevation	Not applicable	
Peak values		
Normalization		
Causes of spurious results	Not applicable	
Additional info	Anti-HER2 therapies (e.g., trastuzumab, lapatinib) often given if positive	

FISH = fluorescence in situ hybridization; HER2 = human epidermal growth factor receptor 2; IHC = immunohistochemistry.

QUICKVIEW | BCR-ABL

PARAMETER	DESCRIPTION	COMMENTS
Common reference range		
Adults	Not applicable	This is an abnormal fusion gene that results from a genetic translocation producing a fusion mRNA normally not present in any significant amount unless a malignancy is present
Pediatrics	Not applicable	
Critical value	Not applicable	
Inherent activity	When present, causes abnormal growth of cells	Translocation results in an abnormal fusion protein with increased tyrosine kinase activity continually signaling cells to grow
Location	Chromosome 22 resulting from t(9;22) translocation	Also present in small amounts in urine and blood; level should decline after birth
Production	Not applicable	
Storage	Not applicable	
Secretion/excretion	Not applicable	
Causes of abnormal values		
High	Cancer	
Low	Not applicable	
Signs and symptoms		
High level	Not applicable	
Low level	Not applicable	
After event, time to....		
Initial elevation	Not applicable	Rising levels of BCR-ABL mRNA correlate with increasing disease activity whereas falling levels are consistent with response to therapy
Peak values		
Normalization		
Causes of spurious results	Not applicable	
Additional info	Called the Philadelphia chromosome; levels of BCR-ABL mRNA should decrease with therapy, and failure to do so indicates treatment failure; patients should be tested for T315I mutations upon diagnosis and additional mutations if they relapse	

mRNA = messenger RNA.

QUICKVIEW | EGFR Mutation (exon 19 and 21)

PARAMETER	DESCRIPTION	COMMENTS
Common reference range		
Adults	Not applicable	This is a gene that codes for a transmembrane receptor; it does not normally contain any mutations
Pediatrics	Not applicable	
Critical value	Not applicable	
Inherent activity	When present, causes abnormal growth of cells	Mutation in lung cancer cells leads to perpetual signaling
Location	Located on chromosome 7p12—region of interest is exon 19 and 21h	
Production	Not applicable	
Storage	Not applicable	
Secretion/excretion	Not applicable	
Causes of abnormal values		
High	Not applicable	
Low	Not applicable	
Signs and symptoms		
High level	Not applicable	
Low level	Not applicable	
After event, time to....		
Initial elevation	Not applicable	
Peak values		
Normalization		
Causes of spurious results	Not applicable	
Additional info	The presence of a mutation in exon 19 or 21 in lung cancer indicates a higher likelihood of response to erlotinib	

QUICKVIEW | KRas Mutation

PARAMETER	DESCRIPTION	COMMENTS
Common reference range		
Adults	Not applicable	This is a gene that codes for a GTPase that is a binary switch in cell signaling; it does not normally contain any mutations—when mutations are not present it is referred to as WT
Pediatrics	Not applicable	
Critical value	Not applicable	
Inherent activity	When present, causes abnormal growth of cells	Mutation in colorectal cancer cells leads to perpetual signaling and resistance to monoclonal antibodies targeting EGFR
Location	Chromosome 12p12— region of interest is exon 1 (codon 12 and 13)	
Production	Not applicable	
Storage	Not applicable	
Secretion/excretion	Not applicable	
Causes of abnormal values		
High	Mutation common in lung adenocarcinoma, mucinous adenoma, ductal carcinoma of the pancreas, and colorectal carcinoma	
Low	Not applicable	
Signs and symptoms		
High level	Not applicable	
Low level	Not applicable	
After event, time to....		
Initial elevation	Not applicable	
Peak values		
Normalization		
Causes of spurious results	Not applicable	
Additional info	Cetuximab and panitumumab should only be used for patients with colorectal cancer with WT KRas tumors	

EGFR = epidermal growth factor receptor; KRas = V-Ki-ras2 Kirsten rat sarcoma viral oncogene homolog; WT = wild type.

QUICKVIEW | BRAF Mutation

PARAMETER	DESCRIPTION	COMMENTS
Common reference range		
Adults	Not applicable	This is a gene that codes for a kinase involved in cell signaling through the MAP kinase pathway; it does not normally contain any mutations
Pediatrics	Not applicable	
Critical value	Not applicable	
Inherent activity	When present, causes abnormal growth of cells	Mutation in cancer cells leads to perpetual signaling
Location	Chromosome 7q34—mutation of interest is at amino acid 600 (BRAF V600E)	
Production	Not applicable	
Storage	Not applicable	
Secretion/excretion	Not applicable	
Causes of abnormal values		
High	Mutation common in non-Hodgkin lymphoma, colorectal cancer, malignant melanoma, thyroid carcinoma, non-small-cell lung carcinoma, and adenocarcinoma of lung	
Low	Not applicable	
Signs and symptoms		
High level	Not applicable	
Low level	Not applicable	
After event, time to....		
Initial elevation	Not applicable	
Peak values		
Normalization		
Causes of spurious results	Not applicable	
Additional info	Patients with malignant melanoma should receive only vemurafenib if they have a tumor with the V600E mutation	

MAP = mitogen-activated protein.

QUICKVIEW | ALK Mutation

PARAMETER	DESCRIPTION	COMMENTS
Common reference range		
Adults	Not applicable	This is a fusion gene between EML4- and ALK; the resulting protein promotes cancer growth through increased kinase signaling activity; cells do not normally contain this gene fusion
Pediatrics	Not applicable	
Critical value	Not applicable	
Inherent activity	When present, causes abnormal growth of cells	Mutation in cancer cells leads to increased signaling
Location	Chromosome 2 contains the genes for EML4 and ALK—mutation of interest is translocation/fusion gene EML4-ALK	
Production	Not applicable	
Storage	Not applicable	
Secretion/excretion	Not applicable	
Causes of abnormal values		
High	Mutation most commonly found in adenocarcinoma of the lung carcinoma in nonsmokers	
Low	Not applicable	
Signs and symptoms		
High level	Not applicable	
Low level	Not applicable	
After event, time to....		
Initial elevation	Not applicable	
Peak values		
Normalization		
Causes of spurious results	Not applicable	
Additional info	Patients with metastatic non-small-cell lung cancer should receive only crizotinib if they have a tumor with the ALK rearrangement	

ALK = anaplastic lymphoma kinase.

CHAPTER 20

INTERPRETING PEDIATRIC LABORATORY DATA

DONNA M. KRAUS

Objectives

After completing this chapter, the reader should be able to

- Define the various pediatric age group terminology

- Discuss general pediatric considerations as they relate to blood sampling

- Describe how pediatric reference ranges are determined

- Discuss the age-related physiologic differences that account for variations by age in the normal reference ranges for serum sodium, potassium, bicarbonate, calcium, phosphorus, and magnesium

- List common pediatric causes of abnormalities in the electrolytes and minerals listed above

- Explain why age-related differences in serum creatinine (SCr) and kidney function tests occur

- Discuss the age-related differences that occur in serum albumin, liver enzyme tests, and bilirubin

- Describe what is meant by the physiologic anemia of infancy and explain how it occurs

The interpretation of laboratory data in the pediatric patient population can be complex. Compared to adults, the pediatric population is much more dynamic. Alterations in body composition, organ function, and physiologic activity accompany the normal processes of maturation and growth that occur from birth through adolescence. These alterations can result in different normal reference ranges in pediatric patients for various laboratory tests. Pediatric patients not only have different normal laboratory values compared to adults, but normal laboratory values may differ in various pediatric age groups. It is important for the clinician to understand the reasons for these different, commonly accepted reference ranges and to use age-appropriate reference ranges when providing pharmaceutical care to pediatric patients.

The measurement of substances in neonates, infants, and young children is further complicated by the patient's smaller physical size and difficulty in obtaining blood and urine samples. The smaller blood volume in these patients requires blood samples to be smaller and, thus, special microanalytical techniques must be used. Additionally, in the neonate, substances that normally occur in higher amounts in the blood—such as bilirubin, lipids, and hemoglobin—may interfere with certain assays. This chapter will briefly review pertinent general pediatric principles and focus on the different age-related factors that must be considered when interpreting commonly used laboratory data in pediatric patients.

GENERAL PEDIATRIC CONSIDERATIONS

Knowledge of pediatric age group terminology is important to better understand age-related physiological differences and other factors that may influence the interpretation of pediatric laboratory data. These terms are defined in Table 20-1 and will be used throughout this chapter.[1,2]

The interpretation of any patient's laboratory data must be viewed in light of the patient's clinical status. This includes the patient's symptoms, physical signs of disease, and physiologic parameters, such as respiratory rate, heart rate, and blood pressure. For example, an elevated $PaCO_2$ from an arterial blood gas may be clinically more significant in a patient who is extremely tachypneic (perhaps indicating impending respiratory failure) compared to a patient whose respiratory rate is mildly elevated. Thus, it is important to know the relative differences in physiologic norms that occur in the various pediatric age groups.

Normal respiratory rates are higher in neonates and young infants compared to children, adolescents, and adults. The average respiratory rate of a newborn is 60 breaths/min at 1 hour after birth, but 30–40 breaths/min at greater than 6 hours after birth. Mean respiratory rates of infants and young children <2 years of age (25–30 breaths/min) continue to be higher than in children 3–9 years of age (20–25 breaths/min) and adolescents (16–20 breaths/min).[1]

Normal heart rates follow a similar pattern with higher heart rates in neonates and young infants, which then slowly decrease with increasing age through adolescence. For example, the mean heart rate of a newborn is 120–160 beats/min and that of a 1-month-old infant is 145 beats/min, while the mean heart rate for a 1-year-old is 120 beats/min and that of a 12-year-old is 85 beats/min.[3]

TABLE 20-1. Definition of Age Group Terminology[a]

Gestational age (GA)	The time from conception until birth; more specifically, GA is defined as the number of weeks from the first day of the mother's LMP until the birth of the baby; GA at birth is assessed by the date of the LMP and by physical exam (Dubowitz score)
Postnatal age (PNA)	Chronological age since birth
Postmenstrual age (PMA)	Postmenstrual age is calculated as gestational age plus postnatal age (PMA = GA + PNA)
Neonate	A full-term newborn 0–28 days PNA; this term may also be applied to a premature neonate whose PMA is 42–46 weeks
Premature neonate	Neonate born at <38 weeks GA
Full-term neonate	Neonate born at 38–42 weeks (average ~40 weeks) GA
Infant	1 month (>28 days) to 1 yr of age
Child/children	1–12 yr of age
Adolescent	13–18 yr of age
Adult	>18 yr of age

LMP = last menstrual period.

[a]The term postconceptional age (PCA; age since conception) is no longer recommended for use in clinical pediatrics.[2] However, the use of this term may occur in pediatric literature. Traditionally, PCA was defined as GA + PNA. Since the exact time of conception is not generally known (except in cases of assisted reproductive technology) and GA is calculated as above (according to the mother's LMP), PMA is considered a more accurate term to use. When PCA is used in the pediatric literature, it should be defined within the article where it is used.

Source: Reproduced, with permission, from reference 1.

In pediatric patients, normal blood pressure values vary according to age, gender, and percentile height of the patient.[4,5] Blood pressures are lower in neonates and increase throughout infancy and childhood. For example, typical blood pressures for a full-term newborn would be in the range of 65–95 systolic and 30–60 diastolic. The normal blood pressure (blood pressure <90th percentile) for a 1-year-old girl of average height (50th percentile height) would be less than 100/54, while that of a 15-year-old girl of average height would be less than 123/79. Blood pressures are slightly different for girls compared to boys and are higher in taller children. Appropriate references should be consulted to obtain normal blood pressure values when providing clinical care to pediatric patients.[1,4,5]

In addition to age-related physiologic differences in respiratory rates, heart rates, and blood pressures, age-related changes in body composition (e.g., fluid compartments), cardiac output, organ perfusion, and organ function also exist. These age-related changes may result in different normal laboratory values for pediatric patients compared to adults. For example, age-related changes in fluid compartments affect normal laboratory values for serum electrolytes, as discussed in the Serum Electrolytes and Minerals section below. Being aware of the normal laboratory values for age is important for proper monitoring of efficacy and toxicity of pediatric drug therapy.

Pediatric Blood Sampling

The smaller physical size of pediatric patients makes it more difficult to obtain blood samples. In general, venipuncture techniques used in adults can be utilized in older children and adolescents. However, vacuum containers used for blood sampling may collapse the small veins of younger children and are not recommended in these patients.[6] Capillary puncture (also called *microcapillary puncture* or *skin puncture*) is used in patients with small or inaccessible veins. Thus, it is the blood sampling method of choice for premature neonates, neonates, and young infants. Since this method also helps preserve total blood volume, it may also be beneficial to use in infants and small children who require multiple blood tests.[7]

The physical sites that are used for capillary puncture include the heel, finger, great toe, and ear lobe.[6,7] The preferred site in neonates is the medial or lateral portion of the plantar surface of the heel. The medial surface of the great toe may also be used. The central area of the foot is avoided because of the risk of damage to the calcaneus bone, tendons, nerves, and cartilage. Heelsticks (capillary puncture of the heel) are often used in neonates and younger infants, while fingersticks may be used in children and adults. The earlobe is never used for capillary puncture for neonates and infants but may be used as a "site of last resort" in older children and adults.[7]

Since capillary and venous blood are similar in composition, the capillary puncture method may be used to obtain samples for most chemistry and hematology tests.[7] However, differences may occur between venous and capillary blood for certain substances such as glucose, calcium, potassium, and total protein. For example, glucose concentrations may be 10% higher when the sample is collected by capillary puncture compared to venipuncture.[6] In addition, improper capillary puncture sample collection may result in hemolysis or introduction of interstitial fluid into the specimen. This may result in higher concentrations for potassium, magnesium, lactate dehydrogenase, and other substances. Therefore, using the proper procedure to collect blood by the capillary puncture method is essential. It is also important that the site of capillary puncture be warmed prior to sample collection, especially for blood gas determinations.[6] Complications of capillary puncture include infection, hematoma, and bruising.

TABLE 20-2. Total Blood Volume by Age Group

AGE	EXAMPLE WEIGHT (kg) [AGE]	APPROXIMATE TOTAL BLOOD VOLUME (mL/kg)[a]	ESTIMATED TOTAL BLOOD VOLUME (mL)
Premature infant	1.5	89–105	134–158
Term newborn	3.4	78–86	265–292
1–12 months	7.6 [6 months]	73–78	555–593
1–3 yr	12.4 [2 yr]	74–82	918–1017
4–6 yr	18.2 [5 yr]	80–86	1456–1565
7–18 yr	45.5 [13 yr]	83–90	3777–4095
Adults	70.0	68–88	4760–6160

[a]Approximate total blood volume information compiled from reference 8.

Source: Reproduced, with permission, from reference 1.

The size of the blood sample is an important issue to the pediatric clinician. Compared to adults, pediatric patients have a much smaller total blood volume (Table 20-2). For example, a full-term newborn of average weight (3.4 kg) has an approximate total blood volume of 78–86 mL/kg, or about 265–292 mL total.[1,8] However, a 70-kg adult has an estimated total blood volume of 68–88 mL/kg or 4760–6160 mL total. If a standard 10-mL blood sample were to be drawn from a pediatric patient, it would represent a much higher percent of total blood volume compared to an adult. Therefore, the smaller total blood volume in pediatric patients requires blood sample sizes to be smaller. This issue is further complicated in newborns because their relatively high hematocrit (approximately 60% or higher) decreases the yield of serum or plasma from the amount of blood collected. Microanalytical techniques have reduced the required size of blood samples. However, critically ill, pediatric patients may require multiple or frequent blood sample determinations. Thus, it is essential to plan pediatric laboratory tests, especially in the neonate and premature neonate, to avoid excessive blood drawing.

Substances that normally occur in higher amounts in the blood of neonates, such as bilirubin, lipids, and hemoglobin, may interfere with certain assays. Hyperbilirubinemia may occur in premature and term neonates. High bilirubin concentrations may produce falsely low creatinine or cholesterol values when measured by certain analytical instruments.[6] Neonates, especially those that are born prematurely, may have lipemia when receiving intravenous (IV) fat emulsions. Lipemia may interfere with spectrophotometric determinations of any substance or with flame photometer determinations of potassium and sodium. Newborns have higher hemoglobin values and hemoglobin may interfere with certain assays. For example, hemolysis and the presence of hemoglobin may interfere with bilirubin measurements. Therefore, it is important to ensure that the assay methodology selected for measurement of substances in neonatal serum or plasma is not subject to interference from bilirubin, lipids, or hemoglobin.

Pediatric Reference Ranges

Various methods can be used to determine reference ranges, and each method has its own advantages and disadvantages. In adults, reference ranges are usually determined by obtaining samples from known healthy individuals. The frequency distribution of the obtained values are assessed and the extreme outliers (e.g., 0–2.5th percentile and 97.5–100th percentile) are excluded. This leaves the values of the 2.5–97.5th percentiles to define the reference range.[9] However, it also labels the 0–2.5th percentile and 97.5–100th percentile values from the healthy individuals as being outside of the reference range. If the frequency distribution of the obtained values fall in a bell-shaped or Gaussian distribution, then the mean (or average) value plus or minus two standard deviations (SDs) can then be used to define the reference range. The mean value plus or minus 2 SDs includes 95% of the sample. This method labels 5% of the healthy individuals as having values that fall outside of the reference range.

In the pediatric population, however, one cannot easily obtain blood samples from known healthy individuals. Large sample sizes of healthy pediatric individuals that include an appropriate age distribution from birth to 18 years of age would be required. Furthermore, it may be considered unethical to obtain blood samples from healthy pediatric patients when these individuals cannot legally give informed consent and there is no direct benefit to these individuals of obtaining the blood sample. Therefore, many pediatric reference ranges are determined by using results of tests from hospitalized sick pediatric patients and applying special statistical methods.[9] The statistical methods are designed to remove outliers and to distinguish the normal values from the values found in the sick patients. Obviously, problems in determining the true reference range may arise, especially when overlap between values from the diseased and nondiseased population occurs.

As in adults, many factors can influence the pediatric reference range including the specific assay methodology used, type of specimen analyzed, specific population studied, nutritional status of the individual, time of day the sample is obtained, timing of meals, medications taken, and specific patient demographics (age, sex, height, weight, and body surface area [BSA]). These factors, if not properly identified, may also influence the determination of reference ranges. In addition, since pediatric reference ranges are typically established in hospitalized patients, concomitant diseases may also influence the determination of the specific reference range being studied.

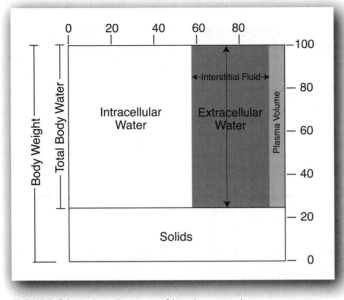

FIGURE 20-1. Distribution of body water in a term newborn infant. (Reproduced, with permission, from Bell EF, Oh W. Fluid and electrolyte management. In: MacDonald MG, Seshia MMK, Mullett MD, eds. *Avery's Neonatology: Pathophysiology and Management of the Newborn*. 6th ed. Philadelphia, PA: Lippincott Williams & Wilkins; 2005:363.)

All of these factors, plus the greater heterogeneity (variance) observed in the pediatric population makes the determination of pediatric reference ranges more complex.

Pediatric studies that define reference ranges may not always give detailed information about factors that may have influenced the determination of the specific pediatric reference range. Furthermore, due to the variation in influencing factors, most published pediatric reference ranges are not in exact agreement with each other.[1,3,9-17] Some studies report reference ranges by age for each year, others by various age groups, and others only by graphic display. Thus, it makes it very difficult to ascertain standard values for pediatric reference ranges and to apply published pediatric reference ranges to one's own patient population.

The reference ranges listed in this chapter reflect a compilation from various sources and are meant to be general guidelines. Clinicians should consult with their institution's laboratory to determine the specific age-appropriate pediatric reference ranges to be used in their patient population.

Pediatric Clinical Presentation

In general, the clinical symptoms of laboratory abnormalities in pediatric patients are similar to those symptoms observed in adults. However, certain manifestations of symptoms may be different in pediatric patients. For example, central nervous system irritability due to electrolyte imbalances (such as hypernatremia) may manifest as a high-pitched cry in infants. Hypocalcemia is more likely to manifest as seizures in neonates and young infants (compared to adults) due to the immaturity of the central nervous system. Neonates may also

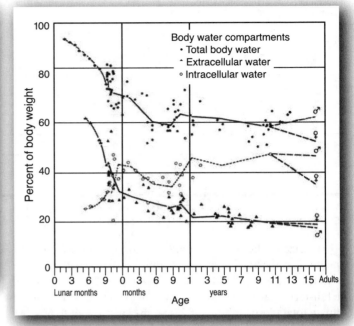

FIGURE 20-2. Changes in body water from early fetal life to adult life. (Reproduced, with permission, from Friis-Hansen B. Water distribution in the foetus and newborn infant. *Acta Paediatr Scand.* 1983;305:8.)

have nonspecific or vague symptoms for many disorders. For example, neonates with sepsis, meningitis, or hypocalcemia, may have poor feedings, lethargy, and vomiting. In addition, young pediatric patients are unable to communicate symptoms they may be experiencing. Thus, although symptoms of laboratory abnormalities in pediatric patients are important, oftentimes the correct diagnosis relies on the physical exam and appropriate laboratory tests.

SERUM ELECTROLYTES AND MINERALS

The homeostatic mechanisms that regulate fluid, electrolyte, and mineral balance in adults also apply to the pediatric patient. However, several important age-related differences exist. Compared to adults, neonates and young infants have alterations in body composition and fluid compartments; increased insensible water loss; immature (decreased) renal function; and variations in the neuroendocrine control of fluid, electrolyte, and mineral balance.[18] In addition, fluid, electrolyte, and mineral intake are not controlled by the individual (i.e., the neonate or young infant) but are controlled by the individual's caregiver. These age-related physiologic differences can result in alterations in the pediatric reference range for several electrolytes and minerals and can influence the interpretation of pediatric laboratory data.

A large percent of the human body is comprised of water. Total body water (TBW) can be divided into two major compartments: intracellular water (ICW) and extracellular water (ECW). The ECW compartment consists of the interstitial water and the intravascular water (or plasma volume) (see Figure 20-1). Both TBW and ECW, when expressed as

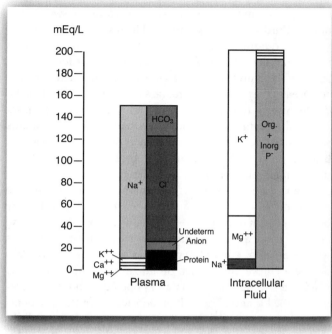

FIGURE 20-3. Ion distribution in the blood plasma, which represents extracellular fluid, and in the intracellular fluid compartment. (Reproduced, with permission, from Bell EF, Oh W. Fluid and electrolyte management. In: MacDonald MG, Seshia MMK, Mullett MD, eds. *Avery's Neonatology: Pathophysiology and Management of the Newborn.* 6th ed. Philadelphia, PA: Lippincott Williams & Wilkins; 2005:364.)

a percentage of body weight, are increased in the fetus and the newborn (especially the premature neonate) and decrease during childhood with increasing age (Figure 20-2).[19,20] The TBW of a fetus is 94% during the first month of gestation and decreases to 75% in a full-term newborn. The TBW of a preterm newborn may be 80%. The TBW decreases to approximately 60% by 6–12 months of age and to 55% in an adult. ECW is about 44% in a full-term newborn, 30% in a 3–6-month-old infant, 25% in a 1-year-old, and 19% in an adult.[19,20] The decrease in TBW that is seen after birth is largely due to a contraction (or mobilization) of the ECW compartment. This mobilization is, most likely, the result of an increase in renal function that is seen after birth. The ICW compartment is lower at birth, increases slowly after birth, and is greater than ECW by about 3 months of age. It is important to note that the intake of water and electrolytes can influence these postnatal changes in TBW and the distribution between ECW and ICW.[18]

The electrolyte composition of ECW versus ICW is very different (Figure 20-3). Sodium is the major cation found in intravascular water (plasma volume) of the ECW. Potassium, calcium, and magnesium make up a much smaller amount of the intravascular cations. Chloride is the primary intravascular anion and bicarbonate, protein, and other anions comprise the balance. The electrolyte composition of the interstitial component of ECW is similar to the intravascular composition, but protein content is lower. Potassium and magnesium are the major cations found in ICW. Phosphate (organic and

inorganic) is the primary intracellular anion, and bicarbonate makes up a smaller amount.[18]

These compositional differences in ECW and ICW, along with the age-related differences in the amounts of these water compartments, can result in maturational differences in the amount of electrolytes per kg of body weight. For example, since premature neonates have a larger ECW compartment and ECW contains a higher amount of sodium and chloride, premature neonates contain a higher amount of sodium and chloride per kilogram of body weight compared to term neonates.[18] These principles are important to keep in mind when managing neonatal fluid and electrolyte therapy. One must also remember that the management of fluid and electrolyte therapy in the mother during labor can result in alterations in the newborn's fluid and electrolyte status. For example, if the mother is given too much fluid (i.e., too much free water) during labor, the newborn may be born with hyponatremia.[21]

Insensible water loss is the water that is lost via evaporation from the skin and through the respiratory tract.[18] Knowledge of the factors that influence insensible water loss in pediatric patients is important to estimate appropriate water intake and to assess electrolyte imbalances that may occur. Compared to adults, neonates and young infants have an increase in the amount of insensible water loss. This is primarily due to their increased surface area to body weight ratio and higher respiratory rate. Smaller newborns and those born at a younger gestational age (GA) have an even higher insensible water loss. This is related to their immature (thinner) skin, greater skin blood flow, and larger TBW. Many other factors increase insensible water loss, such as the environmental and body temperature, radiant warmers, phototherapy, motor activity, crying, and skin breakdown or injury. Congenital skin defects, such as gastroschisis, omphalocele, or neural tube defects will also increase insensible water loss. The use of high inspired or ambient humidity, plastic heat shields or blankets, occlusive dressings, and topical waterproof agents will decrease insensible water loss.

The primary functions of the kidney (glomerular filtration, tubular secretion, and tubular reabsorption) are all decreased in the newborn, especially in the premature newborn, compared to adults. These functions increase with GA at birth and with postnatal age (PNA). The decreased glomerular and tubular functions in the neonatal kidney result in differences in how the neonate handles various electrolyte loads and differences in the normal reference ranges for several electrolytes, as described below.

Sodium

Normal range[22] for premature neonates (at 48 hr of life):
   128–148 mEq/L or 128–148 mmol/L
   newborns: 133–146 mEq/L or 133–146 mmol/L
   infants: 139–146 mEq/L or 139–146 mmol/L
   children: 138–145 mEq/L or 138–145 mmol/L
   adults: 136–142 mEq/L or 136–142 mmol/L

Sodium is primarily excreted via the kidneys, but it is also excreted via stool and sweat.[23] Usually, unless diarrhea occurs, sodium loss in the stool is minimal. In children with cystic fibrosis, aldosterone deficiency, or pseudohypoaldosteronism, the sodium concentration in sweat is increased and higher sweat losses may contribute to or cause sodium depletion.

In neonates and young infants, the renal handling of sodium is altered compared to adults.[24,25] Differences in tubular reabsorption, aldosterone concentrations, and patterns of renal blood flow help to maintain a positive sodium balance, which is required for growth. In the neonate, sodium reabsorption is decreased in the proximal tubule, but increased in the distal tubule. Aldosterone increases sodium reabsorption in the distal tubules, and plasma concentrations of renin, angiotensin II, and aldosterone are all increased in neonates. This increase in aldosterone may be a compensatory mechanism to help increase sodium reabsorption in the distal tubule. The pattern of renal blood flow is also different in the neonate. In adults, a larger amount of renal blood flow goes to the cortical area of the kidneys. However, in the neonate, the majority of renal blood flow goes to the medullary area, which is more involved with sodium conservation than excretion. These factors help the neonatal kidney to retain sodium, but also result in the neonate having a decreased ability to excrete a sodium load. Therefore, if an excessive amount of sodium is administered to a neonate, it will result in sodium retention with subsequent water retention and edema.

Although most infants are in a positive sodium balance, very low birth weight infants (birth weight <1.5 kg) are usually in a negative sodium balance.[24] This is due to their very immature kidneys and the larger amounts of sodium that are lost in the urine. These infants are at a higher risk of sodium imbalance and may require higher amounts of sodium, especially during the first weeks of life.

Compared to adults, pediatric patients may be more susceptible to imbalances of sodium and water. This may be due to their higher amount of TBW and the common pediatric occurrence of causative factors such as diarrhea and dehydration.

Hyponatremia

In infants and children, *hyponatremia* is defined as a serum sodium less than 135 mEq/L, although slightly lower values would be considered acceptable for premature neonates and newborns.[23] As in adults, hyponatremia occurs in pediatric patients when the ratio of water to sodium is increased. This may occur with low, normal, or high amounts of sodium in the body; likewise, the amount of water in the body may be low (hypovolemic), normal (euvolemic), or high (hypervolemic). The causes of hyponatremia in pediatric patients are the same as in adults. However, certain causes may be more commonly seen in children.

In hypovolemic hyponatremia, both sodium and water have been lost from the body, but a higher proportion of sodium has been lost. The most common cause of hypovolemic hyponatremia in children is diarrhea due to gastroenteritis.[23] Emesis can also cause hyponatremia if hypotonic fluids are administered, but most children with emesis have either a normal serum sodium or hypernatremia. In addition to gastrointestinal (GI) losses, hypovolemic hyponatremia may also occur from losses of sodium through the skin (e.g., excessive sweating or burns), third space losses, and renal losses.

Renal sodium loss can occur in the pediatric population from a number of causes including thiazide or loop diuretics, osmotic diuresis, cerebral salt wasting, and hereditary or acquired kidney diseases. Cerebral salt wasting is thought to be due to hypersecretion of atrial natriuretic peptide, which causes renal salt wasting. This condition is usually seen in patients with central nervous system disorders such as head trauma, brain tumors, hydrocephalus, cerebral vascular accidents, neurosurgery and brain death.[26] Hereditary kidney diseases that can cause hypovolemic hyponatremia include juvenile nephronophthisis, autosomal recessive polycystic kidney disease, proximal (type II) renal tubular acidosis, 21-hydroxylase deficiency, and pseudohypoaldosteronism type I. Patients with congenital adrenal hyperplasia due to 21-hydroxylase deficiency have an absence of aldosterone. Aldosterone is needed for sodium retention and potassium and acid excretion in the kidneys. The lack of aldosterone in these patients produces hyponatremia, hyperkalemia, and metabolic acidosis. Patients with pseudohypoaldosteronism have elevated aldosterone serum concentrations, but the kidneys do not respond properly to aldosterone. A lack of response to aldosterone by the renal tubules may also occur in children with a urinary tract obstruction and/or acute urinary tract infection and result in hyponatremia.[23]

In euvolemic hyponatremia, patients have no real evidence of volume depletion or volume overload.[23] Usually, these patients have a slight decrease in total body sodium with an excess of TBW. Although some patients may have an increase in body weight (indicating volume overload), patients often appear clinically normal or have subtle signs of fluid overload. Causes of euvolemic hyponatremia include the syndrome of inappropriate antidiuretic hormone (SIADH), glucocorticoid deficiency, hypothyroidism, and water intoxication. Although SIADH is not common in children, it may occur in patients with central nervous system disorders or lung disease and tumors. Certain medications can cause an increase in antidiuretic hormone (ADH) secretion and are reviewed in Chapter 6: Electrolytes, Other Minerals, and Trace Elements.

Dilutional hyponatremia may commonly occur in hospitalized children who receive relatively large amounts of free water (e.g., hypotonic IV solutions). This may even occur when medications are diluted in 5% dextrose in water, for example, and administered as 50- or 100-mL IV rider bags or piggyback riders. Neonates and young infants are more prone to this water overload (due to their lower glomerular filtration rate [GFR] and limited ability to excrete water), and, thus, should receive medications diluted in smaller volumes of IV fluid. Other causes of hyponatremia due to water intoxication in pediatric patients include administration of diluted infant formula, tap water enemas, infant swimming lessons, forced water intake (child abuse), and psychogenic polydipsia.[23] (See Minicase 1.)

Hypernatremia

In general for pediatric patients, *hypernatremia* is defined as a serum sodium concentration greater than 145 mEq/L. As in

MINICASE 1

A Case of Hyponatremia and Seizures

HUNTER N., A 3-DAY-OLD MALE, is currently in the neonatal ICU being treated with antibiotics for suspected sepsis. This morning Hunter. N. began having rhythmic clonic twitching of his lower extremities, fluttering of his eyelids, and repetitive chewing movements, consistent with seizure activity. Hunter N. was born at 39 weeks of gestation to a mother with prolonged rupture of membranes (>72 hours). On the day of his birth, Hunter N. was admitted to the neonatal ICU with an elevated temperature, tachycardia (HR 166), and low WBC count (3.2 × 10^3 cells/mm³). Blood and urine cultures were obtained and antibiotics were started to treat his possible sepsis. Culture results are still pending. Medications include ampicillin 85 mg IV in 25 mL D5W as IV rider q 8 hr (75 mg/kg/day) and gentamicin 8.5 mg IV in 25 mL D5W as IV rider q 12 hr (5 mg/kg/day).

Hunter N.'s vital signs include BP 76/46 mm Hg, HR 129 beats/min, RR 35 breaths/min, and temperature 98.8°F. Length is 49 cm (50th percentile for age), and weight is 3.4 kg (50th percentile for age). Laboratory data includes sodium 119 mEq/L, potassium 3.8 mEq/L, chloride 99 mEq/L, total CO_2 20 mEq/L, BUN 9 mg/dL, SCr 0.7 mg/dL, and glucose 87 mg/dL.

Question: What is the most likely cause of Hunter N.'s seizure activity and electrolyte imbalance? What other laboratory tests should be obtained to further assess his seizure disorder?

Discussion: Electrolyte imbalance is a common cause of neonatal seizures. As in adults, hyponatremia may cause seizure activity in neonates and occurs when the ratio of water to sodium is increased. The total body content of sodium in patients with hyponatremia may be low, normal, or high, and the volume status may be hypovolemic, euvolemic, or hypervolemic. There are many causes of hyponatremia, but the most

likely cause in Hunter N. is the extra D5W that he received with his antibiotics. Dilutional hyponatremia may occur in neonates and young infants when medications are administered in excess fluids, such as IV riders of 5% dextrose in water. These patients are more prone to water overload due to their lower GFR and their limited ability to excrete water. Medications for these patients should be diluted in smaller amounts of IV fluid, so that excess fluid is not administered. To better define Hunter N.'s sodium and volume status, his total fluid intake and output, type of IV fluids administered, changes in body weight, and other laboratory data need to be assessed. In addition, other causes of hyponatremia, such as meningitis and SIADH, should be ruled out. It should be noted that a low WBC count, as observed in Hunter N., often occurs in neonates with a serious bacterial infection (see section on White Blood Cell Count). Although the most likely cause of Hunter N.'s seizure activity is his low serum sodium, his serum calcium, phosphorous, and magnesium levels should also be assessed, as other electrolyte abnormalities can also cause seizure activity.

In hypervolemic hyponatremia, both sodium and water are increased in the body, but there is a greater increase in water than sodium. Hypervolemic hyponatremia is typically observed in patients with congestive heart failure (CHF), cirrhosis, nephrotic syndrome, and chronic renal failure. It may also occur in patients with hypoalbuminemia or in patients with capillary leak syndrome due to sepsis.[23] These conditions decrease the patient's effective blood volume, either due to poor cardiac function or third spacing of fluid. The compensatory mechanisms in the body sense this decrease in blood volume; ADH and aldosterone are secreted and cause retention of water and sodium in the kidneys. A decrease in serum sodium occurs because the intake of water in these patients is greater than their sodium intake and ADH decreases water excretion.

---

adults, hypernatremia occurs in pediatric patients when the ratio of sodium to water is increased. This may occur with low, normal, or high amounts of sodium in the body. Hypernatremia may occur with excessive sodium intake, excess water loss, or a combination of water and sodium loss when the water loss exceeds the sodium loss.[23]

Excessive sodium intake or sodium intoxication may occur due to improperly mixed infant formulas, excess sodium bicarbonate administration, IV hypertonic saline solutions, intentional salt poisoning (e.g., child abuse), and ingestion of sodium chloride or seawater.[23] Neonates, especially premature newborns, and young infants can develop hypernatremia from excessive sodium due to the decreased ability of immature kidneys to excrete a sodium load. This becomes a problem especially in the premature neonate when IV sodium bicarbonate is used to correct a metabolic acidosis.

Excess water loss resulting in hypernatremia may occur in pediatric patients due to diabetes insipidus, increased insensible water losses, or inadequate intake. Diabetes insipidus can be of central or nephrogenic origin and either type can be acquired or congenital. Also, certain drugs may cause diabetes insipidus (see Chapter 6: Electrolytes, Other Minerals, and Trace Elements).

Neonates may be predisposed to hypernatremia from increased insensible water losses, especially during the first few days of life. A normal physiologic contraction of the ECW occurs after birth, resulting in a net loss of water and sodium. In term infants, this may result in a weight loss of 5% to 10% during the first week of life. In premature newborns, the weight loss may be 10% to 20%. This water loss, plus the relatively large and variable insensible water loss in neonates, can complicate the assessment of fluid and sodium balance. More premature newborns may be at higher risk for hypernatremia, as they have a more pronounced contraction of ECW and higher insensible water loss.[27] The use of radiant warmers and phototherapy (used to treat hyperbilirubinemia) will further increase insensible water loss.

Inadequate water intake can also cause hypernatremia in pediatric patients. This may be due to the caregiver not administering enough fluids (e.g., child neglect or abuse, or ineffective breast-feeding). Ineffective breast-feeding may result in severe hypernatremic dehydration. Rarely, inadequate intake may be due to adipsia (absence of thirst).[23]

Hypernatremia, due to water losses greater than sodium losses, occurs in patients with water and sodium losses through the GI tract (e.g., diarrhea, emesis, nasogastric suctioning, and osmotic cathartics), skin (e.g., burns and excessive sweating), and kidneys (e.g., diabetes mellitus, chronic kidney disease, osmotic diuretics, and acute tubular necrosis [polyuric phase]). Hypernatremia is most likely to occur in infants or children with diarrhea who also have inadequate fluid intake due to anorexia, emesis, or lack of access to water.

It should be noted that due to the immaturity of the blood vessels in their central nervous system, premature neonates are especially vulnerable to the adverse effects of hypernatremia (e.g., intracranial hemorrhage). These patients are also at greater risk of adverse central nervous system effects if an elevated serum sodium is corrected too rapidly. Thus, maintaining a proper sodium balance in these patients is extremely important.

Potassium

Normal range[11,22] for premature neonates (at 48 hr of life):
  3.0–6.0 mEq/L or 3.0–6.0 mmol/L
  newborns: 3.7–5.9 mEq/L or 3.7–5.9 mmol/L
  infants: 4.1–5.3 mEq/L or 4.1–5.3 mmol/L
  children: 3.4–4.7 mEq/L or 3.4–4.7 mmol/L
  adults: 3.8–5.0 mEq/L or 3.8–5.0 mmol/L

Potassium is the major intracellular cation, and less then 1% of total body potassium is found in the plasma.[23] However, small changes in serum potassium can have large effects on cardiac, neuromuscular, and neural function. Thus, appropriate homeostasis of extracellular potassium is extremely important. Insulin, aldosterone, acid–base balance, catecholamines, and renal function all play important roles in the regulation of serum potassium. Serum potassium can be lowered quickly when potassium shifts intracellularly or more slowly via elimination by the kidneys.

The kidney is the primary organ that regulates potassium balance and elimination. Potassium undergoes glomerular filtration and almost all filtered potassium is then reabsorbed in the proximal tubule. Urinary excretion of potassium, therefore, is dependent on distal potassium secretion by the collecting tubules. Neonates and young infants, however, have a decreased ability to secrete potassium via the collecting tubules. Thus, the immature kidneys tend to retain potassium. This results in a positive potassium balance, which is required for growth (potassium is incorporated intracellularly into new tissues).[24,25] Potassium retention by the immature kidneys also results in higher serum potassium concentrations compared to the adult.[25]

Hypokalemia

Hypokalemia is defined as a serum potassium concentration <3.5 mEq/mL. As in adults, a low serum potassium may occur in pediatric patients due to an intracellular shift of potassium, decreased intake, or increased output (from renal or extrarenal losses). An intracellular shift of potassium may be seen with alkalosis, beta-adrenergic stimulation, or insulin treatment. Endogenous beta-adrenergic agonists (such as epinephrine released during stress) and exogenously administered beta-agonists (such as albuterol) stimulate the cellular uptake of potassium. Other causes of an intracellular shift of potassium

seen in pediatric patients include overdoses of theophylline, barium intoxication, and glue sniffing (toluene intoxication). A falsely low potassium concentration can be reported in a patient with a very elevated white blood cell (WBC) count (e.g., a patient with leukemia) if the plasma sample is inappropriately stored at room temperature. This allows the WBCs to uptake potassium from the plasma resulting in a falsely low measurement.[23]

Most cases of hypokalemia in children are related to extrarenal losses of potassium due to gastroenteritis and diarrhea.[23] Hypokalemia due to diarrhea is usually associated with a metabolic acidosis, since bicarbonate is also lost in the stool. Adolescent patients with eating disorders may be hypokalemic due to inadequate intake of potassium, for example, in patients with anorexia nervosa. Adolescents with bulimia or laxative abuse may also have significant extrarenal losses of potassium.

Many causes of hypokalemia due to renal potassium loss exist. Medications commonly used in the pediatric population that are associated with hypokalemia due to renal potassium loss include loop and thiazide diuretics, corticosteroids, amphotericin B, and cisplatin (see Chapter 6: Electrolytes, Other Minerals, and Trace Elements). Cushing syndrome, hyperaldosteronism, and licorice ingestion may also cause hypokalemia via this mechanism.

In the pediatric population, other causes of increased renal potassium loss, such as hereditary diseases, must be considered. Remember that many hereditary diseases are first diagnosed during infancy and childhood. Renal tubular acidosis (both distal and proximal types) may present with hypokalemia and metabolic acidosis. Patients with cystic fibrosis have greater losses of chloride in sweat. This may lead to metabolic alkalosis, low urine chloride, and hypokalemia. Certain forms of congenital adrenal hyperplasia may also lead to increased renal potassium excretion and hypokalemia. Other inherited renal diseases that are due to defects in renal tubular transporters, such as Bartter syndrome, may result in metabolic alkalosis, hypokalemia, and high urine chloride. Thus, unlike the adult population, hereditary diseases need to be considered when certain electrolyte abnormalities are not explained by common causes.

Hyperkalemia

In infants, children, and adults, *hyperkalemia* is defined as a serum potassium greater than 5.0 mEq/L. Since a normal serum potassium is slightly higher in neonates and preterm infants, hyperkalemia is defined as a serum potassium greater than 6.0 mEq/L in these patients. Hyperkalemia is one of the most alarming electrolyte imbalances because it has the potential to cause lethal cardiac arrhythmias.

As in adults, hyperkalemia in pediatric patients may be due to increased intake, an extracellular shift of potassium, or decreased renal excretion. Factitious hyperkalemia is very common in pediatric patients, due to the difficulty in obtaining blood samples. Hemolysis often occurs during blood sampling and potassium is released from red blood cells (RBCs) in sufficient amounts to cause falsely elevated test results. This may especially happen with improperly performed heelsticks (see section on Pediatric Blood Sampling). Potassium may also be released locally from muscles after prolonged tourniquet application or from fist clenching, which may also result in false elevations of measured potassium. A falsely elevated serum potassium can also be observed in patients with leukemia or extremely elevated WBC counts (usually >200,000/mm³) due to the release of potassium from WBCs. Prompt analysis with measurement of a plasma sample usually avoids this problem.[23]

Hyperkalemia may occur due to extracellular shifts of potassium. During a metabolic acidosis, hydrogen ions move into the cells (down a concentration gradient), and in exchange, potassium ions move out of the cells into the extracellular (intravascular) space. This shift leads to a significant increase in serum potassium.

In older patients with fully developed (normal) renal function, hyperkalemia rarely results from increased intake alone. However, this may occur in patients receiving large amounts of oral or IV potassium or in patients receiving rapid or frequent blood transfusions (due to the potassium content of blood).[23] In patients with immature renal function or in those with renal failure, increased intake of potassium can also lead to hyperkalemia due to decreased potassium excretion.

Decreased renal excretion of potassium is the most common cause of hyperkalemia. Decreased potassium excretion occurs in patients with immature renal function, renal failure, primary adrenal disease, hyporeninemic hypoaldosteronism, renal tubular disease, and with certain medications.[23] Hyperkalemia is the most common life-threatening electrolyte imbalance seen in neonates. Due to the decreased ability of immature kidneys to excrete potassium, neonates, particularly premature neonates, may be predisposed to hyperkalemia. These patients also cannot tolerate receiving extra potassium. Hyperkalemia can be seen in premature infants, during the first 3 days of life, even when exogenous potassium is not given and when renal dysfunction is absent.[27] A rapid elevation in serum potassium is seen within the first day of life in more immature newborns. This hyperkalemia, which can be life-threatening, may be due to a shift of potassium from the intracellular space to the extracellular (intravascular) space, immaturity of the distal renal tubules, and a relative hypoaldosteronism.[28]

Acute or chronic renal failure in pediatric patients will decrease potassium excretion and may result in hyperkalemia. Several inherited disorders may also cause decreased potassium excretion and hyperkalemia in pediatric patients including certain types of congenital adrenal hyperplasia (e.g., 21-hydroxylase deficiency), aldosterone synthase deficiency, sickle cell disease, and pseudohypoaldosteronism (types I and II).[23] Medications used in pediatric patients that may also cause hyperkalemia include angiotensin-converting enzyme inhibitors, beta$_2$-adrenergic antagonists, potassium-sparing diuretics, nonsteroidal anti-inflammatory agents, heparin, trimethoprim, and cyclosporine.

Serum Bicarbonate (Total Carbon Dioxide)

Normal range[22,25] *for*
preterm infants: 16–20 mEq/L or 16–20 mmol/L

full-term infants: 19–21 mEq/L or 19–21 mmol/L
infants–children 2 yr of age: 18–28 mEq/L or 18–28 mmol/L
children >2 yr and adults: 21–28 mEq/L or 21–28 mmol/L

The *total carbon dioxide concentration* actually represents *serum bicarbonate*, the basic form of the carbonic acid–bicarbonate buffer system (i.e., a low serum bicarbonate may indicate an acidosis). In addition to the buffer systems, the kidneys also play an important role in acid–base balance. The proximal tubule reabsorbs 85% to 90% of filtered bicarbonate. The distal tubule is responsible for the net secretion of hydrogen ions and urinary acidification.[29] Compared to adults, neonates have a decreased capacity to reabsorb bicarbonate in the proximal tubule, and, therefore, a decreased renal threshold for bicarbonate (the renal threshold is the serum concentration at which bicarbonate appears in the urine). The mean renal threshold for bicarbonate in adults is 24–26 mEq/L but only 18 mEq/L in the premature infant and 21 mEq/L in the term neonate. The renal threshold for bicarbonate increases during the first year of life and reaches adult values by about 1 year of age. Neonates also have decreased function of the distal tubules to secrete hydrogen ions and to acidify urine. The ability to acidify urine increases to adult values by about 1–2 months of age.[25,29] The neonate's decreased renal capacity to reabsorb bicarbonate and excrete hydrogen ions results in lower normal values for serum bicarbonate and blood pH. In addition, the neonate is less able to handle an acid load or to compensate for acid–base abnormalities.

It should be noted that for multiple reasons, the full-term newborn is in a state of metabolic acidosis immediately after birth (arterial pH 7.11–7.36). The blood pH increases to more normal values within 24 hours, mostly due to increased excretion of carbon dioxide via the lungs.[25]

Calcium

Total serum calcium—normal range[12] *for newborns:*
3–24 hr old: 9.0–10.6 mg/dL or 2.3–2.65 mmol/L
24–48 hr old: 7.0–12.0 mg/dL or 1.75–3.0 mmol/L
4–7 days old: 9.0–10.9 mg/dL or 2.25–2.73 mmol/L
children: 8.8–10.8 mg/dL or 2.2–2.7 mmol/L
adolescents and adults: 8.4–10.2 mg/dL or 2.1–2.55 mmol/L

Ionized calcium—normal range for newborns:
3–24 hr old: 4.3–5.1 mg/dL or 1.07–1.27 mmol/L
24–48 hr old: 4.0–4.7 mg/dL or 1.00–1.17 mmol/L
infants, children, adolescents, and adults:
  4.5–4.92 mg/dL or 1.12–1.23 mmol/L

Calcium plays an integral role in many physiologic functions including muscle contraction, neuromuscular transmission, blood coagulation, bone metabolism, and regulation of endocrine functions. The great majority of calcium in the body (99%) is found in the bone, primarily as hydroxyapatite. Due to the growth that occurs during infancy and childhood, bone mass increases faster than body weight.[30] This increase in bone mass requires a significant increase in total body calcium. The increased calcium requirement is reflected in the higher recommended daily allowances (per kg body weight) in pediatric patients compared to adults.

Calcium regulation in the body has two main goals.[30] First, serum calcium must be tightly regulated to permit the normal physiologic functions in which calcium plays a role. Second, calcium intake must be adequate to permit appropriate bone mineralization and skeletal growth. It is important to remember that bone mineralization may be sacrificed (i.e., calcium may be released from the bone) in order to allow maintenance of a normal serum calcium concentration.

As in adults, serum calcium in pediatric patients is regulated by a complex hormonal system that involves vitamin D, serum phosphate, parathyroid hormone (PTH), and calcitonin. Briefly, calcium is absorbed in the GI tract, primarily via the duodenum and jejunum.[30] Although some passive calcium absorption occurs when dietary intake is high, most GI absorption of calcium occurs via active transport that is stimulated by 1,25-dihydroxyvitamin D. This occurs especially when dietary intake is low. Calcium excretion is controlled by the kidneys and influenced by multiple hormonal mediators (e.g., PTH, 1,25-dihydroxyvitamin D, and calcitonin). In the mature kidneys, approximately 99% of filtered calcium is reabsorbed by the tubules with the majority (>50%) absorbed by the proximal tubules. Calcium is also absorbed in the loop of Henle, distal tubule, and collecting ducts.

During the first week of life, urinary calcium excretion is inversely related to GA (i.e., more premature infants will have a greater urinary calcium excretion).[25] Compared to adults, urinary calcium excretion is higher in neonates and preterm infants. The urinary calcium-to-creatinine ratio is 0.11 in adults but may be greater than 2 in premature neonates and ranges from 0.05–1.2 in full-term neonates during the first week of life. This high rate of calcium excretion may be related to the immaturity of the renal tubules and may contribute (along with other factors) to neonatal hypocalcemia. In addition, certain medications that are commonly administered to neonates and premature infants, such as furosemide, dexamethasone, and methylxanthines, further increase urinary calcium excretion. These medications may also increase the risk for hypocalcemia as well as nephrocalcinosis and nephrolithiasis.[25]

Measurement of Calcium

Total serum calcium measures all three forms of extracellular calcium: complex bound, protein bound, and ionized. However, ionized calcium is the physiologically active form. Usually a parallel relationship exists between the ionized and total serum calcium concentrations. However, in patients with alterations in acid–base balance or serum proteins, the ionized serum calcium and total serum calcium are affected, respectively, and measurements of total serum calcium may no longer reflect the ionized serum concentration. Neonates have lower serum concentrations of protein (including albumin) and may be acidotic. This results in a lower total serum calcium concentration for a given ionized plasma concentration.[27] Although equations exist to adjust total serum calcium measurements for low concentrations of serum albumin, these equations have limitations and may not be precise. Therefore, ionized calcium should be measured in neonates (if micro-techniques are available) and other pediatric patients with hypoalbuminemia or acid–base disorders.

Hypocalcemia

As in adults, *hypocalcemia* may occur in pediatric patients due to a variety of causes including inadequate calcium intake, hypoparathyroidism, vitamin D deficiency, renal failure, redistribution of plasma calcium (e.g., hyperphosphatemia and citrated blood transfusions), and hypomagnesemia. Hypocalcemia may also occur due to lack of organ response to PTH (e.g., pseudohypoparathyroidism) and in the neonate due to other specific causes.

In the pediatric population, hypocalcemia most commonly occurs in neonates. *Early neonatal hypocalcemia* occurs during the first 72 hours of life and may be due to several factors. During fetal development, a transplacental active transport process maintains a higher calcium concentration in the fetus compared to the mother. After birth, this transplacental process suddenly stops. Serum calcium concentrations then decrease, even in healthy full-term newborns, reaching a nadir at 24 hours.[30] The high serum calcium concentrations in utero may also suppress the fetus' parathyroid gland. Thus, early neonatal hypocalcemia may also be due to a relative hypoparathyroidism in the newborn. In addition, newborns may have a decreased response to PTH.

Early neonatal hypocalcemia is more likely to occur in premature and low birth weight newborns. It also occurs more commonly in infants of diabetic mothers, infants with intrauterine growth retardation, and in newborns that have undergone prolonged difficult deliveries. Inadequate calcium intake in critically ill newborns also contributes to hypocalcemia.

Late neonatal hypocalcemia, which usually presents during the first 5–10 days of life, is caused by a high phosphate intake. It is much less common than early neonatal hypocalcemia, especially since the phosphorus content of infant formulas was decreased. It may, however, still occur if neonates are inappropriately given whole cow's milk. Cow's milk has a high phosphate load, which can cause hyperphosphatemia and secondary hypocalcemia in the neonate.

Hypocalcemia may also occur in neonates born to mothers with hypercalcemia. The maternal hypercalcemia is usually due to hyperparathyroidism. In utero suppression of the fetal parathyroid gland can lead to hypoparathyroidism and hypocalcemia in the neonate.

Hypocalcemia due to inadequate dietary calcium intake rarely occurs in the United States, but can occur if infant formula or breast milk is replaced with liquids that contain lower amounts of calcium. Hypocalcemia may be iatrogenically induced if inadequate amounts of calcium are administered in hyperalimentation solutions. Adequate amounts of calcium and phosphorus may be difficult to deliver to preterm neonates due to their high daily requirements and limitations of calcium and phosphorus solubility in hyperalimentation solutions. Certain pediatric malabsorption disorders, such as celiac disease, may also cause inadequate absorption of calcium and vitamin D.

Hypoparathyroidism can be caused by many genetically inherited disorders, such as the DiGeorge syndrome, X-linked hypoparathyroidism, or PTH gene mutations.[30] These and other syndromes must be considered when pediatric patients present with hypoparathyroidism.

In pediatric patients with vitamin D deficiency, hypocalcemia occurs primarily due to decreased intestinal absorption of calcium. The lower amounts of calcium in the blood stimulate the release of PTH from the parathyroid gland. Parathyroid hormone then prevents significant hypocalcemia via several different mechanisms. It causes bone to release calcium, increases urinary calcium reabsorption, and increases the activity of 1-alpha-hydroxylase in the kidneys (the enzyme that converts 25-hydroxyvitamin D into 1, 25-dihydroxyvitamin D, the active form of vitamin D). Hypocalcemia only develops after these compensatory mechanisms fail. In fact, most children with vitamin D deficiency present with rickets before they develop hypocalcemia.[30] In addition to elevated PTH concentrations, children with vitamin D deficiency will have an elevated serum alkaline phosphatase concentration (due to increased osteoclast activity) and a low serum phosphorus (secondary to decreased intestinal absorption and decreased reabsorption in the kidneys), all due to the effects of PTH.

Vitamin D deficiency may be due to several factors including inadequate intake, lack of exposure to sunlight, malabsorption, or increased metabolism of vitamin D (e.g., from medications such as phenobarbital and phenytoin). Generally, patients may have more than one of these factors. For example, institutionalized children (who are not exposed to sunlight) receiving chronic anticonvulsant therapy may be at a greater risk for developing vitamin D deficiency and rickets. Vitamin D deficiency may also occur with liver disease (failure to form 25-hydroxyvitamin D in the liver) and with renal failure (failure to form the active moiety, 1,25-dihydroxyvitamin D, due to a loss of activity of 1-alpha-hydroxylase in the kidneys).

Genetic disorders, such as vitamin D-dependent rickets, may also cause hypocalcemia. The absence of the enzyme, 1-alpha-hydroxylase, in the kidneys occurs in children with vitamin D-dependent rickets type 1. Therefore, these children cannot convert 25-hydroxyvitamin D to its active form. Children with vitamin D-dependent rickets type 2 have a defective vitamin D receptor, which prevents the normal response to 1,25- dihydroxyvitamin D.[30] (See Minicase 2.)

Hypocalcemia also occurs when patients receive citrated blood transfusions or exchange transfusions (citrate is used to anticoagulate blood). Citrate forms a complex with calcium and decreases the ionized calcium concentration. This may result in symptoms of hypocalcemia. Pediatric patients at highest risk include those receiving multiple blood transfusions or exchange transfusions, such as neonates treated for hyperbilirubinemia and older children treated for sickle cell crisis. It should be noted that the total serum calcium concentration in these patients can be normal or even elevated, because the calcium-citrate complex is included in the measurement.[30]

Hypercalcemia

Hypercalcemia is an uncommon pediatric electrolyte disorder. As in adults, it may be caused by excess PTH, excess vitamin D, excess calcium intake, excess renal reabsorption of calcium, increased calcium released from the bone, and miscellaneous factors, such as hypophosphatemia or adrenal insufficiency.[30] Causes of hypercalcemia that are of particular interest in pediatric patients include neonatal hyperparathyroidism, hypervitaminosis D, excessive calcium intake, malignancy associated hypercalcemia, and immobilization. Also, several genetic syndromes and disorders may cause hypercalcemia.

Neonatal hyperparathyroidism, an autosomal recessive disorder, can be severe and life-threatening.[30] Typically, these patients have defective calcium sensing receptors in the parathyroid gland. Normally, high serum calcium concentrations would be sensed by the parathyroid gland, and PTH levels would then decrease. In these patients, however, the parathyroid gland cannot sense the high serum calcium concentrations, and PTH continues to be released. This further increases serum calcium concentrations. Transient secondary neonatal hyperparathyroidism occurs in neonates born to mothers with hypocalcemia. Maternal hypocalcemia leads to hypocalcemia in the fetus with secondary hyperparathyroidism. These neonates may be born with skeletal demineralization and bone fractures. Hypercalcemia in these patients usually takes days to weeks to resolve.

Excessive intake of vitamin D or calcium may also cause hypercalcemia. Typically, this may occur in children who are being treated with vitamin D and calcium with excessive doses. Excess calcium in hyperalimentation solutions commonly results in hypercalcemia.

Compared to adults, hypercalcemia from immobilization occurs more frequently in children, especially adolescents.[30] This is due to a higher rate of bone remodeling in these patients. Immobilization of children and adolescents may be required due to specific injuries such as leg fractures, spinal cord paralysis, burns, or other severe medical conditions. In children with leg fractures requiring traction, hypercalcemia usually occurs within 1–3 weeks. Immobilization may also result in isolated hypercalciuria, which may result in nephrocalcinosis, kidney stones, or renal insufficiency.

Phosphorus

Normal range[23] *for newborns:*
0–5 days old: 4.8–8.2 mg/dL or 1.55–2.65 mmol/L
1–3 yr: 3.8–6.5 mg/dL or 1.25–2.10 mmol/L
4–11 yr: 3.7–5.6 mg/dL or 1.20–1.80 mmol/L
12–15 yr: 2.9–5.4 mg/dL or 0.95–1.75 mmol/L
16–19 yr: 2.7–4.7 mg/dL or 0.90–1.50 mmol/L
adults: 2.3–4.7 mg/dL or 0.74–1.52 mmol/L

Phosphorus is the primary intracellular anion and plays an integral role in cellular energy and intracellular metabolism. It is also a component of phospholipid membranes and other cell structures. The great majority of phosphorus in the body (85%) is found in the bone, while <1% of phosphorus is found in the plasma. Like calcium, phosphorus is essential for bone mineralization and skeletal growth. During infancy and childhood,

MINICASE 2

Rickets in a Child

RACHEL C., AN 8-YEAR-OLD FEMALE, was admitted to the emergency room from a local pediatric long-term care facility with c/o pain, tenderness, and decreased movement to her right leg. Rachel C. sustained a fall at the long-term care facility when she was being moved from her bed to her wheel chair. Born at term, Rachel C. suffered a traumatic birth with severe perinatal asphyxia. She subsequently developed seizures that were controlled by the combined anticonvulsant therapy of phenobarbital and phenytoin. As a result of her asphyxia at birth, Rachel C. developed spastic cerebral palsy and severe neurodevelopmental delay. She was transferred to the long-term care facility at 6 months of age and has remained on phenobarbital and phenytoin since that time. Two years ago, Rachel C. was diagnosed with gastroesophageal reflux disease (GERD), which has been controlled with antacids. Medications include phenobarbital elixir 40 mg (10 mL) PO BID; phenytoin suspension 50 mg (2 mL) PO TID; and Alternagel® 5 mL PO QID.

Rachel C.'s vital signs include BP 105/69 mm Hg; HR 90/min; RR 22/min; and temperature 98.6°F. Her height is 124 cm (25th percentile for age) and weight is 20 kg (<5th percentile for age). Rachel C.'s physical exam of her chest is significant for a pigeon breast deformity and slightly palpable enlargement of costochondral junctions. She has redness in her right leg, 10 cm below the knee, and pain on movement. The preliminary x-ray findings reveal a fracture of her right tibia with osteomalacia and bone changes consistent with rickets.

Significant laboratory data includes calcium 7.9 mg/dL (normal for children: 8.8–10.8 mg/dL); ionized calcium: 4.0 mg/dL (normal for infants–adults: 4.5–4.92 mg/dL); phosphorus: 2.2 mg/dL (normal for 4–11 years: 3.7–5.6 mg/dL); magnesium: 1.8 mg/dL (normal for 2–14 years: 1.5– 2.3 mg/dL); albumin 2.8 g/dL (normal for children 7–19 years: 3.7–5.6 g/dL); ALT: 58 units/L (normal 10–40 units/L); AST: 68 units/L (normal for children 7–9 years: 15–40 units/L); alkaline phosphatase: 682 units/L (normal for children 2–10 years: 100–320 units/L).

Question: What evidence exists that Rachel C. has rickets? How did her medications affect her serum phosphorus, calcium, and liver enzymes, and how would you modify her drug therapy?

Discussion: Rickets is diagnosed by both radiologic and chemical findings. The preliminary x-ray findings and the physical findings of the pigeon breast deformity (i.e., the sternum and adjacent cartilage appear to be projected forward) and the palpable enlargement of costochondral junctions (rachitic rosary sign) are compatible with the diagnosis of rickets. Serum calcium may be low or normal in patients with rickets, depending on the etiology. The primary causes of rickets in the United States are vitamin D deficiency (with secondary hyperparathyroidism), primary phosphate deficiency, and end-organ resistance to 1,25-dihydroxyvitamin D. In patients with vitamin D deficiency, serum calcium concentrations can be normal or low, phosphorus concentrations are

usually low, and alkaline phosphatase activity is elevated. In patients with primary phosphate deficiency, serum calcium is normal, serum phosphorus is low, and alkaline phosphatase is elevated. In patients with end-organ resistance to 1,25-dihydroxyvitamin D, serum calcium is low, serum phosphorus may be low or normal, and serum alkaline phosphatase is elevated.

In Rachel C., ionized calcium and serum phosphorus are both low and serum alkaline phosphatase is high, all of which are consistent with a diagnosis of rickets. Serum magnesium is normal for age; ALT and AST are slightly elevated. The serum magnesium was obtained since hypomagnesemia may also cause hypocalcemia. She also has hypoalbuminemia. A total serum calcium measures all three forms of extracellular calcium: complex bound, protein bound, and ionized. In patients with low albumin, the concentration of ionized calcium will be increased for a given total serum calcium concentration. Equations can be used to "correct" total serum calcium measurements for low concentrations of serum albumin, but these equations have limitations and may not be precise. Thus, in patients with low albumin (like Rachel C.), an ionized serum calcium should be obtained.

Rachel C.'s medications affected her laboratory tests. She is receiving an aluminum-containing antacid, which binds phosphorus in the GI tract. This resulted in decreased absorption of phosphorus and contributed to Rachel C.'s low serum phosphorus. Enzyme-inducing anticonvulsants, such as phenobarbital and phenytoin, will increase the metabolism of vitamin D and may result in a deficiency of vitamin D with resultant anticonvulsant-induced osteomalacia and rickets. Both the aluminum-containing antacid and the anticonvulsants contributed to Rachel C. developing rickets, and thus, to the elevated serum alkaline phosphatase. In addition, due to her other medical conditions, she is nonambulatory and resides at a long-term care facility. Thus, she may have a lack of exposure to sunlight and, therefore, a lack of vitamin D. This lack of vitamin D would also contribute to the development of rickets.

For treatment of her rickets, Rachel C. should be started on oral supplements of calcium, phosphorous, and vitamin D. However, modifications in Rachel C.'s preadmission medications should be made. The aluminum-containing antacid (Alternagel®) should be discontinued and replaced with a calcium-containing antacid (e.g., calcium carbonate). The amount of calcium in this new antacid should then be subtracted from any calcium supplement that would be started in the hospital, so that the total daily dose of calcium stays the same. Alternatively, the total dose of calcium supplement can be given as calcium carbonate. Discontinuing the aluminum-containing antacid will result in a greater amount of phosphorus absorbed enterally. This will then require a decrease in the oral supplement of phosphate (depending on serum phosphorus concentrations). Once Rachel C. is stable, her neurologist should be consulted to see if other anticonvulsants that have less of an enzyme-inducing effect could be used to treat her seizures.

a positive phosphorus balance is required for proper growth to allow adequate amounts of phosphorus to be incorporated into bone and new cells. The higher phosphorus requirement that is needed to facilitate growth may help explain the higher serum concentrations seen in the pediatric population compared to adults.

The kidney is the primary organ that regulates phosphorus balance. Approximately 90% of plasma phosphate is filtered by the glomerulus with the majority being actively reabsorbed at the proximal tubule. Some reabsorption also occurs more distally, but phosphate is not significantly secreted along the nephron.[23] Unlike other active transport systems, phosphate reabsorption, both proximal and distal, is greater in the neonatal kidney compared to adults.[25,29] Thus, the neonatal kidney tends to retain phosphate, perhaps as a physiologic adaptation to the high demands for phosphate that are required for growth. Neonatal renal phosphate reabsorption may be regulated by growth hormone.[29]

Hypophosphatemia

As in adults, *hypophosphatemia* may occur in pediatric patients due to several causes including increased renal excretion, decreased phosphate or vitamin D intake, or intracellular shifting. Causes of excessive renal phosphorus excretion in pediatric patients include hyperparathyroidism, metabolic acidosis, diuretics, glucocorticoids, glycosuria, IV fluids and volume expansion, kidney transplantation, and inherited disorders such as hypophosphatemic rickets.

Inadequate dietary phosphate intake is an unusual cause of hypophosphatemia in adults. However, infants are more predisposed to nutritional hypophosphatemia due to their higher phosphorus requirements.[23] The phosphorus requirements of premature infants are even higher due to their rapid skeletal growth. If premature infants are fed regular infant formula (instead of premature infant formula that contains additional calcium and phosphorus), phosphorus deficiency and rickets may occur. Phosphorous deficiency and rickets can also occur in pediatric patients who receive aluminum hydroxide containing antacids, which bind dietary and secreted phosphorous and prevent its absorption from the GI tract. Inadequate vitamin D intake and genetic causes of vitamin D deficiency (e.g., vitamin D-dependent rickets type 1) can also result in hypophosphatemia in pediatric patients.

Hypophosphatemia due to intracellular shifting of phosphorus occurs with processes that stimulate intracellular phosphorus utilization. For example, high serum levels of glucose will stimulate insulin. Insulin then enables glucose and phosphorus to move into the cell, where phosphorus is used during glycolysis. Intracellular shifting of phosphorus also occurs during anabolism, for example, in patients receiving hyperalimentation and during refeeding in those with protein-calorie malnutrition (e.g., severe anorexia nervosa). The high anabolic (growth) rate in infants (especially premature infants) and children make them more susceptible to hypophosphatemia when adequate amounts of phosphate are not supplied in the hyperalimentation solution. Hypophosphatemia, due to refeeding malnourished children, usually occurs within 5 days of refeeding. It may be prevented by a more gradual increase in nutrition and with phosphate supplementation.[23]

Hyperphosphatemia

Hyperphosphatemia in pediatric patients may be caused by decreased excretion of phosphorus, increased intake of phosphate or vitamin D, or a shift of intracellular phosphate to extracellular fluid. The most common cause of hyperphosphatemia in the pediatric population is decreased excretion of phosphorus due to renal failure. Excessive phosphorus intake in pediatric patients (especially in those with renal dysfunction or in neonates whose renal function is normally decreased due to immaturity) is a common cause of hyperphosphatemia.[23] Hyperphosphatemia may also occur if neonates are inappropriately given whole cow's milk. As previously mentioned, cow's milk contains a high phosphate load, which can cause hyperphosphatemia and secondary hypocalcemia in the neonate. Administration of sodium phosphorus laxatives or enemas to infants and children may also result in excessive phosphate intake. In addition, the pediatric dosing of phosphate supplements may be confusing to some due to the multiple salts available and multiple units of measure. This may result in unintentional overdoses with resultant hyperphosphatemia.

Magnesium

Normal range[12] for newborns:
0–6 days old: 1.2–2.6 mg/dL or 0.49–1.07 mmol/L
7 days–2 yr: 1.6–2.6 mg/dL or 0.66–1.07 mmol/L
2–14 yr: 1.5–2.3 mg/dL or 0.62–0.95 mmol/L

Magnesium plays an important role in neuromuscular function and is a required cofactor for many enzymatic systems in the body. Approximately 50% of magnesium is located in bone with one-third being slowly exchangeable with extracellular fluid. About 45% of magnesium is found in the intracellular fluid with only 5% in extracellular fluid. The kidney is the primary organ responsible for magnesium excretion. Approximately 95% to 97% of filtered magnesium is reabsorbed; 15% in the proximal tubule, 70% in the thick ascending limb of Henle, and 5% to 10% in the distal tubule.[23] In the neonate, reabsorption of magnesium may be increased in the proximal tubule. Thus, the immature neonatal kidney tends to retain magnesium compared to adults.[25] This results in slightly higher normal values for serum magnesium in neonates and infants compared to older children and adults. In fact, serum magnesium concentrations in the newborn have been shown to be inversely related to GA at birth and postmenstrual age (PMA). In other words, more immature neonates will have slightly higher serum magnesium concentrations.[31,32]

Hypomagnesemia

Hypomagnesemia occurs in pediatric patients due to excessive renal or GI losses, decreased GI absorption, decreased intake, and specific neonatal causes.[23] Hypomagnesemia may occur in neonates due to several maternal causes. Maternal diuretic use, laxative overuse or abuse, diabetes, or decreased intake due to vomiting during pregnancy may cause maternal hypomagnesemia and lead to hypomagnesemia in the newborn.[33] Hypomagnesemia also commonly occurs in neonates with intrauterine growth retardation (due to deficient placental transfer of magnesium) and in neonates who receive exchange transfusions with citrated blood.

Excessive renal losses of magnesium may be due to a variety of reasons. Of particular pediatric concern is the use of medications (e.g., diuretics, amphotericin, and cisplatin) that may cause magnesium wasting. Hypomagnesemia may also occur due to rare hereditary renal magnesium-losing syndromes, such as Bartter syndrome and autosomal recessive renal magnesium–wasting syndrome.

Excessive GI losses of magnesium may occur in pediatric patients with diarrhea or large losses of gastric contents (e.g., emesis or nasogastric suction). Decreased GI absorption of magnesium may occur in patients with short gut syndrome. These patients have had a portion of their small bowel removed, which results in poor intestinal absorption. Other important pediatric GI diseases that may result in hypomagnesemia include cystic fibrosis, inflammatory bowel disease, and celiac disease.[23]

Poor magnesium intake may also result in hypomagnesemia. Although this rarely occurs in children fed orally, it may occur in hospitalized children receiving inadequate amounts of magnesium in IV fluids or hyperalimentation. Hypomagnesemia can also occur during the refeeding of children with protein-calorie malnutrition (e.g., severe anorexia nervosa). These patients have low magnesium reserves but a high requirement of magnesium during cellular growth during refeeding.[23]

Hypermagnesemia

As in adults, the most common cause of *hypermagnesemia* in pediatric patients is renal dysfunction. However, in neonates, the most common cause is the IV infusion of magnesium sulfate in the mother for the treatment of preeclampsia or eclampsia.[23,33] The high levels of magnesium in the mother are delivered transplacentally to the fetus. Neonates and young infants are also more prone to hypermagnesemia, due to their immature renal function. Thus, these patients cannot easily tolerate a magnesium load. Other common pediatric causes of hypermagnesemia include excessive intake due to magnesium-containing antacids, laxatives, or enemas.

AGE-RELATED DIFFERENCES IN KIDNEY FUNCTION TESTS

Serum Creatinine

Jaffe Method:
Normal range[34] *for*
newborns: 0.3–1.0 mg/dL or 27–88 μmol/L
infants: 0.2–0.4 mg/dL or 18–35 μmol/L
children: 0.3–0.7 mg/dL or 27–62 μmol/L
adolescents: 0.5–1.0 mg/dL or 44–88 μmol/L
adult males: 0.6–1.2 mg/dL or 53–106 μmol/L
adult females: 0.5–1.1 mg/dL or 44–97 μmol/L

Isotope Dilution Mass Spectrometry (IDMS)-Traceable Enzymatic Method:
Normal range[12] *for*
Newborns – 4 yr: 0.03-0.50 mg/dL or 2.65-44.2 μmol/L
4–7 yr: 0.03-0.59 mg/dL or 2.65-52.2 μmol/L
7–10 yr: 0.22-0.59 mg/dL or 19.4-52.2 μmol/L
10–14 yr: 0.31-0.88 mg/dL or 27.4-77.8 μmol/L
>14 yr: 0.50-1.06 mg/dL or 44.2-93.7 μmol/L

Serum creatinine (SCr) is a useful indicator of renal function and can be used to estimate GFR. Creatinine is generated from the metabolism of creatine and creatine phosphate, a high-energy biochemical important in muscle activity. Creatinine is produced in muscles, released into the extracellular fluid, and excreted by the kidneys. Excretion of creatinine is primarily via glomerular filtration, but a smaller amount undergoes tubular secretion. The amount of creatinine that is secreted by the tubules increases in patients as GFR decreases. Thus, creatinine clearance (CrCl) will overestimate the actual GFR in patients with renal insufficiency.[35]

In pediatric patients, three major factors influence the SCr concentration: the patient's muscle mass per unit of body size, their GFR, and (in newborns) the exogenous (maternal) creatinine load.[36] At birth, the newborn's SCr reflects the maternal SCr. Since SCr crosses the placenta, if a pregnant woman has an elevated SCr, then the concentration of creatinine in the fetus will also be elevated. In fact, the plasma creatinine concentration of umbilical cord blood is almost equal to the creatinine concentration in the mother.[27] In full-term newborns, SCr may increase slightly, shortly after birth, due to the contraction of the ECW compartment.[36] Serum creatinine then decreases over the first few days of life and usually reaches 0.4 mg/dL (Jaffe method) by about 10 days of age.[25,36] The apparent half-life of this postnatal decrease in SCr is about 2.1 days in normal full-term infants and is due to the ongoing maturation of the kidneys and progressive increase in GFR. Serum creatinine is higher at birth in premature newborns compared to full-term newborns, and the postnatal decrease in SCr may occur more slowly. This is due to the preterm newborn's more immature kidneys and lower GFR.[27,37]

Compared to adults, pediatric patients have a lower muscle mass per unit of body size. Since the production of creatinine is dependent on muscle mass, this results in significantly lower normal values for SCr for neonates, infants, and children. The percentage of muscle mass differs with various pediatric age groups and increases with age from birth through young adulthood.[36] This increase in muscle mass accounts for the increase in the normal values for SCr with increasing age (see normal values for SCr above).

Creatinine excretion is dependent on GFR and, as in adults, SCr will become elevated in pediatric patients with renal dysfunction. For example, an infant with a SCr as measured by the Jaffe method of 0.8 mg/dL (twice the normal value for age) will have approximately a 50% decrease in GFR. Using the age-appropriate normal values to interpret SCr is essential. In the above example, a SCr of 0.8 mg/dL (which would be considered normal in an adult) denotes significant renal dysfunction in younger patients. Correct interpretation of SCr values is extremely important because the doses of fluids, many electrolytes, and medications that are renally eliminated will need to be adjusted. Misinterpretation of SCr (e.g., not recognizing renal dysfunction) can result in serious and potentially fatal fluid and electrolyte imbalances and overdosing of medications.

Reliable and accurate measurement of SCr is clinically important in order to properly assess renal function. Historically, SCr was measured by the alkaline picrate-based method, also known as the *Jaffe method*. However, substances that interfere with the measurement of creatinine by this method (i.e., noncreatinine chromogens such as uric acid, glucose, fructose, and acetone) can cause an overestimation of SCr and, thus, an underestimation of kidney function. In addition, certain medications and endogenous substances (e.g., bilirubin, lipemia, and hemolysis) may interfere with the determination of SCr by this method.[6,11] This interference may especially be a problem in the neonatal population, since neonates often have hyperbilirubinemia or lipemia, and blood sampling in neonates often results in hemolysis.

Inaccuracies of the Jaffe method and other methodologies, have lead the National Kidney Disease Education Program to recommend a recalibration and standardization of SCr measurements.[38] This has resulted in implementation of improved methods of SCr determinations, such as an enzymatic assay with an IDMS-traceable international standard. It is important to know what methodology your laboratory is using, because measurement by newer assays will result in lower SCr determinations. Thus, the normal value of SCr for a specific patient will depend on the assay method being used and the age of the patient (see normal values for SCr above). Further information about laboratory measurement and reporting of SCr can be found in Chapter 8: The Kidneys.

Age-Related Physiologic Development of Renal Function

Compared to adults, a newborn's kidneys are anatomically and functionally immature. The primary functions of the kidney (glomerular filtration, tubular secretion, and tubular reabsorption) are all decreased in the full-term newborn. These renal functions are even further decreased in the premature infant. After birth, glomerular and tubular renal function increase (i.e., mature) with PNA. During the first 2 years of life, kidney function matures to adult levels and in the following order: (1) glomerular filtration, (2) tubular secretion, and (3) tubular reabsorption. The interpretation of pediatric kidney functions tests can be better understood if one knows how each function of the kidneys matures during the first 2 years.

Glomerular filtration. In the fetus, nephrogenesis (i.e., the formation of new nephrons) begins at 8 weeks of gestation and continues until about 36 weeks of gestation.[39] Although the number of adult nephrons (~1 million) is reached at this time, the nephrons are smaller and not as functionally mature as the nephrons found in an adult kidney.[24] After 36 weeks of gestation, no new nephrons are formed. However, renal mass continues to increase due to the increase in renal tubular growth. Glomerular filtration rate is very low in the young fetus but gradually increases during gestation (Figure 20-4). Before 36 weeks of gestation, the increase in GFR is primarily due to nephrogenesis and the increase in the number of new glomeruli. From 36 weeks of gestation until birth, a much smaller increase in GFR occurs as renal mass and kidney function increase.[40]

At birth, GFR increases dramatically compared to what it was in utero (Figure 20-4). This dramatic increase in GFR, which occurs at birth and continues during the early postnatal period, is due to several important hemodynamic and physiologic changes. Cardiac output and systemic blood pressure increase

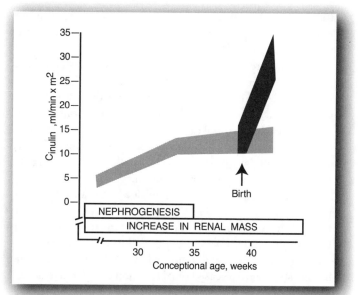

FIGURE 20-4. Maturation of GFR in relation to conceptional age. (Reproduced, with permission, from Guignard JP. The neonatal stressed kidney. In: Gruskin AB, Norman ME, eds. *Pediatric Nephrology: Proceedings of the Fifth International Pediatric Nephrology Symposium.* Presented at The Fifth International Pediatric Nephrology Symposium; October 6–10, 1980; Philadelphia, PA; The Hague: Martinus Nijhoff Publishers; 1981:507.)

at birth and a significant decrease in renal vascular resistance occurs. These changes result in an increase in renal blood flow and effective glomerular filtration pressure. In addition, alterations in the pattern of renal blood flow distribution occur and the permeability of the glomerular membrane and surface area available for filtration increase.[24,39,40] All of these changes help to increase GFR.

Despite the increase in GFR that occurs during this time, GFR is still very much decreased in comparison to adults. As determined by creatinine or inulin clearance, the GFR in a full-term newborn is only 10–15 mL/min/m^2 (2–4 mL/min). Glomerular filtration rate then doubles by 1–2 weeks of age to 20–30 mL/min/m^2 (8–20 mL/min).[39] Adult values of GFR are approached by about 6–12 months of age (70–90 mL/min/m^2). Compared to full-term newborns, GFR in premature newborns is much lower at birth (5–10 mL/min/m^2 or 0.7–2 mL/min) and increases at a less dramatic rate during the first 1–2 weeks after birth (10–12 mL/min/m^2 or 2–4 mL/min).[39] After the first postnatal week, the rate of increase in GFR is comparable in preterm and full-term infants, but the actual GFR value is still lower in preterm infants.

Renal tubular function. Tubular secretion and reabsorption are both decreased in the full-term newborn. This is due to the small size and mass of the renal tubules, decreased peritubular blood flow, and immature biochemical processes that supply energy for active transport. In addition, full-term newborns have a limited ability to concentrate urine and have lower urinary pH values.[39] In the preterm newborn, renal tubular functions are further decreased. Limitations of the newborn's tubular function with respect to the renal handling of serum electrolytes are listed above within the discussion section of each serum electrolyte.

Tubular secretion transports certain electrolytes and medications from the peritubular capillaries into the lumen of the renal tubule. At birth, tubular secretion is only 20% to 30% of adult values and slowly matures by about 8 months of age. Tubular reabsorption, which is also decreased at birth, may not fully mature until 1–2 years of age. Thus, during infancy, a glomerulotubular imbalance occurs, with GFR maturing at a faster rate than renal tubular function.

The decreased renal function in newborns and the maturational changes in GFR and tubular function that occur throughout early infancy have important implications for the interpretation of laboratory data. For example, one must remember that even with a normal SCr for age, neonates and infants still have decreased renal function compared to adults. This decreased renal function must be taken into account, especially in the very young, when dosing electrolytes or medications that are eliminated by the kidneys. In addition, as in adults, certain medications, diseases, and medical conditions (such as hypoxic events that may occur in newborns) may cause further decreases in renal function.

Standardization of Creatinine Clearance

Creatinine clearance (CrCl) can be expressed using several different units of measure, including mL/min, mL/min/m², or mL/min/1.73 m². To better compare the CrCl of patients of different body sizes, CrCl is most commonly standardized to the BSA of an average-sized adult (1.73 m²). Thus, CrCl is most commonly measured as mL/min/1.73 m². Using these units is especially helpful in pediatric patients where a large range of body sizes occur. For example, the average BSA ranges from 0.25 m² in a full-term newborn to 1.34 m² in a 12-year-old.[1] Expressing CrCl in mL/min or even mL/min/m² over this wide of a range of BSAs would give an extremely wide range of values. (See Minicase 3.)

Estimating Body Surface Area in Pediatric Patients

Body surface area (BSA) can be estimated using several different methods. In pediatrics, BSA is most commonly estimated using standard nomograms or equations and the patient's measured height and weight.[1] Two equations are commonly used in pediatrics, an older equation (the DuBois formula)[41]:

$$\text{BSA (m}^2\text{)} = \text{Wt (kg)}0.425 \times \text{Ht (cm)}0.725 \times 0.007184 \quad (1)$$

and a more simplified equation[42]

$$\text{BSA (m}^2\text{)} = \text{the square root of ([Ht (cm)} \times \text{Wt (kg)]}/3600) \quad (2)$$

Estimation of the patient's BSA is required in order to calculate CrCl from a urinary collection.

Determination of CrCl from a Urinary Creatinine Collection

The same equation that is used in adults can be used in pediatric patients to calculate CrCl from a timed urine collection. The following equation is used:

$$\text{CrCl} = (\text{UV/P}) \times (1.73/\text{BSA}) \quad (3)$$

where CrCl is in units of mL/min/1.73 m²; U is the urinary creatinine concentration in mg/dL; V (mL/min) is the total urine volume collected in milliliters divided by the duration of the collection in minutes; P is the SCr concentration in mg/dL; and BSA is the patient's BSA in m².

Ideally, urine should be collected over a 24-hour period. However, a full 24-hour collection period is very difficult in pediatric patients, especially in those who do not have full control over their bladder and do not have a urinary catheter in place. Thus, shorter collection periods (e.g., 8 or 12 hours) are sometimes used. Urinary specimen bags can be placed to collect urine in neonates and infants, but incomplete collection due to leakage of urine often occurs. The incomplete collection of urine will result in an inaccurate calculation of CrCl.

With any urine collection for creatinine determination, it is important to have the patient empty their bladder and discard this specimen before beginning the urine collection. All urine during the time period should be collected, including the urine that would be voided at the end of the collection period. A SCr is usually obtained once during the urinary collection period (ideally at the midpoint) if the patient has stable renal function. If the patient's renal function is changing, then two SCr samples (one at the beginning of the urine collection and one at the end of the urine collection) may be obtained. The average SCr can then be used in the above equation.[3]

Due to the inherent problems of collecting a 24-hour urine sample from pediatric patients and receiving inaccurate calculations, CrCl (or GFR) is often estimated using prediction equations that consider the patient's age, height, gender, and SCr (see below). In fact, using a 24-hour timed urine specimen to calculate CrCl has been shown to be no more reliable (and often less reliable) than using equations based on SCr.[43] Therefore, the National Kidney Foundation recommends that GFR should be estimated in children and adolescents using prediction equations, such as the one by Schwartz.[36] A timed urine collection (e.g., 24-hour sample) may be useful for (1) estimations of GFR in patients with decreased muscle mass (e.g., muscle wasting, malnutrition, or amputation) or in those receiving special diets (e.g., vegetarian diets or creatine supplements); (2) assessments of nutritional status or diets; and (3) evaluations for the need to start dialysis.[43]

Estimating CrCl from Serum Creatinine

Several methods (for example, the Cockcroft-Gault equation) are used in adults to estimate CrCl from a SCr. These equations cannot be used in pediatrics because pediatric patients have a different ratio of muscle mass to SCr. In addition, the amount of pediatric muscle mass per body weight changes over time. Adult equations are based on adult muscle mass and adult urinary creatinine excretion rates. Thus, the use of adult equations in pediatric patients will result in erroneous calculations.

Several predictive equations have been developed to estimate CrCl in pediatric patients. One simple equation was developed for use in children 1–18 years of age with stable SCr[44]:

$$\text{CrCl (mL/min/1.73 m}^2\text{)} = 0.48 \times \text{Height (cm)/SCr(mg/dL)} \quad (4)$$

TABLE 20-3. Mean Values of k by Age Group

AGE GROUP	MEAN k VALUE
Low birth weight infants ≤1 yr	0.33
Full-term infants ≤1 yr	0.45
Children 2–12 yr	0.55
Females 13–21 yr	0.55
Males 13–21 yr	0.70

Source: Modified from reference 36.

This equation was found to be clinically useful in predicting CrCl in children. However, it may be less accurate in children with a height <107 cm.[45]

Another equation, developed by Schwartz, is more commonly used to estimate GFR in pediatric patients,

$$GFR(mL/min/1.73\ m^2) = k \times Length(cm)/SCr(mg/dL) \quad (5)$$

where k is a constant of proportionality.[36] In patients with stable renal function, k is directly related to the muscle component of body weight, which correlates well with the daily rates of urinary creatinine excretion. Since the percentage of muscle mass per body weight varies for different age groups, a different value for k must be used for different age groups. In addition to age, the value of k will be affected by body composition; thus, the values for k listed in Table 20-3 should be used in pediatric patients with average build.

It is important to remember that these two equations were developed using the Jaffe method to assay SCr. Values for SCr as measured by newer methods (e.g., the IDMS-traceable enzymatic method) will be lower than those measured by the Jaffe method (especially at low concentrations of SCr). This will result in an overestimation of GFR if these equations and constants are used when SCr is measured by the newer assays. In fact, use of the Schwartz equation and constants may overestimate GFR by approximately 20% to 30%.[46] Therefore, revised constants for the Schwartz equation must be determined to better estimate GFR when SCr is measured by newer assays using IDMS-based reference standards.

Recently, an "updated" Schwartz bedside equation, based on SCr measured by a newer enzymatic method, was developed in children 1–16 years of age.[47]

$$GFR\ (mL/min/1.73\ m^2) =$$
$$0.413 \times Height\ (cm)/SCr\ (mg/dL) \quad (6)$$

The pediatric patients in which this equation was developed had mild-to-moderate chronic kidney disease (95% of measured GFR values were between 21–76 mL/min/1.73 m²) and were short in stature for their age and gender. Thus, further studies of this equation in children with higher GFRs and a more normal body habitus are needed before it can be widely applied to the pediatric population.

The above equations may not be accurate in certain pediatric populations, including those patients with unstable renal function, abnormal body habitus (e.g., obesity or malnutrition), decreased muscle mass (e.g., cardiac patients), severe chronic renal failure, or insulin dependent diabetes.[36,48] If

MINICASE 3

Vancomycin Dose Determination Based on Estimated Creatinine Clearance in a Child

MORGAN R., A 4-YEAR-OLD FEMALE, is currently in the PICU recovering from cardiac surgery (postoperative day 7). Morgan R.'s blood culture today is positive for methicillin-resistant *Staphylococcus aureus* and vancomycin therapy is to be initiated. Vital signs include BP 95/62 mm Hg, HR 142 beats/min, RR 27 breaths/min, and temperature 101.2°F. Her height is 101 cm (50th percentile for age); weight is 16 kg (50th percentile for age); BSA is 0.67 m². Laboratory data includes sodium 140 mEq/L, potassium 3.8 mEq/L, chloride 102 mEq/L, total CO_2 28 mEq/L, BUN 42 mg/dL, SCr 2.4 mg/dL (Jaffe method), and glucose 109 mg/dL.

Question: Knowing the following information, what dose of vancomycin would you recommend for Morgan R.?

The normal dose of vancomycin used at this hospital for a child of this age is 40 mg/kg/day divided q 6 hr. The recommended dosing adjustment for patients with renal dysfunction is as follows[50]:

CrCl 70–89 mL/min/1.73 m²: administer the normal dose q 8 hr

CrCl 46–69 mL/min/1.73 m²: administer the normal dose q 12 hr

CrCl 30–45 mL/min/1.73 m²: administer the normal dose q 18 hr

CrCl 15–29 mL/min/1.73 m²: administer the normal dose q 24 hr

Discussion: Vancomycin is primarily eliminated by glomerular filtration in the kidney; 80% to 90% of a dose is excreted in the urine as unchanged drug. Morgan R.'s BUN and SCr are elevated indicating that she has renal impairment. Thus, the dose of vancomycin must be adjusted for her renal dysfunction. In order to recommend an appropriate dose, Morgan R.'s CrCl needs to be calculated. Since this laboratory used the Jaffe method to measure SCr, an estimation of CrCl from Morgan R.'s SCr and height can be obtained by using equation (5) and the k value of 0.55 for children 2–12 years of age (Table 20-3). Morgan R.'s estimated CrCl is 23 mL/min/1.73 m². To determine the appropriate dose of vancomycin, one must first calculate the normal dose (i.e., as if the patient did not have any renal dysfunction), and then adjust the dose according to the given guidelines. Since Morgan R. weighs 16 kg, the normal dose of vancomycin would be 160 mg q 6 hr (40 mg/kg/day divided q 6 hr). Since Morgan R.'s CrCl is 23 mL/min/1.73 m², she should receive 160 mg q 24 hr. Appropriate therapeutic drug monitoring should be performed to adjust this initial dosing regimen. It should be noted that if SCr was measured by a newer enzymatic assay using IDMS-based reference standards, then equation (6) should be used to estimate CrCl. If equation (5) and the constants from Table 20-3 were used, it would result in an overestimation of CrCl by approximately 20% to 30%. Additionally, almost all drug dosage guidelines for patients with renal impairment (including those recommended by pharmaceutical manufacturers) were developed using SCr as measured by older assay methodologies. Thus, estimated CrCl values may not correlate well with these dosage guidelines. These limitations further emphasize the need for appropriate therapeutic drug monitoring and followup dosage adjustment.

clinically indicated, CrCl should be determined by a timed urine collection in these patients.

Estimating GFR from Serum Cystatin C

In order to improve calculated estimations of GFR, other endogenous markers of renal function have been investigated. Cystatin C is a cysteine protease inhibitor that is produced by all nucleated cells at a relatively constant rate; it is freely filtered by the kidneys. Its rate of production is so constant that serum cystatin C levels are not thought to be influenced by muscle mass, gender, body composition, and age (after 12 months). Reciprocal values of serum cystatin C have been correlated to measured GFR values in adults and children.[46] However, serum cystatin C alone may not accurately estimate GFR in renal transplant patients, patients with high C-reactive protein, diabetes with ketonuria, or thyroid dysfunction. Thus, other equations have been developed which incorporate multiple patient parameters and endogenous markers of renal function. One such pediatric equation includes terms for the ratio of height to SCr, the reciprocals of serum cystatin C and BUN, a factor for gender, and a separate factor for height alone.[47] This complex equation is not clinically friendly but is being further investigated in the National Institutes of Health sponsored Chronic Kidney Disease in Children study. Results of this investigation may yield a more accurate equation to estimate GFR in pediatric patients. Unfortunately at this time, serum cystatin C assays are not readily available at many institutions.

AGE-RELATED DIFFERENCES IN LIVER FUNCTION TESTS

Serum Albumin

Normal range[9] for newborns:
0–5 days old, body weight <2.5 kg: 2.0–3.6 g/dL or
*   20–36 g/L*
0–5 days old, body weight >2.5 kg: 2.6–3.6 g/dL or
*   26–36 g/L*
1–3 yr: 3.4–4.2 g/dL or 34–42 g/L
4–6 yr: 3.5–5.2 g/dL or 35–52 g/L
7–19 yr: 3.7–5.6 g/dL or 37–56 g/L

Serum proteins, including albumin, are synthesized by the liver. Thus, measurements of serum total protein, albumin, and other specific proteins are primarily a test of the liver's synthetic capability. Maturational differences in the liver's ability to synthesize protein help determine the normal range for serum albumin concentrations. The liver of the fetus is able to synthesize albumin beginning at approximately 7–8 weeks of gestation. However, the predominant serum protein in early fetal life is alpha-fetoprotein. As gestation continues, the concentration of albumin increases, while alpha-fetoprotein decreases. At approximately 3–4 months of gestation, the fetal liver is able to produce each of the major serum protein classes. However, serum concentrations are much lower than those found at maturity.[49]

At birth, the newborn liver is anatomically and functionally immature. Due to immature liver function and a decreased ability to synthesize protein, full-term neonates have decreased concentrations of total plasma proteins, including albumin, gamma globulin, and lipoproteins. Concentrations in premature newborns are even lower, with serum albumin levels as low as 1.8 g/dL.[12]

Adult serum concentrations of serum albumin (~3.5 g/dL) are reached only after several months of age. Conditions that cause abnormalities in serum albumin in pediatric patients are the same as in adults and can be reviewed in Chapter 12: Liver and Gastroenterology Tests.

Liver Enzymes

Alanine aminotransferase (ALT, also called SGPT)—
*   normal range[3] for neonates and infants: 13–45 units/L*
adult males: 10–40 units/L
adult females: 7–35 units/L

Aspartate aminotransferase (AST, also called SGOT)—
*   normal range for newborns: 25–75 units/L*
infants: 15–60 units/L
children 1–3 yr: 20–60 units/L
children 4–6 yr: 15–50 units/L
children 7–9 yr: 15–40 units/L
children 10–11 yr: 10–60 units/L
adolescents 12–19 yr: 15–45 units/L

Alkaline phosphatase—normal range for infants:
*   150–420 units/L*
children 2–10 yr: 100–320 units/L
males 11–18 yr: 100–390 units/L
females 11–18 yr: 100–320 units/L
adults: 20–130 units/L

Lactate dehydrogenase—normal range for neonates 0–4 days:
*   290–775 units/L*
neonates 4–10 days: 545–2000 units/L
infants 10 days–24 months: 180–430 units/L
children 24 months–12 yr: 110–295 units/L
adolescents >12 yr: 100–190 units/L

The normal reference ranges for liver enzymes are higher in pediatric patients compared to adults. This may be due to the fact that the liver makes up a larger percentage of total body weight in infants and children compared to adults. For certain enzymes, such as alkaline phosphatase, the higher normal concentrations in childhood represent higher serum concentrations of an isoenzyme from other sources, specifically bone. Approximately 80% of alkaline phosphatase originates from liver and bone. Smaller amounts come from the intestines, kidneys, and placenta. Normally, growing children have higher osteoblastic activity during the bone growth period and an influx into serum of the alkaline phosphatase isoenzyme from bone.[11] Thus, the higher normal concentrations of alkaline phosphatase in childhood primarily represent a higher rate of bone growth. After puberty, the liver is the primary source of serum alkaline phosphatase.

One must keep these age-related differences in mind when interpreting liver enzyme test results. For example, an isolated increase in alkaline phosphatase in a rapidly growing adolescent—whose other liver function tests are normal—would not indicate hepatic or biliary disease, but merely a rapid increase in bone growth.

As in adults, increases in AST and ALT in pediatric patients are associated with hepatocellular injury, while elevations of alkaline phosphatase are associated with cholestatic disease. Cholestasis and bone disorders (such as osteomalacia and rickets) are common causes of elevated serum alkaline phosphatase concentrations in pediatric patients.

Bilirubin

Total bilirubin, premature neonates—normal range[3] for
0–1 day old: <8 mg/dL or <137 µmol/L
1–2 days old: <12 mg/dL or <205 µmol/L
3–5 days old: <16 mg/dL or <274 µmol/L
>5 days old: <2 mg/dL or <34 µmol/L

Total bilirubin, full-term neonates—normal range for
0–1 day old: <8.7 mg/dL or <149 µmol/L
1–2 days old: <11.5 mg/dL or <197 µmol/L
3–5 days old: <12 mg/dL or <205 µmol/L
>5 days old: <1.2 mg/dL or <21 µmol/L
adults: 1–1.2 mg/dL or 2–21 µmol/L

Conjugated bilirubin—normal range for neonates:
<0.6 mg/dL or <10 µmol/L
infants and children: <0.2 mg/dL or <3.4 µmol/L

To better understand the age-related differences in serum bilirubin concentrations, a brief review of bilirubin metabolism is needed. *Bilirubin* is a breakdown product of hemoglobin. Hemoglobin, which is released from senescent or hemolyzed RBCs, is degraded by heme oxygenase into iron, carbon monoxide, and biliverdin. Biliverdin undergoes reduction by biliverdin reductase to bilirubin. Unconjugated bilirubin then enters the liver and is conjugated with glucuronic acid to form conjugated bilirubin, which is water soluble. Conjugated bilirubin is excreted in the bile and enters the intestines, where is it broken down by bacterial flora to urobilinogen. However, conjugated bilirubin can also be deconjugated by bacteria in the intestines and reabsorbed back into the circulation.[51]

Compared to adults, newborns have higher concentrations of bilirubin. This results from a higher production of bilirubin in the neonate and a decreased ability to excrete it. A higher rate of production of bilirubin occurs in newborns due to the shorter life span of neonatal RBCs and the higher initial neonatal hematocrit. The average RBC life span is only 65 days in very premature neonates and 90 days in full-term neonates, compared to 120 days in adults.[52] In addition, full-term neonates have a mean hematocrit of about 50%, compared to adult values of approximately 44%. The shorter RBC life span plus the higher hematocrit both increase the load of unconjugated bilirubin to the liver. Newborn infants, however, have a decreased ability to eliminate bilirubin. The activity of

neonatal uridine diphosphate glucuronosyltransferase, the enzyme responsible for conjugating bilirubin in the liver, is decreased. In addition, newborns lack the intestinal bacteria needed to breakdown conjugated bilirubin into urobilinogen. However, the newborn's intestine does contain glucuronidase, which can deconjugate bilirubin and allow unconjugated bilirubin to be reabsorbed back into the circulation (enterohepatic circulation). This enterohepatically reabsorbed bilirubin further increases the unconjugated bilirubin load to the liver.

Due to these limitations in bilirubin metabolism, a "physiologic jaundice" commonly occurs in newborns. Typically in full-term neonates, high serum bilirubin concentrations occur in the first few days of life, with a decrease over the next several weeks to values seen in adults. High bilirubin concentrations may occur later in premature newborns, up to the first week of life, and are usually higher and persist longer than in full-term newborns.

Pathologic jaundice may occur in newborns due to many reasons, including increased production of bilirubin, decreased uptake of unconjugated bilirubin into the liver, decreased conjugation of bilirubin in the liver, and increased enterohepatic circulation of bilirubin.[51] Increased production of bilirubin may occur with RBC hemolysis due to blood group incompatibilities, enzyme deficiencies of the erythrocytes, erythrocyte structural defects (e.g., spherocytosis), or in infants of certain racial or ethnic groups (e.g., Asian, Native American, and Greek islander). Certain genetic disorders may cause neonatal hyperbilirubinemia. For example, patients with Gilbert syndrome have decreased hepatic uptake of bilirubin and infants with Crigler-Najjar syndrome have a deficiency of uridine diphosphate glucuronosyltransferase, the enzyme that is responsible for conjugation of bilirubin in the liver. Breast-feeding is also associated with neonatal hyperbilirubinemia and jaundice. Newborns who are exclusively breast-fed, not feeding well, or not being enterally fed (i.e., newborns who are not taking anything by mouth) may have increased intestinal reabsorption of bilirubin that can cause or worsen hyperbilirubinemia. Breast-feeding may also increase bilirubin concentrations by other mechanisms. Breast milk may contain substances that decrease the conjugation of bilirubin by inhibiting the enzyme, uridine diphosphate glucuronosyltransferase.

Appropriate monitoring of serum bilirubin is very important in neonates, as high concentrations of unconjugated bilirubin can cause bilirubin encephalopathy or kernicterus (i.e., deposits of bilirubin in the brain). The neurotoxic effects of bilirubin are serious and potentially lethal. Clinical features of acute kernicterus include poor sucking, stupor, seizures, fever, hypotonia, hypertonia, opisthotonus, and retrocollis. Neonates who survive may develop mental retardation, delayed motor skills, movement disorders, and sensorineural hearing loss. Phototherapy and exchange transfusion are common treatments for neonatal hyperbilirubinemia.[51]

AGE-RELATED DIFFERENCES IN HEMATOLOGIC TESTS

Erythrocytes

Mean values and lower limit of normal (minus 2 standard deviations)[53]

Red Blood Cell Count

Birth (cord blood): 4.7 (3.9) x 10[12] cells/L

newborns 1–3 days old: 5.3 (4.0) x 10[12] cells/L

1 week: 5.1 (3.9) x 10[12] cells/L

2 weeks: 4.9 (3.6) x 10[12] cells/L

1 month: 4.2 (3.0) x 10[12] cells/L

2 months: 3.8 (2.7) x 10[12] cells/L

3–6 months: 3.8 (3.1) x 10[12] cells/L

0.5–2 yr: 4.5 (3.7) x 10[12] cells/L

2–6 yr: 4.6 (3.9) x 10[12] cells/L

6–12 yr: 4.6 (4.0) x 10[12] cells/L

12–18 yr, female: 4.6 (4.1) x 10[12] cells/L

12–18 yr, male: 4.9 (4.5) x 10[12] cells/L

18–49 yr, female: 4.6 (4.0) x 10[12] cells/L

18–49 yr, male: 5.2 (4.5) x 10[12] cells/L

Hemoglobin

Birth (cord blood): 16.5 (13.5) g/dL

newborns 1–3 days old: 18.5 (14.5) g/dL

1 week: 17.5 (13.5) g/dL

2 weeks: 16.5 (12.5) g/dL

1 month: 14.0 (10.0) g/dL

2 months: 11.5 (9.0) g/dL

3–6 months: 11.5 (9.5) g/dL

0.5–2 yr: 12.0 (10.5) g/dL

2–6 yr: 12.5 (11.5) g/dL

6–12 yr: 13.5 (11.5) g/dL

12–18 yr, female: 14.0 (12.0) g/dL

12–18 yr, male: 14.5 (13.0) g/dL

18–49 yr, female: 14.0 (12.0) g/dL

18–49 yr, male: 15.5 (13.5) g/dL

Hematocrit

Birth (cord blood): 51 (42)%

1–3 days old: 56 (45)%

1 week: 54 (42)%

2 weeks: 51 (39)%

1 month: 43 (31)%

2 months: 35 (28)%

3–6 months: 35 (29)%

0.5–2 yr: 36 (33)%

2–6 yr: 37 (34)%

6–12 yr: 40 (35)%

12–18 yr, female: 41 (36)%

12–18 yr, male: 43 (37)%

18–49 yr, female: 41 (36)%

18–49 yr, male: 47 (41)%

TABLE 20-4. Red Blood Cell Indices by Age: Mean Values and Lower Limits of Normal (minus 2 standard deviations)

	MCV fL	MCH pg/cell	MCHC g/dL
Birth (cord blood)	108 (98)	34 (31)	33 (30)
1–3 days	108 (95)	34 (31)	33 (29)
1 week	107 (88)	34 (28)	33 (28)
2 weeks	105 (86)	34 (28)	33 (28)
1 month	104 (85)	34 (28)	33 (29)
2 months	96 (77)	30 (26)	33 (29)
3–6 months	91 (74)	30 (25)	33 (30)
0.5–2 yr	78 (70)	27 (23)	33 (30)
2–6 yr	81 (75)	27 (24)	34 (31)
6–12 yr	86 (77)	29 (25)	34 (31)
12–18 yr			
Female	90 (78)	30 (25)	34 (31)
Male	88 (78)	30 (25)	34 (31)
18–49 yr	90 (80)	30 (26)	34 (31)

MCV = mean corpuscular volume; MCH = mean corpuscular hemoglobin; MCHC = mean corpuscular hemoglobin concentration.
Source: Adapted from reference 53.

Compared to adults, normal newborn infants have higher hemoglobin and hematocrit values. For example, the mean hemoglobin value in a full-term newborn on the first day of life is 18.5 g/dL, compared to 15.5 g/dL in adult males. Hemoglobin and hematocrit start to decrease within the first week of life and reach a minimum level at 8–12 weeks in term infants and by 6 weeks of age in premature infants.[54] This normal decrease in hemoglobin and hematocrit is called the *physiologic anemia of infancy.* This physiologic anemia is normochromic and microcytic and is accompanied by a low reticulocyte count. Physiologic anemia of infancy does not require medical treatment.

The age-related changes in hemoglobin that occur during the first few months of life are due to several reasons. In utero, a low arterial pO_2 exists, which stimulates the production of erythropoietin in the fetus. This results in a high rate of erythropoiesis and accounts for the high levels of hemoglobin and hematocrit that exist at birth. At birth, pO_2 and oxygen content of blood significantly increase with the newborn's first breaths. The higher amount of oxygen that is available to the tissues will down-regulate erythropoietin production and decrease the rate of erythropoiesis.[55] Without the stimulation of erythropoietin to produce new RBCs, hemoglobin concentrations decrease as aged RBCs are removed from the circulation. The shorter life span of neonatal RBCs (90 days versus 120 days in adults) also contributes to the decline in hemoglobin.

Hemoglobin continues to decline in full-term infants until 8–12 weeks of age when values reach 9–11 g/dL. These levels of hemoglobin result in lower amounts of oxygen delivery to the tissues. Usually at this point, oxygen requirements exceed

TABLE 20-5. White Blood Cell Differential by Age

	MEAN VALUES			
	NEUTROPHILS	LYMPHOCYTES	EOSINOPHILS	MONOCYTES
Birth	61%	31%	2%	6%
2 weeks	40%	63%	3%	9%
3 months	30%	48%	2%	5%
0.5–6 yr	45%	48%	2%	5%
7–12 yr	55%	38%	2%	5%
Adult	55%	35%	3%	7%

Source: Adapted from reference 57.

oxygen delivery and the relative hypoxia stimulates the production of erythropoietin. Erythropoiesis then increases and the reticulocyte count and hemoglobin concentrations begin to rise.

It is important to remember that the iron from the aged RBCs that were previously removed from the circulation has been stored. The amount of this stored iron is usually adequate to meet the requirements of hemoglobin synthesis.

In premature infants, the physiologic anemia occurs at 3–6 weeks of age (sooner than in full-term infants) and the nadir of the hemoglobin concentrations is lower (e.g., 7–9 g/dL).[55] This can be explained by the even shorter life span of the premature infant's RBCs (40–60 days versus 90 days in full-term newborns) and by the inadequate synthesis of erythropoietin in response to anemia. Thus, anemia of prematurity may require treatment with recombinant human erythropoietin and iron.

Differences in RBC indices also exist for different pediatric ages. For example, compared to adults, newborns have larger erythrocytes (mean corpuscular volume [MCV] of 108 fL, compared to an adult value of 90 fL). Mean values and the lower limits of normal for RBC indices according to different ages are listed in Table 20-4.

Causes of the various types of anemias in pediatric patients are similar to the causes in adults. Of particular note is the iron deficiency anemia that occurs in infants who are fed whole cow's milk. The iron in whole cow's milk is less bioavailable and may cause inadequate iron intake. Typically infants with iron deficiency anemia from whole cow's milk have chronically consumed large amounts of cow's milk (>24 ounces per day) and foods that are not supplemented with iron. Some infants receiving whole cow's milk develop severe iron deficiency due to chronic intestinal blood loss. The blood loss is thought to be due to intestinal exposure to a specific heat-labile protein found in whole cow's milk. Breast feeding, delaying the introduction of whole cow's milk until 12 months of age, and decreasing the amount of whole cow's milk to <24 ounces per day, have been recommended to decrease the loss of blood.[56]

In pediatric patients with anemia, genetic disorders that produce inadequate RBC production (e.g., Diamond-Blackfan anemia), hemolytic anemias (e.g., hereditary spherocytosis), or hemoglobin disorders (e.g., sickle cell disease) must also be considered.

Leukocytes

White Blood Cell Count

Normal range[57] for newborns at birth:
9.0–30.0 x 10³ cells/mm³
2 weeks: 5.0–21.0 x 10³ cells/mm³
3 months: 6.0–18.0 x 10³ cells/mm³
0.5–6 yr: 6.0–15.0 x 10³ cells/mm³
7–12 yr: 4.5–13.5 x 10³ cells/mm³
adults: 4.4–11.0 x 10³ cells/mm³

Normal WBC counts are higher in neonates and infants compared to adults. Typically in adults, an elevated WBC may indicate infection. However, in neonates and infants with a systemic bacterial infection, the WBC count may be increased, decreased, or within the normal range. Neonates have a lower storage pool of neutrophils and an overwhelming infection (for example, neonatal sepsis) may deplete this pool and cause neutropenia. Therefore, while an increase in WBCs is a nonspecific finding in neonates (i.e., it may occur in many conditions other than sepsis), neutropenia is a highly significant finding and may be the first abnormal laboratory result that indicates neonatal bacterial infection.[54] Not recognizing that neutropenia in neonates indicates a serious infection could result in a delay in treatment and significant morbidity or even mortality for the patient.

In addition to the age-related differences in total WBC count, the age-related differences in WBC differential also need to be taken into consideration when interpreting laboratory results (Table 20-5). After the newborn period and up until 5–6 years of age, lymphocytes represent the most prevalent circulating WBC type. Subsequent to this, neutrophils predominate in the blood for the remainder of life.

Platelets

Platelet Count

Normal range for newborns[12]: 84,000–478,000/mm³
neonate >1 week, infants, children, adolescents, and adults:
150,000–400,000/mm³

Compared to adults, the normal platelet count in the newborn may be lower. Adult values are reached after 1 week of age, although platelet counts may range higher in children (up to 600,000/mm³) than in adults. Platelet counts are discussed in detail in the Chapter 15: Hematology: Red and White Blood Cell Tests.

SUMMARY

Interpreting pediatric laboratory data can be complex. Age-related differences in normal reference ranges occur for many common laboratory tests. These differences may be due to changes in body composition and the normal anatomic and physiologic maturation that occurs throughout childhood. Changes in various body compartments, the immature function of the neonatal kidney, and the increased electrolyte and mineral requirements necessary for proper growth, help to explain many age-related differences in serum electrolytes and minerals. Alterations in skeletal muscle mass and the pattern of kidney function maturation account for the various age-related differences in SCr and kidney function tests. Neonatal hepatic immaturity and subsequent maturation help to explain the age-related differences in serum albumin, liver enzymes, and bilirubin. Likewise, the immature hematopoietic system of the newborn and its maturation account for the age-related differences in various hematologic tests.

This chapter also reviews several general pediatric considerations including differences in physiologic parameters, pediatric blood sampling considerations, and the determination of pediatric reference ranges. Interpretation of pediatric laboratory data must take into account the various age-related differences in normal values. If these differences are not taken into consideration, inappropriate diagnoses and treatment may result.

Learning Points

1. **Would the dose of a medication that is primarily excreted by the kidney ever have to be adjusted in a patient with a SCr of 0.8 mg/dL?**

   Answer: The age of the patient must be taken into consideration when interpreting laboratory tests, especially SCr. In addition, the methodology used to assay SCr needs to be considered. For the Jaffe method, a SCr of 0.8 mg/dL indicates significant renal dysfunction in an infant whose normal SCr should be 0.2–0.4 mg/dL and mild or moderate renal dysfunction in a child whose normal SCr should be 0.3–0.7 mg/dL. However, a SCr of 0.8 mg/dL in an adolescent or adult would be considered within the normal range. Thus, medications that are primarily excreted by the kidney would need to have a dosage adjustment in infants and children with a SCr of 0.8 mg/dL as measured by the Jaffe method. For the IDMS-traceable enzymatic method, measured SCr values and normal values for age will be lower than with the Jaffe method. A SCr of 0.8 mg/dL indicates significant renal dysfunction in an infant or young child (newborn to 4 years of age) whose normal SCr should be 0.03–0.5 mg/dL and mild-to-moderate renal dysfunction in a child 4–7 years of age whose normal SCr should be 0.03–0.59 mg/dL or in a child 7–10 years of age whose normal SCr should be 0.22–0.59 mg/dL. However, a SCr of 0.8 mg/dL in an adolescent or adult would be considered within the normal range.

2. **Are there any concerns with using ceftriaxone in a neonate?**

   Answer: Ceftriaxone has been shown in vitro to displace bilirubin from its albumin binding sites. Thus, ceftriaxone should not be used in hyperbilirubinemic neonates, especially premature neonates, since displacement of bilirubin from albumin-binding sites may lead to bilirubin encephalopathy. Ceftriaxone may also cause sludging in the gallbladder and cholelithiasis. In addition, fatal reactions have been recently reported in neonates due to ceftriaxone–calcium precipitates in the lungs and kidneys when ceftriaxone and calcium-containing IV solutions were coadministered. In some of these cases the ceftriaxone and calcium-containing solutions were administered in different infusion lines and at different times. Therefore, ceftriaxone must not be administered to neonates who are also receiving calcium-containing IV solutions.[1,58]

3. **Would a hemoglobin of 9.5 g/dL in a 10-week-old infant who was born at full term require initiation of iron therapy?**

   Answer: No. Iron therapy would not be required because this anemia would be considered a normal physiologic anemia of infancy. In full-term infants, hemoglobin values of 9–11 g/dL normally occur at 8–12 weeks of age. After this time, the reticulocyte count and hemoglobin concentration should begin to rise. If an infant's hemoglobin concentration remained at 9.5 g/dL after 12 weeks of age, a further workup of the infant's anemia would be required. If the anemia was found to be due to an iron deficiency, then iron therapy would be required. Dietary causes of iron deficiency, such as consuming large amounts of whole cow's milk, would also need to be considered.

REFERENCES

1. Taketomo CK, Hodding JH, Kraus DM. *Pediatric and Neonatal Dosage Handbook*. 18th ed. Hudson, OH: Lexi-Comp Inc; 2011.

2. Engle WA, American Academy of Pediatrics Committee on Fetus and Newborn. Age terminology during the perinatal period. *Pediatrics*. 2004;114:1362-1364.

3. Tschudy MM, Arcara KM, eds. *The Harriet Lane Handbook*. 19th ed. Philadelphia, PA: Elsevier Mosby; 2012.

4. Task Force on Blood Pressure Control in Children. Report of the second task force on blood pressure control in children—1987. *Pediatrics*. 1987;79:1-25.

5. National High Blood Pressure Education Program Working Group on High Blood Pressure in Children and Adolescents. The fourth report on the diagnosis, evaluation, and treatment of high blood pressure in children and adolescents. *Pediatrics*. 2004;114:555-576.

6. Hicks JM. Pediatric clinical biochemistry: why is it different? In: Soldin SJ, Rifai N, Hicks JM, eds. *Biochemical Basis of Pediatric Disease*. 2nd ed. Washington DC: AACC Press; 1995:1-17.

7. Malarkey LM, McMorrow ME. Specimen collection procedures. In: *Nurses Manual of Laboratory Tests and Diagnostic Procedures*. 2nd ed. Philadelphia, PA: W.B. Saunders; 2000:16-36.

8. Nathan DG, Orkin SH, eds. *Nathan and Oski's Hematology of Infancy and Childhood*. 5th ed. Philadelphia, PA: WB Saunders; 1998.

9. Soldin SJ, Brugnara C, Wong EC, eds. *Pediatric Reference Intervals*. 5th ed. Washington DC: AACC Press; 2005.

10. Malarkey LM, McMorrow ME. *Nurses Manual of Laboratory Tests and Diagnostic Procedures*. 2nd ed. Philadelphia, PA: WB Saunders; 2000.

11. Jacobs DS, DeMott WR, Oxley DK. *Laboratory Test Handbook*. 5th ed. Hudson, OH: Lexi-Comp Inc; 2001.

12. Lo SF. Reference intervals for laboratory tests and procedures. In: Kliegman RM, Stanton BF, et al., eds. *Nelson Textbook of Pediatrics*. 19th ed. Philadelphia, PA: Saunders Elsevier; 2011.

13. Siparsky G, Accurso FJ. Chemistry & hematology reference intervals. In: Hay WW, Levin MJ, Sondheimer JM, et al, eds. *Current Diagnosis and Treatment: Pediatrics*. 20th ed. New York, NY: McGraw-Hill; 2011.

14. Gomez P, Coca C, Vargas C, et al. Normal reference-intervals for 20 biochemical variables in healthy infants, children, and adolescents. *Clin Chem*. 1984; 30:407-412.

15. Burritt MF, Slockbower JM, Forsman RW, et al. Pediatric reference intervals for 19 biological variables in healthy children. *Mayo Clin Proc*. 1990;65:329-336.

16. Jagarinec N, Flegar-Mestric Z, Surina B, et al. *Clin Chem Lab Med*. 1998;36:327-337.

17. Cherian AG, Hill JG. Percentile estimates of reference values for fourteen chemical constituents in sera of children and adolescents. *AJCP*. 1978;69:24-31.

18. Bell EF, Oh W. Fluid and electrolyte management. In: MacDonald MG, Seshia MMK, Mullett MD, eds. *Avery's Neonatology: Pathophysiology and Management of the Newborn*. 6th ed. Philadelphia, PA: Lippincott Williams & Wilkins; 2005.

19. Friis-Hansen B. Water distribution in the foetus and newborn infant. *Acta Paediatr Scand*. 1983;305:7-11.

20. Friis-Hansen B. Changes in body water compartments during growth. *Acta Paediatr*. 1957;110(suppl):1-68.

21. Tarnow-Mordi WO, Shaw JC, Liu D, et al. Iatrogenic hyponatremia of the newborn due to maternal fluid overload: a prospective study. *Br Med J*. 1981; 83:639-642.

22. Malarkey LM, McMorrow ME. Serum electrolytes. In: *Nurses Manual of Laboratory Tests and Diagnostic Procedures*. 2nd ed. Philadelphia, PA: W.B. Saunders; 2000:82-103.

23. Greenbaum LA. Electrolyte and acid-base disorders. In: Kliegman RM, Stanton BF, et al.,eds. *Nelson Textbook of Pediatrics*. 19th ed. Philadelphia, PA: Saunders Elsevier; 2011.

24. Blackburn ST. Renal function in the neonate. *J Perinat Neonatal Nurs*. 1994;8:37-47.

25. Nafday SM, Brion LP, Benchimol C, et al. Renal disease. In: MacDonald MG, Seshia MMK, Mullett MD, eds. *Avery's Neonatology: Pathophysiology and Management of the Newborn*. 6th ed. Philadelphia, PA: Lippincott Williams & Wilkins; 2005.

26. Breault DT, Majzoub JA. Other abnormalities of arginine vasopressin metabolism and action. In: Kliegman RM, Stanton BF, et al., eds. *Nelson Textbook of Pediatrics*. 19th ed. Philadelphia, PA: Saunders Elsevier; 2011.

27. Lorenz JM. Assessing fluid and electrolyte status in the newborn. *Clinical Chemistry*. 1997;43:205-210.

28. Papageorgiou A, Pelausa E, Kovacs L. The extremely low birth weight infant. In: MacDonald MG, Seshia MMK, Mullett MD, eds. *Avery's Neonatology: Pathophysiology and Management of the Newborn*. 6th ed. Philadelphia, PA: Lippincott Williams & Wilkins; 2005.

29. Jones DP, Chesney RW. Development of tubular function. *Clinics in Perinatology*. 1992;19:33-57.

30. Greenbaum LA. Electrolytes and acid-base disorders. In: Behrman RE, Kliegman RM, Jenson HB, eds. *Nelson Textbook of Pediatrics*. 17th ed. Philadelphia, PA: WB Saunders; 2004.

31. Stigson L, Kjellmer I. Serum levels of magnesium at birth related to complications of immaturity. *Acta Paediatr*. 1997;86: 991-994.

32. Ariceta G, Rodriguez-Soriano J, Vallo A. Magnesium homeostasis in premature and full-term neonates. *Pediatr Nephrol*. 1995;9:423-427.

33. Geven WB, Monnens LA, Willems JL. Magnesium metabolism in childhood. *Mimer Electrolyte Metab*. 1993;19:308-313.

34. Pesce MA. Reference ranges for laboratory tests and procedures. In: Kliegman RM, Behrman RE, et al., eds. *Nelson Textbook of Pediatrics*. 18th ed. Philadelphia, PA: Saunders Elsevier; 2007.

35. Pan CG, Avner ED. Introduction to glomerular diseases. In: Kliegman RM, Stanton BF, et al., eds. *Nelson Textbook of Pediatrics*. 19th ed. Philadelphia, PA: Saunders Elsevier; 2011.

36. Schwartz GJ, Brion LP, Spitzer A. The use of plasma creatinine concentration for estimating glomerular filtration rate in infants, children, and adolescents. *Pediatric Clinics of North America*. 1997;34:571-590.

37. Bueva A, Guignard JP. Renal function in preterm neonates. *Pediatric Research*. 1994;36:572-577.

38. Meyers GL, Miller WG, Coresh J, et al. Recommendations for improving serum creatinine measurement: a report from the Laboratory Working Group of the National Kidney Disease Education Program. *Clin Chem*. 2006;52:5-18.

39. Alcorn J, McNamara PJ. Ontogeny of hepatic and renal systemic clearance pathways in infants: part 1. *Clin Pharmacokinet*. 2002;41:959-998.

40. Guignard JP. Renal function in the newborn infant. *Pediatr Clin North Am*. 1982;29:777-790.

41. DuBois D, Dubois EF. A formula to estimate the approximate surface area if height and weight be known. *Arch Intern Med*. 1916;17:863-871.

42. Mosteller RD. Simplified calculation of body-surface area. *New Engl J Med*. 1987;317:1098.

43. Hogg RJ, Furth S, Lemley KV, et al. National Kidney Foundation's kidney disease outcomes quality initiative clinical practice guidelines for chronic kidney disease in children and adolescents: evaluation, classification, and stratification. *Pediatrics*. 2003;111:1416-1421.

44. Traub SL, Johnson CE. Comparison of methods of estimating creatinine clearance in children. *Am J Hosp Pharm*. 1980;37:195-201.

45. DeAcevedo LH, Johnson CE. Estimation of creatinine clearance in children: comparison of six methods. *Clin Pharm*. 1982;1:158-161.

46. Schwartz GJ, Work DF. Measurement and Estimation of GFR in Children and Adolescents. *Clin J Am Soc Nephrol* 2009; 4:1832-1843.

47. Schwartz GJ, Munoz A, Schneider MF, et al. New Equations to Estimate GFR in Children with CKD. *J Am Soc Nephrol* 2009;20:629-637.

48. Waz WR, Feld LG, Quattrin T. Serum creatinine, height, and weight do not predict glomerular filtration rate in children with IDDM. *Diabetes Care*. 1993;16:1067-1070.

49. Miethke AG, Balistreri WF. Morphogenesis of the liver and biliary system. In: Kliegman RM, Stanton BF, et al., eds. *Nelson Textbook of Pediatrics*. 19th ed. Philadelphia, PA: Saunders Elsevier; 2011.

50. Taketomo CK, Hodding JH, Kraus DM. *Pediatric Dosage Handbook*. 16th ed. Hudson, OH: Lexi-Comp Inc; 2009.

51. Dennery PA, Seidman DS, Stevenson DK. Neonatal hyperbilirubinemia. *N Engl J Med*. 2001;344:581-590.

52. Lockitch G. Beyond the umbilical cord: interpreting laboratory tests in the neonate (review). *Clin Biochem*. 1994;27:1-6.

53. Osberg IM. Chemistry and hematology reference (normal) ranges. In: *Current Pediatric Diagnosis and Treatment*. 16th ed. New York, NY: Lange Medical Books/McGraw-Hill; 2003.

54. Blanchette V, Dror Y, Chan A. Hematology. In: MacDonald MG, Seshia MMK, Mullett MD, eds. *Avery's Neonatology: Pathophysiology and Management of the Newborn*. 6th ed. Philadelphia, PA: Lippincott Williams & Wilkins; 2005.

55. Lerner NB. Physiologic anemia of infancy. In: Kliegman RM, Stanton BF, et al., eds. *Nelson Textbook of Pediatrics*. 19th ed. Philadelphia, PA: Saunders Elsevier; 2011.

56. Lerner NB, Sills R. Iron-deficiency anemia. In: Kliegman RM, Stanton BF, et al., eds. *Nelson Textbook of Pediatrics*. 19th ed. Philadelphia, PA: Saunders Elsevier; 2011.

57. Glader B. The anemias. In: Kliegman RM, Behrman RE, Jenson HB, et al., eds. *Nelson Textbook of Pediatrics*. 18th ed. Philadelphia, PA: Saunders Elsevier; 2007

58. Rocephin˚ [product information]. South San Francisco, CA: Genentech USA Inc; November 2010.

CHAPTER 21

Women's Health

MICHELLE J. WASHINGTON, CANDACE S. BROWN

ANATOMY AND PHYSIOLOGY

The reproductive cycle depends on the complex cyclic interaction between hypothalamic gonadotropin-releasing hormone (GnRH), the pituitary gonadotropins follicle-stimulating hormone (FSH) and luteinizing hormone (LH), and the ovarian sex steroid hormones estradiol and progesterone.[1] Through positive and negative feedback loops, these hormones stimulate ovulation, facilitate implantation of the fertilized ovum, or induce menstruation. Feedback loops between the hypothalamus, pituitary gland, and ovaries are depicted in Figure 21-1. If the levels or relationship of any one (or more) of the above hormones become altered, the reproductive cycle becomes disrupted, and ovulation and/or menstruation cease.

MENSTRUAL CYCLE

The reproductive cycle is divided into three phases: menstruation and the follicular phase, ovulation, and the luteal phase.[1] These three phases referring to the status of the ovary during the reproductive cycle are depicted in Figure 21-2.[1] The endometrium has the proliferative and secretory phases.

Phase I. Menstruation and the follicular phase. The first day of menstrual bleeding is considered day 1 of the typical 28 day menstrual cycle. During menstruation, the endometrium is sloughed in response to progesterone withdrawal. This is accompanied by the development of a new follicle during the follicular phase, with renewal of the endometrial lining of the uterus in preparation for implantation of an embryo. Women usually menstruate for 3–5 days.

Menstruation marks the beginning of the follicular phase of the cycle. With the beginning of menstruation, plasma concentrations of estradiol, progesterone, and LH reach their lowest point. In response to this reduction in negative feedback at the pituitary gland, FSH is increased at the beginning of menstruation. The increase in FSH begins approximately 2 days before the onset of menstruation. Under the influence of FSH, the granulosa cells begin to secrete estradiol.

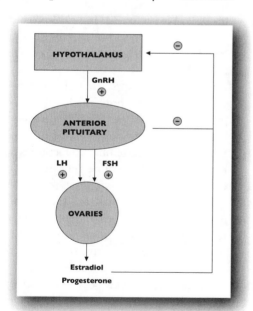

FIGURE 21-1. Hypothalamic-pituitary-ovarian axis (GnRH = gonadotropin-releasing hormone; LH = luteinizing hormone; FSH = follicle-stimulating hormone; (+) = stimulation of hormone secretion; (-) = inhibition of hormone secretion).

Estradiol begins to rise in plasma by the fourth day of the cycle. Estradiol stimulates LH receptors on the theca cells, further increasing secretion of androgen precursors, which are converted by aromatase to estradiol in granulosa cells. The upregulation of LH receptors and hormone production prepares the granulosa and theca cells for progesterone synthesis after ovulation.

With rising estradiol levels, there is negative feedback to the pituitary gland to decrease the release of FSH and positive feedback to the pituitary gland to increase the release of LH. During the early follicular phase of the cycle, the FSH:LH ratio is <1; as the cycle progresses, the FSH:LH ratio becomes >1, demonstrating both positive and negative feedback effects of estradiol on the pituitary gland.

Phase II. Ovulation. As the dominant follicle secretes more and more estradiol, there is marked positive feedback to the pituitary gland to secrete LH. By days 11 to 13 of the normal cycle, an LH surge occurs, which triggers ovulation. Ovulation occurs within 30–36 hours of the LH surge, causing the oocyte to be expelled from the follicle and the follicle to be converted into corpus luteum to facilitate progesterone production during the remainder of the cycle. In addition, there is a slight increase in the basal body temperature (BBT) after ovulation.

Phase III. Luteal phase. The luteal phase of the menstrual cycle is characterized by a change in secretion of sex steroid hormones from estradiol predominance to progesterone predominance. As FSH rises early in the cycle, stimulating production of estradiol, additional LH receptors are created in the granulosa cells and then theca cells. With the LH surge at the time of ovulation, LH facilitates production of progesterone.

The production of progesterone begins approximately 24 hours before ovulation and rises rapidly thereafter. A maximum production of progesterone occurs 3–4 days after ovulation and is maintained for approximately 11 days following ovulation. If fertilization and implantation do not occur, progesterone production diminishes rapidly, initiating events leading to the beginning of a new cycle.

Adequate progesterone production is necessary to facilitate implantation of the fertilized oocyte into the endometrium and to sustain pregnancy into the early first trimester. If the initial rise in FSH is inadequate and the LH surge does not achieve maximal amplitude, an "inadequate luteal phase" can occur, resulting in progesterone production that is inadequate to facilitate implantation of a fertilized oocyte or to sustain pregnancy.

The corpus luteum has a fixed life span of 13–14 days unless pregnancy occurs. If the oocyte becomes fertilized and implants within the endometrium, the early pregnancy begins secreting human chorionic gonadotropin (hCG), which sustains the corpus luteum for another 6–7 weeks.

Physiologic plasma levels of progesterone exert negative feedback on pituitary secretion of both FSH and LH. During the luteal phase of the cycle, both FSH and LH are suppressed to low levels. As the corpus luteum fails and progesterone secretion diminishes, FSH begins to rise to prepare a woman for the next reproductive cycle.

AMENORRHEA

Amenorrhea is the absence or abnormal cessation of the menses.[2] Primary and secondary amenorrhea describe the occurrence of amenorrhea before and after menarche, respectively. Primary amenorrhea can be diagnosed if a patient has normal secondary sexual characteristics but no menarche by 16 years of age.[3] Secondary amenorrhea is the absence of menses for 3 months in women with previously normal menstruation and for 9 months in women with previous oligomenorrhea (scant menses). Secondary amenorrhea is more common than

TABLE 21-1. Medical History Associated with Amenorrhea

PATIENT HISTORY	ASSOCIATIONS
Acne, greasy or oily skin, hirsutism, obesity	PCOS
History of chemotherapy	Ovarian failure
History of radiation therapy	Ovarian failure
History of diabetes mellitus, Addison disease, or thyroid disease	Ovarian failure (autoimmune etiology)
Galactorrhea	Hyperprolactinemia
Weight loss, excessive exercise, severe dieting	Functional amenorrhea
Sexual activity	Pregnancy
Cessation of menstruation followed by hot flashes, vaginal dryness, dyspareunia, or mood swings	Menopause
Rapid progression of hirsutism	Adrenal or ovarian androgen-secreting tumor
Bodybuilder	Exogenous androgen use
Medication history	Amenorrhea secondary to medication use (e.g., danazol, medroxyprogesterone [Depo-Provera], LHRH agonists, LHRH antagonists, oral contraceptives)
Constipation, hoarseness, loss of hair, memory impairment, sensation of cold, weakness, weight gain	Hypothyroidism
Headache, neurological symptoms, visual field defect	CNS lesion (hypothalamic or pituitary)
History of PID, endometriosis, or D&C	Asherman syndrome
History of cautery for cervical intraepithelial neoplasia or obstructive cervical malignancy	Cervical stenosis
Debilitating illness	Functional amenorrhea

CNS = central nervous system; D&C = dilation and curettage; LHRH = luteinizing hormone-releasing hormone; PID = pelvic inflammatory disease; PCOS = polycystic ovary syndrome.
Source: Adapted from references 3 and 5.

primary amenorrhea.[4] The reader is referred to other texts for the evaluation of primary amenorrhea.

The prevalence of amenorrhea not due to pregnancy, lactation, or menopause is approximately 3% to 4%.[2,4] History, physical examination, and measurement of FSH, thyroid-stimulating hormone (TSH), and prolactin will identify the most common causes of amenorrhea. Table 21-1 illustrates how symptoms elicited from a patient history assist in diagnosing the cause of amenorrhea.[3,5]

During the physical examination, the clinician should note the presence of galactorrhea, thyromegaly, or other evidence of hypothyroidism or hyperthyroidism, hirsutism, acne, or signs of virilization.[6] In addition, the patient's body mass index (BMI) should be calculated. A BMI >20 may indicate hypothalamic ovulatory dysfunction, such as occurs with anorexia or other eating disorders. The presence of breast development suggests there has been previous estrogen activity. Excessive testosterone secretion is suggested most often by hirsutism and rarely by increased muscle mass or signs of virilization.

The combination of amenorrhea and galactorrhea strongly correlates with hyperprolactinemia. The history and physical examination should include a thorough assessment of the external and internal genitalia. Table 21-2 illustrates how

TABLE 21-2. Physical Examination Findings Associated with Amenorrhea

FINDINGS	ASSOCIATIONS
Bradycardia	Hypothyroidism, physical or nutritional stress
Coarse skin, coarseness of hair, dry skin, edema of the eyelids, weight gain	Hypothyroidism
Galactorrhea	Hyperprolactinemia
Bradycardia, cold extremities, dry skin with lanugo hair, hypotension, hypothermia, minimum of body fat, orange discoloration of skin (hypercarotenemia)	Anorexia nervosa
Painless enlargement of parotid glands, ulcers or calluses on skin of dorsum of fingers or hands	Bulimia
Signs of virilization: clitoromegaly, frontal balding, increased muscle bulk, severe hirsutism	Adrenal or ovarian androgen-secreting tumor
Centripetal obesity, hirsutism, hypertension, proximal muscle weakness, striae	Cushing syndrome
BMI, hirsutism, acne	PCOS
Transverse vaginal septum, imperforate hymen	Uterine outflow tract obstruction

BMI = body mass index; PCOS = polycystic ovary syndrome.
Source: Adapted from references 3 and 5.

physical examination findings assist in diagnosing the cause of amenorrhea.[3,5]

Hypothyroidism. Although other clinical signs of thyroid disease are usually noted before amenorrhea presents, abnormal thyroid hormone levels can affect prolactin levels. Treatment of hypothyroidism should restore menses, but this may take several months.[7] Table 21-3 provides differential diagnoses of anovulatory disorders and associated serum laboratory findings.[8]

Hyperprolactinemia. A patient with markedly elevated prolactin levels, galactorrhea, headaches, or visual disturbances should receive imaging tests to rule out a pituitary tumor. Adenomas are the most common cause of anterior pituitary dysfunction.[9] A prolactin level more than 100 ng/mL suggests a prolactinoma, and a magnetic resonance imaging (MRI) should be performed. If tumor is excluded as the cause, medications (e.g., oral contraceptive pills, antipsychotics, antidepressants, antihypertensives, histamine (H_2) blockers, and opiates) are the next most common cause of hyperprolactinemia. Medications usually increase prolactin levels to >100 ng/mL.[9]

In most amenorrheic women with hyperprolactinemia, prolactin levels do not decline without treatment, and the

MINICASE 1

Amenorrhea Secondary to Anorexia Nervosa

KIMBERLY M., A 20-YEAR-OLD WOMAN, comes into office for a urine pregnancy test due to no menses for about 2 months. Kimberly M. has no significant past medical history. Further questioning reveals she has lost a total of 30 pounds over the past 4 months and complains of recent acne. Her blood pressure is 100/63; her heart rate is 55 BPM; her temperature is 96.8° F; and her weight is 116 lb. Laboratory tests are as follows: urine hCG negative, FSH 1 million International Units/mL (5–25 million International Units/mL, follicular phase, LH 3 million International Units/mL (5–25 million International Units/mL, follicular phase), prolactin 20 ng/mL (1–25 ng/mL), testosterone 20 ng/dL (20-60 ng/dL).

Question: What is the most likely diagnosis?

Discussion: Kimberly M. complains of amenorrhea. Pregnancy is not a cause of amenorrhea because her urine hCG is negative. She has hypotension, bradycardia, and hypothermia—all indicative of anorexia. Also, she reports significant weight loss in a relatively short period of time.

Treatment of hypothalamic amenorrhea depends on the etiology. Women with excessive weight loss should be screened for eating disorders and treated if anorexia nervosa or bulimia nervosa is diagnosed. Menses usually will return after a healthy body weight is achieved.[15] With young athletes, menses may return after a modest increase in caloric intake or a decrease in athletic training. Women with hypothalamic amenorrhea are also susceptible to the development of osteoporosis.[16] Unless the primary cause can be easily treated, cyclic estrogen-progestin therapy or oral contraceptive pills should be initiated to prevent excessive bone loss.

TABLE 21-3. Differential Diagnosis of Amenorrhea and Associated Serum Laboratory Findings[a]

CONDITION	FSH	LH	PROLACTIN	TESTOSTERONE
Extreme exertion or rapid weight changes	↔	↔	↔	↔
Premature ovarian failure	↑↑↑	↑↑↑↑	↔	↔
Pituitary adenoma	↓	↓	↑↑	↔
Progestational agents	↓	↓	↔	↔
Hypothyroidism	↔	↔	↔/↑	↔
Eating disorders	↓↓	↓↓	↔	↔
PCOS	↔/↓	↑↑	↔/↑	↔/↑↑
CAH	↔	↔	↔	↔/↑

CAH = congenital adrenal hyperplasia; FSH = follicle-stimulating hormone; LH = luteinizing hormone; PCOS = polycystic ovary syndrome.
[a]Normal = ↔; mildly reduced = ↓; moderately reduced = ↓↓; significantly reduced = ↓↓↓; mildly elevated = ↑; moderately elevated = ↑↑; significantly elevated = ↑↑↑
Source: Adapted from reference 8.

amenorrhea does not resolve as long as the prolactin levels remain elevated.[9] In the absence of another organic condition, dopamine agonists (e.g., bromocriptine) are the preferred treatment of hyperprolactinemia with or without a pituitary tumor.[2,10,11]

Uterine outflow obstruction. The most common cause of outflow obstruction in secondary amenorrhea is Asherman syndrome (intrauterine scarring usually from curettage or infection).[3] Certain gynecologic procedures can help diagnose Asherman syndrome. Other causes of outflow tract obstruction include cervical stenosis and obstructive fibroids or polyps.

Functional (hypothalamic) amenorrhea. Functional disorders of the hypothalamus or higher centers are the most common reason for chronic anovulation. Psychogenic stress, weight changes, undernutrition, and excessive exercise are frequently associated with functional hypothalamic amenorrhea, but the pathophysiologic mechanisms are unclear. More cases of amenorrhea are associated with weight loss than with anorexia, but amenorrhea with anorexia nervosa is more severe.[11] (See Minicase 1.) Women involved in competitive sports activities have a threefold higher risk of primary or secondary amenorrhea than others, and the highest prevalence is among long-distance runners.[14]

Ovarian failure. Approximately 1% to 5% of women have premature ovarian failure, a condition where persistent estrogen deficiency and elevated FSH levels occur prior to the age of 40 years, resulting in amenorrhea.[17] Ovarian failure is confirmed by documenting an FSH level persistently in the menopausal range.[2] Iatrogenic causes of premature ovarian failure, such as chemotherapy and radiation therapy for malignancy, have a potential for recovery. Ovarian function may fluctuate, with an increasingly irregular menstrual cycle before permanent ovarian failure. The resulting fluctuations in gonadotropin levels account for the lack of accuracy associated with a single FSH value.[18] Women with ovarian failure should be offered estrogen and progestin treatment to promote and maintain secondary sexual characteristics and reduce the risk of developing osteoporosis.

Menopause represents a type of "physiologic" ovarian failure, which is defined as the cessation of menses for at least 12 months. The climacteric or perimenopause are the periods of waning ovarian function before menopause (i.e., the transition from the reproductive to the nonreproductive years).[1] The average age for menopause in the United States is between 50 and 52 years of age (median 51.5), with 95% of women experiencing this event between the ages of 44 and 55.[1] (See Minicase 2.)

During perimenopause, the ovarian follicles diminish in number and become less sensitive to FSH.[1] The process of ovulation becomes increasingly inefficient, less regular, and less predictable than in earlier years. Initially, a woman may notice a shortening of the cycle length. With increasing inefficiency

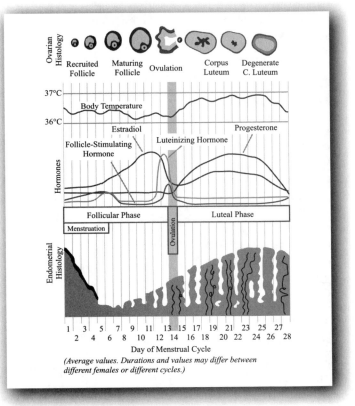

FIGURE 21-2. The menstrual cycle.

MINICASE 2

Premature Menopause

BECCA T., A 38-YEAR-OLD WOMAN, returns for further testing due to complaints of irregular menses over the past 8 months, loss of sexual desire, vaginal dryness, and episodes of warmth and sweating throughout the day. Her past medical history includes breast cancer, for which she underwent chemotherapy and radiation. On examination, her blood pressure is 120/68, her heart rate is 90 BPM, and her temperature is 100°F. The thyroid gland is normal to palpation. Cardiac and lung examinations are unremarkable. Breast examination reveals symmetrical breasts, without masses or discharge. Examination of the external genitalia does not reveal any masses. Her laboratory values were obtained on day 3 of menses and are as follows: FSH 23 million International Units/mL (5–25 million International Units/mL, follicular phase), LH 96 million International Units/mL (5–25 million International Units/mL, follicular phase).

Question: What is the most likely diagnosis?

Discussion: Becca T. complains of irregular menses, vaginal dryness, and intermittent sensations of warmth and sweating. This constellation of symptoms is consistent with the premature menopause. Elevated FSH and LH levels confirm the diagnosis. Due to this woman's age and

medical history, premature menopause is likely. However, even when gonadotropins are in the menopausal range, as in this case, ovulation can still be occurring, albeit irregularly and unpredictably. Thus, it is best to draw FSH and LH levels during the follicular phase because they reach their lowest point during this phase. Hot flushes, which are typical vasomotor changes due to decreasing estrogen levels, are associated with skin temperature elevation and sweating lasting for 2–4 minutes. The low estrogen concentration also has an effect on the vagina by decreasing the epithelial thickness, leading to atrophy and dryness. Although this woman's estradiol level would mostly likely be low, it is not a reliable indicator of menopausal transition because estradiol levels are prone to cyclical fluctuations, as shown in Figure 21-2. Thus, it is not necessary to draw an estradiol level.

Treatment for hot flashes includes hormone therapy with estrogen. Certain antidepressants, such as venlafaxine, can help with vasomotor symptoms as well.[53] When the woman still has her uterus, the addition of progestin to estrogen replacement is important for preventing endometrial cancer. Because of significant increased risks of breast cancer, heart disease, pulmonary embolism, and stroke are associated with hormone therapy, estrogens are not the best treatment for vasomotor symptoms for Becca T.[20,21]

TABLE 21-4. Reference Ranges for Serum Hormones According to Age

CATEGORY	FSH (MILLION INTERNATIONAL UNITS/mL)	LH (MILLION INTERNATIONAL UNITS/mL)	ESTRADIOL (ng/dL)	PROGESTERONE (ng/dL)
Children	5–10	5–10	<2	
Adult women				
Follicular phase	5–25	5–25	1.8–2.4	37–57
Midcycle	20–30	40–80	16.6–23.2	Rising
Luteal phase	5–25	5–25	6.3–7.3	332–1198
Menopausal women	40–250	>75	<1.5	10–22

FSH = follicle-stimulating hormone; LH = luteinizing hormone.

Source: Adapted from reference 19.

TABLE 21-5. Steroid Hormone Serum Concentrations in Premenopausal Women, Postmenopausal Women, and Women After Oophorectomy

HORMONE	PREMENOPAUSAL (NORMAL RANGE IN PARENTHESIS)	POSTMENOPAUSAL	POST-OOPHORECTOMY
Testosterone (ng/dL)	32 (20–60)	23	11
Androstenedione (ng/dL)	150 (50–300)	80–90	80–90
Estrone (pg/mL)	30–200	25–30	30
Estradiol (pg/mL)	35–500	10–15	15–20

Source: Adapted from reference 8.

TABLE 21-6. Suggested Diagnostic Criteria for PCOS

CLINICAL FEATURES

Amenorrhea, oligomenorrhea, or dysfunctional uterine bleeding

Anovulatory infertility

Central obesity

Hirsutism and/or acne

ENDOCRINE ABNORMALITIES ON LABORATORY TESTS

Elevated androgen (i.e., testosterone) levels

Elevated LH

Insulin resistance with hyperinsulinemia

LH-to-FSH ratio >3

Decreased FSH

RADIOLOGIC ABNORMALITIES ON ULTRASOUND EXAMINATION

Increased ovarian stromal density and/or volume

Multiple (nine or more) subcortical follicular cysts

EXCLUSION OF OTHER ETIOLOGIES

CAH

Cushing syndrome

Prolactinoma

Virilizing adrenal or ovarian tumors

CAH = congenital adrenal hyperplasia; FSH = follicle-stimulating hormone; LH = luteinizing hormone; PCOS = polycystic ovary syndrome.
Source: Adapted from reference 8.

MINICASE 3

Polycystic Ovary Syndrome

SARAH T., A 23-YEAR-OLD UNMARRIED WOMAN, presents with a complaint of an increased need to wax her upper lip and chin. Her history includes several irregular menstrual cycles with occasional amenorrhea. She is on hydrochlorothiazide for hypertension, is not sexually active, and otherwise feels well. She is concerned about the irregularity of her menses and future fertility. Pelvic ultrasound reveals a solid appearing right ovary 5–6 cm in diameter. Laboratory findings on day 5 of her menstrual cycle are as follows: urine hCG negative, FSH 15 million International Units/mL (5–25 milliunits/mL, follicular phase), LH 50 million International Units/mL (5–25 milliunits/mL, follicular phase), prolactin 35 ng/mL (1–25 ng/mL), total testosterone 75 ng/dL (20–60 ng/dL).

Question: What is the most likely cause of her symptoms?

Discussion: Polycystic ovary syndrome is the most common cause of Sarah T.'s complaints. The increased hair growth revealed androgen excess in general are symptoms consistent with those of PCOS. Testosterone levels are elevated, LH and prolactin are slightly increased, and the LH to FSH ratio is 3:1, all suggestive of PCOS. Urine hCG ruled out pregnancy. Prolactinoma was not a causative factor because the prolactin level was only mildly elevated. It was not necessary to obtain dehydroepiandrosterone sulfate (DHEAS) levels to determine the presence of a virilizing adrenal tumor because the testosterone level was <200 ng/dL. In order to check for glucose intolerance and the prevention of cardiovascular disease, a glucose level, glucose tolerance test, and lipid profile should be obtained in Sarah T.

---

of the reproductive cycle, the follicular phase shortens, but the luteal phase is maintained at normal length. With the passing of time, some cycles become anovulatory. As menopause approaches, the remaining follicles become almost totally resistant to FSH. The process of ovulation ceases entirely, and cyclic hormone production ends with menopause.

Serum FSH levels begin to rise with diminishing ovarian function; the elevation is first detected in the follicular phase. This early follicular phase rise in FSH has been developed into an endocrine test of ovarian functional reserve in which one draws an FSH level on cycle day 3. With a further decrease in ovarian function, the FSH level will be elevated consistently throughout the menstrual cycle in perimenopausal women and in women after oophorectomy. Table 21-4 depicts serum hormones according to age.[19]

The postmenopausal ovary is not quiescent. Under the stimulation of LH, androgens (i.e., testosterone and androstenedione) are secreted. Testosterone concentrations decline after menopause but remain 2 times higher in menopausal women with intact ovaries than in those with ovaries removed (oophorectomy). Estrone is the predominant endogenous estrogen in postmenopausal women and is termed *extragonadal estrogen* because the concentration is directly related to body weight and androstenedione is converted to estrone in adipose tissue. Table 21-5 compares concentrations of androgens and estrogens in premenopausal women, postmenopausal women, and women after oophorectomy.[1]

Polycystic ovary syndrome. PCOS affects approximately 6% of women of reproductive age and is the most frequent cause of anovulatory infertility.[22,23] Clinical signs include those associated with a hyperandrogenic anovulatory state, including hirsutism and acne. Approximately 70% of affected women manifest growth of coarse hair in androgen-dependent body regions (e.g., sideburn area, chin, upper lip, periareolar area, chest, lower abdominal midline and thigh) as well as upper-body obesity with a waist-to-hip ratio of >0.85.[8] Patients usually retain normal secondary sexual characteristics and rarely exhibit virilizing signs such as clitoromegaly, deepening of the voice, temporal balding or masculinization of body habitus. Suggested diagnostic criteria for PCOS are provided in Table 21-6.[8] (See Minicase 3.)

Women with PCOS often develop polycystic ovaries as a function of a prolonged anovulatory state. Follicular cysts are observed on ultrasound in more than 90% of women with PCOS, but they are also present in up to 25% of normal women.[23-26] Although PCOS is primarily a clinical diagnosis, some debate exists about whether the diagnosis should be based on assays of circulating androgens rather than clinical signs and symptoms of hirsutism and/or acne, as well as glucose abnormality. This is because a substantial number of women with PCOS have no overt clinical signs of androgen excess.[8]

TABLE 21-7. Suggested Laboratory and Radiologic Evaluation of PCOS

17-OHP level[a]

DHEAS level[a]

Dexamethasone suppression test[a]

Fasting glucose level

FSH level

Lipid profile (total, low-density, and high-density lipoproteins)

LH level

Pelvic ultrasound examination[a]

Prolactin level

Testosterone level

hCG level

17-OHP = 17 alpha-hydroxyprogesterone; DHEAS = dehydroepiandrosterone sulfate; FSH = follicle-stimulating hormone; hCG = urine human chorionic gonadotropin; LH = luteinizing hormone; PCOS = polycystic ovary syndrome.
[a]Suggested only in selected patients.
Source: Adapted from reference 8.

Gonadotropin abnormalities in PCOS include elevated levels of testosterone and LH or an elevated LH-to-FSH ratio, an increased LH pulse frequency and altered diurnal rhythm of LH secretion. The LH-to-FSH ratio is used to facilitate diagnosis, and many researchers consider an LH-to-FSH ratio of 3:1 or greater diagnostic of the syndrome.[28] Although serum testosterone levels are mildly-to-moderately elevated in women with PCOS, testosterone levels are also measured to rule out virilizing tumors. Prolactin levels are usually measured to exclude a possible prolactinoma. Suggested laboratory and radiologic evaluation for PCOS is provided in Table 21-7.[8]

Women with PCOS should also be screened for abnormal glucose metabolism because of an association with glucose intolerance. To aid in the possible prevention of cardiovascular disease, lipid abnormalities and blood pressure should be monitored annually.

The primary treatment for PCOS is weight loss through diet and exercise. Modest weight loss can lower androgen levels, improve hirsutism, normalize menses, and decrease insulin resistance.[28] Use of oral contraceptive pills or cyclic progestational agents can help maintain a normal endometrium. The optimal cyclic progestin regimen to prevent endometrial cancer is unknown, but a monthly 10- to 14-day regimen is recommended.[28] Insulin sensitizing agents such as metformin can reduce insulin resistance and improve ovulatory function.[28,29]

Hyperandrogenism. Significantly elevated testosterone or DHEAS levels may also indicate an androgen-secreting tumor (ovarian or adrenal). Levels of 17 alpha-hydroxyprogesterone (17-OHP) can help diagnose adult-onset congenital adrenal hyperplasia (CAH).[28] Cushing syndrome is rare; therefore, patients should only be screened when characteristic signs and symptoms (e.g., striae, buffalo hump, significant central obesity, easy bruising, hypertension, proximal muscle weakness) are present.[28]

Estrogen status. If TSH and prolactin levels are normal, a progesterone challenge test can help detect endogenous estrogen that is affecting the endometrium. A withdrawal bleed usually occurs 2–7 days after the challenge test.[3] A negative progesterone challenge test signifies inadequate estrogenization, and requires further followup for other underlying causes.

HIRSUTISM AND VIRILIZATION

Hirsutism is defined as the presence of excess terminal hair in androgen-dependent areas of a woman's body and occurs in up to 8% of women.[30-32] The disorder is a sign of increased

---

MINICASE 4

Hirsutism Secondary to Adnexal (Ovarian) Tumor

KELLY S., A 45-YEAR-OLD PAROUS WOMAN, has noticed increasing hair growth on her face and abdomen over the past 6 months. She denies using steroid medications, weight change, or a family history of hirsutism. Her menses has been monthly with the exception of the past 3 months. Her past medical and surgical histories are unremarkable. On examination, her thyroid is normal to palpation. She has excess facial hair and male pattern hair on her abdomen. Acne is noted on the face. She also notes increased sweating and some thinning of her hair. Cardiac and pulmonary examinations are normal. Abdominal examination reveals no masses or tenderness. Examination of the external genitalia reveals possible clitoromegaly. Pelvic examination shows a normal uterus and cervix and an 8 cm, right adnexal mass. Her laboratory values obtained on the 4th day of her menstrual cycle are as follows: LH 10 (5–25 million International Units/mL, follicular phase), FSH 7(5–25 million International

Units/mL, follicular phase), total testosterone 85 ng/dL (20–60 ng/dL), prolactin 13 ng/mL (1–25 ng/mL).

Question: What is the mostly likely diagnosis?

Discussion: Kelly S. has onset of excess male-pattern hair over the past 6 months, as well as features of virilism (clitoromegaly). This is evidence of excess androgens. The rapid onset suggests a tumor. Adrenal or ovarian tumors are possibilities. She has a large adnexal mass, so the diagnosis is straightforward. She has irregular menses because of an inhibition of ovulation by androgens. Kelly S. does not have the presentation of Cushing syndrome, such as hypertension, buffalo hump, abdominal striae, and central obesity. Likewise, she does not take any medications containing anabolic steroids (e.g., oxymetholone). Although PCOS is probably the most common cause of hyperandrogenism, it does not fit her clinical presentation because it usually presents with a gradual onset of hirsutism and irregular menses since menarche. Also, she does not have an LH:FSH ratio <3.

TABLE 21-8. Causes of Hirsutism and Associated Laboratory Findings[a]

DIAGNOSIS	TESTOSTERONE	17-OHP	LH/FSH	PROLACTIN	DHEAS	CORTISOL
CAH	↔/↑	↑	↔	↔	↔/↑	↔/↓
PCOS	↔/↑	↔	↔/↑ LH	↔/↑	↔/↑	↔
			↔/↓ FSH			
Ovarian tumor	↑	↔	↔	↔	↔	↔
Adrenal tumor	↑	↔	↔	↔	↑	↔/↑
Pharmacologic agents[b]	↔	↔	↔	↔	↔	↔
Idiopathic	↔	↔	↔	↔	↔	↔
Familial	↔	↔	↔	↔	↔	↔

17-OHP = 17 alpha-hydroxyprogesterone; CAH = congenital adrenal hyperplasia; DHEAS = dehydroepiandrosterone sulfate; FSH = follicle-stimulating hormone; LH = luteinizing hormone; PCOS = polycystic ovary syndrome.
[a]Normal = ↔; decreased = ↓; increased = ↑.
[b]Pharmacologic agents: androgens (e.g., testosterone, danazol), anabolic steroids (e.g., oxymetholone), metoclopramide, methyldopa, phenothiazines (e.g., prochlorperazine), progestins (e.g., medroxyprogesterone).
Source: Adapted from reference 30.

androgen action on hair follicles from increased circulating levels of androgens (endogenous or exogenous) or increased sensitivity of hair follicles to normal levels of circulating androgens.

Infrequently, hirsutism may signal more serious pathology, and clinical evaluation should differentiate benign causes from tumors or other conditions that require specific treatment. Hair growth varies widely among women and distinguishing normal variations of hair growth from true hirsutism is important.

While 60% to 80% of women with hirsutism have increased levels of circulating androgens, degrees of hirsutism correlate poorly with androgen levels.[33] The ovary is the major source of increased levels of testosterone in women who have hirsutism.[30] Dehydroepiandrosterone sulfate is an androgen that arises almost exclusively from the adrenal gland but is an uncommon cause of hirsutism. Nearly all circulating testosterone is bound to sex hormone binding globulin (SHBG) and albumin, with free testosterone being the most biologically active form. When elevated insulin levels are present, SHBG levels decrease while free testosterone levels increase. (See Minicase 4.)

When evaluating hirsutism, it is important to remember that it is only one sign of hyperandrogenism. Other abnormalities associated with excessive levels of androgen include acne, alopecia, android obesity, cardiovascular disease, and dyslipidemia, glucose intolerance/insulin resistance.[30] There are a number of causes of hirsutism. Table 21-8 lists the types of hirsutism according to diagnosis and the associated laboratory findings.[30]

Medications that may cause hirsutism include anabolic steroids (e.g., oxymetholone), danazol, metoclopramide, methyldopa, phenothiazines, and progestins.[30] Increased androgen effect that results in hirsutism can be familial; idiopathic; or caused by excess androgen secretion by the ovary (e.g., tumors, PCOS), excess secretion of androgens by adrenal glands (e.g., CAH, Cushing syndrome, tumor), or exogenous pharmacologic sources of androgens.

Idiopathic hirsutism is common and often familial.[30] It is a diagnosis of exclusion and thought to be related to disorders in peripheral androgen activity. Onset occurs shortly after puberty with slow progression. Patients with idiopathic hirsutism generally have normal menses and normal levels of testosterone, 17-OHP, and DHEAS.

As mentioned previously, PCOS is represented by chronic anovulation and hyperandrogenemia. Patients often report menstrual irregularities, infertility, obesity, and symptoms associated with androgen excess, and diagnosis usually is based on clinical rather than laboratory findings. Up to 70% of patients with PCOS have signs of hyperandrogenism.[30]

Congenital adrenal hyperplasia is a spectrum of inherited disorders of adrenal steroidogenesis, with decreased cortisol production resulting in overproduction of androgenic steroids.[30] The serum 17-OHP measurement is a screening test for adult-onset CAH. Common signs in postadolescent women with adult-onset CAH are hirsutism, acne, and menstrual irregularity. As many as 25% of women with adult-onset CAH also exhibit LH hypersecretion. Serum levels of 17-OHP should be drawn at 8 a.m. in the morning. Basal follicular-phase serum 17-OHP levels above 5 ng/mL suggest adult-onset CAH caused by 21-hydroxylase deficiency. In contrast, serum 17-OHP levels are normal in women with PCOS.[35]

Hirsutism may result from use of exogenous pharmacologic agents, including danazol, anabolic steroids (e.g., oxymetholone), and testosterone. Oral contraceptives containing levonorgestrel, norethindrone, and norgestrel tend to have stronger androgen effects, while those with ethynodiol diacetate, norgestimate, and desogestrel are less androgenic.[30]

Androgen-secreting tumors of the ovary or adrenal are usually heralded by *virilization* (e.g., development of male characteristics in women) and rapid progression of hirsutism and cessation of menses. Androgen-secreting ovarian tumors are more common than adrenal tumors, and are associated with a better prognosis.[30] Virilization occurs in >1% of patients with hirsutism. Signs of virilization are shown in Table 21-9.[30]

A thorough history and physical examination are essential to evaluate women with hirsutism to determine which patients need additional diagnostic testing. Family history is

TABLE 21-9. Signs of Virilization

Acne

Clitoromegaly

Deepening of voice

Hirsutism

Increased libido

Increased muscle mass

Infrequent/absent menses

Loss of breast tissue or normal female body contour

Malodorous perspiration

Temporal hair recession/balding

Source: Adapted from reference 30.

TABLE 21-10. Medical History and Physical Examination in Women with Infertility

HISTORY	PHYSICAL EXAMINATION
Coital practices	Breast formation
Medical history (e.g., genetic disorders, endocrine disorders, PID)	Galactorrhea
	Genitalia (e.g., patency, masses, tenderness, discharge)
Medications (e.g., hormone therapy)	Hyperandrogenism (e.g., hirsutism, acne, clitoromegaly)
Menstrual history	
Sexually transmitted diseases, genital inflammation (e.g., vaginal discharge, dysuria, abdominal pain, fever)	
Previous fertility	
Substance abuse, including caffeine	
Surgical history (e.g., genitourinary surgery)	
Toxin exposure	

PID = pelvic inflammatory disease.
Source: Adapted from reference 41.

important, as 50% of women with hirsutism have a positive family history of the disorder.[30] Physical examination should distinguish normal amounts of hair growth from hirsutism. Diagnosis often can be made on clinical assessment alone or by limited laboratory testing. Virilization should be noted and abdominal and pelvic examinations should be performed to exclude any masses.

Identification of serious underlying disorders is the primary purpose of laboratory testing and should be individualized. About 95% of these patients have PCOS or idiopathic hirsutism.[36] History and physical examination can exclude most underlying disorders, and full hormonal investigation is usually warranted only in those patients with rapid progression of hirsutism, abrupt symptom onset, or virilization.

In patients with hirsutism of peripubertal onset and slow progression, regular menses, otherwise normal physical examination, and no virilization, the likelihood of an underlying neoplasm is small. Whether laboratory investigation in these patients is warranted is controversial; however, some experts recommend routine testing to exclude underlying ovarian and/ or adrenal tumors and adult-onset adrenal hyperplasia.[32] For diagnostic purposes, serum levels of testosterone and 17-OHP are usually sufficient.[30]

For patients with irregular menses, anovulation, PCOS, late-onset adrenal hyperplasia, and idiopathic hirsutism, prolactin levels and thyroid function tests are suggested to identify thyroid dysfunction and pituitary tumors. Testing of glucose, testosterone, and 17-OHP levels should be considered, along with careful breast examination to rule out galactorrhea.

Hirsutism outside of the perimenarchal period, rapid progression of hirsutism, or signs of Cushing syndrome or virilization should indicate the possibility of an ovarian or adrenal neoplasm. Diagnostic testing should examine levels of serum testosterone, 17-OHP, and DHEAS. Levels of serum testosterone >200 ng/dL and/or DHEAS >700 ng/mL are strongly indicative of virilizing tumors.[37] For patients with this degree of hormonal elevation or those whose history suggests a neoplasm, additional diagnostic imaging, including abdominal computed tomography to assess the adrenals, should be performed.

Pharmacologic treatment for hirsutism aims at blocking androgen action at hair follicles or suppression of androgen production. Classes of pharmacologic agents used include oral contraceptives, antiandrogens (e.g., cyproterone), glucocorticoids, GnRH agonists (e.g., leuprolide), antifungal agents (e.g., ketoconazole), topical hair growth retardants (e.g., depilatory agents), and insulin sensitizing agents (e.g., metformin). Response to pharmacologic agents is slow, occurring over many months.

INFERTILITY

Infertility, occurring in 10% to 15% of couples in the United States, is defined as 1 year of frequent, unprotected intercourse during which pregnancy has not occurred.[6,38] Many of these couples present first to their primary care clinician, who may initiate evaluation and treatment. Infertility can be attributed to any abnormality in the female or male reproductive system and is distributed fairly equally among male factors, ovarian dysfunction, and tubal factors. A smaller percentage of cases are attributed to endometriosis, uterine or cervical factors, or other causes. In approximately one-fourth of couples, the cause is uncertain, and the etiology is multifactorial for some couples. The reader is referred to other texts for the evaluation of male infertility. (See Minicase 5.)

The medical history should include details of the menstrual cycle to determine whether the cycles are ovulatory or anovulatory. A menstrual cycle length of 22–35 days suggests ovulatory cycles, as does the presence of mittelschmerz and premenstrual symptoms.[41] During review of the woman's substance use history, caffeine intake should be assessed, as high levels have been associated with lower fertility rates.[41] Table 21-10 describes important elements in obtaining a medical history

Infertility Secondary to Gonorrhea

OLIVIA B., A 35-YEAR-OLD woman who presents with a 3-year history of infertility. She states that her menses began at age 14 years and cycles occur at 28-day intervals. A biphasic BBT chart is recorded. She admits to a past diagnosis of gonorrhea, and a hysterosalpingogram (HSG) shows patent tubes and a normal uterine cavity. Her husband is 37 years old, and his semen analysis is normal.

Question: What is the most likely etiology?

Discussion: Olivia B. has secondary infertility. In approaching infertility, there are five basic factors to examine: (1) ovulatory, (2) uterine, (3) tubal, (4) male factor, and (5) peritoneal (gonorrhea). Olivia B. has regular monthly menses. That in itself argues strongly for regular ovulation; the biphasic BBT chart is further evidence for regular ovulation. Uterine and tubal factors are normal based on the normal HSG. The male factor is not

an issue based on the normal semen analysis. Therefore, the remaining factor not addressed is the peritoneal factor. If the patient had prior cryotherapy to the cervix, the examiner might be directed to consider cervical factor (rare).[12] Similarly, if Olivia B. had symptoms of endometriosis (e.g., dysmenorrhea, dyspareunia), then the examiner would be pointed toward the peritoneal factor. Because there is evidence of a past sexually-transmitted disease, the clinician should consider pelvic inflammatory disease (PID) as a result of the infection.

In general, an infertility evaluation is initiated after 12 months of unprotected intercourse during which pregnancy has not been achieved.[39] Earlier investigation may be considered when historical factors, such as previous PID or amenorrhea, suggest infertility, or when the female partner is older than 35 years, because fertility rates decrease and spontaneous miscarriage and chromosomal abnormality rates increase with advancing maternal age.[40]

and performing a physical examination in women with infertility.[41]

Basal body temperature charting is a simple and inexpensive means of documenting ovulation.[42] In recent years, BBT charting for documentation of ovulation has largely been replaced by use of the less cumbersome urinary LH prediction kit. During ovulatory cycles, an LH surge can be detected in the urine 14–48 hours before ovulation.[43] Additionally, a single midluteal progesterone level, measured at the midpoint between ovulation and the start of the next menstrual cycle, can provide further confirmation as well as information about the adequacy of the luteal phase. A level >6 ng/mL implies ovulation and normal corpus luteal production of progesterone.[44] Of the three tests, the urinary LH kit provides the greatest accuracy in predicting ovulation.[44]

If ovulatory dysfunction is suspected based on the results of initial evaluation, focused laboratory investigation and other testing can help determine the underlying cause. Testing in patients with amenorrhea, irregular menses, or galactorrhea should involve checking FSH, prolactin, and TSH levels.[39,45] Low or normal FSH levels are most common in patients with PCOS and hypothalamic amenorrhea.[39] The presence or absence of obesity and androgenization, generally occurring in women with PCOS, can be used to distinguish between the two disorders.[39] A high FSH level suggests possible ovarian failure.[39] Evaluation of a prolactin level is useful to rule out pituitary tumor, and measurement of TSH is necessary to rule out hypothyroidism.[39] Measurement of 17-OHP and serum testosterone levels is helpful in evaluating patients with hyperandrogenism or late-onset CAH and androgen-secreting tumors.[46] Table 21-11 describes the key laboratory evaluations and specialized tests that should be formed in a woman with infertility.[41]

Women older than 35 years may benefit from testing of FSH and estradiol levels on day 3 of their menstrual cycle to assess ovarian reserve.[40] An FSH level of >10 million International Units/mL, combined with estradiol level of >80 pg/mL,

suggests favorable follicular potential.[40] The clomiphene citrate challenge test, in which the FSH level is obtained on day 3 of the cycle, then again on day 10 after administration of clomiphene citrate 100 mg/day on days 5 to 9, also can be helpful in assessing ovarian reserve.[40] Normal and abnormal values vary by laboratory.

If the initial history and physical examination suggest tubal dysfunction or a uterine abnormality, or if other testing has failed to reveal an etiology, hysterosalpingography (HSG), a radiologic study in which dye is placed into the uterine cavity via a transcervical catheter), is indicated.[39,45] The contour of the uterine cavity, including the presence or absence of any abnormalities, as well as tubal patency can be assessed. Other gynecologic procedures can be performed to further detect tubal or uterine abnormalities.

TABLE 21-11. Laboratory Evaluation in Women with Infertility

DOCUMENT OVULATION
Measurement of midluteal progesterone level
Urinary LH using home prediction kit
BBT charting
DETERMINE ETIOLOGY IF OVULATORY DYSFUNCTION SUSPECTED
Measurement of FSH, prolactin, TSH, 17- OHP, and testosterone (if hyperandrogenism suspected)
ASSESS OVARIAN RESERVE (WOMEN OLDER THAN 35 YEARS)
Measurement of FSH and estradiol levels on day 3 of the menstrual cycle
Clomiphene citrate (Clomid) challenge test

17-OHP = 17 alpha-hydroxyprogesterone; BBT = basal body temperature; FSH = follicle-stimulating hormone; LH = luteinizing hormone; TSH = thyroid-stimulating hormone.
Source: Adapted from reference 41.

Management of infertility involves treating the couple, treating the male partner (if infertile) and treating the female (if infertile). Couple management includes reviewing coital frequency, the "fertile window," use of ovulation kits, and emotional support. For men, they should be referred to a fertility specialist for evaluation of possible semen abnormalities. Women should be treated according to the underlying etiology, whether it is ovulatory dysfunction, tubal/uterine/pelvic disease, or unexplained infertility.

In women with anovulation resulting from a specific condition such as thyroid dysfunction, the underlying cause should be corrected if possible.[39] Women with hyperprolactinemia can be treated with dopaminergic agents (e.g., bromocriptine), which may restore ovulation.[47] Insulin-sensitizing agents, such as metformin, have been shown to increase ovulation and pregnancy rates in patients with PCOS.[48] In other women with ovulatory dysfunction without evident cause or that is not otherwise correctable, the condition can be managed with the use of oral ovulation-inducing agents such as clomiphene citrate and aromatase inhibitors such as letrozole.[49]

Tubal disease may be treated with tubal reparative surgery or with in vitro fertilization (IVF).[41,50] Patients with endometriosis may benefit from laparoscopic ablation or ovulation induction with or without IVF.[51]

LABORATORY TESTS

Follicle-Stimulating Hormone (FSH)[19]

Children = 5–10 million International Units/mL

Adult women, early in cycle = 5–25 million International Units/mL

Adult women, midcycle = 20–30 million International Units/mL

Adult women, luteal phase = 5–25 million International Units/mL

Menopausal women = 40–250 million International Units/mL

Follicle-stimulating hormone is a glycoprotein pituitary hormone produced and stored in the anterior pituitary. It is under complex regulation by hypothalamic GnRH and by the gonadal sex hormones estrogen and progesterone. Normally, FSH increases occur at earlier stages of puberty, 2–4 years before LH reaches comparable levels. In females, FSH stimulates follicular formation in the early stages of the menstrual cycle; then the midcycle surge of LH causes ovulation of the FSH-ripened ovarian follicle.

This test may be helpful in determining whether a gonadal deficiency is of primary origin or is secondary to insufficient stimulation by the pituitary hormones. Decreased FSH levels may occur in feminizing and masculinizing ovarian tumors (when FSH production is inhibited because of increased estrogen secretion); pituitary adenomas; neoplasm of the adrenal glands (which influences secretion of estrogen or androgens); and PCOS.[52] Increased FSH levels occur in premature ovarian failure and in menopause.[52]

TABLE 21-12. Drugs Affecting Plasma Laboratory Test Values of FSH

INCREASE FSH (OR CAUSE FALSE-POSITIVE VALUES)	DECREASE FSH (OR CAUSE FALSE-NEGATIVE VALUES)
Phenytoin	Anabolic steroids (e.g., danazol)
Dopamine agonists (bromocriptine, levodopa)	Carbamazepine
Cimetidine	Diethylstilbestrol
GnRH agonists	Digoxin
Growth hormone-releasing hormone antagonists	Estrogen/oral contraceptives
Ketoconazole	Megestrol
Naloxone	Phenothiazines (e.g., promethazine)
Pravastatin	Pravastatin
Spironolactone	Tamoxifen
Tamoxifen	Testosterone

FSH = follicle-stimulating hormone; GnRH = gonadotropin-releasing hormone.
Source: Adapted from reference 52.

The date of the last menstrual period (LMP) should be considered when interpreting FSH in premenopausal women. Sometimes multiple blood specimens are necessary because of episodic releases of FSH from the pituitary gland. An isolated sample may not indicate the actual activity; therefore, multiple single blood specimens may be required.

Interfering factors include recently administered radioisotopes, hemolysis of the blood sample, pregnancy, and drugs, such as estrogens or oral contraceptives or testosterone. Table 21-12 provides a detailed list of drugs affecting plasma laboratory test values of FSH.[52]

Luteinizing Hormone (LH)[19]

Children = 5–10 million International Units/mL

Adult women, early in cycle = 5–25 million International Units/mL

Adult women, midcycle = 40–80 million International Units/mL

Adult women, luteal phase = 5–25 million International Units/mL

Menopausal women = >75 million International Units/mL

Like FSH, *luteinizing hormone* is a glycoprotein pituitary hormone produced and stored in the anterior pituitary that is under complex regulation by hypothalamic-releasing hormone and by estrogen and progesterone. The midcycle surge of LH causes ovulation.

Decreased LH and FSH occur in pituitary adenomas and eating disorders, while elevated levels are found in ovarian failure and menopause.[52] Elevated basal LH with an LH/FSH ratio of 3 or more and some increase of ovarian androgen in an essentially anovulatory adult woman is presumptive evidence of PCOS.[52]

TABLE 21-13. Drugs Affecting Plasma Laboratory Test Values of LH

INCREASE LH (OR CAUSE FALSE-POSITIVE VALUES)	DECREASE LH (OR CAUSE FALSE-NEGATIVE VALUES)
Anticonvulsants (e.g., phenytoin)	Anabolic steroids (e.g., danazol)
Dopamine agonists (bromocriptine)	Anticonvulsants (e.g., carbamazepine)
Clomiphene	Corticotropin-releasing hormone
GnRH agonists	Diethylstilbestrol
Growth hormone-releasing hormone antagonists	Digoxin
Ketoconazole	Dopamine agonists
Mestranol	Estrogen/oral contraceptives
Spironolactone	Megestrol
	Phenothiazines (e.g., thioridazine)
	Pravastatin
	Progesterone
	Tamoxifen
	Testosterone

GnRH = gonadotropin-releasing hormone; LH = luteinizing hormone.
Source: Adapted from reference 52.

TABLE 21-14. Drugs Affecting Plasma Laboratory Test Values of Progesterone

INCREASE PROGESTERONE (OR CAUSE FALSE-POSITIVE VALUES)	DECREASE PROGESTERONE (OR CAUSE FALSE-NEGATIVE VALUES)
Valproic acid	Ampicillin
Clomiphene	Anticonvulsants (carbamazepine, phenytoin)
Corticotropin	Danazol
Ketoconazole	GnRH agonists (e.g., leuprolide)
Progesterone	Oral contraceptives
Tamoxifen	Pravastatin

GnRH = gonadotropin-releasing hormone.
Source: Adapted from reference 52.

The date of the LMP should be considered in premenopausal females. Interfering factors include recently administered radioisotopes, hemolysis of the blood sample, pregnancy, and estrogens or oral contraceptives or testosterone.[52] A detailed list of drugs that affect plasma laboratory test values of LH are listed in Table 21-13.[52]

Estradiol[19]

Children = <2 ng/dL
Adult women, early in cycle = 1.8–2.4 ng/dL
Adult women, midcycle = 16.6–23.2 ng/dL
Adult women, luteal phase = 6.3–7.3 ng/dL

Together with the FSH levels, *estradiol* is useful in evaluating menstrual and fertility problems, as well as estrogen-producing tumors. Estradiol (E_2) is the most active of the endogenous estrogens. Estriol (E_3) levels in both plasma and urine rise as pregnancy advances; significant amounts are produced in the third trimester. E_3 is no longer considered useful for detection of fetal distress.[52]

Estradiol levels are increased by estrogen-producing tumors, during menstruation, before ovulation and during the 23rd to 41st weeks of pregnancy. Estradiol levels are decreased in premature ovarian failure and in menopause.

Normal estradiol values vary widely between women and in the presence of pregnancy, the menopausal state, or the follicular, ovulatory, or luteal stage of the menstrual cycle.

The number of weeks of gestation should be considered if the patient is pregnant when interpreting estradiol levels. The number of days into the menstrual cycle must be documented

and considered for a nonpregnant woman. Interfering factors include radioactive pharmaceuticals and oral contraceptives.

Progesterone[19]

Adult women, early in cycle = 37–57 ng/dL
Adult women, midcycle = rising
Adult women, luteal phase = 332–1198 ng/dL
Menopausal women = 10–22 ng/dL

Progesterone is primarily involved in the preparation of the uterus for pregnancy and its maintenance during pregnancy. The placenta begins producing progesterone at 12 weeks of gestation. Progesterone level peaks in the midluteal phase of the menstrual cycle. In nonpregnant women, progesterone is produced by the corpus luteum. Progesterone on day 21 is the single best test to determine whether ovulation has occurred.

This test is part of a fertility workup to confirm ovulation, evaluate corpus luteum function, and assess risk for early spontaneous abortion. Testing of several samples during the cycle is necessary. Ovarian production of progesterone is low during the follicular (first) phase of the menstrual cycle. After ovulation, progesterone levels rise for 2–5 days and then fall. During pregnancy, there is a gradual increase from week 9 to week 32 of gestation, often to 100 times the level in the nonpregnant woman. Levels of progesterone in twin pregnancy are higher than in a single pregnancy.

Increased progesterone levels are associated with CAH and some ovarian tumors. Decreased progesterone levels are associated with threatened spontaneous abortion and hyperprolactinemia.

The date of the LMP and/or length of gestation should be recorded. No radioisotopes should be administered within 1 week before the test. Drugs that affect plasma laboratory test values of progesterone are listed in Table 21-14.[52]

Prolactin[19]

Children = 1–20 ng/mL
Adult women = 1–25 ng/mL
Menopausal women = 1–20 ng/mL

Prolactin is a pituitary hormone essential for initiating and maintaining lactation. The gender difference in prolactin does not occur until puberty, when increased estrogen production results in higher prolactin levels in females. A circadian change in prolactin concentration in adults is marked by episodic fluctuation and a sleep-induced peak in the early morning hours.[52]

This test may be helpful in the diagnosis, management, and followup of prolactin-secreting tumors, including the effectiveness of surgery, chemotherapy, and radiation treatment. Levels >100 ng/mL in a nonlactating female indicates a prolactin-secreting tumor; however, a normal prolactin level does not rule out pituitary tumor. In addition to pituitary adenomas, increased prolactin levels are associated with hypothyroidism (primary), PCOS, and anorexia nervosa, and are helpful in the differential diagnosis of infertility.

The patient should be fasting for 12 hours before testing. Specimens should be procured in the morning, 3–4 hours after awakening. Interfering factors occur in a number of circumstances. Increased values are associated with newborns, pregnancy, the postpartum period, stress, exercise, sleep, nipple stimulation, and lactation. Drugs, such as estrogens, methyldopa, phenothiazines, and opiates, may increase values. Dopaminergic drugs inhibit prolactin. Administration of dopaminergic agents can normalize prolactin levels in patients with galactorrhea, hyperprolactinemia, and pituitary tumor. Table 21-15 provides a comprehensive list of drugs affecting plasma laboratory test values of prolactin.[52]

Testosterone[19]

Children = 0.12–0.16 ng/mL
Adult women = 0.20–0.60 ng/mL
Menopausal women = 0.21–0.37 ng/mL

The adrenal glands and ovaries in women secrete *testosterone*. Excessive production virilizes women. Testosterone exists in serum as both unbound (free) fractions and fractions bound to albumin, sex hormone binding globulin (SHBG), and testosterone-binding globulin. Unbound (free) testosterone is the active portion. Testosterone serum levels undergo large and rapid fluctuations; levels peak in early morning.[52]

This test is useful in the detection of ovarian tumors and virilizing conditions in women. It may also be part of a fertility workup. Increased total testosterone levels occur in adrenal neoplasms, CAH, and ovarian tumors (benign or malignant). Increased free testosterone levels are associated with female hirsutism, PCOS, and virilization.

Blood should be drawn in the early morning (between 6–10 a.m.) to obtain the highest levels. Multiple pooled samples drawn at different times throughout the day may be necessary for more reliable results. No radioisotopes should be administered within 1 week before the test.

A number of drugs interfere with test results, including estrogen, androgens, and steroids, which decrease testosterone levels. Other drugs that interfere with interpreting laboratory values of testosterone are provided in Table 21-16.[52]

TABLE 21-15. Drugs Affecting Plasma Laboratory Test Values of Prolactin

INCREASE PROLACTIN (OR CAUSE FALSE-POSITIVE VALUES)	DECREASE PROLACTIN (OR CAUSE FALSE-NEGATIVE VALUES)
Antihistamines	Calcitonin
Calcitonin	Carbamazepine
Cimetidine	Clonidine
Danazol	Cyclosporin A
Diethylstilbestrol	Dexamethasone
Estrogens/oral contraceptives	Dopamine agonists (apomorphine, bromocriptine, levodopa)
Fenfluramine	Ergot alkaloid derivatives
Furosemide	Metoclopramide
GnRH agonists	Nifedipine
Growth hormone-releasing hormone antagonists	Opiates (morphine)
Haloperidol	Pergolide
Histamine antagonists	Ranitidine
Insulin	Rifampin
Interferon	Secretin
Labetalol	Tamoxifen
Loxapine	
Megestrol	
Methyldopa	
Metoclopramide	
Monoamine oxidase inhibitors	
Molindone	
Nitrous oxide	
Opiates (e.g., morphine)	
Parathyroid hormone	
Pentagastrin	
Phenothiazines (e.g., chlorpromazine)	
Phenytoin	
Ranitidine	
Reserpine	
Thiothixene	
Thyrotropin-releasing hormone	
Tumor necrosis factor	
Verapamil	

GnRH = gonadotropin-releasing hormone.
Source: Adapted from reference 52.

TABLE 21-16. Drugs Affecting Plasma Laboratory Test Values of Testosterone

INCREASE TESTOSTERONE (OR CAUSE FALSE-POSITIVE VALUES)	DECREASE TESTOSTERONE (OR CAUSE FALSE-NEGATIVE VALUES)
Anabolic steroids (e.g., danazol)	Alcohol
Anticonvulsants (e.g., phenytoin, barbiturates, rifampin)	Anticonvulsants (e.g., carbamazepine)
Cimetidine	Androgens
Clomiphene	Cimetidine
Dopamine agonists (e.g., bromocriptine)	Corticosteroids (e.g., dexamethasone)
Gonadotropin	Cyclophosphamide
Pravastatin	Diazoxide
Tamoxifen	Diethylstilbestrol
	Digoxin
	Estrogens/oral contraceptives
	Ketoconazole
	GnRH agonists (e.g., leuprolide)
	Magnesium sulfate
	Medroxyprogesterone
	Phenothiazines (e.g., thioridazine)
	Pravastatin
	Spironolactone
	Tetracycline

GnRH = gonadotropin-releasing hormone.
Source: Adapted from reference 52.

SUMMARY

Knowledge of the HPO axis is key to understanding the normal reproductive cycle throughout a woman's lifespan, including pubertal development, menstruation, pregnancy, and menopause. Changes in the gonadotropic hormones FSH and LH, and the ovarian steroid hormones estradiol and progesterone are also essential in identifying underlying causes of amenorrhea, hirsutism, and infertility. Moreover, pharmacologic treatments are often based on alteration of the HPO axis.

Learning Points

1. **What laboratory abnormalities are useful in the differential diagnosis of secondary amenorrhea?**

   Answer: In addition to history and physical examination, FSH, TSH, and prolactin will identify the most common causes of amenorrhea.[2] When the physical examination is normal, the initial investigations should exclude pregnancy and FSH and prolactin concentrations should be assessed. Measurement of TSH is useful to rule out subclinical hypothyroidism, even in the absence of thyroid-related symptoms. If the serum prolactin is persistently elevated, and there is no history of medication or drug use that may elevate prolactin, a pituitary tumor should be considered. When FSH values are normal or low, the problem is most often PCOS, or hypothalamic amenorrhea, such as in anorexia or extreme exercise. Conversely, an elevated FSH would indicate premature ovarian failure or menopause.

2. **What laboratory abnormalities can be used to determine the potential cause of hirsutism or identify suspected PCOS?**

   Answer: A thorough history and physical examination are essential to evaluate women with PCOS and hirsutism to determine which patients need additional laboratory testing. About 95% of these patients will have either possible PCOS or idiopathic hirsutism.[30] A full hormonal investigation is usually warranted only in those patients with rapid progression of hirsutism, abrupt symptom onset, or virilization. Measurement of 17-OHP, testosterone, and DHEAS levels are helpful in evaluating patients with hyperandrogenism, late-onset CAH, and androgen-secreting adrenal and ovarian tumors.

3. **What laboratory evaluations can be done to detect women with ovulatory infertility?**

   Answer: Ovulation disorders constitute 40% of cases of female infertility.[41] To document ovulation, midluteal progesterone levels can be obtained in addition to urinary LH using home prediction kits and BBT charting. If ovulatory dysfunction is suspected based on results of initial evaluation, focused laboratory investigation can help determine the underlying cause. FSH, prolactin, TSH and testosterone levels should be done to identify hypothalamic amenorrhea, pituitary tumor, thyroid disease, and adrenal disease. Low or normal FSH levels are most common in patients with PCOS and hypothalamic amenorrhea, such as occurs with extreme exertion or in eating disorders. Elevated FSH can identify premature ovarian failure. To assess ovarian reserve, measurement of FSH and estradiol levels on day 3 of the menstrual cycle or the clomiphene citrate challenge test may be done.

REFERENCES

1. Beckmann CRB, Ling FW, Smith RP, et al. *Obstetrics and Gynecology.* 5th ed. Philadelphia, PA: Lippincott Williams & Wilkins; 2006.

2. The Practice Committee of the American Society for Reproductive Medicine. Current evaluation of amenorrhea. *Fertil Steril.* 2006;86(suppl 4):S148-S155.

3. Master-Hunter T, Heiman DL. Amenorrhea: Evaluation and treatment. *Am Fam Physician.* 2006;73:1374-1382, 1387.

4. Pettersson F, Fries H, Nillius SJ. Epidemiology of secondary amenorrhea. I. Incidence and prevalence rates. *Am J Obstet Gynecol.* 1973;117:80-86.

5. Desai SP. *Clinician's Guide to Laboratory Medicine.* 3rd ed. Hudson, OH: Lexi-Comp Inc; 2004.

6. American College of Obstetricians and Gynecologists. *Management of infertility caused by ovulatory dysfunction* (Practice Bulletin 34). Washington, DC: ACOG; 2002.

7. Kairo B. Impaired fertility caused by endocrine dysfunction in women. *Endocrinol Metab Clin North Am.* 2003;32:573-592.

8. Hunter MH, Sterrett JJ. Polycystic ovary syndrome: It's not just infertility. *Am Fam Physician.* 2000;62:1079-1088, 1090.

9. Pickett CA. Diagnosis and management of pituitary tumors: recent advances. *Prim Care.* 2003;30:765-789.

10. American College of Obstetrician and Gynecologists. *Management of anovulatory bleeding* (Practice Bulletin 14). Washington, DC: ACOG; 2000.

11. Schlechte J, Dolan K, Sherman B, et al. The natural history of untreated hyperprolactinemia: a prospective analysis. *J Clin Endocrinol Metab.* 1989;68:412-418.

12. Toy EC, Baker B, Ross J, Gilstrap LC, eds. *Case Files: Obstetrics and Gynecology.* 2nd ed. New York, NY: Lange Medical Books/McGraw-Hill; 2007.

13. Lucas AR, Crowson CS, O'Fallon WM, et al. The ups and downs of anorexia nervosa. *Int J Eat Disord.* 1999;26:397-405.

14. Warren MP, Goodman LR. Exercise-induced endocrine pathologies. *J Endocrinol Invest.* 2003;26:873-878.

15. Mitan LA. Menstrual dysfunction in anorexia nervosa. *J Pediatr Adolesc Gynecol.* 2004;17:81-85.

16. Davies MC, Hall ML, Jacobs HS. Bone mineral loss in young women with amenorrhoea. *BMJ.* 1990;301:790-793.

17. Van Campenhout J, Vauclair R, Maraghi K. Gonadotropin-resistant ovaries in primary amenorrhea. *Obstet Gynecol.* 1972;40:6-12.

18. Conway GS, Kaltsas G, Patel A, et al. Characterization of idiopathic premature ovarian failure. *Fertil Steril.* 1996;65:337-341.

19. Sacher R, McPherson RA, Campos J. Reproductive, endocrinology (Chapter 17). In: Sacher R, McPherson RA, Campos J, eds. *Widman's Clinical Interpretation of Laboratory Tests.* 11th ed. Philadelphia, PA: FA Davis Co; 2000:825-870.

20. Dehn B. Care of the menopausal patient: A nurse practitioner's view. *J Amer Acad Nurse Practitioners.* 2007;19:427-437.

21. Writing Group for the Women's Health Initiative Investigators. Risks and benefits of estrogen plus progestin in healthy postmenopausal women. *JAMA.* 2002;288:321-333.

22. Franks S. Polycystic ovary syndrome. *N Engl J Med.* 1995;333:853-861. (Published erratum appears in *N Engl J Med.* 1995;333:1435.)

23. Stein IF, Leventhal ML. Amenorrhea associated with bilateral polycystic ovaries. *Am J Obstet Gynecol.* 1935;29:181-191.

24. Guzick D. Polycystic ovary syndrome: symptomatology, pathophysiology, and epidemiology. *Am J Obstet Gynecol.* 1998;179:S89-S93.

25. Adams J, Franks S, Polson DW, et al. Multifollicular ovaries: clinical and endocrine features and response to pulsatile gonadotropin releasing hormone. *Lancet.* 1985;2(8469/70):1375-1379.

26. Polson DW, Adams J, Wadsworth J, et al. Polycystic ovaries—a common finding in normal women. *Lancet.* 1988;1(8590):870-872.

27. Lobo RA, Granger L, Goebelsmann U, et al. Elevations in unbound serum estradiol as a possible mechanism for inappropriate gonadotropin secretion in women with PCO. *J Clin Endocrinol Metab.* 1981;52:156-158.

28. American College of Obstetricians and Gynecologists. *Polycystic ovary syndrome* (Practice Bulletin 41). Washington, DC: ACOG; 2002.

29. Kolodziejczyk B, Duleba AJ, Spaczynski RZ, et al. Metformin therapy decreases hyperandrogenism and hyperinsulinemia in women with polycystic ovary syndrome. *Fertil Steril.* 2000;73:1149-1154.

30. Hunter MH, Carek PJ. Evaluation and treatment of women with hirsutism. *Am Fam Physician.* 2003;67:2565-2572.

31. Knochenhauer ES, Key TJ, Kahsar-Miller M, et al. Prevalence of the polycystic ovary syndrome in unselected black and white women in the southeastern United States: a prospective study. *J Clin Endocrinol Metab.* 1998;83:3078-3082.

32. Redmond GP, Bergfeld WF. Diagnostic approach to androgen disorders in women: acne, hirsutism, and alopecia. *Cleve Clin J Med.* 1990;57:423-427.

33. Carmina E, Lobo RA. Peripheral androgen blockade versus glandular androgen suppression in the treatment of hirsutism. *Obstet Gynecol.* 1991;78(5 Pt 1):845-849.

34. Deaton MA, Glorioso JE, McLean DB. Congenital adrenal hyperplasia: not really a zebra. *Am Fam Physician.* 1999;59:1190-1196.

35. Goudas VT, Dumestic DA. Polycystic ovary syndrome. *Endocrinol Metab Clin North Am.* 1997;26:893-912.

36. Rittmaster RS. Clinical relevance of testosterone and dihydrotestosterone metabolism in women. *Am J Med.* 1995;98(1A):17S-21S.

37. American College of Obstetricians and Gynecologists. *Evaluation and treatment of hirsute women* (Technical Bulletin 203). Washington, DC: ACOG; 1995.

38. Mosher WD, Bachrach CA. Understanding U.S. fertility: continuity and change in the National Survey of Family Growth, 1988–1995. *Fam Plann Perspect.* 1996;28:4-12.

39. Practice Committee of the American Society for Reproductive Medicine. Optimal evaluation of the infertile female. *Fertil Steril.* 2004;82(suppl 1):S169-S72.

40. Practice Committee of the American Society for Reproductive Medicine. Aging and infertility in women. *Fertil Steril.* 2004;82(suppl 1):S102-S106.

41. Jose-Miller AB, Boyden JW, Frey KA. Infertility. *Am Fam Physician.* 2007;75:849-856, 857-858.

42. McCarthy JJ Jr, Rockette HE. Prediction of ovulation with basal body temperature. *J Reprod Med.* 1986;31(8 suppl):742-747.

43. Miller PB, Soules MR. The usefulness of a urinary LH kit for ovulation prediction during menstrual cycles of normal women. *Obstet Gynecol.* 1996;87:13-717.

44. Guermandi E, Vegetti W, Bianchi MM, et al. Reliability of ovulation tests in infertile women. *Obstet Gynecol.* 2001;97:92-96.

45. Rowe PJ. *WHO Manual for the Standardized Investigation and Diagnosis of the Infertile Couple.* New York, NY: Cambridge University Press; 1993.

46. Azziz R, Zacur HA. 21-Hydroxylase deficiency in female hyperandrogenism: screening and diagnosis. *J Clin Endocrinol Metab.* 1989;69:577-584.

47. Crosignani PG. Management of hyperprolactinemia in infertility. *J Reprod Med.* 1999;44(12 suppl):1116-1120.

48. Nestler JE, Stovall D, Akhter N, et al. Strategies for the use of insulin-sensitizing drugs to treat infertility in women with polycystic ovary syndrome. *Fertil Steril.* 2002;77:209-215.

49. Practice Committee of the American Society for Reproductive Medicine. Use of clomiphene citrate in women. *Fertil Steril.* 2004;82(suppl 1):S90-S96.

50. Lavy G, Diamond MP, DeCherney AH. Ectopic pregnancy: its relationship to tubal reconstructive surgery. *Fertil Steril.* 1987;47:543-556.

51. Practice Committee of the American Society for Reproductive Medicine. Endometriosis and infertility. *Fertil Steril.* 2004;82(suppl 1):S40-S45.

52. Fischbach F. Chemistry Studies, Chapter 6. In: Fischbach F, ed. *A Manual of Laboratory and Diagnostic Tests.* 6th ed. Philadelphia, PA: Lippincott, Williams & Wilkins; 2000:418-498.

53. Evans ML, Pritts E, Vittinghoff E, et al. Management of postmenopausal hot flushes with venlafaxine hydrochloride: a randomized, controlled trial. *Obstet Gynecol.* 2005 Jan;105(1):161-166.

QUICKVIEW | FSH

PARAMETER	DESCRIPTION	COMMENTS
Reference range		
Children	5–10 million International Units/mL	Sometimes multiple blood specimens are necessary because of episodic increases of FSH
Adult women, early cycle	5–25 million International Units/mL	
Adult women, midcycle	20–30 million International Units/mL	Document date of LMP
Adult women, luteal phase	5–25 million International Units/mL	
Menopausal women	40–250 million International Units/mL	
Critical values	Not established	Extremely high or low values should be reported quickly
Natural substance?	Yes	
Inherent action?	Yes	
Major causes of...		
High results		
Associated signs and symptoms	Premature ovarian failure	Hot flashes/night sweats
	Menopause	Hot flashes/night sweats
Low results		
Associated signs and symptoms	Ovarian tumors	Virilization
	Pituitary adenoma	Galactorrhea/visual change
	Adrenal tumors	Virilization
	PCOS	Hirsutism/acne/obesity
	Eating disorders	Cachetic/decreased BMI
After insult, time to...	Not applicable	
Initial evaluation		
Peak values		
Normalization		
Diseases monitored with test	Infertility	FSH >10 million International Units/mL on day 3 of the menstrual cycle suggests normal ovarian reserve
Drugs monitored with the test	Clomiphene challenge test	Compares FSH before and after clomiphene administration to determine ovarian reserve
Significant interferences with laboratory tests	Recently administered radioisotopes	
	Hemolysis of blood sample	
	Estrogens, oral contraceptives, testosterone, progestational agents (see Table 21-12)	
	Pregnancy	

BMI = body mass index; FSH = follicle-stimulating hormone; LMP = last menstrual period; PCOS = polycystic ovary syndrome.

QUICKVIEW | LH

PARAMETER	DESCRIPTION	COMMENTS
Reference range		
Children	5–10 million International Units/mL	Often measured with FSH to determine hormonally-related functions/disorders
Adult women, early cycle	5–25 million International Units/mL	
Adult women, midcycle	40–80 million International Units/mL	Document date of LMP
Adult women, luteal phase	5–25 million International Units/mL	
Menopausal women	>75 million International Units/mL	
Critical values	Not established	Extremely high or low values should be reported quickly
Natural substance?	Yes	
Inherent action?	Yes	
Major causes of...		
High results		
Associated signs and symptoms	Premature ovarian failure	Hot flashes/night sweats
	Menopause	Hot flashes/night sweats
	PCOS	Hirsutism/acne/obesity
Low results		
Associated signs and symptoms	Pituitary adenoma	Galactorrhea/visual changes
	Eating disorders	Cachetic/low BMI
After insult, time to...		
Initial evaluation	Not applicable	
Peak values		
Normalization		
Diseases monitored with test	None	
Drugs monitored with the test	None	
Significant interferences with laboratory tests	Recently administered radioisotopes	
	Hemolysis of blood sample	
	Estrogens or oral contraceptives	
	Progestational agents, testosterone (see	
	Table 21-13)	
	Pregnancy	

BMI = body mass index; FSH = follicle-stimulating hormone; LMP = last menstrual period; LH = luteinizing hormone.

QUICKVIEW | ESTRADIOL

PARAMETER	DESCRIPTION	COMMENTS
Reference range		
Children	<2 ng/dL	Estradiol is most active of endogenous estrogens
Adult women, early cycle	1.8–2.4 ng/dL	
Adult women, midcycle	16.6–23.2 ng/dL	Document date of LMP and/or length of gestation
Adult women, luteal phase	6.3–7.3 ng/dL	
Critical values	Not established	Extremely high or low values should be reported quickly
Natural substance?	Yes	
Inherent action?	Yes	
Major causes of...		
High results		
Associated signs and symptoms	Estrogen-producing tumors	
	Menstruation/pre-ovulatory	
	23rd to 41st weeks of pregnancy	
Low results		
Associated signs and symptoms	Menopause	Hot flashes/night sweats
	Premature ovarian failure	Hot flashes/night sweats
After insult, time to...	Not applicable	
Initial evaluation		
Peak values		
Normalization		
Diseases monitored with test	Fertility	Estradiol >80 pg/mL on day 3 suggests adequate ovarian reserve
Drugs monitored with the test	None	
Significant interferences with laboratory tests	Radioactive pharmaceuticals and oral contraceptives	

LMP = last menstrual period.

QUICKVIEW | PROGESTERONE

PARAMETER	DESCRIPTION	COMMENTS
Reference range		
Adult women, early cycle	37–7 ng/dL	Document LMP and/or length of gestation
Adult women, midcycle	Rising	
Adult women, luteal phase	332–1198 ng/dL	
Menopausal women	10–22 ng/dL	
Critical values	Not established	Extremely high or low values should be reported quickly
Natural substance?	Yes	
Inherent action?	Yes	
Major causes of...		
High results		
Associated signs and symptoms	CAH	↑17-OHPb, ↑DHEASc, ↓cortisol, hirsutism/acne
	Ovarian tumor	Virilization, rapid progression of symptoms
Low results		
Associated signs and symptoms	Spontaneous abortion	Vaginal bleeding
After insult, time to...	Not applicable	
Initial evaluation		
Peak values		
Normalization		
Diseases monitored with test	Infertility	Midluteal progesterone >6 ng/mL suggests ovulation
Drugs monitored with the test	None	
Significant interferences with laboratory tests	Drugs may affect test outcome (see Table 21-14)	

17-OHP = 17 alpha-hydroxyprogesterone; CAH = congenital adrenal hyperplasia; DHEAS = dehydroepiandrosterone sulfate; LMP = last menstrual period.

QUICKVIEW | PROLACTIN

PARAMETER	DESCRIPTION	COMMENTS
Reference range		
Children	1–20 ng/mL	Obtain 12-hr fasting samples in the morning
Adult women	1–20 ng/mL	
Menopausal women	1–20 ng/mL	
Critical values	Levels >100 ng/mL in nonlactating female may indicate a prolactin-secreting tumor	Extremely high or low values should be reported quickly
Natural substance?	Yes	
Inherent action?	Yes	
Major causes of...		
High results		
Associated signs and symptoms	Pituitary adenoma	Galactorrhea/visual changes
	Hypothyroidism (primary)	Coarse skin and hair
	PCOS	Hirsutism/acne/obesity
	Anorexia nervosa	Cachetic/low BMI
Low results		
Associated signs and symptoms	No common disorders	
After insult, time to...	Not applicable	
Initial evaluation		
Peak values		
Normalization		
Diseases monitored with test	Pituitary adenoma	
Drugs monitored with the test	Dopaminergic drugs	To monitor effect on prolactin levels in pituitary adenoma
Significant interferences with laboratory tests	Increased values are associated with newborns, pregnancy, postpartum period, stress, exercise, sleep, nipple stimulation, and lactation	
	Drugs (estrogens, methyldopa, phenothiazines, opiates) may increase values (see Table 21-15)	

BMI = body mass index; PCOS = polycystic ovary syndrome.

QUICKVIEW | TESTOSTERONE

PARAMETER	DESCRIPTION	COMMENTS
Reference range		
Children	0.12–0.16 ng/mL	Unbound (free) testosterone is active form
Adult women	0.20–0.60 ng/dL	Draw levels between 6–10 a.m.
Menopausal women	0.21–0.37 ng/dL	
Critical values	Testosterone >200 ng/dL indicates virilizing tumor	Extremely high or low values should be reported quickly
Natural substance?	Yes	
Inherent action?	Yes	
Major causes of...		
High results		
Associated signs and symptoms	Adrenal neoplasms	Virilization, ↑DHEAS, ↑cortisol, rapid progression of symptoms
	CAH	↑17-OHP, ↑DHEAS, ↓cortisol, hirsutism
	Ovarian tumors	Virilization, rapid progression of symptoms
	PCOS	Hirsutism/acne/obesity, ↑DHEAS
	Cushing syndrome	Buffalo hump/obesity/striae
Low results		
Associated signs and symptoms	No common disorders	
After insult, time to...	Not applicable	
Initial evaluation	Rapid progression of symptoms indicative of ovarian or adrenal tumor	
Peak values		
Normalization		
Diseases monitored with test	None	
Drugs monitored with the test	None	
Significant interferences with laboratory tests	Estrogen therapy increases testosterone levels (see Table 21-16)	
	Many drugs, including androgens and steroids, decrease testosterone levels (see Table 21-16)	

17-OHP = 17 alpha-hydroxyprogesterone; CAH = congenital adrenal hyperplasia; DHEAS = dehydroepiandrosterone sulfate; PCOS = polycystic ovary syndrome.
Source: Adapted from references 19 and 52.

CHAPTER 22

COMMON MEDICAL DISORDERS OF AGING MALES—CLINICAL AND LABORATORY TEST MONITORING

MARY LEE, ROOHOLLAH SHARIFI

This chapter focuses on laboratory and clinical tests used to evaluate several common medical disorders in aging males—androgen deficiency, erectile dysfunction, benign prostatic hyperplasia (BPH), prostate cancer, and prostatitis. Tumor markers for assessing testicular cancer and labs for diagnosis of urinary tract infection and venereal diseases are discussed in other chapters.

HYPOGONADISM

Hypogonadism refers to medical conditions when the testes or ovaries fail to produce adequate amounts of testosterone or estrogen, respectively, to meet the physiologic needs of the patient. For the purposes of this chapter on men's health disorders, hypogonadism will refer to conditions when testicular production of testosterone is inadequate. When compared to the usual serum testosterone levels observed in adult men, age 20 years old, the estimated prevalence of hypogonadism is 2% to 5% in men age 40 years old, 15% to 25% in men age 50 years old, and 30% to 70% in men age 70 years old.[1] A consistent observation is that increasing patient age is associated with a greater percentage of men with serum testosterone levels that are below the normal range.

Testosterone Production and Physiologic Effects

The principal androgen in males is *testosterone,* and it is produced by the testes. Testosterone comprises approximately 90% of circulating androgens. Dehydroepiandrosterone, produced by the adrenal glands, has little androgenic activity and is converted to androstenedione to exert physiologic effects. Androgens enter the bloodstream, which delivers the hormones to target cells in muscle, bone, brain, reproductive and genital organs.[1] At some targets, testosterone itself appears to be physiologically active (e.g., central nervous system). However, at other targets where 5-alpha reductase enzyme is expressed (e.g., prostate, scalp) testosterone is activated intracellularly by 5-alpha reductase to dihydrotestosterone, which has at least twice the potency of testosterone. Two separate forms of 5-alpha reductase enzymes exist: Type I and Type II. Each enzyme type tends to predominate in a particular tissue. Type I enzyme concentrates in the skin, liver, and sebaceous glands of the scalp. Type II 5-alpha reductase predominates in the prostate and hair follicles of the scalp, and dihydrotestosterone in these tissues causes the development of BPH and alopecia, respectively.[2,3]

In nontarget tissue, including the liver and adipose tissue, the aromatase enzyme can convert excess androgen to estrone and estradiol. In males, excess estrogen or a higher ratio of serum estrogen to androgen can result in gynecomastia and decreased libido.

Testosterone is responsible for various age-related physiologic effects in males, but most notably, it is responsible for development of secondary sexual characteristics in males (Table 22-1).

In young men, 4–10 mg of testosterone is produced each day. Testosterone secretion follows a circadian pattern, such that the highest secretion occurs at 7:00 a.m. and the lowest secretion occurs at 8:00 p.m. Testosterone circulates in three different forms: free (unbound) testosterone; albumin-bound testosterone; and sex hormone-binding globulin (SHBG)-bound testosterone. These forms comprise

TABLE 22-1. Physiologic Effects of Testosterone and Dihydrotestosterone[2-4]

STAGE OF LIFE OF MALE	PHYSIOLOGIC EFFECT
In utero	Normal differentiation of male internal and external genitalia
At puberty	Male body habitus, deepening of voice, male hair distribution, enlargement of testes, penis, scrotum, and prostate; increased sexual drive and bone growth
In adult	Sexual drive, muscle strength and mass, bone mass, prostate enlargement, male hair growth and distribution, spermatogenesis

approximately 2%, 54%, and 44% of circulating testosterone levels, respectively. Free testosterone is physiologically active. While albumin-bound testosterone is inactive, testosterone can be easily released from albumin, which has low affinity for the androgen. Therefore, albumin-bound testosterone has the potential to be bioavailable and become physiologically active.[4] Total bioavailable testosterone is about 50% of circulating serum testosterone. In contrast, SHBG has high affinity for testosterone, and SHBG-bound testosterone is physiologically inactive. The production of SHBG in the liver is increased by estrogen and thyroid hormone and decreased by androgens and corticosteroids.

Testosterone secretion is regulated by the hypothalamic-pituitary gonadal axis. The hypothalamus secretes gonadotropin-releasing hormone (GnRH). This acts on anterior pituitary receptors to stimulate the release of luteinizing hormone (LH) and follicle-stimulating hormone (FSH). Luteinizing hormone stimulates testicular Leydig cells to produce testosterone. Testosterone is then released into the bloodstream. Once the serum level of testosterone increases into the normal physiological range, it triggers a negative feedback loop, which inhibits GnRH release from the hypothalamus. Pituitary LH release is inhibited, too, but generally less so than GnRH. Follicle-stimulating hormone acts on testicular Sertoli cells to stimulate spermatogenesis.

Hormonal Changes Associated with Primary, Secondary, and Tertiary Hypogonadism

Primary hypogonadism occurs when the testicles are absent or surgically removed or when they are nonfunctional secondary to an acquired disease (e.g., mumps orchitis). *Secondary hypogonadism* occurs when the pituitary fails to release adequate amounts of LH, and thus, the testes are not stimulated to produce adequate amounts of testosterone. *Tertiary hypogonadism* refers to a disorder of the hypothalamus such that there is inadequate release of GnRH, and a subsequent decrease in release of LH from the pituitary and testosterone from the testes (Table 22-2).

Late-Onset Hypogonadism

Late-onset hypogonadism, also known as *andropause* or *androgen deficiency in aging males (ADAM)*, refers to the biochemical changes associated with age-related alterations in the hypothalamic-pituitary-gonadal axis, which may or may not be associated with clinically significant symptoms and signs.[4,5] As testosterone levels decline, some men develop symptoms including decreased libido, erectile dysfunction, mood changes, difficulty in coping with stress, lack of motivation, inability to concentrate, a diminished sense of well-being,

TABLE 22-2. Comparison of Laboratory Test Results in Patients with Primary, Secondary, and Tertiary Hypogonadism[5,6]

	PRIMARY	SECONDARY	TERTIARY
Common causes	Klinefelter syndrome	Kallmann syndrome	Infectious or infiltrative diseases of the hypothalamus (e.g., tuberculosis, sarcoidosis, infectious abscess)
	Cryptorchidism	Pituitary adenoma or infarction	
	Mumps orchitis	Prolactinoma	
	Orchiectomy	Medications: estrogens, LHRH agonists (e.g., leuprolide, goserelin), LHRH antagonists (e.g., degarelix), prolonged course of high dose corticosteroids, megestrol acetate, medroxyprogesterone, long-acting opioids	
	Irradiation of testes		
	Traumatic injury to the testes		
	5-α reductase deficiency		
	Aging		
	Autoimmune disorders (e.g., Hashimoto thyroiditis or Addison disease)		
	Medications: high dose ketoconazole, cytotoxins		
Serum testosterone level	Decreased	Decreased	Decreased
LH level	Increased	Decreased	Decreased
GnRH level	Increased	Increased	Decreased

GnRH = gonadotropin-releasing hormone; LH = luteinizing hormone ; LHRH = luteinizing hormone–releasing hormone.

TABLE 22-3. Characteristics of Late-Onset Hypogonadism in Aging Males Versus Menopause in Aging Females[6,7]

	LATE-ONSET HYPOGONADISM	MENOPAUSE
Time period over which gonadal function decreases	Decades, beginning at age 30–40 years[3]	4–6 years, beginning at approximately age 50–52 years old
Fertility is maintained	Yes	No
Symptoms	Decreased libido, erectile dysfunction, gynecomastia, weight gain, moodiness, decreased sense of well-being, muscle aches, weight gain, osteoporosis	Menstrual cycles become progressively heavier and lighter, shorter and longer, and then stop; hot flashes, weight gain, vaginal dryness, dyspareunia, and hair loss
Symptoms and signs are linked to serum level of gonadal hormone	No	Yes

generalized muscle aches, decreased muscle strength, increased body fat, gynecomastia, and decreased bone mineral density.[4] However, other men with decreased testosterone levels do not complain of their symptoms or have vague, nonspecific symptoms (e.g., malaise or decreased energy) for which they do not seek medical treatment.[5] Although late-onset hypogonadism is often compared to the menopause in aging females, these conditions are different (Table 22-3). In males gonadal function decreases over decades, and symptoms develop slowly and often are not attributed to decreasing hormone levels. In females, gonadal function decreases over a comparatively shorter time period of 4–6 years, and symptoms are closely associated with decreasing hormone levels.

Hormonal Changes Associated with Late-Onset Hypogonadism[4-6]

Low serum testosterone levels in patients with late-onset hypogonadism are due to multiple physiologic changes including[4,5]

1. Increased sensitivity of the hypothalamus and pituitary gland to negative feedback. Thus, even low circulating testosterone levels stimulate the negative feedback loop.
2. Irregular, nonpulsatile secretion pattern of LH
3. Loss of usual circadian secretion pattern of testosterone from Leydig cells; smaller difference in peak and trough serum concentrations during the day when compared to young adult males
4. Increased production of SHBG, which increases the plasma concentration of physiologically-inactive SHBG-bound testosterone[3]
5. Decreased number of functioning Leydig cells, which results in an age-related decrease in testicular production of testosterone. As mentioned previously, the decrease in testicular production occurs over decades. Starting at age 40, serum testosterone levels decrease by 1% to 2% annually. At age 80, the mean serum testosterone declines by approximately 40% of that typically observed in men at age 40.[7]

Of importance, late-onset hypogonadism was once thought to be a type of primary hypogonadism. However, multiple alterations in the hypothalamic pituitary gonadal axis suggest that late-onset hypogonadism can present as either primary or secondary hypogonadism in individual patients. This phenomenon occurs in the face of a wide range of serum (total)

testosterone and bioavailable testosterone levels among elderly males. Whereas some symptomatic elderly males have levels that are below the normal physiological range, others have levels that are decreased but are still within the normal range.[8]

A male patient, age 50 years or older, who presents with symptoms of hypogonadism (e.g., decreased libido, unexplained mood changes) or signs of hypogonadism (e.g., gynecomastia, testicular atrophy) should undergo evaluation for late-onset hypogonadism. However, this is a diagnosis of exclusion, which is made after all other causes of low serum concentrations of testosterone have been ruled out. To assess symptom severity, the patient is commonly asked to complete a validated self-assessment questionnaire at baseline and at regular intervals after treatment is started. For example, the St. Louis University Androgen Deficiency in Aging Males questionnaire includes 10 questions to which the patient responds either "yes" or "no."[9,10] An affirmative response to at least three questions on the survey is considered significant. A similar alternative self-assessment instrument is the Aging Male Symptom Scale.[11] These surveys are sensitive but not specific for hypogonadism. Rather than being used for diagnostic purposes, they are used prior to and during treatment to monitor the effectiveness of treatment.[2,4,5]

Late-onset hypogonadism should be treated with testosterone supplements if the patient has both symptoms of hypogonadism and an unequivocal serum testosterone level of 230 ng/dL or less, based on at least two separate serum testosterone measurements on different days, and provided that the patient has no contraindications for androgen supplementation.[5,12] In addition to relieving symptoms and potentially preventing osteoporosis and bone fracture from long-term hypogonadism, treatment may decrease the prevalence of prostate cancer, which tends to occur more frequently in men with hypogonadism.[13] For a patient with symptoms of hypogonadism and a serum testosterone level of 230–350 ng/dL, the treatment of late-onset hypogonadism should be decided after assessing the benefits versus the risks of androgen supplementation by the physician and patient. Controversy exists on the value of testosterone replacement in this subset of patients.[12,14] As long as the serum testosterone level is in the normal physiologic range, some physicians will not prescribe testosterone supplements. This is because some evidence suggests that administration of exogenous androgens to increase the serum testosterone level from one end of the normal range to a higher point within the normal range does not improve or increase sexual drive or energy.[15,16] Rather than prescribe testosterone supplements, the physician will treat individual symptoms with specific nonandrogen treatments. For example, if the patient is moody or depressed, psychotherapy may be beneficial. If the patient has erectile dysfunction, then a phosphodiesterase inhibitor may be indicated. On the other hand, there is evidence that suggests that signs and symptoms of hypogonadism respond to different levels of serum testosterone; libido may be restored at the lower end of the normal physiologic range, whereas increased bone mineralization is observed when serum testosterone is at the higher end of the normal physiologic range.[4,16] For this reason, some physicians will prescribe testosterone replacement to patients who have serum testosterone levels at the low end of the normal range. Patients with symptoms of hypogonadism and a serum testosterone level of 350 ng/dL or more should not receive testosterone supplements.

Once a testosterone replacement regimen is initiated, the patient should return for assessment of the efficacy and safety of treatment every 3 or 4 months during the first year.[14,16] A minimum clinical trial of a testosterone supplement is 3 months.[4,5] Within the normal serum testosterone range, an adult male will generally have appropriate sexual drive and feel energetic.

Assessments of efficacy should include serum testosterone levels, which should return to the normal range by the third month. The target serum testosterone level when the patient is receiving testosterone replacement is 400–500 ng/dL.[4] Other assessments include a persistent reduction of symptoms of hypogonadism as assessed by medical history and the patient's responses to the self-assessment questionnaire. Since testosterone can theoretically stimulate prostate enlargement and is a cocarcinogen in the development of prostate cancer, the patient should also annually undergo a digital rectal exam of the prostate and PSA testing. Finally, since excess androgen is converted to estrogen, which can induce breast cancer or gynecomastia, the patient should also undergo breast examination prior to the start of and periodically during treatment.

Testosterone, Total

Normal range, adult male: 280–1100 ng/dL or 9.7–38.14 nmol/L
Normal range, age-related:
Male, 6–9 yr old: 3–30 ng/dL or 0.10–1.04 nmol/L
Male, pubertal: 265–800 ng/dL or 9.19–27.74 nmol/L

A routine serum testosterone level reflects the total concentration of testosterone in the bloodstream, in all three of its forms: free, albumin-bound, and SHBG-bound. Testosterone secretion follows a circadian pattern such that morning levels are approximately 20% higher than evening levels, which is a difference of approximately 140 ng/dL between the peak and nadir serum levels. In addition, intrapatient variability in measured testosterone levels is characteristic from day to day, from week to week, and seasonally.[17] Thus, when obtaining serum testosterone levels, it is recommended that

TABLE 22-4. Common Causes of Decreased and Increased Total Testosterone Levels[6,15]

TOTAL TESTOSTERONE LEVELS	
DECREASED	**INCREASED**
Primary or secondary hypogonadism	Hyperthyroidism
Primary or secondary hypopituitarism	Adrenal tumors
	Adrenal hyperplasia
Klinefelter syndrome	Testicular tumors
Orchiectomy	Precocious puberty
Traumatic injury to testicles	Excessive testosterone use
Testicular maldescent	Anabolic steroids
Mumps	
Sickle cell disease	
Hepatic cirrhosis	
Late stage kidney disease	
Immobilization	
Malnutrition	
Acute illness	
Age greater than 50 years	
Hyperprolactinemia	
Hypothyroidism	
Excessive exercise	
Abiraterone	
Estrogens	
Corticosteroids, high doses	
LHRH agonists	
LHRH antagonists	
Digoxin	
Cyclophosphamide	
Ketoconazole	
Opiates	

LHRH = luteinizing hormone-releasing hormone.

blood samples be obtained between 8:00 a.m. to 11:00 a.m. Furthermore, to confirm a low serum testosterone level, it is also recommended that a second sample be obtained usually at least 1 week apart. If the patient has a medical disorder or is taking medication that can alter serum testosterone levels, it is recommended that testing for serum testosterone levels be deferred until the medical disorder resolves or the medication is discontinued. Common causes of decreased and increased serum testosterone levels are listed in Table 22-4.

The normal range is wide for serum testosterone levels and is based on lab results for young adult males. Although this normal range is applied to interpretation of serum testosterone levels in elderly males, no single threshold serum testosterone value has been identified to be pathognomonic for hypogonadism in this age group.[16,18] When treating patients with prostate

TABLE 22-5. Comparison of the Percentage of Serum Bioavailable Testosterone in Young Versus Old Male[6]

	YOUNG MALE	OLDER MALE
% of total testosterone, which is free testosterone	2	2
% of total testosterone, which is bound to albumin	38	20
% of total testosterone, which is bound to SHBG	60	78
% of bioavailable testosterone (% free + % albumin-bound)	40	22

SHBG = sex hormone-binding globulin.

cancer with LHRH agonists or antagonists, medical castration is induced. The target serum testosterone level is 50 ng/dL or less.

Testosterone levels are commonly determined using radioimmunoassay, nonradioactive immunoassays, or chemiluminescent detection methods. However, these methods exhibit significant performance variability in the normal range.[19,20] Thus, some experts recommend that a normal range of serum testosterone be determined for each clinical laboratory that runs the assay.[21] Such a determination would require measurement of serum testosterone in approximately 40 normal, healthy men, aged 20–40 years.[4,6] The U.S. Centers for Disease Control and Prevention has initiated a program to standardize testosterone assays, which involves providing reference material to calibrate immunoassays. This should reduce the variability of testosterone lab results among laboratories.[15] Alternatively, stable isotope dilution liquid chromatography using benchtop tandem mass spectrometry has improved accuracy over radioimmunoassay and is simple and fast.[22]

Free Testosterone

Normal age-related range, adult male:
10–15 ng/dL, age 20–29 yr
9–13 ng/dL, age 30–39 yr
7–11 ng/dL, age 40–49 yr
6–10 ng/dL, age 50–59 yr
5–9 ng/dL, age >60 yr

Free testosterone levels are the best reflection of physiologically-active androgen. When compared to young adult males, elderly males experience an almost 20% decrease in albumin-bound testosterone and an almost 20% increase in SHBG-bound testosterone in the circulation. Since free testosterone is in equilibrium with albumin-bound testosterone, the amount of bioavailable testosterone is decreased in elderly males, and therefore, elderly males may develop symptoms of hypogonadism despite having serum total testosterone levels near the normal range (Table 22-5).

Free testosterone levels are altered by the concentration of SHBG. Thus, free testosterone levels are preferred in patients with diseases or taking medications, which increase or decrease levels of SHBG (Table 22-6), or when the patient has symptoms of hypogonadism but has a serum total testosterone in the normal physiologic range.[23]

The most accurate assay method to measure free testosterone is by centrifugal ultrafiltration or equilibrium dialysis technique. However, such assays are not routinely available and are expensive. Thus, many laboratories offer radioimmunoassay for free testosterone levels. Although inexpensive, this method is associated with less accurate results.[24] Saliva specimens using a direct luminescence immunoassay can be used to measure free testosterone but is rarely done.[25]

If free testosterone levels cannot be measured using an assay, the level may be estimated (a commonly used calculator is available at http://www.issam.ch/freetesto.htm; last accessed March 2, 2012). By inserting serum levels of albumin, SHBG, and total testosterone into the online calculator, the patient's free testosterone level is derived. Estimated values are comparable to measured values by equilibrium dialysis.[23]

Bioavailable Testosterone

Normal age-related range, adult male:
83–257 ng/dL, age 20–29 years
72–235 ng/dL, age 30–39 years
61–213 ng/dL, age 40–49 years
50–190 ng/dL, age 50–59 years
40–168 ng/dL, age 60–69 years
Not established, age greater than 70 years
Also expressed as percentage of total serum testosterone
Normal range, adult male: 12.3% to 63%

Bioavailable testosterone levels measure the concentration of free testosterone and albumin-bound testosterone in a serum sample. Since albumin has low affinity for testosterone, reversible binding of testosterone to albumin allows an equilibrium to be established between free and albumin-bound testosterone fractions. Thus, these two forms of circulating testosterone are considered bioavailable and physiologically-active.[4,6] As men age, bioavailable testosterone levels decrease as serum SHBG levels increase. Similar to free testosterone levels, which are dependent on SHBG levels, bioavailable testosterone levels may be preferred when assessing testosterone activity in patients with significant alterations of SHBG (Tables 22-5 and 22-6).

An ammonium sulfate precipitation assay is used to measure bioavailable testosterone. It is expensive and technically challenging to perform. For this reason, this test is not commonly available in clinical labs. If bioavailable testosterone levels cannot be measured using an assay, the level may be estimated. (A commonly used calculator is available at http://www.issam.ch/freetesto.htm; last accessed March 2, 2012.) By inserting serum levels of albumin, SHBG, and total testosterone into the online calculator, the patient's bioavailable testosterone level is derived.

ERECTILE DYSFUNCTION

Erectile dysfunction is the consistent inability over a minimum duration of 3 months to achieve a penile erection sufficient for sexual intercourse.[26] The prevalence of erectile dysfunction increases with increasing patient age. According to the

TABLE 22-6. Medical Conditions and Drugs That Alter SHBG Concentrations

	INCREASED SHBG	DECREASED SHBG
Medical conditions that produce an alteration of SHBG concentration	Hepatic cirrhosis	Hypothyroidism
	HIV disease	Nephrotic syndrome
	Anorexia nervosa	Obesity
	Hyperthyroidism	Acromegaly
	Aging males	Cushing syndrome
	Prolonged stress	
Drugs that produce an alteration of SHBG concentration	Estrogens	Testosterone supplements, excessive doses
	Phenytoin	
		Corticosteroids
		Progestins

HIV = human immunodeficiency virus; SHBG = sex hormone-binding globulin.

TABLE 22-7. Comparison of Organic and Psychogenic Erectile Dysfunction[26]

	ORGANIC	PSYCHOGENIC
Patient age	Older male	Younger male
Onset	Gradual, unless erectile dysfunction is due to traumatic injury	Sudden and complete loss of erectile function
Linked to a particular event in the patient's life	No	Yes (e.g., divorce, job-related stress financial stress)
Patient has a normal libido	Yes	No
Patient has nocturnal erections, which are reflex reactions	No	Yes
Patient has erections on awakening	No	Yes
Patient has erections with masturbation	No	Yes
Patient has erections with foreplay	No	Yes
Patient has concurrent medical illnesses that could contribute to erectile dysfunction	Yes	No
Patient's partner is perceived to be a problem in the relationship prior to the onset of erectile dysfunction	No	Yes
Patient has performance anxiety prior to the onset of erectile dysfunction	No	Yes

Massachusetts Male Aging Study, the prevalence of moderate erectile dysfunction increases in men from the 4th decade of life to the 6th decade of life, from 12% to 46%, respectively.[27] In the health professional study of men, age 50 years or older, the overall prevalence of erectile dysfunction was 33%, with an increased prevalence in patients with risk factors, including cigarette smoking, excessive alcohol intake, sedentary lifestyles, and obesity.[28,29] However, advancing age is not considered an independent risk factor for erectile dysfunction.

The causes of erectile dysfunction are broadly divided into two types: *organic* and *psychogenic*.[26,30] Most patients with erectile dysfunction have the organic type, in which concurrent medical illnesses interfere with one or more physiologic components essential for a penile erection (Table 22-7).[30] That is, the patient has one or more medical illnesses that impairs vascular flow to the corpora cavernosa; impairs central or peripheral innervation necessary for a penile erection; or is associated with testosterone insufficiency, in which case the patient develops erectile dysfunction secondary to a decreased libido (Table 22-8). Psychogenic erectile dysfunction is commonly situational in that the patient is unable to have an erection with a particular person, has performance anxiety, or is recovering from a major life stress (e.g., loss of a job, divorce, death in the family, etc.) (Table 22-7).[30]

Because current first choice treatment for erectile dysfunction is effective in up to 70% of treated patients, independent of the etiology, the diagnostic assessment of these patients has been streamlined. These patients are commonly diagnosed in primary care clinics with a comprehensive sexual history to identify the particular type of sexual dysfunction that the patient has (e.g., decreased libido, erectile dysfunction, or ejaculation disorder). Details on onset of symptoms are obtained, a patient's self-assessment of the severity of the problem using a validated, reliable questionnaire (e.g., International Index of Erectile Function, Sexual Health Inventory for Men [SHIM], Brief Male Sexual Function Inventory) is completed, and information on the patient's expectations for improved sexual function are collected from the patient and from the spouse or significant other.[31,32]

A comprehensive medical history is then performed to identify treatable underlying diseases, which may be contributing to erectile dysfunction (Table 22-8).[26] In addition, because erectile dysfunction may be the first presenting symptom of underlying cardiovascular or metabolic diseases, the clinician will investigate thoroughly for such conditions.[33] Blood pressure is measured and, if elevated, is treated. The patient is instructed to discontinue smoking, if applicable. A physical exam is completed to check for signs of hypogonadism (e.g., gynecomastia, small testes, decreased body hair). Peripheral pulses are palpated to assess vascular integrity (which would suggest adequate blood flow to the corpora cavernosa). A thorough urological examination to evaluate the integrity of the lower urinary tract and functional status of the bladder, urethra, and external genitalia is mandatory. A digital rectal

TABLE 22-8. Common Causes of Organic Erectile Dysfunction[26,30]

IMPAIRMENT	HOW IT CAUSES ERECTILE DYSFUNCTION	EXAMPLE DISEASES/CONDITIONS ASSOCIATED WITH THIS TYPE OF IMPAIRMENT
Vascular	Decreased arterial flow to the corpora cavernosa	Hypertension
		Congestive heart failure
		Coronary artery disease
		Arteriosclerosis
		Smoking
		Obesity
		Peripheral vascular disease
		Chronic, heavy smoking
		Drugs that cause hypotension: antihypertensives, central and peripheral sympatholytic agents
Neurologic	Decreased central processing of sexual stimuli or impaired peripheral nerve transmission, which decreases erectogenic reflex responses to tactile stimuli	Stroke
		Diabetes mellitus
		Chronic alcoholism
		Postradical prostatectomy in which pelvic nerve injury has occurred
		Epilepsy
		Multiple sclerosis
		Parkinson disease
		Psychosis
		Major depression
		Pelvic trauma with nerve injury
		Spinal cord injury
		Drugs with anticholinergic effects: antispasmodics, phenothiazines, tricyclic antidepressants, first generation antihistamines, etc.
Hormonal	Decreased serum testosterone, increased serum estrogen, increased ratio of serum estrogen to serum testosterone, or hyperprolactinemia results in decreased libido; erectile dysfunction is secondary to the decrease in libido	Late-onset hypogonadism
		Primary or secondary hypogonadism
		Hypo/hyperthyroidism
		Hyperprolactinemia
		Adrenal gland disorders
		Drugs with estrogenic effects: diethylstilbestrol, LHRH superagonists, LHRH antagonists
Anatomic	Penile deformity or curvature when erect	Peyronie disease
		Traumatic injury to the penis

LHRH = luteinizing hormone–releasing hormone.

exam is conducted on patients who are 50 years of age or older. This checks for anal sphincter tone, which indicates adequacy of sacral nerve innervation to the corpora cavernosa; prostate enlargement, which could obstruct urinary flow and lead to incontinence (which has been linked to erectile dysfunction); and a nodular or indurated prostate, which is suggestive of prostate cancer. Finally, an examination of the external genitalia identifies the presence of penile deformity or tissue scarring, which may contribute to erectile dysfunction.

For those patients who are over the age of 50 years and who have a life expectancy of at least 10 years, a blood test for prostate specific antigen (PSA) is obtained. If the medical or medication history suggests that the patient has concurrent medical illnesses that may contribute to erectile dysfunction, laboratory tests should be obtained to determine if these medical illnesses require more aggressive treatment. Such laboratory tests include a fasting blood glucose for diabetes mellitus, a lipid profile for hypercholesterolemia, a urinalysis to check for genitourinary tract disorders, serum testosterone levels for hypogonadism, a serum prolactin level if the patient has erectile dysfunction, decreased libido, and gynecomastia. Specialized clinical testing to identify surgically correctable causes of erectile dysfunction is reserved for those patients who do not respond to drug therapy, which includes oral phosphodiesterase

TABLE 22-9. Specialized Diagnostic Testing for Erectile Dysfunction[26,33]

TEST	DESCRIPTION	PURPOSE OF TEST
CIS testing	A single dose of alprostadil, papaverine, and/ or phentolamine is administered as an intracavernosal injection	Allows visual assessment of vascular integrity of penile arterial and venous flow
Duplex ultrasonography	CIS is performed, then ultrasound and Doppler imaging of arterial flow to the corpora cavernosa is done	Allows assessment of the flow through the main dorsal artery and the cavernous artery

CIS = combined intracavernous injection and stimulation.

inhibitors (e.g., sildenafil), intracavernosal alprostadil, intraurethral inserts, and vacuum erection devices (Table 22-9).

International Index of Erectile Function

The *International Index of Erectile Function (IIEF)* is a validated self-assessment questionnaire that includes 15 questions. The patient assesses the presence and severity of decreased libido, erectile or ejaculatory dysfunction, diminished orgasm, and his overall satisfaction with his sexual performance for the past month.[31] The questionnaire takes approximately 10–15 minutes to complete. Total scores can range from 0–25 and various score ranges are associated with symptom severity (Table 22-10).

Two shorter self-assessment questionnaires that are also used include the abridged IIEF, which includes four of the 15 questions from the original survey that focus on erectile dysfunction and the last question concerning the patient's overall satisfaction with his sexual performance and the Male Sexual Function Scale.[32,33] Some clinicians consider these shorter questionnaires to be more practical to use than the original IIEF. The IIEF is used at baseline to assist the physician in determining the severity of erectile dysfunction. Once treatment is initiated, the patient is asked to complete the IIEF questionnaire again so that the physician can assess the level of improvement in erectile function.

Prolactin

Normal range, adult males: 0–15 ng/mL or 0–15 mcg/L
Prolactin is secreted by the anterior pituitary gland in multiple pulses during the day. The normal daily production rate is 200–536 mcg per m[2] total body surface area. Although some prolactin circulates in inactive dimeric form (also known as "big prolactin") or in a less active form complexed to immunoglobin (also known as "big, big prolactin"), the majority exists as active hormone. Its pulsatile secretion is predominately controlled by prolactin inhibitory factor, which is believed to be a dopamine$_2$-like substance secreted by the hypothalamus in response to high levels of prolactin in the systemic or hypophyseal portal circulation. A prolactin stimulatory factor may also

TABLE 22-10. Interpretation of International Index of Erectile Function Scores[31]

SCORE	INTERPRETATION
22–25	No erectile dysfunction
17–21	Mild erectile dysfunction
12–16	Mild to moderate erectile dysfunction
8–11	Moderate erectile dysfunction
0–7	Severe erectile dysfunction

regulate prolactin secretion; however, its chemical structure still needs to be identified. Prolactin follows a diurnal pattern of secretion with highest serum levels occurring when the patient sleeps at night. Nadir levels occur between 10:00 a.m. and 12:00 p.m. The precise role of prolactin in males is unclear; however, it has been hypothesized that high circulating prolactin levels suppress LH and FSH, thereby decreasing testosterone production and spermatogenesis. Prolactin is excreted renally.

Hyperprolactinemia occurs in 1% to 2% of men who present with erectile dysfunction and is typically associated with symptoms of hypogonadism. Medical conditions and medications that can produce hyperprolactinemia are included in Table 22-11. They can be broadly classified as disorders of the hypothalamus or pituitary gland, neoplastic conditions, metabolic disorders, or drug causes. Whereas hypothalamic (e.g., craniopharyngioma), pituitary (e.g., prolactinoma), and neoplastic conditions (e.g., paraneoplastic syndromes) can cause significant increases in serum prolactin levels exceeding 250 ng/mL, physiologic and pharmacologic factors, including medications, sleep, pain, or meals, cause only smaller increases in serum prolactin level that rarely exceed 200 ng/mL. It should be noted that decreased prolactin levels in men is a rare condition. The clinical significance of this finding is unknown as it is associated with no symptoms or disease.

Indications for assessing serum prolactin levels include (1) a patient who is less than 50 years of age who complains of decreased libido and gynecomastia, or who has low serum testosterone levels; (2) a patient who is more than 50 years of age who complains of gynecomastia; or (3) a patient with late-onset hypogonadism and erectile dysfunction, whose symptoms are not corrected with a testosterone replacement regimen that restores serum testosterone to the normal range. Prolactin levels should not be routinely obtained in patients who present with erectile dysfunction. (See Minicase 1.)

Assay techniques for prolactin measurement include immunoassays using chemiluminescent, fluorescent, or radioactive labels. To minimize interference of prolactin assays by meals and stress, both of which can cause increased prolactin levels, it is recommended that blood specimens be collected 3 or 4 hours after the patient has awakened and fasted overnight. Prior to the blood draw, it is recommended that the patient rest for at least 20 minutes. Big prolactin and big, big prolactin, which are the less active forms of prolactin, crossreact with prolactin in immunoassays. To eliminate this interference, polyethylene glycol extraction and centrifugal ultrafiltration assay methods

TABLE 22-11. Medical Conditions and Medications Associated with Increased or Decreased Prolactin Levels[34–36]

INCREASED PROLACTIN LEVELS	DECREASED PROLACTIN LEVELS
Pituitary adenoma (nonprolactinoma)	Panhypopituitarism
Pituitary prolactinoma	Pituitary infarction
Acromegaly	Medications: carbamazepine, phenytoin, valproic acid, bromocriptine, clonidine, ergot alkaloids, levodopa, pergolide, nifedipine, rifampin, tamoxifen
Severe head trauma	
Craniopharyngioma	
Paraneoplastic syndrome with ectopic production of prolactin	
Primary hypothyroidism	
Renal failure, chronic	
Liver cirrhosis	
Addison disease	
Idiopathic pituitary hyperprolactinemia	
Stress	
Sarcoidosis	
Chest wall trauma	
Seizures	
Epilepsy	
Anorexia nervosa	
Medications: phenothiazines, thioxanthenes, buspirone, olanzapine, risperidone, haloperidol, loxapine, pimozide, tricyclic antidepressants, molindone, monoamine oxidase inhibitors, oral contraceptives, estrogens, megestrol, morphine, opiates, cocaine, antihistamines, ranitidine, cimetidine, metoclopramide, pimozide, reserpine, methyldopa, verapamil, labetolol	

can be employed.[36] Extremely high serum levels of prolactin may saturate the ability of immunoassays to measure correct levels. Therefore, in patients with prolactinomas, it may be necessary to dilute the specimen to 1:100 before assaying.

BENIGN PROSTATIC HYPERPLASIA

Benign prostatic hyperplasia (BPH) is an enlargement of the prostate gland that occurs in all males as they age. The histologic disease prevalence is 80% in men aged 70–79 years.[37] Furthermore, 50% of men with a histologic diagnosis of BPH develop clinical symptoms of at least moderate severity.[38] Beginning at approximately age 40 years in males, the prostate

gland undergoes a second growth spurt and the prostate grows from a normal adult size of 15–20 g to a much larger size that can exceed 100 g. The local complications of BPH include obstructive and irritative voiding symptoms. Collectively, these symptoms are often referred to as *lower urinary tract symptoms (LUTS)*; however, LUTS are not specific for BPH and may be due to other genitourinary tract disorders (e.g., neurogenic bladder, prostate cancer, urethral stricture, prostatitis, and urinary tract infection).[38] Obstructive symptoms include a slow urinary stream, difficulty emptying urine out of the bladder, hesitancy, dribbling, a sensation of incomplete bladder emptying, and straining to void. Such symptoms can be due to the enlarged prostate, which produces an anatomical block of the bladder neck. Irritative symptoms include urinary frequency, nocturia, and urgency, which may progress to urinary incontinence. Such symptoms are due to the long-term effects of obstruction on the detrusor muscle of the bladder. That is, an enlarged prostate results in partial obstruction of the bladder outlet. In time this causes hypertrophy of the bladder muscle and increased intravesical pressure, which translates to urgency, frequency, nocturia, and urge incontinence. If untreated, progressive increased resistance at the bladder outlet will result in decompensation and residual urine, and then total urinary retention and overflow incontinence. Other complications of untreated, severe BPH include recurrent urinary tract infection, urosepsis, urolithiasis (primarily bladder stones), and chronic renal disease.

The symptoms of BPH are most often the driver that brings the patient to medical attention. Nocturia (which interferes with sleeping) and urgency-associated incontinence (which curbs social activity) can significantly reduce quality of life. Thus symptom assessment is crucial in evaluating the disorder. Symptom assessment is typically completed by having the patient use a validated questionnaire such as the American Urological Association Symptom Score or the International Prostate Symptom Score instrument.

Signs of disease are evaluated by the physician using clinical procedures that can be performed easily in the outpatient setting. A careful medical history is taken to identify any concurrent medical illnesses or medications that may be causing LUTS or worsening LUTS. A physical examination should be performed to check for bladder distention and neurologic innervation of the lower urinary tract. A digital rectal exam is performed to assess prostate gland size, shape, and consistency, and anal sphincter tone. The latter is maintained by the pudendal nerve, which is also responsible for bladder contraction and emptying. In addition, to rule out other common causes of urinary frequency and urgency, physicians should obtain a urinalysis. Microscopic examination of the spun sediment for white blood cells and bacteria, and a dipstick check for leukocyte esterase and nitrite help identify urinary tract infection as a cause for the patient's symptoms. If gross or microscopic hematuria is present and the patient has a past or current history of smoking, urine is sent for cytological assessment. Bladder neoplasms typically shed cancer cells into the urine. For patients in whom the urinalysis is suspicious

MINICASE 1

A Patient with Erectile Dysfunction and Low Serum Testosterone Levels

TERENCE T. IS A 70-YEAR-OLD, AFRICAN-AMERICAN MALE who complains of erectile dysfunction and no sexual drive. He feels like he is disappointing his sexual partner because he has no desire for sexual intercourse and cannot seem to perform adequately. He attributes all of this to getting older and wonders if a pill can "make him better."

Cc: Terence T. has erectile dysfunction and decreased libido.

HPI: Terence T. reports that the problem has been getting worse over the past 5 years. Initially, he had periodic erectile dysfunction. Now, he has no nocturnal erections and can't get an erection when he needs it.

PMH: Essential hypertension

Medications: Hydrochlorothiazide and diltiazem

Allergies: None

Physical exam:

ROS: Well-developed, well-nourished African-American male with mild nocturia and some urinary hesitancy, particularly in the morning

Vital signs: BP 140/85, HR 65, RR 16, T 98.6°F, weight 75 kg, height 6'

Genitourinary tract: Normal penis, no curvature; testes, mildly atrophic; anal sphincter tone intact and within normal limits; digital rectal exam reveals mildly enlarged prostate; pedal pulses, PSA 1.9 ng/mL

Assessment: Suspect late-onset hypogonadism with erectile dysfunction and BPH

Question: A serum total testosterone level is ordered. The result is 275 ng/dL. Is testosterone supplementation indicated?

Discussion: Terence T.'s decreased libido and erectile dysfunction are consistent with late-onset hypogonadism. His serum testosterone is at the low-end of the normal range. However, in older men, SHBG serum levels increase. Once bound to SHBG, testosterone is inactive. Therefore, a serum free testosterone or bioavailable testosterone level should be obtained to confirm the diagnosis of hypogonadism before testosterone supplementation is started. Measurement of LH, FSH, and prolactin would also be helpful in confirming the diagnosis. Both LH and FSH should be elevated in patients with late-onset hypogonadism, where the primary defect is decreased testicular production of testosterone.

Question: A serum free testosterone level is 5 ng/dL. Interpret this laboratory result. Is testosterone supplementation indicated?

Discussion: Terence T. has a low serum free testosterone level (normal range is 5–9 ng/dL). This laboratory test result, along with his symptoms of no libido and erectile dysfunction, confirm the diagnosis of late-onset hypogonadism. Testosterone supplementation can improve his libido and lift his mood. An adequate clinical trial of testosterone supplementation is 3 months. If testosterone supplementation does not improve his erectile function after 3 months, additional treatment for erectile dysfunction (i.e., a phosphodiesterase inhibitor) should be started.

for renal impairment (e.g., casts are detected on microscopic examination) or in whom surgical treatment of BPH is being considered, specialized testing is performed. Serum creatinine may be assessed to check for evidence of chronic renal disease. If present, such patients have a higher risk of postoperative complications than patients with normal renal function, 25% versus 17%, respectively, and of worsening renal function due to radiographic contrast media, if used during intravenous pyelography to assess renal function and anatomy.[38] In such high-risk patients, a renal ultrasound would be a better test for evaluation of renal anatomy.

Other specialized tests include uroflowmetry, postvoid residual urine volume, transrectal ultrasound of the prostate, and cystoscopy. Uroflowmetry and postvoid residual urine volume, which are quantitative tests, are discussed below. Transrectal ultrasound of the prostate entails insertion of an ultrasound probe into the rectum. Ultrasound waves are bounced off the prostate through the rectal mucosa and images are produced. These images allow identification of stones, abscesses, or other changes in echogenicity in the prostate, and also provide an estimate of prostate size, which is more accurate than digital rectal exam. During cystoscopy an endoscope is passed transurethrally so that the urologist can visualize the urethra, bladder neck, and bladder. In patients with BPH, the classic findings are changes in the bladder mucosa secondary to prolonged bladder neck obstruction, and obstruction of the urethral lumen and bladder neck by an enlarged prostate. This gives the appearance that the three side-walls of the prostatic urethra bulge out and appear to kiss each other.

American Urological Association (AUA) Symptom Score and International Prostate Symptom Score (IPSS)

This validated survey instrument is administered to the patient, who responds to a series of seven questions about the severity of his obstructive and irritative voiding symptoms. For each question, the patient rates symptom severity on a scale of 1 to 5, where 0 is not bothersome and 5 is severely bothersome. Thus, the lowest total score is 0 and the maximum total score is 35. Scores are interpreted according to the following ranges:

- Mild symptoms, score of 0–7
- Moderate symptoms, score of 8–19
- Severe symptoms, score of 20–35

The AUA Symptom Score Survey is administered to establish a baseline and then is repeated at regular intervals for patients with mild symptoms to determine if symptoms are worsening over time and deserve medical or surgical treatment. Similarly, once specific treatment for BPH is initiated, the AUA Symptom Score Survey is repeated several weeks after treatment is started to determine if the treatment is effective in relieving symptoms.

An effective treatment should reduce the AUA Symptom Score by 30% to 50% or decrease the score by at least three points.

The International Prostate Symptom Score Survey is a symptom survey instrument, which includes all seven questions in the AUA Symptom Score survey plus one additional question about the impact of the patient's voiding symptoms on overall quality of life. The last question is not included in the total score. Therefore, the total score ranges from 0 to 35, with 0 suggesting that the patient has no symptoms and 35 suggesting that the patient has severe symptoms.

Both the AUA and the International Prostate Symptom Score may not correlate with the actual severity of the patient's obstruction. This is partly because some patients deny the presence of LUTS and attribute their symptoms to getting older. Furthermore, the AUA and International Prostate Symptom Score do not always correlate with prostate gland size, urinary flow rate, or postvoid residual urine volume. However, patients with high AUA and International Prostate Symptom Scores generally show significant improvement with surgical treatment for BPH.[42]

Digital Rectal Exam of the Prostate

Because of its location below the urinary bladder, the prostate is difficult to examine directly. Instead, it must be examined indirectly by having a physician insert a gloved index finger into the anus and then digitally palpating the prostate through the rectal wall. This is a simple physical examination procedure, which can be performed without any local anesthetic or bowel preparation. The prostate is assessed for its size, shape, consistency, and mobility. A normal prostate is 15–20 g in size, is heart-shaped and symmetric, has a soft consistency similar to the thenar eminence of the hand with no areas of nodularity or induration, and should be moveable when pushed with the finger. Patients with BPH have an enlarged, symmetric, rubbery, mobile gland with a smooth surface. In contrast, a patient with prostate cancer could have a variable size (normal-sized or enlarged), asymmetric gland with a nodular or indurated surface on palpation. If the cancer has locally extended to surrounding periprostatic tissue, the prostate becomes fixed in place and is no longer mobile.

The physician will estimate the size of the gland based on the degree to which the examiner's finger can reach up to the base and over the border of the prostate gland. The accuracy of the prostate size assessment by digital rectal exam is dependent on the expertise of the physician who is conducting the exam. Due to skill variability among clinicians for this physical assessment technique, a transrectal or transabdominal ultrasound is often performed to better assess the size of an enlarged gland.[43]

An accurate prostate size assessment is useful for identifying patients at high risk for developing complications of BPH, who would most benefit from treatment with finasteride and dutasteride. These agents are most effective in patients with prostates that are least 40 g in size and treatment can reduce the risk for acute urinary retention, slow BPH progression, and delay the need for surgery. In addition, the size of the prostate helps determine the best surgical approach for large prostate glands.[44,45]

Estimated prostate size does not correlate with the severity of voiding symptoms, degree of bladder neck obstruction, or the need for treatment.[38,46] This can be explained by the existence of at least two mechanisms for obstructive voiding symptoms in patients with BPH. In some patients, the obstructive voiding symptoms are due to the anatomic blockade of the urethra caused by the enlarged prostate gland. However, in other patients, obstructive voiding symptoms may be due to excessive alpha adrenergic stimulation of receptors in the smooth muscle fibers of the prostate and bladder neck, which decreases the caliber of the urethral lumen. In these patients, despite the absence of a significantly enlarged prostate gland, the patient may develop significant symptoms. Alternatively, some patients with BPH have enlargement of the median lobe of the prostate, which grows inside the bladder and produces a ball-valve obstruction of the bladder neck. In this case, the enlarged gland is not palpable on digital rectal exam, but must be identified by transrectal ultrasound of the prostate or cystoscopy.

Peak Urinary Flow Rate

Peak urinary flow rate, normal range:
≥25 mL/sec, in young male
≥10–15 mL/sec, minimum, in older males

The urinary flow rate refers to the speed with which urine is emptied out of a full bladder. Urinary flow rate is assessed as a simple outpatient procedure. The patient is instructed to drink water until his bladder is full, and then is instructed to urinate into the uroflowmetry measuring device until he feels empty. The peak urinary flow rate is the maximum flow rate using the time period limited to the interval when the bladder volume was at least 150 mL.[46] The average urinary flow rate is calculated from the total volume (mL) of urine collected divided by the total time (seconds) that it took to empty his bladder.

A low peak urinary flow rate is suggestive of bladder outlet obstruction, particularly when the peak urinary flow rate is less than 10–12 mL/sec. In addition, a patient with a peak urinary flow rate of less than 10 mL/sec is more likely to benefit from surgical correction of BPH than a patient with a higher flow rate.[38] However, there is no direct correlation between voiding symptom severity and urinary flow rate. Again, this is likely due to patient's attribution of voiding difficulty to advancing age (and not due to a prostate disorder), or a patient's denial of the presence of symptoms.[38]

There is no standardized cutoff point for urinary flow rate that identifies a patient with clinically significant urinary obstruction requiring medical or surgical treatment.[47] In patients with BPH, the urinary flow rate is typically used along with the patient's AUA symptom score and the absence or presence of complications secondary to bladder neck obstruction to assess the severity of the patient's disease.[46] As mentioned, a patient may have a low urinary flow rate, but may not consider his symptoms severe. In this case, the perceived severity of the patient's symptoms will impact on

TABLE 22-12. Typical Actions Taken Depending on PSA and Digital Rectal Exam Screening Results[51–53]

IF THE RESULTS SHOW:

PSA	DIGITAL RECTAL EXAM RESULT	NEXT STEP IN DIAGNOSIS
Normal	Normal	Have the patient return in 1 yr for repeat testing
Normal	Abnormal	Have the patient undergo prostate needle biopsy
Abnormal	Normal	Repeat the PSA; if it remains elevated, have the patient undergo prostate needle biopsy
Abnormal	Abnormal	Have the patient undergo prostate needle biopsy

PSA = prostate specific antigen.

the ultimate choice of therapy for the patient rather than the urinary flow rate.

A limitation of uroflowmetry testing is that there is intra-patient variability of results from test to test. That is, even if repeated on the same day, the urinary flow rate may not be the same in the same patient.[38] Also a low flow rate is not specific for BPH. Low flow rates may be due to urethral stricture, meatal stenosis, or neurogenic bladder secondary to detrusor muscle hypotonicity.[46,47] The latter occurs in patients with diabetes mellitus, peripheral neuropathy, or spinal cord injury.[47] Finally, the uroflowmetry test requires a minimal urine volume of 150 mL, which may be difficult for some patients to attain (i.e., they balk at consuming so much fluid in a short period of time).

Postvoid Residual Urine Volume

Normal range: <50 mL

Postvoid residual urine volume refers to the amount of urine left in the bladder after a patient empties his bladder and voids a minimum volume of 120–150 mL. In a normal person, the postvoid residual urine volume should be zero, range 0.09–2.24 mL. However, in patients with BPH, the enlarged prostate at the bladder neck causes an obstruction that makes it difficult to empty urine completely from the bladder. Chronic retention of large volumes of urine increases the risk of urinary tract infections in men with BPH and can lead to decompensation of the detrusor muscle fibers of the urinary bladder, which can result in urinary frequency, overflow incontinence, or acute urinary retention.

Traditionally to assess the postvoid residual urine volume, the patient is asked to empty his urinary bladder. Then a small bore urethral catheter is inserted up the urethra and into the urinary bladder to drain any residual urine. The urine is collected and the volume is measured. This method is invasive and is associated with some risk of urethral injury and pain secondary to catheter insertion. More recently, noninvasive determination of the postvoid residual urine volume with abdominal ultrasonography is commonly used.

A specific postvoid residual urine volume has not been identified as a critical value that necessitates treatment, although in clinical practice, a persistent postvoid residual urine volume of 50 mL or more is cause for concern.[38] Although a high postvoid residual urine volume correlates with decreased peak urinary flow rate, the former may not correlate with the patient's reported symptom severity.[48,49] However, effective drug or surgical treatment that improves symptoms of BPH generally reduces a high postvoid residual urine volume. As a result, clinicians generally evaluate elevated postvoid residual urine volumes in the context of the patient's medical history of recurrent urinary tract infections.

A high postvoid residual urine volume is not specific for BPH. An enlarged prostate due to prostate cancer can be associated with an increased postvoid residual urine volume. Also, a hypotonic detrusor muscle, which lacks contractile force to empty the bladder, as occurs in patients with peripheral neuropathies secondary to severe diabetes mellitus, spinal cord injury, or chronic alcoholism, can be associated with a high postvoid residual urine volume.

Transrectal Ultrasound of the Prostate

Normal prostate size: <15–20 cm³

In this outpatient procedure, after application of a local anesthetic jelly to the rectal mucosal surface, biplanar ultrasound probes are inserted into the rectum. Ultrasound waves are bounced through the rectal wall to assess the size, shape, and echogenicity of the prostate. *Transrectal ultrasound* of the prostate is more accurate in estimating prostate size than digital rectal exam and helps inform the urologist of the best approach for surgical removal of an enlarged prostate gland.

Transrectal ultrasound of the prostate is also used to assess indurated or nodular areas of the prostate or an elevated PSA, which are suspicious for prostate cancer. A transrectal ultrasound of the prostate may reveal hyper-, hypo-, and isoechoic areas of the prostate. By so doing, different sites for prostate needle biopsy can be better identified.[50]

PROSTATE CANCER

Prostate cancer is the most common cancer of American men, and the second leading cause of cancer-related death among American men. The prevalence is highest in males aged 50 years or more. Approximately 11% of men present with advanced disease at the time of first diagnosis, and unfortunately, there is no cure for advanced disease at this time. The clinical presentation of prostate cancer is heterogeneous. In some patients, prostate cancer is slow growing and may or may not be associated with localized symptoms, such as voiding difficulty. Such patients are more likely to die from other concurrent medical illnesses, and not prostate cancer. In other patients, prostate cancer spreads quickly, follows a progressive

TABLE 22-13. Clinical Tests Used to Stage Prostate Cancer[51]

CHECKING FOR METASTASES IN	INITIAL CLINICAL TEST	ADDITIONAL CLINICAL TESTS IF INITIAL CLINICAL TEST IS POSITIVE
Bone	Bone scan	Bone survey (radiograph of entire boney skeleton)
Lung	Chest x-ray	Chest CT scan
Liver	Liver function tests	CT scan of the abdomen
Lymph nodes	PSA greater than 20 ng/mL or Gleason score of 8–10; or peripheral edema on physical exam	CT scan of the pelvis
Periprostatic tissue (e.g., seminal vesicles, fat tissue)	Digital rectal exam of the prostate, transrectal ultrasound of the prostate	

CT = computerized axial tomography; PSA = prostate specific antigen.

course, and produces many systemic symptoms. Such patients are more likely to die from complications of prostate cancer and its treatment.

The symptoms of prostate cancer are associated with cancer invasion of the prostate gland or tumor spread to metastatic sites. Tumor in the prostate gland generally causes hardness, nodularity, induration, asymmetry, and may also be associated with glandular enlargement, which can lead to obstructive voiding symptoms (e.g., decreased force of urinary stream, inability to completely empty the bladder, and overflow urinary incontinence, similar to BPH). Tumor spread to the lungs can cause dyspnea; to the bone it can cause bone pain and anemia; to the vertebral bodies it can cause peripheral neuropathies, urinary or fecal incontinence, or difficulty walking; to the lymph nodes it can cause lymphadenopathy, lower extremity peripheral edema, or ureteral obstruction; and to the rectum it can cause rectal bleeding.[51]

As recommended by the American Cancer Society and the American Urological Association, screening for prostate cancer is recommended for a patient age 50 years or older and who has a life expectancy of at least 10 years. Screening includes both a digital rectal exam (described above in the section on BPH) and a blood test for PSA. In patients with risk factors for prostate cancer, including African Americans and those with a family history of first-degree relatives with prostate cancer, screening with a digital rectal exam and PSA is recommended beginning at age 45 and 40 years, respectively.[52] Four common scenarios may result (Table 22-12).

It should be noted that the value of PSA screening for prostate cancer has been questioned by the American College of Preventative Medicine and the U.S. Preventative Services Task Force.[53,54] PSA has several limitations as a screening tool. Despite the widespread use of PSA for screening, only a 20% decrease in prostate cancer-related mortality has been attributed to PSA screening alone. Although PSA has produced a 70% increase in the diagnosis of patients with prostate cancer, many of these patients are at low risk of significant morbidity or mortality from their disease but yet are treated aggressively with surgery, radiation therapy, or medically.[55,56] Treatment is expensive and is associated with many adverse effects. Finally, there is no threshold PSA which guarantees the absence of

prostate cancer. In the Prostate Cancer Prevention Trial, men with PSAs ≤0.5 ng/mL, 0.6–1.0 ng/mL, 1.1–2.0 ng/mL, 2.1–3.0 ng/mL, and 3.1–4.0 ng/mL had a 6.6%, 10%, 17%, 23.9%, and 26.9% prevalence of histologically confirmed prostate cancer, respectively. Of these cases, 10% to 25% had high-grade tumors, which generally carry a worse prognosis than low grade ones.[57] For these reasons, the U.S. Preventative Services Task Force recommends that physicians candidly discuss with each patient the option of routine screening versus not screening with PSA and give full consideration to the patient's age, the patient's willingness to live with cancer, the risk of side effects of treatment if prostate cancer is diagnosed, and the patient's overall health in determining the use of PSA for screening.[54]

In scenarios where the patient undergoes a prostate needle biopsy and it yields a positive pathologic result, the tissue-diagnosis of prostate cancer confirms the presence of the tumor. Based on the Gleason score of the tumor specimen, PSA, digital rectal exam, and transrectal ultrasound of the prostate, a clinical stage of disease can be determined and a risk assessment can be performed. If the patient is thought to have disease confined to the prostate and is considered to be at low risk of tumor recurrence, no further testing is done. If the patient is thought to have disease that has spread locally or is metastatic, and is considered to be at intermediate or high risk of tumor recurrence, the patient will undergo clinical staging to determine the presence and the location of tumor spread. A variety of clinical tests are performed. If initial tests are positive, additional tests are run to assess tumor burden and degree of spread of the cancer in the patient, and hence, to determine the stage of disease (Table 22-13). Current clinical tests to stage prostate cancer fail to identify approximately one-third of patients with prostate cancer that has spread outside of the prostate gland.[51] Thus, the search continues for improved diagnostic tools. For example, ProstaScint® is a type of scan that uses indium-111 capromab pendetide, a monoclonal antibody against prostate specific membrane antigen, to detect prostate cancer cells, which may have spread to soft tissue outside of the prostate gland.[59] Initial evaluation shows that ProstaScint may be useful for detecting tumor recurrence or for identifying those patients with disease which has spread locally outside the prostate. However, its role as a tumor marker must be further defined.

Prostate Specific Antigen

Non-age-related normal range: <4 ng/mL
Age-related normal ranges:
Men, age 40–49 yr, 0–2.5 ng/mL
Men, age 50–59 yr, 0–3.5 ng/mL
Men, age 60–69 yr, 0–4.5 ng/mL
Men, age 70+yr, 0–6.5 ng/mL

Prostate specific antigen (PSA) is a glycoprotein produced by the glandular epithelial cells in the transition zone of the prostate gland. Small amounts are also produced by breast tissue, parotid gland, and periurethral glands. In normal, healthy males, 20–45 years of age, mean plasma PSA levels are undetectable or at the low end of the normal range, usually less than 1.14 ng/mL in Caucasians and less than 1.37 in African Americans. This is because PSA is carried out of the prostate through ducts to the urethra, where it is passed out of the body in the ejaculate during coitus. Prostate specific antigen liquefies semen after ejaculation. However, once the prostate gland becomes cancerous, the duct system in neoplastic tissue is inadequate. As the gland grows, PSA production increases and leaks into the circulation; this results in elevated plasma PSA levels.

In the bloodstream, PSA exists in two forms: free PSA (fPSA) and complexed PSA (cPSA). Of the total PSA in plasma, 30% to 40% is fPSA, and 50% to 70% of the total PSA is complexed to alpha 1-antichymotrypsin (ACT) and alpha 2-macroglobulin (A2M).[60] Free PSA is renally excreted, while cPSA is hepatically catabolized. The plasma half-life of PSA is 2–3 days. Because of daily intrapatient variation in PSA measurements, it is recommended to confirm an increased PSA value by repeating it.[60] A PSA level measures both fPSA and PSA complexed to ACT. Prostate specific antigen complexed to A2M is not detected by immunoassay.

In the bloodstream, fPSA exists in several forms. ProPSA is the inactive precursor of PSA and is associated with prostate cancer.[61] It may be modified or clipped to produce two different inactive forms; however, most of it is converted to active PSA. Active PSA can be converted to inactive PSA (iPSA) or benign PSA (BPSA), which is produced by BPH tissue, as opposed to normal prostate tissue. High levels of BPSA are associated with high-volume BPH and obstructive voiding symptoms.[61] Preliminary studies are being conducted to evaluate the diagnostic usefulness of measuring ProPSA, clipped forms of ProPSA, and BPSA. Currently, these forms of fPSA are largely used as research tools. Whether these will replace PSA as a tumor marker is not known at this time.

Prostate specific antigen serum levels are affected by several patient factors.[62,63] Decreased PSA levels are associated with obesity. It has been postulated that obese patients have larger circulating plasma volumes, which dilutes PSA concentrations in the bloodstream.[64] Decreased PSA is also seen with hypogonadism. This is probably because hypogonadism results in shrinkage of the prostate gland, the major site of PSA production. Increased PSA levels are observed in elderly patients probably because BPH occurs with a high prevalence. Also, increased PSA normal range levels are reported in African-American patients less than 60 years of age.[65] The reason for this is unknown.

As a tumor marker, PSA has several uses: as a diagnostic screening test for prostate cancer; to determine the spread of the disease; and to assess the patient's response to treatment. As a diagnostic screening test, PSA has high sensitivity (70% to 80%), but low specificity (50%) for prostate cancer when used alone. The positive predictive value of PSA to diagnose prostate cancer is directly related to the PSA value such that the higher the PSA value, the higher the positive predictive value. In the range of 2.5–4 ng/mL, PSA has a positive predictive value of 18%. In the range of 4–10 ng/mL, PSA has a positive predictive value of 20%. Above 10 ng/mL, PSA has a positive predictive value of 42% to 64%.[66] Prostate specific antigen should be used in combination with a digital rectal examination of the prostate for prostate cancer screening because either test alone has inadequate sensitivity and specificity as a diagnostic test. When used in combination with a digital rectal exam, the sensitivity of PSA is increased to 85% to 90%, and the positive predictive value of a PSA cutoff of 4 ng/mL to diagnose prostate cancer is increased from 32% to 49%.[67] With the use of PSA screening, patients with prostate cancer are diagnosed 5–13 years earlier in the course of their disease when the tumor burden is less. Thus, fewer patients present with advanced stage disease at the time of initial diagnosis.[68]

When used for prostate cancer screening, a common interpretation of test results follows if the PSA normal range is assumed to be <4 ng/mL:

0–3.9 ng/mL	Normal range
4–9 ng/mL	A biopsy is recommended (the probability of detecting prostate cancer is 25% to 30%).
≥10 ng/mL	A biopsy is recommended (the probability of prostate cancer is at least 50%).

Prostate specific antigen can be used as a laboratory test to determine the spread of prostate cancer. Although the amount of PSA produced increases with the size of the tumor, there is a poor correlation between the PSA level and the actual size of the prostate tumor. However, a semiquantitative relationship exists between the PSA level and the degree of prostate cancer spread such that a PSA level less than 10 ng/mL suggests that tumor is confined to the prostate, a PSA level of greater than 20 ng/mL suggests the possibility of extracapsular spread, and a PSA level of greater than or equal to 80 ng/mL suggests advanced disease.

When used to assess the patient's response to treatment for prostate cancer, an elevated PSA prior to treatment should be reduced to the normal range, or at least exhibit a two-fold reduction in PSA level, with effective treatment. In addition, pretreatment PSA is used along with the Gleason score of prostate tissue and the clinical stage of disease to predict the prognosis of patients in terms of their low-, medium-, or high-risk of post-treatment disease recurrence.[69] This information is then used to guide treatment selection for individual patients.[29] Although multiple risk stratification schemes have been devised, no one system is considered the standard.[70]

TABLE 22-14. Diseases, Procedures and Medications That Increase (total) PSA[52,60,71a]

BPH

Prostatitis

Prostate trauma (e.g., massage, biopsy)

Prostate surgery

Acute urinary retention

Ejaculation

Exercising on an exercise bicycle for 30 min

Medications: testosterone supplements

BPH = benign prostatic hyperplasia; PSA = prostate specific antigen.
[a]Procedures that have minimal effect on (total) PSA: digital rectal exam, transrectal ultrasound of the prostate, cystoscopy, and urethral catheterization.[71]

As previously mentioned, using a cutoff value of 4 ng/mL, PSA is 70% to 80% sensitive in screening for prostate cancer but has low specificity. Many noncancerous conditions can increase PSA (Table 22-14), which could trigger a clinical decision for an unnecessary prostate biopsy. For example, almost 30% of men with BPH have PSA values of 4 ng/mL or higher. Also, as previously mentioned, some high-grade prostate tumors do not produce PSA. Thus, this cutoff value for PSA potentially misses up to 27% of patients with prostate cancer confined to the prostate gland, which is curable.[60] Therefore, various alternative strategies have been employed to improve the usefulness of PSA as a tumor marker for prostate cancer screening including the following:

1. Consider the normal value of total PSA to be less than 2.5 ng/dL, particularly in men less than 60 years of age. Thus, patients with a total PSA of 2.5 ng/dL or greater would undergo a prostate needle biopsy. This should avoid missing that subgroup of patients with organ confined prostate cancer who have PSA values in the range of 2.5–4.0 ng/dL.[72,73] However, lowering the normal value of PSA also is likely to increase the number of biopsies that are negative.[52,74]

2. Consider age-related normal value ranges.[75] Using the current cutoff value of 4 ng/mL, the specificity of PSA decreases as men age.[67] This is because PSA normally increases as men age and develop BPH. Thus, to minimize the risk of interpreting an increased PSA as due to prostate cancer, when it is due to BPH, age-related normal value ranges, which have been further delineated for Asians and African Americans, as listed below, are

often provided by clinical laboratories (Table 22-15).[76,77] An advantage of age-related normal value ranges is that they increase the likelihood of disease detection in young men. However, a disadvantage is that they delay biopsies in older men, which can delay the diagnosis of prostate cancer.[60,77]

The total PSA range of 4–10 ng/mL is considered to be a gray-zone range because the increase in PSA in many cases is due to BPH and not prostate cancer. Thus, to improve the usefulness of total PSA in the range of 4–10 ng/mL as a screening test or to assess prognosis of patients, the following strategies have been recommended by some investigators:

1. **PSA density (PSAD).** The PSAD is thought to be increased in patients with prostate cancer as compared to patients with BPH. The PSAD is calculated by dividing the total PSA by the prostate volume as determined by transrectal ultrasound of the prostate (TRUS). A normal PSAD is less than 0.15 ng/mL/cm^3. If the PSAD is 0.15 ng/mL/cm^3 or more, it suggests that the patient's increased PSA is due to prostate cancer, and this patient should undergo additional diagnostic testing. However, this cutoff value has only 50% sensitivity, and it misses many patients with prostate cancer.[77,78] In addition, to derive PSAD, a TRUS must be performed. This adds an extra cost to the patient and is uncomfortable for the patient. Finally, a TRUS measurement of prostate volume is difficult to reproduce in the same patient.[60]

2. **PSA velocity.** The PSA velocity refers to the rate of increase in PSA values over time and is based on the concept that a faster rate of rise is suggestive of the presence of prostate cancer. To determine PSA velocity, the patient must have three PSA values performed, each one is at least 1 year apart; or alternatively the patient must have three PSA values performed over a 1.5-year period.[78] If the PSA velocity is greater than 0.75 ng/mL/year, this suggests that the patient has prostate cancer and should undergo additional diagnostic testing. Prostate specific antigen velocity has 95% specificity as a screening test for prostate cancer, which is much better than total PSA. In men less than age 60 years, whose lifespans are potentially more severely impacted by aggressive prostate cancer, it is suggested that a PSA velocity greater than 0.4 ng/mL/year be used as a threshold value.[79] Prostate specific antigen velocity is affected by the intrapatient variation of PSA values. That is, a PSA value may fluctuate 10% to 25% from day-to-day in the same patient. For this reason, it may be difficult to de-

TABLE 22-15. Age-Specific Median and Normal Value Ranges for PSA in Adult Males of Various Races[76]

PATIENT AGE (YEARS)	OVERALL MEDIAN (ng/mL)	CAUCASIANS (ng/mL)	ASIANS (ng/mL)	AFRICAN AMERICANS (ng/mL)
40–49	0.7	0–2.5	0–2.0	0–2.0
50–59	0.9	0–3.5	0–3.0	0–4.0
60–69	1.3	0–4.5	0–4.0	0–4.5
>70	1.7	0–6.5	0–5.0	0–5.5

TABLE 22-16. Estimated Probability of Prostate Cancer Depending on the Percentage of Free PSA[81,82]

% FREE PSA RANGE	% PROBABILITY OF PROSTATE CANCER
0–10	56
10–15	28
15–20	20
20–25	16
>25	8

rive a consistent PSA velocity value for a patient. Thus, some recommend that the trend of an increase in PSA values over a 1.5-year period should be considered as suggestive of prostate cancer in place of the 0.75 ng/mL/yr cutoff.[60] In addition, the long period of time needed to collect enough PSA measurements to determine PSA velocity is a significant disadvantage of using this parameter.

A related alternative strategy is to evaluate PSA doubling time or the length of time it takes for the PSA level to double. The preoperative PSA doubling time has been used to predict cancer recurrence after surgical intervention for the disease. A preliminary study suggests that a PSA doubling time of less than 10 months indicates that the patient probably has tumor recurrence.[80] A disadvantage to using PSA doubling time is that there is no accepted standard for the minimum number of PSA values to use or the time interval between PSA values.

3. **Percentage of free PSA (% fPSA).** Prostate cancer is associated with an increased fraction of cPSA as opposed to fPSA in the plasma. Therefore, the fPSA level is inversely related to the risk of prostate cancer in a patient. Thus, if the percentage of fPSA is less than 25% of the total PSA, and depending on the actual percentage of fPSA, the patient has up to a 56% probability of having prostate cancer (Table 22-16).[81,82] The use of fPSA to screen for prostate cancer when the total PSA is less than 4 ng/mL has not been well-studied, but preliminary evaluation suggests that the percentage of fPSA may be a good screen for prostate cancer.[60] One study showed that in the (total) PSA range of 2.5–10 ng/mL, the fPSA cutoff of 25% had greater than 90% sensitivity for screening for organ-confined prostate cancer.[82]

Assessing the percentage of fPSA helps the clinician determine if the elevated PSA is due to prostate cancer or BPH. Thus, prostate needle biopsy would be reserved for those patients with an fPSA less than 25%. Free PSA is renally excreted; therefore, in patients with renal failure, the fPSA level will be increased, and the percentage of fPSA will increase.[83] Free PSA increases after digital rectal exam of the prostate, prostate needle biopsy, and after ejaculation. Finasteride and dutasteride also decrease free and complexed PSA but do not affect the ratio of the two; therefore, fPSA percentages are not affected by these medications. Free PSA blood specimens are subject to degradation if stored for long periods of time at ambient temperature. It is recommended that specimens for fPSA be stored at –70°C or assayed within 3 hours of specimen collection.

4. **cPSA.** As previously mentioned prostate cancer is associated with an increased fraction of cPSA. With this assay, the concentration of PSA complexed to ACT is measured. Using the PSA normal value of 4 ng/mL, the cPSA normal value is 3.1 ng/mL. Although cPSA assays appear to be comparable in sensitivity and specificity to PSA assays, cPSA assays have not replaced PSA assays.[84]

Medications may alter PSA levels. Of importance, the 5-alpha reductase inhibitors (e.g., finasteride (Proscar®) and dutasteride (Avodart®), generally produce an average 50% reduction in PSA after 6 months of continuous treatment. This has been reported with usual daily doses of both drugs (5 mg finasteride daily and 0.5 mg dutasteride daily) for treatment of BPH, and also with 1 mg finasteride (Propecia®) daily used for androgenetic alopecia.[85-87] To preserve the usefulness of PSA as a tumor marker in patients who are taking 5-alpha reductase inhibitors, it is essential to obtain a pretreatment PSA as a baseline. After at least 6 months of treatment, when PSA levels are repeated, it is recommended to double the measured PSA level before interpreting it. If a patient has a PSA level that is significantly higher than baseline after 6 months of treatment, it is recommended that the patient be evaluated for causes of the abnormal PSA level, including prostate cancer. If the patient has not experienced a 50% decrease in measured PSA level after 6 months of treatment, it is recommended that the patient be questioned as to his adherence with the prescribed regimen. These agents cause a variety of adverse effects, including sexual dysfunction, which may be a reason for a patient to discontinue the drug against medical advice.

Another interesting aspect of the effect of finasteride on PSA levels is that when finasteride was used to prevent prostate cancer, it appeared to increase the sensitivity of PSA as a screening test for prostate cancer, and to improve the ability of the prostate needle biopsy to detect prostate cancer.[84,88] To minimize the impact of noncancerous conditions on PSA (Table 22-14), it is recommended to allow an adequate interval after the condition has resolved before measuring PSA. Consideration of the 2–3 day plasma half-life of PSA along with the time it takes the condition to resolve affects the time interval to allow. For example, following transurethral prostatectomy, it is recommended to wait 6 weeks before obtaining a PSA, whereas, following ejaculation, it is recommended to wait only 2 days. Also, in a patient with PSA levels in the gray zone of 4–10 ng/mL who has a normal digital rectal exam and no evidence of infection on urinalysis, a short 3-week treatment course of antibiotics (to treat a presumptive prostate infection) has been used before repeating the PSA. In some cases, the PSA returns to the normal range. This strategy has been used to avoid unnecessary biopsy of the patient; however, it is considered a controversial measure at this time.[89]

A 20% biological variation in measured PSA levels has been documented when the PSA ranges from 0.1–20 ng/mL. For this reason, it is common practice to repeat a single elevated PSA and not to take action based on a single elevated value.[86]

MINICASE 2

Interpreting PSA in a Patient with Prostate Cancer

ROBERT R. IS A 60-YEAR-OLD WHITE MALE with newly diagnosed adenocarcinoma of the prostate cancer. He is undergoing cancer staging and risk assessment to determine the next step in his management.

Cc: Robert R. is anxious and concerned about his diagnosis. He has a 10-year-old daughter and an 8-year-old son and expresses fear that he "will not be around" as they grow older.

HPI: On a routine annual physical exam, Robert R. had an abnormal digital rectal exam. The prostate was enlarged and symmetric. A small nodule was palpated and subsequently biopsied, which showed adenocarcinoma, Gleason grade 8 in 60% of the biopsy specimens. Two PSA tests, which were conducted 1 week apart before the prostate needle biopsy, were 25 ng/mL and 28 ng/mL. Liver function tests, BUN, and serum creatinine were all normal.

PMH: Hypertension; leg cramps occasionally at night

Medications: Lisinopril 20 mg orally once a day; aspirin 325 mg orally once a day

Allergies: None

Vital signs: BP 140/85, HR 80, RR 16, weight 200 lb

Question: What does Robert R.'s PSA suggest about the stage of Robert R.'s disease? What additional tests should be performed to confirm the stage of prostate cancer in him?

Discussion: Because Robert R.'s PSA is >20 ng/mL and the prostate cancer is a Gleason grade 8 in a majority of the specimen, he is at high risk of tumor recurrence, and his cancer has likely spread outside of the prostate. To determine the sites of tumor spread, additional testing should include a bone scan, transrectal ultrasound of the prostate, computerized axial tomography (CT) scan of the pelvis, and chest radiograph.

Question: Let us assume that the bone scan shows no boney metastatic sites, the chest radiograph shows no lung metastases, and the CT scan of the pelvis shows no lymphatic invasion. However, the digital rectal exam

PSA and the transrectal ultrasound of the prostate suggest direct extension of the prostate through the prostatic capsule to the periprostatic tissues, including the seminal vesicles. Robert R. has clinical stage T3 prostate cancer. How would this information be used in a risk assessment?

Discussion: Assessment of the risk of tumor recurrence is used to guide treatment selection. Although no single risk assessment tool has been accepted as a standard, most risk assessments are similar in that they are based on the prostate cancer disease stage, PSA, and Gleason score of the tumor. One commonly used risk assessment is depicted below.[39]

As an example, for the low-risk category, a patient with stage T1C or T2A disease, a PSA less than 10 ng/mL or a Gleason score <6, could be offered active surveillance if his life expectancy is less than 10 years, or radiation therapy or radical prostatectomy if his life expectancy is 10 years or more. The selection of a particular treatment should be individualized based on Robert R.'s life expectancy, patient's preference, and patient's ability to deal with potential adverse effects or complications of various treatment options. Active surveillance has no adverse effects and entails PSA monitoring every 6 months and an annual prostate needle biopsy. Such close monitoring will allow the physician to detect early tumor progression to a higher stage or higher grade. Radiation therapy can be delivered as external beam or internally with seed implants into the prostate. As an adjuvant to external beam radiation therapy, androgen deprivation therapy with a combination of an LHRH agonist and an antiandrogen has been shown to be more effective in prolonging tumor-free survival over external beam radiation therapy alone for stage T2 and T3 prostate cancer.[40,41] A radical prostatectomy, which includes removal of the prostate, prostatic urethra, pelvic lymph nodes, and periprostatic tissues is an effective treatment modality for localized prostate cancer and lowers the likelihood of disease recurrence and decreases cancer-related mortality. However, perioperative complications include bleeding and infection. Late complications include urinary incontinence and erectile dysfunction.

Based on Robert R.'s disease stage, Gleason score, and PSA, he is considered at high risk of tumor recurrence and the best treatment option would be external radiation with adjuvant androgen deprivation therapy.

RISK CATEGORY	STAGE OF PROSTATE CANCER[a]	PSA (ng/mL)	GLEASON SCORE	TREATMENT OPTIONS
Low	T1C or T2A	<10	6 or less	Active surveillance if life expectancy <10 yr; radiation therapy or surgery if life expectancy >10 yr
Intermediate	T2B	10–20	7	Active surveillance if life expectancy <10 yr; radiation therapy with or without androgen deprivation therapy or surgery if life expectancy >10 yr
High	T2C or T3A or T3B or T3C	>20	8–10	External radiation with androgen deprivation therapy; or surgery in selected cases

[a]Stage T1 and T2 are localized to the prostate. Stage T3 refers to cancer that has directly extended to periprostatic tissue. Stage T4 is metastatic to lymph nodes, bone, or soft tissues distant from the prostate. The alphabetic letter refers to the volume of the prostate cancer tissue. A refers to one focus; B refers to two foci; and C refers to multiple foci of tumor.

TABLE 22-17. National Institutes of Health Categories of Types of Prostatitis[97]

CATEGORY	SYMPTOMS/SIGNS	% OF PROSTATITIS CASES	INFECTIOUS ETIOLOGY	RESULTS OF 4-GLASS SPECIMEN COLLECTION METHOD
Acute bacterial prostatitis	Acute onset of urinary frequency, urgency, dysuria; perineal or suprapubic pain; and urinary retention; may be associated with fever, chills, nausea, vomiting, malaise, myalgia, lower abdominal or suprapubic discomfort, prostate is swollen, warm, tender on palpation; urinalysis shows significant white blood cells and bacteria; blood cultures are often positive	2–5	Yes	VB1 and/or VB2 are positive for infection
Chronic bacterial prostatitis	History of recurrent urinary tract infection; episodes of perineal, penile, suprapubic pain; frequency, urgency, and dysuria, which are separated by asymptomatic periods; symptoms are present for a minimum of 3 months in duration; prostate may be normal on digital rectal exam, may be mildly tender and boggy, or focally indurated with crepitation; urinalysis shows significant white blood cells	2–5	Yes	EPS and VB3 are positive for infection
Chronic pelvic pain syndrome	Waxing and waning dull aching symptoms of perineal, suprapubic, scrotal or penile pain; pain on ejaculation, may be associated with frequency, urgency, and dysuria; minimum of 3 months in duration; digital rectal exam is unremarkable; this is stratified into inflammatory and noninflammatory disease	90–95	No	All specimens are negative for infection; patients with inflammatory disease have white blood cells, but no bacteria, in EPS and VB3; patients with noninflammatory disease have no white blood cells or bacteria in EPS and VB3
Asymptomatic inflammatory prostatitis	No symptoms; this is incidentally diagnosed on histological review of a prostate tissue biopsy specimen; digital rectal exam is unremarkable	Unknown	No	White blood cells in EPS and/ or VB3

EPS = expressed prostatic secretion; VB1 = first 10 mL of urine voided; VB2 = midstream urine collection; VB3 = first 5–10 mL of urine after prostate massage.

A radioimmunoassay is commonly used to measure total and free PSA levels. Assays are quick to perform and commonly available. Newer commercially available assay kits allow for measurement of PSA concentrations that are less than 0.1 ng/mL. Several different immunoassays are available and results are not interchangeable among them. Therefore, it is recommended that the same assay methodology be used when interpreting serial PSA results.[91]

Prostate Needle Biopsy

A needle biopsy of the prostate is used to establish a tissue diagnosis of prostate cancer. It may be performed transrectally in one of two ways: digitally guided or guided by TRUS.

As a digitally-guided procedure, a biopsy needle is passed over the index finger of the urologist into the rectum and is directed to the site in the prostate where induration or a nodule was palpated. The needle is inserted through the rectal mucosa into the prostate to obtain a core of suspicious tissue. In addition, the urologist obtains four to six other biopsy specimens from the base, lateral mid portion, and apex of the prostate gland. The false-negative rate with this technique is 20%

to 25%.[92] Alternatively, a biopsy gun is used along with transrectal ultrasound for guidance. Local anesthesia is required. To reduce the false-negative rate, the number of random biopsy specimens is increased from 6 or 8–20.[93,94] With the increase in tissue sampling, the false-negative rate is only 4%.[95]

All biopsy specimens are sent to the pathologist for examination. If prostate cancer is detected microscopically, the sample is graded histologically. The Gleason scoring system is used to grade the pattern of glandular differentiation of the prostate tumor. Two grades are assigned: one for the dominant pattern of glandular differentiation and a second for the less prevalent pattern. Uniform, round well-formed glands would be graded as 1 or 2, whereas solid sheets of tumor cells without gland formation would receive a grade of 5. Transition between these two extremes would be graded as 3 or 4. Two grades are assigned if two patterns of infiltration are identified; or, if only one pattern of infiltration is evident, the same number is assigned twice. The two numbers are then added to give the Gleason score, which can range from 2–10. The Gleason score correlates with progression of the tumor and the patient's prognosis; the higher the score the worse the prognosis. A single, tissue specimen score of 4 or more, or a total score of 7 or higher suggests that the patient is at intermediate or high risk of developing metastatic disease.[96] Along with other parameters, the Gleason score has been incorporated into various formulae to predict the prognosis of patients. (See Minicase 2.)

Prostate needle biopsy is an invasive procedure. It can be painful and result in minor bleeding and infection. However, severe adverse effects requiring hospitalization occur in less than 1% of patients.[50]

PROSTATITIS

Prostatitis is the most common genitourinary tract disorder among men less than 50 years of age. The lifetime prevalence is 16%. Prostatitis is an inflammatory condition of the prostate gland due to infection or a noninfectious cause. The National Institutes of Health (NIH) has stratified patients with prostatitis into four unique categories (Table 22-17). Of these, only the first two categories—acute and chronic prostatitis—have infection as the etiology and are generally responsive to antibiotic treatment. For the other two categories—chronic pelvic pain syndrome and asymptomatic inflammatory prostatitis—the etiology is unclear, which accounts for the low response rates to existing treatments. Chronic pelvic pain syndrome can be inflammatory or noninflammatory (i.e., inflammation is evidenced by the presence of white blood cells in the expressed prostate secretion (EPS), semen, or in tissue removed from the prostate during prostatectomy or biopsy).[97,98]

Differentiation among the types of prostatitis is largely determined by clinical presentation of the patient, digital rectal exam of the prostate, and the laboratory analysis of EPS. Digital exam of the inflamed prostate is described as boggy or having a softer consistency than usual. Patients with acute bacterial prostatitis are symptomatic of their infection with fever, nausea, vomiting, urinary frequency, urgency, and dysuria. They may also develop acute urinary retention. Because of the concern that prostate massage could expel bacteria from the prostate into the bloodstream, prostate massage is not performed in patients with suspected acute prostatitis. Instead symptoms and blood and urine cultures are used to diagnose the disease. Expressed prostatic secretion is key for diagnosing chronic bacterial prostatitis, chronic pelvic pain syndrome, and asymptomatic inflammatory prostatitis, and it is collected after a prostate massage, in which the prostate is stroked from side to side and then from top to bottom during a digital rectal exam for 2–3 minutes (the resulting fluid is collected as it drips out of the urethral meatus).[98,99]

To assess symptoms and their severity, the NIH has devised a symptom index, which is a self-assessment tool comprised of nine questions that focus on the quality of the patient's pain, urinary voiding symptoms, and impact of the symptoms on the patient's quality of life. The total score ranges from 0–43; the higher the score the worse the symptoms. This tool is used for a baseline assessment and then repeated at regular intervals during the course of the patient's care. This symptom survey is considered a reliable and valid instrument and is commonly used in practice.[97,100]

4-Glass Versus 2-Glass Method of Specimen Collection

The classic method for collecting a specimen to diagnose chronic prostatitis is the 4-glass specimen collection method.[97,101] The specimens include the following:

- **Glass 1 or voided bladder (VB1) specimen (first 10 mL of urine)**—This represents the urethral specimen.
- **Glass 2 or VB2 specimen (a midstream urine collection)**—This represents the bladder specimen.
- **Glass 3 or EPS**—After a 1- to 3-minute prostate massage, EPS will drip out of the urethra over the next few minutes. This represents the prostate specimen.
- **Glass 4 or VB3 (first 5–10 mL of urine after the prostate massage)**—This sample will include any residual EPS in the urethra. This represents the prostate specimen as well.

Although the 4-glass specimen collection method has been considered the standard for diagnosis, it should be noted that the method has not been validated for accuracy.[102] The diagnosis of chronic bacterial prostatitis is made when the bacterial culture in EPS or urine specimen after the prostate massage (VB3) has a 10-fold greater bacterial count as compared to the urethral (VB1) and bladder specimens (VB2).

Because of the complexity and time-consuming nature of the 4-glass specimen collection method, many clinicians use only a 2-glass method, collecting a VB2 and VB3 specimen pre- and post-massage, respectively. The 2-glass method produces results that are comparable to the 4-glass method, and the former has a sensitivity and specificity of at least 90%, and is 96% to 98% as accurate as the 4-glass method.[100,102]

In addition to sending all specimens for bacterial culture, EPS and VB3 are checked for the presence of white blood cells. A drop of EPS is applied to a glass side, a cover slip is placed on top, and the specimen is examined under high power on the microscope. VB3 specimens are typically centrifuged for 5 minutes first, and the sediment is examined in a similar fashion. The presence of more than 5–10 white blood cells per high power field is considered significant of inflammation.[97] Finally, it should be noted that when chronic prostatitis is strongly suspected, but EPS cultures are negative, semen specimens have been used as a substituted for EPS.

SUMMARY

This chapter reviews common clinical tests and laboratory tests used for diagnosing and monitoring treatment for common urologic disorders in elderly males including ADAM, erectile dysfunction, BPH, prostate cancer, and prostatitis. Many of these disorders are managed with tests other than laboratory tests.

Learning Points

1. What is the differentiation between serum total testosterone levels and free testosterone levels?

Answer: Testosterone circulates in the bloodstream in several forms: free testosterone and testosterone bound to proteins, specifically SHBG and albumin. Most protein-bound testosterone is bound to SHBG and only a small portion is bound to albumin. The free testosterone fraction is physiologically active. Typically, when a clinician orders a testosterone serum level, the level reflects the total testosterone concentration in the bloodstream, which includes free and protein-bound testosterone. A free testosterone serum level reflects only the unbound portion of testosterone in the bloodstream. Free testosterone serum levels may be indicated in patients in whom the concentration of SHBG is decreased or increased. In such patients, a free testosterone serum level will be a better indicator of the concentration of physiologically active testosterone. Increased SHBG is associated with cirrhosis, hyperthyroidism, old age, and drug treatment with estrogens or anticonvulsants. Decreased SHBG is associated with hypothyroidism, obesity, and drug treatment with excessive doses of testosterone supplements.

2. Why does the AUA Symptom Score not correlate with the findings on digital rectal exam or peak urinary flow rate in a patient with BPH?

Answer: The AUA Symptom Score is derived from a patient's self-reporting and self-assessment of the bothersomeness of obstructive and/or irritative voiding symptoms due to BPH. Thus, it is a subjective assessment. It is well-known that many elderly patients with BPH may deny the presence of bothersome voiding symptoms and may attribute their symptoms to their advancing age. Thus, some patients think that their problems are a normal part of the aging process and should not be treated. Other patients will make lifestyle changes (e.g., drink less fluids, take naps during the day because it is impossible to sleep through the night) to try to ameliorate their symptoms. Thus, the AUA Symptom Score may not correlate with the size of the prostate as assessed by digital rectal exam, the decrease in peak urinary flow rate, or the degree of bladder neck obstruction on cystoscopy, which are usual objective findings in patients with BPH.

3. Should a serum prolactin level be obtained routinely in patients with erectile dysfunction?

Answer: Hyperprolactinemia occurs in only 1% to 2% of men with erectile dysfunction; therefore, serum prolactin levels should not be routinely obtained in patients who present with erectile dysfunction. However, in patients with late-onset hypogonadism and erectile dysfunction, whose symptoms are not corrected with a testosterone replacement regimen that restores serum testosterone to the normal range, it is reasonable to check serum prolactin levels.

4. Why are digital rectal exam and PSA used together to screen for prostate cancer?

Answer: As a single screening test, the digital rectal exam has insufficient sensitivity and specificity for prostate cancer. Some prostate tumors develop in an area of the prostate, which is not easy to palpate. In addition, some of the physical changes associated with prostate cancer (e.g., glandular enlargement or changes in prostate consistency) can be due to noncancerous diseases of the prostate. Finally, the quality of the exam is highly dependent on the expertise of the clinician who is performing the test. Prostate specific antigen has high sensitivity but low specificity for prostate cancer. Many noncancerous conditions of the prostate are associated with increased PSA levels. This includes prostatitis, BPH, manipulation of the prostate (including biopsy, transrectal ultrasonography, massage, etc.), urethral catheterization, prostate surgery, acute urinary retention, etc. In addition, use of an exercise bicycle or ejaculation can elevate PSA. A PSA in the normal range is found is 27% of patients with prostate cancer. Using a digital rectal exam and PSA together to screen for prostate cancer increases the sensitivity and specificity of both tests. Successful early screening for prostate cancer results in earlier diagnosis of prostate cancer in patients and a reduction in the number of patients with advanced stage disease on first presentation for medical care.

REFERENCES

1. Morley JE, Perry HM. Andropause: an old concept in new clothing. *Clin Geriatr Med.* 2003;19:507-528.

2. Bain J. Testosterone and the aging male: to treat or not to treat. *Maturitas.* 2010;66:16-22.

3. Roehrborn CG, Boyle P, Nickel JC, et al. Efficacy and safety of a dual inhibitor of 5-alpha reductase types 1 and 2 (dutasteride) in men with benign prostatic hyperplasia. *Urology.* 2002;60:434-441.

4. Bassel N, Late-onset hypogonadism. *Med Clin N Am.* 2011;95:507-523.

5. Corona G, Rastrelli G, Forti G, et al. Update on testosterone for men. *J Sex Med* 2011;8:639-654.

6. Lombardo F, Lupini C, Meola A, et al. Clinical and laboratoristic strategy in late onset hypogonadism. *Acta Biomed.* 2010;81 (suppl 1):85-88.

7. Jockenhovel F. Testosterone therapy-what, when, and to whom? *Aging Male.* 2004;7:319-324.

8. Brand T, Canby-Hagino E, Thompson IM. Testosterone replacement therapy and prostate cancer: a word of caution. *Curr Urol Rep.* 2007;8:185-189.

9. Morley JE, Perry HM 3rd, Kevorkian RT, et al. Comparison of screening questionnaires for the diagnosis of hypogonadism. *Maturitas.* 2006;53:424-429.

10. Morley JE, Charlton E, Patrick P, et al. ADAM: validation of a screening questionnaire for androgen deficiency in aging males. *Metabolism.* 2000;49:1239-1242.

11. Heinemann LA, Saad F, Heinemann K, et al. Can results of the Aging Males' Symptoms (AMS) scale predict those of screening scales for androgen deficiency? *Aging Male.* 2004;7:211-218.

12. Wang C, Nieschlag E, Swerdloff R, et al. Investigation, treatment, and monitoring of late onset hypogonadism in males. *J Androl.* 2009;30:1-9.

13. Morgentaler A, Rhoden EL. Prevalence of prostate cancer among hypogonadal men with prostate-specific antigen levels of 4.0 ng/mL or less. *Urology.* 2006; 68:1263-1267.

14. American Association of Clinical Endocrinologists. AACE Medical Guidelines for Clinical Practice for the evaluation and treatment of hypogonadism in adult male patients-2002 update. *Endocr Pract.* 2002;8:440-456.

15. Rosner W, Vesper H on behalf of The Endocrine Society and the endorsing organizations. Toward excellence in testosterone testing. A consensus statement. *J Clin Endocrinol Metab.* 2010;95:4542-4548.

16. Wu FC. Tajar A. Beynon JM, et al. Identification of late onset hypogonadism in middle-aged and elderly men. *N Engl J Med.* 2010;363:123-135.

17. Diver MJ. Analytical and physiologic factors affecting the interpretation of serum testosterone concentrations in men. *Ann Clin Biochem.* 2006;43(part 1):3-12.

18. Swerdloff R, Wang C. Testosterone treatment of older men-why are controversies created? *J Clin Endocrinol Metab.* 2011;96:62-65.

19. Goncharov N, Katsya G, Dobracheva A, et al. Serum testosterone measurement in men: evaluation of modern immunoassay technologies. *Aging Male.* 2005;8:194-202.

20. Wang C, Catlin DH, Demers LM, et al. Measurement of total serum testosterone in adult men: comparison of current laboratory methods versus liquid chromatography-tandem mass spectrometry. *J Clin Endocrinol Metab.* 2004;89:534-543.

21. Rosner W, Auchus RJ, Azziz R, et al. Position statement: utility, limitations, and pitfalls in measuring testosterone: an Endocrine Society position statement. *J Clin Endocrinol Metab.* 2007;92:405-413.

22. Cawood ML, Field HP, Ford CG, et al. Testosterone measurement by isotope-dilution liquid chromatography-tandem mass spectrometry: validation of a method for routine clinical practice. *Clin Chem.* 2005;51:1472-1479.

23. Bhasin S, Cunningham GR, Hayes FJ, et al. Testosterone therapy in men with androgen deficiency syndromes: an Endocrine Society Clinical Practice Guideline. *J Clin Endocrinol Metab.* 2010;95:2536-59.

24. Van Uytfanghe K, Stockl D, Kaufman JM, et al. Validation of 5 routine assays for serum free testosterone with a candidate reference measurement procedure based on ultrafiltration and isotope dilution-gas chromatography-mass spectrometry. *Clin Biochem.* 2005;38:253-261.

25. Goncharov N, Katsya G, Dobracheva A, et al. Diagnostic significance of free salivary testosterone measurement using a direct luminescence immunoassay in healthy men and in patients with disorders of androgenic status. *Aging Male.* 2006;9:111-122.

26. NIH Consensus Conference. Impotence. NIH Consensus Development Panel on Impotence. *JAMA.* 1993;270:83-90.

27. Feldman HA, Goldstein I, Hatzichristou DG, et al. Impotence and its medical and psychosocial correlates: results of the Massachusetts Male Aging Study. *J Urol.* 1994;151:54-61.

28. Bacon CG, Mittleman MA, Kawachi I, et al. Sexual function in men older than 50 years of age: results from the health professionals follow-up study. *Ann Intern Med.* 2003;139:161-168.

29. Bacon CG, Mittleman MA, Kawachi I, et al. A prospective study of risk factors for erectile dysfunction. *J Urol.* 2006;176:217-221.

30. McVary KT. Erectile dysfunction. *New Engl J Med.* 2007;357:2472-2481.

31. Rosen RC, Riley A, Wagner G, et al. The international index of erectile function (IIEF): a multidimensional scale for assessment of erectile function. *Urology.* 1997;49:822-830.

32. Rosen RC, Capelleri JC, Smith MD, et al. Development and evaluation of an abridged, 5-item version of the International Index of Erectile Function as a diagnostic tool for erectile function. *Int J Impot Res.* 1999;11:319-326.

33. Lue TF, Basson R, Rosen R, et al. *Sexual Medicine: Sexual Dysfunction in Men and Women.* Paris: Health Publications; 2004.

34. Haddad PM, Wieck A. Antipsychotic-induced hyperprolactinemia: mechanisms, clinical features, and management. *Drugs.* 2004;64:2291-2314.

35. Volovka J, Czobor P, Cooper TB, et al. Prolactin levels in schizophrenia and schizoaffective disorder patients treated with clozapine, olanzapine, risperidone, or haloperidol. *J Clin Psych.* 2004;65:57-61.

36. Hackett G, Kell P, Ralph D, et al. British Society for Sexual Medicine guidelines on the management of erectile dysfunction. *J Sex Med.* 2008;5:1841-1865.

37. Arrighi HM, Metter EJ, Guess HA, et al. Natural history of benign prostatic hyperplasia and risk of prostatectomy: the Baltimore Longitudinal Study of Aging. *Urology.* 1991;38(1 suppl):4-8.

38. AUA Practice Guideline Committee. AUA guidelines on management of benign prostatic hyperplasia: 2003. Chapter 1: diagnosis and treatment recommendations. *J Urol.* 2003;170:530-547.

39. Mohler J, Bahnson RR, Boston B, et al. NCCN clinical practice guidelines in oncology: prostate cancer. *J Natl Comp Canc Netw.* 2010;8:162-200.

40. Carter HB. Management of low (favourable)-risk prostate cancer. *BJU Int.* 2011;108:1684-1695.

41. Jones CU, Hunt D, McGowan DG, et al. Radiotherapy and short term androgen deprivation for localized prostate cancer. *N Engl J Med.* 2011;365:107-118.

42. Bosch JLHR, Hop WCJ, Kirkels WJ, et al. The international prostate symptom score in a community sample of men between 55 and 74 years of age: prevalence and correlation of symptoms with age, prostate volume, flow rate, and residual urine volume. *Br J Urol.* 1995;75:622-630.

43. Roehrborn CG, Germain CJ, Rhodes T, et al. Correlation between prostate size estimated by digital rectal examination and measured by transrectal ultrasound. *Urology.* 1997;49:548-557.

44. McConnell JD, Roehrborn CG, Bautista OM, et al. The long-term effect of doxazosin, finasteride, and combination therapy on the clinical progression of benign prostatic hyperplasia. *N Engl J Med.* 2003;349:2387-2398.

45. Roehrborn CG, Barkin J, Siami P, et al. Clinical outcomes after combined therapy with dutasteride plus tamsulosin or either monotherapy in men with benign prostatic hyperplasia (BPH) by baseline characteristics: 4-year results from the randomized double-blind Combination of Avodart and Tamsulosin (CombAT) trial. *BJU Int.* 2011;107:946-954.

46. Beckman TJ, Mynderse LA. Evaluation and medical management of benign prostatic hyperplasia. *Mayo Clin Proc.* 2005;80:1356-1362.

47. Lam JS, Cooper MD, Kaplan SA. Changing aspects in the evaluation and treatment of patients with benign prostatic hyperplasia. *Med Clin North Am.* 2004;88:281-308.

48. McConnell JD, Barry MJ, Bruskewitz RC. Benign prostatic hyperplasia: diagnosis and treatment. Agency for Health Care Policy and Research. *Clinical Practice Guide Quick Reference Guide.* 1994;8:1-17.

49. McNeill SA, Hargreave TB, Geffriaud-Ricouard C, et al. Postvoid residual urine in patients with lower urinary tract symptoms suggestive of benign prostatic hyperplasia: pooled analysis of eleven controlled studies with alfuzosin. *Urology.* 2001;57:459-465.

50. Coley CM, Barry MJ, Fleming C, et al. Early detection of prostate cancer. Clinical guideline. Part 1. *Ann Intern Med.* 1997;126:394-406.

51. Hernandez J, Thompson IM. Diagnosis and treatment of prostate cancer. *Med Clin North Am.* 2004;88:267-279.

52. Carroll P, Albertson PC, Greene K, et al. American Urological Association prostate specific antigen best practice statement 2009 update (updated January 11, 2011). Available at http://www.auanet.org/content/guidelines.and.quality.care/clinical-guidelines/main.

53. Lim LS, Sherin K. Screening for prostate cancer in U.S. men. ACPM position statement on preventative practice. *Am J Prev Med.* 2008;34:164–170.

54. U.S. Preventative Services Task Force. Screening for prostate cancer: US Preventative Task Force recommendation statement. *Ann Intern Med.* 2009;149:185–191.

55. Schroder FH, Hugosson J, Roobol MJ, et al. Screening and prostate cancer mortality in a randomized European study. *N Engl J Med.* 2009;360:1320–1328.

56. Catalona WJ. The United States Preventative Services Task Force recommendation against prostate specific antigen screening— counterpoint. *Cancer Epidemiol Biomarkers Prev.* 2012;21:395–397.

57. Thompson IM, Pauler DK, Goodman PJ, et al. Prevalence of prostate cancer among men with a prostate-specific antigen level ≤4.0 ng per milliliter. *N Engl J Med.* 2004;350:2239–2246.

58. Catalona WJ, Richie JP, Ahmann FR, et al. Comparison of digital rectal examination and serum prostate specific antigen in the early detection of prostate cancer: results of a multicenter clinical trial of 6,630 men. *J Urol.* 1994;151:1283–1290.

59. Reiter WJ, Keane TE, Ahlman MA, et al. Diagnostic performance of In-11 capromab pendetide SPEC/CT in localized and metastatic prostate cancer. *Clin Nucl Med.* 2011;36(1):872–878.

60. Gjertson CK, Albertsen PC. Use and assessment of PSA in prostate cancer. *Med Clin North Am.* 2011;95:191–200.

61. Shariat SF, Semjnonow A, Lilja H, et al. Tumor markers in prostate cancer I: blood-based markers. *Acta Oncol.* 2011;50(suppl 1):61–75.

62. Oesterling JE, Jacobsen SJ, Chute CG, et al. Serum prostate specific antigen in a community-based population of healthy men: establishment of age-specific reference ranges. *JAMA.* 1993;270:860–864.

63. Gelmann EP, Chia D, Pinsky PF, et al. PLCO screening trial investigators: relationship of demographic and clinical factors to free and total prostate specific antigen. *Urology.* 2001;58:561–566.

64. Banez LL, Hamilton RJ, Partin AW, et al. Obesity-related plasma hemodilution and PSA concentration among men with prostate cancer. *JAMA.* 2007;298:2275–2280.

65. Fowler JE Jr, Bigler SA, Kilambi NK, et al. Relationships between prostate-specific antigen and prostate volume in black and white men with benign prostate biopsies. *Urology.* 1999;53:1175–1178.

66. American College of Physicians. Screening for prostate cancer. Clinical guideline: Part III. *Ann Intern Med.* 1997;126:480–484.

67. Catalona WJ, Richie JP, Ahmann FR. Comparison of digital rectal examination and serum prostate specific antigen in the early detection of prostate cancer: results of a multicenter clinical trial of 6,630 men. *J Urol.* 1994;151:1283–1290.

68. Jemel A, Siegal R, Xu J, et al. Cancer statistics, 2010. *CA Cancer J Clin.* 2010;60:277–300.

69. Humphrey PA. Gleason grading and prognostic factors in carcinoma of the prostate. *Mod Pathol.* 2004;17:292–306.

70. Montironi R, Egevad L, Bjartell A, et al. Role of histopathology and molecular markers in the active surveillance of prostate cancer. *Acta Oncol.* 2011;50 (suppl 1):56–60.

71. Tchetgen MB, Song JT, Stawderman M, et al. Ejaculation increases the serum prostate specific antigen concentration. *Urology.* 1996;47:511–516.

72. Catalona WJ, Smith DS, Ornstein DK. Prostate cancer detection in men with serum PSA concentrations of 2.6–4.0 ng/mL and benign prostate examination: enhancement of specificity with free PSA measurements. *JAMA.* 1997;277:1452–1455.

73. Punglia RS, D'Amico AV, Catalona WJ. Effect of verification bias on screening for prostate cancer by measurement of prostate specific antigen. *N Engl J Med.* 2003;349:335–342.

74. Stephan C, Miller K, Jung K. Is there an optimal prostate specific antigen threshold for prostate biopsy. *Expert Rev Anticancer Ther.* 2011;11:1215–1221.

75. Oesterling JE, Jacobsen SJ, Cooner WH. The use of age-specific reference ranges for serum prostate specific antigen in men 60 years old or older. *J Urol.* 1995;153:1160–1163.

76. Loeb S, Roehl Ka, Antenor JA, et al. Baseline prostate specific antigen compared with median prostate specific antigen for age group as predictor of prostate cancer risk in men younger than 60 years old. *Urology.* 2006;67:316–320.

77. Catalona WJ, Southwick PC, Slawin KM, et al. Comparison of percent free PSA, PSA density, and age-specific PSA cutoffs for prostate cancer detection and staging. *Urology.* 2000;56:255–260.

78. Routh JC, Leibovich BC. Adenocarcinoma of the prostate: epidemiological trends, screening, diagnosis, and surgical management of localized disease. *Mayo Clin Proceed.* 2005;80:899–907.

79. Loeb S, Roehl Ka, Catalona WJ, et al. Prostate specific antigen velocity threshold for predicting prostate cancer in young men. *J Urol.* 2007;177:899–902.

80. Cannon GM Jr, Walsh PC, Partin AW, et al. Prostate specific antigen doubling time in the identification of patients at risk for progression after treatment and biochemical recurrence for prostate cancer. *Urology.* 2003;62(suppl 2B):2–8.

81. Catalona WJ, Smith DS, Wolfert RL, et al. Evaluation of percentage of free serum prostate specific antigen to improve specificity of prostate cancer screening. *JAMA.* 1995;274:1214–1220.

82. Catalona WJ, Partin AW, Slawin KM, et al. Use of the percentage of free prostate specific antigen to enhance differentiation of prostate cancer from benign prostatic disease: a prospective multicenter clinical trial. *JAMA.* 1998;279:1542–1547.

83. Pruthi RS. The dynamics of prostate-specific antigen in benign and malignant diseases of the prostate. *BJU Intern.* 2000;86:652–658.

84. Stenman UH. Leinonen J, Alfthan H, et al. A complex between prostate-specific antigen and alpha 1-antichymotrypsin is the major form of prostate-specific antigen in serum of patients with prostate cancer: assay of the complex improves clinical sensitivity for cancer. *Cancer Res.* 1991;51:222–226.

85. Andriole GL, Marberger M, Roehrborn CG. Clinical usefulness of serum prostate specific antigen for the detection of prostate cancer is preserved in men receiving dual 5a-reductase inhibitor dutasteride. *J Urol.* 2006;175:1657–1662.

86. Soletormos G, Semjenow A, Sibley PE, et al. Biological variation of total prostate specific antigen: a survey of published estimates and consequences for clinical practice. *Clin Chem.* 2005;51:1342–1351.

87. D'Amico AV, Roehrborn CG. Effect of 1 mg/d finasteride on concentrations of serum prostate specific antigen in men with androgenic alopecia: a randomized controlled trial. *Lancet Oncol.* 2007;8:21–25.

88. Thompson IM, Chi C, Ankerst DP. Effect of finasteride on the sensitivity of PSA for detecting prostate cancer. *J Natl Cancer Inst.* 2006;98:1128–1133.

89. Kaygisiz O, Ugurlo O, Kosan M, et al. Effects of antibacterial therapy on PSA change in the presence and absence of prostatic inflammation in patients with PSA levels between 4 and 10 ng/mL. *Prostate Cancer Prostatic Dis.* 2006;9:235–238.

90. Scardino PT. The responsible use of antibiotics for an elevated PSA level. *Nat Clin Pract Urol.* 2007;4:1.

91. Stephen C, Klaas M, Muller C, et al. Interchangeability of measurements of total and free prostate specific antigen in serum with 5 frequently used assay combinations: an update: *Clin Chem.* 2006;52:59–64.

92. Stroumbakis N, Cookson MS, Reuter VE, et al. Clinical significance of repeat sextant biopsies in prostate cancer patients. *Urol.* 1997;49:113–118.

93. Presti JC Jr, Chang JJ, Bhargava V et al. The optimal systematic prostate biopsy strategy scheme should include 8 rather than 6 biopsies: results of a prospective clinical trial. *J Urol.* 2000;163:163–167.

94. Yamamoto S, Ito T, Aizawa T, et al. Does transrectal ultrasound guided eight-core prostate biopsy improve cancer detection rates in patients with prostate-specific antigen levels of 4.1–10 ng/mL? *Int J Urol.* 2004;11:386–391.

95. Descazeaud A, Rubin M, Chemama S, et al. Saturation biopsy protocol enhances prediction of pT3 and surgical margin status on prostatectomy specimen. *World J Urol.* 2006;24:676–680.

96. Epstein JI, Partin AW, Sauvageot J, et al. Prediction of progression following radical prostatectomy: a multivariate analysis of 721 men with long-term follow-up. *Am J Surg Pathol.* 1996;20:286–292.

97. Litwin MS, McNaughton Collins M, Fowler FJ Jr, et al for the Chronic Prostatitis Collaborative Research Network: The National Institutes of Health Chronic Prostatitis Symptom Index: development and validation of a new outcome measure. *J Urol.* 1999;162:369–375.

98. Lipsky BA, Byren I, Hoey CT. Treatment of bacterial prostatitis. *Clin Infect Dis.* 2010;50:1641–1652.

99. Nickel JC, Alexander RB, Schaeffer AJ, et al. Leukocytes and bacteria in men with chronic prostatitis/chronic pelvic pain syndrome compared to asymptomatic controls. *J Urol.* 2003;170:818–822.

100. Touma NJ, Nickel JC. Prostatitis and chronic pelvic pain syndrome in men. *Med Clin N Am.* 2011;95:75–86.

101. Benway BM, Moon TD. Bacterial prostatitis. *Urol Clin N Am.* 2008;35:23–32.

102. Nickel JC, Shokses D, Wang Y, et al. How does the pre-massage and post-massage 2-glass test compare to pain syndrome? *J Urol.* 2006;176:119–124.

QUICKVIEW | Testosterone

PARAMETER	DESCRIPTION	COMMENTS
Reference range		
Adult, males	280–1100 ng/dL	Normal range exhibits variability lab-to-lab
		This is largely due to the assay method used
		It is recommended that each lab establish its own normal range
Critical values	<230 ng/dL (generally associated with symptomatic hypogonadism)	Extremely high or low values should be reported quickly
	≤50 ng/dL is associated with surgical or medical castration	
	Residual serum testosterone levels reflect continuing adrenal androgen production	
Inherent action?	Yes	Exerts different physiologic effects at different stages of life in males (Table 22-1)
Location		
Production	Testosterone is produced in the testes	The testes produce 90% of circulating androgen; the rest is produced by the adrenal glands
Storage	It is not stored	
Secretion/excretion	Testosterone is activated to dihydrotestosterone intracellularly in some target tissues by 5α reductase; in adipose tissue, excess testosterone is converted to estrogen	In some target tissues (e.g., brain) testosterone is active; in other target tissues (e.g., prostate and scalp) testosterone must be activated to dihydrotestosterone to exert an effect; peripheral conversion of testosterone to estrogen results in gynecomastia
Causes of abnormal values		
High	Hyperthyroidism, adrenal tumors, adrenal hyperplasia, testicular tumors, precocious puberty, anabolic steroids, excessive testosterone supplementation	
Low	Primary or secondary hypogonadism, late-onset hypogonadism, primary or secondary hypopituitarism, Klinefelter syndrome, orchiectomy, traumatic injury to testicles, mumps, maldescent of testicles, hepatic cirrhosis, excessive exercise, hyperprolactinemia, hypothyroidism, high-dose corticosteroids, LHRH antagonists, LHRH agonists, estrogens	
Signs and symptoms		
High level	Increased libido, mood swings	
Low level	Absent or depressed libido, lack of energy, decreased sense of well being, erectile dysfunction, gynecomastia, small testicles, decreased body hair	

LHRH = luteinizing hormone–releasing hormone.

QUICKVIEW | Testosterone (cont'd)

PARAMETER	DESCRIPTION	COMMENTS
After event, time to...		
Initial evaluation	After orchiectomy, serum testosterone levels decrease to ≤50 ng/dL in several hours	Orchiectomy is indicated for symptomatic management of metastatic prostate cancer
Peak values	After depot LHRH superagonist injection, serum testosterone levels decrease to ≤50 ng/dL in 2–3 weeks	LHRH superagonists are alternatives to orchiectomy for symptomatic management of metastatic prostate cancer
Normalization	With testosterone supplementation for late-onset hypogonadism an adequate clinical trial is 3 months in length; after supplementation is started, serum testosterone should be repeated every 3–4 months during the first year; a low baseline serum testosterone level should return to the normal range with adequate supplementation	Depending on the dosage formulation of testosterone supplement, supraphysiologic serum testosterone concentrations may be produced after administration This occurs with intramuscular depot injections In contrast, with other dosage formulations (e.g., testosterone transdermal patches or buccal patch systems), only physiologic serum testosterone concentrations are produced after drug administration The clinical significance of this difference is not known
Causes of spurious results	Excessive testosterone supplementation	
Additional information	Testosterone bound to SHBG is inactive; therefore, conditions which significantly alter the concentration of SHBG can increase or decrease the concentration of free testosterone, which is physiologically active (see Table 22-6 for a listing of such conditions)	In such patients, a free testosterone level would be preferred over a total serum testosterone level

LHRH = luteinizing hormone-releasing hormone; SHBG = sex hormone-binding globulin.

QUICKVIEW | PSA[a]

PARAMETER	DESCRIPTION	COMMENTS
Reference range		
Adult, males	<4 ng/mL	This cutoff value misses 20% to 25% of patients with organ-confined prostate cancer; as a result, some experts recommend using age-related normal ranges (Table 22-15), % fPSA, or PSA velocity instead
Critical values	≥10 ng/mL is highly suggestive of prostate cancer	Extremely high values should be reported to the physician quickly
Inherent action?	Yes	Responsible for liquefying semen after ejaculation
Location		
Production	PSA is produced by the prostate	
Storage	It is not stored	
Secretion/ excretion	PSA normally passes out of the body in the ejaculate; it liquefies semen	Blood levels of PSA are usually very low; however, in patients with prostate cancer or other diseases of the prostate, the normal prostatic architecture of ducts is not intact
		Instead of passing out of the body, PSA enters the bloodstream, which results in elevated blood levels
Causes of abnormal values		
High	Prostate cancer	Noncancerous causes of high results include BPH, prostatitis, prostate trauma, prostate surgery, acute urinary retention, ejaculation, exercise bicycling, exogenous testosterone supplements
Low	Low lab results are normal.	
Signs and symptoms		
High level	This disease is commonly asymptomatic until the prostate cancer is large enough to cause voiding symptoms, or until the tumor has metastasized; in the latter case, the patient may complain of bone pain, shortness of breath, or leg weakness due to bone, lung, or spinal cord metastases, respectively	
Low level	Not applicable	
After insult, time to...		
Initial evaluation	After prostate manipulation, the PSA levels will increase within hours and remain elevated for the duration of the prostatic inflammation; for example, after prostate massage, PSA may return to the normal range within days, whereas after transurethral prostatectomy, it may take weeks	
Peak values		
Causes of spurious results		
	As patients age, PSA normally increases	
	BPH and organ-confined prostate cancer show overlap in PSA levels	
	(See Table 22-14 for other conditions that increase PSA)	

BPH = benign prostatic hyperplasia; PSA = Prostate specific antigen.
[a]Percentage of fPSA, PSA velocity, and PSA density are additional types of PSA tests that are used to improve the usefulness of PSA as a tumor marker for prostate cancer screening and to monitor treatment response.

1,25 dihydroxycholecalciferol—most potent form of vitamin D, which is a result of both hepatic and renal activation of precursor. It enhances intestinal absorption of calcium, enhances parathyroid hormone-induced bone resorption, and enhances calcium reabsorption in the proximal renal tubules. Overall, vitamin D is important for maintaining serum calcium levels in the normal range.

5α reductase—intracellular enzyme in some target tissues for testosterone, which converts testosterone to an active metabolite, dihydrotestosterone. Two types of 5α reductase exist. Type I is mostly found in the skin, liver, and sebaceous glands. Type II is mostly found in urogenital tissue, including the prostate, and hair follicles.

Achiral—a drug that exists in only one form such that the molecules are superimposable on their mirror images.

Acrodermatitis enteropathica—a rare inherited disorder of infants and young children characterized by skin eruptions around the mouth and other body orifices, alopecia, and diarrhea. The disorder is caused by zinc deficiency.

Action potential—changes in electrical potential across muscle or nerve cell when triggered by an appropriate stimulus leading to cellular contraction.

Adipsia—absence of thirst.

ADME—refers to absorption, distribution, metabolism, and excretion of drugs, which are all related to pharmacokinetic handling of drugs by the human body.

Agglutination—the clumping or aggregation of cells (e.g., erythrocytes) in a solution.

Airway resistance—the degree of ease with which air can pass through the airways. It is expressed as the change in pressure divided by the change in flow.

Allele—an alternate form of the gene that is located at a particular chromosomal location. One allele is inherited from our mother and one from our father.

Alpha fetoprotein—also known as *AFP*, this glycoprotein is produced by the liver, gastrointestinal tract, and fetal yolk sac. Elevated serum levels may occur in patients with hepatocellular carcinoma, nonseminomatous germ cell tumors, and cancers of the pancreas, stomach, lung, and colon. For this reason, AFP is used as a tumor marker.

Amenorrhea—absence of menstrual bleeding, which may be primary or secondary.

Amylin—a peptide hormone, cosecreted with insulin, that slows gastric emptying after eating, decreases gastrointestinal glucose absorption, and promotes satiety. Amylin helps reduce postprandial increases in serum glucose levels.

Analyte—the substance measured by the laboratory assay.

Anion gap—this calculated value is used to identify potential causes of metabolic acidosis. The anion gap is estimated by subtracting the sum of serum chloride and venous bicarbonate concentrations from the serum sodium concentration.

Anisocytosis—variability in the size of erythrocytes (red blood cells).

Antibiogram—a cumulative report describing the in vitro antimicrobial susceptibility results of the most common bacterial strains isolated at a particular institution/healthcare setting during the time period of the report (usually annually).

Anticyclic citrullinated peptide (anti-CCP) antibodies—also known as *anti-citrulline antibody* or *citrulline antibody*. These antibodies bind to the nonstandard amino acid citrulline and are highly specific for rheumatoid arthritis when present in serum.

Antidiuretic hormone—also known as *arginine vasopressin*. This hormone regulates renal handling of free water. It is secreted by the hypothalamus in response to hypovolemia, thirst, increased serum osmolality, and angiotensin II.

Antineutrophil cytoplasmic antibodies (ANCAs)—antibodies directed against neutrophil cytoplasmic antigens. Testing for ANCAs is important for diagnosis and classification of various forms of vasculitis.

Antinuclear antibodies (ANA)—autoantibodies directed against components of the cell nucleus, such as DNA, RNA, and histones.

Antiphospholipid antibodies—these antibodies react with proteins in the blood that are bound to phospholipid. Antiphospholipid antibodies interfere with the normal function of blood vessels by causing narrowing and irregularity of the vessel, thrombocytopenia, and thrombosis. Examples of these antiphospholipid antibodies include lupus anticoagulant and anticardiolipin antibodies.

Apophysis—an offshoot.

Apoptosis—noninflammatory cell death via autolysis.

Asherman syndrome—development of intrauterine scar tissue after intrauterine surgery, which can lead to amenorrhea.

Atrial natriuretic factor—also known as *atrial natriuretic peptide*, is a vasodilatory hormone synthesized and primarily released by the right atrium. It is secreted in response to plasma volume expansion as a result of increased atrial stretch and results in a global down regulation of renin, aldosterone, and ADH. A net increase in sodium excretion is achieved.

B-RAF—mutated B-RAF proteins have elevated kinase activity. The proteins are controlled by a B-RAF gene. Vemurafenib is a serine-threonine protein kinase B-RAF inhibitor indicated for patients with advanced melanoma harboring the B-RAF gene.

Beta-lactamases—enzymes produced by some bacteria that are capable of breaking the chemical ring structure, deactivating antibacterial properties, and mediating resistance to selected beta-lactam antibiotics.

Biomarker—an objectively measured indicator of normal biological or pathogenic processes or pharmacologic responses used to diagnose and stage disease, assess disease progress, or assess response to therapeutic interventions.

Biosensor system—a bioreceptor molecule, which recognizes a target analyte and either generates a specific molecular species or results in a physiochemical change that can be measured by electro-chemical methods.

Blastoconidia—bud produced by asexual reproduction of fungus.

Brain natriuretic peptide—also known as *B-type natriuretic peptide*. It is principally produced and secreted by the ventricles of the brain (brain natriuretic peptide regulates natriuresis). An increase in blood volume or pressure enhances BNP secretion, which increases natriureis and to a lesser extent, diuresis.

Bronchial alveolar lavage—after inserting a bronchoscope into the lumen of the airways, sterile normal saline solution is flushed into the airways and then removed by aspiration. The solution is then sent for cellular and chemical analysis.

Bulemia—illness characterized by periods of overeating or binging followed by purging and vomiting.

Calcitonin—a hormone secreted by the C-cells of the thyroid gland. It inhibits osteoclastic activity, thereby inhibiting bone resorption. It also decreases calcium reabsorption in the renal proximal tubules.

Calcium-phosphorus product—the multiplication product of serum calcium and phosphorus concentrations, expressed as mg/dL. Insoluble calcium-phosphorus complex is likely to be formed when the product is high. In patients with chronic kidney disease, dietary restriction and pharmacotherapy are used to maintain the calcium-phosphorus product no higher than 50.

Capillary puncture—blood sampling method for premature neonates, neonates, and young infants who have small or inaccessible veins. Blood sampling is done at the heel, fingertip, or great toe. Also known as *microcapillary puncture* or *skin puncture.*

Carcinoembryonic antigen—also known as *CEA,* this protein is normally found in fetal intestine, pancreas, and liver. Elevated serum levels of CEA are found in patients with colon, breast, gastric, thyroid, or pancreatic cancer. For this reason, CEA is used as a tumor marker.

Cast—masses of glycoproteins that conform to the shape of the renal tubular lumen. Casts are detected by microscopic evaluation of the urine. The cellular composition of some casts are suggestive of the presence of various types of renal disorders.

Cholestasis—deficiency of the excretory function of the liver.

Cholesterol—a substance of dietary origin or synthesized in the liver and intestines that serves as a structural component of cell wall membranes and is a precursor for the synthesis of steroid hormones and bile acids.

Coagulation—process by which blood forms clots.

Cockcroft-Gault equation—this equation is used to estimate creatinine clearance in patients with stable renal function. The equation requires that the patient's gender, age, total body weight, and serum creatinine are known.

Codon—three base pairs that specify an amino acid. Because of redundancy in the genetic code, a change in one base pair may or may not change the amino acid coded by the codon.

Colonization—the presence of microorganisms, including potential pathogens, at a body site (i.e., oropharynx, skin, colon, vagina, surfaces of wounds) that are not causing infection.

Complement—a cascade system of at least 17 different plasma proteins that interacts to provide a defense mechanism against microbial invaders and serves as an adjunct or "complement" to humoral immunity. The complement cascade can be activated via the classical, alternative, or lectin pathways.

Congenital adrenal hyperplasia—a rare inherited disease of the adrenal glands in which cortisol and aldosterone production are impaired but androgen production is excessive.

Corpora cavernosa—one of two channels on the dorsal side of the penis, which is comprised of sinusoidal tissues. During a penile erection, the sinuses fill with arterial blood. In the flaccid state, the sinuses are empty.

Corrected serum calcium concentration—in patients with low plasma binding of calcium, often as a result of hypoalbuminemia, the "effective" serum calcium concentration must be assessed. The measured serum calcium concentration has to be corrected according to the serum albumin concentration. The corrected serum calcium concentration better reflects the amount of physiologically active calcium, which is the free (unbound) moiety.

Costochondral junction—the point where the ribs connect to the cartilage in the sternum (breast bone). Palpable enlargement of the costochondral junctions is called the rachitic rosary sign and is compatible with the diagnosis of rickets.

C-peptide—proinsulin, a precursor of insulin, is comprised of C-peptide and insulin. C-peptide must be cleaved from insulin for insulin to function. Elevated C-peptide levels in the blood stream is consistent with increased insulin levels.

C-reactive protein—plasma protein of the acute-phase response to injury or infection. The precise physiologic function of c-reactive protein is unknown, but it is known to participate in activation of the complement pathway and interact with cells in the immune system.

Creatinine—an endogenous substance produced by muscle cells. The production rate varies little day-to-day in patients with stable kidney function. Creatinine is freely filtered at the glomerulus with little reabsorbed or secreted. It is commonly used for assessing kidney function.

Creatinine clearance—a practical method of assessing kidney function to monitor kidney disease or dose medication (can be derived by measuring creatinine concentration via a urine collection or by using the serum creatinine concentration in the Cockcroft-Gault equation).

Crigler-Najjar syndrome—rare genetic disorder in which bilirubin cannot be conjugated by the liver. If not treated, bilirubin accumulates in the blood stream resulting in kernicterus.

Critical value—a result far enough out of the reference range that it indicates impending morbidity.

Cryptorchidism—failure of one or both testicles to descend through the inguinal canal into the scrotum after birth. As a result, the undescended testicle is at high risk for twisting on its spermatic cord, decreasing spermatogenesis, and developing testicular cancer.

Cystatin C—protease inhibitor that is filtered by the glomerulus but not reabsorbed or secreted. Cystatin C serum concentrations are used in various formulae to estimate glomerular filtration rate.

Cystic fibrosis—a genetic disorder that primarily affects the lungs and gastrointestinal tract. Patients with cystic fibrosis produce very thick mucus that can clog the airways of the lungs and cause severe lung infections that can be life-threatening. The mucus also obstructs the outflow tract of the pancreas and stops pancreatic enzymes from helping to break down and absorb nutrients. The sweat of patients with cystic fibrosis contains a high amount of sodium chloride.

D-dimer—a neoantigen formed when plasmin digests fibrin. When present on blood testing, D-dimer indicates the presence of thrombosis.

Depolarization—an electrical phenomenon that represents the decrease in the differential ionic charges across muscle or nerve cell membranes from the resting state to the excited state. The intracellular space becomes more positively charged than the extracellular space leading to cellular activation and contraction.

Diabetes insipidus—a condition in which the kidneys are not able to reabsorb water (back into the body). Central diabetes insipidus is caused by a lack of pituitary secretion of antidiuretic hormone (ADH). Nephrogenic diabetes is caused by failure of the kidneys to respond to ADH.

Diffusion—the process in which gases in the alveoli equilibrate from areas of high concentration to areas of low concentration.

Dihydropyrimidine dehydrogenase—this enzyme metabolizes 5-fluorouracil. A genetically-mediated enzyme deficiency is associated with increased 5-fluorouracil toxicity.

Direct bilirubin—this is formed when the liver conjugates bilirubin by linking it to glucuronic acid. This creates a water soluble form of bilirubin, which is excreted into bile and eliminated in feces. Direct bilirubin can also be excreted in urine.

Dubin-Johnson syndrome—autosomal recessive disease in which hepatocytes fail to secrete conjugated bilirubin into bile. As a result, patients develop high serum levels of conjugated bilirubin and mild jaundice.

Dynamic spirometry—a pulmonary breathing test that is based on time and, therefore, is more dependent on flow and "forced."

Dysgeusia—impaired sense of taste.

Dyspareunia—painful intercourse.

Eclampsia—a condition that occurs in pregnant women when preeclampsia is not treated. In addition to the symptoms of preeclampsia, women may experience seizures and coma. Eclampsia is a serious condition, as death of the mother and baby may occur.

EGFR-TKI—epidermal growth factor receptor tyrosine kinase inhibitor. An example drug is erlotinib. Increased sensitivity to EGFR-TKIs has been linked to the presence of EGFR activating mutations in the tumor, mostly exons 18 and 21 of the EGFR gene. EGFR testing has been used for non-small cell lung cancer and other tumors.

Electrocardiography—the recording of the electrical activity of the heart on an electrocardiogram.

Enantiomer—one of a pair of nonsuperimposable mirror image molecules. Enantiomers of a chiral drug may have different effects.

Enthesitis—inflammation of the sites where tendons or ligaments attach to bone.

Epidermal growth factor receptor—also known as *EGFR, HER1,* or *C-ERB B1.* When activated, this receptor supports tumor growth. The gene that encodes for EGFR is most commonly found in adenocarcinoma of the lungs in nonsmokers.

Esophageal varix—an engorged, superficial vein in the lumen of the esophagus (pl. = varices).

Etest (Epsilometer test)—quantitative method of antimicrobial susceptibility testing based on the diffusion of a continuous concentration gradient of an antibiotic from a plastic strip into an agar medium for the determination of minimum inhibitory concentration (MIC) values.

Euvolemic—refers to patients with normal plasma volume.

Exon—sequence of gene that is translated into mRNA and protein.

Extracellular water compartment—the extracellular water compartment consists of interstitial water and circulating plasma volume. The extracellular water compartment and intracellular water compartment comprise total body water.

Extrahepatic cholestasis—anatomic obstruction of macroscopic bile ducts.

FE$_{NA}$ or fractional excretion of sodium—percent of filtered sodium that is ultimately excreted in the urine.

Ferritin—intracellular form of stored iron. Iron is bound to a storage protein.

Fibrinolysis—mechanism by which formed thrombi are lysed through the dissolution of fibrin to prevent excessive clot formation and vascular occlusion.

Fibroids—the most common benign tumor of the uterus.

Fibromyalgia—a syndrome of pain, fatigue, sleep disturbances, and other medical problems. According to the American College of Rheumatology, an individual must have a history of chronic widespread pain and tenderness at 11 or more of 18 specific tender points sites on physician examination.

Fingerstick—a way of obtaining venous blood by pricking the fingertip with a lancet.

Fistula—an abnormal communication, opening, or passage from one hollow organ or abscess to another organ or to the skin. This could be due to infection, congenital malformation, or other disease.

Fluorescence in situ hybridization (FISH)—a laboratory technique used to look at genes or chromosomes in cells and tissues. Pieces of DNA that contain a fluorescent dye are made in the laboratory and used as probes. These DNA probes light up when they bind to specific genes or chromosomes and are viewed under a microscope with ultraviolet light.

Follicular phase—early portion of the menstrual cycle during which the ovarian follicle matures.

Forced vital capacity—total volume of air, measured in liters, forcefully and rapidly exhaled in one breath.

Galactorrhea—secretion of a milky discharge from the breast other than when breastfeeding.

Gastroschisis—a defect in the wall of the abdomen, which occurs during fetal development (i.e., a congenital malformation or birth defect). It allows the intestines (and sometimes other organs) to develop outside of the abdominal cavity. Having the internal organs outside of the abdominal wall will increase insensible water loss.

Gestational age—as it refers to a newborn, the gestational age is defined as the number of weeks from the first day of the mother's last menstrual period until the birth of the baby.

Gilbert syndrome—rare, hereditary deficiency of glucuronyltransferase, which normally conjugates bilirubin in the liver. As a result, patients develop high serum levels of unconjugated bilirubin and jaundice.

Glabrous—refers to hairless parts of the body, including palms of hands and soles of feet.

Glucagon—peptide hormone secreted by the pancreas, which increases serum glucose concentration by stimulating gluconeogenesis and glycogenolysis in the liver.

Glycogenolysis—breakdown of glycogen in muscle and liver to glucose and glucose-1-phosphate.

Glycosylated hemoglobin—also known as *glycated hemoglobin.* Glucose combines irreversibly with hemoglobin in red blood cells to form glycosylated hemoglobin. Increased glycosylated hemoglobin serum levels are indicative of poor long-term glucose control.

Granulocyte—also known as *polymorphonuclear leukocyte,* category of white blood cell that has phagocytic activity. Granulocytes include neutrophils, eosinophils, and basophils.

Haplotype—a set of alleles from a single chromosome that tends to be inherited as a unit.

Hashimoto thyroiditis—chronic progressive thyroid disease where functioning thyroid tissue is replaced by lymphoid or scar tissue. The patient may develop a goiter and has hypothyroidism.

Heelstick—capillary puncture of the heel. A blood drawing technique used in pediatric patients with small or inaccessible veins. It is the blood sampling method of choice for premature neonates, neonates, and young infants.

Hemostasis—a complex relationship among substances that promotes clot formations, inhibits coagulations, and dissolves formed clots.

Hepatic encephalopathy—diffuse metabolic dysfunction of the brain, which may occur in acute or chronic liver failure. Clinically it ranges from subtle changes in personality to coma and death.

Hepatitis—histologic pattern of inflammation of hepatocytes.

HER2—human epidermal growth factor receptor 2 protein is overexpressed in approximately 25% of breast cancers. When semiquantitative tests show that HER2 overexpression is present, the patient is more likely to respond to trastuzumab.

Hirsutism—excess hair growth in women due to excessive androgen stimulation. Excessive hair may appear in sideburn area, chin, upper lip, periareolar area of breast, chest, lower abdominal midline, and thighs.

Human chorionic gonadotropin—also known as *HCG,* this glycoprotein is normally produced by the placenta during pregnancy. Elevated HCG levels are seen in patients with some tumors of the testes and ovaries. For this reason, serum levels of HCG are used as a tumor marker.

Hyperosmolar hyperglycemic state—also known as *hyperosmolar hyperglycemia nonketotic state.* Patients have severe hyperglycemia, generally greater than 600 mg/dL, but do not have ketosis. Hyperglycemia causes water to shift from the intracellular to vascular compartment. This occurs in type 2 diabetes mellitus, when the patient is stressed by a concurrent medical illness (e.g., infection).

Hyposmia—decreased sense of smell.

Ileus—obstruction of the bowel that leads to nausea, vomiting, and abdominal pain. It could be due to a physical obstruction or due to absence of peristalsis (also known as *paralytic ileus*).

Immunohistochemistry (IHC)—the process of obtaining tissue from a biopsy and fixing it onto a glass slide. Antibodies to the antigen thought to be in the biopsy specimen are added and bind to the antigen. The antibodies that are bound to the antigen stain the biopsy and are then read by a pathologist to determine the amount of staining present on the biopsy specimen tested.

Incretin—gut hormones that enhance insulin secretion when serum glucose levels rise after meals. Two major incretins are glucagon-like peptide and glucose dependent insulotropic peptide.

In vitro (literally)—this refers to a reaction or process that occurs inside a test tube.

In vivo (literally)—this refers to a reaction or process that occurs inside the body of a plant or animal, or inside cells that are inside the body.

Indirect bilirubin—unconjugated bilirubin. Is water insoluble. Must be converted to direct bilirubin by the liver in order to be excreted.

Infant—refers to a baby that is 1 month to 1 year of age.

Infarction—the death of part or whole of an organ secondary to obstruction of blood flow by a blood clot (thrombus) or an embolus in the supplying artery.

Informatics—the use of collected data for the purposes of problem solving and healthcare decision-making.

Inotropic—related to the contraction of heart muscle (e.g., positive inotropic agents increase the force of contractions of the heart muscle).

Intermediate (I)—interpretive category for in vitro susceptibility testing of bacteria where the resulting MIC is equivocal (i.e., MIC is higher than those interpreted as susceptible but lower than those interpreted as resistant). The organism/infection may be eradicated if the antimicrobial agent achieves high concentrations at the site of infection or maximum doses of the antimicrobial agent are utilized.

International normalized ratio (INR)—the PT ratio that would result if the World Health Organization (WHO) international reference thromboplastin were used to test a blood sample.

Intrahepatic cholestasis—disorders of hepatocytes and microscopic bile ducts.

Intron—gene sequence between exons that is excised before mRNA is translated into protein. Introns are historically called "junk" DNA. However, it is increasingly being realized that introns contain gene sequences that do have functional importance.

Inulin—an inert carbohydrate that is filtered by the glomerulus but not reabsorbed or secreted by the renal tubule. It is used to measure glomerular filtration rate.

Ischemia—an inadequate blood flow to a part of the body secondary to constriction or blockage of the supplying artery.

Kernicterus—hyperbilirubinemia-induced brain damage in infants.

Km (The Michaelis constant)—the concentration of substrate at which an enzymatic reaction rate is half its maximal value.

KRAS—when present, this gene is strongly associated with primary resistance to the anti-EGFR monoclonal antibodies, panitumumab, and cetuximab.

Lacrimal fluid tears—ultrafiltrate of plasma that is secreted by lacrimal glands in the eye.

Lanugo hair—down-like, fine, soft hair usually on the ears, forehead, or flank of adult humans.

Laparoscopy—medical procedure that allows visualization of the abdominal and pelvic organs.

Leukocyte esterase—this enzyme is released from white blood cells and can be detected in urine by dipstick testing. When present, it indicates the presence of white blood cells in the urine, which suggest either infection or inflammation of the urinary tract.

Lower urinary tract symptoms (also known as *LUTS*)—This term refers to a collection of urinary obstructive and irritative voiding symptoms, which impacts negatively on a patient's quality of life.

Luteal phase—the part of the menstrual cycle in which the secretion of progesterone, rather than estradiol, predominates.

MDRD equation—refers to Modification of Diet in Renal Disease formula for estimating glomerular filtration rate in patients with chronic kidney failure. The patient's serum creatinine, age, African-American status, and gender are included in the formula. The MDRD equation tends to underestimate the level of renal function in those with normal or higher levels of renal function.

Mean corpuscular hemoglobin concentration—also known as *MCHC*, the average amount of hemoglobin in a red blood cell. A decreased MCHC value implies hypochromic red cells and suggests iron deficiency anemia.

Mean corpuscular volume—also known as *MCV*, average volume of a red blood cell. If the MCV is high, the cells are known as *macrocytic*. This is associated with vitamin B_{12} or folate deficiency. If the MCV is low, the cells are known as *microcytic*. This is associated with iron deficiency.

Menkes syndrome—also known as *kinky-* or *steely-hair syndrome*. This is an X-linked disorder associated with defective copper absorption, which results in growth and mental retardation, defective keratinization and pigmentation of hair, hypothermia, and degenerative changes in the aortic elastin and neurons. Children with this genetic disorder are often deceased by age 3.

Menses—bloody discharge that occurs during menstrual cycles.

Michaelis-Menten—behavior that describes a drug metabolism process that is saturable.

Minimum bactericidal concentration (MBC)—lowest concentration of a specific antimicrobial agent that kills 99.9% of the inoculum of the organism under a standardized set of in vitro conditions.

Minimum inhibitory concentration (MIC)—lowest concentration of a specific antimicrobial agent that prevents visible growth of the organism after 24 hours under a standardized set of in vitro conditions.

Mittelschmerz—lower abdominal and pelvic pain that occurs midway through the menstrual cycle.

Modification of diet in renal disease (MDRD)—the original MDRD study was undertaken to assess if reduction in protein intake had beneficial effects on progression of kidney disease. The study used iothalamate clearances to assess glomerular filtration rates. The data was used to develop alternative equations (the MDRD equations) to better identify and treat patients with chronic kidney disease.

Mutation—variation in genomic DNA that occurs in less than 1% of the population. Mutations may be rare or unique to an individual. The types of variation include single-base pair changes, insertions/deletions, repeats, and chromosomal arrangements.

Myocardium—the muscular tissue of the heart.

Myoglobin—low molecular weight heme protein found in cardiac and skeletal muscle.

Myopathy—elevations in creatine phosphokinase accompanied by muscle pain or tenderness.

Nanotechnology—the emerging clinical science involving the interactions of cellular and molecular components, specifically clusters of atoms, molecules, and molecular fragments.

Neonate—a full term newborn of 0–28 days postnatal age or a premature neonate whose postmenstrual age is 41–46 weeks.

Nephrogenesis—development of the kidney.

Nephrotic syndrome—a condition caused by damage to the glomeruli of the kidneys and characterized by large amounts of protein in the urine (proteinuria), low amounts of protein in the blood (hypoproteinemia), edema, and high amounts of cholesterol in the blood (hypercholesterolemia).

Nonlinear kinetics—see *Michaelis-Menten*.

Normal flora—natural colonization of several anatomic sites by bacteria that do not typically cause infection but may become pathogenic under certain circumstances. Normal flora colonization commonly provides defense against invasion by other bacterial or fungal organisms by occupying space, competing for nutrients, and stimulating antibody production.

Oligoarthritis—arthritis affecting one to four joints during the first 6 months of disease.

Oligomenorrhea—infrequent or very light menstruation in women with previously normal periods.

Omphalocele—a defect in the wall of the abdomen at the umbilical ring, which occurs during fetal development (i.e., a congenital malformation or birth defect). It allows the intestines (and sometimes other organs) to protrude into the base of the umbilical cord. Thus, the intestines and other organs are outside of the abdominal cavity enclosed in a clear membranous sac. Having the internal organs outside of the abdominal wall will increase insensible water loss.

Oncogene—a gene that normally directs cell growth. If altered, an oncogene can promote or allow the uncontrolled growth of cancer. Alterations can be inherited or caused by an environmental exposure to carcinogens.

Opisthotonus—spasm of the axial muscles of the spinal column results in this extrapyramidal movement in which the head, neck, and spine of the patient assume an arch- or bridge-like position. This is a classic presentation of tetanus.

Orchiectomy—surgical removal of the testes.

Osteomalacia—bone disorder in which bones are soft and weak due to deficiency of vitamin D, calcium, and phosphorus. In children, this is also known as *rickets*.

P wave—the electrocardiogram recording of the electrical activity of the heart leading to atrial depolarization and contraction.

Paget disease—bone disorder associated with excessive bone resorption and excessive bone formation, which leads to thickened, softened bone. Also known as *osteitis deformans*.

Panhypopituitarism—disease cause by absent or deficient anterior pituitary gland function, which results in deficiency in growth hormone, luteinizing hormone, follicle-stimulating hormone, adrenocorticotropin, and thyroid-stimulating hormone. A patient may present with clinical symptoms and signs due to one or more hormone deficiencies. This disorder may be due to a disorder of the hypothalamus or the pituitary gland.

Pathogen—microorganism that is capable of damaging host tissues and eliciting specific host responses and symptoms consistent with an infectious process.

Patient self-management—for patients on chronic warfarin therapy. Patients test their own INR and adjust their own therapy, usually based off of an algorithm, which offers more patient autonomy and control over their dosage regimen.

Patient self testing—for patients on chronic warfarin therapy. A patient will test his or her own INR but relies on a clinician for interpretation of results and any modifications to the current regimen.

Peak expiratory flow rate—maximum airflow rate on exhalation. It is measured using a hand-held peak flow meter. If the peak expiratory flow rate is low, it indicates large airway obstruction or that asthma is severe.

Perfusion—the movement of blood through the lungs.

Pharmacoenhancer—a drug that, when coadministered with another drug, increases its serum levels with the objective of increasing and prolonging its effect.

Pharmacogenetics—translational science of correlating inter-individual genetic variation with variability in drug response. This science has the potential to provide personalized medicine selection and dosing to individual patients.

Philadelphia (Ph) chromosome—an abnormality of chromosome 22 in which part of chromosome 9 is translocated to it. Bone marrow cells that contain the Philadelphia chromosome are often found in chronic myelogenous leukemia. See *translocation.*

Pica—abnormal food craving.

Plethysmography—as it refers to pulmonary assessments, plethysmography measures lung volumes (or amount of gas contained in the lungs) at various stages of inflation.

Poikilocytosis—variability in the circular, biconcave shape of erythrocytes.

Point-of-care testing—analysis of specimens, involving portable analyzers, that takes place in physician's office, in emergency rooms, or at the bedside in a patient's home.

Polymerase chain reaction (PCR)—clinical laboratory technique involving the in vivo replication and amplification of DNA fragments, thus allowing identification of the source of the hereditary material.

Polymorphism—variation in DNA that occurs in at least 1% of the population. Examples of types of polymorphisms include single nucleotide polymorphism (SNP) (single base pair substitutions), insertion/deletions (In/Del) (regions of the genome that are inserted or deleted), tandem repeats (a small number of base pairs that are repeated a variable number of times, e.g., TA repeat), and copy number variants (CNVs) (large regions of the genome or whole genes that occur with variable repetition throughout the genome).

Polyps—small growths in the lining of the uterus.

Positron emission tomography (PET)—nuclear imaging technique that measures blood flow and cellular metabolism in an organ.

Prealbumin—a plasma protein similar to albumin but with a shorter half-life. It is synthesized in the liver and is regarded as the best laboratory test of protein malnutrition.

Preanalytic variable—a substance present in the laboratory specimen that interferes with laboratory analytic methods. Examples of such substances include certain drugs, hemolyzed red blood cells, bilirubin, and high lipid concentrations.

Preeclampsia—a condition that occurs in pregnant women characterized by hypertension, edema, and large amounts of protein in the urine. Preeclampsia may lead to eclampsia (an even more serious condition).

Premature neonate—neonate born at less than 38 weeks gestational age.

Prerenal azotemia—kidney dysfunction caused by a reduced perfusion to the kidney, which could be due to volume depletion (diuretics), hypotension, heart failure, and emboli to the renal arteries.

Primary biliary cirrhosis—chronic disease involving progressive destruction of small intrahepatic bile ducts leading to cholestasis and progressive fibrosis over a period of decades.

Prolactinoma—a pituitary that secretes prolactin.

Prostacyclin—this protein produced by cells of blood vessel walls inhibits platelet aggregation.

Protected specimen brush—refers to an invasive procedure to obtain sputum from the lung. A plastic tube that contains a retractable brush is inserted down the throat to the lungs to avoid contaminating the brush with bacteria in the mouth and throat.

Proteinuria—the loss of protein in the urine, which is usually characteristic of glomerular disease.

Pulmonary compliance—the degree of elasticity or stiffness in the lung expressed as the change in volume divided by the change in pressure.

QRS complex—the electrocardiogram recording of the electrical activity of the heart leading to ventricular depolarization and contraction.

Red blood cell distribution width—also known as *RDW*, this lab test indicates the variability in the size of red blood cells. A high RDW indicates a large variability in size, which often occurs in nutritional anemias and thalessemias.

Reference range—a statistically-derived numerical range of values obtained by testing a sample of individuals assumed to be healthy; represents the range of values where 95% of individuals within the reference population fall.

Renal tubular acidosis—a condition in which the kidney tubules are not able to adequately remove acids from the blood in order to be excreted in the urine. This decreased ability of the kidney to excrete acids results in a build up of acids in the blood (metabolic acidosis) and electrolyte imbalances.

Repolarization—an electrical phenomenon that represents the recovery of the resting state electrical potential across muscle or nerve cell. The intracellular space becomes more negatively charged than the extracellular space leading to cellular relaxation.

Resistant (R)—interpretive category for in vitro susceptibility testing of bacteria where the MIC of the bacteria is high, and the organism is not likely to be inhibited or eradicated by standard doses of the antimicrobial because the MIC is higher than what can be achieved using maximum doses of the antibiotic.

Reticulocyte—premature red blood cell.

Retrocollis—a dystonia in which sustained muscle contraction causes the head to tilt backward.

Rhabdomyolysis—condition characterized by breakdown of skeletal muscle tissue with release of myoglobin, enzymes, and electrolytes from cells.

Rheumatoid factors—immunoglobulins directed against the Fc region of immunoglobulin G that are found in the serum of patients with rheumatoid arthritis and other rheumatic diseases.

Rickets—bone disease caused by chronic vitamin D deficiency and calcium deficiency. Bones become soft and weak.

RT-PCR (reverse-transcriptase polymerase chain reaction)—a very sensitive molecular genetic test for finding specific DNA sequences, such as those occurring in some cancers. The RNA strand is first reverse transcribed into complementary DNA, followed by amplification of the resulting DNA using a polymerase chain reaction.

Sarcoidosis—also known as *sarcoid,* a systemic granulomatous disease affecting many organs. Small nodules of tissue composed of lymphocytes and macrophages appear in skin, lungs, joints, and lymph nodes. Patients may be asymptomatic or develop complications such as pericarditis or meningitis. The etiology is unknown. The disease may or may not be chronic.

Sensitivity—when referring to a test, it is the ability of the test to show positive results in patients who actually have the disease (true positive rate). For a test with high sensitivity for a diagnosis of a disease, a patient with a negative test result probably doesn't have the disease.

Specificity—when referring to a test, it is the ability of the test to show negative results in patients who do not have the disease (true negative rate). For a test with high specificity for diagnosis of a disease, a patient with a positive test result has a high probability of having the disease.

Specimen—the sample used for laboratory analysis (e.g., whole blood, arterial blood, urine, stool).

Spirometry—a type of pulmonary function test that measures the maximum amount of air that is exhaled by a patient after complete inhalation.

Sporangiophore—a threadlike structure of a fungus that has sporangia (asexual spores) at the tip.

Static spirometry—a pulmonary breathing test that is volume-based and slow.

Susceptible (S)—interpretive category for in vitro susceptibility testing of bacteria where the organism is readily inhibited based on the MIC of the antibiotic; the organism/infection will most likely be eradicated using standard dosing of the antimicrobial agent for that infection type since concentrations of the antibiotic in the serum and at the site of infection readily exceed the MIC.

Syndrome of inappropriate antidiuretic hormone secretion—also known as *SIADH,* these patients have excessively high levels of antidiuretic hormone, which results in increased water reabsorption and dilutional hyponatremia.

Synovial fluid—joint fluid, this fluid lubricates and nourishes the articular cartilage.

T wave—the electrocardiogram recording of the electrical activity of the heart leading to ventricular repolarization and relaxation.

Tachyzoites—a rapidly reproducing stage of Toxoplasma gondii, associated with acute infections.

Thalessemia—a genetic hemoglobinopathy in which the patient has difficulty producing intact hemoglobin inside red blood cells. As a result, the red blood cell is degraded more rapidly and has a shorter lifespan than usual. Thalessemia results in anemia.

Thiopurine methyltransferase (TPMT)—enzyme responsible for in vivo conversion of azathioprine and 6-mercaptopurine to inactive metabolites. Genetic variants to the TPMT gene can result in deficient or absent TPMT activity, which can lead to increased hematologic adverse effects of azathioprine or 6-mercaptopurine.

Thrombocytopenia—reduction in the platelet count.

Thrombocytosis—elevation in the platelet count.

Thromboxane—this protein produced by platelets is essential for platelet aggregation.

Thyrotoxicosis—the patient has excessive thyroid hormone.

Transferrin—an iron transporting protein in the blood stream. The percentage of iron-binding sites of transferrin, which are occupied by iron, is known as *transferrin saturation.* This is used as an indirect measure of circulating iron levels.

Translocation—movement of part of one chromosome that has broken off to another chromosome.

Triglycerides—esterified form of glycerol and fatty acids that constitute the main form of lipid storage in humans to be used as fuel for gluconeogenesis or for direct combustion as an energy source.

Troponin—protein that regulates calcium-mediated interaction of actin and myosin, essential for contraction of cardiac muscle.

Tumor marker—substances produced by tumor cells or by other cells of the body in response to cancer. These substances can be found in the blood, in the urine, in the tumor tissue, or in other tissues. Some tumor marker levels can also be altered in patients with noncancerous conditions, which limit their usefulness for cancer screening.

Tyrosine kinase—an intracellular enzyme that transfers a phosphate group from ATP to a tyrosine residue in a protein. Phosphorylation of proteins by kinases is an important mechanism in signal transduction (and cell growth) and often becomes dysregulated in cancer.

Ultrafiltrate—a solution that has passed through a semipermeable membrane with very small pores.

Urethral stricture—scarring of the urethra, due to infection, inflammation, or instrumentation, that results in narrowing of the urethral lumen. A patient will then have difficulty passing urine from the bladder through the narrowed urethral lumen.

VKORC1—this gene encodes for vitamin K epoxide reductase complex subunit 1, the enzyme responsible for activating vitamin K. Various VKORC1 genotypes affect the daily dose of warfarin and potential of bleeding with warfarin in patients. Uncommonly, a VKORC1 genotype is associated with warfarin resistance.

Von Willebrand factor—this circulating protein binds to other circulating proteins and is essential for platelet adhesion.

Ventilation—the movement of air in and out of the lungs.

Vmax—the maximum rate of a drug's metabolism by a particular enzyme system in the liver.

Wilson disease—an autosomal recessive disease state of improper copper storage. It is associated with elevated urinary copper loss; low plasma ceruloplasmin; low copper concentrations; and copper deposition in the liver, brain, and cornea.

APPENDIX A. Therapeutic Ranges of Drugs in Traditional and SI Units[a]

DRUG	TRADITIONAL RANGE	CONVERSION FACTOR[b]	SI RANGE
Acetaminophen	>5 mg/dL toxic	66.16	>330 μmol/L toxic
N-acetylprocainamide	4–10 mg/L	3.606	14–36 μmol/L
Amitriptyline	75–175 ng/mL	3.605	270–630 nmol/L
Carbamazepine	4–12 mg/L	4.230	17–51 μmol/L
Chlordiazepoxide	0.5–5.0 mg/L	3.336	2–17 μmol/L
Chlorpromazine	50–300 ng/mL	3.136	150–950 nmol/L
Chlorpropamide	75–250 mcg/mL	3.613	270–900 μmol/L
Clozapine	250–350 ng/mL	0.003	0.75–1.05 μmol/L
Cyclosporine	100–200 ng/mL[c]	0.832	80–160 nmol/L
Desipramine	100–160 ng/mL	3.754	375–600 nmol/L
Diazepam	100–250 ng/mL	3.512	350–900 nmol/L
Digoxin	0.9–2.2 ng/mL	1.281	1.2–2.8 nmol/L
Disopyramide	2–6 mg/L	2.946	6–18 μmol/L
Doxepin	50–200 ng/mL	3.579	180–720 nmol/L
Ethosuximide	40–100 mg/L	7.084	280–710 μmol/L
Fluphenazine	0.5–2.5 ng/mL	2.110	5.3–21 nmol/L
Glutethimide	>20 mg/L toxic	4.603	>92 μmol/L toxic
Gold	300–800 mg/L	0.051	15–40 μmol/L
Haloperidol	5–15 ng/mL	2.660	13–40 nmol/L
Imipramine	200–250 ng/mL	3.566	710–900 nmol/L
Isoniazid	>3 mg/L toxic	7.291	>22 μmol/L toxic
Lidocaine	1–5 mg/L	4.267	5–22 μmol/L
Lithium	0.5–1.5 mEq/L	1.000	0.5–1.5 μmol/L
Maprotiline	50–200 ng/mL	3.605	180–720 μmol/L
Meprobamate	>40 mg/L toxic	4.582	>180 μmol/L toxic
Methotrexate	>2.3 mg/L toxic	2.200	>5 μmol/L toxic
Nortriptyline	50–150 ng/mL	3.797	190–570 nmol/L
Pentobarbital	20–40 mg/L	4.419	90–170 μmol/L
Perphenazine	0.8–2.4 ng/mL	2.475	2–6 nmol/L
Phenobarbital	15–40 mg/L	4.306	65–172 μmol/L
Phenytoin	10–20 mg/L	3.964	40–80 μmol/L
Primidone	4–12 mg/L	4.582	18–55 μmol/L
Procainamide	4–8 mg/L	4.249	17–34 μmol/L
Propoxyphene	>500 ng/mL toxic	2.946	>1500 ng/mL

APPENDIX A. Therapeutic Ranges of Drugs in Traditional and SI Units[a], cont'd

DRUG	TRADITIONAL RANGE	CONVERSION FACTOR[b]	SI RANGE
Propranolol	50–200 ng/mL	3.856	190–770 nmol/L
Protriptyline	100–300 ng/mL	3.797	380–1140 nmol/L
Quinidine	2–6 mg/L	3.082	5–18 μmol/L
Salicylate (acid)	15–25 mg/dL	0.072	1.1–1.8 mmol/L
Theophylline	10–20 mg/L	5.550	55–110 μmol/L
Thiocyanate	>10 mg/dL toxic	0.172	>1.7 mmol/L toxic
Valproic acid	50–100 mg/L	6.934	350–700 μmol/L

[a]Also see Table 5-3 in Chapter 5.
[b]Traditional units are multiplied by conversion factor to get SI units.
[c]Whole blood assay.

APPENDIX B. Nondrug Reference Ranges for Common Laboratory Tests in Traditional and SI Units[a]

LABORATORY TEST	REFERENCE RANGE TRADITIONAL UNITS	CONVERSION FACTOR	REFERENCE RANGE SI UNITS	COMMENT
Alanine aminotransferase (ALT)	0–30 International Units/L	0.01667	0–0.50 μkat/L	SGPT
Albumin	3.5–5 g/dL	10	35–50 g/L	
Ammonia	30–70 mcg/dL	0.587	17–41 μmol/L	
Aspartate aminotransferase (AST)	8–42 International Units/L	0.01667	0.133–0.700 μkat/L	SGOT
Bilirubin (direct)	0.1–0.3 mg/dL	17.10	1.7–5 μmol/L	
Bilirubin (total)	0.3–1.0 mg/dL	117.10	5–17 μmol/L	
Calcium	8.5–10.8 mg/dL	0.25	2.1–2.7 mmol/L	
Carbon dioxide (CO_2)	24–30 mEq/L	1.000	24–30 mmol/L	Serum bicarbonate
Chloride	96–106 mEq/L	1.000	96–106 mmol/L	
Cholesterol (HDL)	>40 mg/dL	0.026	>1.05 mmol/L	Desirable
Cholesterol (LDL)	<130 mg/dL	0.026	<3.36 mmol/L	Desirable
Creatine kinase (CK)	25–90 International Units/L (males)	0.01667	0.42–1.50 μkat/L	Males
	10–70 International Units/L (females)		0.17–1.17 μkat/L	Females
Creatinine clearance (CrCl)	90–140 mL/min/1.73 m²	0.017	1.53–2.38 mL/sec/1.73 m²	
Folic acid	150–540 ng/mL	2.266	340–1020 nmol/L	
Gamma-glutamyl transpeptidase	0–30 units/L (but varies)	0.01667	0–0.50 μkat/L (but varies)	GGT/GGTP
Globulin	2–3 g/dL	10.00	20–30 g/L	
Glucose (fasting)	70–110 mg/dL	0.056	3.9-6.1 mmol/L	Fasting
Hemoglobin (Hgb)	14–18 g/dL (males)	0.622	8.7–11.2 mmol/L	Males
	12–16 g/dL (females)		7.4–9.9 mmol/L	Females
		10	140–180 g/L	Males
			120–140 g/L	Females
Iron	50–150 mcg/dL	0.179	9–26.9 μmol/L	
Iron-binding capacity (total)	250–410 mcg/dL	0.179	45–73 μmol/L	TIBC

APPENDIX B. Nondrug Reference Ranges for Common Laboratory Tests in Traditional and SI Units[a], cont'd

LABORATORY TEST	REFERENCE RANGE TRADITIONAL UNITS	CONVERSION FACTOR	REFERENCE RANGE SI UNITS	COMMENT
Lactate dehydrogenase	100–210 International Units/L	0.01667	1667–350 nmol/L, 1.7–3.2 μkat/L	LDH
Magnesium	1.5–2.2 mEq/L	0.500	0.75–1.1 mmol/L	
5' nucleotidase	1–11 units/L (but varies)	0.01667	0.02–0.18 μkat/L (but varies)	
Phosphate	2.6–4.5 mg/dL	0.3229	0.85–1.48 mmol/L	
Potassium	3.5–5.0 mEq/L	1.000	3.5–5.0 mmol/L	
Serum creatinine (SCr)	0.7–1.5 mg/dL	88.40	62–133 μmol/L	Adults
Serum lactate (arterial)	0.5–2.0 mEq/L	1.000	0.5–2.0 mmol/L	
Serum lactate (venous)	0.5–1.5 mEq/L	1.000	0.5–1.5 mmol/L	Lactic acid
Sodium	136–145 mEq/L	1.000	136–145 mmol/L	
Total serum thyroxine (T_4)	4–12 mcg/dL	12.86	51–154 nmol/L	Total T_4
Triglycerides	<150 mg/dL	0.0113	<1.26 mmol/L	Adults >20 yr
Total serum triiodothyronine (T_3)	78–195 ng/dL	0.0154	1.2–3.0 nmol/L	Total T_3
Urea nitrogen, blood	8–20 mg/dL	0.357	2.9–7.1 mmol/L	BUN
Uric acid (serum)	3.4–7 mg/dL	59.48	202–416 μmol/L	

[a]Some laboratories are maintaining traditional units for enzyme tests.

APPENDIX C. Blood Collection Tubes: Color Codes, Additives, and Appropriate Sample Volumes[a,b]

CAP COLOR	ADDITIVE(S)[c]	NUMBER OF TUBE INVERSIONS AT COLLECTION	LABORATORY USE AND COMMENTS[d]
Brown	Sodium heparin	8	For lead determinations; inversions prevent clotting
Gold	Clot activator and gel for serum separation	5	Serum separator tube for serum determinations in chemistry; inversions ensure mixing of clot activator with blood and clotting within 30 min
Gray	Potassium oxalate/sodium fluoride	8	For glucose, lactate, alcohol, and bicarbonate determinations; glycolytic inhibitors stabilize glucose for 24 hr at room temperature (iodoacetate) and for 3 days with fluoride; oxalate and heparin give plasma samples— without them, samples are serum; for lactate (on ice)
	Sodium fluoride	8	
	Lithium iodoacetate	8	
	Lithium iodoacetate/heparin	8	
	Heparin sodium	8	
Green	Heparin sodium	8	For plasma determinations in chemistry; inversions prevent clotting; used for arterial blood gases, ammonia (on ice), and electrolytes
	Lithium heparin	8	
	Ammonium heparin	8	
Lavender	Liquid potassium EDTA	8	For whole-blood hematology determinations; inversions prevent clotting
	Freeze-dried sodium EDTA	8	

APPENDIX C. Blood Collection Tubes: Color Codes, Additives, and Appropriate Sample Volumes[a,b], cont'd

CAP COLOR	ADDITIVE(S)[c]	NUMBER OF TUBE INVERSIONS AT COLLECTION	LABORATORY USE AND COMMENTS[d]
Light blue	0.105 M sodium citrate 3.2%	8	For coagulation determinations on plasma; inversions prevent clotting; some tests may require chilling
	0.129 M sodium citrate 3.8%	8	
Light green	Lithium heparin and gel for plasma separation	8	Plasma separation tube for plasma determinations in chemistry; inversions prevent clotting
Orange	Thrombin	8	For stat serum determinations in chemistry; inversions ensure clotting within 5 min
Red	None	0	For serum determinations in chemistry, serology, and blood banking
Royal blue	Heparin sodium	8	For trace element, toxicology, and nutrient determinations; not for chromium, manganese, aluminum, and selenium
	Sodium EDTA	8	
	None	0	
Yellow	Sodium polyanethole sulfonate (SPS)	8	For blood culture specimen collections in microbiology; inversions prevent clotting
	ACD solution B of trisodium citrate		For blood banking and histocompatibility testing

EDTA = ethylenediaminetetraacetic acid; NA = not applicable.

[a]Compiled from (1) 1990 company literature (Becton Dickinson, Rutherford, NJ 07070) on Vacutainer collection systems; (2) Jacobs DS, Kasten BL Jr, Demott WR, et al., eds. *Laboratory Test Handbook.* St. Louis, MO: Lexi-Comp/Mosby;1988; (3) National Committee for Clinical Laboratory Standards. Procedures for handling and processing of blood specimens, H18-A. Villanova, PA: 1989; and (4) editor's experience.

[b]Colors and additives are specific only for vacutainer tubes with Hemogard closure or stoppers from Becton Dickinson. Other types and brands may vary.

[c]If known, the Becton Dickinson vacutainer blood collection tubes are designed to collect specimens, which are within ± the draw volume stated on the tube. This avoids spurious results due to an inappropriate ratio of anticoagulant to specimen. In general, tubes with liquid additives should be filled.

[d]In general, specimens should not be chilled before delivery to the laboratory unless specified otherwise. Exceptions include lactic acid, blood gases, pyruvate, gastrin, ammonia, parathyroid hormone, catecholamines, and possibly activated partial thromboplastin time. Stoppers should not be removed outside the laboratory, because specimens may be oxidized, volatile, or contaminated by bacteria. Serum or plasma should be separated from contact with cells within 2 hr of collection unless specified otherwise.

*Page numbers in *italics* indicate a figure; page numbers in **boldface** indicate a list, a Quickview Chart, or a table.

---

*Page numbers in *italics* indicate a figure; page numbers in **boldface** indicate a list, a Quickview Chart, or a table.

*Page numbers in *italics* indicate a figure; page numbers in **boldface** indicate a list, a Quickview Chart, or a table.

---

*Page numbers in *italics* indicate a figure; page numbers in **boldface** indicate a list, a Quickview Chart, or a table.

---

*Page numbers in *italics* indicate a figure; page numbers in **boldface** indicate a list, a Quickview Chart, or a table.

---

*Page numbers in *italics* indicate a figure; page numbers in **boldface** indicate a list, a Quickview Chart, or a table.

*Page numbers in *italics* indicate a figure; page numbers in **boldface** indicate a list, a Quickview Chart, or a table.

*Page numbers in *italics* indicate a figure; page numbers in **boldface** indicate a list, a Quickview Chart, or a table.

*Page numbers in *italics* indicate a figure; page numbers in **boldface** indicate a list, a Quickview Chart, or a table.

---

*Page numbers in *italics* indicate a figure; page numbers in **boldface** indicate a list, a Quickview Chart, or a table.

---

*Page numbers in *italics* indicate a figure; page numbers in **boldface** indicate a list, a Quickview Chart, or a table.

---

*Page numbers in *italics* indicate a figure; page numbers in **boldface** indicate a list, a Quickview Chart, or a table.

---

*Page numbers in *italics* indicate a figure; page numbers in **boldface** indicate a list, a Quickview Chart, or a table.

---

*Page numbers in *italics* indicate a figure; page numbers in **boldface** indicate a list, a Quickview Chart, or a table.

---

*Page numbers in *italics* indicate a figure; page numbers in **boldface** indicate a list, a Quickview Chart, or a table.

---

*Page numbers in *italics* indicate a figure; page numbers in **boldface** indicate a list, a Quickview Chart, or a table.

---

*Page numbers in *italics* indicate a figure; page numbers in **boldface** indicate a list, a Quickview Chart, or a table.

*Page numbers in *italics* indicate a figure; page numbers in **boldface** indicate a list, a Quickview Chart, or a table.

*Page numbers in *italics* indicate a figure; page numbers in **boldface** indicate a list, a Quickview Chart, or a table.

---

*Page numbers in *italics* indicate a figure; page numbers in **boldface** indicate a list, a Quickview Chart, or a table.

---

*Page numbers in *italics* indicate a figure; page numbers in **boldface** indicate a list, a Quickview Chart, or a table.

*Page numbers in *italics* indicate a figure; page numbers in **boldface** indicate a list, a Quickview Chart, or a table.

---

*Page numbers in *italics* indicate a figure; page numbers in **boldface** indicate a list, a Quickview Chart, or a table.

---

*Page numbers in *italics* indicate a figure; page numbers in **boldface** indicate a list, a Quickview Chart, or a table.

---

*Page numbers in *italics* indicate a figure; page numbers in **boldface** indicate a list, a Quickview Chart, or a table.